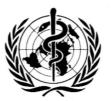

World Health Organization Classification of Tumours

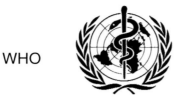

WHO   OMS

International Agency for Research on Cancer (IARC)

4th Edition

WHO Classification of Tumours of the Digestive System

Edited by

Fred T. Bosman

Fátima Carneiro

Ralph H. Hruban

Neil D. Theise

International Agency for Research on Cancer

Lyon, 2010

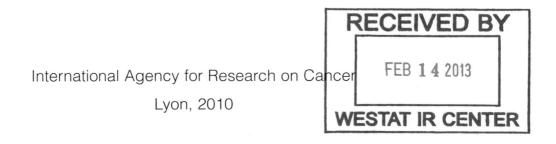

World Health Organization Classification of Tumours

Series Editors   Fred T. Bosman, M.D.
Elaine S. Jaffe, M.D.
Sunil R. Lakhani, M.D.
Hiroko Ohgaki, Ph.D.

WHO Classification of Tumours of the Digestive System

Editors   Fred T. Bosman, M.D., Ph.D.
Fátima Carneiro, M.D., Ph.D.
Ralph H. Hruban, M.D.
Neil D. Theise, M.D.

Technical Editor   Heidi Mattock, Ph.D.

Layout   Sébastien Antoni
Alberto Machado

Printed by   Participe Présent
69250 Neuville sur Saône, France

Publisher   International Agency for
Research on Cancer (IARC)
69008 Lyon, France

This volume was produced with support from the

MEDIC Foundation

The WHO Classification of Tumours of the Digestive System
presented in this book reflects the views of a Working Group
that convened for an Editorial and Consensus Conference at the
International Agency for Research on Cancer (IARC), Lyon
December 10–12, 2009.

Members of the Working Group are indicated
in the List of Contributors on pages 338–344

Published by the International Agency for Research on Cancer (IARC),
150 cours Albert Thomas, 69372 Lyon Cedex 08, France

Distributed by
WHO Press, World Health Organization, 20 Avenue Appia, 1211 Geneva 27, Switzerland
(Tel: +41 22 791 3264; Fax: +41 22 791 4857; e-mail: bookorders@who.int).

First print run (10 000 copies)

Format for bibliographic citations:
Bosman F.T., Carneiro F., Hruban R.H., Theise N.D. (Eds.):
WHO Classification of Tumours of the Digestive System.
IARC: Lyon 2010

IARC Library Cataloguing in Publication Data

WHO classification of tumours of the digestive system - 4th edition / edited by Fred T. Bosman ... [et al.]

(World Health Organization classification of tumours)

1. Digestive System Neoplasms – classification 2. Digestive System Neoplasms – genetics
3. Digestive System Neoplasms – pathology
I. Bosman, F.T. II. Series

ISBN 978-92-832-2432-7   (NLM Classification: WI 15)

Contents

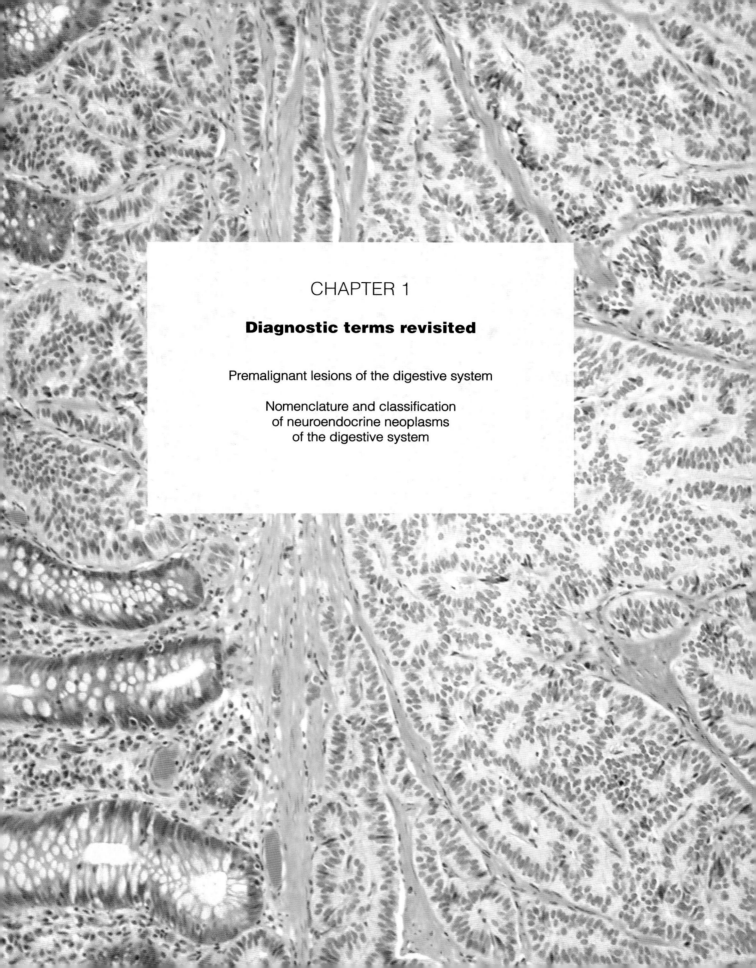

CHAPTER 1

Diagnostic terms revisited

Premalignant lesions of the digestive system

Nomenclature and classification
of neuroendocrine neoplasms
of the digestive system

Premalignant lesions of the digestive system

R.D. Odze
R.H. Riddell
F.T. Bosman
F. Carneiro
J.-F. Fléjou
K. Geboes
R.M. Genta
T. Hattori
R.H.Hruban

J.H. van Krieken
G.Y. Lauwers
G.J.A. Offerhaus
M. Rugge
M. Shimizu
T. Shimoda
N.D. Theise
M. Vieth

Introduction and historical perspective

Pathologists are often confronted with biopsies of the digestive system that show architectural and/or cytological features of precursors of invasive neoplasia, either squamous or columnar. Historically, noninvasive neoplasia of the digestive system has been termed "dysplasia" by pathologists when obvious, unambiguous, architectural and/or cytological alterations of epithelium normally associated with neoplastic growth are present, without evidence of infiltration into the lamina propria {2674}.

In 1982, Riddell et al. proposed a classification system for dysplasia in the tubal gut, which provided a meaningful method of estimating the risk of progression to cancer in patients with inflammatory bowel disease (IBD) {2674}. This "IBD dysplasia-grading system" was accepted quite readily, at least in the USA and in most European countries, as the "standard" method of assessing cancer risk in patients with IBD. The system was adopted by clinicians and was subsequently adapted for other, noninvasive neoplastic conditions of the gastrointestinal tract, such as those that occur in Barrett oesophagus, chronic gastritis and colorectal adenomas {2654, 2752, 962}. In addition, it was used to classify squamous neoplastic lesions of the oesophagus {2742A}.

As use of this grading system spread to other regions of the world, such as Japan, a number of limitations became evident {2841}. Such limitations stem from increasing recognition of the morphological and clinical heterogeneity of precursor lesions of invasive neoplasia of the digestive system, lack of reproducibility in the grading of dysplasia among pathologists worldwide, lack of universally accepted diagnostic criteria for each distinct grade of dysplasia, and lack of universal agreement on the definition of invasive carcinoma, in particular, between pathologists in North America and Europe and those in Japan {2841}.

Controversies regarding terminology

In the previous (3rd) edition of the WHO Classification of Tumours of the Digestive Tract (2000) an attempt was made to clarify some of these issues by introducing the term "intraepithelial neoplasia" as a synonym for lesions classified morphologically as dysplasia.

Furthermore, in 2000, a group of gastrointestinal pathologists convened in Vienna, Austria, for the purpose of developing a new system for the classification of dysplasia that would help to address the limitations discussed above {2842, 3090}. The goal of the "Vienna system", as it was termed, was to minimize the widely recognized discrepancies in morphological interpretation of precursor lesions of invasive neoplasia among pathologists in North America and Europe and those in Japan, and to reach consensus on the nomenclature. Ultimately, the Vienna grading system is very similar to the one proposed by Riddell et al., except that the former uses the term "noninvasive neoplasia", which is a synonym of intraepithelial neoplasia, instead of "dysplasia" and also uses the term "suspicious for invasive carcinoma" for lesions that show equivocal cytological and/or architectural features of tissue invasion. Differences in use of the term "carcinoma" are due to the fact that pathologists in North America and Europe typically define this lesion as one that has histological evidence of invasive growth, whereas most Japanese pathologists diagnose carcinoma solely on the basis of the architectural and cytological changes observed, without requiring morphological evidence of invasive growth.

Not surprisingly, modification of the nomenclature has not resolved the high level of intra- and interobserver variability with regard to the pathological classification of neoplastic precursor lesions, and particularly for epithelial lesions that reveal borderline features between regeneration and neoplasia {2841, 2135, 3090}. This is not surprising since precursor lesions of invasive neoplasia develop on a continuum, and thus, there will always be a certain lack of consistency when this is artificially translated into discrete categories. One repercussion of the Vienna grading system is that it recommended a change in terminology from "dysplasia" to "intraepithelial neoplasia." However, pathologists from the USA and some European countries continue to use the term "dysplasia," whereas

Table 1.01 Precursor lesions of invasive neoplasia (intraepithelial neoplasia) of the tubal gut.

Oesophagus
Barrett-associated dysplasia
  Adenomatous
  Non-adenomatous
    Foveolar
    Serrated
Squamous dysplasia

Stomach
Gastritis-associated dysplasia
  Adenomatous (type 1)
  Foveolar (type 2)
Adenoma
  Intestinal type
  Pyloric-gland type
  Foveolar type
Fundic gland polyp-associated dysplasia

Small intestine
Crohn disease-associated dysplasia
Adenoma
  Intestinal type
  Brunner gland
Hamartoma-associated dysplasia

Colon
Inflammatory bowel disease-associated dysplasia
  Adenomatous
  Serrated
  Villous hypermucinous
Adenoma
  Conventional
  Traditional serrated
Sessile serrated adenoma/polyp
  Without dysplasia
  With dysplasia
Hamartoma-associated dysplasia

Anus
Squamous dysplasia (anal intraepithelial neoplasia)
HPV/condyloma-associated dysplasia
Bowen disease (perianal squamous intraepithelial neoplasia)

most Japanese pathologists use the term "intraepithelial neoplasia". This has led to much confusion among pathologists and, particularly, clinicians with regard to the meaning of the terms "dysplasia" and "intraepithelial neoplasia." Furthermore, since the publication of the Vienna grading system, precursor lesions of invasive neoplasia have been identified and characterized in other gastrointestinal organs, such as the pancreas and anus, in which the term "intraepithelial neoplasia" has been used instead of "dysplasia" e.g. pancreatic intraepithelial neoplasia (PanIN), anal canal intraepithelial neoplasia (ACIN) {1083, 2979, 2851A}.

Thus, at the current time, two different terms are used among pathologists to describe precursor lesions of invasive neoplasia of the gastrointestinal tract. In some organs, such as the oesophagus, stomach and colon, the term "dysplasia" is used by some and "intraepithelial neoplasia" by others. Such differences may be institutional or geographical. On the other hand, in some organs there is better agreement on usage. For instance, although the term "intraepithelial neoplasia" is exclusively used for anal lesions, in the pancreas, the term "intraepithelial neoplasia" is used for some lesions (PanINs), but "dysplasia" is used for others (mucinous cystic neoplasms and intraductal papillary mucinous neoplasms).

Current WHO classification and definitions

The consensus meeting that preceded the publication of the 4th edition of the WHO classification did not lead to an agreement on one term for noninvasive neoplasia for several reasons. First, specific cytological and/or architectural abnormalities of precursor lesions of invasive neoplasia differ considerably according to anatomical location/organ, and the histology of the native epithelium and their biological characteristics, and malignant potential, vary substantially among different organ sites. Second, recent advancements in our understanding of the timing, type, and sequence of molecular events that lead to neoplastic transformation, have made clear that clonal, molecular abnormalities that lead to dysregulation of cell proliferation and differentiation, and an increasing risk for subsequent neoplastic progression, may occur without typical morphological characteristics of noninvasive neoplasia. Examples are aneuploidy and mutations in *TP53* and *CDKN2A*, that precede the development of morphological features of

dysplasia in Barrett oesophagus and IBD {3539A, 1838A, 936A, 3274, 1277}, and sessile serrated adenomas/polyps (SSA/P) in the colon which contain few, if any, dysplastic features, but are now recognized as a contributor to colon cancer {3274, 1277, 1400, 2993}.

Tables 1.01 and 1.02 highlight some of the major types of precursor lesions of invasive neoplasia of the gastrointestinal tract, liver, biliary tract and pancreas. The following definitions and guidelines are offered:

Neoplasia

One classical definition of neoplasia is the following: "A neoplasm is an abnormal mass of tissue, the growth of which exceeds and is uncoordinated with that of normal tissue, and persists in the same excessive manner after cessation of any stimulus that may have evoked the change" {2163A, 2052A, 736A, 2867A}. However, not all neoplastic conditions lead to a mass. Furthermore, as indicated above, difficulties arise when morphological features that define a specific type of neoplasia are not present.

Intraepithelial neoplasia

Intraepithelial neoplasia is a term used to describe lesions that generally display cytological or architectural alterations perceived to reflect underlying molecular abnormalities that may lead to invasive carcinoma. However, molecular alterations are not invariably reflected in the presence of such cytological/architectural atypia. Thus, "intraepithelial neoplasia" includes morphologically recognizable lesions with such atypia (for example, IBD-associated dysplasia) or without (for example sessile serrated andenoma/polyp). The types of intraepithelial neoplasia, and the morphological characteristics associated with these presursor lesions of invasive neoplasia differ per organ (Tables 1.01 and 1.02). Key elements of the definition of intraepithelial neoplasia are that all lesions are morphologically identifiable, have the potential to become malignant and are noninvasive.

Dysplasia

Traditionally, dysplasia is defined as histologically unequivocal neoplastic epithelium without evidence of tissue invasion. The term is distinct from intrepithelial neoplasia since it refers to the presence of morphological features of neoplasia.

Table 1.02 Precursor lesions of invasive neoplasia (intraepithelial neoplasia) of the gallbladder, biliary tract, pancreas and liver.

Gallbladder/biliary tree
BilIN 1–3
Intraductal (bile ducts) or intracystic (gallbladder) papillary neoplasms with intraepithelial neoplasia
Mucinous cystic neoplasm with intraepithelial neoplasia
Adenoma
Pancreas/ampulla
PanIN 1–3
Intraductal papillary mucinous neoplasms with dysplasia
Mucinous cystic neoplasm with dysplasia
Ampullary adenoma
Noninvasive pancreaticobiliary papillary neoplasm
Flat intraepithelial neoplasia (dysplasia)
Liver
Large and small cell change
Dysplastic nodules
Liver cell adenoma (rare)

Carcinoma in situ

The term "carcinoma *in situ*" has been used to refer to cytologically malignant lesions in squamous or columnar epithelium that do not show invasive growth. Although valid from a biological point of view, use of the term "carcinoma *in situ*" in pathology reports is strongly discouraged, particularly for columnar precursor lesions of invasive neoplasia. Lesions with these features are encompassed within the terms "high-grade dysplasia" (or "high-grade intraepithelial neoplasia") since neither type of lesions show invasive growth, and the clinical implications and treatment regimens are similar. However, one exception is in the setting of hereditary diffuse gastric carcinoma (HDGC) where the term "*in situ* signet ring cell carcinoma" has become standard.

Intramucosal adenocarcinoma

The definition of intramucosal carcinoma varies in different parts of the world {2841, 2842}. In the USA and in most European countries, the term is applied to lesions that show histological evidence of invasion into the lamina propria or muscularis mucosa, but not into the submucosa. Histological evidence of invasion includes, but is not limited to, infiltration of the stroma by single cells, or small clusters of cells, atypical or complex glandular arrangements that are beyond that present in normal mucosa, presence of a stromal response such as desmoplasia, and evidence of lymphovascular invasion. In some circumstances, such as in Barrett oesophagus-associated dysplasia and chronic gastritis-associated dysplasia, it is difficult to determine with certainty whether a high-grade lesion has invaded the lamina propria and, therefore, there is significant interobserver variability with regard to separating high-grade dysplasia from intramucosal adenocarcinoma {2353}. As a result, in some parts of the world, such as Japan, the term "noninvasive carcinoma" is used to reflect lesions that show cytological and/or architectural features of "carcinoma" regardless of whether invasion into the lamina propria can be documented histologically.

Epithelial atypia

In diagnostic pathology, the term "atypia" has been loosely used both as a descriptive term, to capture cytological and/or architectural features of potentially neoplastic epithelium, but also as a diagnostic term to define epithelial lesions that differ from normal, but do not quite reach the histological threshold of true neoplasia. As a diagnostic term, it lacks general consensus among pathologists worldwide, clinicians find it ambiguous, and as such, its use is to be avoided in digestive-tract, liver, biliary tract and pancreas pathology. In the tubal gut, the term "indefinite for dysplasia (intraepithelial neoplasia)" is used instead of "atypia" to describe lesions that raise concerns for, but are not diagnostic of, neoplasia.

Summary

With improvements in our understanding of the molecular alterations involved in carcinogenesis, particularly related to conditions in which chronic inflammation is the main stimulus for oncogenesis, and with the advent of studies that intend to establish correlation between genotype and phenotype, pathologists now recognize a broad spectrum of precursor lesions of invasive carcinoma, including lesions that do not necessarily show morphological abnormalities typical of neoplasia.

Therefore, in the current (4th) edition of the WHO classification, the term intraepithelial neoplasia is used to encompass all precursor lesions of invasive neoplasia, regardless of the presence or absence of traditional morphological features of neoplasia. The term "dysplasia" is used in pathology reports for some forms of preinvasive neoplasia, such as those that arise in chronic inflammatory conditions of the oesophagus, stomach, and colon. However, the term "intraepithelial neoplasia" is also acceptable in these settings. For the anus, only the term "intraepithelial neoplasia" is used. For preinvasive neoplastic lesions in the pancreas and biliary tract, both terms are used but depending on the specific type of lesion.

In the subsequent chapters of the current edition of the WHO classification of tumours of the digestive system, the specific terminology, classifications, and histological features of these lesions are described in detail.

Nomenclature and classification of neuroendocrine neoplasms of the digestive system

G. Rindi
R. Arnold
F.T. Bosman
C. Capella

D.S. Klimstra
G. Klöppel
P. Komminoth
E. Solcia

Introduction

One of the major problems in the management of patients with gastrointestinal (neuro)endocrine tumours (NETs) is the lack of universally accepted standards, both for nomenclature (i.e. the clinical significance of current definitions) and for staging of disease {2114}. Based on a wealth of evidence, the most recent WHO classification of 2000 {3013} provided a rational approach to the nomenclature and classification of NETs of the digestive system, developing a coherent terminology and allowing the prognostic stratification of these neoplasms. This WHO classification has served as a basis for establishing criteria for practical management, as reflected in the guidelines of many scientific societies {2343–2345, 2567, 2621}. However, while most institutions in the European Union (EU) adhere to the WHO 2000 classification scheme, the scheme has not achieved widespread acceptance in diagnostic practice in the United States of America (USA). The reasons for this include: (1) the embedding of stage-related information within a grading system; (2) the complicated clinical–pathological classification schemes; and (3) the category "uncertain behaviour," which has met with resistance from both clinicians and pathologists {850}. In addition, the continued widespread use of the term "carcinoid," with its largely incorrect benign connotation, hampered universal acceptance of this classification system. Taking into account the considerations stated above, the European Neuroendocrine Tumor Society (ENETS) has recently proposed two complementary classification tools – a grading classification and a site-specific staging system {2684, 2685}. The intention was to improve the WHO 2000 classification by strengthening its appreciation of the following concepts: (1) tumour heterogeneity, i.e. tumours differ according to the site of origin; (2) tumour differentiation i.e. tumours differ according to tumour cell differentiation status; and (3) malignancy, i.e. long-term follow-up indicates that NETs as a category are malignant.

Such concepts stem from evidence that biological characteristics and stage at diagnosis largely determine the clinical behaviour of NETS. As it does for other epithelial neoplasms, the ENETS grading and staging system formally recognizes the malignant potential of NETs and organizes their classification according to grade and stage.

WHO 2010 classification

In the present volume of the WHO classification of tumours, we attempt to bridge the above-mentioned classification gap by introducing a grading scheme and applying the terms NET and NEC as widely accepted and used by clinicians in both the EU and USA. The term "neuroendocrine" is adopted here to indicate the expression of neural markers in neoplastic cells with otherwise exquisitely endocrine properties and phenotype. The term "neuroendocrine neoplasm" can be used synonymously with "neuroendocrine tumour".

Grading classification

Grading is performed on the basis of morphological criteria (see individual chapters) and the assessment of proliferation fraction according to the ENETS scheme {2684, 2685}. Evidence that the proliferation fraction has prognostic significance is available for NETs of foregut origin, including stomach and pancreas {250, 850, 1705, 2514, 2676, 2682, 2686}. The proposed grading based on proliferation has three tiers (G1, G2, G3) with the following definitions of mitotic count and Ki67 index:
– G1: mitotic count, < 2 per 10 high power fields (HPF) and/or ≤ 2% Ki67 index;
– G2: mitotic count 2–20 per 10 HPF and/or 3–20% Ki67 index;
– G3: mitotic count > 20 per 10 HPF and/or > 20% Ki67 index.

The grading requires mitotic count in at least 50 HPFs (1 HPF = 2 mm^2) and Ki67 index using the MIB antibody as a percentage of 500–2000 cells counted in areas of strongest nuclear labelling ("hot spots"). If grade differs for mitotic count compared with Ki67 index, it is suggested that the higher grade be assumed. Evidence to support this grading scheme is available for the stomach, duodenum and pancreas NETs {772, 868, 1705, 2449}, but is still lacking for NETs of the intestine.

Table 1.03 Transition scheme for the new classification (WHO 2010) including previous definitions for neuroendocrine neoplasms of the digestive system (WHO 1980 and 2000).

WHO 1980	WHO 2000	WHO 2010
I Carcinoid	1. Well-differentiated endocrine tumour (WDET)[a]	1. NET G1 (carcinoid)[b]
	2. Well-differentiated endocrine carcinoma (WDEC)[a]	2. NET G2[b]
	3. Poorly differentiated endocrine carcinoma/small cell carcinoma (PDEC)	3. NEC (large cell or small cell type)[b,c]
II Mucocarcinoid III Mixed forms carcinoid-adenocarcinoma	4. Mixed exocrine-endocrine carcinoma (MEEC)	4. Mixed adenoneuroendocrine carcinoma (MANEC)
IV Pseudotumour lesions	5. Tumour-like lesions (TLL)	5. Hyperplastic and preneoplastic lesions

{1106, 3013, 3516}
G, grade (for definition, see text); NEC, neuroendocrine carcinoma; NET, neuroendocrine tumour.
[a] The difference between WDET and WDEC was defined according to staging features in the WHO 2000 classification. G2 NET does not necessarily translate into WDEC of the WHO 2000 classification.
[b] Definition in parentheses for the International Classification of Diseases for Oncology (ICD-O) coding.
[c] "NET G3" has been used for this category but is not advised, since NETs are by definition well-differentiated.

Site-specific staging system

Grading is combined with a site-specific staging system to improve prognostic strength. Since the grading and staging schemes are still evolving, it is expected that the grade definitions as well as site-specific definitions of TNM (tumour, node, metastasis) stage {2996} may need adjustment in the future, following accumulation of additional follow-up or molecular data. We feel that the introduction of an approach that combines the classification of grade and stage provides a framework that can be applied to NETs in all body organs. Furthermore, distinction of grading and staging allows prognostically relevant grading information to be applied to NETs in metastatic sites whereas, previously, all such NETs were grouped together in the classification system. The TNM staging classifications are presented in each relevant chapter, together with other histopathological variables with recognized prognostic value. In addition, the WHO 2010 classification system reports in brackets the WHO 2000 definitions linked to the codes for the International Classification of Disease Oncology (ICD-O) {904A} (Table 1.03).

Definition of neuroendocrine neoplasms

Definition of neuroendocrine tumour (NET)

A NET is defined as a well-differentiated, neuroendocrine neoplasm composed of cells with features similar to those of the normal gut endocrine cell, expressing general markers of neuroendocrine differentiation (usually diffuse and intense chromogranin A and synaptophysin) and hormones (usually intense but not necessarily diffuse) according to site, with mild-to-moderate nuclear atypia and a low number of mitoses (< 20 per 10 HPF); grade G1 and G2 are defined according to proliferation fraction and histology. This definition encompasses neoplasms termed "carcinoid tumour" in the WHO 2000 classification {3013, 3516} (Table 1.03).

Definition of neuroendocrine carcinoma (NEC)

A NEC is a poorly differentiated, high-grade malignant neoplasm composed of small cells or large to intermediate cells, sometimes with organoid features resembling NET, diffusely expressing the general markers of neuroendocrine differentiation (diffuse expression of synaptophysin; faint or focal staining for chromogranin A), with marked nuclear atypia, multifocal necrosis and a high number of mitoses (> 20 per 10 HPF); high grade (G3) defined according to the proliferation fraction and histology. This definition refers to neoplasms previously classified as small cell carcinoma, large cell (neuro)endocrine carcinoma, or poorly differentiated (neuro)endocrine carcinoma {1106, 3013} (Table 1.03).

Definition of mixed adenoneuroendocrine carcinoma (MANEC)

MANECs have a phenotype that is morphologically recognizable as both gland-forming epithelial and neuroendocrine, and are defined as carcinomas since both components are malignant and should be graded. A component of squamous cell carcinoma is rare. Arbitrarily, at least 30% of either component should be identified to qualify for this definition. The identification in adenocarcinoma of scattered neuroendocrine cells by immunohistochemistry does not qualify for this definition.

Reporting of NETs

Minimum requirements for the reporting of NETs are the exact site and size and the distance from the resection margins (for resection specimens; see specific chapters for site-specific requirements) {1599, 1608}.

Microscopically, the number of mitoses counted per 10 HPF, the number of HPF assessed and the Ki67 index are essential. Assessment of endocrine function should be provided upon specific clinical request. The diagnosis should contain: (1) the classification of the lesion (NET or NEC); (2) the grade (G1, G2 or G3); (3) the relevant TNM stage (for resection specimens; see specific chapters); and (4), upon specific request the cell type and functional activity. One may add in parentheses the WHO 2000 definitions according to staging (well-differentiated endocrine tumour [WDET], well-differentiated endocrine carcinoma [WDEC] or poorly differentiated endocrine carcinoma [PDEC]).

Finally, the suffix "oma" following the name of a hormone (e.g. somatostatinoma, gastrinoma) is only appropriate when there is a clinical syndrome related to excess production of that hormone. In case of immunohistochemical evidence only, terms such as somatostatin-producing NET or gastrin-producing NET are not encouraged; rather, the staining result may be apended to the broad NET diagnostic category (e.g. NET with immunohistochemically demonstrated gastrin production).

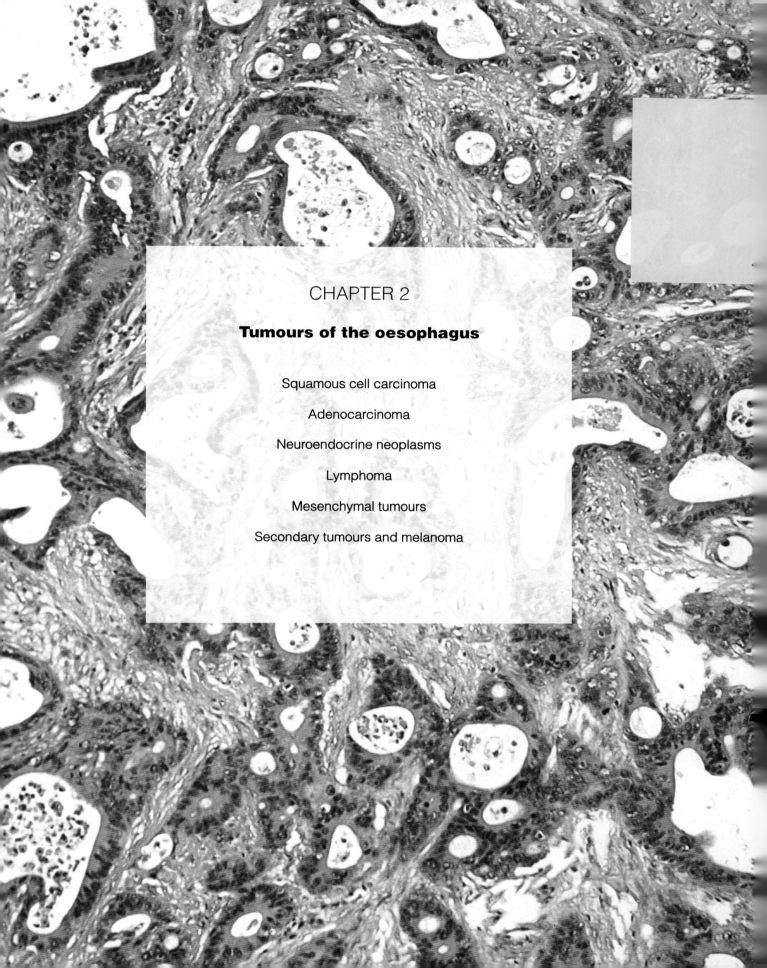

CHAPTER 2

Tumours of the oesophagus

Squamous cell carcinoma

Adenocarcinoma

Neuroendocrine neoplasms

Lymphoma

Mesenchymal tumours

Secondary tumours and melanoma

WHO classification[a] of tumours of the oesophagus

Epithelial tumours

Premalignant lesions

Squamous
   Intraepithelial neoplasia (dysplasia), low grade   8077/0*
   Intraepithelial neoplasia (dysplasia), high grade   8077/2

Glandular
   Dysplasia (intraepithelial neoplasia), low grade   8148/0*
   Dysplasia (intraepithelial neoplasia), high grade 8148/2

Carcinoma

Squamous cell carcinoma	8070/3
Adenocarcinoma	8140/3
Adenoid cystic carcinoma	8200/3
Adenosquamous carcinoma	8560/3
Basaloid squamous cell carcinoma	8083/3
Mucoepidermoid carcinoma	8430/3
Spindle cell (squamous) carcinoma	8074/3
Verrucous (squamous) carcinoma	8051/3
Undifferentiated carcinoma	8020/3

Neuroendocrine neoplasms[b]

Neuroendocrine tumour (NET)
   NET G1 (carcinoid)   8240/3
   NET G2   8249/3
Neuroendocrine carcinoma (NEC)   8246/3
   Large cell NEC   8013/3
   Small cell NEC   8041/3
Mixed adenoneuroendocrine carcinoma   8244/3

Mesenchymal tumours

Granular cell tumour	9580/0
Haemangioma	9120/0
Leiomyoma	8890/0
Lipoma	8850/0
Gastrointestinal stromal tumour	8936/3
Kaposi sarcoma	9140/3
Leiomyosarcoma	8890/3
Melanoma	8720/3
Rhabdomyosarcoma	8900/3
Synovial sarcoma	9040/3

Lymphomas

Secondary tumours

---

[a] The morphology codes are from the International Classification of Diseases for Oncology (ICD-O) {904A}. Behaviour is coded /0 for benign tumours, /1 for unspecified, borderline or uncertain behaviour, /2 for carcinoma *in situ* and grade III intraepithelial neoplasia, and /3 for malignant tumours.
[b] The classification is modified from the previous (third) edition of the WHO histological classification of tumours {691} taking into account changes in our understanding of these lesions. In the case of neuroendocrine neoplasms, the classification has been simplified to be of more practical utility in morphological classification.
* These new codes were approved by the IARC/WHO Committee for ICD-O at its meeting in March 2010.

TNM classification[a] of carcinoma of the oesophagus

T - Primary tumour
TX   Primary tumour cannot be assessed
T0   No evidence of primary tumour
Tis   Carcinoma *in situ*/high-grade dysplasia
T1   Tumour invades lamina propria, muscularis mucosae, or submucosa
   T1a   Tumour invades lamina propria or muscularis mucosae
   T1b   Tumour invades submucosa
T2   Tumour invades muscularis propria
T3   Tumour invades adventitia
T4   Tumour invades adjacent structures
   T4a   Tumour invades pleura, pericardium, or diaphragm
   T4b   Tumour invades other adjacent structures such as aorta, vertebral body, or trachea

N - Regional lymph nodes
NX   Regional lymph nodes cannot be assessed
N0   No regional lymph-node metastasis
N1   Metastasis in 1 to 2 regional lymph nodes
N2   Metastasis in 3 to 6 regional lymph nodes
N3   Metastasis in 7 or more regional lymph nodes

M - Distant metastasis
M0   No distant metastasis
M1   Distant metastasis

Anatomic stage grouping – All carcinomas[b]

Stage	T	N	M
Stage 0	Tis	N0	M0
Stage IA	T1	N0	M0
Stage IB	T2	N0	M0
Stage IIA	T3	N0	M0
Stage IIB	T1, T2	N1	M0
Stage IIIA	T4a	N0	M0
	T3	N1	M0
	T1, T2	N2	M0
Stage IIIB	T3	N2	M0
Stage IIIC	T4a	N1, N2	M0
	T4b	Any N	M0
	Any T	N3	M0
Stage IV	Any T	Any N	M1

Prognostic grouping

Squamous cell carcinoma[c]

Group	T	N	M	Grade[c]	Location[c]
Group 0	Tis	0	0	1	Any
Group IA	1	0	0	1, X	Any
Group IB	1	0	0	2, 3	Any
	2, 3	0	0	1, X	Lower, X
Group IIA	2, 3	0	0	1, X	Upper, middle
	2, 3	0	0	2, 3	Lower, X
Group IIB	2, 3	0	0	2, 3	Upper, middle
	1, 2	1	0	Any	Any
Group IIIA	1, 2	2	0	Any	Any
	3	1	0	Any	Any
	4a	0	0	Any	Any
Group IIIB	3	2	0	Any	Any
Group IIIC	4a	1, 2	0	Any	Any
	4b	Any	0	Any	Any
	Any	3	0	Any	Any
Group IV	Any	Any	1	Any	Any

Adenocarcinoma

Group	T	N	M	Grade[d]
Group 0	Tis	0	0	1
Group IA	1	0	0	1, 2, X
Group IB	1	0	0	3
	2	0	0	1, 2, X
Group IIA	2	0	0	3
Group IIB	3	0	0	Any
	1, 2	1	0	Any
Group IIIA	1, 2	2	0	Any
	3	1	0	Any
	4a	0	0	Any
Group IIIB	3	2	0	Any
Group IIIC	4a	1, 2	0	Any
	4b	Any	0	Any
	Any	3	0	Any
Group IV	Any	Any	1	Any

---

[a] {762, 2996}
[b] The TNM classification and stage grouping for oesophageal GISTs can be found on page 47.
[c] Other carcinomas, apart from adenocarcinomas, can be grouped by the scheme for squamous cell carcinoma.
[d] X, value unknown.

A help desk for specific questions about the TNM classification is available at http://www.uicc.org.

Squamous cell carcinoma of the oesophagus

E. Montgomery
J.K. Field
P. Boffetta
Y. Daigo
M. Shimizu
T. Shimoda

Definition

Squamous cell carcinoma (SCC) of the oesophagus is a malignant epithelial tumour with squamous-cell differentiation, microscopically characterized by keratinocyte-like cells with intercellular bridges and/or keratinization.

ICD-O codes

Intraepithelial neoplasia (dysplasia)
Low grade   8077/0
High grade   8077/2
Squamous cell carcinoma   8070/3
Basaloid squamous cell carcinoma
                     8083/3
Spindle cell (squamous) carcinoma
                     8074/3
Undifferentiated carcinoma   8020/3
Verrucous (squamous) carcinoma
                     8051/3

Epidemiology

The geographical distribution of oesophageal cancer is characterized by wide variations within relatively small areas. High rates (> 50 per 100 000 population) are recorded in men and women in the north of the Islamic Republic of Iran and various provinces of eastern China, (Henan, Jiangsu, Shanxi), in certain areas of Kazakhstan and among men from Zimbabwe. Intermediate rates in men (10–50 per 100 000 population) occur in eastern Africa, southern Brazil, the Caribbean, most of China (with the exception of southern provinces such as Hunan, Guangxi, Guizhou and Yunnan), regions of central Asia, northern India, and southern Europe {634}. In areas with a high risk of developing cancer of the oesophagus, SCC is the predominant histological type. It has been suggested that ethnic factors are involved in susceptibility to this cancer; populations at higher risk in central Asia are of Turkish or Mongolian (not Caucasian) origin, and rates in African-Americans are two- to threefold those in Caucasian Americans, regardless of sex. Incidence rates are 2–10 times higher in men than in women. In many high-risk areas, a decrease in the incidence of oesophageal SCC has occurred during recent decades, in tandem with a sharp increase in oesophageal adenocarcinomas in low-risk populations (northern Europeans and Caucasians in the USA).

Etiology

Tobacco. Tobacco-smoking is a major risk factor for oesophageal SCC {285}. The increased risk in heavy smokers, relative to nonsmokers, is of the order of four- to eightfold. A strong dose–risk relationship has been shown for smoking duration and average consumption. Quitting smoking substantially reduces the risk of oesophageal cancer: the relative risk declines within 5 years after cessation and approaches that of never-smokers within 10–20 years. Smoking black tobacco, high-tar and hand-rolled cigarettes and pipes might exert a stronger effect than smoking other products. Chewing tobacco-containing products is an important risk factor in India and southern Africa, but is of unconfirmed relevance in central Asia. In the latter region, use of opium (smoking and eating) might have (or at least might have in the past) contributed to the high incidence of this cancer.

Alcohol. Alcohol consumption is another important risk factor for oesophageal SCC {293}. It is unclear whether there are differences in the carcinogenic potency of various alcoholic beverages. It has been suggested that there is a reduction in the excess risk of oesophageal SCC after cessation of alcohol drinking, but only after 15–20 years. The effect of alcohol is independent from that of tobacco, but the interaction between the two exposures is synergistic. Together, tobacco-smoking and alcohol consumption account for > 90% of cases of oesophageal SCC in western Europe and North America; however, this proportion is lower in developing countries, particularly in selected areas of Asia and South America where risk is very high.

Hot beverages. Intake of hot maté, an herbal beverage, is an important risk factor for this neoplasm in northern

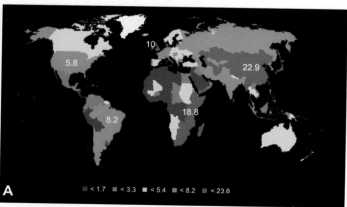

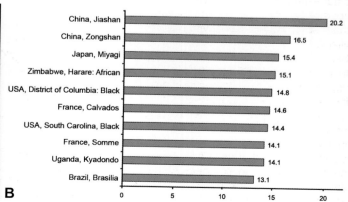

Fig. 2.01 A Age-standardized incidence (per 100 000) of oesophageal cancer in men. Numbers on the map indicate regional average values {842A}. **B** Selected highest age-standardized incidence (per 100 000) of oesophageal cancer in men (1998–2002) {842}.

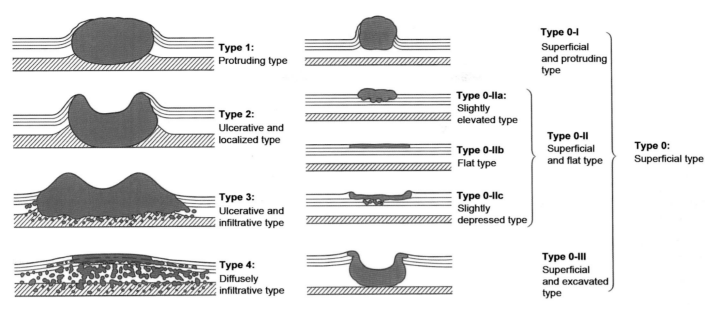

Fig. 2.02 Macroscopic classification of squamous cell carcinoma of the oesophagus. From: Japanese Esophageal Cancer Society, *Japanese Classification of Esophageal Cancer*, 10th edition, 2009 {1388}.

Argentina, southern Brazil and Uruguay. The effect appears to relate to the high temperature of this beverage: studies from other areas suggest that intake of hot beverages (e.g. hot tea in the Islamic Republic of Iran, Japan and Singapore; hot coffee in Puerto Rico; and hot drinks or soups in China, Hong Kong Special Administrative Region) increases the risk of oesophagitis and oesophageal SCC, although the evidence is less consistent than for maté.

Dietary factors. Dietary factors probably play a role in the etiology of oesophageal SCC {3548}. Low intake of fresh fruits and vegetables, fresh or frozen meat or fish, and dairy products and high intake of barbecued meat may all increase the risk; however, the available data do not allow establishment of a preventive role of specific micronutrients, and prevention trials with retinol, riboflavin, selenium, vitamin E and zinc have failed to show a benefit.

In several areas of China, intake of pickled vegetables has been associated with an increased risk of oesophageal SCC. The active carcinogens might be mycotoxins or *N*-nitroso compounds. Mycotoxins, including fumonisin B1, have been detected in mouldy corn from high-risk areas in China and southern Africa. In Japan, eating bracken fern has been associated with an elevated risk of oeso-phageal cancer.

Other factors. Oesophageal cancer is related to ionizing radiation, particularly in women who have undergone radiotherapy for breast cancer.

Other environmental agents that are suspected but not proven to cause oeso-phageal cancer are infection by human papilloma virus (HPV) and combustion fumes.

Patients with Plummer-Vinson syndrome, a sideropenic dysphagia caused by deficiency of iron, riboflavin and other vitamins, show an increased incidence of oesophageal and hypopharyngeal cancers. The risk of oesophageal cancer is also increased among patients with coeliac disease. Patients with achalasia are also at increased risk for carcinoma {1371, 1794, 3677}.

Localization
Oesophageal SCC is located most commonly in the middle third followed by the lower and upper third, respectively, of the oesophagus {1832, 2938}.

Clinical features
The most common symptoms of advanced oesophageal cancer are dysphagia, weight loss, retrosternal or epigastric pain, and regurgitation caused by strictures {798}. Superficial SCC usually has no specific symptoms, but is sometimes associated with a tingling sensation and, therefore, is sometimes detected during endoscopy of the upper gastrointestinal tract {791, 3152}.

Endoscopy and chromoendoscopy
Superficial oesophageal cancer is commonly observed as a slight elevation or shallow depression on the mucosal surface, a minor morphological change compared with advanced cancer.

Macroscopically, three types can be distinguished: polypoid, flat, and ulcerated. Chromoendoscopy using toluidine blue or Lugol iodine spray may be of value. Toluidine blue, a metachromatic stain from the thiazine group, has affinity for RNA and DNA, and stains areas that are richer in nuclei than the normal mucosa. Lugol solution reacts with glycogen in normal squamous epithelium, whereas precancerous and cancerous lesions (but also inflamed areas and gastric heterotopia) are not stained. However, superficially invasive carcinomas cannot be clearly recognized by simple endoscopy. A newer technique called endocytoscopy is based on the technology of light-contact microscopy and can be used together with vital staining, allowing real-time assessment of nuclei, reducing the number of biopsies required for diagnosis {1676}. Confocal endomicroscopy, in which a confocal microscope is affixed to an endoscope, also can be used to improve targeting of biopsy sites {688, 2508}. Narrow-band imaging has also been used to facilitate the detection of early lesions {1684}. Endoscopic ultrasonography is used to evaluate the depth of tumour infiltration and para-oesophageal lymph-node involvement {2046, 2535}. Oesophageal carcinoma often

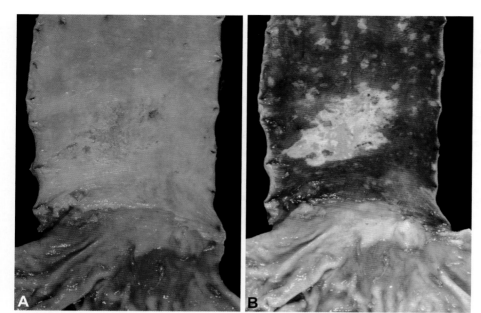

Fig. 2.03 Squamous cell carcinoma of the oesophagus, superficial type (subtype 0-IIc according to the guidelines of the Japanese Esophageal Society). **A** Fresh specimen: slight mucosal depression with irregular margin. **B** With Lugol iodine solution, the carcinoma remains unstained.

presents on endosonography as a circumscribed or diffuse wall-thickening with a predominantly echo-poor or echo-inhomogeneous pattern. As a result of tumour penetration through the wall and into surrounding structures, the endosonographic wall layers are destroyed.

Computed tomography and magnetic resonance imaging

In advanced carcinomas, computed tomography (CT) and magnetic resonance imaging (MRI) give information on local and systemic spread. Tumour growth is characterized as swelling of the oesophageal wall, with or without direct invasion to surrounding organs {2549}. Lymph-node enlargement can be assessed. Three-dimensional CT or MRI images may effectively demonstrate lesions of stage T2, T3 and T4, but not T1. The combination of the metabolic information from 18-fluoro-2-deoxyglucose-positron emission tomography (FDG-PET) with the anatomical information from CT in integrated PET/CT scanners can be valuable for staging oesophageal carcinoma by combining metabolic and anatomical information in a single imaging study {872, 2104, 2710}.

Macroscopy

The gross appearance of oesophageal SCC varies according to the depth of invasion, and is classified by the Japanese Esophageal Society into major superficial type (which is early stage) and advanced type. Superficial type (0 type) indicates that tumour invasion limited to the mucosa or submucosa, and advanced type (types 1–5) extends into and beyond the muscularis propria {1388}. The superficial type is subclassified as follows: 0-I (protruding type) is polypoid or plaque-like; 0-II (superficial and flat type) is either slightly elevated (subtype 0-IIa), completely flat (subtype 0-IIb), or slightly depressed (subtype 0-IIc). Type 0-III is described as a superficial and excavated type. Type 0-II is often an obscure or occult lesion {294} that shows unstained areas using Lugol iodine solution. Type 0-I and 0-II lesions can be managed by endoscopic mucosal resection or endoscopic submucosal dissection {1697}.

For the classification of advanced oesophageal SCC, Ming has proposed three major types: fungating, ulcerative and infiltrating {2084}. On the other hand, the Japanese guidelines for clinical and pathological studies of carcinoma of the oesophagus propose the following types: type 1: protruding; type 2: ulcerative localized; type 3: ulcerative infiltrating; type 4: diffuse infiltrating; and type 5: unclassified. Type 1 has a predominantly exophytic growth pattern, while type 2 is well-demarcated and shows an intramural growth pattern and central surface ulceration. Type 3 has as an ill-defined tumour margin with intramural extension and deep ulceration. Types 2 and 3 correspond to the ulcerative type described in the Ming classification. Type 4, which is the least common, is characterized by wide intramural infiltration of tumour cells with only a small mucosal defect or ulceration and thickness and stiffness of the oesophageal wall. Type 5 is an unclassified type showing mixed patterns.

Tumour spread and staging

Oesophageal SCC invades both horizontally and vertically. When invasion is restricted to the mucosa or the submucosa, irrespective of the presence of regional lymph-node metastases, the lesion is referred to as "superficial oesophageal carcinoma" {294, 3170}. The term "early oesophageal carcinoma" is also used in China and Japan, and is defined as intramucosal carcinoma regardless of the presence of lymph-node metastases {1038, 3170}. In several studies from Japan, superficial carcinomas accounted for 10–20% of all resected carcinomas, whereas in North America and European countries, superficial carcinomas are much less frequently reported {905}.

The term "advanced oesophageal carcinoma" is used for a tumour that invades beyond the muscularis propria.

The TNM (tumour, node, metastasis) system used by the American Joint

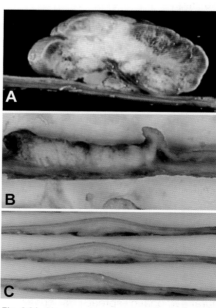

Fig. 2.04 Macroscopic appearance of squamous cell carcinoma of the oesophagus (cut surfaces). **A** Type 0-I (superficial, protruding). **B** Type 2 (advanced), ulcerative localized. **C** Type 4 (advanced), diffuse infiltrating. Classified according to the guidelines of the Japanese Esophageal Society.

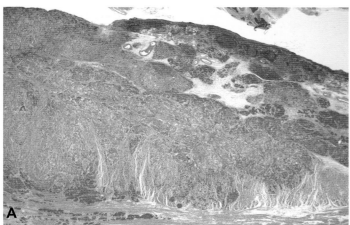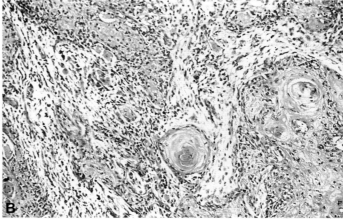

Fig. 2.05 Squamous cell carcinoma of the oesophagus with intramural invasion. **A** Low-power view: intramural invasion is evident. **B** Medium-power view: displaying a well- to moderately differentiated carcinoma.

Committee on Cancer (AJCC) and the International Union against Cancer (UICC) is the most widely accepted staging system {762, 2996}. The 2009 seventh edition AJCC (but not the UICC) has incorporated prognostic groupings in addition to purely anatomical ones for staging oesophageal SCC. These include the addition of grade (G1–G4; well-differentiated, moderately differentiated, poorly differentiated, and undifferentiated, respectively) and location in the oesophagus (upper, middle or lower third) as well as depth of invasion, based on data that show that squamous carcinomas in the upper and middle oesophagus and those that are not well-differentiated are more aggressive than those in the lower oesophagus or are well-differentiated. The number of positive nodes determines the N stage rather than the location of involved nodes. "Tis" is defined as "high-grade dysplasia" by the AJCC, which is considered equivalent to carcinoma *in situ* and non-invasive carcinoma. In both the UICC and AJCC systems, T1 and T4 have been subdivided as of 2009 to provide additional information.

Metastases are usually to regional lymph nodes, found in about 60% of patients at the time of diagnosis. The frequency of lymph-node metastasis correlates with depth of invasion (about 5% for intramucosal carcinoma and about 40% for submucosal carcinoma) {112, 1823}. Intramural metastasis (also called intramural lymphatic spread) is common, being seen in up to 16% of cases {1497, 1696}. It is associated with advanced stage and shortened survival.

Tumours of the upper third of the oesophagus commonly spread to the cervical or upper mediastinal lymph nodes, while carcinomas of the middle and the lower third metastasize to the lower mediastinal or perigastric lymph nodes {56, 112}. Skip-node metastasis can be encountered.

The most common sites for haematogenous metastases include the liver, lungs, adrenals and kidneys, and occasionally the central nervous system (CNS) {1971, 3022}.

Treatment groups. Following clinical staging, two treatment groups are considered. One is for potentially curative treatment (e.g. surgery, radiotherapy, multimodal therapy) for locoregional disease, and the other is palliative treatment; e.g. radio- and/or chemotherapy; for advanced SCC {1031}. Oesophageal early-stage SCC and high-grade intraepithelial neoplasia (dysplasia) can be treated by endoscopic mucosal resection or endoscopic submucosal dissection {2404, 2946}.

Histopathology

Oesophageal SCC is defined as a squamous neoplasm that penetrates the epithelial basement membrane into the lamina propria or deeper tissue layers. Depending on tumour grade, variable amounts of keratinization are seen, manifested by cells showing brightly eosinophilic opaque cytoplasm. Invasion into the lamina propria is initiated by the proliferation of rete-like projections of neoplastic squamous epithelium with pushing borders. Both horizontal and vertical spread is observed. Tumours commonly penetrate vertically through the oesophageal wall and invade intramural lymphatic channels and veins. Invasion of mucosal and submucosal lymphatic channels is also common, and the frequency of lymphatic and blood-vessel invasion increases with increasing depth of invasion {2806}. SCC invades the muscularis propria and extends into the adventitia, from where it may spread to adjacent tissues or organs, such as the trachea, bronchi, aorta, lung, and pericardium; it may cause mediastinitis, pleural fistulas, and tracheo-oesophageal fistulas {3022}. Advanced oesophageal SCC spreads either with an expansive or infiltrative growth pattern. The former pattern comprises a solid mass with a smooth, broad edge, while the latter contains isolated tumour cells or small nests with an irregular invasion front. Occasionally, a desmoplastic stromal reaction or prominent lymphocytic infiltration can be observed {527}.

Additionally, invasive SCC can spread into adjoining non-neoplastic squamous surface epithelium, ducts, or even gastric mucosa in a pattern that appears similar to that of intraepithelial neoplasia. This pattern has been termed "intraepithelial spread" {3167, 3172}. In some instances, the intraepithelial spread involves only the basal half of the replaced non-neoplastic squamous epithelium {3167}.

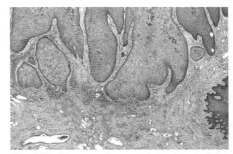

Fig. 2.06 Verrucous (squamous) carcinoma of the oesophagus: highly differentiated keratinized cells with minimal cytological atypia and a pushing pattern of invasion.

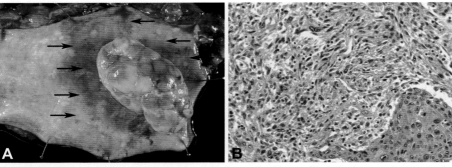

Fig. 2.07 Spindle cell carcinoma of the oesophagus. **A** The large polypoid mass of the lesion is surrounded by extensive intraepithelial neoplasia (arrows). **B** The transition from an area of conventional cells to an area of spindle cells.

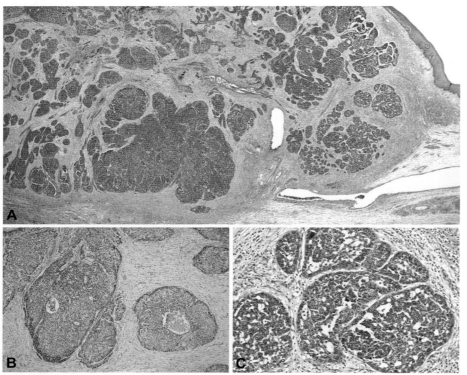

Fig. 2.08 Basaloid squamous cell carcinoma of the oesophagus showing a solid growth pattern. **A** Solid growth pattern. **B** Comedo-like necrosis. **C** Small gland-like structures.

osseous, cartilaginous and skeletal-muscle differentiation {1115}. In immunohisto-chemical and ultrastuctural studies, most cases display various degrees of epithelial differentiation and a transition between epithelial and sarcomatous differentiation. However, there remains a possibility of two independent malignant cell clones {1763}.

Basaloid squamous cell carcinoma

Basaloid SCC is a distinct, unusual variant that occurs more commonly in the upper aerodigestive tract {187, 3298}. It is more common in older men, who present with dysphagia. Microscopically, it consists of basaloid cells with oval to round nuclei, open pale chromatin, and scant baso-philic cytoplasm. It is arranged in solid or cribriform lobules with comedonecrosis {1621A}. Areas of squamous intraepithelial neoplasia or conventional SCC are commonly observed {3429}. Adenoid cystic carcinoma and basaloid squamous cell carcinoma should be distinguished: ade-noid cystic carcinoma is less aggressive {1838}.

Precursor lesions

The development of oesophageal SCC is thought to be a multistep process, progress-ing from normal squamous epithelium, intraepithelial neoplasia (dysplasia), to invasive carcinoma {616, 661, 2608}.

Most data regarding squamous precursor lesions originate from the Far East, where the term "intraepithelial neoplasia" is favoured over "dysplasia". The term "intraepithelial neoplasia" is thus used herewith.

Intraepithelial neoplasia is classified as low-grade (LGIEN) or high-grade (HGIEN). Epidemiologically, LGIEN is associated with a low risk of invasive carcinoma, whereas HGIEN is associated with a high risk {661, 2946}. Morphologically, intraepithelial neo-plasia shows both architectural and cytological abnormalities. Architectural abnormalities include cellular disorganiza-tion/loss of polarity and downward growth of the epithelium {2945, 3168}. Cytological abnormalities include hyperchromasia, increased nucleus : cytoplasm ratio and mitotic activity. In LGIEN, the abnormalities are confined to the lower half of the epithe-lium. In HGIEN, the abnormalities involve the upper half, and cytological alterations are greater than those in LGIEN. In the Far East, the terms "squamous cell carcinoma *in situ*" and "noninvasive carcinoma" are used for HGIEN in which the full thickness of the ep-ithelium is involved. {2839, 2842, 2946, 3170}.

Verrucous (squamous) carcinoma

Verrucous carcinoma is an extremely rare, distinct, highly differentiated variant of SCC. It is usually associated with chronic oesophagitis, achalasia, diverticular disease, or gastro-oesophageal reflux disease {1502}. Grossly, it is an exophytic, papillary, or warty mass. Microscopically, it consists of highly differentiated keratin-ized cells with minimal cytological atypia. Papillary projections are prominent. The tumour shows a pushing rather than an infiltrating margin {2413}, growing slowly and invading locally. Metastases are uncommon.

Spindle cell (squamous) carcinoma

Spindle cell carcinoma is an SCC with a variable spindle-cell component. Synonyms include carcinosarcoma, sarcomatoid carcinoma, pseudosarcomatous SCC, polypoid carcinoma, metaplastic carci-noma, SCC with a spindle-cell component, and carcinoma with mesenchymal stroma {1763}. Grossly, it is polypoid, usually involving the middle and lower third of the oesophagus. Microscopically, it is biphasic with epithelial and spindle cells. The epithelial element is typically well- to mod-erately-differentiated SCC or exclusively carcinoma *in situ*. The spindle-cell compo-nent is usually high-grade. It may show

Basal cell hyperplasia

Basal cell hyperplasia has been defined histologically as involvement of > 15% of the thickness of the squamous epithelium {2198}. The upper limit of the basal cell layer can be defined as the level above which the nuclei are separated by a distance greater than the nuclear diameter {863}. Basal cell hyperplasia is a reactive change in response to inflammation. Endoscopically, this lesion does not retain Lugol iodine applied to the mucosa at endoscopy {2198, 2232}. The presence of multiple unstained areas in the mucosa is a risk factor for multicentric SCCs of the head and neck {3643}. In the oesophagus, several studies have shown that some patients who have multiple unstained mucosal areas also have genetic polymorphisms {3643}. However, the role of basal cell hyperplasia in the development of SCC is controversial.

Grading

Grading oesophageal SCCs is traditionally based on mitotic activity, nuclear atypia and degree of squamous differentiation. However, although incorporated into the 2009 AJCC prognostic groupings {762}, grading is controversial as a means of determining prognosis {2804}.

Well-differentiated carcinoma. There is prominent keratinization and a minor component of nonkeratinizing basal-like cells. The keratinized component shows squamous pearl formation akin to the appearance of non-neoplastic squamous epithelium (normal oesophageal squamous epithelium does not keratinize). Tumour cells are arranged in sheets and mitotic counts are typically low compared with those for moderately and poorly differentiated tumours.

Moderately differentiated SCC. This is the most common histological type, demonstrating variable histological features ranging from parakeratotic to poorly keratinized lesions. Generally, pearl formation is absent. However, definite histological criteria for moderately differentiated SCC are not established and grading is thus affected by inter-observer variability.

Poorly differentiated SCC. This consists predominantly of basal-like cells forming large and small nests with frequent central necrosis. The nests consist of sheets or pavement-like arrangements of tumour cells, and are occasionally punctuated by small numbers of parakeratotic or keratinized cells.

Undifferentiated carcinoma. This lacks definite microscopic features of squamous differentiation. The tumour cells form nests and sheet-like arrangements. Immunohistochemically, tumours express squamous epithelial markers. Such neoplasms must be distinguished from neuroendocrine/small cell NEC. Immunohistochemically, undifferentiated carcinoma is negative for neuroendocrine markers.

Genetic susceptibility

Familial predisposition to oesophageal cancer has been studied predominantly in association with focal non-epidermolytic palmoplantar keratoderma (NEPPK or tylosis) {1262, 2156, 2157}. This autosomal dominantly inherited disorder of the palmar and plantar skin surfaces segregates with oesophageal cancer in three pedigrees, two of which are extensive {784, 1169, 3077}. The causative locus is known as the tylosis oesophageal cancer (*TOC*) gene and maps to 17q25 between the anonymous microsatellite markers D17S1839 and D17S785 {1516, 2690, 2691}.

The genetic defect is thought to be in a molecule involved in the physical structure of stratified squamous epithelia, whereby loss of gene function may alter oesophageal integrity, thereby increasing susceptibility to environmental mutagens. Several candidate genes, including envoplakin (*EVPL*), integrin b4 (*ITGB4*) and plakoglobin, have been excluded as the *TOC* gene following integration of the genetic and physical maps of this region {2692}.

Linkage and haplotype analysis have mapped the *TOC* locus to a 42.5 kb region that contains the promoter of one gene (FLJ22341), the entire cytoglobin gene (*CYGB*) and the 5' end of an uncharacterized gene that completely overlaps *CYGB* in the opposite orientation {1739}. Sequencing of genomic DNA from affected and unaffected TOC family members has identified two putative disease-specific alterations, but they are located in regions of no known function. However, it has been shown that the expression of *CYGB* in oesophageal biopsies from tylotic patients is reduced by 70% compared with normal oesophagus. As this is an autosomal disease, it has been argued that these results exclude haploinsufficency as a mechanism for the disease and suggests a novel *trans*-allele interaction. The mechanism by which the downregulation of *CYGB* may cause the TOC phenotype is unclear, as the function of *CYGB* is unknown {2030};

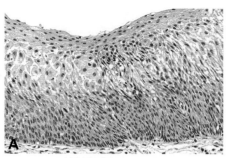
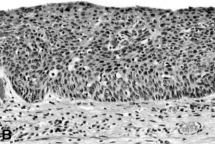

Fig. 2.09 Intraepithelial neoplasia of the oesophagus. **A** Low-grade (LGIEN): an increased number of basal cells and mild cytological atypia are displayed. **B** High-grade (HGIEN): architectural disarray, loss of polarity and cellular atypia (much greater than in A) are evident.

however, some authors suggest that, as the TOC pathology occurs in epithelia, it is likely that an epithelial–mesenchymal interaction is involved in this disease.

The genomic region containing the *TOC* gene also associates with sporadic oesophageal SCCs {1372, 2895, 3411}, adenocarcinoma of the oesophagus {751} and primary breast cancers {918} in studies of loss of heterozygosity (LOH). The *CYGB* gene also plays a role in lung and head and neck cancer {2157, 2912, 3569}.

In Asians, polymorphisms in *ALDH1B1* and *ALDH2*, the genes encoding aldehyde dehydrogenase, are associated with oesophageal SCC {340, 629}. The effects of these polymorphisms are synergistic with alcohol use and smoking. Additionally, some polymorphisms in *ALDH1*, result in accumulation in acetaldehyde, which causes flushing upon ingestion of alcohol ("Asian flush") {340} in about one third of east Asians (Chinese, Japanese and Koreans).

Molecular pathology

Mutation in the *TP53* gene (17p13) is an early event, sometimes detectable in intraepithelial neoplasia. The frequency and type of mutation varies by geographic region, suggesting that some *TP53* mutations may occur as the result of exposure to exogenous risk factors. However, even in SCCs from western Europe, *TP53* does not show the same tobacco-associated mutations as in lung cancers {2134}. Amplification of cyclin D1 (11q13) occurs in 20–40% of SCCs and is frequently detected in cancers that retain expression of the Rb protein, supporting the notion that these two factors cooperate within the same pathway {1428}. Inactivation of CDKN2A, either by homozygous deletion or de novo methylation, appears to be associated with advanced cancer. Other potentially important genetic alterations include transcriptional inactivation of the FHIT gene (fragile histidine triad, a presumptive tumour suppressor on 3p14) by methylation of 5' CpG islands, and deletion of the TOC gene on 17q25 {2132, 3411}. Furthermore, analysis of clones on 3p21.3 and 9q32, where frequent LOH occurs in oesophageal cancer {2152}, led to the identification of the novel genes DLEC1 (deleted in lung and esophageal cancer-1) and DEC1 (deleted in esophageal cancer-1) {645, 1809, 2306, 3616}. Although the function of these genes remains to be clarified, reverse-transcriptase-polymerase chain reaction (RT-PCR) experiments indicate that 33–53% of primary oesophageal cancers lack functional transcripts, and introduction of DLEC1 or DEC1 cDNA into cancer cell lines suppresses cell growth. Recent evidence suggests frequent silencing of LRP1B (low density lipoprotein receptor-related protein 1B) and CRABP1 (cellular retinoic acid binding protein 1) expression by genetic and/or epigenetic mechanisms in primary oesophageal cancers {3020, 3184}. Amplification of several proto-oncogenes has also been reported: FGF4 (HST1), FGF6 (HST2), EGFR, MYC {2134}. Analyses of genome-wide gene expression profiles and proteomic approaches have identified candidate tumour suppressor genes, oncogenes, and cancer-related microRNAs {644, 1086, 2602, 3576}. The mechanisms by which these various genetic events correlate with phenotypical changes and cooperate in the sequence of events leading to SCC remain unknown.

Prognosis and predictive factors

Overall, the prognosis for oesophageal SCC is poor; 5-year survival rates are about 10%. A cure can only be anticipated in patients with superficial cancer. The probability of survival depends upon the patient's general health (performance status, weight loss, haemoglobin level), TNM stage at diagnosis, treatment (radicality of surgical resection [R0] or radiological and endoscopic response to chemoradiation therapy), and morphological and molecular features of the tumour {278, 1858}.

Morphological factors. The extent to which the carcinoma has spread is the most important prognostic factor; the TNM classification is the most widely-used staging system.

Staging. All studies indicate that the depth of invasion and the presence of nodal or distant metastases are independent predictors of survival {1305, 1496, 1905}. In particular, any lymph-node involvement, regardless of the extent of the primary tumour, indicates poor prognosis {1542, 3128, 3152}. Other histopathological features associated with a poor prognosis include vascular and/or lymphatic invasion {1305, 2806} and an infiltrative growth pattern of the primary tumour {2804}.

Differentiation. Although most (but not all {1196, 1305}) studies have not shown a significant influence of tumour grade on survival {764, 2699, 2804, 3121}, tumour-grade has nonetheless been incorporated into the 2009 AJCC TNM classification as a factor affecting prognostic grouping {762}.

Assessment of early-stage carcinoma for endoscopic treatment. In many cases, early-stage oesophageal SCCs are moderately and poorly differentiated. Well-differentiated early SCC is rare {1388}. Since early-stage carcinomas can often be managed by endoscopic resection or endoscopic submucosal dissection {1388}, additional factors can be assessed to better stratify risk and identify patients who do not require additional post-endoscopy treatment (surgery or chemoradiation) {769, 1387, 2945, 2946}. Lesions that can be managed endoscopically include those with: (1) invasion confined to the mucosa with downward growth from the epithelium or submucosal invasion to a depth of 200 µm or less from the muscularis mucosae {1387}; (2) expansive growth of neoplastic cells without small nests or scattered cells infiltrating into stroma; and (3) no lymphovascular invasion {3155}.

Lymphocytic infiltration. Intense lymphocytic response to the tumour has been associated with a better prognosis {764, 2804}.

Cell proliferation. The cancer-cell proliferation index, determined immunohistochemically by antibodies to proliferating cell nuclear antigen (PCNA) or Ki67 is not an independent prognostic factor {1313, 1730, 2803, 3661}.

DNA ploidy. Aneuploidy of cancer cells, as determined by flow cytometry or image analysis, has been identified in 55–95% of oesophageal SCCs {1591}. Patients with diploid tumours usually survive longer than those with aneuploid tumours; however, a prognostic impact independent of tumour stage (TNM) has not been confirmed in the majority of studies {729, 2010, 1591, 1823}.

Extent of resection. The frequency of locoregional recurrence is negatively correlated with the distance of the primary tumour from the proximal resection margin {1766, 3176}.

Molecular factors. The TP53 gene is mutated in 35–80% of oesophageal SCCs {2134}. Some studies have indicated a negative prognostic influence for nuclear accumulation of p53 {485, 2937}, but this has not been observed consistently {575, 1313}. Other potential prognostic factors include growth factors and their receptors {1578}, proto-oncogenes (e.g. ERBB2, FGF3/INT2) {1312}, cell-cycle regulators (e.g. cyclin D1 {2185, 2951}), tumour-suppressor genes {3166}, redox defence-system components (e.g. metallothionein and heat-shock proteins {1508}), E-cadherin {123}, VEGF {2934} and matrix proteinases {2194, 3278, 3590}. Molecular classification using these single biomarkers plus novel markers identified through genomic and proteomic approaches were shown to be independent prognostic parameters {1201, 1358, 3182, 3334, 3577}; however, none of the factors tested so far is indicated for use in clinical practice.

Adenocarcinoma of the oesophagus

J.-F. Fléjou
R.D. Odze
E. Montgomery
P. Chandrasoma
H. Höfler
P. Boffetta
S.J. Spechler

Definition
A malignant epithelial tumour of the oesophagus with glandular differentiation. These tumours arise predominantly from columnar ("Barrett") mucosa in the lower third of the oesophagus. Rarely, adenocarcinoma originates from heterotopic gastric mucosa in the upper oesophagus, or from mucosal and submucosal glands.

ICD-O codes
Dysplasia (intraepithelial neoplasia)
Low grade	8148/0
High grade	8148/2
Adenocarcinoma	8140/3
Adenoid cystic carcinoma	8200/3
Adenosquamous carcinoma	8560/3
Mucoepidermoid carcinoma	8430/3

Epidemiology
In high-resource countries, the incidence and prevalence of oesophageal adenocarcinoma has risen during the last decades of the 20th century {1720}. Population-based studies in the United States of America (USA) and several European countries indicate that the incidence of oesophageal adenocarcinoma doubled between the early 1970s and late 1980s and continues to increase at a rate of about 5% per year {285, 1720}. This is paralleled by rising rates of adenocarcinoma of the oesophagogastric junction (OGJ) and of the proximal stomach, reducing the likelihood that this increase is attributable to changes in the classification of anatomically close lesions. In the early 2000s, the incidence of oesophageal adenocarcinoma was estimated at 1–5 per 100 000 population per year in Europe and North America, exceeding that of squamous cell oesophageal cancer. The countries with the highest incidence were the United Kingdom UK), Australia, the Netherlands and the USA. Relatively lower rates of incidence are reported from eastern Europe and Scandinavia. In Latin America, Asia and Africa, oesophageal adenocarcinoma is uncommon, but increases have also been reported.

In addition to increases in incidence, adenocarcinoma of the oesophagus and of the oesophagogastric junction share some epidemiological characteristics that clearly distinguish these neoplasms from squamous cell oesophageal carcinoma and adenocarcinoma of the distal stomach. These include a high male : female ratio (between 4 : 1 and 7 : 1) and a higher incidence among whites and groups with higher socioeconomic status {285}.

Etiology
Hereditary factors
Although familial association has been reported, population-based studies have shown that the influence of genetic factors is limited, consistent with the rapid changes in incidence rates observed in many populations over a very short period {1720}.

Barrett oesophagus and gastro-oesophageal reflux
The epidemiological features of adenocarcinoma of the oesophagus and OGJ match those of patients with known intestinal metaplasia in the distal oesophagus, i.e. Barrett oesophagus {3507}, which has been identified as the single most important precursor lesion and risk factor for oesophageal adenocarcinoma, irrespective of the length of the segment with intestinal metaplasia. Intestinal metaplasia of the oesophagus develops when the squamous oesophageal epithelium is replaced by columnar epithelium during the process of healing after repetitive injury, and is typically associated with gastro-oesophageal reflux disease (GORD) {3036}. Intestinal metaplasia can be detected in most patients with oesophageal adenocarcinoma {1557}.

The relative risk of oesophageal adenocarcinoma in patients with Barrett oesophagus is in the order of 30–60 {1720},

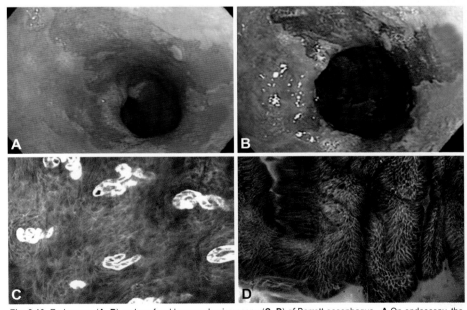

Fig. 2.10 Endoscopy (**A**, **B**) and confocal laser endomicroscopy (**C**, **D**) of Barrett oesophagus. **A** On endoscopy, the pink metaplastic columnar mucosa extends both circumferentially and with "tongues." **B** On narrow band imaging, the distinction between columnar mucosa and squamous mucosa is enhanced. **C** Squamous mucosa (the confocal laser endomicroscope is placed en face on the mucosa). The capillaries are accentuated by fluorescein, administered intravenously to the patient. **D** Barrett mucosa without dysplasia. Note the regular cell borders and empty areas within individual cells (corresponding to goblet cells).

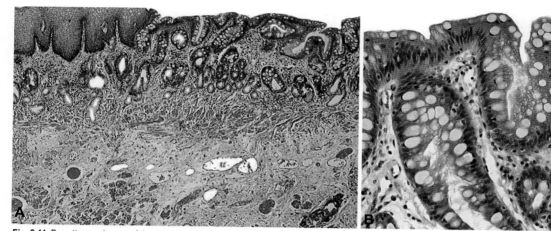

Fig. 2.11 Barrett oesophagus. **A** Intestinal metaplasia adjacent to squamous epithelium (low power). **B** Typical metaplastic mucosa with a villiform pattern, and with goblet cells and columnar cells (high power).

with approximately 5% of patients having a previous diagnosis of Barrett oesophagus {747}. A meta-analysis of studies in patients with Barrett oesophagus has shown an incidence of oesophageal adenocarcinoma of the order of 6.1 per 1000 person-years, which reduced to 3.9 per 1000 person-years when only high-quality studies were considered {3660}. This translates into a life-time risk of about 10% in these patients.

The biological significance of so-called "ultra-short" Barrett oesophagus or intestinal metaplasia just beneath a normal Z line has yet to be clarified {2251}. Whether adenocarcinoma of the OGJ or proximal stomach is also related to foci of intestinal metaplasia at or immediately below the OGJ {1207, 2907, 3033} is discussed in Chapter 3. There is need for an evaluation of the impact of periodic endoscopic screening of Barrett oesophagus patients on mortality from oesophageal adenocarcinoma.

Chronic GORD is the usual underlying cause of the repetitive mucosal injury and also provides an abnormal environment during the healing process that predisposes to intestinal metaplasia {3036}. The relative risk of oesophageal adenocarcinoma in persons with recurrent reflux symptoms, compared with persons without such symptoms, is in the order of 5–10 {164, 823, 1721, 3555, 3629}. The more frequent, more severe, and longer-lasting the symptoms of reflux, the greater the risk. In a Swedish study, the risk of oesophageal adenocarcinoma was increased by 40-fold in persons with long-standing and severe symptoms {1721}. Factors predisposing for the development of Barrett oesophagus and adenocarcinoma

in patients with GORD include a markedly increased duration of oesophageal exposure to refluxed gastric and duodenal contents owing to a defective barrier function of the lower oesophageal sphincter and ineffective clearance function of the tubular oesophagus {3067}. Experimental and clinical data indicate that combined oesophageal exposure to gastric acid and duodenal contents (bile acids and pancreatic enzymes) appears to be more detrimental than isolated exposure to gastric juice or duodenal contents alone {3068}. Combined reflux is thought to increase cancer risk by promoting cellular proliferation, and by exposing the oesophageal epithelium to potentially genotoxic gastric and intestinal contents, e.g. nitrosamines {3068}.

Tobacco-smoking

Smoking has been identified as another major risk factor for oesophageal adenocarcinoma, the relative risk for ever-smokers vs never-smokers being in the order of 2 {1333}. Tobacco-smoking may account for as many as 40% of cases. The risk of oesophageal adenocarcinoma remains elevated up to 30 years after smoking cessation {3556}, suggesting that tobacco-smoking acts through an early-stage carcinogenic effect.

Overweight and obesity

An association between risk of oesophageal adenocarcinoma and overweight and obesity has been observed in many populations and it is considered to be causal {3548}. In meta-analyses, the risk was increased 1.5–1.9-fold among overweight individuals and 2.4–2.8-fold among obese individuals, compared with

individuals of normal weight {1111, 1669}. The pathogenetic basis of the association with obesity is not fully elucidated, but one of the mechanisms may be through central obesity, which may increase intra-abdominal pressure, promoting GORD and Barrett oesophagus {780}.

Alcohol

In contrast to squamous-cell oesophageal carcinoma, there is no association between alcohol consumption and oesophageal adenocarcinoma {285}.

Diet

The evidence linking specific dietary factors (including foods that may cause the lower oesophageal sphincter to relax {3223}) to risk of oesophageal adenocarcinoma is inconsistent {285}.

Helicobacter pylori

Case–control studies have reported a reduced risk of oesophageal adenocarcinoma among individuals infected with *Helicobacter pylori*, in particular of CagA type {285}. A similar protective association has been observed for GORD {1048}. The mechanism may involve reduction of the amount of gastric acid that is refluxed into the oesophagus.

Medications

Several studies have observed an increased risk of oesophageal adenocarcinoma following use of medications that lower stomach acidity and relax the gastro-oesophageal sphincter, e.g. H2-receptor antagonists, proton-pump inhibitors, tricyclic antidepressants, calcium-channel blockers and anti-asthma agents {285}. However, the available evidence points towards a role of the underlying medical conditions. It has been suggested that the use of non-steroidal anti-inflammatory drugs (NSAIDs) is protective {1090}, but confounding by indication may also be responsible for the observed effect in this case.

Localization
Adenocarcinoma may occur anywhere in a segment of columnar-lined oesophagus. It develops most often (but not always) in areas of mucosa with intestinal metaplasia (goblet cells) most commonly in the distal region of the columnar-lined segment {3232}. Adenocarcinoma in a short segment of Barrett oesophagus is easily mistaken for adenocarcinoma of the OGJ. Since adenocarcinomas originating from the distal oesophagus may infiltrate the OGJ and carcinoma of the proximal stomach may grow into the distal oeso-phagus, these entities are frequently diffi-cult to distinguish. However, it is now considered that adenocarcinomas that cross the OGJ should be called adeno-carcinomas of the OGJ, regardless of where the bulk of the tumour lies {2963}; it is therefore very likely that a significant proportion of those OGJ cancers are indeed Barrett adenocarcinomas origi-nating from a metaplastic oesophageal mucosa (see Chapter 3).

Exceptionally, adenocarcinoma also oc-curs in the middle or proximal third of the oesophagus, in the latter usually from a congenital islet of heterotopic columnar mucosa, present in up to 10% of the population.

Barrett oesophagus
Symptoms and signs
Barrett oesophagus as the precursor of most adenocarcinomas is clinically silent in up to 90% of cases. The symptomatology of Barrett oesophagus, when present, is that of GORD {1733, 2896, 3034}.

Endoscopy
The endoscopic analysis of the squamo-columnar junction aims at the detection of columnar metaplasia in the distal oesoph-agus according to anatomical landmarks. If the length of the columnar lining in this distal oesophagus is > 3 cm, it is termed "long-segment" Barrett oesophagus. When the length is < 3 cm, it is termed "short-segment" Barrett oesophagus. Single or multiple finger-like (1–3 cm) protrusions of columnar mucosa are classified as short-segment type. The Prague C and M

criteria, a new system for categorizing Barrett oesophagus, identify both the circumferential extent (C) and the maximum extent (M) of Barrett metaplasia {2904}. The risk of developing adenocarcinoma is reported to be lower in patients with short-segment Barrett oesophagus, than in those with long-segment Barrett oesophagus {2905}.

Histopathology
In North America and parts of Europe, the diagnosis of Barrett oesophagus is restricted to columnar epithelium with goblet cells {2354, 3447}. However, some authorities accept columnar epithelium without goblet cells as part of the definition {478, 2675, 2906, 3169}.

Barrett epithelium shows a variety of cell types such as goblet cells ("specialized"), mucinous columnar cells, enterocytes, Paneth cells, neuroendocrine cells, and epithelium with mixed features (multi-layered epithelium with squamous and columnar features) {997}. The underlying glands may be mucous, oxyntic or both. Duplication of the muscularis mucosae is a common feature {1827}.

Intraepithelial neoplasia in Barrett oesophagus
General comments
Adenocarcinoma in Barrett oesophagus develops through a progressive sequence of morphologically identifiable premalig-nant lesions termed "dysplasia". Worldwide, there are two classification systems used for dysplasia in Barrett oesophagus: the system proposed by the Inflammatory Bowel Disease (IBD) Dysplasia Morphology Study Group, which classifies dysplasia as negative, indefinite, or positive (low- or high-grade) and the Vienna classification system, which does not use the term

dysplasia, but instead categorizes epithe-lial alterations as negative, indefinite, non-invasive low- or high-grade intraepithelial neoplasia, and invasive neoplasia {2654, 2674, 2842}. In the Vienna system, the non-invasive high-grade epithelial neoplasia category is separated into "high-grade ade-noma/dysplasia", "noninvasive carcinoma (carcinoma in situ)" and lesions considered "suspicious for invasive carcinoma". The invasive neoplasia category is separated into intramucosal and submucosal adeno-carcinoma {2842}.

Macroscopy
Grossly, dysplasia may be undetectable or appear as flat, irregular, plaque-like, nodular, polypoid, eroded, or ulcerated mucosa {147, 387, 1195, 2136, 2653, 2654, 3245}. The risk of malignancy is de-pendent on the macroscopic appearance of the lesion. For instance, patients with at least one macroscopically detectable lesion are more likely to develop high-grade dysplasia or cancer {1195}. The presence of mucosal nodules or ulcers has been associated with a higher risk of high-grade dysplasia or adenocarcinoma {387, 2136}. Dysplastic epithelium may appear as a well-defined adenoma-like polyp, but these lesions show a high association with high-grade dysplasia and adenocarcinoma within adjacent flat mucosa {147, 3245}. Thus, the preferred term is "polypoid dysplasia arising in Barrett oesophagus" rather than "adenoma" {3245}.

Histopathology
Dysplasia is diagnosed by the presence and degree of cytological and architectural atypia {2135, 2353, 2654, 2842}.
Negative for dysplasia. This term is applied to cases that show metaplastic columnar epithelium, either with or without

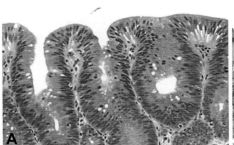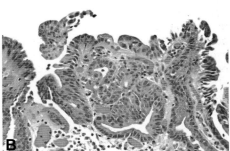

Fig. 2.12 Dysplasia in Barrett oesophagus. **A** Low-grade dyplasia. The nuclei are elongated and crowded with mild pleomorphism, while the crypt architecture is relatively preserved. **B** High-grade dyplasia. The nuclei in the glands are enlarged and hyperchromatic and the changes extend to the surface. In the glands and on the surface, the nuclei have lost their polarity.

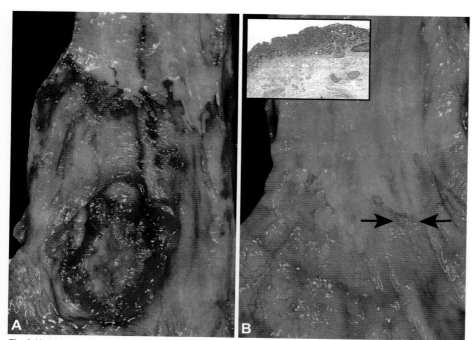

Fig. 2.13 Adenocarcinoma in Barrett oesophagus. **A** Large ulcerated tumour in the lower part of a long-segment Barrett oesophagus. **B** Short-segment Barrett oesophagus with an occult intramucosal adenocarcinoma (arrows and inset).

goblet cells, with regenerative changes. Regenerating Barrett oesophagus may show a slight degree of crypt budding and branching, atrophy, and even cystic change, particularly adjacent to or underneath ulcers. The nuclei may be slightly enlarged, hyperchromatic, show prominence of nucleoli and mild nuclear stratification, particularly at the bases of the crypts.

Indefinite for dysplasia. The "indefinite" category is used most often where technical issues render the interpretation of atypia difficult, where atypia approaches but does not quite attain dysplasia, particularly when it is related to inflammation and ulceration, and atypical (dysplasia-like) changes present in the bases of the crypts, but without surface involvement {1889, 2353}. However, recent evidence suggests that this represents true "early" dysplasia {1889}. In general, the presence of an abrupt transition from non-atypical to atypical epithelium is suggestive of true neoplasia. For inflammation-associated atypia, increased anti-GORD therapy is recommended, followed by repeat biopsies after 3–6 months in order to re-evaluate the atypical area.

Low-grade dysplasia. This is characterized by crypts with relatively preserved architecture, or only minimal distortion, containing cells with atypical pencil-shaped nuclei limited to the basal portion

of the cell cytoplasm. The nuclei are elongated, enlarged, crowded, hyperchromatic, show an irregular contour, a dense chromatin pattern either with or without multiple inconspicuous nucleoli, mild pleomorphism and mild loss of polarity, mucin depletion and increased mitoses.

High-grade dysplasia. This is diagnosed by the presence of marked cytological abnormalities and/or significant architectural complexity of the glands. Cytological abnormalities of high-grade dysplasia include marked nuclear pleomorphism and loss of polarity, irregularity of nuclear contour, increased nucleocytoplasmic ratio, increased number of atypical mitoses particularly in the upper levels of the crypts, and full-thickness nuclear stratification in the crypts and the surface epithelium. Architectural abnormalities of high-grade changes include crypt budding, branching, marked crowding, or villiform contour of the epithelium and, rarely, intraluminal papillae, bridges or a cribriform growth pattern.

Intramucosal adenocarcinoma. High-grade dysplasia can be difficult to distinguish from intramucosal adenocarcinoma, the latter being defined by the presence of invasion of the lamina propria. Observer agreement in separating high-grade dysplasia from intramucosal adenocarcinoma

is modest at best {740}. Previously published criteria of intramucosal adenocarcinoma include: (1) single cells or small clusters of compact back-to-back glands within the lamina propria; (2) a cribriform or solid pattern of growth with expansion and distortion of the adjacent crypts; and (3) a highly distorted/irregular glandular proliferation not explained by the presence of preexisting glands. The presence of necrosis and/or desmoplasia also favours adenocarcinoma, although these features are rarely present in carcinomas limited to the mucosa and, in fact, may not be present in submucosal invasive carcinomas either {2409}. Intraluminal necrosis was shown to be predictive of carcinoma at the time of resection in one study {3717}.

Other cases. Some cases of dysplasia show cuboidal-shaped cells, with round- to oval-shaped nuclei and high nucleocytoplasmic ratio, but without nuclear stratification, which has been termed "non-adenomatous" dysplasia {2747}. Foveolar dysplasia, indicating the presence of neoplastic epithelial cells rich in mucin, is rare in Barrett oesophagus. In the early stages of development, dysplasia may be limited to the crypt bases, without surface involvement {1889, 3702}. These cases are often associated with traditional full-length crypt dysplasia in biopsies elsewhere in the oesophagus.

The diagnostic reproducibility of dysplasia is highly dependent on the level of expertise of the observer, and is less pronounced at the two extremes of the spectrum (negative and high-grade) than it is for lesions in the middle (indefinite and low-grade) {2135, 2654}. The American College of Gastroenterology strongly recommends that all diagnoses of dysplasia be confirmed by an expert gastrointestinal pathologist before patient management {3447}.

Adenocarcinoma
Symptoms and signs
Symptoms of advanced adenocarcinoma are similar to those of squamous cell carcinoma {798}. Superficial adenocarcinoma has no specific symptoms. It can be discovered in patients presenting with symptoms of GORD, or during the surveillance of patients with Barrett oesophagus {2896}.

Endoscopy

Areas with high-grade dysplasia are often multicentric and occult. Therefore systematic tissue sampling has been recommended when no abnormality is evident macroscopically {817}. The endoscopic aspect has poor reliability in the prediction of invasive or noninvasive neoplasia {124}. The addition of indigo carmine chromoendoscopy, acetic acid chromoendoscopy, narrow-band imaging, and confocal laser endomicroscopy has been proposed to improve detection of early neoplasia in Barrett oesophagus {636, 749, 1538, 3538}. The endoscopic pattern of the early stages of the tumour may be that of a small polypoid adenomatous-like lesion, but is more often flat, depressed, elevated or occult {1732, 1733}. The usual pattern of advanced adenocarcinoma as seen by endoscopy is that of an axial, and often tight, stenosis in the distal third of the oesophagus; with a polypoid tumour; bleeding occurs on contact.

Radiology

Today, barium studies are helpful mostly for the analysis of stenotic segments; they are less efficient than endoscopy for the detection of flat abnormalities. Computed tomography (CT) will detect distant thoracic and abdominal metastases.

Endoscopic ultrasonography

At high frequency, some specificities in the echoic pattern of the mucosa and submucosa of the columnar-lined oesophagus are displayed. However, the procedure is only suitable for the staging of tumours previously detected at endoscopy; the tumour is hypoechoic. Lymph nodes adjacent to the oesophageal wall can also be visualized by this technique {2507, 2726}.

Macroscopy

The cancer may arise anywhere within Barrett oesophagus, although early cancers are often contiguous with the squamous epithelium. Adjacent to the tumour, the typical salmon-pink mucosa of Barrett oesophagus may be evident, especially in early carcinomas. At early stages, the gross findings of Barrett adenocarcinoma may be subtle, with irregular mucosal bumps or small plaques. At the time of diagnosis, most tumours are advanced, with deep infiltration of the oesophageal wall. The advanced carcinomas are predominantly flat and ulcerated with only

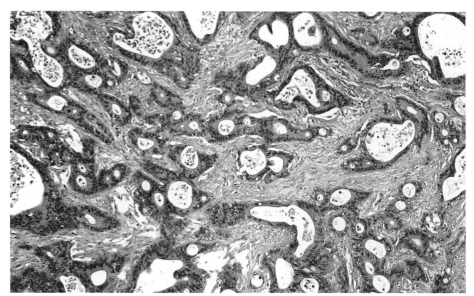

Fig. 2.14 Adenocarcinoma of the oesophagus, well- to moderately differentiated ("low-grade").

one third having a polypoid or fungating appearance. Occasionally, multifocal tumours may be present {1823, 2991}. The rare adenocarcinomas arising independently of Barrett oesophagus from ectopic gastric glands and oesophageal glands display predominantly ulceration and polypoid gross features, respectively. These tumours are also found in the upper and middle third of the oesophagus, but are infrequent {494, 1479}.

Histopathology

Oesophageal adenocarcinomas are typically papillary and/or tubular. A large majority of cases belong to the intestinal type according to the Laurén classification {2802}. A few tumours are of the diffuse type and show rare glandular formations, and sometimes signet-ring cells {2460, 2991}. Differentiation may result in neuroendocrine cells, Paneth cells and squamous cells. Mucinous adenocarcinomas, i.e. tumours with > 50% of the lesion consisting of mucin, also occur.

Grading

Most adenocarcinomas are well or moderately differentiated {2460, 2802}. In biopsy specimens of well-differentiated tumours, the infiltrating component may be difficult to recognize as invasive {1823}. Glandular structures are only slightly formed in poorly differentiated adenocarcinomas and absent in undifferentiated tumours.

Tumour spread and staging

Adenocarcinomas spread first locally and deeply within the oesophageal wall. Distal spread to the stomach may occur. Like squamous cell carcinoma, tumours limited to the mucosa or submucosa are called superficial adenocarcinomas. A specific issue for adenocarcinomas is the almost constant presence of a double muscularis mucosae in Barrett oesophagus. Cancers infiltrating between the inner and outer muscularis mucosae are still considered to be intramucosal cancer, but they have a higher frequency of angiolymphatic invasion and lymph-node metastases compared with those that are limited to the original lamina propria {9, 1969}. Extension through the oesophageal wall into adventitial tissue, and then into adjacent organs or tissues is similar to squamous cell carcinoma. Common sites of local spread comprise the mediastinum, tracheobronchial tree, lung, aorta, pericardium, heart and spine {1823, 3022}. Barrett adenocarcinoma metastasizes to para-oesophageal and paracardial lymph nodes, and those of the lesser curvature of the stomach and the coeliac nodes. Distant metastases occur late. The TNM classification used for squamous cell carcinoma is applicable to Barrett adenocarcinoma and provides prognostically significant data {762, 2996, 3277}.

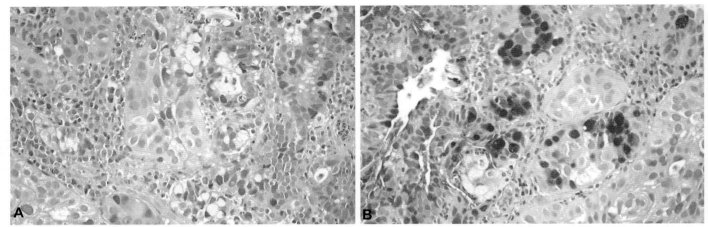

Fig. 2.15 Adenosquamous carcinoma of the oesophagus. **A** The lesion displays glands and islands with intercellular bridges typical of squamous differentiation. **B** On Alcian blue staining (pH 2.5), droplets of acid mucin are apparent in some of the cells in the glandular component, but not in the squamous component.

Other carcinomas

Adenosquamous carcinoma

This carcinoma has mixed elements of adenocarcinoma and squamous cell carcinoma, which remain clearly distinguishable within the tumour.

Mucoepidermoid carcinoma

This rare carcinoma shows an intimate mixture of squamous cells, mucus-secreting cells and cells of an intermediate type {3180}.

Adenoid cystic carcinoma

This neoplasm is also infrequent and believed to arise, like the mucoepidermoid variant, from oesophageal glands {1479}. Both lesions tend to be of salivary gland type with a generally favourable prognosis. Basaloid squamous cell carcinoma has a similar appearance to adenoid cystic carcinoma but is more aggressive {1838}. The presence of associated squamous carcinoma *in situ* is a strong argument for the diagnosis of basaloid carcinoma. Oesophageal adenocarcinoma can also arise from ectopic gastric glands, or oesophageal glands {494, 811}.

Genetic susceptibility

Several lines of evidence suggest genetic susceptibility to oesophageal adenocarcinoma arising from Barrett oesophagus. The striking predominance in white males and the early age of onset of Barrett oesophagus in some families support the involvement of genetic factors {467, 1425}. Several reports describe familial clustering of Barrett oesophagus, adenocarcinoma and reflux symptoms in up to three generations, a subset with an autosomal dominant inheritance pattern {796, 809, 814, 958, 1433, 2592, 2720, 3295}. However, typical risk factors, such as obesity, may potentiate risk in susceptible family members {466}.

Linkage analysis in families has not been reported. However, increased susceptibility to oesophageal adenocarcinoma in persons with polymorphisms in genes in various pathways that govern inflammatory response and nucleic acid repair is known. The first reported was an association between a variant of the *GSTP1* (glutathione *S*-transferase P1) gene and Barrett oesophagus and adenocarcinoma {3367}. Other variants of the GST gene (*GSTM1* and *GSTT1*) may augment the smoking-associated risk for adenocarcinoma {453}.

Other polymorphisms alter risk, but none are suitable for routine clinical testing. Examples of these include increased risk in persons with poly A tracts involving the xeroderma pigmentosum group C (*XPC*) gene, the cyclin D1 polymorphism (G870A) {451}, and polymorphisms of the cyclooxygenase 2 (*PTGS2/COX2*) gene {841, 2139}, epidermal growth factor (*EGF*) gene {1742} and matrix metalloprotein genes {320}, and an apparent protective effect with Lys751Gln homozygous variant of xeroderma pigmentosum group D (*ERCC2/XPD*), *XRCC1* (X-ray repair cross-complementing 1) Arg399Gly homozygous variant {452}, and NAD(P)H:-quinine oxireductase 1 (NQO1 TT) C609T polymorphism {715}.

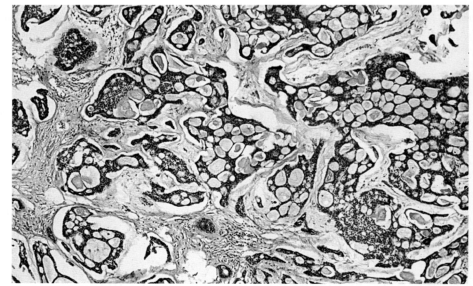

Fig. 2.16 Adenoid cystic carcinoma of the oesophagus showing a typical cribriform pattern and thus resembling its counterpart in the salivary gland.

Molecular pathology

Multiple genetic alterations are involved in the development and progression of Barrett oesophagus to oesophageal adenocarcinoma. Genetic alterations in tumour suppressor genes, oncogenes, growth factor receptors or enzymes that play important roles in diverse cellular functions such as cell-cycle control, apoptosis, cell signalling, cell adhesion and genetic stability, signal transduction or DNA repair have been identified.

Loss and gains of several chromosomal loci have been identified. The majority of studies demonstrate gains in the region of 8q (*MYC* region) and 20q, and losses at 3p (*FHIT*), 4q, 5q (*APC*) and 18q (*SMAD4*, *DCC*), with an increasing number of chromosomal alterations in the metaplasia–intraepithelial neoplasia–carcinoma sequence {1651}.

The frequency and type of the main genetic alterations described in oeso-phageal adenocarcinoma are presented in Table 2.01. Of these, only *TP53* gene mutation and ensuing p53 protein over-expression, and *AMACR* expression, have been suggested as potentially useful to strengthen a diagnosis of dysplasia.

There is evidence for an increasing role of epigenetic alterations in the carcinogenesis of oesophageal adenocarcinomas and gene silencing by promoter methylation has been demonstrated frequently for the E-cadherin, *APC*, *CDKN2A/p16*, *MGMT*, and *TMEFF2/HPP1* genes {2819}.

Prognosis and predictive factors
Prognostic factors after surgery

Prognosis is dependent on the depth of mural invasion and the presence of lymph-node or distant metastases, as summarized in the current TNM (tumour, node, metastasis) and American Joint Committee on Cancer/International Union Against Cancer (AJCC/UICC) staging system. The staging of carcinoma of the oesophagus has undergone important modifications between the sixth and seventh editions of TNM: T1 was subdivided in order to distinguish mucosal (T1a) and submucosal (T1b) depth of invasion, and T4 was divided according to the adjacent structures that were invaded between T4a (pleura, pericardium, or diaphragm) and T4b (other adjacent structures such as aorta, vertebral body, or trachea); regional lymph nodes are subdivided by number involved rather than by location; distant metastases has been simplified to M1 rather than subdivided by location.

Table 2.01. Frequency of the most common genetic alterations found in oesophageal adenocarcinomas and their precursor lesions.

Gene	Alteration	Frequency and timing	References
CDKN2A (p16)	Promoter methylation, LOH	80%, early occurrence	{2144, 2502}
TP53	Mutation, LOH	40–80%, increases from LGD to HGD and cancer	{996, 1415, 1525, 1740, 2195, 3610, 3655}
CCND1	Overexpression	30% in metaplasia 90% in cancer	{138, 186, 1740, 2931}
ERBB2	Overexpression, amplification	0–70%, late occurrence	{138, 1718, 1740, 2638, 3431}
EGFR	Overexpression, mutation (rare)	30–60%	{1700, 1718, 1740}
KRAS	Mutation	21%	{3016A}
PTGS2 (COX2)	Upregulation	79%, correlated with expression of VEGFA, VEFGC	{383, 3415}
AMACR	Overexpression	72–96%, progressive increase from low-grade dysplasia	{736, 2836}
IMP3 (insulin-like growth factor II mRNA binding protein)	—	Sensitive and specific for HGD and adenocarcinoma	{1904}

HGD, high-grade dysplasia; LGD, low-grade dysplasia; LOH, loss of heterozygosity.

Stage grouping has been divided into: (1) purely anatomical stages applicable to all types of carcinomas; and (2) prognostic groups that separate squamous from adenocarcinoma {762, 2996}.

On a molecular level, considerable negative prognostic impact has been demonstrated for *ERBB2*/Her2-neu amplification or overexpression, *TP53* mutations, expression of *COX2*, *PRAP1/UPA*, and *MMP1* and DNA ploidy (4N) {1718}. *NFκB* expression is also associated with negative clinical outcome {1375}.

Prognostic factors after preoperative (radio)chemotherapy and surgery

Surgery plays a central role in the treatment of oesophageal adenocarcinoma. Advanced-stage tumours are also treated with preoperative radiochemotherapy and chemotherapy {630A, 955A}. Assessment of histopathological tumour regression grade (TRG) after preoperative treatment provides highly valuable prognostic information. A three-tiered classification system (complete tumour regression: 0% residual tumour; subtotal or partial tumour regression: 1–50% residual tumour; minor or no tumour regression: > 50% residual tumour) has been shown to be the best reflection of tumour response to preoperative treatment {1971A, 528A, 3561A, 1739B, 3145A, 2714A, 480A}. Complete tumour regression {235A, 3145A, 1739B} and absence of lymph-node involvement and metastatic disease {4569} are recognized to be the strongest prognostic factors.

Factors for prediction of response to chemotherapy on pretreatment biopsies

The identification of biomarkers (e.g. enzymes related to 5-fluorouracil metabolism or multidrug resistance) for prediction of response to preoperative treatment in clinical practice is a subject of ongoing intense research, as is profiling of differential expression of genes involved in apoptosis, calcium homeostasis, stress response and the epidermal differentiation complex in responders and nonresponders to preoperative therapy {1917B, 1917A, 1739A}. However, data generated from these studies should at present be regarded as preliminary.

Neuroendocrine neoplasms of the oesophagus

R. Arnold
C. Capella
D.S. Klimstra
G. Klöppel
P. Komminoth
E. Solcia
G. Rindi

Definition
Neoplasms with neuroendocrine differentiation including well-differentiated (low- to intermediate-grade) neuroendocrine tumours (NETs) and poorly differentiated (high-grade) neuroendocrine carcinomas (NECs) arising in the oesophagus. Mixed adenoneuroendocrine carcinomas (MANECs) have an exocrine and an endocrine component, with one component exceeding 30%.

ICD-O codes
Neuroendocrine tumour (NET)
    NET G1 (carcinoid)   8240/3
    NET G2   8249/3
Neuroendocrine carcinoma (NEC) 8246/3
    Large cell NEC   8013/3
    Small cell NEC   8041/3
Mixed adenoneuroendocrine
carcinoma (MANEC)   8244/3

Synonyms
Synonyms for oesphageal NETs include: carcinoid, well-differentiated endocrine tumour/carcinoma {3013}. Synonyms for NECs include: poorly differentiated endocrine carcinomas, high-grade neuroendocrine carcinoma, small cell and large cell endocrine carcinomas.

Classification
NETs and NECs of the oesophagus are classified on the basis of criteria common to all gastrointestinal and pancreatic neuroendocrine neoplasms (see Chapter 1). Most oesophageal neuroendocrine neoplasms are NECs or MANECs, with either an adenocarcinoma or a squamous cell carcinoma component, usually of large size and located in the lower part of the oesophagus.

Epidemiology
Oesophageal neuroendocrine neoplasms are exceedingly rare. About 100 cases have been reported, the majority being NECs (poorly differentiated neuroendocrine carcinomas) {1221, 1320, 2116, 2150, 3171}. In an earlier analysis of 8305 NETs ("carcinoid tumours") at different anatomical sites, only 3 (0.04%) were reported in the oesophagus {2115}. Most NECs arise in males, the male-to-female ratio being 6 : 1 or higher. Age at presentation is widely variable, ranging from 30 to 82 years, but reported cases occur most frequently in the sixth and seventh decades of life {1993, 2116}. The reported frequency of these neoplasms as a proportion of all oesophageal cancers ranges between 0.05% and 7.6% {335, 728, 1288, 1765, 1993}. MANECs are observed in males in their sixth or seventh decades of life {448, 537, 1993}.

Etiology
Patients with oesophageal NECs often have a history of heavy smoking. An individual case was associated with long standing achalasia {158, 2594}. Co-existing Barrett oesophagus is frequently reported, both in pure NETs or NECs and in MANECs {335, 1616, 1993, 2777, 2829}.

Localization
Most neuroendocrine neoplasms of the oesophagus are typically located in the lower third of the oesophagus, paralleling the increase in endocrine cell number in the distal oesophagus {448, 2116, 2259, 2642, 2962}. Most of the rare true NETs (carcinoids) are found in the lower oesophagus in association with Barrett oesophagus and adenocarcinoma. Oesophageal NETs may also occur as rare incidental findings associated with heterotopic oxyntic mucosa {1616}. Of the more frequent NECs and MANECs, almost all occur in the distal half of the oesophagus {335, 728, 1993}. In a recent retrospective series of 40 cases, only one was reported in the proximal oesophagus, and five in the middle oesophagus {1993}.

Clinical features
NETs are often incidental findings. In NECs and MANECs, dysphagia, gastro-oesophageal reflux disease (GORD), severe weight loss and sometimes chest pain and blood in stool/haematemesis are the main symptoms. Patients with NECs or MANECs often present at an advanced stage {1288, 1765}. Inappropriate antidiuretic hormone

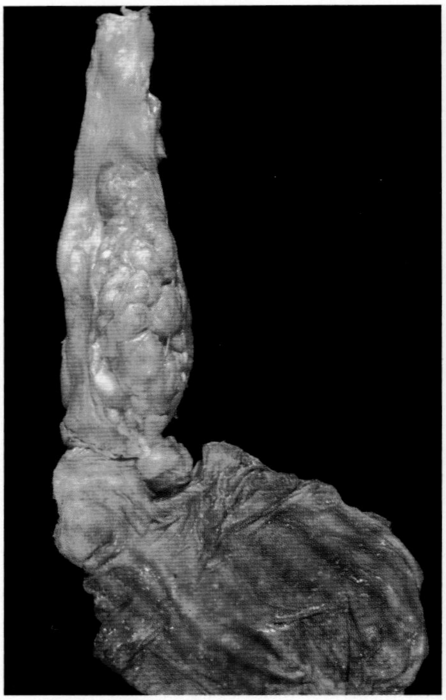

Fig. 2.17 Neuroendocrine carcinoma (NEC) of the oesophagus.

syndrome and hypercalcemia have been reported {728}. In addition, in the older literature, a case of watery diarrhoea, hypokalaemia-achlorhydria (WDHA) syndrome, attributable to ectopic production of vasoactive intestinal peptide (VIP) by a MANEC (small cell/squamous cell carcinoma) and a case of carcinoid syndrome have been described {338, 3469}. Oesophago-gastroscopy with multiple biopsies is the initial diagnostic procedure to evaluate the background of dysphagia as the leading tumour symptoms. Staging includes endoscopic ultrasound, multiphasic computed tomography (CT) and/or magnetic resonance imaging (MRI) of the chest and evaluation of distant metastases. Whether radiolabelled somatostatin analogue scintigraphy [Octreoscan(R)] or 68-Gallium PET may be relevant staging procedures for these mostly poorly differentiated, high-grade malignant neoplasms remains to be established.

Macroscopy

NETs are small, polypoid and rarely ulcerated. They are often associated with Barrett oesophagus and adenocarcinoma {1616}. Most oesophageal NECs and MANECs are large (4–10 cm in diameter), present as fungating or ulcerated masses and deeply infiltrate the oesophageal wall {1616, 2259, 2642, 2962}.

Histopathology

NET

G1 NETs are very rare in the oesophagus (for appropriate grading, see Chapter 1). Most of these neoplasms are polypoid and are small lesions found as incidental findings in association with Barrett oesophagus and adenocarcinomas. Histologically, oesophageal NETs are characterized by uniform bland, tumour cells with an insular growth pattern and solid to cribriform structures. Besides positive staining for chromogranin A and synaptophysin, strong immunoreactivity for vesicular monoamine transporter 2 (VMAT2) was reported in two oesophageal NETs associated with heterotopic oxyntic mucosa, indicating an enterochromaffin-like cell (ECL-cell) phenotype {448, 1616}.

G2 NETs are probably more frequent. Indeed most oesophageal "carcinoids" reported in the older literature are malignant, large, ulcerated lesions, deeply invasive, often with synchronous metastases {2642}, and display a solid-nest, acinar or trabecular structure, with evident mitoses, reported as "abundant" or "considerable", and with focal necrosis {2259, 2642, 2962}.

NEC

Oesophageal NECs (poorly differentiated neuroendocrine carcinomas) are aggressive, deeply infiltrative neoplasms, with synchronous metastases {1616, 1993, 2642}. In the older literature, these neoplasms may still have been called "carcinoids" {2259, 2642, 2962}.

Microscopically, they display either large-cell or small-cell features. Large cell NECs are more frequent, being reported in 27 out of 40 cases recently investigated, and often associate with Barrett oesophagus {1993}.

Large cell NECs. Also defined as "atypical carcinoid" in the older literature {2642}, these neoplasms may show an organoid pattern, with solid nests or acinar structures, focal necrosis and high mitotic rate,

fitting the present G3 class (see Chapter 1). Similar to their counterparts in the lung {3288}, the cells of these neoplasms are large to intermediate in size, with a low nucleus-to-cytoplasm ratio, nuclei with evident nucleoli and vesicular chromatin, and often abundant eosinophilic cytoplasm. Large cell NECs are positive for chromogranin A, synaptophysin, Grimelius silver impregnation, and neuron-specific enolase and may display characteristic membrane-bound neurosecretory granules at ultrastructural examination {2962}.

Small cell NECs. Small cell NEC of the oesophagus is indistinguishable from its counterpart in the lung on the basis of histological and immunohistochemical features or clinical behaviour {3288}. The cells may be small with dark nuclei of round or oval shape and scanty cytoplasm, or larger with more cytoplasm (intermediate cells) forming solid sheets and nests. Foci of squamous cell or adenocarcinoma and/or mucoepidermoid carcinoma may also be observed, a finding that raises the possibility of an origin from pluripotent cells present in the squamous epithelium or ducts of the submucosal glands {3171}. Argyrophylic granules can be demonstrated by Grimelius stain, and small dense-core granules are always detected by electron microscopy {1320}. Immunohistochemistry for chromogranin A, synaptophysin, NCAM1/CD56, B3GAT1/Leu7 and neuron-specific enolase is usually positive, synaptophysin being reported to be the most sensitive

diagnostic marker {1993, 2909, 3664}. Positive staining for thyroid transcription factor 1 (TTF1) has also been observed in 2 out of 6 and 15 out of 21 cases, respectively, investigated in two different studies {3594, 3664}. Some cases were reported to be positive for calcitonin and adrenocorticotropic hormone (ACTH), although in the absence of any hyperfunctional syndrome {2150}. Staining for periodic-acid Schiff and keratin 5/6 or p63 may help to distinguish areas of adeno- or squamous differentiation {1993}.

MANEC

Oesophageal MANECs with a NET component are exceedingly rare and reported in association with Barrett oesophagus and adenocarcinoma {448}. Oesophageal MANECs usually combine a NEC component with a gastrointestinal-type adenocarcinoma or, more rarely, a squamous cell carcinoma component {448, 537}. In oesophageal MANECs, the adenocarcinoma component seems to be more frequently observed. In a recent series of 40 oesophageal NECs and MANECs, adenocarcinoma was reported in 15 out of 16 MANECs {1993}. A squamous cell carcinoma component appears to be more present in oesophageal MANECs from Chinese and Japanese series {2150, 3594, 3664}. The NEC component displays the morphology and the immunophenotype described for pure NECs.

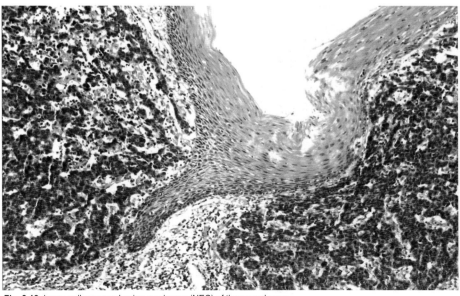

Fig. 2.18 Large cell neuroendocrine carcinoma (NEC) of the oesophagus.

Prognosis and predictive factors

In contrast to other gastrointestinal sites {2684, 2685}, there is no proposal for a TNM/staging classification for neuroendocrine neoplasms of the oesophagus. The relative rarity of oesophageal NETs and NECs may account for this. For practical purposes the staging of oesophageal NECs may be performed according to the TNM/staging classification for oesophageal carcinomas {762, 2996}.

Despite the limited statistics on survival available for oesophageal NETs and NECs, prognosis correlates reasonably with the grade and stage of the disease {2116}. Oesophageal NETs are rarely associated with lymph-node metastases and have an excellent prognosis. Eleven patients with primary oesophageal NETs were all alive and disease-free at 1–23 years after surgical excision {554, 1616}. Two out of three oesophageal NETs from the analysis of 8305 cases of "carcinoid tumours" {2115} were associated with distant metastases.

In contrast, the overall survival of patients with NECs is short and reported in the older literature as < 6 months {1765}. Prognosis largely depends on stage and tumour type. In a recent retrospective series of 40 oesophageal NECs and MANECs, better survival was reported for patients with locoregional disease vs patients with distant metastases {1993}. Survival was better for patients with MANEC than for patients with pure NEC, most likely because of the higher stage observed in pure NECs compared with MANECs.

No difference in survival was observed between small cell and large cell NECs. Interestingly, however, large cell pure NECs are associated with Barrett oesophagus.

Established treatment recommendations cannot be expected for this rare entity. As for neuroendocrine neoplasms elsewhere, surgery is the treatment of choice. Most reports indicate that the preferred surgical intervention is oesophagectomy, or subtotal variants with gastro-oesophageal anastomosis, associated with preoperative neoadjuvant therapy as described for adenocarcinoma or squamous cell carcinoma in patients with MANECs. Small lesions (< 1.5 cm in size) may by treated curatively by endoscopic resection.

Lymphoma of the oesophagus

H.K. Müller-Hermelink
J. Delabie
Y.H. Ko
E.S. Jaffe
S. Nakamura

Definition

Primary lymphoma of the oesophagus is defined as an extranodal lymphoma arising in the oesophagus, with the bulk of disease localized to this site {1341}. Contiguous lymph-node involvement may be seen, but peripheral and mediastinal lymph nodes, spleen or liver should not be affected and chest radioimaging and leukocyte count should be normal. Thus, by exclusion of any other site, the primary clinical presentation is in the oesophagus and therapy is directed at this site.

Most frequently, primary oesophageal lymphomas are diffuse large B-cell lymphoma (DLBCL) {2769} or extranodal marginal-zone lymphoma of mucosa-associated lymphoid tissue (MALT lymphoma) {1246, 1582, 2106}. Presentation of classical Hodgkin lymphoma has also been reported in the oesophagus, but is considered an extension of nodal disease {596, 1441}. Primary oesophageal T-cell lymphoma has been described, but is exceedingly rare {914}. Involvement of the oesophagus in widespread primary intestinal T-cell lymphoma has also been reported {46}.

ICD-O codes

Diffuse large B-cell lymphoma 9680/3
Marginal zone lymphoma of mucosa-associated lymphoid tissue (MALT lymphoma) 9699/3

Epidemiology

The oesophagus is a very uncommon primary site, accounting for < 1% of patients with lymphoma {2364}. Oesophageal involvement is more common as a secondary either from mediastinum, from nodal disease or from a primary gastric location. Less than 30 cases of *bona fide* primary oesophageal lymphoma have been described as single case reports or as small series of two cases. Patients are frequently male and usually aged > 50 years. MALT lymphomas of the oesophagus are mostly reported from Asian countries.

Immunodeficiency associated with infection with HIV {3480} and chronic immunosuppression {1023} appear to be risk factors.

Clinical features

Tumours predominantly occur in the intermediate and lower portion of the oesophagus and may cause dysphagia {1089}.

Macroscopy

The macroscopic appearance is nonspecific, ranging from small polypoid masses that can be removed by mucosectomy {1246} to larger nodular or tumorous lesions, ulcerated tumours or more extensive sometimes multifocal involvement.

Histopathology

The morphological and cytological features of reported cases are typical of the respective lymphoma subtypes found elsewhere in the gastrointestinal tract.

Secondary involvement of the oesophagus may occur in the dissemination of any type of lymphoma but is rare.

Data on molecular pathology are not available owing to the rarity of these tumours.

Mesenchymal tumours of the oesophagus

M. Miettinen
C.D.M. Fletcher
L.-G. Kindblom
W.M.S. Tsui

Definition

A group of nonepithelial tumours with variable histogenesis, including smooth muscle, stromal/Cajal cell, fibroblastic/-myofibroblastic, endothelial, and Schwannian origin, although the latter are, in a strict sense, of neuroectodermal and not mesenchymal origin.

ICD-O codes

Granular cell tumour	9580/0
Haemangioma	9120/0
Leiomyoma	8890/0
Lipoma	8850/0
Gastrointestinal stromal tumour	8936/3
Kaposi sarcoma	9140/3
Leiomyosarcoma	8890/3
Rhabdomyosarcoma	8900/3
Synovial sarcoma	9040/3

Leiomyoma

Leiomyoma, the most common mesenchymal tumour of the oesophagus, occurs over a wide range of ages from childhood onwards and is twice as frequent in males as in females. Leiomyomas are typically located in the distal to middle oesophagus and often manifest as dysphagia. The tumour varies from a minimal intramural nodule to a larger mural nodule to an externally extending mediastinal mass, but most are 1–3 cm in size {1135, 2073, 2879}. Grossly, oesophageal leiomyomas form firm to hard greyish-white masses. Histologically they are composed of irregularly oriented bundles of well-differentiated smooth-muscle cells. Cytoplasmic eosinophilic inclusions are often present, and calcification and infiltration by eosinophilic granulocytes are not uncommon. Mitotic activity is scant, if present. Immunohistochemical positivity for smooth muscle actin (SMA) and desmin is typical; desmin labels cytoplasmic inclusions. In contrast to gastrointestinal stromal tumours (GIST), leiomyomas are negative for KIT and DOG1/ANO1.

Childhood (and adult) cases include patients with familial Alport syndrome who, in addition to renal glomerular disease, may have longitudinally extending complex intramural oesophageal leiomyomas, often referred to as "leiomyomatosis". This syndrome is caused by germline deletions in the collagen IV subunit genes, among them *COL4A5* and *COL4A6,* found at chromosome Xq22 {1151}. For forms of leiomyomatosis that involve these genes, inheritance is X-linked, causing a more severe syndromic phenotype in men. Somatic deletions in the same genes have been identified in sporadic leiomyomas, suggesting a common pathogenesis {1150}.

Leiomyosarcoma

Malignant smooth-muscle tumours are very rare in the oesophagus. They are recognized by a histological resemblance to smooth muscle, nuclear atypia, mitotic activity, and immunohistochemical presence of SMA and desmin. Many reported examples have presented as polypoid intraluminal masses, and prognosis has been poor {2073}.

Gastrointestinal stromal tumour (GIST)

For definition, terminology, incidence, clinical and pathological features, we refer to the sections on gastric and small-intestinal GISTs (Chapters 4 and 6). GISTs are very rare in the oesophagus and comprise 10–20% of the combined group of smooth-muscle and stromal tumours. Most are clinically detected as intraluminal distal oesophageal masses causing dysphagia, but externally extending oesophageal GISTs can manifest as mediastinal tumours. Occasional examples have been incidentally detected during radiological screening or surveillance studies, and such tumours can have a good prognosis, an exception among this group of tumours, among which sarcomas predominate.

Most of these GISTs are spindle-cell tumours with sarcomatoid features including significant mitotic activity, but occasional epithelioid examples have also been reported {287, 2073}. Oesophageal GISTs are KIT-positive, and *KIT* mutations reported are similar to those identified in gastric GISTs. The pathological and genetic features of these tumours are described in more detail in Chapter 4.

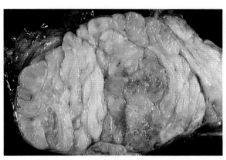

Fig. 2.19 Oesophageal leiomyoma. Grossly, this tumour often forms a demarcated mass with a grey, trabeculated or whorled cut surface.

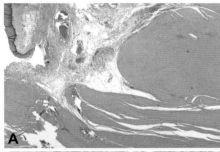

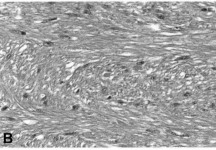

Fig. 2.20 Oesophageal leiomyoma, arising as a demarcated intramural nodule. Histologically, this tumour is composed of relatively paucicellular, well-differentiated smooth-muscle cells. Note the eosinophilic cytoplasmic inclusions, especially in the centre.

Granular cell tumour

Granular cell tumours are usually incidental endoscopic findings in the distal oesophagus and measure < 1 cm. Rare larger examples can cause dysphagia. Incidence is higher in African Americans, and tumour multiplicity is common, as has been previously observed for granular cell tumours in soft tissue.

Most cases lack nuclear atypia and mitotic activity, and immunohistochemical

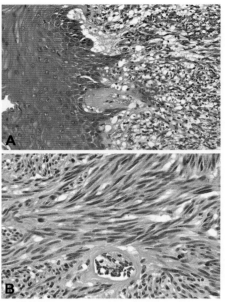

Fig. 2.21 Oesophageal gastrointestinal stromal tumour (GIST). **A** The tumour involves the wall beneath the squamous epithelium. **B** Moderately cellular spindle cell GIST with dilated capillaries.

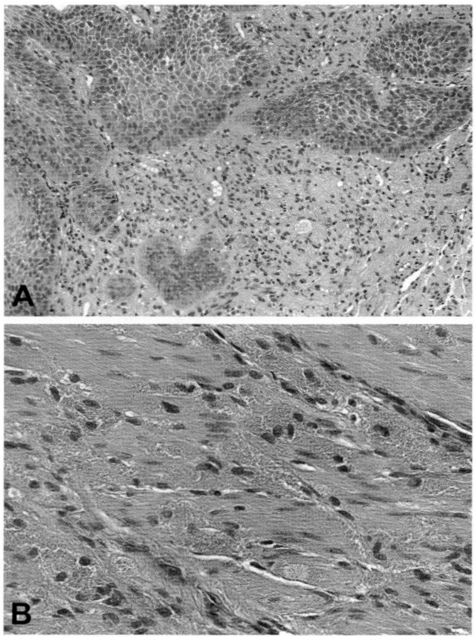

Fig. 2.22 Granular cell tumour of the oesophagus. **A** Pseudoepitheliomatous hyperplasia is often elicited in the overlying squamous epithelium. **B** In the muscularis propria, it intermingles with the smooth-muscle elements.

myogenic regulatory proteins (MyoD1 or myogenin) is required for diagnosis.

Synovial sarcoma
Isolated cases of biphasic synovial sarcomas have been reported in the upper oesophagus. These have mostly occurred in children and young adults. Grossly, they formed polypoid intraluminal masses, and were histologically similar to synovial sarcomas in soft tissue with glandular elements that were positive for keratin and epithelial membrane antigen (EMA) {259, 281}.

Other mesenchymal tumours
Glomus tumours, lipomas, and schwannomas similar to those more commonly seen in the stomach and intestines are very rare in the oesophagus. Kaposi sarcoma occurs with some frequency in patients with HIV/AIDS and post-transplant patients. For description of these entities, we refer to the section on mesenchymal tumours of the stomach and colon (Chapters 4 and 8).

detection of S100 protein is a consistent finding. Pseudoepitheliomatous hyperplasia of the squamous epithelia may be present in mucosally extending lesions. Presence of nuclear atypia and mitotic activity raise the concern of biological potential necessitating documented complete excision and follow-up in such cases {1013}.

Haemangioma
Most reported oesophageal haemangiomas have been polypoid intraluminal lesions measuring 1–3 cm that have occurred in older adults, with an apparent predominance in males. Histologically they have been variably characterized as capillary (the majority of cases) or cavernous. Endoscopic polypectomy has been the usual treatment {3003}.

Lymphangioma
Lymphangiomas vary from small mucosal lesions to pedunculated polyps and large masses that may involve surrounding structures extending into the mediastinum. Most have occurred in older adults, arising in the middle and lower third underneath an intact mucosa, and many have been characterized as cavernous lymphangiomas. Some cystic lymphangiomas of the neck in infants have involved the upper oesophagus {2833}.

Rhabdomyosarcoma
Only a small number of well-documented rhabdomyosarcomas (of embryonal type) have been reported in the oesophagus. These tumours have occurred in the distal oesophagus in older adults {3381}. Immunohistochemical demonstration of desmin and nuclear expression of

Secondary tumours and melanoma of the oesophagus

C. Iacobuzio-Donahue
G.M. Groisman

Definition
Tumours of the oesophagus that originate from an extra-oesophageal neoplasm or that are discontinuous with a primary tumour elsewhere in the oesophagus.

Epidemiology
In a series of 4198 cases of malignant oesophageal disease, 114 (2.7%) were metastases from non-oesophageal primary neoplasms {2625}. A higher frequency (6.1% of autopsy cases) was reported in Japan {2108}. Malignant melanoma (ICD-O code, 8720/3) of the oesophagus is an extremely rare neoplasm with < 300 cases reported {2792, 3373}.

Origin of metastases
After exclusion of pharyngeal carcinomas, gastric carcinomas and malignant mediastinal neoplasms involving the oesophagus by direct extension, metastatic neoplasms may reach the oesophagus by haematogenous or lymphatic dissemination. Any primary neoplasm is a potential source of haematogenous spread to the oesophagus, whereas lymphatic spread is mainly seen in association with breast and lung tumours. The most common origins of oesophageal metastases are breast and lung carcinomas, followed by melanoma {1844, 2108, 3461}. Metastasis from carcinomas of the thyroid, cervix, ovary, prostate and kidney have also been reported {594, 1777, 2108, 2227, 3291}.

Localization
The most common site of haematogenous metastases is the middle third of the oesophagus.

Clinical features
Metastatic lesions typically form symptomatic or asymptomatic submucosal nodules, but may also produce large symptomatic, obstructive tumours {2971}. The most common symptom is dysphagia; achalasia, haematemesis, weight loss and anaemia are less commonly seen {167, 2625, 2995}. The development of new-onset dysphagia in a patient with a known malignancy may suggest an oesophageal metastasis. Although all modes of imaging have value when evaluating oesophageal metastases, endoscopic ultrasound is used most often to define the extent of oesophageal involvement. Minimally invasive thoracoscopy may facilitate the diagnosis of carcinosis of the oesophagus caused by breast cancer {2625, 2971, 2995}.

Melanoma
Cases of melanoma of the oesophagus typically arise in the middle or distal oesophagus of older adults {1829, 2792}. The most common clinical complaint is dysphagia. At endoscopy, the neoplasms are polypoid and melanin pigmentation is seen in almost all cases {889, 2792}.

Histopathology
The histopathology of oesophageal metastases will be most similar to the primary neoplasm of origin. A pertinent clinical history, the submucosal distribution of the lesion, the absence of epithelial surface involvement and the presence of adenocarcinoma in the wall of the squamous lined oesophagus is generally sufficient to distinguish metastatic from primary oesophageal carcinoma. Difficulty may arise when a metastatic squamous cell carcinoma involves the oesophageal mucosa or a metastatic adenocarcinoma infiltrates the lower oesophageal mucosa. In those instances, clinical history and immunohistochemical stains including "organ-specific" markers may help in reaching the diagnosis.

Melanoma
Histologically, the tumours are composed of spindle and/or epithelioid cells, similar to their cutaneous counterparts. An *in situ* component, which helps to establish the diagnosis of primary melanoma, is seen in the majority of cases {2792}. Immunohistochemistry (S100 protein, Melan A, HMB45) helps to confirm the diagnosis.

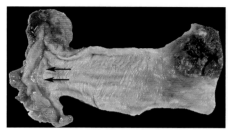

Fig. 2.23 Primary melanoma of the oesophagus. The oesophagogastric junction is on the left (arrows).

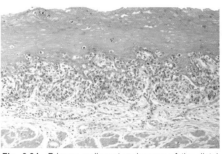

Fig. 2.24 Primary malignant melanoma of the distal oesophagus. The diagnosis is supported by the fact that the zone of atypical junctional proliferation of melanocytes is located adjacent to the invasive tumour.

Prognosis and predictive factors
Oesophageal metastasis is a sign of advanced disease, but the outcome is better when the growth rate of the primary tumour is slow {2382} or when systemic therapy is employed, as for metastatic breast cancer {167, 2625}.

Melanoma
The preferred therapy is total or near-total oesophagectomy followed by radiotherapy and/or chemotherapy {139, 1829, 3410}. The prognosis is poor. Median survival is between 8 and 24 months {1829, 2792}.

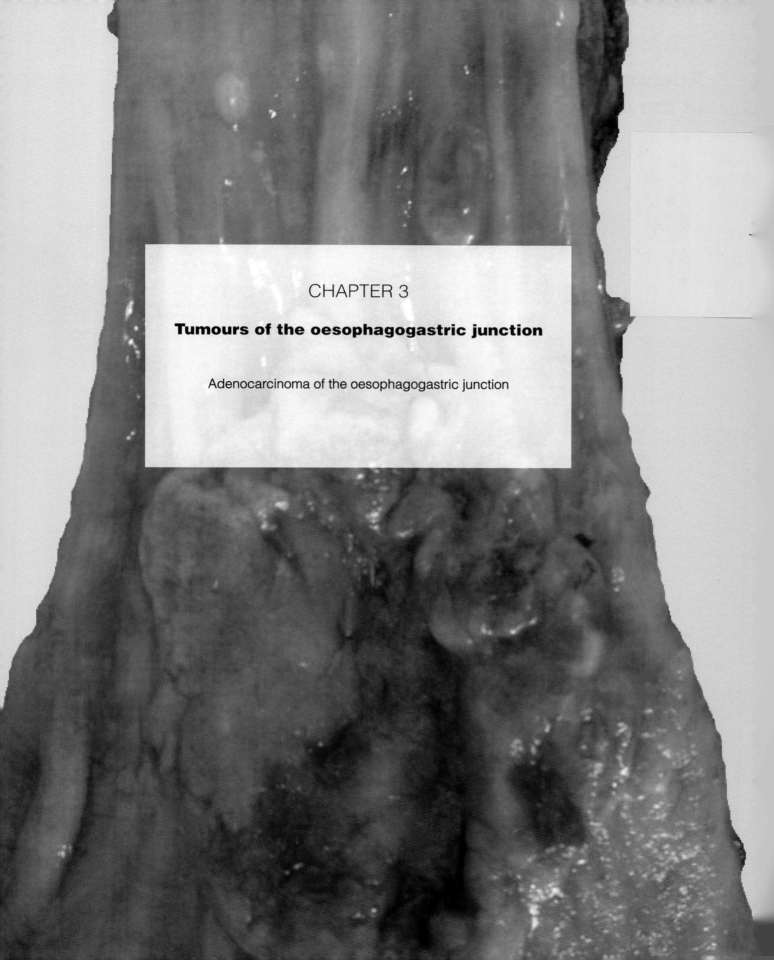

CHAPTER 3

Tumours of the oesophagogastric junction

Adenocarcinoma of the oesophagogastric junction

Adenocarcinoma of the oesophagogastric junction

R.D. Odze
J.-F. Fléjou
P. Boffetta
H. Höfler
E. Montgomery
S.J. Spechler

Definition

Adenocarcinomas that straddle the junction of the oesophagus and stomach are designated as tumours of the oesophagogastric junction (OGJ). This definition includes many tumours formerly called cancers of the gastric "cardia". Squamous cell carcinomas that occur at the OGJ are considered to be carcinomas of the distal oesophagus, even if they cross the OGJ.

ICD-O code   8140/3

Definition of the oesophagogastric junction

Conceptually, the OGJ is defined as the point at which the oesophagus ends and the stomach begins. Practically, there are no universally accepted and clearly reproducible landmarks that identify the OGJ with precision. Different criteria are used by anatomists, radiologists, physiologists, surgeons and endoscopists {3036}. For instance, in the normal patient, the OGJ can be defined by many criteria: the end of the tubular oesophagus, the squamo-columnar junction, the peritoneal reflection, the angle of His, the proximal limit of gastric rugal folds, the distal limit of squamous epithelium, the proximal limit of gastric oxyntic mucosa, the distal limit of the lower oesophageal sphincter, and the distal limit of palisading vessels. When the oesophagus is damaged by gastro-oesophageal reflux disease (GORD), most of these landmarks are destroyed. Few studies have addressed this issue specifically and, in the absence of a validated landmark, the accuracy of any criterion cannot be assessed meaningfully.

Systems proposed for the classification of these tumours, such as the Siewert classification, used in some parts of the world as a surgical guide {1462, 2963}, have generally been based on the location of the epicentre of the tumour in relation to the OGJ, but the authors of these systems often do not provide specific criteria for identifying the OGJ.

For the treatment of patients with tumours that cross the border between the oesophagus and the stomach, great precision in identification of the OGJ is not usually an important clinical issue. For investigators intent on determining the origin of those tumours, however, such precision can be critical.

Endoscopists in North America and Europe generally identify the OGJ as the most proximal extent of the gastric folds {2018}. *In vivo*, the location of the proximal extent of the gastric folds is affected by respiration, gut motor activity and the degree of distention of the oesophagus and stomach, all of which can vary from moment to moment. In resected specimens that include the OGJ, the level of the proximal extent of the gastric folds is affected by traction on the oesophagus, which is often a function of how the specimen is mounted. Bulky tumours at the OGJ also may completely obliterate the tops of the gastric folds. Endoscopists in Asia often use the distal extent of the palisade vessels (fine longitudinal veins in the lamina propria of the distal oesophagus) as their landmark for the OGJ because of difficulty in identifying gastric folds in a population with a high prevalence of chronic atrophic gastritis {535, 2233, 3402}. Furthermore, the level at which the palisade vessels terminate can be irregular and difficult to localize with precision, and this is not a practical landmark for routine use in surgical specimens.

The choice of the "best" landmark for the OGJ is necessarily arbitrary. Adenocarcinomas that straddle the OGJ, wherever that is, are likely to have originated either from Barrett oesophagus or from the proximal stomach. Since the majority of published studies on Barrett oesophagus conducted over the past 20 years have used the proximal extent of the gastric folds as the landmark for the OGJ and, in the absence of compelling data for the use of alternative markers, it seems reasonable to use that landmark despite its considerable shortcomings.

The proximal stomach is often referred to as the "cardia", but the histology of this region is controversial. Some authorities suggest that the "cardia" is composed of pure oxyntic glands, while others propose that it is composed of pure mucous

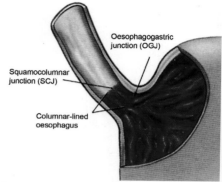

Fig. 3.01 Topography of the oesophagogastric junction and proximal stomach {3033}.

glands or a mixture of mucous glands and oxyntic glands. Regardless, this represents an extremely short segment of mucosa and is probably of little consequence in terms of cancer risk {479, 480, 2352}.

Diagnostic criteria

Various diagnostic criteria have been used to classify tumours in the region of the OGJ as either oesophageal or gastric {567, 1079, 1152, 1292, 1462, 2093, 2149}. In most of these classification systems, the anatomical location of the epicentre, or predominant mass of the tumour, is used to determine whether the neoplasm is oesophageal or gastric in origin. The use of endoscopic criteria, as in North America and Europe, suggests that many gastric "cardia" cancers actually represent distal oesophageal cancers secondary to Barrett oesophagus. This correlates well with epidemiological data that show a similar incidence rate, over the last four decades, with oesophageal adenocarcinoma, and an etiological association with GORD in some studies. Owing to the use of divergent classification systems, the patient populations used in studies on cancers of the proximal stomach are heterogeneous. Some include patients with gastric tumours and others with tumours of oesophageal origin. The following guidelines are based on the definition of the OGJ described above: (1) adenocarcinomas that cross the OGJ are considered adenocarcinomas of the OGJ, regardless of where the bulk of the tumour lies; (2) adenocarcinomas located entirely above the OGJ, as defined above, are considered to represent oesophageal carcinomas; and (3) adenocarcinomas located entirely below the OGJ are considered to be gastric in origin. For the latter group, use of the ambiguous and often misleading term "carcinoma of the gastric cardia" is discouraged in favour of the term "carcinoma of the proximal stomach".

Epidemiology

The epidemiology of adenocarcinoma of the OGJ shares many characteristics with that of adenocarcinoma of the distal oesophagus in particular, and also with those of the proximal stomach. Reliable population-based data on the incidence of adenocarcinoma of the OGJ are not available because cancer registries typically distinguish adenocarcinomas of the distal oesophagus only from those of the proximal stomach.

Incidence rates of OGJ adenocarcinomas are higher among Caucasians, in men compared with women, and in the middle-aged and elderly {1512}. The incidence of OGJ adenocarcinoma has increased markedly in the second half of the 20th century {3706}. In 1985–1989, incidence rates in Connecticut were 3.0 per 100 000 in men and 0.6 per 100 000 in women {3706}. The incidence of adenocarcinoma of the OGJ appears to be rising in parallel with that of adenocarcinoma of the lower oesophagus {347, 2521}.

Etiology

The risk factors for development of adenocarcinoma of the OGJ mainly parallel those of adenocarcinoma of the lower oesophagus {1512}. GORD and intestinal metaplasia have been strongly and consistently associated with an increased risk of adenocarcinoma of the OGJ {402, 547, 1721}. Although difficult to determine because of variation in the definitions used in previous studies, the risk of adenocarcinoma may be lower in patients with intestinal metaplasia of the proximal stomach than in patients with intestinal metaplasia of the distal oesophagus (Barrett oesophagus) {402, 567}.

Increasing body weight and obesity play a role in adenocarcinoma of the OGJ independent from GORD {546, 1722}.

Tobacco-smoking has been associated with an increased risk of adenocarcinoma of the OGJ, although the data are weaker than for oesophageal adenocarcinoma {3556}. The role of alcohol, dietary factors and medication has not been fully established {1512}. Some case–control studies have reported a reduced risk of Barrett oesophagus and oesophageal adenocarcinoma among individuals who are positive for *Helicobacter pylori*, particularly those infected with the cag A type {285}. A similar protective association has been observed for GORD {1048}. However, there are no data on the effect of infection with *H. pylori* on OGJ cancers.

Clinical features

Patients with adenocarcinomas that straddle the OGJ comprise a heterogeneous population of those with Barrett cancer, which is associated with GORD, and those with gastric cancer, which is associated with *H. pylori* infection {3035}.

Thus, some patients with OGJ tumours describe a prior history of GORD symptoms, whereas others may describe a history of peptic ulcer disease. Both in the oesophagus and stomach, intestinal metaplasia caused by chronic inflammation appears to predispose to the development of adenocarcinoma. However, metaplastic epithelium *per se* does not cause symptoms. Patients with adenocarcinomas of the OGJ generally present with symptoms of dysphagia, weight loss, and abdominal pain. Early OGJ cancers infrequently cause symptoms, and the presence of dysphagia, weight loss or abdominal pain usually indicates that the tumour is bulky and incurable. Uncommonly, cancers of the OGJ are discovered at an early, curable stage during endoscopic surveillance of patients known to have Barrett oesophagus {2896}.

Endoscopy and imaging

OGJ adenocarcinomas are typically diagnosed by endoscopic examination and biopsy sampling. The OGJ is identified endoscopically as the most proximal extent of the gastric folds. Large circumferential tumours may obliterate this anatomical landmark, obliging the endoscopist to estimate the location of the OGJ. The endoscopist should attempt to identify whether there is columnar-lined (Barrett) oesophagus (see *Adenocarcinoma of the oesophagus*), and obtain biopsy specimens of the oesophageal columnar lining. The finding of dysplastic columnar epithelium in the oesophagus of a patient with an OGJ tumour is strong evidence

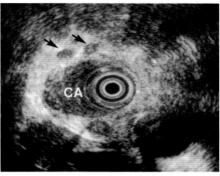

Fig. 3.02 Adenocarcinoma (CA) with deep infiltration at the oesophagogastric junction and several lymph nodes with metastases (arrows), as visualized by endoscopic ultrasonography.

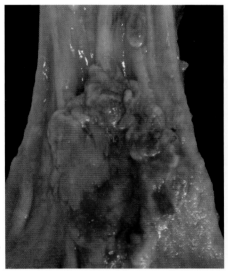

Fig. 3.03 Adenocarcinoma of the oesophagogastric junction.

that the cancer arose from Barrett oesophagus. If possible, the proximal stomach should be examined by retroflexion of the endoscope in order to assess the extent of gastric involvement. Computed tomography (CT) is used to detect distant metastases (M staging) in the chest and abdomen. For assessment of tumour depth (T staging) and local/regional lymph node involvement (N staging), endoscopic ultrasonography is the diagnostic modality of choice {275}. Occasionally, it can be difficult to distinguish reactive (inflammatory) changes from metastases in lymph nodes by ultrasonographic criteria, especially for ulcerated tumours. In these cases, endoscopic ultrasonography can be used to guide fine needle aspiration of the suspicious lymph node.

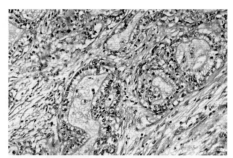

Fig. 3.04 Adenocarcinoma of the proximal stomach ("pylorocardiac type").

Tumour spread and staging

Currently, staging of carcinomas of the OGJ is based on the following TNM (tumour; node; metastasis) criteria: a tumour whose centre is located within 5 cm of the OGJ and which also extends into the oesophagus is staged according to the scheme for oesophageal carcinoma. Tumours with an epicentre in the stomach > 5 cm from the OGJ, or those within 5 cm of the OGJ without extension in the oesophagus, are staged according to the scheme for gastric carcinoma {762, 2996}. The main clinical differences between staging for the oesophagus versus the stomach is that: (1) oesophageal cancer incorporates tumour grade as a significant prognostic variable; and (2) metastasis in 7 or more regional lymph nodes (N3) is divided into N3a (7 to 15 nodes) and N3b (16 or more nodes) for gastric carcinomas. In addition, for lesions classified as oesophageal cancer, T1 and T4 are further subdivided in order to provide greater information for imaging and management, regional lymph nodes (N) are subdivided by the number involved rather than by their location, and distant metastasis (M) is indicated as M1 and is not subdivided by location. Stages are now divided into: (1) purely anatomical stages that are applicable to both oesophageal and gastric carcinomas; and (2) are also divided into separate prognostic groups based on tumour grade, as mentioned above. For oesophageal adenocarcinomas, distinction between well- and moderately-differentiated (G1 and G2) and poorly-differentiated (G3) cancers is important for stage groupings IA, IB and IIA {762, 2996}.

Adenocarcinomas located at the OGJ have a proclivity for proximal spread mainly via lymphatics in the submucosa of the oesophagus. For this reason, intraoperative frozen-section examination of the proximal oesophageal resection margin is recommended for these cases. Proximal spread can also involve lower mediastinal nodes. Lymphatic spread from proximal gastric cancers frequently extend distally to lymph nodes in the oesophagogastric angles, and also to those surrounding the left gastric artery, and also may involve para-coeliac and para-aortic lymph nodes {47, 1624}.

Histopathology

Adenocarcinoma

Most cancers that arise at the OGJ are adenocarcinomas {3023}. Histologically, several types are recognized: papillary, tubular, mucinous, signet ring cell and other poorly cohesive non-signet ring cell carcinomas, and mixed carcinomas (see Chapter 4). The relative proportion of well-differentiated, gland-forming carcinomas is significantly lower for tumours that arise in the OGJ compared with pure oesophageal carcinomas {2802}. Signet ring carcinomas are far less common in the proximal than in the distal stomach, and are not usually accompanied by atrophic gastritis {3444}. Well-differentiated "tubular" adenocarcinomas may present considerable difficulty for diagnosis since the neoplastic tubules may reveal a deceptively bland and regular appearance, and are thus easily mistaken for benign hyperplasia or dysplasia {2315}.

Pylorocardiac carcinoma

Mulligan et al. {3101} termed neoplastic lesions that resemble normal pyloric glands "pylorocardiac carcinomas". Such lesions are typically located in the proximal stomach, contain tall epithelial cells with clear or pale cytoplasm and basal or centrally located nuclei. However, this pattern of growth is difficult to distinguish reliably from other types of gland-forming adenocarcinomas, so the significance of this subtype is unclear {3101}. For instance, "clear cell" adenocarcinoma of the proximal stomach probably represents a similar histological subtype {972}.

Adenosquamous carcinoma

Adenosquamous carcinoma has mixed elements of adenocarcinoma and squamous cell carcinoma. The diagnosis rests on the finding of a mixture of neoplastic glandular and squamous elements, and not merely the presence of benign metaplastic squamoid foci in an otherwise typical adenocarcinoma. The latter is a frequent finding in tumours at this site. Adenosquamous carcinoma should be distinguished from mucoepidermoid carcinoma of the oesophagus, which is believed to develop from mucus glands and is similar to such tumours that develop from the salivary glands {3180}. Although the term "mucoepidermoid" was used in the past synonymously with adenosquamous carcinomas {2495}, the latter are distinguished by the presence of marked nuclear pleomorphism, occasional keratin pearls, and the anatomical separation of the two components within the tumour. It is generally accepted that this malignancy results from divergent differentiation of malignant cells rather than a collision of two tumour types.

Small cell carcinoma

Small cell carcinoma can also occur at this site. The prognosis is poor, although after radiochemotherapy some cases show favourable behaviour {255, 1667} (see Neuroendocrine tumours of the oesophagus).

Grading

Adenocarcinomas of the OGJ are graded as well-, moderately, or poorly differentiated. Unfortunately, interobserver agreement on tumour grading is poor. Nevertheless, tumour grading is now incorporated into separate prognostic categories that are used for TNM staging of oesophageal cancers (tumours in which the epicentre is located within 5 cm of the OGJ and with involvement of oesophagus) {1362, 2672}. Blomjous et al. {282} reported that 3.6% of gastric "cardiac" cancers were well-differentiated, 31% were moderately differentiated, and 43% were poorly differentiated, but other investigators have revealed a greater proportion of well-differentiated cancers, particularly when "early" carcinomas are included in the analysis {2149, 2302, 3206}.

Precursor lesions

Regardless of the precise anatomical site of origin (oesophagus vs proximal stomach), many, but not all, adenocarcinomas of the OGJ develop via a precursor stage of intestinal metaplasia. Tumours may arise in endoscopically visible segments of Barrett oesophagus or in short or ultrashort segments of oesophageal columnar metaplasia that are difficult, if not impossible, to identify endoscopically. The prevalence of intestinal metaplasia in a biopsy obtained from this region is variable. In patients with a visible segment of columnar epithelium in the distal oesophagus measuring > 3 cm, the prevalence of intestinal metaplasia is 90%. For patients with < 3 cm length of columnar epithelium, the prevalence of intestinal metaplasia is close to 30%. The incidence of intestinal metaplasia in endoscopically normal patients varies by 5–15% in different studies {3036A}. There are limited data on cancer progression of intestinal metaplasia when it is found in a biopsy from the OGJ region, but it is believed that the risk is higher when it occurs in the distal oesophagus than in the proximal stomach {2907}.

Careful examination of the type of epithelium in which intestinal metaplasia occurs, and its pathological associations, suggests the following: when intestinal metaplasia is found in a biopsy from visible columnar-lined oesophagus and the length is < 3 cm, this is considered "short-segment" Barrett oesophagus. The risk of cancer associated with short-segment Barrett oesophagus is believed to be similar to, or only slightly less, than that associated with "long-segment" Barrett oesophagus {615, 953}. When intestinal metaplasia is detected in a biopsy from the OGJ in a patient with an endoscopically normal oesophagus, there are several possibilities. One is that intestinal metaplasia is occurring in an area of "ultra-short" (microscopic) Barrett oesophagus (< 1 cm), which is the most common scenario for intestinal metaplasia in this region. These patients have no evidence of chronic atrophic gastritis in distal biopsies. However, intestinal metaplasia may also occur in gastric oxyntic mucosa as part of chronic atrophic pan-gastritis. This usually results either from infection with *H. pylori* or from autoimmune gastritis and is easily recognized by the fact that chronic inflammation, atrophy and intestinal metaplasia are present in both the proximal and distal stomach. This scenario is common in populations in which the prevalence of infection with *H. pylori* is high. Finally, intestinal metaplasia may develop in pure mucus or mixed mucus/oxyntic glands in the OGJ region, in association with chronic atrophic pan-gastritis. In this case, it is difficult to determine whether the intestinal metaplasia developed in metaplastic oesophageal columnar mucosa or metaplastic gastric oxyntic mucosa with atrophy and pseudopyloric metaplasia. The risk of cancer associated with these different scenarios has not been established, partly owing to paucity of data as a result of management guidelines that discourage biopsies in endoscopically normal patients. However, dysplasia and adenocarcinomas of the OGJ region are not frequently associated with chronic atrophic gastritis, which suggests strongly that most of these tumours arise in metaplastic oesophageal mucosa (i.e. ultra-short segment Barrett oesophagus).

Molecular pathology

Adenocarcinomas of the OGJ share many similarities at the molecular level with adenocarcinomas of the oesophagus and distal stomach. Unfortunately, delineating specific genetic alterations of OGJ tumours is difficult owing to the use of disparate and inconsistent clinical and pathological criteria for these tumours in the literature. Nevertheless, both loss and gain of chromosomal loci have been identified in "gastric cardia" adenocarcinomas and in adenocarcinomas of the distal oesophagus. The most prevalent gains (> 40% of tumours), with inclusion of assigned candidate genes, were found at 1q, 7p (*EGFR*), 7q, 8q (*MYC*), 17q (*ERBB2*), 19q, 20pq. Losses are most frequently observed at 3p, 4q, 5q (*APC, MCC* at 5q21, α-catenin at 5q31), 9p, and 18q (*SMAD4, DCC*) and on the Y chromosome in males {3352, 3353}. A detailed analysis of the amplicon at chromosome 7q21 identified the gene encoding the cell-cycle regulator Cdk6 as the target of recurrent high-level amplifications at 7q21 {3354}.

Mutations in *TP53* are the most frequent alterations in OGJ tumours. *TP53* abnormalities have been reported in 31–63% of "gastric cardia" tumours and 50–79% of oesophageal tumours {996, 3195}. The prevalence of *TP53* mutations is considerable higher in "gastric cardia" adenocarcinomas than in antral adenocarcinomas (42% vs 25%) {874}. In one study, the prevalence of *TP53* mutations was similar in adenocarcinomas of the oesophagus (53%) and "cardia" adenocarcinomas (58%), but not "non-cardia" gastric adenocarcinomas (17%) {1339}. Loss of heterozygosity (LOH) of *TP53* at chromosome 17p13 was found in 83% of "cardia" carcinomas {996} and in 63% of

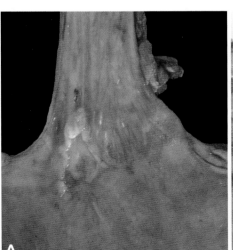
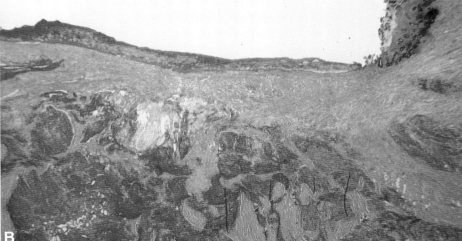

Fig. 3.05 Regression of adenocarcinoma of the oesophagogastric junction after radiochemotherapy. **A** The photo of the gross specimen shows ulceration, but no mass lesion. **B** Histologically, there is ulceration and underlying neoplastic mucin lakes, but no viable epithelium.

"non-cardia" gastric tumours, compared with 46% in oesophageal adenocarcinomas in other studies {3610}.

Other abnormalities detected in "cardia" cancers include overexpression of ERBB2 (about 20%) and increased expression of CDX2 (about 41%) {382, 3028}. In one study, proteome analysis of a small number of "gastric cardia" adeno-carcinomas revealed 23 differentially expressed proteins {518}.

Promoter methylation of the RAS-association domain family 1A (RASSF1A) gene was detected in 59% of "gastric cardia" adenocarcinomas in one study {3353}. There are considerable differences between oesophageal, "cardia" and "non-cardia" gastric adenocarcinomas in pro-moter methylation of the APC and CDKN2A (p16) genes (APC: 78% vs 32% vs 84%, respectively; and CDKN2A: 54% vs 36% vs 10%, respectively) {2805}.

Prognosis and predictive factors

The completeness of resection, lymph-node status and the presence of post-surgical complications are the most important prognostic factors for patients with adenocarcinoma of the OGJ {2417, 2964}. TP53 mutations were associated with more advanced disease and poor prognosis in one study, which included adenocarcinomas of the oesophagus and of the proximal stomach {1339}. Correlation between elevated expression of COX2 (PTGS2) and reduced survival has been found for adenocarcinomas of the oeso-phagus, but not the proximal stomach {382}. The yTNM staging system is recom-mended for patients treated with neoadju-vant chemotherapy {762, 2996}.

Histopathological response categorized by the three-tiered system proposed for gastric and oesophageal cancers has limitations {219}. An early metabolic response defined by 18-fluoro-2-deoxy-glucose-PET (FDG-PET) has been shown to be predictive of both survival and histopathological response {1898}. Factors predictive of response to neoadjuvant therapy have been studied in oeso-phageal or gastric adenocarcinomas, but not specifically in OGJ tumours {820, 1223}. Decreased expression of thymidylate synthase, a key enzyme in the metabolism of 5-fluorouracil (5FU) has been shown to be associated with a positive response in a study that included OGJ tumours {87}. However, no molecular markers are currently used in clinical practice to guide the treatment of patients with carcinomas of the OGJ.

CHAPTER 4

Tumours of the stomach

Gastric carcinoma

Hereditary diffuse gastric cancer

Neuroendocrine neoplasms

Lymphoma

Mesenchymal tumours

Secondary tumours

WHO classification[a] of tumours of the stomach

Epithelial tumours

Premalignant lesions

Adenoma	8140/0
Intraepithelial neoplasia (dysplasia), low grade	8148/0*
Intraepithelial neoplasia (dysplasia), high grade	8148/2*

Carcinoma

Adenocarcinoma	8140/3
Papillary adenocarcinoma	8260/3
Tubular adenocarcinoma	8211/3
Mucinous adenocarcinoma	8480/3
Poorly cohesive carcinoma (including signet ring cell carcinoma and other variants)	8490/3*
Mixed adenocarcinoma	8255/3
Adenosquamous carcinoma	8560/3
Carcinoma with lymphoid stroma (medullary carcinoma)	8512/3
Hepatoid adenocarcinoma	8576/3
Squamous cell carcinoma	8070/3
Undifferentiated carcinoma	8020/3

Neuroendocrine neoplasms[b]

Neuroendocrine tumour (NET)	
NET G1 (carcinoid)	8240/3
NET G2	8249/3

Neuroendocrine carcinoma (NEC)	8246/3
Large cell NEC	8013/3
Small cell NEC	8041/3
Mixed adenoneuroendocrine carcinoma	8244/3
EC cell, serotonin-producing NET	8241/3
Gastrin-producing NET (gastrinoma)	8153/3

Mesenchymal tumours

Glomus tumour	8711/0
Granular cell tumour	9580/0
Leiomyoma	8890/0
Plexiform fibromyxoma	8811/0*
Schwannoma	9560/0
Inflammatory myofibroblastic tumour	8825/1
Gastrointestinal stromal tumour	8936/3
Kaposi sarcoma	9140/3
Leiomyosarcoma	8890/3
Synovial sarcoma	9040/3

Lymphomas

Secondary tumours

---

[a] The morphology codes are from the International Classification of Diseases for Oncology (ICD-O) {904A}. Behaviour is coded /0 for benign tumours, /1 for unspecified, borderline or uncertain behaviour, /2 for carcinoma *in situ* and grade III intraepithelial neoplasia, and /3 for malignant tumours; [b] The classification is modified from the previous WHO histological classification of tumours {691} taking into account changes in our understanding of these lesions. In the case of neuroendocrine neoplasms, the classification has been simplified to be of more practical utility in morphological classification; *These new codes were approved by the IARC/WHO Committee for ICD-O at its meeting in March 2010.

TNM classification[a] of tumours of the stomach

Carcinoma of the stomach

T – Primary tumour
TX   Primary tumour cannot be assessed
T0   No evidence of primary tumour
Tis   Carcinoma *in situ*: intraepithelial tumour without invasion of the lamina propria, high-grade dysplasia
T1   Tumour invades lamina propria, muscularis mucosae, or submucosa
  T1a   Tumour invades lamina propria or muscularis mucosae
  T1b   Tumour invades submucosa
T2   Tumour invades muscularis propria
T3   Tumour invades subserosa
T4   Tumour perforates serosa or invades adjacent structures
  T4a   Tumour perforates serosa (visceral peritoneum)
  T4b   Tumour invades adjacent structures[b,c,d]

N – Regional lymph nodes
NX   Regional lymph nodes cannot be assessed
N0   No regional lymph-node metastasis
N1   Metastasis in 1 to 2 regional lymph nodes
N2   Metastasis in 3 to 6 regional lymph nodes
N3   Metastasis in 7 or more regional lymph nodes
  N3a   Metastasis in 7 to 15 regional lymph nodes
  N3b   Metastasis in 16 or more regional lymph nodes

M – Distant metastasis
M0   No distant metastasis
M1   Distant metastasis

Stage grouping

Stage	T	N	M
Stage 0	Tis	N0	M0
Stage IA	T1	N0	M0
Stage IB	T2	N0	M0
	T1	N1	M0
Stage IIA	T3	N0	M0
	T2	N1	M0
	T1	N2	M0
Stage IIB	T4a	N0	M0
	T3	N1	M0
	T2	N2	M0
	T1	N3	M0

Stage	T	N	M
Stage IIIA	T4a	N1	M0
	T3	N2	M0
	T2	N3	M0
Stage IIIB	T4b	N0, N1	M0
	T4a	N2	M0
	T3	N3	M0
Stage IIIC	T4a	N3	M0
	T4b	N2, N3	M0
Stage IV	Any T	Any N	M1

Carcinoid of the stomach[e]

T – Primary tumour[f]

TX   Primary tumour cannot be assessed

T0   No evidence of primary tumour

Tis   Carcinoid *in situ*/dysplasia (tumour less than 0.5 mm, confined to mucosa)

T1   Tumour confined to mucosa and 0.5 mm or more but no greater than 1 cm in size; or invades submucosa and is no greater than 1 cm in size

T2   Tumour invades muscularis propria or is more than 1 cm in size

T3   Tumour invades subserosa

T4   Tumour perforates visceral peritoneum (serosa) or other organs or adjacent structures

N – Regional lymph nodes

NX   Regional lymph nodes cannot be assessed

N0   No regional lymph-node metastasis

N1   Regional lymph-node metastasis

M – Distant metastasis

M0   No distant metastasis

M1   Distant metastasis

Stage grouping

Stage	T	N	M
Stage 0	Tis	N0	M0
Stage I	T1	N0	M0
Stage IIA	T2	N0	M0
Stage IIB	T3	N0	M0
Stage IIIA	T4	N0	M0
Stage IIIB	Any T	N1	M0
Stage IV	Any T	Any N	M1

Gastrointestinal stromal tumour (GIST)

T – Primary tumour

TX   Primary tumour cannot be assessed

T0   No evidence for primary tumour

T1   Tumour 2 cm or less in greatest dimension

T2   Tumour more than 2 cm but not more than 5 cm

T3   Tumour more than 5 cm but not more than 10 cm

T4   Tumour more than 10 cm in greatest dimension

N – Regional lymph nodes

NX   Regional lymph nodes cannot be assessed[g]

N0   No regional lymph-node metastasis

N1   Regional lymph-node metastasis

M – Distant metastasis

M0   No distant metastasis

M1   Distant metastasis

G – Histopathological grading

Grading for GIST is dependent on mitotic rate[h]

   Low mitotic rate: 5 or fewer per 50 hpf

   High mitotic rate: more than 5 per 50 hpf

Stage grouping for gastric GIST[i]

Stage	T	N	M	Mitotic rate
Group IA	T1, T2	N0	M0	Low
Group IB	T3	N0	M0	Low
Group II	T1, T2	N0	M0	High
	T4	N0	M0	Low
Group IIIA	T3	N0	M0	High
Group IIIB	T4	N0	M0	High
Group IV	Any T	N1	M0	Any rate
	Any T	Any N	M1	Any rate

Stage grouping for small-intestinal GIST[i]

Stage	T	N	M	Mitotic rate
Group I	T1, T2	N0	M0	Low
Group II	T3	N0	M0	Low
Group IIIA	T1	N0	M0	High
	T4	N0	M0	Low
Group IIIB	T2, T3, T4	N0	M0	High
Group IV	Any T	N1	M0	Any rate
	Any T	Any N	M1	Any rate

[a] {762, 2996};   [b] The adjacent structures of the stomach are the spleen, transverse colon, liver, diaphragm, pancreas, abdominal wall, adrenal gland, kidney, small intestine, and retroperitoneum;   [c] Intramural extension to the duodenum or oesophagus is classified by the depth of greatest invasion in any of these sites, including stomach;   [d] Tumour that extends into gastrocolic or gastrohepatic ligaments or into greater or lesser omentum, without perforation of visceral peritoneum, is T3;   [e] Neuroendocrine tumour (NET) or well-differentiated neuroendocrine tumour/carcinoma;   [f] For any T, add (m) for multiple tumours;   [g] NX: Regional lymph-node involvement is rare for GISTs, so that cases in which the nodal status is not assessed clinically or pathologically could be considered N0 instead of NX or pNX;
[h] The mitotic rate of GIST is best expressed as the number of mitoses per 50 high power fields (hpf) using the 40× objective (total area, 5 mm^2 in 50 fields);
[i] Staging criteria for gastric tumours can be applied in primary, solitary omental GISTs. Staging criteria for intestinal tumours can be applied to GISTs in the oesophagus, colon, rectum, and mesentery.

A help desk for specific questions about the TNM classification is available at http://www.uicc.org.

Gastric carcinoma

G.Y. Lauwers
F. Carneiro
D.Y. Graham
M.-P. Curado

S. Franceschi
E. Montgomery
M. Tatematsu
T. Hattori

Definition

Gastric carcinomas are malignant epithelial neoplasms. They represent a biologically and genetically heterogeneous group of tumours with multifactorial etiologies, both environmental and genetic. They are characterized by broad morphological heterogeneity with respect to patterns of architecture and growth, cell differentiation and histogenesis.

ICD-O codes

Adenoma	8140/0
Intraepithelial neoplasia (dysplasia)	
Low grade	8148/0
High grade	8148/2
Adenocarcinoma	8140/3
Papillary adenocarcinoma	8260/3
Tubular adenocarcinoma	8211/3
Mucinous adenocarcinoma	8480/3
Poorly cohesive carcinoma	
(including signet ring cell carcinoma	
and other variants)	8490/3
Mixed adenocarcinoma	8255/3
Adenosquamous carcinoma	8560/3
Carcinoma with lymphoid stroma	
(medullary carcinoma)	8512/3
Hepatoid adenocarcinoma	8576/3
Squamous cell carcinoma	8070/3
Undifferentiated carcinoma	8020/3

Epidemiology

Gastric cancer accounts for 7.8% of cancers worldwide {842A}. Areas where incidence is high at > 60 per 100 000 males include eastern Asia (Republic of Korea and Japan), eastern Europe and central and Latin America. Low-incidence areas (< 15 per 100 000 population) include North America, northern Europe, and most countries in Africa and south-eastern Asia {634}. The "intestinal" type of adenocarcinoma (ICD-O code 8144/3) is relatively predominant in high-incidence regions of the world, whereas the "diffuse" type (ICD-O code 8145/3) is relatively more common in low-incidence areas. Cancers of the antrum and pylorus are most common in high-incidence geographical areas, whereas cancers of the proximal stomach ("cardia") occur most commonly where incidence is low {2483}.

Countries with a high incidence of gastric cancer and where asymptomatic patients are screened have a high proportion (30–50%) of early gastric cancer (e.g. Japan) {1210, 2377}, an invasive carcinoma that is limited to the mucosa, or the mucosa and submucosa. In contrast, the proportion of early gastric cancer is much lower (16–24%) in North America and European countries {445, 1057, 1067}.

Time trends

There has been a steady decline in both the incidence and mortality of gastric carcinoma worldwide over the last 15 years. However, the absolute incidence rate continues to

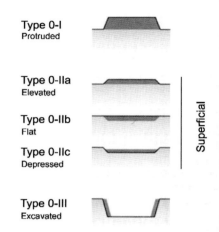

Fig. 4.01 Growth patterns of early gastric carcinoma.

rise, presumably due to the advancing age of the global population {2489}. More specifically, there has been a shift in the proportion of some subtypes. For instance, the incidence of "tubular" adenocarcinoma has decreased mainly in young patients {1471}. Paradoxically, despite the overall decreasing rates of gastric cancer, the incidence of "diffuse" carcinoma localized to the proximal stomach has been increasing {2101}.

Age and sex distribution

Gastric carcinoma is rare in persons aged < 30 years. In general, incidence increases progressively with age in males and females {634}. In young people, tumours

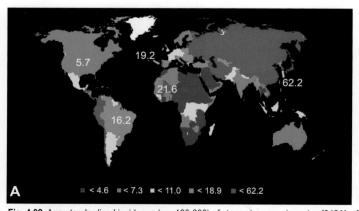

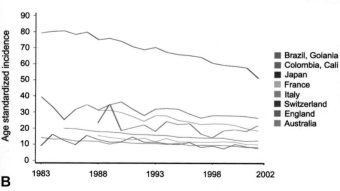

Fig. 4.02 Age-standardized incidence (per 100 000) of stomach cancer in males {842A}. **A** Worldwide incidence. Numbers on the map indicate regional average values. **B** The incidence of stomach cancer is decreasing worldwide, including in countries with a high disease burden.

are more likely to be hereditary, a greater proportion are of the "diffuse" type and females are more frequently affected than males {1471, 2101}.

Etiology
Smoking
An association between smoking and gastric cancer that is not explained by bias or confounding factors has been shown {1025, 1333}. Futhermore, smoking also potentiates the carcinogenic effect of infection with cagA-positive *Helicobacter pylori* {330, 2970, 3680}.

Diet
Certain dietary habits are associated with an increased risk of gastric cancer, especially of "intestinal" type. These include high intakes of salt-preserved and/or smoked foods {1788, 2935} and low intakes of fresh fruit and vegetables, particularly in combination with *H. pylori* infection {773, 799, 1332, 2543, 2935}. High intakes of all meat, red meat, and processed meat have been associated with an increased risk of "non-cardia" cancer {1024}. The true impact of dietary factors is difficult to assess in observational studies owing to insufficient accuracy in the assessment of exposure and in controls for confounding factors {1332}.

Trials of antioxidant supplements
Despite claims for a protective effect associated with high intake of fresh fruit and vegetables {1332}, a recent meta-analysis of randomized trials comparing antioxidant supplements (i.e. β-carotene and vitamins A, C, E and selenium, alone or in combination) with placebo or no intervention did not show a significant protective effect on the incidence of gastric cancer {271}. The results seem, however, to be influenced by whether the trials are performed in well-nourished populations or in those likely to have nutritional deficiencies (in which antioxidants may have a beneficial effect) {2604}. In the latter case, a significant reduction (11%) in mortality is noted in individuals receiving β-carotene, vitamin E and selenium, notably in individuals aged < 55 years {2604}.

Bile reflux
The risk of gastric carcinoma increases 5–10 years after gastric surgery, especially after a Bilroth II operation (which increases bile reflux) has been performed. However, the mechanism (including the role of bile acids) is not well understood, and *H. pylori* is not an important risk factor for stump cancer, its growth being impaired by gastroduodenal reflux {1644, 2978}.

Infection with H. pylori
H. pylori infection, which is commonly acquired during early childhood and persists throughout adult life unless eradicated, is the most important cause of distal gastric carcinoma {316}. In a subset of patients, persistent infection with *H. pylori* for several decades induces a series of phenotypical changes (i.e. chronic gastritis, mucosal atrophy, focal intestinal metaplasia and dysplasia) that occur before the development of "intestinal" type adenocarcinoma {602, 612, 782, 2749, 3467}. Nested case–control studies and prospective cohort studies have underscored the increased relative risk associated with *H. pylori* infection; in a meta-analysis evaluating prospective studies in subjects tested at least 10 years before diagnosis, the odds ratio was 5.9 (95% confidence interval, 3.4–10.3) {882, 1157, 2316, 2491}. The relative risk increases when the most sensitive testing procedures, e.g. immunoblot, are used {2096, 2969}. The preventive role of antibiotic therapy has been noted in patients free of atrophy or metaplasia at baseline {3541}. When considering precancerous lesions as end-points, eradication of *H. pylori* is found to have a significant beneficial effect {1810, 1828, 2051, 3654}. Finally, a randomized controlled trial study of 544 *H. pylori*-positive Japanese patients with early gastric cancer has shown a significant reduction in the recurrence of cancer (from 4% to 1.4%) in the group receiving eradication therapy after endoscopic resection {917}. Factors associated with colonization and pathogenicity of *H. pylori* comprise outer membrane proteins, including BabA, SabA, OipA, AlpA/B, homB {1452, 1953, 2350} as well as the virulence factors cagA in the cag pathogenicity island (cagPAI) and the vacuolating cytotoxin vacA {156, 210, 462}. Polymorphic determinants influencing the expression of vacA cytotoxin include the signal region (s1 and s2), mid-region (m1 and m2), intermediary region (i1 and i2) and d region (d1 and d2) {2312, 2363, 2668}. Strains producing the cagA protein that induce a greater degree of inflammation are associated with gastric precancerous lesions and a greater risk of developing "non-cardia" cancer {2440, 2568, 2609}. Although the risk of gastric cancer in some countries of Europe and North

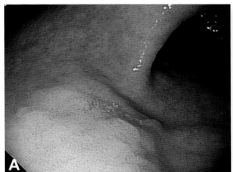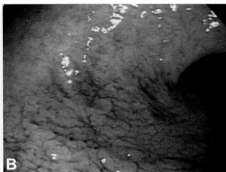

Fig. 4.03 Early gastric carcinoma in the antrum, endoscopic view. **A** Conventional endoscopy. **B** Chromoendoscopy markedly improves the visibility of the lesion.

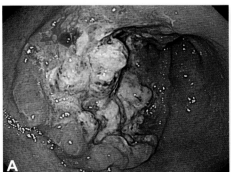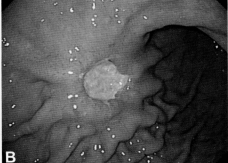

Fig. 4.04 Advanced gastric carcinoma, endoscopic view. **A** Type 2 (fungating). **B** Type 3 (ulcerated).

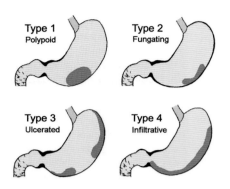

Fig. 4.05 Growth patterns of advanced gastric cancer according to the Borrmann classification.

America has been related to vacA genotype {856, 1293}, such relationships have not been observed in east Asian countries; the consequences of variation in vacuolating activity are apparently dependent on geographical region {2363}.

Ammonia, which stimulates cell replication, is abundantly liberated by the potent urease activity of *H. pylori* bacteria. *H. pylori* also causes increased expression of the inducible isoform of nitric oxide synthetase, with continuous production of oxidants and reactive nitrogen intermediates, including nitric oxide {1973}. Nitrosated compounds are recognized gastric carcinogens in the experimental setting. Free radicals, oxidants and reactive nitrogen species all

cause DNA damage (usually generating point mutations, the commonest being G:C->A:T.) and provoking either DNA repair or apoptosis {604}. *In vivo*, an increase in the formation of micronuclei in peripheral blood lymphocytes {3110}, DNA damage {1716}, and DNA-adduct formation have been noted in individuals infected with *H. pylori*. Infection has also been associated with modified expression of specific oncogenes or tumour-suppressor genes, e.g. *CTNNB1* (β-catenin), *CCND1* (cyclin D1), *TP73 (p73)* and *CDKN1B (p27)* {767, 888, 3481}.

Corpus-predominant gastritis with multifocal gastric atrophy, and hypo- or achlorhydria is seen in approximately 1% of subjects infected with *H. pylori*. As a direct consequence of elevation in gastric pH, there is a change in gastric flora, with colonization by anaerobic bacteria responsible for the formation of carcinogenic nitrosamines {2795}. Finally, the role of bone marrow-derived cells that may contribute to repopulation of the mucosa, in the setting of mucosal damage, may lead to the development of metaplasia and neoplasia {603, 1250}.

The severity and extent of gastritis caused by *H. pylori* are modulated by cytokines. Polymorphisms of the interleukin 1 β (*IL1B*) gene (initiation and amplification of inflammatory response) and the interleukin 1 receptor antagonist gene (*IL1RN*) (modulation of inflammation) are associated with

individual (or familial) susceptibility to carcinogenesis associated with *H. pylori* {777}. It has been suggested that in individuals with alleles that predispose to inflammation, infection with *H. pylori* may cause increased production of gastric interleukin 1 β, leading to severe and sustained inflammation that would increase the risk of developing gastric cancer {104, 776, 778, 855}.

Localization

The most frequent site of "non-cardia" gastric cancer is the antro-pyloric region. Carcinomas of the "cardia" have been most commonly reported in North American and European populations {632}, but this is likely to change subsequent to revision of the classification of adenocarcinomas of the oesophagogastric junction and the TNM (tumour, node, metastasis) classification of 2009 {762, 2996}. According to the TNM classification, if the epicentre of a tumour is within 5 cm of the oesophagogastric junction and extends into the distal oesophagus, the tumour should be staged as an oesophageal carcinoma. Consequently, the gastric antrum is likely to become the most common site of gastric carcinoma in North American and European series, in conformity with the rest of the world. Carcinomas in the body of the stomach are typically located along the greater or lesser curvature.

Clinical features

Endoscopy is a sensitive and specific diagnostic test for gastric cancer. Modern video-endoscopy allows the recognition of subtle changes in colour, relief, and architecture of the mucosal surface. Although detection of lesions associated with early gastric cancer can be improved using chromoendoscopy and narrow-band imaging, a substantial number of such lesions still escape detection {1247}.

Gastric cancers are classified endoscopically according to growth pattern {1390, 2186}. Early gastric cancers are divided into three types: protruded (type 0-I); superficial (type 0-II); and excavated (type 0-III) {1389}. The superficial type accounts for 80% of early gastric cancers and is further subdivided into 0-IIa (elevated type), 0-IIb (flat type), and 0-IIc (depressed type), the latter being the most common {3572}. Histologically, most early gastric cancers have a tubular or papillary architecture.

The risk of deep and multifocal penetration of the submucosa and of lymphatic

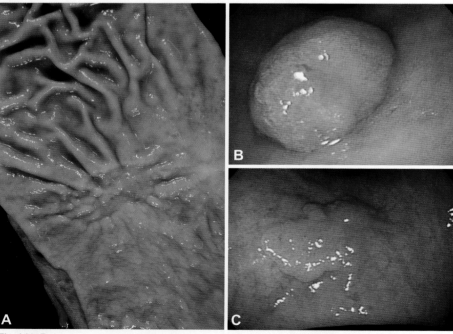

Fig. 4.06 Early gastric cancer, macroscopic features. **A** Type 0-IIc (superficial depressed). **B** Type 0-I (protruded). **C** Type 0-IIa (superficial elevated).

invasion vary according to type, being greater for type 0-IIc. Infiltration of the gastric wall (linitis plastica or "leather bottle") may be suspected if there is limited flexibility of the gastric wall. Since the invasive cells percolate beneath a usually normal mucosa, the diagnosis may require multiple, "jumbo" biopsies. The depth of invasion of the tumour is staged by endoscopic ultrasound. Radiology with barium meal is still used in mass-screening protocols in Japan, followed by endoscopy if an abnormality is detected. Recently, testing for serum pepsinogen has been used as a screening tool to identify high-risk patients and detect early cancers {2080}.

Tumour staging before treatment decision involves endoscopic ultrasound for characterization of the primary tumour, but is less useful for nodal (N) staging, whereas computed tomography (CT) is used to detect lymph-node and liver metastases.

Positron emission tomography (PET) in combination with CT imaging may be superior to either alone for preoperative staging {505, 1854, 2728}. Laparoscopic staging may be the only way to exclude peritoneal seeding in the absence of ascites.

Macroscopy

Noninvasive neoplasia – intraepithelial neoplasia or dysplasia – may present as a flat process that is difficult to detect by conventional endoscopy but may be apparent after dye-staining, or as a polypoid growth (sometimes reported as adenoma), or with an intermediate appearance as a depressed or reddish or discoloured mucosa. The macroscopic type of early gastric carcinoma is classified using criteria similar to those used in endoscopy {1390, 2186}. The gross appearance of advanced carcinoma is described according to the Borrmann classification {308}. Fungating and ulcerated

types are common. Diffuse (infiltrative) tumours (type 4) spread superficially, producing flat, plaque-like lesions, with or without shallow ulcerations. With extensive infiltration, linitis plastica may develop. Mucinous adenocarcinomas appear gelatinous with a glistening cut surface.

Tumour spread and staging

Gastric carcinomas can spread either by direct extension to adjacent organs, metastasis or peritoneal dissemination. Carcinomas of the "intestinal" type preferentially metastasize haematogenously to the liver, whereas carcinomas composed of poorly cohesive cells ("diffuse" type) preferentially metastasize to peritoneal surfaces {432, 2151}. Mixed carcinomas exhibit the metastatic patterns of both types {2151}.

"Diffuse" cancers of the antro-pyloric region have a high frequency of serosal and

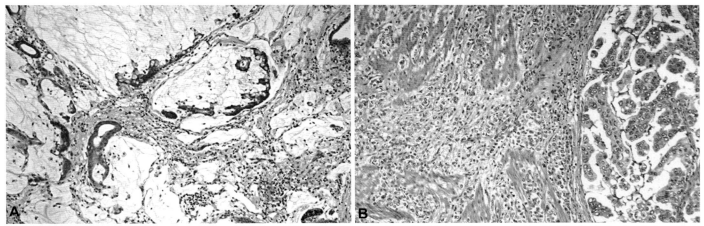

Fig. 4.07 **A** Mucinous carcinoma of the stomach. Irregular cords and clusters of mucus-secreting epithelial elements are readily identified floating in the abundant mucinous material. **B** Mixed carcinoma. The lesion shows both papillary (intestinal) and poorly cohesive (diffuse) components.

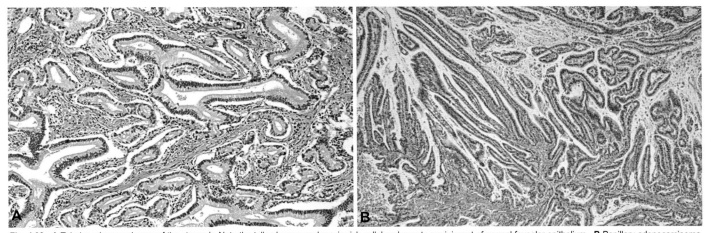

Fig. 4.08 **A** Tubular adenocarcinoma of the stomach. Note the tall columnar and mucin-rich cellular elements reminiscent of normal foveolar epithelium. **B** Papillary adenocarcinoma composed of exophytic projections lined by cuboidal neoplastic cells.

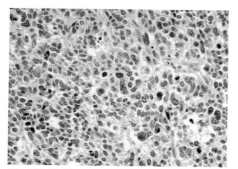

Fig. 4.09 Undifferentiated gastric carcinoma.

lympho-vascular invasion and lymph-node metastases. These tumours also commonly invade the duodenum via submucosal or subserosal routes or via the submucosal lymphatics. Duodenal invasion occurs more frequently than expected on the basis of gross examination and, in practical terms, resection margins should be monitored by intraoperative consultation. When the carcinoma penetrates the serosa, peritoneal implants generally flourish. Bilateral massive involvement of the ovaries (Krukenberg tumour) can result from transperitoneal or haematogenous spread. The principal value of nodal dissection is the detection and removal of metastatic disease and appropriate staging. The accuracy of pathological staging is proportional to the number of regional lymph nodes examined and their anatomical location in relation to the neoplasm. If only nodes that are close to the tumour are assessed, many cancers can be classified incorrectly. Staging for gastric carcinoma was substantially modified in the 2009 classification proposed by the International Union Against Cancer and the American Joint Committee on Cancer (UICC/AJCC): (1) T1 was subdivided to delineate mucosal and submucosal depth of invasion; (2) T2a and T2b were separated into T2 (muscularis propria) and T3 (subserosa); (3) T3 and T4 were changed to T4a (penetrates serosa) and T4b (invades adjacent structures), respectively; (4) The T, N, and M categories are now almost identical to those for the oesophagus (and oesophago-gastric junction) except that N3 (metastasis in 7 or more regional lymph nodes) is divided into N3a (7–15 nodes) and N3b (≥ 16 nodes) for gastric but not oesophageal carcinomas {762, 2996}.

Histopathology

The heterogeneity of gastric carcinomas is reflected in part by the diversity of the various histopathological classification schemes on record. Although the most commonly used are those of WHO and Laurén {1758}, several other schemes have been proposed, including those of Ming {2085}, Nakamura {2214}, Mulligan {2182}, Goseki {1039} and Carneiro {426}.

WHO classification

This is a strictly descriptive scheme that recognizes five main types of gastric adenocarcinoma and rare entities. The major advantage of the WHO classification is the recognition of morphological patterns that are also exhibited by neoplasms in other segments of the gastrointestinal tract, such as the small and large bowel, thus contributing to harmonization of the histological typing of carcinomas of the gut. The main categories are tubular, papillary, mucinous, poorly cohesive (including signet-ring cell type) and mixed carcinomas. The WHO classification, however, does not take into account histogenesis, differentiation or epidemiological data.

Tubular adenocarcinoma

This type is composed of dilated or slit-like and branching tubules of varying diameter. Acinar structures may also be present. Individual neoplastic cells can be columnar, cuboidal, or flattened by prominent intraluminal mucin. A clear cell variant has been recognized. The degree of nuclear atypia varies from low- to high-grade {792, 2301}. There is a poorly differentiated variant, sometimes called solid carcinoma. Tumours with prominent lymphoid stroma are sometimes called carcinoma with lymphoid stroma {3463}, medullary carcinoma {2083}, or lymphoepithelioma-like carcinoma {3445}. The degree of desmoplasia varies and may be conspicuous.

Papillary adenocarcinoma

This is a well-differentiated exophytic carcinoma with elongated finger-like processes lined by cylindrical or cuboidal cells supported by fibrovascular connective tissue cores. The cells tend to maintain their polarity. Some tumours show tubular (papillotubular) differentiation. Rarely, micropapillary architecture is present. The degree of cellular atypia and mitotic index vary; there may be severe nuclear atypia. The invading edge of the tumour is usually sharply demarcated; the tumour may be infiltrated by acute and chronic inflammatory cells.

Mucinous adenocarcinoma

This tumour is composed of malignant epithelium and extracellular mucinous pools. By convention, the tumour shows more than 50% extracellular mucin. Mucinous carcinomas may contain scattered signet-ring cells.

Poorly cohesive carcinomas, including signet ring cell carcinoma and other variants

Poorly cohesive carcinomas are composed of neoplastic cells that are isolated or arranged in small aggregates. These encompass:

Signet-ring cell type is defined as a tumour composed predominantly or exclusively of

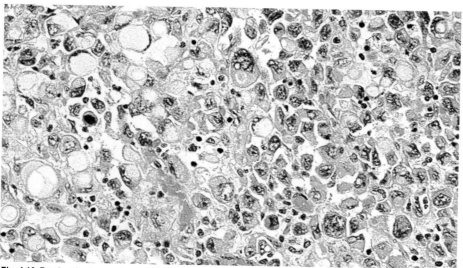

Fig. 4.10 Poorly cohesive carcinoma. This example displays a combined cellular infiltrate, with classic signet ring cells, bizarre/pleomorphic cells and smaller eosinophilic cells.

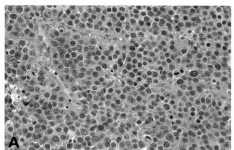
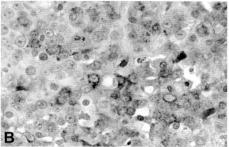

Fig. 4.11 Hepatoid adenocarcinoma of the stomach. **A** The tumour is composed of hepatocyte-like neoplastic cells growing in a sheet-like pattern. **B** Immunohistochemical staining for α-fetoprotein confirms the presence of hepatocytic differentiation.

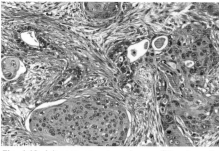

Fig. 4.12 Adenosquamous carcinoma of the stomach: the neoplasm combines adenocarcinoma and squamous cell carcinoma, with a transition between both elements.

signet-ring cells, characterized by a central optically clear, globoid droplet of cytoplasmic mucin with an eccentrically placed nucleus. Malignant signet-ring cells may form a lace-like gland or delicate microtrabecular pattern in the mucosa or be accompanied by marked desmoplasia in deeper levels of the stomach wall. In some cases, signet-ring cells may be restricted to the mucosa in combination with other variants of poorly cohesive cells within the deeper levels of the gastric wall.

Other cellular variants of poorly cohesive carcinoma include tumours composed of neoplastic cells resembling histiocytes or lymphocytes; others have deeply eosinophilic cytoplasm; some poorly cohesive cells may show irregular, bizarre nuclei. A mixture of the different cell types can be present, including few signet-ring cells.

Mixed carcinoma

These carcinomas display a mixture of discrete morphologically identifiable glandular (tubular/papillary) and signet-ring/poorly-cohesive cellular histological components. Any discrete histological component should be reported; although the prognostic relevance of the proportion of each component has not been established, preliminary data suggest that any signet-ring/poorly cohesive cellular histological component is associated with a poor prognosis.

Mixed carcinomas are clonal {447A, 3705} and phenotypic divergence has been attributed to somatic mutation in the E-cadherin gene (*CDH1*), which is restricted to the signet-ring/poorly-cohesive component {1941}.

Other classification schemes

In the Laurén classification, tumours are separated into diffuse (ICD-O code 8145/3), intestinal (ICD-O code 8144/3),

mixed and indeterminate types {1758}. Diffuse carcinomas consist of poorly cohesive cells with little or no gland formation. Intestinal carcinomas form glands with various degrees of differentiation. Tumours containing approximately equal quantities of intestinal and diffuse components are termed "mixed".

Undifferentiated tumours are classified as indeterminate. The Ming classification {2085} is based on patterns of growth and invasion at the advancing edge and divides tumours into expanding and infiltrative types. Nakamura categorizes all tumours as either differentiated or undifferentiated {2214}. The Mulligan system divides tumours into mucus, intestinal, and pyloro-cardiac gland types {2182}. Goseki recognizes four types on the basis of tubular differentiation and intracellular production of mucin {1039}. Finally, the Carneiro system recognizes four categories (glandular, isolated cell, solid and mixed) on the basis of morphology and immunophenotype; thus tumours designated as "intestinal" by the Laurén classification are subclassified into tumours with intestinal, gastric or mixed differentiation {426, 431, 865}. Lines of differentiation can be established using gastric markers (mucins MUC5AC, MUC6, and trefoil peptide TFF1), intestinal markers (MUC2, transcription factor CDX2 and CD10), and others (pepsinogen-1) {426, 1692, 1694, 1938, 1939, 2956, 3312}. Some studies have shown that phenotypic characterization has prognostic value {1113, 1786, 3430}.

Rare histological variants

Uncommon histological variants represent about 5% of gastric cancers. These include adenosquamous carcinoma {2148, 2249, 3648}, squamous cell carcinoma {1994, 3539}, hepatoid adenocarcinoma {1326, 1361, 2169, 2203}, carcinoma with

lymphoid stroma {2008, 2192, 2222, 3445, 3463, 3512, 3600}, choriocarcinoma {1321}, carcinosarcoma {1311, 1463, 2247, 2825}, parietal cell carcinoma {411, 3613}, malignant rhabdoid tumour {2694, 3337}, mucoepidermoid carcinoma {1140}, Paneth cell carcinoma {2405}, undifferentiated carcinoma, mixed adeno-neuroendocrine carcinomas, endodermal sinus tumour, embryonal carcinoma, pure gastric yolk-sac tumour and oncocytic adenocarcinoma {1760}.

Hepatoid adenocarcinoma

Hepatoid adenocarcinoma is composed of large polygonal eosinophilic hepatocyte-like neoplastic cells. α-Fetoprotein (AFP) can be detected *in situ*, but also in the serum. Bile and periodic acid-Schiff (PAS)-positive and diastase-resistant intracytoplasmic eosinophilic globules can be observed. Other rare AFP-producing carcinomas include well-differentiated papillary or tubular-type adenocarcinoma with clear cytoplasm and yolk-sac tumour-like carcinoma {1326, 1361, 2169, 2203}.

Gastric carcinoma with lymphoid stroma

This tumour, also reported as lympho-epithelioma-like carcinoma or medullary carcinoma, is characterized by poorly developed tubular structures associated with a prominent lymphoid infiltration of the stroma. These tumours frequently affect the proximal stomach or gastric stump and are more common in males while > 80% are associated with infection with Epstein-Barr virus (EBV) {2192}. The role of EBV in carcinogenesis is debated, but occurs at an early stage since EBV can be found in adjacent dysplasia. The prognosis for patients with these tumours is reportedly better than that for patients with typical gastric cancers {2008, 2192, 2222, 3445, 3463, 3512, 3600}.

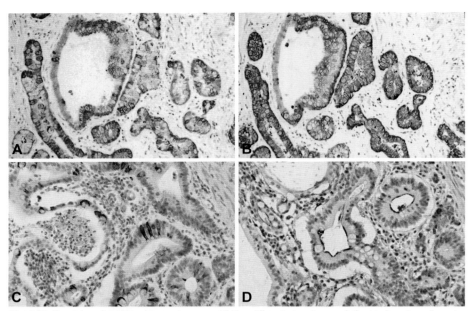

Fig. 4.13 Examples of gastric adenocarcinomas exhibiting different phenotypes. **A** Gastric foveolar cell mucin, MUC5AC(+). **B** Pyloric-gland cell mucin, MUC6(+). **C** Intestinal goblet-cell mucin, MUC2(+). **D** Small-intestinal brush border differentiation, CD10(+).

Gastric choriocarcinoma

Gastric choriocarcinomas usually display syncytiotrophoblast and cytotrophoblast elements admixed with adenocarcinoma. Yolk-sac and hepatoid components can also be seen. Human chorionic gonado-tropin can be detected *in situ* and in the serum. These tumours are frequently associated with haematogenous dissemination and nodal metastases {1321}.

Early gastric cancer

This is an invasive carcinoma that is limited to the mucosa, or the mucosa and submucosa, regardless of nodal status. Most such cancers measure 2–5 cm and are located on the lesser curvature and around the angulus {1822, 2086}. If untreated, most progress over a few months to several years {3313}. Tubular and papillary variants represent 50% and 30%, respectively, of cases. Signet ring cell carcinoma and "poorly differentiated" carcinoma represent 25% and 15% of cases, respectively, and are usually depressed or ulcerated {808, 1822, 3572}.

Stromal reactions

The four common stromal responses to invasive gastric carcinoma are marked desmoplasia, lymphocytic infiltration, stromal eosinophilia and a granulomatous response. The density of tumour-infiltrating lymphocytes, particularly peritumoral regulatory T cells, has been shown to be predictive of regional lymph-node metastasis with improved outcome {1098, 1781, 2109}. Scirrhous stromal reaction has been noted as a predictor of aggressive behaviour and peritoneal seeding {1278}.

Grading

The grading system applies primarily to tubular and papillary carcinomas (not other types). Well-differentiated adenocarcinomas are composed of well-formed glands, sometimes resembling metaplastic intestinal epithelium. Moderately differentiated adenocarcinomas are composed of neoplams that are intermediate between well- and poorly differentiated. Poorly differentiated adenocarcinomas comprise highly irregular glands that are recognized with difficulty. They may also be graded as low-grade (well- and moderately differentiated) or high-grade (poorly differentiated).

Precursor lesions
Gastritis and intestinal metaplasia

Particularly in high-incidence areas, some patients with *H. pylori*-associated chronic gastritis develop atrophy followed by intestinal metaplasia over time. This is the beginning of a sequence of events that may culminate in neoplasia, especially adenocarcinoma of "intestinal" type {601, 602, 1319}.

Gastritis

Classification schemes, such as the Sydney system, have attempted to combine topographic, morphological, and etiological information into a reporting system designed to include both grading and staging of gastritis {726, 2589, 2750, 2751}. Autoimmune gastritis develops secondary to the development of autoantibodies to parietal and chief cells and thus affects the body fundic mucosa. It is associated with the formation of intestinal metaplasia and an increased risk of developing gastric carcinoma, mostly of intestinal type {3014}. A cross-reactive mechanism between *H. pylori* and gastric epithelial antigens that may be responsible for, or at least participate in, the pathogenesis of autoimmune gastritis has been proposed {642}.

Intestinal metaplasia

The two main types of intestinal metaplasia are: "complete" (also designated as "small intestinal type" or type I), and "incomplete" (types IIA/II and IIB/III) {857, 859}. Using newly developed antibodies, an immunohistochemical classification of intestinal metaplasia is possible. Complete-type metaplasia shows decreased expression of "gastric" mucins (MUC1, MUC5AC and MUC6) and expression of MUC2, an intestinal mucin. In contrast, in incomplete intestinal metaplasia, gastric mucins are co-expressed with MUC2. These expression patterns show that incomplete intestinal metaplasia has a mixed gastric and intestinal phenotype reflecting an aberrant differentiation programme {2656}. Some studies (but not all) indicate a positive correlation between the degree of incomplete intestinal metaplasia and the extent of intestinal metaplasia and risk of progression to carcinoma {679, 782, 858, 1473, 2716, 2743, 2988}. Some authors also claim that intestinal metaplasia is a paracancerous not a precancerous lesion {1460}.

In another pattern of metaplasia termed spasmolytic polypeptide-expressing metaplasia (SPEM), the expression of TFF2 spasmolytic polypeptide is associated with oxyntic atrophy. SPEM, which characteristically develops in the gastric body and fundus, appears to share some characteristics with pseudopyloric metaplasia, has a strong association with chronic infection with *H. pylori* and with gastric adenocarcinoma, and may represent another pathway to gastric neoplasia {1094}.

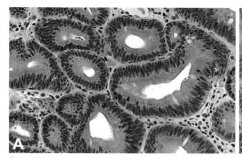
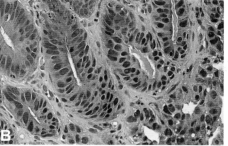

Fig. 4.14 Intraepithelial neoplasia (dysplasia). **A** Low grade: the lesion shows mild cytological atypia with basally located, polarized and pencillate hyperchromatic nuclei. **B** High grade: the neoplastic tubules display enlarged rounded markedly atypical nuclei with stratification and loss of polarization.

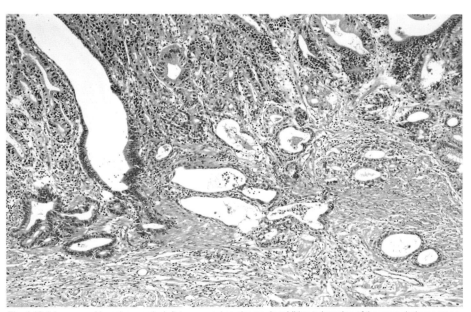

Fig. 4.15 Intraepithelial neoplasia (dysplasia) of gastric phenotype (type II). The cells have a characteristic clear to pale eosinophilic cytoplasm.

Premalignant lesions

In Chapter 1, a historical perspective and an overview of terminology used for premalignant lesions in the present edition are presented, including the definition of intraepithelial neoplasia/dysplasia. Major interpretative problems associated with diagnosing gastric intraepithelial neoplasia (dysplasia) include distinguishing such conditions from reactive or regenerative changes associated with active inflammation, and the distinction between intramucosal and invasive carcinoma {1764, 2840}. Recognizing that the terminology of dysplasia is entrenched in the European and particularly North-American literature, as well as in clinical practice, "intraepithelial neoplasia" and "dysplasia" are acceptable terms. The following three categories should thus be considered:

(1) Negative for intraepithelial neoplasia (dysplasia)

This category includes benign mucosal processes that are inflammatory, metaplastic, or reactive in nature.

(2) Indefinite for intraepithelial neoplasia (dysplasia)

The use of this term represents a pragmatic solution to an ambiguous morphological pattern, but is not a final diagnosis. This category is favoured where there is doubt as to whether a lesion is neoplastic or non-neoplastic (i.e. reactive or regenerative), particularly in small biopsies exhibiting inflammation. In such cases, the dilemma is usually solved by cutting deeper levels, by obtaining additional biopsies, or after correcting for possible etiologies. Foveolar hyperproliferation may be seen, showing irregular and tortuous tubular structures with epithelial mucus depletion, a high nucleus to cytoplasm ratio, and loss of cellular polarity. Large, oval/round, hyperchromatic nuclei associate with prominent mitoses usually located near the proliferative zone in the mucus-neck region. In intestinal metaplasia, areas indefinite for intraepithelial neoplasia may exhibit a hyperproliferative metaplastic epithelium. The glands may appear closely packed and lined by cells with large, hyperchromatic basally located nuclei. The cytoarchitectural alterations tend to decrease from the base of the glands to their superficial portion.

(3) Intraepithelial neoplasia (dysplasia)

This category comprises unequivocally epithelial neoplastic proliferations characterized by variable cellular and architectural atypia, but without convincing evidence of invasive growth.

There are well-known differences between Japanese and European/North American pathologists in categorizing intraepithelial neoplasia {1764, 2840}. For instance, lesions interpreted by the latter as high-grade intraepithelial neoplasia (dysplasia) have been frequently classified by Japanese pathologists as "noninvasive intramucosal carcinoma." In an attempt to resolve this issue, several proposals have been made regarding terminology of the morphological spectrum of lesions ranging from non-neoplastic changes to early invasive cancer, including the Padova and Vienna classifications {2753, 2842, 3090}.

Intraepithelial neoplasia (gastric epithelial dysplasia) can have polypoid, flat, or slightly depressed growth patterns; the flat or slightly depressed patterns may show an irregular appearance on chromoendoscopy or microvasculature anomalies on narrow-band imaging, which are not apparent with conventional white-light endoscopy. In European countries and

Fig. 4.16 Intramucosal invasive neoplasia/intramucosal carcinoma. In addition to invasion of the muscularis mucosae, this lesion is distinguished from high-grade intraepithelial neoplasia (dysplasia) by architectural glandular anomalies, i.e. crowding, excessive branching and budding.

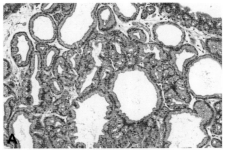
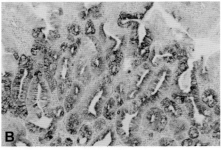

Fig. 4.17 Pyloric-gland adenoma. **A** The lesion is characterized by closely packed pyloric gland-type tubules lined with cuboidal to low columnar epithelial cells containing round nuclei and pale to eosinophilic cytoplasm. **B** Immunoexpression of MUC6 (marker of pyloric-gland mucin) is characteristic.

North America, the term "adenoma" has been applied when the neoplastic proliferation produces a discrete, protruding lesion. In Japan, however, "adenomas" include all gross types (i.e. flat, elevated, and depressed). In the stomach, most cases of intraepithelial neoplasia (dysplasia) have an intestinal phenotype (adenomatous; type I) resembling colonic adenomas with crowded, tubular glands lined by atypical columnar cells with overlapping, pencillate, hyperchromatic and/or pleomorphic nuclei, with pseudostratification and inconspicuous nucleoli, mucin depletion, and lack of surface maturation {1396}. Other variants include a gastric phenotype (foveolar or pyloric phenotype; type II) in which the cells are cuboidal or low-columnar, with clear or eosinophilic cytoplasm, and show round to oval nuclei {1396}. The two types may be distinguished by expression of mucin, CD10, and CDX2 (intestinal/adenomatous: MUC2, CD10, and CDX2; gastric/foveolar: MUC5AC, absence of CD10 and low expression of CDX2) {2311, 2468, 2471}, as well as by background changes in the gastric mucosa {13}. Cases with hybrid differentiation may also occur {2468}.
Intraepithelial neoplasia (dysplasia) is stratified into two grades, low or high.

Low-grade intraepithelial neoplasia (dysplasia). Shows minimal architectural disarray and only mild-to-moderate cytological atypia. The nuclei are elongated, polarized, and basally located, and mitotic activity is mild-to-moderate. For polypoid lesions, the term "low-grade adenoma" has been used {2842}.

High-grade intraepithelial neoplasia (dysplasia). Comprises neoplastic cells that are usually cuboidal, rather than columnar, with a high nucleus to cytoplasm ratio, prominent amphophilic nucleoli, more pronounced architectural disarray, and numerous mitoses, which can be atypical. Importantly, the nuclei frequently extend into the luminal aspect of the cell, and nuclear polarity is usually lost. For polypoid lesions, the term "high-grade adenoma" has been used {2842}.

Intramucosal invasive neoplasia/intramucosal carcinoma

This term defines carcinomas that invade the lamina propria and are distinguished from intraepithelial neoplasia (dysplasia) not only by desmoplastic changes that can be minimal or absent, but also by distinct structural anomalies, such as marked glandular crowding, excessive branching, and budding. Intraluminal necrotic debris is common. Single infiltrating cells can also be seen within the lamina propria in the absence of desmoplasia. The neoplastic cells in intramucosal invasive neoplasia are usually cuboidal with a high nucleus to cytoplasm ratio. Round nuclei with prominent nucleoli and marked loss of polarity are common. Mitoses are usually numerous and atypical mitoses can be identified.
The diagnosis of intramucosal carcinoma indicates that there is an increased risk of lymphatic invasion and lymph-node metastasis. In some circumstances, novel endoscopic techniques can allow treatment of the patient without open surgery, particularly for lesions of < 2 cm in size and for those that are well-differentiated {2211}.

Invasive neoplasia

This terminology defines carcinomas that show invasion beyond the lamina propria. In the stomach, the diagnosis of invasive neoplasia is associated with a varying risk of nodal and distant metastasis and overall prognosis. Surgical resection, sometimes with neoadjuvant therapy, is recommended.

Gastric polyps
Neoplastic polyps

Neoplastic polypoid lesions in the stomach encompass carcinoma (primary or secondary), neuroendocrine tumours (addressed in separate chapters of this volume), adenomatous polyps (intestinal type), gastric-type adenomas (pyloric-gland adenomas and foveolar-type adenomas), and fundic gland polyps.

Adenomatous polyps

Adenomatous polyps usually show evidence of intestinal-type differentiation (absorptive cells, goblet cells, endocrine cells, or even Paneth cells), express intestinal markers (MUC2 and CD10), and are negative for gastric mucins (MUC5AC and MUC6) {1694, 2467}. The risk of malignant transformation is related to size (> 2 cm) and presence of high-grade dysplasia {2470}. However, the importance of the phenotype (intestinal-type versus gastric) is debated {13, 2468}.
Gastric-type adenomas. These encompass pyloric-gland adenoma and foveolar-type adenomas. Pyloric-gland adenoma is a rare neoplasm with gastric epithelial differentiation characterized by closely packed pyloric gland-type tubules with a monolayer of cuboidal to low columnar epithelial cells containing round nuclei and pale to eosinophilic cytoplasm {515, 1694, 2467}. Foveolar-type adenomas are rare in general but more common in patients with familial adenomatous polyposis (FAP) {13, 1694}, and predominantly express MUC5AC without MUC6 {515}. Whether they are low-risk lesions or not is debated {13, 2468}

Fundic-gland polyps

Fundic-gland polyps may occur sporadically, in patients with FAP {2467}, or as a familial condition confined to the stomach without polyposis coli {3306} and also affect patients receiving long-term treatment with proton-pump inhibitors {96, 883}.
Sporadic fundic-gland polyps have very weak malignant potential, and the frequency of dysplasia is very low {1381, 3092}. Patients with FAP may develop dysplasia (in up to 48% of cases) in fundic-gland polyps, but carcinomas are extremely rare {16, 159}.
The frequent finding of genetic alteration involving the APC/β-catenin pathway, either sporadic or arising in the setting of FAP, suggests that fundic-gland polyps may be neoplastic {14, 15, 3272}.

Non-neoplastic polyps

Non-neoplastic polyps of the stomach encompass hyperplastic polyps, hamartomatous polyps (Peutz-Jeghers polyp, juvenile polyp, Cronkhite-Canada syndrome-associated polyp), and miscellaneous lesions with polypoid growth pattern {425, 2467}).

Hyperplastic polyps

Hyperplastic polyps are the second most common gastric polyps and typically arise in previously damaged gastric mucosa {17, 425, 2467}, arising in a background of *H. pylori* gastritis or autoimmune gastritis. Malignant transformation, although rare, is well-documented {427, 433, 3089, 3685}.

Polyposis syndromes

Peutz-Jeghers polyps, juvenile polyps, and Cowden polyps generally do not occur sporadically, but rather as part of hereditary polyposis syndromes. Some cases of juvenile polyposis may affect the stomach only {750}. Gastric Peutz-Jeghers polyps are characterized histologically by branching bands of smooth muscle derived from muscularis mucosae, and hyperplasia, elongation and cystic change of foveolar epithelium; the deeper glandular components tend to show atrophy. However, syndromic gastric polyps can be difficult to distinguish from hyperplastic polyps.

Genetic susceptibility

Familial diffuse gastric cancer with autosomal dominant inheritance, caused by germline mutation of the E-cadherin gene was reported in 1998 {1081}. This new syndrome, hereditary diffuse gastric cancer, is described in the next chapter of this volume.
The risk of gastric cancer is also increased in dominantly inherited cancer-predisposition syndromes such as FAP and Lynch syndrome {415, 1930}, and also in Li-Fraumeni syndrome with germline mutation of *TP53* {3379}. It was reported recently that among patients with Peutz-Jeghers, those with frameshift mutations in the *STK11* gene develop aggressive gastric cancers {2950}. Carriers of mutations in *MSH2* also have an increased risk of gastric cancer {3387}. Furthermore, a novel germline mutation of the *LKB1* gene has been reported in a patient with sporadic Peutz-Jeghers with early-onset gastric cancer {3159}.

Table 4.01 Frequency of the most common genetic alterations found in gastric carcinomas of "intestinal" and "diffuse" types.

Gene	Alteration	Frequency[a]		References
		"Intestinal" carcinoma	"Diffuse" carcinoma	
APC	LOH, mutation	30–40%	< 2%	{1784, 2245A, 3178}
BCL2	Overexpression	—	10–30%	{168, 1782}
CDH1	Mutation, hypermethylation, LOH	—	> 50%	{151, 220, 470, 1082, 1408, 1937, 1940, 2014}
CDKN1B	Reduced expression	40–50%[b]		{1543, 3566, 3627}
CTNNB1	Mutation	17–27%		{3450}
Cyclin E	Overexpression	15–20%[b]		{50}
DCC	LOH	60%	< 1%	{ 2307, 3329}
ERBB2	Amplification	10–15%	< 1%	{204, 2348, 3378}
FGFR2	Amplification	—	35%[c]	{1136, 2990}
KRAS	Mutation	1–28%[d]	< 1%	{331, 1552, 2393, 3559}
MET	Amplification	20–40%[b]		{1678}
MYC	Overexpression	40–45%[b]		{395, 1661}
PTEN	LOH, mutation	20–30%[e]		{1839}
RB1	Reduced expression	—	30%[b]	{828}
TP53	Mutation, LOH	25–40%[f]	0–21%[f]	{1314, 1459, 3644}

LOH, loss of heterozygosity
[a] The frequencies are presented according to the two major histotypes of the Lauren classification, i.e., "intestinal" and "diffuse" (roughly corresponding to the "well-differentiated" and "poorly differentiated" carcinomas of the Japanese classification), as reported in the relevant cited literature.
[b] Correlates with prognosis and/or more advanced disease.
[c] Present only in advanced cases.
[d] Mostly occuring in carcinomas with microsatellite instability.
[e] Associated with invasion and metastasis.
[f] Frequent in aneuploid (60–70%) but rare in diploid carcinoma.

Finally, susceptibility to carcinogens and their precursors varies among individuals. A role for polymorphisms of genes encoding for glutathione *S*-transferase enzymes (known to metabolize tobacco-related carcinogens) and *N*-acetyltransferase 1 {2767, 3500} has been suggested.

Molecular pathology

Gastric cancers are characterized by genetic and epigenetic changes that affect oncogenes, tumour suppressor genes, and DNA mismatch repair (MMR). Consequently, deregulation of cellular proliferation, adhesion, differentiation, signal transduction, telomerase activity, and DNA repair has been reported. Different genetic pathways have been described for various histological types of gastric cancer.

Promoter methylation, acetylation and demethylation

Aberrant CpG island promotor methylation of several genes has been described in gastric cancer. *CDKN2A* (p16) gene hypermethylation is seen in 12–30% of gastric carcinomas. Reduced expression of *CDKN2A* correlates with depth of invasion and metastasis in some studies {221}. Hypermethylation with reduced expression of the retinoic acid receptor β (*RARB*) gene is observed in 60–65% of "intestinal" carcinomas, but not in "diffuse" carcinomas {1141}. Hypermethylation of *RUNX3* (a member of the RUNX family that plays a role in TGF-β signalling) is observed in 45–65% of gastric cancers, sometimes accompanied by reduced expression of *RUNX3* in adjoining non-neoplastic gastric mucosa {2241}. Biallelic inactivation of *RUNX3* can also be caused by homozygous deletion and, rarely, by mutation {1835}.
Aberrant acetylation is frequently detected in H3 and H4 histone genes, in both the promoter and coding regions, and is associated with reduced expression of *CDKN1A* in gastric carcinoma {2094}. Demethylation of some genes, such as melanoma antigen family (MAGE) and

synuclein-γ (*SNCG*) has been described in gastric cancer. Demethylation of the *MAGEA1* and *MAGEA3* promoters is more frequently observed in advanced adenocarcinoma and is associated with a worse prognosis {1233}. *SNCG* methylation is more frequent in cancers with lymph-node metastasis {3609}.

Microsatellite instability (MSI)

The MSI or mutator phenotype is caused by defects in the MMR system responsible for the correction of mismatches that occur during DNA replication. In gastric cancer, MSI is mainly caused by epigenetic silencing (promoter methylation) of the *MLH1* gene {429}. Somatic mutations of MMR genes are very rare in sporadic gastric cancer {2553}. MSI is observed in 5–10% of "diffuse" carcinomas and in 15–40% of "intestinal" carcinomas. Gastric carcinomas with a high level of MSI (MSI-high) are characterized by antral location, "intestinal" phenotype and expanding growth pattern. MSI-high tumours show a better prognosis than do MSI-low {223, 536, 737, 1783, 3558}. Several reports have shown a relation between MSI and tumour multiplicity {536, 1783}.

Prognosis and predictive factors

Early gastric cancer

Early gastric cancers have a low incidence of vessel invasion and lymph-node metastasis and a good prognosis (about 90% of patients survive 10 years). Various multivariate analyses have identified submucosal invasion; tumour diameter > 3.0–3.5 cm; the presence of vascular invasion; the presence of lymphatic permeation; depressed or ulcerated lesions and undifferentiated histology as independent risk factors for nodal metastasis.

For patients meeting these criteria, endoscopic resection is likely to be an ineffective therapeutic modality and surgery should be considered {1041, 2384, 2766}. However, some authors claim that small intramucosal gastric cancers of undifferentiated histology, measuring < 20 mm in size and without lymphovascular invasion have a negligible risk of lymph-node metastasis and could also be considered for endoscopic resection {1200}.

Staging of advanced gastric cancer

The stage of gastric cancer with special reference to extension to the serosa and lymph nodes (summed up in the TNM staging system) remains the strongest prognostic indicator. Five-year survival is 60–80% for patients with tumours that invade the muscularis propria, but 50% for those with tumours invading the subserosa {1354, 3651}. Unfortunately, at the time of diagnosis most patients with advanced carcinoma already have lymph-node metastases for which only palliative surgery can be envisaged {853}. Often seen in advanced cases, lymphatic and vascular invasion specifically carry a poor prognosis. Reported data support the value of a number-based classification scheme for reporting nodal involvement in gastric cancer {2702}. In patients with involvement of 1–6 lymph nodes, the 5-year survival rate is 46% compared with 30% in patients with 7–15 lymph nodes involved. The extent of regional lymphadenectomy performed and quality of lymph-node evaluation have also been stressed significantly. Patients undergoing a "curative" gastrectomy but limited lymph-node dissection (D1/D0) have an overall 5-year survival of only 23% versus > 50% for those undergoing more aggressive lymphadenectomy (D2) {1476}.

Histological typing

The value of histological typing of the tumour in predicting tumour prognosis is controversial. Whether the prognosis for "diffuse" carcinoma (Laurén classification) is or is not worse than that for "intestinal" carcinoma is debated {1989, 3019}. Recently, it has been suggested that "diffuse" carcinomas encompass lesions with different prognosis, i.e. a low-grade desmoplastic subtype (with no or scarce angio-lympho-neuroinvasion) and a high-grade subtype (with anaplastic cells) {525}. The prognosis for patients with poorly cohesive carcinoma is particularly bad for children and young adults, for whom diagnosis is often delayed {2613, 3343} and who are likely to fit into the category of hereditary diffuse gastric cancer. Some investigators have found that only the Goseki classification {1989} added additional prognostic information to the TNM stage {1989, 3019} with 5-year survival of patients with mucus-rich (Goseki II and IV) T3 tumours being significantly worse than that for patients with mucus-poor (Goseki I and III) T3 tumours (18% versus 53%; $p < 0.003$) {1989}. The scheme proposed by Carneiro *et al.* is also believed to have prognostic value {431}. Some patients with medullary carcinoma have a better prognosis than those with other histological types {737}, some being in Lynch-syndrome kindreds with MSI-high, a feature associated with better survival. Not all studies agree that stromal inflammatory response and pushing margins predict a better prognosis {1989, 3019}.

Hereditary diffuse gastric cancer

F. Carneiro
A. Charlton
D.G. Huntsman

Definition

Hereditary diffuse gastric cancer (HDGC) is an autosomal-dominant cancer-susceptibility syndrome that is characterized by signet ring cell (diffuse) gastric cancer and lobular breast cancer. The genetic basis for this syndrome was discovered in 1998 by Guilford *et al.* {1081}, who identified germline mutations of the E-cadherin (*CDH1*) gene (MIM No. 192090) by linkage analysis and mutation screening in three Maori kindreds with multigenerational, diffuse gastric cancer in New Zealand.

MIM No.   137215

Diagnostic criteria

In families with an aggregation of gastric cancer, the histopathology of the tumours is often unknown; these cases are designated as familial gastric cancer (FGC). When the histopathological type of one or more gastric cancers is known, discrete syndromes/diseases can be diagnosed; these include HDGC, familial diffuse gastric cancer (FDGC) and familial intestinal gastric cancer (FIGC) {397}.

On the basis of clinical criteria, the International Gastric Cancer Linkage Consortium (IGCLC) in 1999 defined families with the HDGC syndrome as those fulfilling one of the following features:

(1) Two or more documented cases of diffuse gastric cancer in first- or second-degree relatives, with at least one being diagnosed before the age of 50 years; or (2) Three or more cases of documented diffuse gastric cancer in first- or second-degree relatives, independent of age of diagnosis {397}. Women in these families also have an elevated risk of lobular breast cancer {341, 1501, 1513, 2855, 3136}. IGCLC criteria for genetic testing, updated in 2009 {871} are shown in Table 4.02. An alternative genetically-based nomenclature, proposed by the New Zealand group, in which the term "HDGC" is restricted to families with germline mutations in the *CDH1* gene {1081, 1082}.

The IGCLC definition for HDGC will be used for the remainder of this section {871}.

Epidemiology

The vast majority of gastric cancers are sporadic, but approximately 1–3% result from an inherited predisposition {870, 2396, 2439}.

The prevalence of HDGC is uncertain, partly due to the recent identification of this syndrome. In a review of 439 families with aggregation of gastric cancer {2395}, *CDH1* mutations were preferentially observed in families fulfilling the clinical criteria for HDGC (36.4%). In FDGC, the frequency of germline mutations in *CDH1*

was much lower (12.5%) {2395}. *CDH1* mutations have not been found in families with weaker histories of gastric cancer; however, mutation rates of up to 10% have been described in individuals with no family history but DGC diagnosed at less than age 35 years, from populations with a low incidence of gastric cancer {1501, 3136}. There are striking population-specific differences regarding the fraction of families with aggregation of gastric cancer and frequency of *CDH1* germline mutations. In countries with a low incidence of gastric cancer, the frequency of germline alterations in the *CDH1* gene is > 40%, while in countries with a moderate or high incidence of gastric cancer, the frequency of alterations in *CDH1* is about 20% {2396}. These observations in moderate- or high-incidence countries are probably related to clustering of gastric cancer attributable to environmental risk factors (lifestyle, diet) and/or variation in genes conferring a weak susceptibility {2396}.

Localization

Most index cases with HDGC present with cancers that are indistinguishable from sporadic diffuse gastric cancer, often with linitis plastica, which can involve all topographic regions within the stomach. Systematic complete mapping of total gastrectomies from asymptomatic carriers

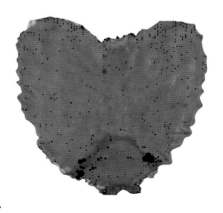
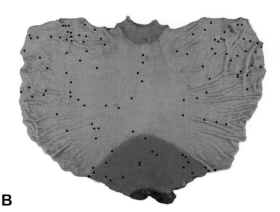

- ● Squamous
- ● Fundic/body
- ● Body/antral transitional zone
- ● Antrum
- ● Duodenum
- ● Signet-ring cell carcinoma

A   **B**

Fig. 4.18 Mapping of gastric mucosal zones (semi-opaque colours) and location of foci of stage T1a signet ring cell (diffuse) carcinoma (black circles) on photos of two stomachs. Adapted from Charlton *et al.* {493}. **A** Asymptomatic *CDH1*-mutation carrier, aged 15 years; the map indicates the location of 318 foci and mucosal zones. **B** Asymptomatic *CDH1*-mutation carrier, aged 19 years, from the same family; the map indicates the location of 115 foci and mucosal zones.

Table 4.02 Criteria for testing for *CDH1* mutation: updated recommendations from the International Gastric Cancer Linkage Consortium (IGCLC).[a]

1. Two or more documented cases of gastric cancer in first-degree relatives, with at least one documented case of diffuse gastric cancer diagnosed before the age of 50 years

2. Three or more cases of documented diffuse gastric cancer in first- or second-degree relatives, independent of age of onset

3. Diffuse gastric cancer before the age of 40 years without a family history

4. Families with diagnoses of both diffuse gastric cancer and lobular breast cancer, with one case before the age of 50 years

[a] In addition, in cases where expert pathologists detect carcinoma *in situ* adjacent to diffuse-type gastric cancer, genetic testing should be considered since this is rarely, if ever, seen in sporadic cases.

of *CDH1* mutations show microscopic, usually multiple, foci of intramucosal signet ring cell (diffuse) carcinoma in almost all cases {195, 276, 428, 493, 1148, 1290, 2322, 2712}. These foci of carcinoma can involve any topographic region of the stomach and are limited to the gastric mucosa. As all regions of the gastric mucosa can be affected, pathological examination of the resected specimen should include confirmation of the presence of a complete cuff of proximal squamous oesophageal mucosa and distal duodenal mucosa.

Clinical features
Age at clinical manifestation
Before the advent of genetic identification of carriers of *CDH1* mutations, and the subsequent implementation of risk-reduction strategies, patients presented with clinically detected gastric cancer, usually at an advanced stage. The age at onset of clinically significant diffuse gastric cancer may be extremely variable (range, 14–85 years), even within families. In one large Maori kindred (Family A), the youngest individual to die from gastric cancer was aged 14 years, but the oldest known asymptomatic mutation-carrier was aged 75 years {276, 1501, 2541}.

Genetic testing
Probands from populations with a low or moderate incidence of gastric cancer, who fulfil the criteria listed in Table 4.02, are offered genetic testing. The age at which to offer testing to at-risk relatives should take into consideration the earliest age of onset of cancer in that family. Testing from late adolescence or in the early 20s occurs in families with early onset gastric cancer {566, 1501}.
The guidelines of the IGCLC recommend that asymptomatic carriers of *CDH1* mutations be offered prophylactic gastrectomy or annual endoscopic surveillance (in selected groups) as risk-reduction strategies.

Endoscopic surveillance
Since the foci of T1a carcinoma are small (many < 1 mm), and are located beneath a normal surface epithelium, without distortion of the pit or gland architecture, it is not surprising that endoscopic detection is difficult in asymptomatic *CDH1*-mutation carriers. In most cases, multiple endoscopic biopsies carried out before gastrectomy fail to detect the multiple foci of stage T1a carcinoma identified by histopathological examination of the resected stomach {195}. Chromoendoscopy was shown to increase the likelihood of detecting T1a foci of > 4 mm when compared with white-light endoscopy {2910}, but this technique has been discontinued owing to concerns over the toxicity of Congo red {566}. The likelihood of obtaining positive biopsies is improved by increasing the number of biopsies to 24 or more {195}, and by the cumulative experience of the same endoscopist regularly performing HDGC endoscopy {566, 2910}. Experience with chromoendoscopy has led to an appreciation that pale areas are visible with standard endoscopy, but they are subtle and would be easily overlooked by most endoscopists {566}.
Endoscopic surveillance is recommended for individuals aged < 20 years, individuals aged > 20 years who elect to delay surgery, or for whom prophylactic gastrectomy (biopsy-negative) is unacceptable, but gastrectomy with curative intent (biopsy-positive) is acceptable, and those with mutations of undetermined significance (e.g. missense) {1501, 2910}.

Prophylactic/curative total gastrectomy
Total gastrectomy is recommended in at-risk family members aged > 20 years, who have a *CDH1* mutation {276}. In biopsy-positive individuals, a curative total gastrectomy is advised, regardless of age. Recent data show that pregnancy can be carried to full term following a prophylactic gastrectomy {1500}. Prophylactic gastrectomy has an estimated mortality rate of up to 2% {1931}.

Breast cancer
Breast cancer occurs with an increased frequency in HDGC families; most cases are lobular. Loss of E-cadherin expression and poorly cohesive morphology is common to both diffuse gastric carcinoma and lobular breast carcinoma. Current estimates of lifetime cumulative risk for female lobular breast cancer are 60% by age 80 years {871}. Gastric cancer, however, is the main cause of mortality in individuals with *CDH1* mutations. Enhanced screening to detect lobular breast carcinoma should be considered {871, 1664}.

Macroscopy
Stomachs from asymptomatic *CDH1*-mutation carriers nearly always appear normal to the naked eye, are normal to

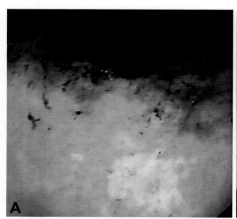
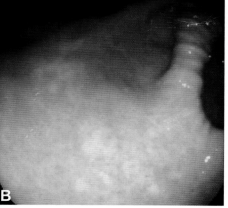

Fig. 4.19 Endoscopic views of intramucosal diffuse carcinoma, confirmed by biopsy, in two different asymptomatic *CDH1*-mutation carriers from the same family. **A** Chromoendoscopic pale area with well defined margins. Adapted from {2910}. **B** A subtle pale area is visible on standard white-light endoscopy.

palpation, and slicing shows normal mucosal thickness. Unlike most sporadic gastric cancers, there is no mass lesion {428, 493, 2712}. In some apparently normal stomachs, close inspection may show white patches after formalin fixation that correspond to intramucosal signet ring cell carcinoma.

Tumour spread and staging

The pathology in asymptomatic *CDH1*-mutation carriers represents a new paradigm in cancer. There is multifocal invasive cancer, without a mass lesion, and without symptoms. Systematic complete pathological mapping of stomachs removed from asymptomatic *CDH1*-mutation carriers show that almost all (96%) {2396} contain multiple foci of intramucosal signet ring cell (diffuse) carcinoma of TNM stage T1a. These T1a tumours are invasive cancers by definition yet may remain indolent for a long time and carry a very low risk for metastasis. Less commonly, larger foci of intramucosal carcinoma can involve superficial and deep mucosa.

Histopathology

Early-stage HDGC in *CDH1*-mutation carriers is characterized by multiple foci of invasive (T1a) signet ring cell (diffuse) carcinoma in the superficial gastric mucosa, with no nodal metastases {276, 493, 558, 1290}. At the neck-zone level, neoplastic cells are small, and usually enlarge towards the surface of the gastric mucosa, with transitional forms between. The foci of intramucosal carcinoma are composed of mitotically inactive neoplastic cells. {276, 1286}. Pathological mapping of the entire gastric mucosa has been performed in many stomachs from kindred with different *CDH1* mutations {195, 276, 428, 493, 1148, 1290, 2322, 2712}. There is wide variation in the number of T1a foci observed in these stomachs, both within and between kindreds, ranging from one focus {428} to hundreds of tiny foci {276, 493}. Histological examination of the entire gastric mucosa is required (one section per block) before the absence of neoplasia can be claimed.

The cause of this variation in number of foci is presently unknown, although both background genetics and environmental factors are probable contributing factors {276}. Early invasive carcinoma is not restricted to any topographic region in the stomach: foci have been identified from the "cardia" to the pre-pyloric region, without evidence of antral clustering {195, 428, 1290, 2712}.

In a large Maori family in New Zealand, the greatest density and largest foci of T1a carcinomas were located in the distal stomach and the body–antral transitional zone in many, but not all stomachs {276, 493}. Individual foci of intramucosal (T1a) signet ring cell (diffuse) carcinoma are small, ranging from 0.1 mm to 10 mm, with most being < 1 mm in diameter {1287, 2712}.

The signet ring cell (diffuse) carcinomas observed in asymptomatic *CDH1*-mutation carriers show absent or reduced staining for E-cadherin {428, 558, 1290}, in keeping with a clonal origin of the cancer foci, indicating that the second *CDH1* allele has been down-regulated or lost. Down-regulation of the second allele in large numbers of widely separated lesions strongly suggests that this "second hit" has occurred as a transcriptional field effect, and not as an independent mutation event in each lesion {276}.

Background changes in the gastric mucosa of prophylactic gastrectomy specimens can encompass mild chronic gastritis, sometimes displaying the features of lymphocytic gastritis. Occasionally, an inflammatory granulomatous reaction is observed at the periphery of some collapsing glands. Foveolar hyperplasia and tufting of surface epithelium, focally with globoid change is also a frequent finding and, in some areas, vacuolization of surface epithelium is striking {428, 430, 2395}. Additionally, erosions and cysts can be observed in non-neoplastic mucosa. Intestinal metaplasia and infection with *H. pylori* are typically absent. The IGCLC has prepared a proforma for reporting the pathology of gastrectomy specimens from patients with HDGC {871}.

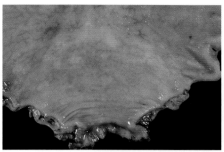

Fig. 4.20 Formalin-fixed stomach showing barely discernible pale patches on the body–antrum transitional zone in the same 15-year-old asymptomatic *CDH1*-mutation carrier as shown in Fig. 4.18A. These correspond to foci of T1a signet ring cell carcinoma.

Precursor lesions

The following precursors to T1a signet ring cell carcinoma are recognized: (1) signet ring cell carcinoma *in situ* (Tis), corresponding to the presence of signet ring cells within the basal membrane, substituting normal epithelial cells, generally with hyperchromatic and depolarized nuclei; (2) a pagetoid spread pattern (not necessarily associated with an invasive carcinoma) of signet ring cells below the preserved epithelium of glands and foveolae, but within the basal membrane {428}. In these lesions, E-cadherin immunoexpression is reduced or absent {428, 2396}. Strictly following criteria for the identification of these precursors will diminish the risk of over-diagnosing nonspecific changes and distinguish precursors from mimics of signet ring cells *in situ*, including telescoped normal glands {3238, 3671}. Confirmation of carcinoma *in situ* (Tis) by an independent histopathologist with experience in this area is

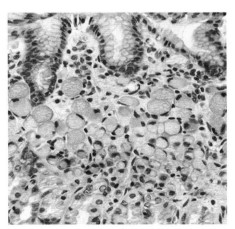

Fig. 4.21 Typical invasive focus of T1a intramucosal signet ring cell (diffuse) carcinoma. The signet ring cells are usually smaller at the neck zone, and larger nearer the surface of the gastric mucosa.

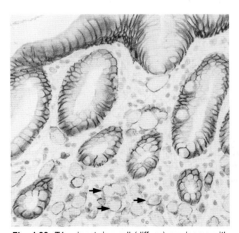

Fig. 4.22 T1a signet ring cell (diffuse) carcinoma with immunostaining for E-cadherin. Signet ring cells show absent or reduced expression of E-cadherin (arrows).

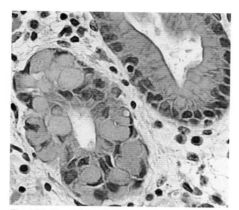

Fig. 4.23 Signet ring cell carcinoma *in situ* (Tis).

strongly recommended. Noteworthy is the discrepancy between the numerous invasive carcinoma (T1a) foci and the low number or absence of carcinoma *in situ* (Tis) lesions, indicating that invasion of the lamina propria by signet ring cells usually occurs without morphologically detectable carcinoma *in situ* {428}. Unlike the usual neoplastic progression sequence from dysplasia to carcinoma, the preinvasive neoplastic precursor, Tis, is absent, or is present in far fewer numbers than T1a invasive carcinoma, and moreover, can be geographically distant from foci of T1a invasive carcinoma.

On the basis of these precursors, a model for the development of diffuse gastric cancer in carriers of deleterious germline *CDH1* mutations has been proposed {428, 430}.

Genetic susceptibility

Mutations in the *CDH1* gene have been identified in families with HDGC from different geographic regions and ethnicities {276, 397, 955, 1082, 1290, 2673}. In clinically defined HDGC, *CDH1* mutations are detected in 30–40% of cases {870, 1501, 2394, 2396}.

The *CDH1* gene is located on the long arm of chromosome 16 (16q22.1), comprises 16 exons transcribed into a 4.5 kb mRNA and encodes E-cadherin {249}. E-cadherin is a transmembrane protein that is predominantly expressed at the basolateral membrane of epithelial cells, where it exerts cell–cell adhesion and invasion-suppression functions {1076, 2206}. The extracellular domain of E-cadherin plays a key role in the correct folding and homo- and heterodimerization of the proteins, as well as in the adhesion mechanism itself. The cytoplasmic domain of the protein interacts with the catenins (α, β, γ, p120ctn) indirectly influencing the organization of the actin cytoskeleton {280}.

Type of CDH1 mutation

Of the identified germline mutations in *CDH1*, 75–80% are truncating (including nonsense, splice-site and frameshift mutations, predicted to produce premature termination codons) and the remaining 20–25% are missense mutations {276, 430}. The latter may have functional effects through alteration of residues critical to protein structure or through alternative splicing {1501, 3134, 3135}. Although a range of different techniques have been used for detecting mutations, direct sequencing is the method of choice.

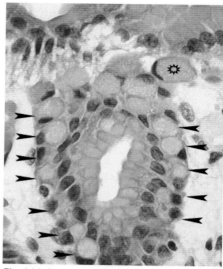

Fig. 4.24 Pagetoid spread of signet-ring cells (arrow heads) representing Tis, and invasion of the lamina propria by a signet-ring cell (empty star), indicating T1a invasive intramucosal signet-ring cell carcinoma.

In addition to point mutations, large germline deletions akin to those described in the Lynch-syndrome genes have been found in 6.5% of HDGC families who tested negative for point mutations {2394}. It is likely that these deletions occur through mechanisms involving mainly nonallelic homologous recombination in Alu repeat sequences {2394}. Such deletions can be detected by multiplex ligation-dependent probe amplification (MLPA). Unlike the somatic mutations in *CDH1* that occur in sporadic gastric cancers and cluster around exons 7 and 8, the germline mutations in *CDH1* in HDGC families span the whole length of the gene and no hot spots have been identified. This means it is necessary to screen all 16 exons of the gene in families that potentially have HDGC, except those from Newfoundland who may carry discrete founder mutations {1501}.

Molecular pathology
Second-hit inactivation mechanism for E-cadherin

As is the case for sporadic diffuse gastric cancers, diffuse gastric cancer developing in germline *CDH1*-mutation carriers generally display abnormal or absent expression of E-cadherin {428, 1286, 1290}, in accordance with the two-hit model of tumour-suppressor gene inactivation. In this regard, sporadic and hereditary cases of DGC are identical and although the use of immunohistochemistry for the

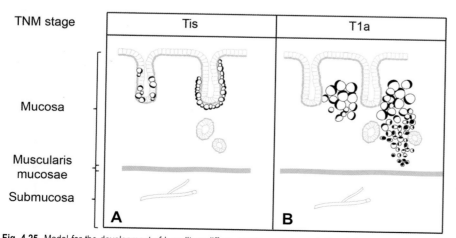

TNM stage	Tis	T1a

Fig. 4.25 Model for the development of hereditary diffuse gastric carcinoma. **A** Signet ring cell carcinoma *in situ*, noninvasive. Single signet-ring cells are shown on the left, pagetoid-spread pattern on the right. **B** Early diffuse gastric cancer. The diagram shows invasion into the lamina propria.

diagnosis of DGC can be useful, it does not allow identification of the subset of cases with germline mutations. In cases of HDGC, the *CDH1* gene can be inactivated by a number of mechanisms. Most frequently, this occurs via promoter methylation (epigenetic modification) and less frequently by loss of heterozygosity (LOH) and *CDH1* mutations {194, 1047, 2397}. An intragenic deletion in the wild-type allele has also been reported {2391}. The second hit in *CDH1* may differ in primary tumours and metastases, epigenetic changes (promoter methylation) being more frequent in HDGC primary tumours and LOH in metastases {2397}.

Alterations in other tumour suppressor genes and oncogenes

Humar *et al.* {1286} have suggested that the initiation of diffuse gastric cancer seems to occur at the proliferative zone of the gastric epithelium and correlates with absent or reduced expression of junctional proteins, activation of the *SRC* (c-src) system, and epithelial–mesenchymal transition. It remains to be seen whether inactivation of c-src kinase marks the development of early diffuse gastric cancer. Identification of the molecular mechanisms underlying disease progression will help to explain why most early intra-

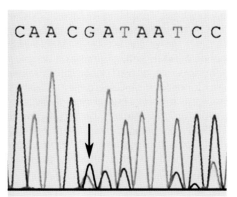

Fig. 4.27 Sequencing of the *CDH1* gene in a patient with hereditary diffuse gastric cancer reveals a frameshift mutation in exon 8.

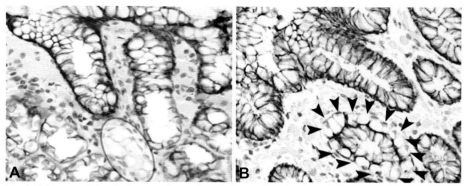

Fig. 4.26 Absence of E-cadherin expression as shown by immunohistochemistry. **A** Signet ring cell carcinoma *in situ* (ellipse). **B** Pagetoid spread of signet ring cells (arrow heads).

mucosal carcinomas remain indolent for undefined periods of time, while a few progress to higher-stage gastric cancer.

Alternative genes in HDGC families that do not show mutations in CDH1

In more than two thirds of cases of HDGC, no *CDH1* germline mutations are identified and the disease remains genetically unexplained. Searching for mutations in genes encoding E-cadherin-binding partners within the adhesion complex, namely the catenins (α, β, γ, p120ctn) has not disclosed any germline mutations, suggesting that catenins are not major susceptibility genes for HDGC {1929}. Germline mutations in *TP53* were detected in two studies of families with gastric cancer and no mutation in *CDH1* {1514, 2392}. Searching for mutations in other candidate genes for HDGC has so far provided no clues for alternative causal genes for this hereditary syndrome {1514, 2392}.

As most HDGC families that show no mutation in *CDH1* have been too small or otherwise not suitable for linkage analysis, whole-genome sequencing using high-throughput methods may ultimately identify the genetic basis of their susceptibility to cancer. This is now practical through the development of massively parallel single-molecule sequencing technologies {126, 2273}.

Prognosis and predictive factors

Presumably, complete silencing of the *CDH1* gene is necessary for disease penetrance or, in other words, for invasive cancer to occur. Based on data from eleven families, Pharoah *et al.* {2541} estimated the cumulative risk of developing clinically significant gastric cancer by age 80 years to be 67% for men and 83% for women. Females were found to have a 39% risk of breast cancer {2541}. Updated analysis in 2008 (unpublished) indicate an estimated risk of more than 80% for the development of gastric cancer and 60% for lobular breast cancer in carriers of germline mutations in *CDH1* {871}.

If foci of carcinoma are limited to the gastric mucosa, prognosis is likely to be excellent after total gastrectomy, although long-term survival with HDGC after gastrectomy remains unknown. It is possible that curative gastrectomies for gastric disease will unmask an additional risk for carcinoma at other sites in HDGC patients. The diagnosis of HDGC offers the opportunity for pre-symptomatic genetic screening for at-risk family members and life-saving cancer risk-reduction surgery for carriers of *CDH1* mutations. In addition to its importance for affected families, HDGC, through the study of prophylactic gastrectomy specimens, has provided a unique window to study the earliest stage of diffuse gastric cancer.

Neuroendocrine neoplasms of the stomach

E. Solcia
R. Arnold
C. Capella
D.S. Klimstra
G. Klöppel
P. Komminoth
G. Rindi

Definition

Neoplasms with neuroendocrine differentiation including neuroendocrine tumours (NET) and neuroendocrine carcinomas (NEC) arising in the stomach. Mixed adeno-neuroendocrine carcinomas (MANEC) have an exocrine and an endocrine component, with one component exceeding 30%.

ICD-O codes

Neuroendocrine tumour (NET)
    NET G1 (carcinoid)   8240/3
    NET G2   8249/3
Neuroendocrine carcinoma (NEC) 8246/3
    Large cell NEC   8013/3
    Small cell NEC   8041/3
Mixed adenoneuroendocrine
  carcinoma (MANEC)   8244/3
EC cell, serotonin-producing NET 8241/3
Gastrin-producing NET (gastrinoma)
                        8153/3

Synonyms

Synonyms for gastric NET include: carcinoid and well-differentiated endocrine tumour/carcinoma {3013}. Synonyms for NEC include: poorly differentiated endocrine carcinomas, high-grade neuroendocrine carcinoma, small cell and large cell endocrine carcinomas.

Classification

Gastric NETs and NECs are classified on the basis of criteria that are common to all gastrointestinal and pancreatic neuroendocrine neoplasms (see Chapter 1). Most neuroendocrine neoplasms of the stomach are NETs – well-differentiated, nonfunctioning enterochromaffin-like (ECL) cell carcinoids (ECL cell NETs) – and arise predominantly in the corpus-fundus region {3013}. Three distinct types are recognized: (1) type I, associated with autoimmune chronic atrophic gastritis (A-CAG); (2) type II, associated with multiple endocrine neoplasia type 1 (MEN1) and Zollinger-Ellison syndrome (ZES); and (3) type III, sporadic (i.e. not associated with A-CAG or MEN1-ZES). Serotonin-producing enterochromaffin (EC) cell,

gastrin cell, ghrelin cell or adrenocorticotrophic hormone (ACTH) cell NETs are very rare and may arise in both the corpus–fundus and antrum.

NECs (poorly differentiated endocrine carcinomas) and MANECs are also rare and may arise in any part of the stomach.

Epidemiology

Incidence and time trends

In the past, gastric NETs were reported to occur with an incidence of 0.002–0.1 per 100 000 population per year and to account for 2–3% of all gastrointestinal NETs {1002} and 0.3% of gastric neoplasms {1935}. However, more recent studies based on endoscopic techniques and increased awareness of such lesions have suggested that the incidence of these tumours might be much higher, reaching 11–41% of all gastrointestinal NETs {2982}. The incidence of gastric NETs is higher in Japan where these neoplasms represent 30% of all gastrointestinal NETs; this may be atributable to the high incidence of chronic atrophic gastritis in this country, as well as to intensive screening by endoscopy {2155}. Recent population-based studies of gastric NETs showed that the annual incidence was 0.18–0.24 per 100 000 among Caucasians and 60% higher among African Americans {1137}. As for NETs at other sites of the gastrointestinal tract, the incidence of gastric NETs shows an incremental trend in the last three decades {3624}.

Age and sex distribution

ECL cell NET. Type-I gastric ECL cell NETs have been reported to represent 74% of all gastric neuroendocrine neoplasms and to occur most often in females (male-to-female ratio, 1 : 2.5), with a mean age at biopsy of 63 years (range, 15–88 years). Type-II ECL cell NETs represent 6% of all gastric neuroendocrine neoplasms and show no sex predilection (male-to-female ratio, 1 : 1) at a mean age of 50 years (range, 28–67 years). Type-III ECL cell NETs account for 13% of all gastric neuroendocrine neoplasms and are observed mainly in males (male-to-female

ratio, 2.8 : 1) at a mean age of 55 years (range, 21–38 years) {2683}. NETs composed of EC, gastrin or ghrelin cells represent less than 1% of all gastric neuroendocrine neoplasms.

NEC and MANEC. NECs (poorly differentiated neuroendocrine carcinomas) account for 6–16% of gastric neuroendocrine neoplasms, are more common in men (male-to-female ratio, 2 : 1) and present at a mean age of 63 years (range, 41–61 years) {2682, 2683}. No specific epidemiological data are available for MANECs.

Etiology

ECL cell NETs

Gastrin has a trophic effect on ECL cells in humans and in experimental animals {305, 1101}. Long-standing hypergastrinaemia, resulting either from unregulated hormone release by a gastrinoma or from a secondary response of antral gastrin cells to achlorhydria, is consistently associated with ECL-cell hyperplasia {305}. Other factors may also be involved in ECL-cell oncogenesis, including mutation or deletion of the multiple endocrine neoplasia I (MEN1) gene at 11q13 in MEN1-ZES patients {683}, and inflammation coupled with severely altered mucosal structure and function in A-CAG patients, with a possible role for several growth factors, including transforming growth factor α (TGFα) and basic growth factor (bFGF) {304, 3343}. The most severe A-type, corpus-predominant, chronic atrophic gastritis, with total loss of parietal cells, achlorhydria, gastrin-cell hypertrophy and hyperplasia and secondary hypergastrinaemia, is usually caused by a T-cell- and antibody-mediated antiparietal cell autoimmune process. Sometimes this process supervenes over a long-standing chronic gastritis caused by Helicobacter pylori {1308}. In a minority (about 20%) of cases, corpus-prevalent subtotal atrophy with a few surviving H. pylori and extensive multifocal intestinal metaplasia were found in association with gastrin-cell hyperplasia, hypergastrinaemia as well as ECL-cell hyperplasia, dysplasia and neoplasm(s) {3014}.

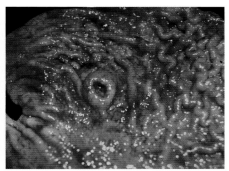

Fig. 4.28 Type III (sporadic) ECL cell NET (carcinoid) of the gastric body. The surrounding mucosa is normal.

ZES results from hypergastrinaemia caused by gastrin-producing neoplasms (gastrinomas) that are preferentially located in the duodenum and pancreas; associated ECL-cell proliferation is usually limited to hyperplastic lesions of the simple linear type {241, 1798, 3009}. MEN1, an inherited neoplasia syndrome, causes a variety of neuroendocrine neoplasms, including gastrinomas. In patients with MEN1-associated ZES (MEN1-ZES), ECL-cell lesions are often dysplastic or overtly neoplastic in nature {3010}. Thus long-standing, severe hypergastrinaemia usually causes only moderate ECL-cell hyperplasia in ZES patients lacking the MEN1 syndrome, whereas in MEN1-ZES patients, ECL-cell hyperplasia progresses to dysplasia in 53% of cases and to formation of neoplasms in 23% of cases {241}.

NEC and MANEC

It is likely that NECs and MANECs share the complex pathogenetic setting of the common gastric adenocarcinoma. The gastrin-promoting role for ECL cell NETs is retained in the exceedingly rare cases of MANECs with an ECL cell NET component that develop in a background of A-CAG {447}.

Localization
NET

ECL cell NETs of types I, II, and III are all located in the mucosa of the body–fundus or body–antrum border of the stomach. The rare gastrin cell NETs are located in the antro-pyloric region, while EC cell tumours may occur in any part of the stomach {2683}. The single functioning ghrelin cell tumour so far described was reported in the corpus {3302}.

NEC and MANEC

NECs and MANECs may arise at any site in the stomach {447, 1555, 2683}.

Clinical features
ECL cell, histamine-producing NET

Of the three types of ECL cell NETs, two, (types I and II), associate with hypergastrinaemia. Type-I ECL cell NETs arise in a background of A-CAG, and predominantly involve the corpus–fundus mucosa. Clinical signs include achlorhydria and, less frequently, pernicious anaemia. Hypergastrinaemia or antral gastrin cell hyperplasia are observed in all cases of A-CAG associated with ECL cell tumour disease {2686}. Type-I NETs are typically small (usually < 1 cm), multiple and multicentric. Hypertrophic-hypersecretory gastropathy and high levels of circulating gastrin are critical diagnostic findings for type-II ECL cell NETs {3010}. ECL-cell hyperplasia and/or dysplasia are invariably present in the fundic peritumoral mucosa {2683}. Type-II NETs are usually multiple and < 1.5 cm in size {2683}.

Type-III (sporadic) ECL cell NETs do not associate with hypergastrinaemia, A-CAG or MEN1-ZES. They are generally solitary growths, arise in a gastric mucosa void of significant pathological lesions except for gastritis and in the absence of ECL-cell hyperplasia/dysplasia. Multiple neoplasms have been observed rarely. Type-III NETs may present either: (1) with symptoms similar to those of an adenocarcinoma, including dyspepsia, gastric haemorrhage, mass obstruction, weight loss and metastasis; or (2) with endocrine symptoms of an "atypical carcinoid syndrome" characterized by red cutaneous flushing in the absence of diarrhoea. The atypical carcinoid syndrome occurs in cases with extensive liver metastases that cause the release of substantial amounts of histamine and 5-hydroxytryptophan {2341, 2696}.

EC cell, serotonin-producing NET

This rare neoplasm is occasionally found in association with a carcinoid syndrome {549}.

Gastrin producing NET (gastrinoma)

NETs that produce gastrin may present in association with ZES due to overproduction of gastrin and may thus be defined as gastrinoma (more frequently occurring in the duodenum). It should be noted that immunohistochemical demonstration of gastrin in the absence of a syndromic condition does not merit use of the term gastrinoma (see Chapter 6).

ACTH-producing NET

This rare neoplasm is associated with Cushing syndrome owing to ectopic secretion of ACTH {1203, 3026}.

NEC and MANEC

These neoplasms usually present with clinically nonspecific symptoms similar to those of conventional gastric cancer, often at an advanced stage, with distant metastases.

Macroscopy
ECL cell, histamine-producing NET

Type-I ECL cell NETs are multiple in approximately 60% of cases {2683}, usually appearing as small, tan-coloured nodules or polyps that reside in the mucosa or, less often, the submucosa. Most neoplasms (77%) are < 1 cm in diameter and 97% of neoplasms are < 1.5 cm. The muscularis propria is involved in only a minority of cases (7%). Patients with type-II NETs have an enlarged stomach with thickened gastric wall (0.6–4.5 cm), due to severe hypertrophic-hypersecretory gastropathy, multiple mucosal-submucosal neoplasms, often larger in size than the average type-I tumour, and < 1.5 cm in 75% of cases {2683}. Type-III ECL cell NETs are usually single and in 33% of cases are > 2 cm in size. Infiltration of the muscularis propria and of the serosa is found in 76% and 53% of cases, respectively {2683}.

NEC and MANEC

NECs (poorly differentiated neuroendocrine carcinomas) may form a large fungating mass deeply infiltrating the gastric wall and often metastatic to lymph nodes and liver {500}. MANECs usually present as conventional gastric cancer.

Histopathology
NET

NETs of the stomach are intensely immunoreactive for chromogranin A and synaptophysin. Most gastric NETs are predominantly composed of ECL cells, stain for the marker vesicular monoamine transporter 2 (VMAT2) and show vesicular secretory granules with characteristic ultrastructure {412, 2686, 2687}. They specifically produce histamine and histidine decarboxylase, which are, however, difficult to demonstrate by immunohistochemical methods in routinely processed specimens {3132}. In the literature, they have been commonly labelled as "ECL carcinoids", although minor cell subpopulations expressing serotonin, ghrelin, gastrin, somatostatin, pancreatic polypeptide (PP), or α-human chorionic gonadotrophin (α-hCG) have been detected {2453, 2686, 2688}.

ECL cell, histamine-producing NET. The majority of type-I and type-II and a minority of type-III ECL cell NETs are characterized by small, microlobular–trabecular aggregates formed by regularly distributed, often aligned cells (mosaic-like pattern), with regular, monomorphic nuclei, usually inapparent nucleoli, and rather abundant, fairly eosinophilic cytoplasm. Mitoses are almost absent, and angioinvasion is infrequent {2682}. Neoplasms with these features fit the current G1 class (for grading, see Chapter 1) and are usually limited to the mucosa or submucosa.

Type-III sporadic ECL cell NETs often display more aggressive features than do types I and II. These neoplasms may show a prevalence of solid, cellular aggregates and large trabeculae, crowding and irregular distribution of round to spindle and polyhedral tumour cells, either with fairly large vesicular nuclei and prominent eosinophilic nucleoli, or with smaller, hyperchromatic nuclei, irregular chromatin clumps and small nucleoli. Scarce necrosis but considerable mitotic activity, sometimes with atypical mitotic images, may be present. Neoplasms with these histological features display a relatively high mitotic rate (mean, 9 per 10 high power fields [HPF]) and a high Ki67-labelling index (mean, about 1000 per 10 HPF) {2682}, fitting the current G2 class (for grading, see Chapter 1). Type-III NETs more frequently express *TP53* (60% of cases) and display lymphatic and vascular invasion than most neoplasms

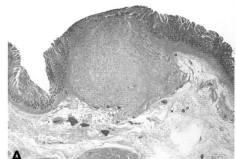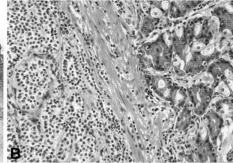

Fig. 4.29 Type-III (sporadic) ECL cell carcinoid (NET). **A** The tumour extends from the mucosa into the submucosa, with a well-delineated inferior border. **B** The carcinoid (left) has round, regular, isomorphic nuclei.

of type I or II, and are often deeply invasive and associated with local and/or distant metastases {2682}.

EC cell, serotonin-producing NET. This is a very rare neoplasm in the stomach {549, 2686}. Its histopathology is similar to that of the ileal NETs. The tumour cells are argentaffin, intensely argyrophilic and immunoreactive for chromogranin A, synaptophysin and anti-serotonin antibodies. The presence of EC cells is confirmed via electron microscopic detection of characteristic pleomorphic, intensely osmiophilic granules similar to those of normal gastric EC cells.

Gastrinoma (gastrin-producing NET). True gastric gastrinomas are very rare {1607}. Well-differentiated gastrin-producing NETs are small, mucosal-submucosal nodules, found incidentally at endoscopy or in a gastrectomy specimen, more frequently in proximity of the pylorus, either on its gastric or, especially, its duodenal slope. They may show a characteristic thin, trabecular–gyriform pattern or a solid nest pattern.

The cells are uniform with scanty cytoplasm and show predominant immunoreactivity for gastrin.

NEC

These highly malignant neoplasms are composed of large, poorly formed trabeculae, nests or sheets of anaplastic round, polyhedral to spindle cells, small to fairly large in size, and immunoreactive for general neuroendocrine markers, including chromogranin A, synaptophysin, neural cell adhesion molecule (NCAM1/-CD56), protein gene product 9.5 (PGP9.5) and/or neuron-specific enolase {1427, 2682, 2686, 2932}. Gastric NECs often show multifocal, abundant necrosis and a high mitotic rate (> 20 mitoses per 10 HPF), thus fitting the current G3 class (for grading, see Chapter 1). Based mainly on nuclear structure and cell size, two subtypes can be identified, small cell and large cell, similar to the corresponding lung cancers. Large cell NECs often show more vesicular nuclei, with more prominent

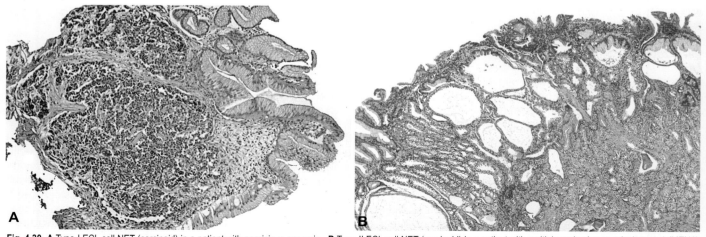

Fig. 4.30 **A** Type-I ECL cell NET (carcinoid) in a patient with pernicious anaemia. **B** Type-II ECL cell NET (carcinoid) in a patient with multiple endocrine neoplasia type 1 (MEN1) and Zollinger-Ellison syndrome (ZES).

nucleoli as well as a more organoid structure, suggestive of moderate neuroendocrine differentiation, as confirmed by more diffuse reactivity for neuroendocrine markers. Mixed neuroendocrine (especially of large-cell type) and non-neuroendocrine cancer may also be found {2932}. This finding parallels the frequent occurrence of foci of ordinary cancer in the intramucosal component of otherwise pure NECs {2686}. Evidence for progression from NET (G1 and G2) to high-grade (G3) NEC has only rarely been obtained. All the evidence indicates that gastric G3 NEC is a distinct, highly malignant cancer that should be clearly distinguished from G1 and G2 NET.

MANEC

Gastric MANECs are mixed carcinomas with a NET-cell component consisting of at least 30% of the whole neoplasm (for definition, see Chapter 1). MANECs are relatively rare in the stomach, despite the frequent occurrence of a minor (< 30%) component of cells with neuroendocrine differentiation in gastric adenocarcinoma, a phenomenon that should not prevent its classification as adenocarcinoma. The neuroendocrine component of the gastric MANEC usually comprises a NEC, often of large-cell type {1427}, and rarely a NET {447, 1555}. The exocrine component is usually an adenocarcinoma with variable grade of differentiation {447, 924, 1427, 1555, 2640}. Gastric MANEC displays a distinct immunophenotype with expression of neuroendocrine markers consistent with that observed in pure neuroendocrine neoplasms restricted to the neuroendocrine component only, possibly also with expression of carcinoembryonic antigen (CEA) in a fraction of cases {447, 924, 1427, 1555, 2640}.

Genetic susceptibility
NET

Information on genetic susceptibility is scant; however, similar to other NETs of the gastrointestinal tract, gastric ECL cell NETs display a relatively small number of genetic abnormalities, the most relevant and frequent being associated with the MEN1 gene {1798, 3010}. In patients with familial MEN1-ZES, type II gastric carcinoids arise in 13–30% of cases, vs exceptional cases in patients with sporadic ZES, despite equally elevated, long-lasting serum levels of gastrin {1418, 1798}. MEN1 is a rare dominantly inherited disorder characterized

by the synchronous or metachronous development of multiple endocrine neoplasms in different endocrine organs by the third decade of life. The parathyroid glands are involved in 90–97%, endocrine pancreas in 30–82%, duodenal gastrinomas occur in 25%, pituitary adenomas in > 60%, and foregut NETs (stomach, lung, thymus) in 5–9% of cases {683}. Other, so-called "non-classical" MEN1 neoplasms, such as cutaneous and visceral lipomas, thyroid and adrenal adenomas, and skin angiofibromas, may occur {683, 2431}.

Molecular pathology
NET

The MEN1 tumour-suppressor gene has been mapped to chromosome 11q13 {181, 477, 683, 1746}. It encodes a 610-amino acid nuclear protein, called multiple endocrine neoplasia I or "menin", whose suppressor function involves direct binding to JunD and inhibition of JunD-activated transcription {42, 477}. High rates of loss of heterozygosity (LOH) at the MEN1 gene locus have been reported in MEN1 syndrome-associated neoplasms, such as endocrine pancreatic, pituitary and parathyroid neoplasms {2612, 3226}. LOH at 11q13 of type-II gastric NETs was found in 9 out of 10 patients with MEN1 investigated {222, 306, 390, 683}. These findings support the concept that gastric NETs are integral components of the MEN1 phenotype, sharing with parathyroid and islet cell neoplasms the highest frequency of LOH at 11q13. In multiple NETs from the same stomach, the deletion size in the wild-type allele differed from one neoplasm to another, suggesting a multiclonal origin {683}.

The role of MEN1 in non-MEN1-associated gastric NETs is more controversial. LOH at 11q13 and 11q14 regions has been reported in less than half of cases {640, 683, 925, 2560}. Mutation of MEN1 is rarely observed in sporadic gastric neuroendocrine neoplasms {909, 1036, 3253}.

Of the other genetic abnormalities investigated, mutations of the REG1A gene involved in ECL cell cycle control have been described in type-I NETs {1191}. X-chromosomal marker loss, with common minimal deletion region restricted to Xq25 and Xq26, has often been demonstrated in gastric NETs and NECs, similar to other neuroendocrine neoplasms of the foregut, but not those of midgut or hindgut origin {171, 639, 2562}.

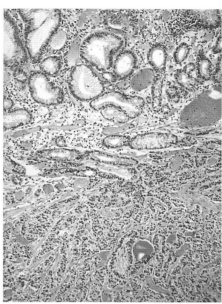

Fig. 4.31 Gastrin-producing NET (gastrinoma) of the pylorus, displaying a trabecular growth pattern.

The association of gastric ECL cell NETs and primary hyperparathyroidism has been recently proposed as a familial syndrome that is independent from MEN1 and still requiring genetic confirmation {550}.

NEC and MANEC

The available data on the genetics of NECs and MANECs are scant; however, gastric NECs, like NECs at other sites of the gastrointestinal tract, display multiple chromosomal abnormalities involving key cell-cycle regulatory genes, including TP53 (the most frequent), FHIT (fragile histidine triad gene) (3p), DCC (deleted in colorectal carcinoma) and SMAD4/-DPC4 (deleted in pancreatic cancer locus 4) (18q) and MEN1, with a higher frequency of allelic imbalances than NETs {925, 2560}. Data on gastric MANEC indicate a relatively higher frequency of chromosomal abnormalities in the NEC vs the adenocarcinoma component; however, shared LOH at chromosome 5q, 11q, 17p and 18q suggested a close genetic relationship and a possible multistep progression from a common precursor lesion {924, 1555}.

Precursor lesions

ECL cell NETs arising in hypergastrinaemic conditions (types I and II) develop through a sequence of hyperplasia–dysplasia–neoplasia that is well-documented {3009}. The successive stages of hyperplasia are termed simple, linear, micronodular, and adenomatoid. Dysplasia is characterized by moderately atypical cells with features of enlarging or fusing micronodules, microinvasion or newly formed stroma. When the nodules increase in size to > 0.5 mm or invade the submucosa, the lesion is classified as microcarcinoid (< 0.5 cm) or plain carcinoid (≥ 0.5 cm). The entire spectrum of ECL cell growth, from hyperplasia to dysplasia and neoplasia has been observed in MEN1-ZES and A-CAG. A similar sequence of lesions has been shown in experimental models of the disease, mostly based on hypergastrinaemia secondary to pharmacological inhibition of acid secretion in rodents {3192}. Linear hyperplasia or more advanced changes have been shown to represent a risk factor for the development of gastric ECL cell tumours in patients with MEN1-ZES {241}, while the presence of dysplastic lesions has been proven to markedly increase the risk of developing ECL cell tumours {121}.

Prognosis and predictive factors

The issue of TNM/staging classification of neuroendocrine neoplasms is as yet unsettled. The classification recently proposed by the American Joint Committee on Cancer (AJCC) and the International Union Against Cancer (UICC) and embraced by WHO is for "carcinoid", i.e. well-differentiated lesions only. By converse, the classification proposed by the European Neuroendocrine Tumor Society (ENETS) is also meant for high-grade neoplasms {2684}. In the stomach, both classifications are substantially in agreement. Lymph-node metastases (N1) are detected in about 5% of cases of type I, 30% of type II and 71% of type III, while distant (liver) metastases (M1) are found in 2.5%, 10% and 69% of cases of type III, respectively {2449, 2682, 2683}. Thus, most ECL cell NETs of type I and II are stage I, i.e. T1 N0 M0, and only a few would be stage IIa or T2 N0 M0. Most ECL cell NETs of type III and NECs (poorly differentiated endocrine carcinomas) fit stages IIa, IIb (T3 N0 M0), IIIa (T4 N0 M0), IIIb (any T N1 M0) or even IV (any T, Any N, M0) {2684}.

The prognosis for patients with gastric NETs is highly variable. A striking difference exists between ECL cell NETs, which are mostly indolent or low-grade malignant, and NECs, which are invariably high-grade malignant. In ECL cell NETs, favourable prognosis associates with growth within mucosa–submucosa, absence of angioinvasion, size < 1 cm, absence of an endocrine syndrome, CAG or MEN1-ZES clinical background. Most type-I, A-CAG associated, NETs have an excellent prognosis, as do the majority of type-II MEN1-ZES NETs {2683, 2686}. Aggressive behaviour of ECL cell NETs associates with invasion of the muscularis propria or beyond, size > 1 cm, angioinvasion, presence of endocrine syndrome, high mitotic activity (G2 grading) and sporadic occurrence {2323, 2682, 2683, 2686}. Only exceptional tumour-related deaths were observed in patients with NETs of type I, while only 1 out of 10 patients died from NETs of type II. Of patients with type-III NETs, mortality was 27%, with a mean survival of 28 months {303, 2683}.

In type-1 ECL cell NETs, antrectomy to remove the main source of gastrin, and removal of as much as possible of the neoplasm (especially if > 1 cm in size), proved to cure about 80% of patients, with sharp regression and disappearance of hyperplastic and neoplastic ECL cell growth {2761}. For ECL cell NETs of < 1 cm, endoscopic surveillance with biopsies has been suggested. Recently, similar results were obtained with long-acting somatostatin analogues {403, 1074}, which also controlled hypergastrinaemia and ECL cell growth {638}. In ECL cell NETs of type 2, surgical removal of the gastrinoma is carried out first {2323} since lifelong treatment with proton-pump inhibitors is very effective in preventing hypersecretion of gastric acid and peptic-ulcer disease, but does not suppress hypergastrinaemia, resulting in the neoplasm becoming aggressive and necessitating surgery {2323}. Therapy with long-acting somatostatin analogues has also proved effective {3257}. ECL cell NETs of type III and of > 1 cm, deeply invasive, G2 and/or associated with the "atypical" carcinoid syndrome, as well as for gastric NETs causing gastrinoma or Cushing syndrome {2761} are generally treated by surgery.

The prognosis for gastric NECs is invariably poor {2004, 2682}, most patients presenting with deeply invasive, advanced-stage disease and short survival. Aggressive surgery and chemotherapy should be considered for any NECs, G3 either small cell or large cell with more organoid, poorly differentiated histology {303, 2004}.

Lymphoma of the stomach

S. Nakamura
H.K. Müller-Hermelink
J. Delabie
Y.H. Ko
J.H. van Krieken
E.S. Jaffe

Definition

Primary gastric lymphomas are defined as lymphomas originating in the stomach. Lymphomas at this site are considered primary if the main bulk of disease is located in the stomach. Any histological subtype can present in the stomach, but the main two histological subtypes (> 90% of cases) are extranodal marginal-zone lymphoma of mucosa-associated lymphoid tissue (MALT lymphoma) and diffuse large B-cell lymphoma (DLBCL). DLBCLs represent about half of gastric lymphomas.

ICD-O codes

Diffuse large B-cell lymphoma   9680/3
Mantle cell lymphoma   9673/3
Marginal zone lymphoma of
   mucosa-associated lymphoid tissue
   (MALT lymphoma)   9699/3

Epidemiology
Incidence

Some 25–50% of all non-Hodgkin lymphomas arise at extranodal sites {2418}, with the gastrointestinal tract being the commonest extranodal site, accounting for about 4–20% of all non-Hodgkin lymphomas in Asian countries, North America and Europe, and up to 25% of cases in the Middle East. Within the gastrointestinal tract, the stomach is the most commonly involved site (50–75% of cases), followed by the small intestine (10–30% of cases) and the large intestine (5–10% of cases) {1622, 2219}.
Lymphoma constitutes 5–10% of all gastric malignancies and incidence is apparently increasing worldwide, although this may be partly due to improvements in diagnostic procedures {530, 1073}. About 30–60% of primary gastric lymphomas are MALT lymphomas {1620, 1622, 2219}, the remainder being primary gastric diffuse large B-cell lymphoma (PG-DLBCL). There is remarkable variation in the incidence of gastric MALT lymphoma, which is only partially related to the incidence of *Helicobacter pylori* infection.

Age and sex distribution

Incidence rates are similar in men and women. The age range is wide, but most patients are aged > 50 years at presentation.

Etiology
Infection with H. pylori

Epidemiological and experimental studies have demonstrated an association between *H. pylori* infection and development of gastric lymphoma {727, 2492, 3551}.

MALT lymphoma

Hussel *et al.* have shown that continued proliferation of gastric MALT lymphoma cells from patients infected with *H. pylori* depends on the presence of T-cells specifically activated by *H. pylori* antigens {1294}. The importance of this stimulation *in vivo* has been clearly demonstrated by the induction of patient remissions in MALT lymphomas confined to the stomach and treated with antibiotics to eradicate *H. pylori*, and confirmed in many studies {3551, 3550, 3563, 3565}.
Initial studies of low-grade gastric MALT lymphoma suggested that the tumour was associated with *H. pylori* infection in > 90% of cases {770, 3551}; subsequent studies have shown a lower incidence (62–77%) {317, 993, 1481, 2223, 3571}, but also that the density and detectability of *H. pylori* infection decreases as the lymphoma evolves from chronic gastritis {2223}.

H. pylori has been shown to be present in 90% of cases limited to the mucosa and submucosa, falling to 76% when deep submucosa is involved, and is present in only 48% of cases with extension beyond the submucosa {2223}. Sequential serological studies {2492} and retrospective studies of archival gastric biopsy material {2217, 3726} have shown that infection by *H. pylori* precedes the development of lymphoma.

DLBCL

H. pylori infection is seen less frequently in DLBCLs with or without a MALT lymphoma component (52–71% and 25–38%, respectively) {317, 847, 993, 1481}. This suggests that some DLBCLs may arise from long-standing *H. pylori*-associated MALT lymphomas. In contrast to early reports, two recent studies showed that eradication of *H. pylori* results in durable histological complete remission in 50–60% of patients with gastric DLBCL with areas of concomitant MALT lymphoma {506, 2147}. These findings suggest that a antigenic drive may remain present in a subset of aggressive gastric lymphomas.

Immunosuppression

In general, lymphomas associated with immunodeficiency show a predilection for extranodal sites, particularly the gastrointestinal tract, irrespective of the cause of the immunodeficiency {1817}.

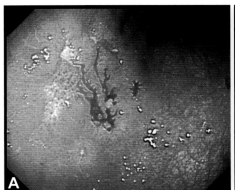 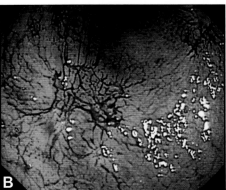

Fig. 4.32 Gastric MALT lymphoma with *H. pylori* infection but not t(11;18)/*BIRC3-MALT1*; the tumour regressed after eradication of *H. pylori*. **A** Endoscopically, a vague superficially depressed lesion with bleeding is visible. **B** The spraying of indigo carmine highlights the depressed lesion and erosions.

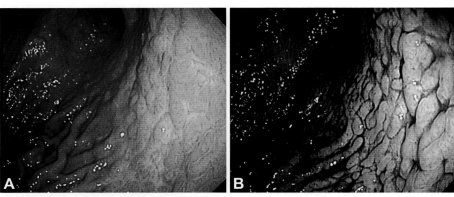

Fig. 4.33 Gastric MALT lymphoma with t(11;18)/*BIRC3-MALT1* but not *H. pylori* infection. **A** Endoscopically, a superficial lesion with small nodules mimicking cobblestones is visible. **B** The spraying of indigo carmine highlights the cobblestone lesion.

The incidence, clinical features and histology of the lesions is indistinguishable from those that develop outside the stomach. Up to 23% of gastrointestinal non-Hodgkin lymphomas arising in patients infected with human immunodeficiency virus (HIV) occur in the stomach and the vast majority of these are diffuse large B-cell or Burkitt lymphomas {218}, although occasional MALT lymphomas have been described {3549}. Aggressive B-cell lymphomas in this setting are almost always associated with Epstein-Barr virus (EBV). Cases of EBV-associated DLBCL without known immunodeficiency are rare and occur predominantly in the elderly, being related to the senescent immune system. This lymphoma shows a more aggressive clinical course than does EBV-negative DLBCL {576, 1789, 2421, 3652}.

Clinical features
Symptoms and signs
Patients with low-grade lymphomas often present with a long history of nonspecific symptoms, including dyspepsia, nausea and vomiting. High-grade lesions may appear as a palpable mass in the epigastrium and can cause severe symptoms, including weight loss. Bone-marrow involvement, elevated lactate dehydrogenase and B symptoms (fever, weight loss, night sweats), are less common in gastric than nodal DLBCL.

Endoscopic appearance
At the time of diagnosis, lymphomas can vary greatly in size and appearance. The tumours can present as superficial-spreading, mass-forming, diffuse-infiltrating, and unclassified types, which are generally related to histological grade {2216}.

Low-grade lymphoma tends to be superficial. High-grade lymphoma is usually associated with more florid lesions, often presents with diffusely infiltrative nodular masses, and may mimic advanced gastric carcinoma. It is often difficult to distinguish lymphoma from carcinoma endoscopically.

Other imaging
Staging work-up for gastric lymphoma includes computed tomography (CT) and endoscopy of the upper gastrointestinal tract. Endoscopic ultrasound is carried out to assess the extent of lymphoma infiltration through the gastric wall and the involvement of perigastric lymph nodes {2504, 3116}. Positron emission tomography (PET) scan using 18-fluoro-2-deoxyglucose (FDG) bears a documented diagnostic value only for DLBCLs, but is controversial for MALT lymphomas, which are frequently reported as FDG-PET-negative owing to their lower metabolism, reflecting indolent clinical behaviour, and small volume of disease {91, 787}.

MALT lymphoma
Definition
Gastric MALT lymphoma is an extranodal lymphoma composed of morphologically heterogeneous small B cells, including marginal zone (centrocyte-like) cells, cells resembling monocytoid cells, small lymphocytes, and scattered immunoblasts and centroblast-like cells. There is plasma-cell differentiation in a proportion of the cases. The lymphoma often grows in the marginal zone surrounding reactive B-cell follicles and extends further into the interfollicular region. The neoplastic cells typically infiltrate the gastric glandular

epithelium, forming lymphoepithelial lesions.

Macroscopy
Grossly, the lesions appear as erosions, ulcers, early cancer-like superficially depressed erosions, discoloured areas, cobblestone lesions (superficial-spreading type), protrusions (mass-forming type), and giant folds (diffuse-infiltrating type) {2216, 2230}.

Histopathology
The lymphoma cells infiltrate around reactive lymphoid follicles, external to a preserved follicle mantle, in a marginal zone pattern. As the lesion progresses, the neoplastic cells erode, colonize and eventually overrun some or most of the follicles (follicular colonization) {1346}.
The characteristic marginal zone B-cells are of intermediate size with pale cytoplasm and a slightly irregular nucleus, resembling those of centrocytes, the term "centrocyte-like" cells being applied to the neoplastic component of MALT lymphomas. The accumulation of more abundant pale-staining cytoplasm may lead to a monocytoid appearance. Alternatively, the marginal zone B cells may more closely resemble small lymphocytes. Plasmacytic differentiation is present in approximately one third of cases and may be very prominent with Dutcher bodies. Large cells resembling centroblasts or immunoblasts are usually present, but are in the minority.
The lymphoma cells infiltrate and destroy adjacent gastric glands to form lymphoepithelial lesions; those that are typical of MALT lymphoma are aggregates of three or more marginal-zone cells with distortion or destruction of the glandular epithelium, often together with eosinophilic degeneration of epithelial cells. Transformed centroblast- or immunoblast-like cells may be present in variable numbers in MALT lymphoma, but when solid or sheet-like proliferations of transformed cells are present, the tumour should be diagnosed as DLBCL and the presence of accompanying MALT lymphoma noted. The term "high-grade MALT lymphoma" should not be used, and the term "MALT lymphoma" should not be applied to a large B-cell lymphoma, even if it has arisen in a MALT site or is associated with lymphoepithelial lesions.

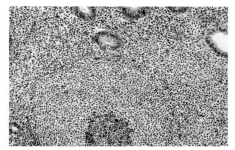

Fig. 4.34 Gastric MALT lymphoma with perifollicular distribution around reactive follicles (lower) and lymphoepithelial lesions (upper).

Immunohistochemistry

The immunophenotype of the cells of gastric MALT lymphoma is similar to that of the marginal zone B cells. They are CD20+, CD79a+, BCL2+, CD5–, CD10–, CD23–, CD43+/–, CD11c+/– (weak) and typically express IgM, less often IgA or IgG and rarely IgD. Immunoglobulin light-chain restriction is most evident in cells showing plasmacytoid differentiation.

There is no specific marker for MALT lymphoma at present. Cyclin D1 and CD10 are useful for distinguishing mantle cell lymphoma from follicular lymphoma, respectively. Immunostaining with anti-keratin antibodies aids the identification of lymphoepithelial lesions. Highlighting follicular dendritic cells with antibodies to CD21, CD23 or CD35 helps to demonstrate underlying follicular dendritic-cell networks in cases in which the lymphoid follicles have been completely overrun by the lymphoma. EBV is rarely associated with MALT lymphomas {1789, 1873, 2416, 3570}.

Molecular pathology

Four translocations – t(11;18)(q21;q21), t(1;14)(p22;q32) and t(14;18)(q32;q21) and t(3;14)(p14.1;q32) – are specifically associated with MALT lymphomas, and result in the production of a chimeric protein (*BIRC3-MALT1*) or in translocational deregulation (*BCL10*, *MALT1*, *FOXP1*) {49, 161, 2226, 2415, 3096, 3097, 3520}. Trisomy of chromosomes 3, 18 or, less commonly, others is a nonspecific but frequent finding in MALT lymphoma. The chromosomal translocations all converge on the activation of the same oncogenic pathway associated with nuclear factor κ-light-chain-enhancer of activated of activated B cells (NF-κB) {821}. The t(11;18)(q21;q21) translocation, which occurs most frequently in gastric MALT lymphomas (15–30% of cases) {161, 2224, 2229}, is not seen in gastritis caused by

H. pylori, is significantly associated with *H. pylori*-negativity and nuclear expression of *BCL10*, and can identify cases that will not respond to eradication of *H. pylori* {1325, 1872, 2226, 2228–2230, 3125}. This translocation is also associated with a low risk of an onset of additional genetic damage and also histological transformation into a large cell aggressive lymphoma {3061}. The translocations t(1;14)/*BCL10-IGH* {3096, 3628}, t(14;18)/*IGH-MALT1* {2657, 3096} and t(3;14)/*FOXP1-IGH* {999, 2224, 2774} are infrequently detected. Extra copies of *MALT1* and *FOXP1*, often suggestive of partial and complete trisomies 18 and 3, are detected in 25% and 17% of cases. The presence of extra copies of *MALT1* is significantly associated with progression or relapse of lymphoma, and is an independent adverse prognostic factor for event-free survival {2224}. Studies of the immunoglobulin genes of MALT lymphoma cells has shown the sequential accumulation of somatic mutations, consistent with ongoing, antigen-driven selection and proliferation {486, 742, 2607}. Study of the third complementary determining region of the immunoglobulin heavy-chain gene shows a pattern of changes associated with the generation of antibody diversity and increased antigen-binding affinity {246}.

Differential diagnosis

The differential diagnosis of MALT lymphoma and gastritis caused by *H. pylori* on the basis of small biopsy specimens may sometimes be difficult. Distinction from reactive processes is based mainly on the presence of destructive infiltrates of extrafollicular B cells, typically with the morphology of marginal zone B cells {3550}. In borderline cases, immunophenotyping or molecular genetic analysis to assess B-cell clonality is necessary to help establish or exclude a diagnosis of

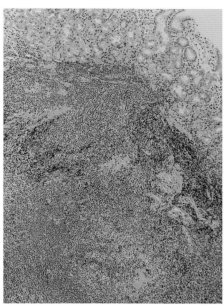

Fig. 4.35 Gastric MALT lymphoma showing a diffuse infiltrate extending into the submucosa.

MALT lymphoma, although molecular studies may also demonstrate clonal B cells in some non-neoplastic MALT proliferations or persistent clonal populations in gastric MALT lymphomas even after histological complete remissions {2128, 3564}. Distinction between MALT lymphoma and other small B-cell lymphomas is based on a combination of the characteristic morphological and immunophenotypical features.

Mantle cell lymphoma
Definition

Mantle cell lymphoma typically involves both spleen and intestines and may present as an isolated mass or as multiple polyps throughout the gastrointestinal tract where it is referred to as multiple lymphomatous polyposis {599}. While gastric involvement is commonly encountered in patients with disseminated nodal mantle

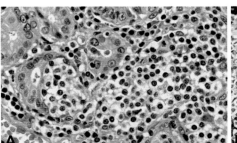
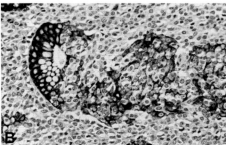

Fig. 4.36 Gastric MALT lymphoma. **A** Lymphoepithelial lesions adjacent to centrocyte-like cells infiltrating grandular epithelium. **B** Immunostaining for keratin highlights lymphoepithelial lesions.

cell lymphoma or multiple lymphomatous polyposis {2330}, primary gastric mantle-cell lymphoma is extremely rare {539, 2611}. Morphologically and immuno-phenotypically, the lymphoma is indistinguishable from mantle cell lymphoma of lymph nodes, with a diffuse and monotonous infiltrate of cells with scanty cytoplasm and irregular nuclei that express B-cell markers and cyclin D1 owing to the t(11;14)(q13;q32) juxtapositioning the cyclin D1 gene and the immunoglobulin heavy-chain gene. Rare cases of mantle cell lymphoma that are negative for cyclin D1 may be identified by overexpression of *SOX11* {2175}.

Diffuse large B-cell lymphoma (DLBCL)

Definition
DLBCL is a neoplasm of large B-lymphoid cells with nuclear size equivalent to or exceeding that of normal macrophage nuclei or more than twice the size that of a normal lymphocyte. The term "primary gastric DLBCL" (PG-DLBCL) is used for tumours that are localized to the stomach at presentation. PG-DLBCL may arise *de novo* or more rarely from transformation of a prior MALT lymphoma. The term "high-grade MALT lymphoma" should be avoided.

Macroscopy
At the time of diagnosis, the tumours vary greatly in size, and often show an ulcerated mass, mimicking advanced gastric carcinomas (mass-forming type) {2216}. The cut section is yellow-to cream-coloured with a "fish-flesh" consistency.

Histopathology
DLBCLs of the stomach are morphologically similar to DLBCLs at other sites. Tumours consist of diffuse sheets of large, blastic lymphoid cells, two to four times

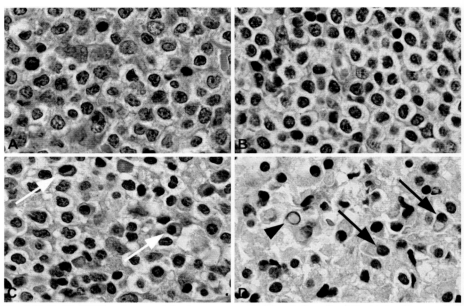

Fig. 4.37 Gastric MALT lymphoma: variation in appearance of centrocyte-like cells. **A** Predominantly monocytoid appearance. **B** Clear cell variant. **C** Lymphoplasmacytoid appearance (arrows). **D** Prominent plasma-cell differentiation (arrows) and Dutcher bodies (arrowhead).

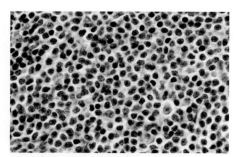

Fig. 4.38 Gastric MALT lymphoma with t(11;18)/*BIRC3-MALT1* shows a relatively monotonous proliferation of centrocyte-like cells with a small number of scattered large cells.

larger than normal lymphocytes, often infiltrating and destroying the gastric glandular architecture. Lymphoepithelial lesions by large cells with vesicular nuclei are infrequent.

About 30–50% of PG-DLBCLs have components of MALT lymphoma {1622, 2219, 2448}, but the extent of this low-grade component varies from only small residual foci to dominant MALT lymphoma with only a small proportion of solid or sheet-like transformed blasts. Tumours with the former characteristics are often indistinguishable from *de novo* PG-DLBCL and should be diagnosed as DLBCL, noting the presence of accompanying MALT lymphoma. The term "high-grade MALT lymphoma" should not be used for tumours with the latter characteristics. The differentiation between transformed MALT lymphoma and *de novo* PG-DLBCL is not clinically important since the two entities behave similarly. The activated B-cell and the germinal-centre types of DLBCL can both present as a primary gastric lymphoma.

Immunohistochemistry
The neoplastic cells are of B-cell phenotype, expressing pan B-cell antigens (CD19, CD20, CD22, CD79a), but may lack one or more of these. Monotypic surface and/or cytoplasmic expression of immunoglobulin light chains can be detected. The reported incidence of

CD10, BCL6 and IRF4/MUM1 varies {512, 2225, 2576, 3164}. Expression of CD10 is found in 20–40%, BCL6 in 40–60%, and IRF/MUM1 in 50–60% of PG-DLBCL cases, implying that both activated B-cell and germinal-centre types exist {1118}. The neoplastic cells express CD5 in < 5% of cases. These CD5+ DLBCL cases usually represent *de novo* DLBCL distinct from Richter syndrome of CLL/SLL and blastoid variant of mantle cell lymphoma {3589}. EBV-positive DLBCL, as revealed by *in situ* hybridization for EBV-encoded mRNA (EBER), occur in 5–10% of cases mainly among the elderly and have a worse clinical course than EBV-negative DLBCL unless treated mildly with rituximab {576, 1789, 2421, 2473, 3652}.

Molecular pathology
Chromosomal translocations involving the immunoglobulin heavy-chain gene locus (*IGH@*) are frequent in DLBCL, and include t(3;14)(q27;q32), t(14;18)(q32;q21) and t(8;14)(q24;q32), resulting in transcriptional dysregulation of *BCL6*, *BCL2*, and *MYC*, respectively {2225}. In PG-DLBC, translocations involving *IGH@* are detected in 32% of cases. The most frequent partner gene is *BCL6* (20–36% of cases), followed by *MYC* and *FOXP1*, but rarely *BCL2*. The t(11;18)/*BIRC3-MALT1* translocation, specific for MALT lymphoma, is infrequently detected in DLBCL with or without MALT lymphoma {242, 3269}. Extra copies of

MALT1/BCL2, FOXP1/BCL6, and MYC, often suggestive of partial or complete trisomies 18, 3, and 8, are identified in 24%, 21%, and 10% of cases, respectively. Genetic aberrations such as deletion of 6q, loss of TP53, amplification of chromosome region 3q27 and the myeloid/lymphoid or mixed-lineage leukaemia gene (MLL) regions have also been reported for PG-DLBCL {3060}.

Burkitt lymphoma
Classical Burkitt lymphomas may be encountered in the stomach {113, 2477}. The morphology is identical to that of Burkitt lymphoma encountered elsewhere, with diffuse sheets of medium-sized cells with scanty cytoplasm and round/oval nuclei containing small nucleoli. Within the sheets there are numerous macrophages, giving a "starry sky" appearance. Mitoses are frequent and apoptotic debris is abundant. The cells express CD10, CD20 and BCL6, but not BCL2. Nearly 100% of nuclei are immunoreactive for Ki67. The cases carry t(8;14). The proportion that are EBV positive varies, being relatively low (15–20%) in sporadic Burkitt lymphoma, and higher in cases associated with immunodeficiency (25–40%).

T-cell lymphoma
Primary gastric T-cell lymphomas are rare and heterogeneous. Adult T-cell leukaemia/lymphoma is common in areas of endemic infection with human T-cell leukaemia virus 1 (HTLV-1) infection, representing up to 7% of gastric lymphomas {2219, 2942}. The lymphoma cells are typically CD4+, CD25+, and CCR4+ in addition to carrying pan T-cell markers. No cytotoxic granule-associated proteins are detected {1134}. In areas where HTLV-1 infection is not endemic, most primary gastric T-cell

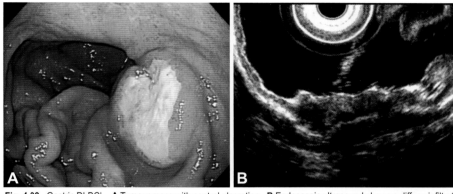
Fig. 4.39 Gastric DLBCL. **A** Tumour mass with central ulceration. **B** Endoscopic ultrasound shows a diffuse infiltrate of lymphoma extending into the submucosa.

lymphomas have a cytotoxic T-cell phenotype, similar to that seen in enteropathy-associated T-cell lymphomas {1789, 3665, 3696}. The neoplastic cells may display features of intraepithelial T-lymphocyte differentiation (e.g. expression of the human mucosal lymphocyte 1 antigen, CD103). These lymphomas may occur sporadically outside the setting of coeliac disease. Extranodal natural killer/T-cell (NK/T-cell) lymphoma of nasal type (EBV+) is also seen in east Asian countries {555, 2942}. Nasal-type NK/T-cell lymphomas and enteropathy-associated T-cell lymphomas have in common the expression of CD56 (NCAM1) and cytotoxic molecules such as granzyme B, TIA1, and perforin in addition to pan-T-cell markers. Therefore, the presence or absence of EBV is mandatory for their distinction. Some of the remainder are similar to peripheral T-cell lymphomas encountered in lymph nodes, including anaplastic large cell lymphoma that expresses anaplastic lymphoma kinase (ALK+).

Hodgkin disease
Classical Hodgkin lymphoma may involve the gastrointestinal tract, but this is usually secondary to nodal disease. Primary gastric classical Hodgkin lymphoma is extremely rare {3722}, and should be differentiated from EBV-positive DLBCL of the elderly {150, 576, 2421, 2473, 3652}.

Prognosis and predictive factors
The Ann Arbor staging system {421} is not easily applied to gastrointestinal lymphomas, therefore alternative staging systems have been proposed. The "Lugano" system {2715} of 1994 is an adaptation of the Ann Arbor staging classification whereas the "Paris" staging

system {2759} of 2003 is a modification of the TNM staging system. The latter takes into account: (1) the depth of tumour infiltration; (2) the extent of nodal involvement; and (3) the extent of local tissue infiltration by lymphoma.

MALT lymphomas have an indolent natural course and eradication of *H. pylori* results in a high rate of complete remission in 60–100% of patients {851, 2552, 2597, 3235, 3550}. The time taken to achieve remission in these patients varies from 4–6 weeks to 18 months. Cases with t(11;18)/BIRC3-MALT1 are associated with resistance to *H. pylori*-eradication therapy. Surgery, radiotherapy, and chemotherapy have been used for PG-DLBCLs alone or in various combinations. Irrespective of treatment modality, patient 5-year survival varies from 60% to 90% {851, 2597}. Younger age, limited clinical stage, and the presence of IGH@/oncogene translocations are indicators for increased overall survival and event-free survival, whereas deep invasion is an adverse prognostic factor, but only for event-free survival {2225}.

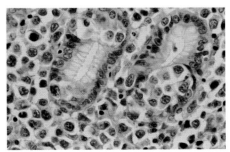
Fig. 4.40 Gastric DLBCL. The neoplastic cells infiltrate the glandular epithelium to form structures reminiscent of lymphoepithelial lesions.

Mesenchymal tumours of the stomach

M. Miettinen
C.D.M. Fletcher
L.-G. Kindblom
W.M.S. Tsui

Definition

A group of nonepithelial tumours of variable mesenchymal cell histogenesis. It is customary to include neuroectodermal tumours, such as Schwann cell tumours, in this category.

ICD-O codes

Glomus tumour	8711/0
Granular cell tumour	9580/0
Leiomyoma	8890/0
Plexiform fibromyxoma	8811/0
Schwannoma	9560/0
Inflammatory myofibroblastic tumour	8825/1
Gastrointestinal stromal tumour	8936/1
Benign (prognostic groups 1, 2, 3a)	8936/0
Uncertain malignant potential (group 4)	8936/1
Malignant (groups 3b, 5, 6a, 6b)	8936/3
Kaposi sarcoma	9140/3
Leiomyosarcoma	8890/3
Synovial sarcoma	9040/3

Gastrointestinal stromal tumour (GIST)

Definition and terminology

GIST is the most common primary mesenchymal tumour of the gastrointestinal tract and spans a clinical spectrum from benign to malignant. It is generally immunohistochemically positive for KIT (CD117), phenotypically paralleling Cajal-cell differentiation, and most examples contain *KIT*- or *PDGFRA*-activating mutations. Most gastric smooth-muscle tumours defined before the current concept of GIST are actually GISTs, as are leiomyoblastomas and tumours formerly designated as gastrointestinal autonomic nerve tumours (GANTs).

Epidemiology

The results of population-based studies in Iceland and Sweden have suggested an annual incidence of GIST of 11–14.5 per 100 000; approximately 60% of these tumours arise in the stomach {2291}. However, minimal GISTs that are detected incidentally are probably more common: a frequency of 10% was reported in a study of specimens from resection of carcinoma of the oesophagogastric junction {10}. We estimate that approximately 25% of gastric GISTs (not counting minimal incidental tumours) are clinically malignant. Surveillance Epidemiology and End Results (SEER) data indicate that GISTs (interpolated from data on leiomyosarcomas) account for 2.2% of all malignant gastric tumours {3237}.

GISTs typically occur in older adults (median age in most series, about 60–65 years) without a distinct difference in incidence between men and women. Rarely, gastric GISTs occur in children, some of whom have Carney triad or Carney-Stratakis syndrome.

Clinical features

The most common presentations include vague abdominal complaints, symptoms related to tumour ulcer, acute and chronic bleeding with or without anaemia, and abdominal mass; gastric-outlet obstruction is rare. These symptoms are also common to other gastric mesenchymal tumours.

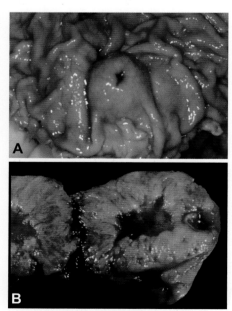

Fig. 4.41 Gross appearance of gastric GISTs. **A** Small tumour with central umbilicated ulcer. **B** Large tumour with a central cystic cavity.

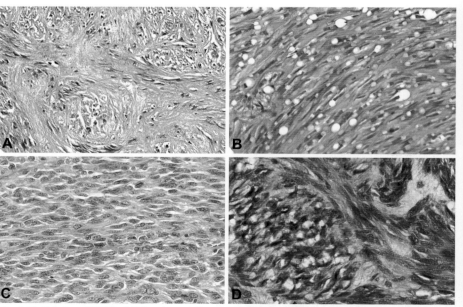

Fig. 4.42 Spindle cell GIST. **A** Sclerosing spindle cell GIST is paucicellular with abundant collagenous matrix. **B** Palisaded-vacuolated GIST contains abundant perinuclear vacuoles and shows nuclear palisading. **C** The hypercellular variant shows dense cellularity with little mitotic activity. **D** Sarcomatous spindle cell GIST with diffuse nuclear enlargement and hyperchromasia, and conspicuous mitotic activity.

Many smaller GISTs are detected incidentally during endoscopy, surgery, or computed tomography (CT) scans. Malignant gastric GISTs spread into the omentum and elsewhere in the abdominal cavity, and metastasize to the liver.

While some malignant GISTs were fatal within 1–2 years before the advent of therapies based on tyrosine-kinase inhibitors, other GISTS may metastasize after a long delay and, in some cases, even patients with liver metastases can survive for a long period. Most GISTs are sporadic, but gastric GISTs can occur rarely in connection with syndromes such as Carney triad (GIST, pulmonary chondroma, paraganglioma) or Carney-Stratakis syndrome (GIST plus paraganglioma). These GISTs occur in younger age groups (including children) and more commonly in women. Carney triad-associated GISTs often have an epithelioid morphology and occur in gastric antrum. Patients with familial GIST syndrome and germline *KIT* mutations can have multiple GISTs throughout the gastrointestinal tract. Approximately 20 such families have been reported. Rarely, gastric GISTs are associated with neurofibromatosis type 1 (NF1), a syndrome conveying increased risk of GIST.

Macroscopy

Gastric GISTs can occur in any part of the stomach. They vary from minimal mural nodules to large complex masses with variably intraluminal and external components. Some GISTs are attached to the gastric wall with a narrow pedicle forming an apparently external mass, sometimes considered "omental" GIST. Gastric GISTs may extend into capsules of liver and spleen, transverse mesocolon, and into the pancreas. On sectioning, GISTs vary in colour from pale to pink tan, and haemorrhage and cystic degeneration are common, especially in larger tumours {2077, 3543}.

Histopathology

Gastric GISTs have a broad morphological spectrum. Most are spindle cell tumours, while epithelioid histology is seen in 20–25% of cases, with a number of cases showing mixed histology. Nuclear pleomorphism is relatively uncommon, and occurs more often in epithelioid tumours. Distinctive histological patterns among spindle cell GISTs include sclerosing type, seen especially in small tumours that often contain calcifications. The palisaded-vacuolated subtype is one of the most common,

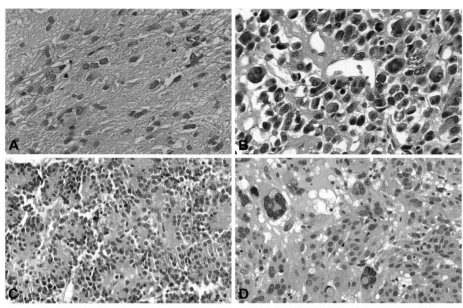

Fig. 4.43 Epithelioid GIST. **A** Sclerosing epithelioid GIST is paucicellular with epithelioid cells in abundant collagenous matrix. **B** Epithelioid GIST with discohesive pattern and nuclear atypia. **C** Cellular epithelioid GIST with a pseudopapillary pattern. **D** Sarcomatoid epithelioid GIST with marked pleomorphism and mitotic activity.

whereas some examples show diffuse hypercellular pattern, and others show sarcomatoid features with significant nuclear atypia and mitotic activity. Epithelioid GISTs may show sclerosing, discohesive, hypercellular, sometimes with pseudopapillary pattern, or sarcomatous morphology with significant atypia and mitotic activity. Myxoid matrix may be present {2077}.

Most gastric GISTs show strong positivity for KIT (CD117), which appears as cytoplasmic, membrane-associated, or sometimes as perinuclear dots. However, a small minority (< 5%), especially GISTs with mutant *PDGFRA*, may have very limited, if any, positivity {2032}. Anoctamin-1 (*ANO1*), a chloride-channel protein detected by DOG1 antibody, is emerging as an equally sensitive and specific marker {805, 2079}. KIT and DOG1 are also expressed in interstitial cells of Cajal, whose stem cell-like subcohort is believed to be the histogenetic

Table 4.03. Prognosis for patients with gastrointestinal stromal tumours (GIST), based on long-term follow-up.

Tumour parameters			Progressive disease during follow-up (% of patients)[a]	
Prognostic group	Size	Mitotic rate per 50 HPFs	Gastric GISTs	Small-intestinal GISTs
1	≤ 2	≤ 5	0	0
2	> 2 ≤ 5	≤ 5	1.9	4.3
3a	> 5 ≤ 10	≤ 5	3.6	24
3b	> 10	≤ 5	12	52
4	≤ 2	> 5	0[b]	50[b]
5	> 2 ≤ 5	> 5	16	73
6a	> 5 ≤ 10	> 5	55	85
6b	> 10	> 5	86	90

HPF, high power field

[a] Based on observation of 1784 patients in studies carried out by the Armed Force Institute of Pathology (AFIP). Intestinal GISTs generally follow the behaviour of small-intestinal GISTs.
[b] Denotes tumour categories with very small numbers of cases. Data based on reference {2066}.

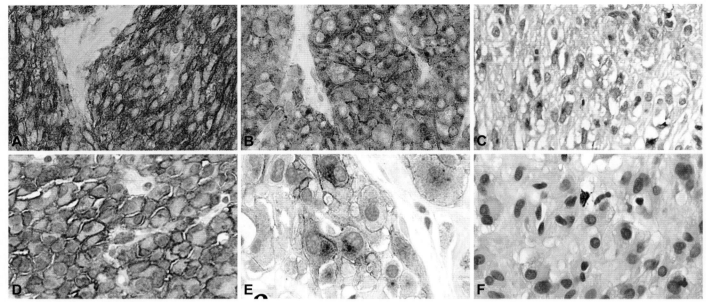

Fig. 4.44 Patterns of KIT immunostaining seen in GISTs. **A** Diffuse strong staining. **B** Strong staining with perinuclear dot pattern. **C** Strong perinuclear dot pattern and weak cytoplasmic staining. **D** Membrane pattern. **E** Focal and delicate positivity in an epithelioid GIST. **F** KIT-negative GIST; only mast cells are positive. This tumour carried a mutation in *PDGFRA* exon 14.

origin for GIST {1206, 1570}. Most spindle cell GISTs are positive for CD34, whereas epithelioid examples are less consistently positive. A minority of gastric GISTs expresses smooth muscle actin (SMA), and rare examples show positivity for desmin, keratins (usually limited to keratin 18), or S100 protein {2066}.

Prognostic factors, grade and stage
The most useful and best studied prognostic factors are tumour size and mitotic activity (typically expressed as number of mitotic figures per 50 high power fields, [HPF]), with a total area of 5 mm². In the TNM classification, grading is based on mitotic rate (< 5 mitoses per 50 HPFs is considered to be a low mitotic rate, while > 5 mitoses per 50 HPFs is considered to be a high mitotic rate). The stage combines tumour size and mitotic activity. Estimates of metastatic rate for prognostic groups defined by tumour size and mitotic rate are shown in Table 4.03. It should be noted that staging criteria are different for gastric and small intestinal GISTs to reflect the more aggressive course of small-intestinal GISTs with similar parameters.

Molecular pathology
KIT-activating mutations, leading to constitutional activation of the KIT signalling pathway, are usually seen in exon 11, and most of these tumours are sensitive to imatinib.

In order of decreasing frequency, the mutation types include in-frame deletions, single-nucleotide substitutions, duplications, and insertions. Complex mutations combining the above types can occur in some cases. Deletions most commonly involve codons 557 and 558. The most common single-nucleotide substitutions lead to V559D, V559A, V560D, W557R, and L576P. Gastric GISTs with exon 11 deletions have a worse prognosis than those with single-nucleotide substitution mutations. Duplications (1–18 codons) typically involve the 3' portion of exon 11 and are usually associated with a more favourable prognosis. *KIT* exons 13 and 17 are rarely involved. Such mutations include K642E and N822K, among others. A subset of gastric GISTs, especially tumours with epithelioid morphology, has mutations in *PDGFRA*, which is closely homologous to *KIT*. Most common of these is exon 18 substitution D842V, and these mutant tumours are notably resistant to imatinib. *PDGFRA* exon 12 deletions and exon 14 substitutions are rare mutations. Most *KIT* mutations are heterozygous, but homozygous mutations can occur (via hemizygosity), and these tumours are often more aggressive than corresponding heterozygous mutants {1750}.
GISTs in children or associated with NF1 do not contain *KIT* or *PDGFRA* mutations {2067, 2585}. Other recurrent genetic changes include deletions/monosomy of

chromosomes 14 and 22 {779, 1153}. GISTs in Carney-Stratakis syndrome (GIST plus paraganglioma) are associated with germline mutations of succinate dehydrogenase subunits B, C, and D. However, the genetic basis for the Carney triad (GIST, paraganglioma, pulmonary chondroma) is unknown {435, 3093}.

Glomus tumour

This rare tumour occurs in adults, especially women. It usually presents as a 2–5 cm intramural mass with symptoms similar to those of gastric GISTs. Histological and immunohistochemical features are similar to those of peripheral glomus tumours. Features that are specific to gastric glomus tumours include plexiform growth within the muscular propria and vascular involvement. The latter has no adverse prognostic significance. Immunohistochemically, there is strong expression of SMA and pericellular laminin/collagen IV, but no KIT, DOG1/ANO1, CD34, or desmin. Focal synaptophysin positivity is not uncommon and should not lead to mistaken diagnosis of a neuroendocrine tumour. Most glomus tumours are benign, but metastasis has been reported in a tumour of > 5 cm in size with mitotic activity {133, 2070}.

Inflammatory myofibroblastic tumour

This tumour is found more commonly in children and young adults. The patient develops gastric or intestinal mural masses that can clinically and grossly simulate a GIST. Some patients have multiple tumours, including extragastrointestinal ones involving the omentum or mesenteries. The tumours vary in size from a few centimetres to > 10 cm. Most are clinically benign, but rare malignant examples have occurred.

Histologically, they typically have a heterogeneous composition with a variably prominent lymphoplasmacytic infiltration and fibrosis. Enmeshed in this background is the neoplastic component: spindled to epithelioid myofibroblast with often abundant amphophilic cytoplasm, with vague resemblance to rhabdomyoblast. While mitotic activity is usually low, high cellularity and mitotic activity occur in malignant examples, although data are insufficient to delineate histological criteria for malignancy. Immunohistochemically, the tumour cells are often positive for anaplastic lymphoma kinase (ALK), and variably for SMA, but negative for KIT and DOG1/ANO1. *ALK* gene rearrangements can often be shown by fluorescent *in situ* hybridization (FISH) or polymerase chain reaction (PCR)-based studies examining *ALK* fusion transcripts; fusion partner genes include 5-aminoimidazole-4-carboxamide ribonucleotide formyltransferase (*ATIC*), clathrin heavy-chain 1 (*CLTC*), Ran-binding protein (*RANBP2*), and tropomyosins 3 and 4 (*TPM3*, *TPM4*) {574, 994, 1485}.

Leiomyoma and leiomyosarcoma

Intramural leiomyoma is rare and, in our experience, is approximately 50 times less common than GIST. These tumours usually occur in older adults and clinically present similarly to GISTs. The tumours vary from minimal mural nodules to masses of > 5 cm in size. However, minimal leiomyomas have been commonly found in oesophagogastric resections for carcinoma {10}. Histologically, these tumours are composed of well-differentiated smooth-muscle cells with no or little atypia and mitotic activity, or isolated mitosis. Immunohistochemically, leiomyomas are positive for SMA and desmin, and are negative for KIT, DOG1/ANO1, and CD34. Smooth-muscle tumours with atypia and mitotic activity are designated leiomyosarcomas, and such tumours are distinctly rare in the stomach. Cases with

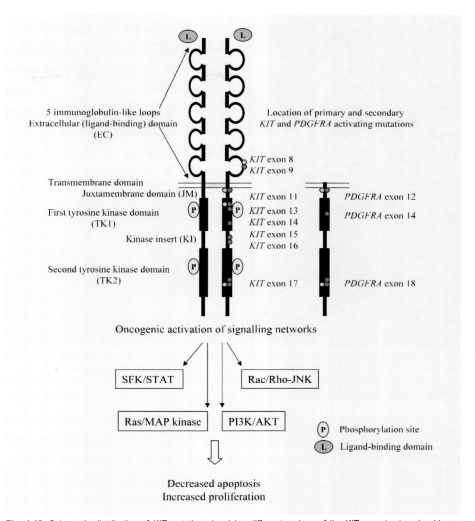

Fig. 4.45 Schematic distribution of *KIT* mutations involving different regions of the KIT receptor tyrosine kinase molecule, and selected downstream effectors in the KIT signalling pathway.

ambiguous criteria of malignancy should be designated as having uncertain malignant potential, and complete excision and follow-up is necessary.

Schwannoma

Schwannoma is rare in the stomach, occurring with a frequency similar to that of leiomyoma. These tumours often occur in older adults, and form intramural masses of 2–10 cm that can ulcerate and present in a manner similar to GIST, gross features included. The behaviour of these tumours is benign and recurrence is exceptional. Histologically typical is a relatively circumscribed mass, often partly surrounded by patches of lymphoid infiltration, sometimes with germinal centres. The tumour is composed of variably organized tumour cells, often arranged in

a microtrabecular pattern in a collagenous background. Focal nuclear atypia is common, but mitotic activity only exceptionally exceeds 5 per 50 HPFs. Immunohistochemically, gastric schwannomas are positive for S100 protein and usually glial fibrillary acidic protein (GFAP), but they can be distinguished from GISTs since they are negative for KIT and DOG1, and usually also for CD34 {646}.

Plexiform fibromyxoma

This very rare, recently described mesenchymal tumour that is apparently specific to stomach, occurs in the antrum and pyloric region, often extending into the duodenal bulb. It occurs over a wide range of ages, from childhood to old age, equally in men and women. Clinically, the tumour manifests similar to GIST, but

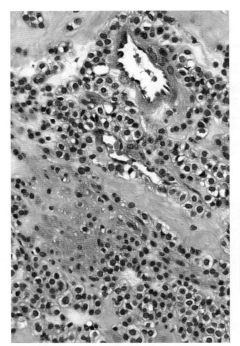

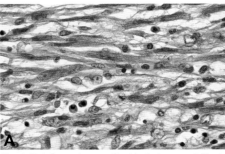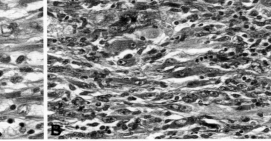

Fig. 4.47 Inflammatory myofibroblastic tumour. **A** The tumour contains an admixture of elongated tumour cells and lymphoplasmacytic infiltration. **B** The cells can also have a more epithelioid, ganglion cell-like morphology.

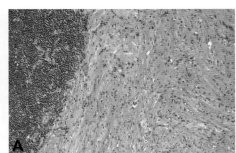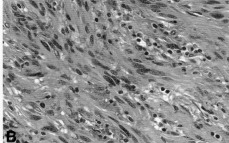

Fig. 4.46 Glomus tumour is composed of uniform cells with round nuclei and clear to eosinophilic cytoplasm, often giving a "fried egg" appearance. The eosinophilic material in the centre is pre-existing gastric smooth muscle.

Fig. 4.48 Schwannoma typically shows a peritumoral lymphoid cuff. Higher magnification typically reveals a microtrabecular pattern of tumour cells.

gastric outlet obstruction is more common. Prognosis is good, and there is no tendency for recurrence. Histologically, the tumour is characterized by a multinodular, plexiform involvement of gastric muscular propria. An extra-gastric non-plexiform component may also be present. The tumour nodules are relatively paucicellular with a prominent capillary pattern, and contain abundant acid mucopolysaccharide-rich myxoid matrix. The tumour cells are bland spindle cells, and mitotic activity is low, generally not exceeding 5 per 50 HPFs. Immunohistochemically, the tumour cells are positive for SMA and CD10 and negative for KIT and DOG1. Desmin-positivity has been reported {2069, 3160}.

Synovial sarcoma

Only a small number of primary synovial sarcomas in the stomach have been reported. These tumours have occurred in young or middle-aged adults. They have varied small (2–3 cm) mucosal or submucosal plaque or cup-like lesions to large transmural masses of > 10 cm. Histologically, most have been monophasic spindle cell tumours, and only isolated biphasic examples have been reported. Detection of keratins and epithelial membrane antigen (EMA) helps to identify monophasic tumours that are negative for KIT and DOG1/ANO1. Prognosis varies, but is good for small tumours, especially in the absence of poorly differentiated, mitotically active histology {259, 1959}.

Kaposi sarcoma

According to screening studies conducted in the 1990s, gastrointestinal Kaposi sarcoma occurred in 38% and 51% of patients in patients with HIV/-AIDS in Italy and Uganda and was most commonly detected in the stomach, being usually multifocal. Many patients showed simultaneous involvement of the colon. Most lesions are incidental small submucosal nodules in asymptomatic patients, but some form larger mural masses and may present with gastrointestinal bleeding and simulate a GIST. These tumours may also occur in immunosuppressed post-transplant patients {2462, 2639}.

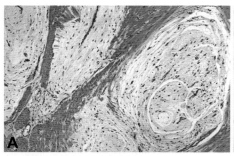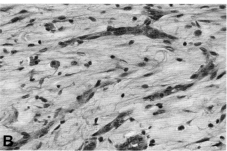

Fig. 4.49 Gastric plexiform fibromyxoma. **A** The tumour involves the gastric wall in a plexiform manner. **B** The tumour shows high vascularity, and the spindled cells are scattered in a myxoid matrix.

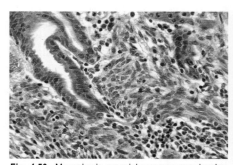

Fig. 4.50 Monophasic synovial sarcoma may involve mucosa. Note uniform spindle cells and high cellularity.

Histologically, this tumour typically appears as a haemorrhagic, vascular spindle-cell proliferation. It may contain focal cytoplasmic eosinophilic hyaline globules. Immunohistochemical demonstration of human herpesvirus-8 (HHV-8) in tumour-cell nuclei is diagnostically helpful. Other typical features include positivity for CD31, CD34, and podoplanin (PDPN/D2-40) {1455}.

Other mesenchymal tumours

Haemangiomas rarely occur in the stomach. They may be associated syndromes such as blue rubber bleb naevus, and mucosal teleangiectasias occur in Osler-Rendu-Weber disease. We have seen isolated examples of haemangioma variants, such as epithelioid haemangioma involving an artery. Lipomas are more common in the colon and are discussed in Chapter 8. In some cases, calcifying fibrous (pseudo)tumour involves the gastric wall, and can also occur in the intestines. Inflammatory fibroid polyps may occur more often in the stomach, but are discussed with tumours of the small intestine, where resection of symptomatic examples seems to be more common (see Chapter 6).

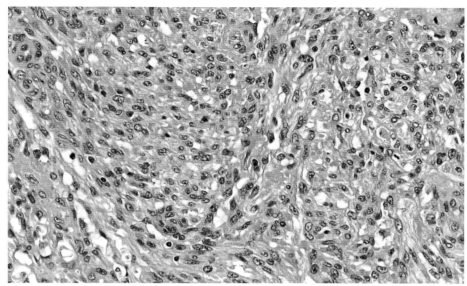

Fig. 4.51 Kaposi sarcoma contains a cellular, haemorrhagic spindle-cell proliferation with little pleomorphism.

Gastric or intestinal involvement of abdominal dedifferentiated liposarcoma should be distinguished from primary mesenchymal tumours because, by their morphological spectrum, these liposarcomas can simulate a wide variety of other mesenchymal tumours, especially GISTs. Gastrointestinal clear cell sarcoma can involve stomach but is more common in small intestine (see Chapter 6). Desmoid fibromatosis can also involve gastric and intestinal walls in some cases simulating gastric tumours such as GIST. Some of these desmoids occur in patients with familial adenomatous polyposis.

Secondary tumours of the stomach

C. Iacobuzio-Donahue
G.M. Groisman

Definition

Tumours of the stomach that originate from an extra-gastric neoplasm or that are discontinuous with a primary tumour elsewhere in the stomach.

Epidemiology

Metastatic disease involving the stomach is unusual. In a series of 771 patients with gastric neoplasms found at endoscopy, only 2.6% were secondary tumours {404}. The incidence of gastric metastasis found in autopsy cases is 0.2–1.4%, whereas that seen in autopsies performed specifically in cancer patients is 1.7–5.4% {658, 725, 1056, 2048, 3211}.

Clinical features

Gastric metastases are symptomatic in half of the patients affected. The most common clinical presentations include anaemia and gastrointestinal bleeding, abdominal pain or dyspepsia {404, 674, 1056, 3560}. The time interval between the diagnosis of a primary neoplasm and its metastasis to the stomach varies according to the tumour type. For example, in most patients with lung or oesophageal carcinomas that had metastasized to the stomach, the metastases were diagnosed within 2 years of diagnosis of the primary malignancy. In contrast, half of melanoma or breast carcinoma metastases to the stomach are diagnosed > 2 years after diagnosis of the primary tumour {674}. In some patients, the development of gastric metastasis leads to the initial diagnosis of their cancer. As metastases to the stomach are frequently limited to the submucosa and seromuscular layers, the results of

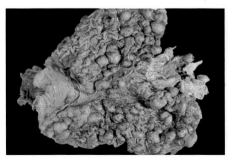

Fig. 4.52 Multiple gastric metastases from rhabdomyosarcoma of the spermatic cord in a boy aged 15 years.

endoscopic evaluation may be normal. The most common endoscopic appearance of a gastric metastasis is of a nodule resembling a submucosal tumour, seen as a mass with a smooth surface, normal-coloured mucosa and a central depression

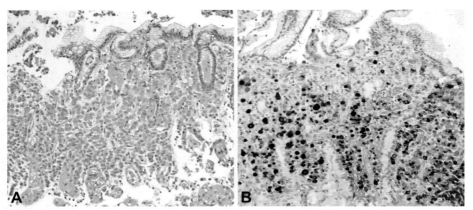

Fig. 4.53 A Metastasis of lobular breast carcinoma to gastric oxyntic mucosa. Differentiation from a primary gastric cancer may be difficult without additional ancillary studies. **B** Immunostaining for gross cystic disease fluid protein (GCDFP) demonstrates strong positive labelling, consistent with origin from a breast primary.

or ulceration ("volcano-like" lesion). In some patients, the presence of metastatic lobular breast cancer may resemble an advanced gastric cancer with features of linitis plastica {674, 1056, 3150}. Imaging is particularly useful in cases of submucosal tumours for which mucosal biopsies give negative results. Radiography – computed tomography (CT) scan and/or double-contrast barium meal – or endoscopic ultrasonography may show pathological thickening of the gastric wall {2894}.

Origin

Cancers can metastasize to the stomach by lymphohaematogenous spread (i.e. melanoma, breast cancer or lung cancer), by direct extension (pancreatic or oesophageal cancer) or by intraperitoneal dissemination (i.e. ovarian cancer) {830}. Although virtually all primary neoplasms can metastasize to the stomach, large series of autopsy studies indicate that gastric metastases most often originate from malignant melanomas or carcinomas of the breast, oesophagus and lung {1056}. In patients who present with gastric metastasis in the clinical setting, the most

common primary neoplasms of origin are also malignant melanomas or carcinomas of the breast, as well as carcinomas of the oesophagus, lung, and pancreas {674, 2346, 3461}. Metastases from primary neoplasms of the kidney, testis, uterus, ovary and colon have also been described {404, 1056}. Two thirds of breast-cancer metastases to the stomach are lobular carcinomas {2028, 3150}.

Macroscopy

Solitary metastases to the stomach are more common than multiple metastases. However, whether single or multiple, most gastric metastases are located in the upper two thirds of the stomach. Metastases are typically seen as a raised nodule covered by normal mucosa that may have a central ulceration. In some instances the metastasis forms a polypoid mass or a necrotic ulcer reminiscent of a primary gastric carcinoma. Metastatic lobular carcinoma of the breast may diffusely infiltrate the wall of the stomach, simulating linitis plastica. Pigmented metastatic melanoma may be seen as small black mucosal spots {404, 674, 1056, 2894}.

Histopathology

The features of metastases to the stomach are similar to those observed in other organs. In most cases the metastasis is located within the submucosal or muscularis propria layers, with little or no involvement of the mucosa. The lack of an *in situ* component within the mucosa may also serve as a clue that the neoplasm is a metastasis. In cases with mucosal involvement, the distinction from a primary adenocarcinoma may be difficult. Immunohistochemistry may help to differentiate between a primary gastric cancer (frequently positive for keratin 7, MUC5AC, MUC2, and CDX2), and metastases from a variety of extra-gastric primary sites, such as metastatic melanoma (positive for Melan A and S100 protein), metastases from ovary and breast (positive for keratin 7, gross cystic disease fluid protein and estrogen/progesterone receptors), lung (positive for keratin 7 and thyroid transcription factor-1 [TTF1] and those from liver, kidney and prostate (negative for keratins 7 and 20 and positive for hepatocyte-paraffin-1 antibody [HepPar1], paired box gene 8 [PAX8] and prostate-specific antigen [PSA] {551, 2335, 2380, 2475, 3267}.

Prognosis and predictive factors

Gastric metastases usually represent a late, disseminated stage of the patient's disease in which other haematogenous metastases may also be found. The prognosis is poor but varies depending on the source of the metastasis. In one series, overall survival after the diagnosis of gastric metastasis from a variety of primary origins ranged from 0 to 14 months, with a median of 4.75 months {404}. In patients with breast carcinoma, the median survival after development of gastric metastasis was 10 months, with 23% of patients surviving > 24 months {3150}.

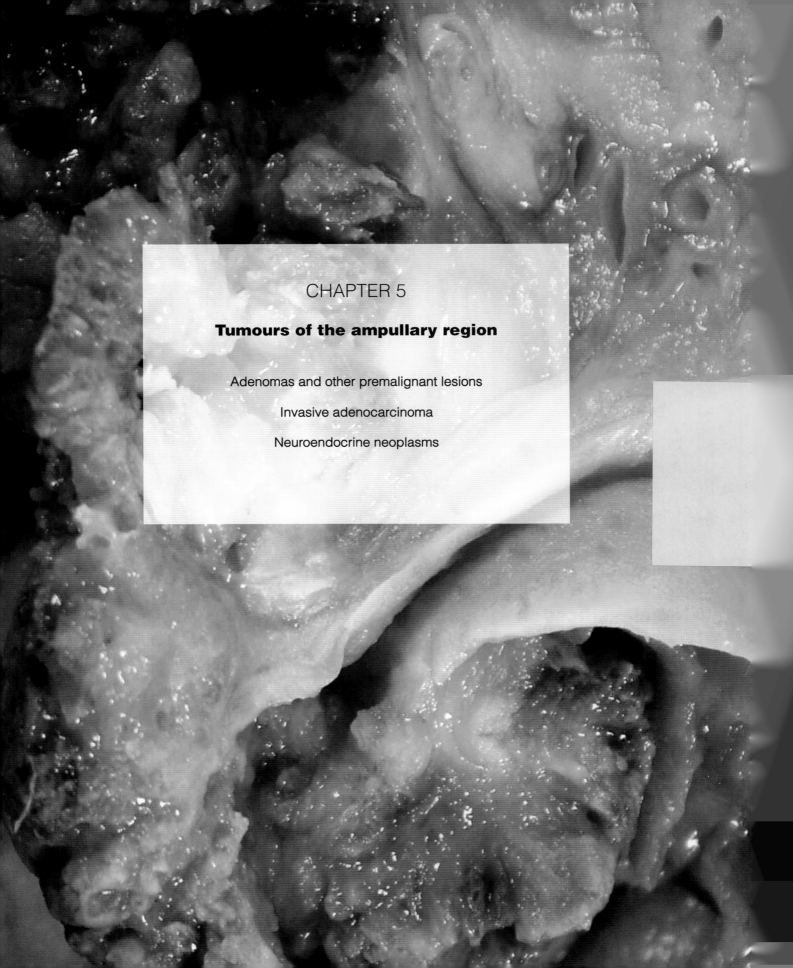

CHAPTER 5

Tumours of the ampullary region

Adenomas and other premalignant lesions

Invasive adenocarcinoma

Neuroendocrine neoplasms

WHO classification[a] of tumours of the ampullary region

Epithelial tumours

Premalignant lesions

Intestinal-type adenoma	8144/0
Tubular adenoma	8211/0
Tubulovillous adenoma	8263/0
Villous adenoma	8261/0
Noninvasive pancreatobiliary papillary neoplasm with low-grade dysplasia (low-grade intraepithelial neoplasia)	8163/0*
Noninvasive pancreatobiliary papillary neoplasm with high-grade dysplasia (high-grade intraepithelial neoplasia)	8163/2*
Flat intraepithelial neoplasia (dyplasia), high grade	8148/2

Carcinoma

Adenocarcinoma	8140/3
Invasive intestinal type	8144/3
Pancreatobiliary type	8163/3*
Adenosquamous carcinoma	8560/3
Clear cell carcinoma	8310/3
Hepatoid adenocarcinoma	8576/3
Invasive papillary adenocarcinoma	8260/3
Mucinous adenocarcinoma	8480/3
Signet ring cell carcinoma	8490/3
Squamous cell carcinoma	8070/3
Undifferentiated carcinoma	8020/3
Undifferentiated carcinoma with osteoclast-like giant cells	8035/3

Neuroendocrine neoplasms[b]

Neuroendocrine tumour (NET)	
NET G1 (carcinoid)	8240/3
NET G2	8249/3
Neuroendocrine carcinoma (NEC)	8246/3
Large cell NEC	8013/3
Small cell NEC	8041/3
Mixed adenoneuroendocrine carcinoma	8244/3
EC cell, serotonin-producing NET	8241/3
Gangliocytic paraganglioma	8683/0
Somatostatin-producing NET	8156/3

Mesenchymal tumours

Secondary tumours

EC, enterochromaffin.

[a] Morphology code of the International Classification of Diseases for Oncology (ICD-O) {904A}. Behaviour is coded /0 for benign tumours, /1 for unspecified, borderline or uncertain behaviour, /2 for carcinoma *in situ* and grade III intraepithelial neoplasia, and /3 for malignant tumours.

[b] The classification is modified from the previous (third) edition of the WHO histological classification of tumours {691} taking into account changes in our understanding of these lesions. In the case of neuroendocrine neoplasms, the classification has been simplified to be of more practical utility in morphological classification.

* These new codes were approved by the IARC/WHO Committee for ICD-O at its meeting in March 2010.

TNM classification[a] of carcinoma of the ampullary region

T - Primary tumour

TX	Primary tumour cannot be assessed
T0	No evidence of primary tumour
Tis	Carcinoma *in situ*
T1	Tumour limited to ampulla of Vater or sphincter of Oddi
T2	Tumour invades duodenal wall
T3	Tumour invades pancreas
T4	Tumour invades peripancreatic soft tissues, or other adjacent organs or structures

N – Regional lymph nodes

NX	Regional lymph nodes cannot be assessed
N0	No regional lymph-node metastasis
N1	Regional lymph-node metastasis

M – Distant metastasis

M0	No distant metastasis
M1	Distant metastasis

Stage grouping

Stage	T	N	M
Stage 0	Tis	N0	M0
Stage IA	T1	N0	M0
Stage IB	T2	N0	M0
Stage IIA	T3	N0	M0
Stage IIB	T1, T2, T3	N1	M0
Stage III	T4	Any N	M0
Stage IV	Any T	Any N	M1

---

[a] {762, 2996}
A help desk for specific questions about the TNM classification is available at http://www.uicc.org.

Adenomas and other premalignant neoplastic lesions

D.S. Klimstra
J. Albores-Saavedra
R.H. Hruban
G. Zamboni

Definition

Preinvasive neoplastic lesions of the ampulla of Vater include intestinal-type adenomas (which are the most common), noninvasive papillary neoplasms of pancreatobiliary type, and flat intraepithelial neoplasia (dysplasia) of the ampullary epithelium. Intestinal-type adenomas are benign epithelial neoplasms exhibiting tubular, villous, or mixed patterns that resemble adenomas of the small and large intestines. Noninvasive papillary neoplasms are exophytic neoplasms with cytological features resembling those of papillary neoplasms of the biliary tree, including architectural complexity and, usually, marked cytological atypia. Flat intraepithelial neoplasia (dysplasia) is a grossly subtle, non-exophytic preinvasive lesion composed of cytologically atypical cells arranged along the native ampullary epithelium. Flat intraepithelial neoplasia (dysplasia) is rarely encountered in the absence of invasive carcinoma.

ICD-O codes

Intestinal-type adenoma	8144/0
Tubular adenoma	8211/0
Tubulovillous adenoma	8263/0
Villous adenoma	8261/0
Noninvasive pancreatobiliary papillary neoplasm with low-grade dysplasia (low-grade intraepithelial neoplasia)	8163/0
Noninvasive pancreatobiliary papillary neoplasm with high-grade dysplasia (high-grade intraepithelial neoplasia)	8163/2
Flat intraepithelial neoplasia (dysplasia), high grade	8148/2

Epidemiology

Adenomas of the small intestine are uncommon, but 80% of them occur in the duodenum near the ampulla {157, 363, 2533, 2765, 3536}. Ampullary adenomas are found at autopsy in 0.04–0.12% of individuals {176, 2901, 2997}. Until recently, most ampullary adenomas were reported to be associated with an invasive adeno-carcinoma at diagnosis {2365, 2729, 3059}, but the increased use of endoscopy

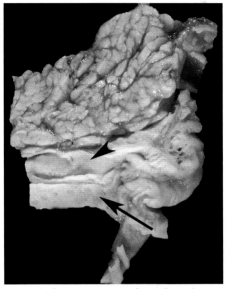

Fig. 5.01 Gross appearance of ampullary adenoma (right). Cut section demonstrates relationship to bile duct (arrow) and pancreatic duct (arrowhead).

means that it is now more common to detect adenomas before the development of invasive carcinoma.

Ampullary adenomas may occur sporadically or in the setting of familial adenomatous polyposis (FAP) (and its variant, Gardner syndrome) {88, 1690, 2916}. The prevalence of ampullary adenomas in patients with FAP is 50–95% {88, 2309, 2351}, and the lifetime risk is nearly 100% {272, 374}. Most patients with sporadic ampullary intestinal-type adenomas are between 33 and 81 years of age (mean, 61 years); females outnumber males by 2.6 : 1 {457, 2365, 2533, 2729, 2997}. Patients with FAP with ampullary adenomas have a mean age of 41 years and men and women are equally affected {88, 2351, 2916}.

Noninvasive papillary neoplasms are uncommon compared with intestinal-type adenomas, and they are rarely encountered in the absence of an associated invasive carcinoma. Only 12% of ampullary carcinomas associated with a noninvasive precursor lesion have components of noninvasive papillary neoplasms; most of the remainder are associated with intestinal-type adenomas {70}. Even fewer (6%)

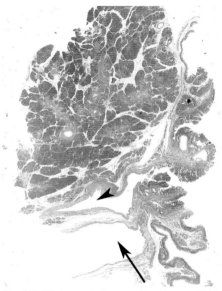

Fig. 5.02 Whole mount of an ampullary adenoma (right) showing relationship to bile duct (arrow) and pancreatic ducts (arrowhead).

predominantly noninvasive neoplasms are noninvasive papillary neoplasms. These neoplasms have not been described in patients with FAP.

Clinical features

Patients with ampullary adenomas generally present with signs and symptoms of biliary obstruction, including jaundice, abdominal pain, weight loss, and occasionally pancreatitis {1825, 2187, 2371, 2575, 2729, 2765, 3498, 3583} accompanied by elevation of serum bilirubin, serum glutamic oxaloacetic transaminase, serum glutamic pyruvic transaminase, and alkaline phosphatase. Some patients also have cholelithiasis or choledocholithiasis {2729, 2997}. Other patients are asymptomatic, and the ampullary adenomas are detected during endoscopic screening. Endoscopic ultrasound is helpful to determine the size of the polyp and to evaluate lesions for an invasive carcinoma {2049}.

In patients with FAP, asymptomatic polyps are frequently found by endoscopic screening after prophylactic colectomy to prevent colorectal adenocarcinoma {2916}; ampullary adenomas in such patients do

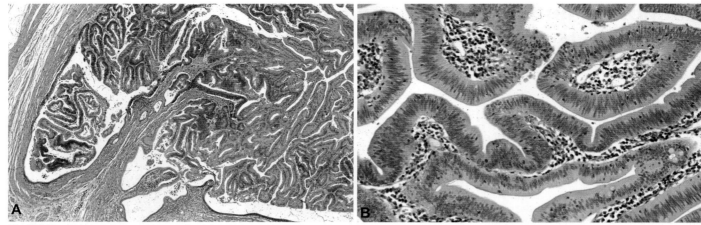

Fig. 5.03 Intestinal-type adenoma of the ampulla. **A** Intestinal-type adenoma extending into peri-ampullary glands. **B** Intestinal-type adenoma with pseudostratified, elongate nuclei.

not usually become symptomatic until 10–15 years after removal of the colon {2351}. Noninvasive papillary neoplasms are rare, and their distinctive clinical features are not well-defined, patients usually presenting in a similar fashion as those with intestinal-type adenomas {70}. Since flat intra-epithelial neoplasia does not produce a mass lesion, it is presumably asymptomatic until invasive carcinoma develops, which explains why few cases of pure flat intraepithelial neoplasia have been detected.

Macroscopy

Sporadic ampullary intestinal-type adenomas generally measure 1–3 cm {3583}; tubular adenomas are smaller than villous adenomas. Intestinal-type adenomas usually arise from the intestinal epithelium covering the papilla, so they often project into the duodenal lumen as a pale soft polyp or plaque {274}. Less commonly the adenoma is confined within the ampulla ("intra-ampullary"), resulting in a prominent bulging papilla covered by intact duodenal mucosa {3583}. Villous adenomas have a feathery appearance whereas tubular adenomas are bosselated. Patients with FAP who undergo endoscopic screening may have a minimally granular or even normal-appearing ampulla that nonetheless exhibits adenomatous changes on biopsy {88, 1309}.

Noninvasive papillary neoplasms presumably arise from the epithelium of the common channel or distal pancreatic and biliary ducts, so they are often grossly intra-ampullary.

Flat intraepithelial neoplasia does not produce a mass lesion but may appear grossly as subtle mucosal granularity, usually adjacent to a frank invasive adenocarcinoma.

Histopathology
Intestinal-type adenoma

Intestinal-type adenomas may arise anywhere within the ampullary region, including from the duodenal-type mucosa of the surface of the papilla, the transitional mucosa within the ampulla itself, and the terminal portions of the pancreatic and biliary ducts {3330}. Commonly, adenomatous epithelium involves more than one of these microanatomic regions {3059}. At the periphery of the polypoid lesion, flat adenomatous changes (flat intraepithelial neoplasia/dysplasia) may extend into the pancreatic and common bile ducts or into the periampullary ductules within the sphincter of Oddi.

Tubular adenomas are usually smaller than villous or tubulovillous adenomas and have a polypoid growth pattern {2533}. They consist of tubular glands resembling the basal portions of the intestinal crypts. Villous adenomas are usually more sessile. The neoplastic cells in villous adenomas line variably long simple or branching papillae that are more exuberant than the normal villi of the duodenal mucosa. Villous adenomas are more likely to have high grade dysplasia or an associated invasive carcinoma than tubular adenomas. By arbitrary definition, tubulovillous adenomas contain more than 25% of both tubular and villous patterns.

In all intestinal-type adenomas, the nuclei are oval, hyperchromatic, and pseudostratified. In adenomas with low-grade dysplasia, the nuclei are located predominantly at the basal aspect of the cells, and the apical cytoplasm is amphophilic. Full-thickness pseudostratification of the nuclei, moderate nuclear atypia, and mild glandular architectural complexity may occur, but

severe nuclear atypia and marked architectural complexity (such as cribriforming) are not found in low-grade dysplasia. Mitotic figures can be frequent and are predominantly basally located.

In high-grade dysplasia, the glandular architecture is more complex, and cribriformed glands are often present. The nuclei are moderately to markedly atypical and are not basally polarized. Mitoses are present at all levels of the epithelium, and some may be atypical. The individual cells may have features indistinguishable from those of invasive carcinoma, although they are still confined within the basement membrane of the mucosa, and there is no stromal reaction and no infiltrative or expansile growth. High-grade dysplasia includes the conceptual category of "carcinoma *in situ*." Most of the columnar cells making up adenomas contain modest amounts of mucin within the apical cytoplasm. True goblet cells are also found, usually in areas of low-grade dysplasia.

Paneth cells and neuroendocrine cells are particularly numerous in intestinal-type adenomas {846, 1637, 2351}.

As in large-bowel adenomas, ampullary adenomas may contain foci in which mucin has "spilled" into the stroma from the glands at the base of the polyp, simulating an invasive mucinous adenocarcinoma. This "pseudoinvasion" is often characterized by an inflammatory reaction to the mucin accompanied by recent or past haemorrhage. No neoplastic cells are found within the mucin.

Noninvasive papillary neoplasm, pancreatobiliary type

Although most noninvasive ampullary neoplasms are intestinal-type adenomas, some more closely resemble a subset of the intraductal papillary neoplasms of the bile ducts and pancreas {929, 1493, 1593, 2252} and are designated noninvasive papillary neoplasms, pancreatobiliary type, of the ampulla {70}. The papillae of pancreatobiliary-type noninvasive papillary neoplasms are complex and arborizing and are usually lined by moderately to markedly atypical cells. The marked architectural complexity may result in intraepithelial lumen formation and cribriforming. The degree of dysplasia (based on the highest grade present) should be specified. Almost all pancreatobiliary-type noninvasive papillary neoplasms have at least focal high-grade dysplasia, and many cases also have an associated invasive carcinoma {70, 929, 1493, 1593, 2252}. The epithelial lining consists of cuboidal cells with round nuclei predominantly arranged in a single layer. Paneth cells are not found, although an endocrine cell component may be detectable by immunohistochemical labelling. The invasive carcinomas arising in association with pancreatobiliary-type noninvasive papillary neoplasms usually have a tubular pattern of growth and are usually also classified as pancreatobiliary-type adenocarcinomas, although some may also be of intestinal type.

Flat intraepithelial neoplasia (dysplasia)

Although most invasive ampullary carcinomas arise from adenomas or pancreatobiliary-type noninvasive papillary neoplasms, some appear to arise from nonpolypoid precursor lesions and this is known as flat intraepithelial neoplasia (dysplasia). Flat intraepithelial neoplasia (dysplasia) may be found in the ampulla, usually in the intra-ampullary or bile duct epithelia, and almost always adjacent to invasive carcinomas {1568}. Microscopically, the dysplastic epithelium can be truly flat or it may have micropapillary projections lacking fibrovascular cores. The minimally pseudostratified cells are cuboidal to columnar and show round to oval nuclei with marked nuclear atypia, mitoses, and loss of nuclear polarity.

Cytopathology

Cytologically, adenomas contain small cluster and sheets of columnar cells. The basally located nuclei are elongated and uniform, with inconspicuous nucleoli and a fine chromatin pattern {3399, 3533}. Although cytoplasmic mucin may be present,

goblet cells are inconspicuous, contrasting with the normal duodenal mucosa. The presence of significant nuclear atypia or an increased ratio of nucleus to cytoplasm raises the possibility of high-grade dysplasia or invasive carcinoma {685}, but making a distinction between high-grade dysplasia and invasive carcinoma on the basis of cytology may be very difficult {196}.

Immunohistochemistry

Intestinal-type adenomas label with antibodies to keratins 7 and 20. They express markers of intestinal differentiation, including MUC2 and CDX2, but not MUC1 {553, 2574}. Immunohistochemistry for carcinoembryonic antigen (CEA) and CA19-9 produces predominantly surface-membrane labelling in adenomas with low-grade dysplasia, but intense cytoplasmic labelling may be found in areas of high-grade dysplasia {3583}. Stains for chromogranin or synaptophysin will highlight scattered neuroendocrine cells.

Pancreatobiliary-type noninvasive papillary neoplasms express keratin 7 and MUC1, but not MUC2, except in scattered goblet cells that may be present. Labelling for keratin 20 and CDX2 is also largely negative in pancreatobiliary-type papillary noninvasive neoplasms {2574}.

Differential diagnosis

The differential diagnosis of ampullary adenomas is particularly problematic when dealing with endoscopic biopsies.

Reactive atypia

The most common lesion to mimic an adenoma is reactive atypia; any condition causing ampullary inflammation (such as lithiasis, ampullary stricture, or prior instrumentation) may induce dramatic reactive epithelial atypia. Reactive atypia is characterized by large nuclei with an open chromatin pattern, thick nuclear membranes, and prominent nucleoli. Full-thickness nuclear pseudostratification is usually not present in reactive atypia. The cytoplasm is often abundant and mucin-rich, in contrast to the more limited, mucin-depleted cytoplasm that often characterizes adenomas. Ampullary adenomas have more elongated nuclei with significant pseudostratification and hyperchromasia. Outside the setting of FAP, it is uncommon to diagnose an ampullary adenoma in the absence of an endoscopically identifiable polypoid lesion, so correlation with endoscopic findings may also be helpful.

Intraductal papillary neoplasms of the bile ducts and pancreatic ducts (intraductal papillary mucinous neoplasms [IPMN]) may grow along the ducts to involve the ampullary epithelium secondarily. These neoplasms may have an intestinal morphology {1493, 2252}, and when they involve the ampulla they are almost indistinguishable from primary ampullary adenomas on the basis of a biopsy. Radiographic and endoscopic correlation is helpful.

Invasive pancreatic and common bile duct adenocarcinomas

These carcinomas can also simulate ampullary adenomas when they invade the ampulla as they have a striking propensity to colonize basement membranes {2574}, including the mucosa of the ampulla or duodenum. Paradoxically, the malignant cells may appear to be better differentiated and morphologically more intestinal than the underlying invasive carcinoma within the stroma, and they can closely simulate an intestinal-type adenoma. Immunolabelling can facilitate the diagnosis, as most pancreatic ductal adenocarcinomas colonizing the ampullary mucosa express keratin 7 and MUC1 and are negative for the intestinal markers keratin 20, MUC2, and CDX2, which are expressed by ampullary adenomas {2574}.

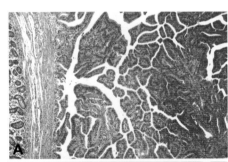
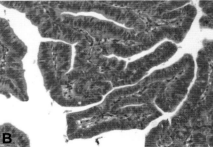

Fig. 5.04 Intestinal-type villous adenoma with high-grade dysplasia arising in the ampulla of Vater. **A** Low-power view showing striking papillary architecture. **B** High magnification: note the complex papillary architecture and considerable cytological atypia.

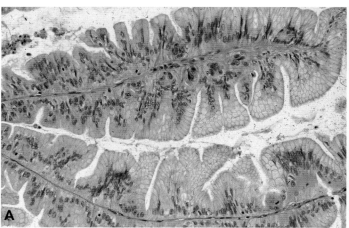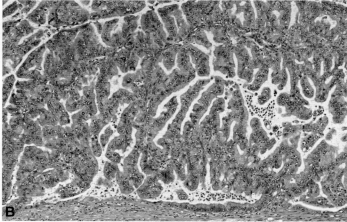

Fig. 5.05 Noninvasive pancreatobiliary-type papillary neoplasm with high-grade dysplasia (high-grade intraepithelial neoplasia). **A** The low-power architecture is markedly complex with numerous micropapillae. **B** The neoplastic cells have abundant mucinous cytoplasm and show focal loss of nuclear polarity.

An ampullary adenoma may be misdiagnosed as invasive carcinoma when adenomatous epithelium extends into peri-ampullary ductules within the smooth muscle of the sphincter of Oddi. This phenomenon is especially troublesome when the adenoma exhibits high-grade dysplasia, or when deep endoscopic biopsies are poorly oriented. The lack of a stromal response around the atypical glands and identification of continuity with benign ductular epithelium help to establish the noninvasive nature of these foci.

Genetic susceptibility

Patients with FAP/Gardner syndrome, an autosomal dominant condition caused by germline mutations in the adenomatous polyposis coli (*APC*) gene on chromosome 5 (5q21–22) {378}, also have a high risk of developing adenomas of the ampulla and periampullary duodenum, and adenomas in patients with FAP are usually multiple {88, 1690, 2916}. Nearly 100% of these patients will develop ampullary adenomas during their lifetime, and progression to ampullary adenocarcinoma is a consequence if the adenomas are not detected and treated in a timely manner.

Molecular pathology

The development of invasive ampullary carcinoma within an adenoma occurs through a sequence of molecular genetic changes that parallel the increasing grades of dysplasia. Although mutations in the *APC* gene contribute to the development of ampullary adenomas, only 17% of sporadic ampullary adenomas have *APC* mutations {23}. Nuclear accumulation of β-catenin is more common in adenomas without *APC* mutations {3428}. Mutations in codon 12 (or, less commonly, codon 13) of the *KRAS* oncogene occur in about 40% of ampullary adenomas {70, 559, 1257, 3428}, with equal frequency in low-grade and high-grade dysplasia {1257}. FAP-associated adenomas appear to have a lower frequency of *KRAS* mutations {3428}. Abnormalities in the *BRAF* gene are uncommon in ampullary adenomas {3428}. *TP53* gene mutations, and nuclear accumulation of p53 protein, may occur in adenomas, generally those with high-grade dysplasia {2832, 3161}. Ampullary adenomas only rarely (9%) have abnormalities in DNA mismatch repair proteins or show microsatellite instability {2748, 3428}.

Prognosis and predictive factors

Ampullary intestinal-type adenomas and pancreatobiliary-type noninvasive papillary neoplasms are preinvasive neoplasms associated with a risk of progression to invasive adenocarcinoma {232, 457, 1663, 2365, 3327, 3536}. Villous adenomas have a greater risk of malignant transformation than tubular adenomas {2533}. The likelihood of finding invasive carcinoma in an ampullary adenoma is greater than the likelihood of finding invasive carcinoma in a colonic adenoma or in an extra-ampullary duodenal adenoma of similar size {2533, 2869}. About 30–50% of ampullary masses showing only adenoma on a biopsy specimen prove to contain invasive carcinoma upon resection {2050, 2765, 2869}. Surgical excision via pancreatoduodenectomy or transduodenal ampullectomy may be indicated if the lesion is too large to be removed endoscopically {3536}.

We do not know how long it takes for an ampullary adenoma to evolve into invasive carcinoma. The natural history of ampullary adenomas in patients with FAP may differ from that of sporadic adenomas. When detected at an early stage, ampullary and periampullary adenomas in patients with FAP are often small (< 0.5 cm) and show no high-grade dysplasia on biopsy. Although complete endoscopic removal may not be possible, these patients can be followed very closely, and most show minimal progression in the size or degree of dysplasia over at least 3 years {61, 375, 2005}. In the familial setting, detection of high-grade dysplasia in a biopsy of an ampullary adenoma suggests that complete surgical removal (including the possibility of pancreatoduodenectomy) should be performed.

Invasive adenocarcinoma of the ampullary region

J. Albores-Saavedra
R.H. Hruban
D.S. Klimstra
G. Zamboni

Definition

A gland-forming malignant epithelial neoplasm, usually with an intestinal or pancreatobiliary phenotype, which originates in the ampulla of Vater. The ampulla may be affected by carcinomas arising from the duodenal mucosa, the distal common bile duct, or the head of the pancreas, but only those carcinomas either centred on the ampulla, circumferentially surrounding it, or demonstrating complete replacement of the ampulla are regarded as "ampullary carcinoma" for the purposes of classification {70, 762}.

ICD-O codes

Adenocarcinoma	8140/3
Invasive intestinal type	8144/3
Pancreatobiliary type	8163/3
Adenosquamous carcinoma	8560/3
Clear cell carcinoma	8310/3
Hepatoid adenocarcinoma	8576/3
Invasive papillary adenocarcinoma	
	8260/3
Mucinous adenocarcinoma	8480/3
Signet ring cell carcinoma	8490/3
Squamous cell carcinoma	8070/3
Undifferentiated carcinoma	8020/3
Undifferentiated carcinoma with	
osteoclast-like giant cells	8035/3

Epidemiology

Carcinoma of the ampulla of Vater is an uncommon and heterogeneous neoplasm. When compared with all other cancer sites in terms of frequency in the USA, this neoplasm ranks as 85th in men and 101st in women. Between 1985 and 2005, the incidence of ampullary carcinoma was 0.7 cases per 100 000 males and 0.4 cases per 100 000 females {1240}. According to the Survey Epidemiology and End Results (SEER) programme of the National Cancer Institute, the incidence of ampullary carcinoma has been increasing annually for the past 32 years in the USA, but this is likely to be related to increased surveillance, especially screening for second cancers after an initial primary colon cancer {78, 654}. Ampullary carcinomas represent 0.5% of all gastrointestinal malignancies {78}. They are less common than ductal carcinomas

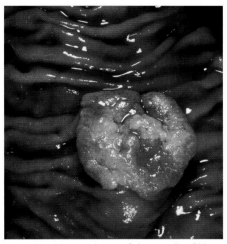

Fig. 5.06 Adenocarcinoma of the ampulla of Vater, luminal view.

of the pancreas and carcinomas of the gallbladder and extrahepatic bile ducts, probably because the relatively small area of mucosa in the ampulla {1172, 1173}. Ampullary carcinomas are more common in men than in women, and are usually diagnosed in patients between the ages of 60 and 80 years (range, 29–85 years). Patients with ampullary adenocarcinomas associated with familial adenomatous polyposis (FAP) or its variant, Gardner syndrome, or neurofibromatosis tend to be younger than those with sporadic tumours {272, 578, 608, 1378, 2359, 2501, 3293}.

Clinical features

The clinical presentation of ampullary carcinoma includes persistent jaundice, abdominal pain, pancreatitis and weight loss {78}. Anaemia due to occult gastrointestinal bleeding occurs in some patients. The classical Courvoisier sign (a distended and palpable gallbladder) is not common. The laboratory data reflect biliary obstruction, with elevated serum levels of bilirubin, glutamic-oxaloacetic transaminase, glutamic pyruvic transaminase and alkaline phosphatase in > 60% of patients. Endoscopic ultrasound, computed tomography (CT), and endoscopic retrograde cholangiopancreatography (ERCP) are useful diagnostic tools and may provide

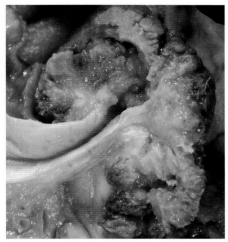

Fig. 5.07 Polypoid mucinous adenocarcinoma of the ampulla of Vater extending along the duodenal mucosa.

preoperative staging information {406, 1670}. While endoscopic biopsy yields a correct histological diagnosis in most patients {3535, 3584}, in cases of adenocarcinoma arising in an adenoma, a superficial biopsy may miss invasive foci and show only the adenoma {3091, 3583}.

Macroscopy

Ampullary carcinomas are classified macroscopically as intra-ampullary, peri-ampullary duodenal, mixed exophytic and mixed ulcerated on the basis of gross appearance and extent of involvement of the ampulla and periampullary duodenum {70}. Microscopic whole-mount sections that include the ampulla, common bile duct, pancreatic duct, and duodenal mucosa are helpful to demonstrate the relationship of the carcinoma to each of these structures. Large (> 4 cm) ampullary carcinomas are difficult to classify grossly because they involve multiple structures. Likewise, large carcinomas of the head of the pancreas, duodenum, or distal common bile duct may extend into the ampulla and closely resemble a primary ampullary carcinoma. When a carcinoma is clearly centred in an adjacent structure and only extends peripherally to involve the ampulla, it is best classified as a

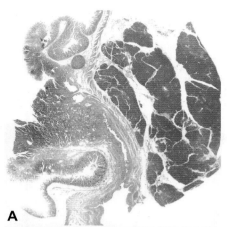

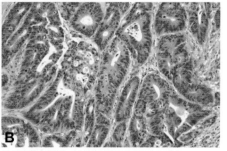

Fig. 5.08 Intestinal-type adenocarcinoma. **A** Low-power view. **B** The neoplastic glands are composed of columnar cells with intestinal phenotype.

primary of the adjacent organ. The term "periampullary carcinoma" has been used for neoplasms for which the site of origin is unclear, but this nonspecific term should be avoided.

Histopathology

The vast majority of invasive carcinomas of the ampulla show a tubular (85–95%) growth pattern. These tumours should be classified according to the predominant component. The remaining carcinomas are morphological variants of adenocarcinomas, or undifferentiated carcinomas. High-grade neuroendocrine carcinomas (large cell neuroendocrine carcinomas and small cell carcinomas) have also been described {1586, 2254, 3119, 3709}. Cytologically, most adenocarcinomas have an intestinal phenotype (50–80%) or a pancreatobiliary phenotype (15–20%) {70, 867, 1566}.

Intestinal-type adenocarcinoma

This type of invasive adenocarcinoma is the most common malignant epithelial tumour of the ampulla and consists of simple or cribriform tubular glands similar to those of adenocarcinomas of the colon.

The glands are lined predominantly by columnar cells with pseudostratified oval or elongated nuclei showing varying degrees of atypia and a variable number of mitotic figures. In some carcinomas, goblet cells are interspersed with the columnar cells. Rarely, Paneth cells and endocrine cells are also present. Dirty-type necrosis as seen in adenocarcinomas of the colon is not as common in ampullary intestinal-type adenocarcinomas. Most of these tumours are associated with an adenoma. Adenocarcinomas arising in adenomas are usually smaller and have a better prognosis than adenocarcinomas unrelated to adenomas.

Pancreatobiliary-type adenocarcinoma

This tubular invasive adenocarcinoma displays a cell phenotype similar to that of pancreatic ductal or extrahepatic bile duct carcinomas. It is composed of simple or branching glands associated with an abundant desmoplastic stroma. The epithelium consists of a single layer of cuboidal or columnar cells, usually without nuclear pseudostratification {70, 3650}. The nuclei are rounder than in intestinal type adenocarcinomas. In general, greater cytological atypia and more mitotic figures are seen in the pancreatobiliary-type adenocarcinoma than the intestinal-type adenocarcinoma. Small solid clusters of neoplastic cells are seen in the less differentiated tumours. A focal micropapillary pattern occurs in < 5% of pancreatobiliary-type adenocarcinomas {1532}. This micropapillary pattern is a marker of clinical aggressiveness in other organs such as the breast and urinary bladder, but its significance in ampullary neoplasms is unknown. Occasionally pancreatobiliary-type adenocarcinomas arise in association with intestinal-type adenomas or noninvasive papillary neoplasms. A small number of invasive carcinomas of the ampulla show a mixed intestinal and pancreatobiliary phenotype.

Cytopathology

Information about the diagnosis of ampullary carcinomas by brush cytology is very limited. In one study of 32 ampullary neoplasms {196}, comparison of cytological and histological diagnoses revealed a sensitivity and specificity of 100%. Carcinomas are characterized by cell clusters, small tubules or isolated cells with a marked degree of atypia. There is considerable variation in nuclear

size and contour with prominent nucleoli. It should be recognized, however, that adenomas with high-grade dysplasia are impossible to distinguish from invasive adenocarcinomas by brush cytology alone.

Immunohistochemistry

Most intestinal-type adenocarcinomas are positive for keratin 20 and only about half are positive for keratin 7, whereas most pancreatobiliary-type adenocarcinomas are keratin 7-positive and keratin 20-negative {754, 1020}. The markers of intestinal phenotype, CDX2 and MUC2, label intestinal-type adenocarcinomas, but are negative in those with a pancreatobiliary phenotype, which are MUC1-positive {553, 867, 3493, 3650}. Because mucinous and signet ring cell carcinomas express CDX2 and MUC2, they are sometimes considered to be variants of intestinal-type adenocarcinomas. Most adenocarcinomas of the ampulla express carcinoembryonic antigen (CEA) and CA19-9, but these markers do not distinguish intestinal-type from pancreatobiliary-type adenocarcinomas {2011, 3584}. In one study, 34% of ampullary carcinomas showed no expression of SMAD4 (DPC4) {2016}.

Ultrastructure

Two types of ampullary carcinomas display distinctive ultrastructural features: the intestinal-type adenocarcinoma and the high-grade neuroendocrine carcinomas. The former is similar to colonic adenocarcinoma and to intestinal-type adenocarcinoma of the gallbladder, extrahepatic bile ducts and pancreas and is composed of columnar cells with abundant organelles and mucin vacuoles, arranged around glandular lumina. The most characteristic ultrastructural feature is the presence of tall microvilli with

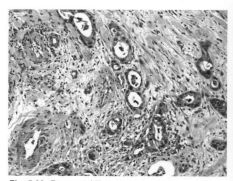

Fig. 5.09 Pancreatobiliary-type adenocarcinoma of the ampulla of Vater, with stromal desmoplasia.

filamentous core rootlets and glycocalyceal bodies {70}. The core microfilaments are continous with the terminal web of the apical cytoplasm. High-grade neuroendocrine carcinomas contain neurosecretory-type granules. Isolated or small clusters of round neurosecretory granules can be identified at the periphery of the cytoplasm of at least some cells. The scant cytoplasm also contains arrays of paranuclear intermediate filaments.

Histological variants
Adenosquamous carcinoma
This unusual neoplasm represents 1% of all ampullary carcinomas and is characterized by a variable combination of two malignant components, one glandular and the other squamous {3017A}. Although the proportion of each component varies, the adenocarcinoma usually predominates, is well- to moderately differentiated, and of pancreatobiliary phenotype. The squamous-carcinoma component is focally keratinizing and by convention should represent at least 25% of the tumour. In contrast, any amount of glandular differentiation suffices to designate a predominantly squamous neoplasm as adenosquamous carcinoma. In some cases, clear cells line the glands and are mixed with the squamous elements. A micropapillary pattern can be seen rarely {1532}. Some adenosquamous carcinomas arise from preexisting adenomas.

Clear cell carcinoma
This exceedingly rare form of ampullary carcinoma has a striking resemblance to metastatic renal cell carcinoma {78, 3391}. Clear cell carcinoma is composed predominantly or exclusively of polygonal cells with abundant clear cytoplasm, well-defined cytoplasmic membranes and centrally placed hyperchromatic nuclei. The cells are arranged in nests, cords or solid sheets and at least some contain cytoplasmic mucin, a useful feature that can distinguish it from renal cell carcinoma. Because of its rarity, the biological behaviour of clear cell carcinoma of the ampulla is unknown.

Hepatoid adenocarcinoma
Fewer than five cases of hepatoid adenocarcinoma of the ampulla have been reported to date {946, 2826}. As its name implies, this neoplasm consists of an adenocarcinoma, usually with an intestinal phenotype, as well as cells closely

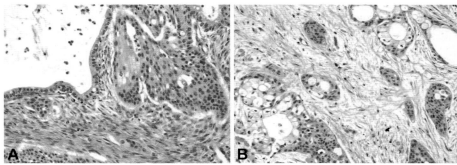

Fig. 5.10 Adenosquamous carcinoma of the ampulla of Vater. **A** Both glandular and squamous differentiation are present. **B** Collections of clear cells are seen in the glands and squamous nests.

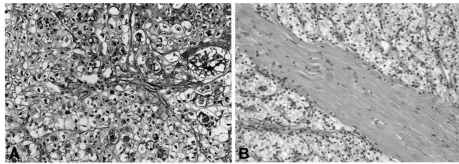

Fig. 5.11 Comparison of: **A** Primary clear cell carcinoma of the ampulla with mucin production; and **B** Metastatic clear cell carcinoma of the kidney.

resembling hepatocytes that grow in sheets or cords. The latter cells are polygonal with abundant eosinophilic cytoplasm are immunoreactive for α-fetoprotein, HepPar1 antibody and polyclonal CEA in a canalicular pattern. Bile pigment has occasionally been identified.

High-grade neuroendocrine carcinoma and mixed carcinomas
Both small cell neuroendocrine carcinoma and large cell neuroendocrine carcinoma can arise in the ampulla {1586, 2254, 3119, 3709} and are regarded as subtypes of neuroendocrine carcinoma, grade 3 (G3). Both can arise in association with intestinal-type adenomas {2254}. The histological features resemble those of their pulmonary counterparts, and the mitotic rate is > 20 per 10 high power fields, by definition.

Mucinous adenocarcinoma
Approximately 5% of the ampullary carcinomas in the SEER database are mucinous adenocarcinomas {78}. The diagnosis of mucinous adenocarcinoma requires that > 50% of the tumour should be composed of stromal mucin that contains small groups of malignant epithelial cells, epithelial strips or ruptured

cystically dilated glands. The strips and glands are lined by columnar cells with an intestinal phenotype, whereas the cells arranged in small groups or clusters may have a signet-ring cell morphology. Some mucinous adenocarcinomas are associated with a component of intestinal adenocarcinoma, a noninvasive papillary neoplasm or an intestinal-type adenoma. Extensive sampling may be needed to demonstrate the neoplastic cells in the mucin pools of some mucinous adenocarcinomas. Some intestinal-type adenocarcinomas contain a focal mucinous component, which is insufficient to classify the tumour as a mucinous adenocarcinoma. Since the vast majority of mucinous adenocarcinomas of the ampulla express the intestinal markers CDX2 and MUC2, these tumours are regarded as variants of intestinal-type adenocarcinomas.

Invasive papillary adenocarcinoma
Exophytic neoplasms with a papillary architecture can occur in the ampulla, similar to those arising in the gallbladder and extrahepatic bile ducts. In the past, these neoplasms have been classified as noninvasive and invasive papillary carcinomas {74, 84, 1215}. Noninvasive lesions

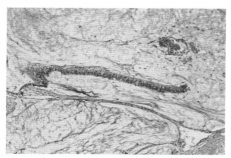

Fig. 5.12 Mucinous adenocarcinoma of the ampulla of Vater. A strip of neoplastic intestinal-type epithelium is surrounded by abundant extracellular mucin.

are now designated "noninvasive papillary neoplasms." When an invasive carcinoma arises in association with a noninvasive papillary neoplasm, the invasive component should be diagnosed, graded, and staged separately from the noninvasive component. In the ampulla, most such invasive carcinomas are of pancreatobiliary or intestinal type. Only rarely does an invasive carcinoma maintain a papillary growth pattern in the invasive elements, and although a descriptive term of "invasive papillary carcinoma" could be used for these neoplasms, most can be more accurately classified on the basis of cellular differentiation and morphology as one of the other histological variants of ampullary carcinoma.

Signet ring cell carcinoma

Signet ring cell carcinoma is a highly malignant neoplasm that represents 2% of all carcinomas of the ampulla {78}. It consists predominantly of epithelial cells with cytoplasmic mucin that pushes the nuclei towards the periphery of the cells {51, 284, 802}). Some neoplastic cells, however, contain little or no cytoplasmic mucin and appear undifferentiated. A minor component of tubular adenocarcinoma and clusters of neuroendocrine cells have been identified in a few signet ring cell carcinomas. Although signet ring cells can be found in mucinous adenocarcinomas, the diagnosis of signet ring cell carcinoma is reserved for those cases with the characteristic diffuse pattern of infiltration, usually without significant extracellular mucin accumulation. Tumours with mild atypia, few mitotic figures and endocrine cells can be confused with goblet cell carcinoid tumours. The infiltrating growth pattern, lack of a nesting pattern, and the mildly atypical neoplastic signet-ring cells favour a diagnosis of signet ring cell carcinoma.

Squamous cell carcinoma

This exceedingly rare ampullary carcinoma is composed entirely of cells with squamous differentiation. Keratinizing and nonkeratinizing types exist {70}. Most ampullary carcinomas with predominant squamous features prove to be adenosquamous carcinomas when extensively sampled and stained for mucin.

Undifferentiated carcinoma

There are two types of undifferentiated carcinoma of the ampulla. The first is composed of small (non-neuroendocrine) cells while in the second type spindle cells predominate and resemble a sarcoma (sarcomatoid carcinoma).

The first type is highly cellular with minimal stroma and is composed of relatively small cells with scant cytoplasm, vesicular nuclei and prominent nucleoli arranged in solid sheets or nests {70, 2124}. There are no glands or signet-ring cells. Numerous mitotic figures and necrosis of variable extent are common. Immunohistochemical stains for neuroendocrine markers are negative.

The second type of undifferentiated carcinoma consists predominantly of fascicles of spindle cells, some of which are keratin-positive, supporting their epithelial phenotype. When extensively sampled, these tumours often contain glandular structures or nests of frank epithelial cells. Considerable cytological atypia including the presence of pleomorphic and anaplastic giant cells may be present in the spindle-cell component. When heterologous elements such as cartilage, bone and skeletal muscle are present, the term "carcinosarcoma" is justified {1539}.

Undifferentiated carcinoma with osteoclast-like giant cells

A very rare form of undifferentiated carcinoma that contains numerous multinucleated osteoclast-like giant cells has been documented in the ampulla {70}. This carcinoma is similar to undifferentiated carcinomas with osteoclast-like giant cells reported in the gallbladder, extrahepatic bile ducts and pancreas {69, 2124, 3493}. The giant cells in these tumours are histiocytic and non-neoplastic and label positively for CD68. In contrast, the neoplastic mononuclear cells may be keratin-positive and are often p53-positive.

Differential diagnosis

The strategic location of the ampulla of Vater at the intersection of the pancreas, duodenum and common bile duct, where malignant neoplasms with similar phenotypes arise, makes establishing the organ of origin of these carcinomas difficult. Carcinomas of the ampulla, pancreas, gallbladder and extrahepatic bile ducts share cell phenotypes, molecular abnormalities and a field effect for carcinogenesis {81, 1172, 1173}, and multiple synchronous or metachronous primaries may involve these sites in an individual patient {43, 826, 1205, 2299, 2319}.

When relatively small pancreatic carcinomas extend into the ampulla and the bulk of the mass is in the pancreas, the neoplasm is recognizable as a pancreatic primary. However, large ductal carcinomas of the pancreas often extend into the ampulla, obliterating this structure and mimicking a primary ampullary carcinoma. Moreover, the histological and immunohistochemical features of pancreatic ductal carcinomas can be identical to those of pancreatobiliary-type ampullary carcinomas {81}. A very useful microscopic feature is the presence of a residual ampullary adenoma or noninvasive papillary neoplasm associated with or adjacent to the invasive carcinoma.

Colonization of the ampullary epithelium by invasive pancreatic ductal adenocarcinoma can simulate a primary ampullary adenoma, but the lesion retains the immunophenotype of pancreatic carcinoma (including MUC1 expression), whereas ampullary adenomas have an intestinal phenotype (positive for keratin 20, MUC2, and CDX2). Carcinomas of the duodenum and common bile duct may also extend into the ampulla and create similar diagnostic problems. Again, the epicentre of the neoplasm is used to define the site of origin.

Metastatic renal cell carcinoma may mimic clear cell carcinoma of the ampulla {3391}. The presence of mucin, immunoreactivity for CEA and lack of reactivity for CD10 and the renal cell carcinoma (RCC) antigen favour a diagnosis of clear cell carcinoma of the ampulla. Signet ring cell carcinomas should be distinguished from goblet cell carcinoids, which have a prominent organoid or nesting pattern; the goblet cells are less atypical and mitotic figures are not seen. In addition, the possibility of secondary involvement from a gastric primary needs to be excluded.

Immunohistochemical lymphoid markers are useful to separate malignant lymphomas from undifferentiated carcinomas. Metastatic malignant melanoma can simulate a primary ampullary carcinoma {3351}; however, the former is immunoreactive for HMB45, Melan A and other melanocytic markers.

Precursor lesions
Ampullary carcinomas may arise in association with intestinal-type adenomas, noninvasive papillary neoplasms, or flat intraepithelial neoplasia (dysplasia).

Genetic susceptibility
Patients with FAP have a 100- to 200-fold increased risk of developing ampullary adenocarcinoma {272, 2359, 2501} with an estimated lifetime incidence of up to 12%. However, a multicentre analysis of 1262 patients with FAP found that ampullary carcinomas occur in only 4% of patients with FAP {3046}. FAP-associated ampullary carcinomas arise in a background of multiple adenomas involving the ampulla and periampullary duodenum. Patients with colorectal carcinoma have an excess risk of developing ampullary cancer, which appears to be part of the spectrum of Lynch syndrome {654}. An excess risk of ampullary adenocarcinomas has also been reported in patients with type 1 multiple neurofibromatosis (von Recklinghausen disease) {578, 608, 1586}.

Molecular pathology
Wide variations in the frequency of genetic abnormalities have been reported in ampullary carcinomas, but little is known about their clinical implications. Moreover, the genetic abnormalities of ampullary carcinomas have not been correlated with intestinal or pancreatobiliary type. Mutations in exons 5, 6 and 7 of the *TP53* gene have been detected in 59–94% of ampullary carcinomas {559, 1586, 2633, 2637, 2831, 3583} and appear to be a late event in carcinogenesis. Mutations in codon 12 (and rarely codon 13) of the *KRAS* oncogene have been recorded in 13–75% of ampullary carcinomas {2633, 2637, 2831}. *KRAS* mutations do not correlate with histological type, grade, stage of disease or prognosis. Loss of expression of the *SMAD4* tumour suppressor gene has been detected in 34% of ampullary carcinomas {2016}. Mutations in the *APC* and β-catenin (*CTNNB1*) genes occur in ampullary carcinomas, but at a

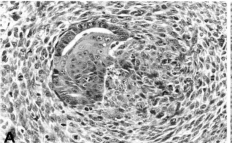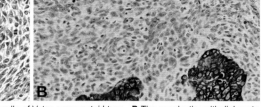

Fig. 5.13 A Undifferentiated carcinoma of the ampulla of Vater, sarcomatoid type. **B** The neoplastic epithelial nests express keratin AE1/AE3. A small number of spindle cells are also positive for keratin.

lower frequency than in colorectal carcinomas. High-level microsatellite instability has been identified in 0–10% of ampullary carcinomas {2748, 2885}. Overexpression of epidermal growth factor (*EGF*) is found in 50–65% of invasive ampullary carcinomas {366, 897, 2660}, and *ERBB2* and *ERBB3* are also overexpressed in ampullary carcinomas {3293}.

Tumour spread and staging
Carcinomas spread directly from the ampullary mucosa through the sphincter of Oddi to the duodenal submucosa and muscularis propria to reach the underlying pancreas or periduodenal soft tissues. The vast majority of carcinomas confined to the ampullary mucosa or sphincter of Oddi do not metastasize, but those that extend to the submucosa do (42% of cases). Nodal metastases occur most commonly in the peripancreatic lymph nodes followed by metastases in the liver, peritoneum, lungs and pleura.
The current American Joint Committee on Cancer and the International Union against Cancer (AJCC/UICC) TNM staging system for ampullary carcinoma {762, 1060, 2996} is widely used.

Prognosis and predictive factors
The prognosis of patients with ampullary carcinoma is determined by tumour stage, histological type, histological grade and presence of pre-existing adenoma {78}. The best predictor of prognosis is stage of disease {78, 179, 1291, 2336, 2603, 2885, 3217}. Based on the SEER data, carcinomas localized to the ampulla have a significantly better 5-year survival rate (45%) than those with regional (31%) extension beyond the ampulla directly into surrounding tissues, or distant disease (4%) (metastasis in distant lymph nodes or in visceral organs). The high mortality rates for patients with ampullary

carcinomas confined to the ampulla, reported in the SEER data, suggests that many of these tumours had in fact extended to the duodenal submucosa (AJCC stage pT2).
Patients with well-differentiated carcinomas do better than those with poorly differentiated carciomas {78}. Carcinomas that arise from adenomas have a more favourable prognosis than adenocarcinomas not associated with adenomas, probably because the former are detected earlier {78}. The intestinal-type ampullary adenocarcinoma has a more favourable prognosis than the pancreatobiliary type, probably because the former usually arises from a pre-existing adenoma {179, 2714, 3535}. The prognosis for patients with ampullary mucinous carcinomas is not better than for those with intestinal- or pancreatobiliary-type adenocarcinomas {78}, in contrast to mucinous carcinomas of the breast and pancreas, and their corresponding ductal carcinomas.
Other negative prognostic factors include a high level of microsatellite instability {2748}, size of the tumour, and vascular and perineural invasion {179, 3113}.

Neuroendocrine neoplasms of the ampullary region

G. Klöppel
R. Arnold
C. Capella
D.S. Klimstra

J. Albores-Saavedra
E. Solcia
G. Rindi
P. Komminoth

Definition

Neoplasms arising in the ampulla of Vater and periampullary region that have predominantly neuroendocrine differentiation. These include well-differentiated (low- to intermediate-grade) neuroendocrine tumours (NETs) and poorly differentiated (high-grade) neuroendocrine carcinomas (NECs). NECs include large cell NEC and small cell NEC. Mixed adenoneuroendocrine carcinoma (MANEC) has exocrine and neuroendocrine components, with each component exceeding 30%.

ICD-O codes

Neuroendocrine tumour (NET)
NET G1 (carcinoid)   8240/3
NET G2   8249/3
Neuroendocrine carcinoma (NEC) 8246/3
Large cell NEC   8013/3
Small cell NEC   8041/3
Mixed adenoneuroendocrine
carcinoma (MANEC)   8244/3
EC cell, serotonin-producing NET 8241/3
Gangliocytic paraganglioma   8683/0
Somatostatin-producing NET   8156/3

Synonyms

Synonyms for ampullary NETs include carcinoid and well-differentiated endocrine tumour/carcinoma {3013}. Synonyms for NEC include poorly differentiated endocrine carcinomas, high-grade neuroendocrine carcinoma, small cell and large cell endocrine carcinomas.

Epidemiology

Ampullary NETs account for approximately 20% of all neuroendocrine neoplasms of the duodenum and for 70% of those of the ampullary-periampullary region {943}. The mean age of diagnosis is 54 years (range, 28–74 years) and the sex ratio is almost one. Approximately 15–25% (in one study up to 50%) of NETs are associated with neurofibromatosis type 1 (NF1), i.e. von Recklinghausen disease {666, 943, 1127}. Gangliocytic paragangliomas account for 20–25% of ampullary-periampullary neuroendocrine neoplasms, presenting at an average age of 54 years and showing an equal sex distribution {372, 943}. NECs account for almost 5% of ampullary-periampullary neoplasms, present at a mean age of 70 years (range, 50–89 years) and affect males more frequently than females {943, 2254, 3670} (see Chapter 6).

Clinical features

Neuroendocrine neoplasms of the ampulla commonly lead to obstructive jaundice, rarely to acute pancreatitis, or haemorrhage. In addition, they may arise in patients with NF1. Hormonal syndromes such as carcinoid syndrome and Zollinger-Ellison (gastrinoma) syndrome are usually absent. The somatostatinoma syndrome (diabetes mellitus, diarrhoea, steatorrhoea, hypohydria or achlorhydria, anaemia and gallstones) is almost never observed {943, 1055}. Some neoplasms, especially those located in the periampullary region, are asymptomatic and often discovered incidentally.

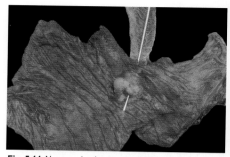

Fig. 5.14 Neuroendocrine tumour (NET) of the ampulla of Vater. A probe is inserted in the bile duct.

Macroscopy

NETs (carcinoid tumours) are mostly 1–2 cm in diameter (mean, 1.8 cm; range, 1.3–5.0 cm). They cause a widening of the papilla of Vater with obstruction of the ampulla by submucosal infiltration {307, 943, 1960}. The overlying mucosa of the ampulla is usually intact and rarely ulcerated. A few neoplasms are infiltrative, intramural nodules of rather large size (up to 5 cm in diameter). Periampullary neoplasms in general do not obstruct the ampulla, but may involve the papilla of Vater. Gangliocytic paragangliomas are mainly found in the periampullary region where they produce polypoid lesions protruding into the duodenal lumen. These neoplasms have a mean diameter of 1.7 cm {413}.
NECs form polypoid and often ulcerated masses in the ampulla and papilla of Vater, with a mean size of 2.5 cm (range, 0.8–4 cm).

Histopathology
NETs

Most NETs of the ampulla have a nested, trabecular or cribriform growth pattern. The uniform neoplastic cells have moderate amounts of cytoplasm and round nuclei with "salt and pepper" chromatin. Mitoses are usually rare (< 2 per 10 high power fields [HPF]). The grading of these neoplasms is detailed in Chapter 1. NETs express chromogranin A, synaptophysin and CD56 (NCAM1).

Somatostatin-producing NET. NETs that produce somatostatin are predominantly composed of tubuloglandular structures admixed with a variable proportion of

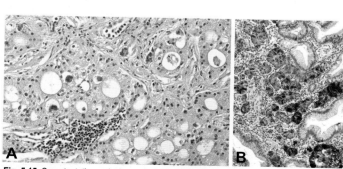

Fig. 5.15 Somatostatin-producing neuroendocrine tumour (NET G1, somatostatinoma) of the ampulla. **A** Tubuloglandular differentiation and psammoma bodies are evident. **B** Immunolabelling for somatostatin.

insular and trabecular structures ("glandular carcinoids"). In about one third of cases, the glands contain psammoma bodies, leading to the alternative descriptor "psammomatous somatostatinoma." They express synaptophysin; chromogranin A is only positive in about 50% of cases. In addition to the somatostatin-producing cells, the neoplasms may have minor cell populations that are positive for gastrin, secretin, calcitonin, pancreatic polypeptide and adrenocorticotropic hormone (ACTH) {413, 666, 943, 1960}. Ultrastructural examination shows large, moderately electron-dense secretory granules, similar to those found in normal somatostatin-producing D cells of the intestinal mucosa {413}.

Gangliocytic paraganglioma. These neoplasms are characterized by their triphasic cellular differentiation, consisting of neuroendocrine cells, spindle-shaped cells with Schwannian differentiation, and ganglion cells, which vary in terms of relative abundance and distribution within each neoplasm. The neuroendocrine cells have an eosinophilic or amphophilic cytoplasm and uniform ovoid nuclei, with low or no mitotic activity. They are arranged in ribbons, solid nests, or pseudoglandular structures that rarely may contain psammoma bodies {943}.

The neuroendocrine cells are immunoreactive for pankeratin, synaptophysin and chromogranin A and often express pancreatic polypeptide, followed in frequency by somatostatin and vasoactive intestinal peptide (VIP) {413, 943, 3055}. The sometimes numerous spindle cells form small fascicles or envelope nerve cells and axons and show intense expression of S100 protein. The ganglion cells may be scattered as single elements or aggregated in clusters and label with antibodies to synaptophysin. In some gangliocytic paragangliomas, the three components intermingle with the normal smooth muscle and small ductules of the ampulla, resulting in a very complex lesion. The complex composition of the gangliocytic paragangliomas suggests that they may be a hamartoma of pancreatic anlage {1105, 2531}. Ultrastructurally, the epithelial cells have abundant cytoplasm packed with dense-core secretory granules, while the ganglion cells are larger and contain a small number of neuroendocrine granules of small size and more numerous secondary lysosomes. The spindle cells are packed with intermediate filaments and resemble either sustentacular cells or Schwann cells {2531}.

NECs

Histologically, there are two types of NEC: one with rather small cells, comparable to small cell NEC of the lung; the other with quite large cells, resembling large cell NEC of the lung. Both types display a diffuse, solid and/or trabecular growth pattern with areas of necrosis. NECs composed of small cells have nuclei with abundant chromatin, but inconspicuous nucleoli; NECs with large cells have vesicular nuclei with a distinct nucleolus. The mitotic rate is high (> 20 per 10 HPF), the proliferative rate ranges from 30% to 80%; NECs are thus histological grade 3 (G3; Chapter 1). A minor component (< 30% of the neoplastic cells) of conventional adenocarcinoma or squamous cell carcinoma may be associated.

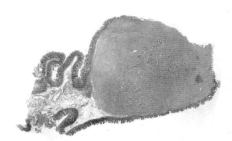

Fig. 5.16 Gangliocytic paraganglioma. Low-power view showing polypoid submucosal tumour.

Deep mural invasion, angioinvasion, and neuroinvasion are common {2254, 3670}.

All NECS are immunoreactive for keratins, especially 7, 8 and 18, and synaptophysin {943, 2254, 3670}. They may also express chromogranin A and CD56, and occasionally p53 and CDKN1B/p27/Kip1. TTF1 is usually not expressed, in contrast to many similar neoplasms in the lung. Some neoplasms are associated with adenomas in the adjacent mucosa of the papilla {2254}.

MANEC

MANECs contain a significant (> 30%) component of mucin-producing adenocarcinoma or rarely squamous cell carcinoma {2254}. The two components may be adjacent or intermingled.

Differential diagnosis

The differential diagnosis for most ampullary NETs (carcinoid tumours) is similar to that for other NETs in the tubular gastrointestinal tract. The glandular pattern and psammoma bodies of somatostatin-producing NETs may cause

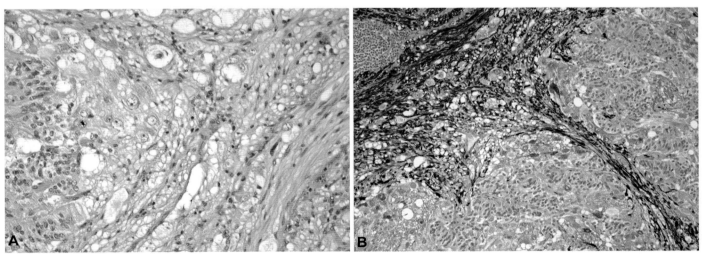

Fig. 5.17 Gangliocytic paraganglioma. **A** Gangliocytic cells, neuroendocrine cells and Schwann cells can be seen. **B** Immunolabelling for S100 protein highlights Schwann cells.

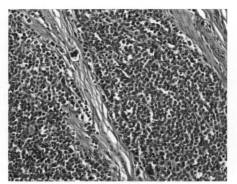

Fig. 5.18 Small cell neuroendocrine carcinoma (NEC) displaying typical cytological features.

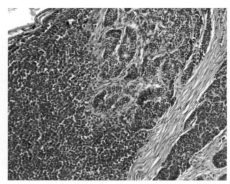

Fig. 5.19 Small cell neuroendocrine carcinoma (NEC) with a solid growth pattern and rosette-like structures (right).

confusion with well-differentiated adeno-carcinoma. Unlike adenocarcinomas, however, the somatostatin-producing NETs are composed of uniform cells with bland nuclei, few mitotic figures and a distinct finely granular eosinophilic cyto-plasm. When the cytoplasm is abundant, these neoplasms can be confused with normal Brunner glands in endoscopic biopsy specimens. Gangliocytic para-gangliomas can be confused with NETs (carcinoid tumours) when the neuro-endocrine component predominates or in the case of primary mesenchymal neo-plasms such as gastrointestinal stromal tumours (GISTs) in which the spindle-cell component is predominant.

Genetic susceptibility

NF1

Patients with von Recklinghausen disease have a significant risk of developing somatostatin-producing ampullary-peri-ampullary NETs {372, 413, 1127}. In addition, these patients may develop other neoplasms, such as GIST {251, 608, 3347}. Some patients with NF1 and ampullary somatostatin-producing NETs also have a phaeochromocytoma involving one or both adrenal glands, a clinical situation that can considerably complicate patient manage-ment. Both gangliocytic paraganglioma and somatostatin-producing NETs have been associated with NF1 {1533, 3076}.

MEN1

MEN1-associated neuroendocrine tumours are frequent in the first part of the duodenum but occur less often in the ampullary region {3055} (see Chapter 6).

Staging, prognosis and predictive factors

The new grading (see Chapter 1) and TNM/staging classifications recently proposed for foregut neuroendocrine tumours (see Chapter 6) should be applied to neuroendocrine neoplasms of the ampulla, as both grade and stage are prognostically important {2449}.

Somatostatin-producing NETs without other hormone expression carry a significant risk of metastasis (> 50%) if they involve the the muscularis propria, are > 2 cm, and have an increased proliferation rate {307, 666, 943, 1295, 1960}. However, even neoplasms with a diameter of 1–2 cm or even smaller can metastasize to paraduo-denal lymph nodes {943, 2003, 2874}. Liver metastases are rare. Complete surgical removal is effective and ensures survival in many patients {943}. In case of recurrence, the liver is the most common site of metastasis {1295}.

Gangliocytic paragangliomas usually fol-low a benign course; however, occasional large neoplasms (size, > 2 cm) may spread to local lymph nodes, mainly man-ifesting as to the neuroendocrine compo-nent of the lesion {358, 1327}.

NECs usually present at advanced stages, i.e. with lymph-node, liver and other re-mote metastases {2254, 3670}. The mean survival time for patients with metastases is 14.5 months {2254, 3670}.

CHAPTER 6

Tumours of the small intestine

Carcinoma

Neuroendocrine neoplasms

B-cell lymphoma

T-cell lymphoma

Mesenchymal tumours

Secondary tumours

WHO classification[a] of tumours of the small intestine

Epithelial tumours

Premalignant lesions

Adenoma	8140/0
Tubular	8211/0
Villous	8261/0
Tubulovillous	8263/0
Dysplasia (intraepithelial neoplasia), low grade	8148/0*
Dysplasia (intraepithelial neoplasia), high grade	8148/2

Hamartomas

Juvenile polyp

Peutz-Jeghers polyp

Carcinoma

Adenocarcinoma	8140/3
Mucinous adenocarcinoma	8480/3
Signet ring cell carcinoma	8490/3
Adenosquamous carcinoma	8560/3
Medullary carcinoma	8510/3
Squamous cell carcinoma	8070/3
Undifferentiated carcinoma	8020/3

Neuroendocrine neoplasms[b]

Neuroendocrine tumour (NET)	
NET G1 (carcinoid)	8240/3
NET G2	8249/3

Neuroendocrine carcinoma (NEC)	8246/3
Large cell NEC	8013/3
Small cell NEC	8041/3
Mixed adenoneuroendocrine carcinoma	8244/3
EC cell, serotonin-producing NET	8241/3
Gangliocytic paraganglioma	8683/0
Gastrinoma	8153/3
L cell, Glucagon-like peptide-producing and PP/PYY-producing NETs	8152/1*
Somatostatin-producing NET	8156/3

Mesenchymal tumours

Leiomyoma	8890/0
Lipoma	8850/0
Angiosarcoma	9120/3
Gastrointestinal stromal tumour	8936/3
Kaposi sarcoma	9140/3
Leiomyosarcoma	8890/3

Lymphomas

Secondary tumours

---

[a] The morphology codes are from the International Classification of Diseases for Oncology (ICD-O) {904A}. Behaviour is coded /0 for benign tumours, /1 for unspecified, borderline or uncertain behaviour, /2 for carcinoma *in situ* and grade III intraepithelial neoplasia, and /3 for malignant tumours.

[b] The classification is modified from the previous (third) edition of the WHO histological classification of tumours {691} taking into account changes in our understanding of these lesions. In the case of neuroendocrine neoplasms, the classification has been simplified to be of more practical utility in morphological classification.

* These new codes were approved by the IARC/WHO Committee for ICD-O at its meeting in March 2010.

TNM classification[a] of tumours of the small intestine[b]

Carcinoma of the small intestine

T – Primary tumour
TX   Primary tumour cannot be assessed
T0   No evidence of primary tumour
Tis   Carcinoma *in situ*
T1   Tumour invades lamina propria, muscularis mucosae or submucosa
    T1a   Tumour invades lamina propria or muscularis mucosae
    T1b   Tumour invades submucosa
T2   Tumour invades muscularis propria
T3   Tumour invades subserosa or nonperitonealized perimuscular tissue (mesentery or retroperitoneum[c]) with extension 2 cm or less
T4   Tumour perforates visceral peritoneum or directly invades other organs or structures (includes other loops of small intestine, mesentery, or retroperitoneum more than 2 cm and abdominal wall by way of serosa; for duodenum only, invasion of pancreas)

N – Regional lymph nodes
NX   Regional lymph nodes cannot be assessed
N0   No regional lymph-node metastasis
N1   Metastasis in 1 to 3 regional lymph nodes
N2   Metastasis in 4 or more regional lymph nodes

M – Distant metastasis
M0   No distant metastasis
M1   Distant metastasis

Stage grouping

Stage	T	N	M
Stage 0	Tis	N0	M0
Stage I	T1, T2	N0	M0
Stage IIA	T3	N0	M0
Stage IIB	T4	N0	M0
Stage IIIA	Any T	N1	M0
Stage IIIB	Any T	N2	M0
Stage IV	Any T	Any N	M1

Carcinoid of the small intestine[d]

T – Primary tumour[e]
TX   Primary tumour cannot be assessed
T0   No evidence of primary tumour
T1   Tumour invades lamina propria or submucosa and is no greater than 1 cm in size[f]
T2   Tumour invades muscularis propria or is greater than 1 cm in size
T3   Jejunal or ileal tumour invades subserosa. Ampullary or duodenal tumour invades pancreas or retroperitoneum
T4   Tumour perforates visceral peritoneum (serosa) or invades other organs or adjacent structures

N – Regional lymph nodes
NX   Regional lymph nodes cannot be assessed
N0   No regional lymph-node metastasis
N1   Regional lymph-node metastasis

M – Distant metastasis
M0   No distant metastasis
M1   Distant metastasis

Stage grouping

Stage	T	N	M
Stage I	T1	N0	M0
Stage IIA	T2	N0	M0
Stage IIB	T3	N0	M0
Stage IIIA	T4	N0	M0
Stage IIIB	Any T	N1	M0
Stage IV	Any T	Any N	M1

[a] {762, 2996}
[b] The TNM classification and stage grouping for small-intestinal GISTs can be found on page 47.
[c] The nonperitonealized perimuscular tissue is, for jejunum and ileum, part of the mesentery and, for duodenum in areas where serosa is lacking, part of the retroperitoneum.
[d] Neuroendocrine tumour (NET, well-differentiated neuroendocrine tumour/carcinoma).
[e] For any T, add (m) for multiple tumours.
[f] Tumour limited to ampulla of Vater for ampullary gangliocytic paraganglioma.

A help desk for specific questions about the TNM classification is available at http://www.uicc.org.

Carcinoma of the small intestine

N.A. Shepherd
N.J. Carr
J.R. Howe
A.E. Noffsinger
B.F. Warren

Definition

A malignant epithelial tumour of the small intestine. Neoplasms of the periampullary region include those of the duodenal mucosa, ampulla of Vater, common bile duct and pancreatic ducts.

ICD-O codes

Adenocarcinoma	8140/3
Mucinous adenocarcinoma	8480/3
Signet ring cell carcinoma	8490/3

Epidemiology

Relative to the length and surface area of the small intestine, adenocarcinomas at this site are remarkably rare {2854}. Data from the United States Surveillance, Epidemiology and End Results (SEER) programme for 1973–2005 show an average annual age-adjusted incidence rate for adenocarcinoma of the small intestine of 6.8 per million; men are affected slightly more often than women, and the incidence in African Americans is about twice that in Whites {2854}. The median age at manifestation is approximately 67 years {3237}.

Etiology

The model of the adenoma–carcinoma sequence is believed to apply to the small intestine as well as the large intestine {2854}.

There is evidence from SEER data that the incidence of adenocarcinoma of the duodenum is increasing at roughly the same rate as colon carcinoma, whereas the incidence of adenocarcinoma of the jejunum and ileum has remained stable {545}. This observation raises the possibility that the risk factors for duodenal and colon carcinomas are similar. Furthermore, patients with carcinoma of the small intestine have a significantly increased risk of developing cancers at other sites, particularly cancer of the colorectum, pancreas, gallbladder and bile ducts, and sarcoma of the soft tissues {2834}.

Chronic inflammation can be associated with the development of small-intestinal adenocarcinoma. In particular, long-standing Crohn disease and coeliac disease are risk factors {990, 2061, 2288, 2626, 2669, 3553}. One study showed that individuals with Crohn disease have an increased risk of adenocarcinoma of the small intestine of 86-fold {1063}. There is also epidemiological evidence that cigarette use and alcohol consumption are risk factors {2269}.

Carcinoma can develop in ileostomies in patients with ulcerative colitis or familial adenomatous polyposis (FAP) subsequent to colonic metaplasia and intraepithelial neoplasia in the ileostomy mucosa {932, 2697}. Carcinoma can also arise in ileal conduits {3305} and in ileal reservoirs, both continent abdominal (Kock) {610} and pelvic {2921, 3403}.

Localization

The duodenum is the main site of occurrence, with more adenocarcinomas arising in the duodenum than in the jejunum and ileum combined {545, 2854, 3237}. In the duodenum, carcinomas are most common around the ampulla of Vater {2797}, possibly owing to biliary or pancreatic effluents. Occasionally, an adenocarcinoma arises in a Meckel diverticulum {1695}.

Clinical features

Symptoms and signs

Small-bowel adenocarcinomas are generally asymptomatic in their early stages, but occult gastrointestinal bleeding may occur, leading to anaemia. As they grow larger, they may cause symptoms of bowel obstruction, with cramp-like abdominal pain, bloating, and emesis. In a review of 172 small-bowel tumours from a single institution, 63% of patients had abdominal pain, 48% had vomiting, 44% had weight loss, 37% had occult blood in the stool, 28% had a palpable mass, and 23% had gastrointestinal bleeding {3173}. Duodenal and ampullary tumours may obstruct the bile duct and cause jaundice. Locally advanced small-bowel tumours may perforate, leading to peritonitis, or be associated with carcinomatosis, leading to bowel obstruction and ascites.

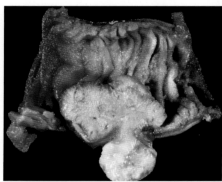

Fig. 6.01 Adenocarcinoma of the small intestine.

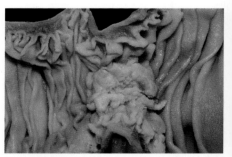

Fig. 6.02 Metastatic colonic carcinoma affecting the small bowel. Mimicry of a primary tumour may be profound, both macroscopically and histologically.

Imaging

The radiological methods that have the highest diagnostic accuracy are spiral computed tomography (CT) scan with contrast medium and enteroclysis; the two methods can be complementary. With enteroclysis, a filling defect, an irregular and circumscribed thickening of the folds with wall rigidity, slowed motility, eccentric passage of the contrast medium, or a clear stenosis may be observed {359}. Small-bowel adenocarcinoma may appear on CT scan as an annular lesion, a discrete nodular mass, or an ulcerative lesion, often with corresponding narrowing of the lumen. CT scan, with global vision of the abdomen, can contribute to staging of the tumour {1034, 1952} Endoscopic methods have the added advantage of being able to obtain a tissue diagnosis at the time of the procedure, but visualization of jejunal and ileal lesions can be challenging owing to the length of the small bowel. Duodenal tumours can be viewed by upper endoscopy, and ampullary tumours are best seen with a side-viewing endoscope. Distal ileal lesions may be seen on colonoscopy, and the proximal small-bowel mucosa may be visualized by push enteroscopy, but this will generally only reach 50–100 cm from the ligament of Treitz; double-balloon endoscopy is another method that allows viewing of the more distal small bowel {2012}. Capsule endoscopy has become a useful means of visualizing the entire length of the small bowel, and has proven an effective noninvasive method of diagnosing these tumours {2520}.

Macroscopy

The macroscopic pathology of small-bowel carcinomas is determined by a number of factors, of which stage and site are the most significant. Many carcinomas of the jejunum and ileum are detected at an advanced stage {334, 663, 3315}. Another determinant is the presence or absence of predisposing factors, namely, an associated adenoma, coeliac disease, Crohn disease, radiotherapy, previous surgery (notably pouch surgery and ileostomy), polyposis syndromes, Meckel diverticulum and intestinal duplication.

Most small-intestinal carcinomas are annular constricting tumours, but they may be protuberant and polypoid on occasion {663}. Jejunal and ileal carcinomas are usually relatively large, annular, constricting tumours with circumferential involvement of the wall of the intestine {334}. Most have already penetrated the muscularis propria at the time of presentation and there is often involvement of the serosal surface {663}. Adenocarcinoma of the ileum may mimic Crohn disease clinically, radiologically, endoscopically and at macroscopic pathological assessment {1245}. Conversely, adenocarcinoma is a recognized complication of small-intestinal Crohn disease, but it may be very difficult to identify the tumour in an area of severe intestinal Crohn disease {664}.

Duodenal carcinomas are usually more circumscribed, with a macroscopically demonstrable adenomatous component in 80% of cases {1663}. Thus, they are often protuberant or polypoid and the central carcinomatous component may show ulceration {663, 2137}. Carcinomas arising at the ampulla of Vater may cause obstructive jaundice before they have

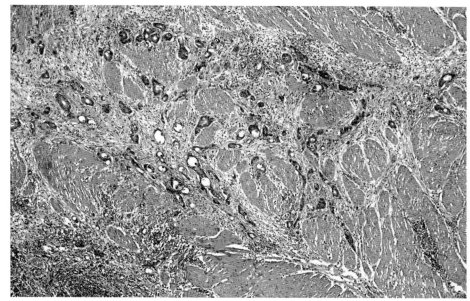

Fig. 6.03 Ileal adenocarcinoma, moderately differentiated, diffusely infiltrating the muscularis propria of the ileum.

reached a large size; they are usually circumscribed nodules measuring not more than 2–3 cm in diameter. They may be within the wall of the duodenum or project into the lumen as a polypoid nodule.

Unusual macroscopic features, such as a lack of ulceration, the predominance of an extramural component and the presence of multicentricity, should alert the pathologist to the possibility that the tumour is a metastasis.

Histopathology

Histologically, small-bowel carcinomas resemble their commoner counterparts in the colon and rectum. However, there are a higher proportion of poorly differentiated tumours {1731} and there is now good evidence that, despite morphological similarities, small-intestinal carcinomas show differing immunophenotypes. This is especially important in view of the difficulties in

differentiating primary small-bowel carcinoma from transcoelomic metastatic spread to the small bowel from a primary carcinoma of the colon. Small-intestinal carcinomas show a different keratin 7/keratin 20 profile, with 50% being positive for keratin 7 and about 40% being positive for keratin 20 {516, 1785}. AMACR/P504S immunostaining may also be helpful as this is commonly expressed in colorectal cancer but not in small-intestinal carcinoma {514}. Accurate diagnosis is important because the small-intestinal mucosa has a particular tendency to mimicry of a pre-existing adenoma, adjacent to invasive adenocarcinoma, when metastatic adenocarcinoma (especially from the colorectum) involves the small intestine. This phenomenon can give rise to the erroneous diagnosis of primary carcinoma of the small intestine {2924}.

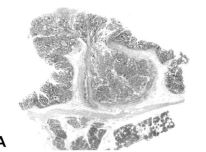
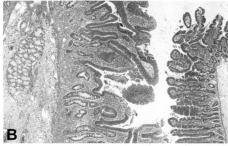

Fig. 6.04 A Tubulovillous adenoma of the duodenum and the ampulla of Vater, which is greatly distended. **B** Villous adenoma of the duodenum adjacent to normal mucosa.

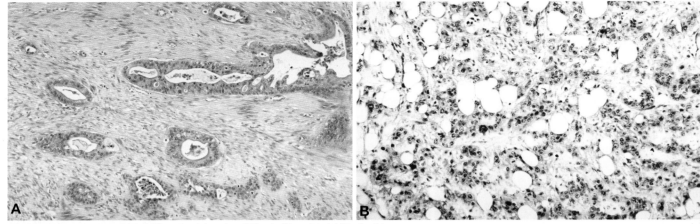

Fig. 6.05 Adenocarcinoma. **A** Well-differentiated, invasive. **B** Poorly differentiated, infiltrating fat.

Tumours arising at the ampulla of Vater display, not surprisingly, either intestinal or pancreaticobiliary phenotypes, both morphologically and immunohistochemically {553, 1091, 2714, 2885}. Immunohistochemical markers such as MUC proteins, trefoil peptides and keratin subtypes, especially keratins 7 and 20, can be used to help differentiate the two phenotypes. This is important for treatment and because the intestinal type has the better prognosis {2714}.

Even rarer types of carcinoma of the small intestine include adenosquamous carcinomas {1064, 2272, 2564}, carcinomas with a prominent neuroendocrine-cell component {1367} and those with tripartite differentiation, namely with glandular, squamous and endocrine components {199, 368}. Primary small cell carcinomas (poorly differentiated endocrine carcinomas) are especially rare {3670}.

Tumour spread and staging
The spread of small-bowel carcinomas is similar to that of the large bowel. Direct spread may cause adherence to adjacent structures in the peritoneal cavity, usually a loop of small intestine, although the stomach, colon or greater omentum may also be involved. Lymphatic spread to regional lymph nodes is common.
Haematogenous and transcoelomic spread also occur. Diffuse involvement of the ovaries, Krukenberg tumour, has been reported {1887}. Staging of carcinomas of the small intestine is by the TNM (tumour, node, metastasis) classification {875, 3534}. A separate TNM classification scheme is used for tumours of the ampulla of Vater because of the complicated anatomy of this site. Alternative staging systems have been proposed {3174}.

Grading
The system by which small-intestinal carcinomas are graded is identical to that used for the large bowel, namely, well-, moderately and poorly differentiated, or high- and low-grade.

Precursor lesions
Adenomas
There is good evidence for an adenoma–adenocarcinoma sequence in the small intestine as for the colon {1457, 2871, 3161}. Residual adenomatous tissue at the margins is seen in 42–65% of duodenal adenocarcinomas {1457, 3161}. Studies performed before the advent of advanced endoscopic techniques showed a high incidence of invasive adenocarcinoma among patients with small-bowel adenomas. For example, one study performed in 1982 reported invasive adenocarcinoma

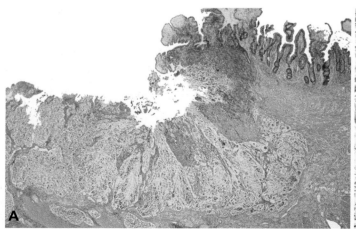
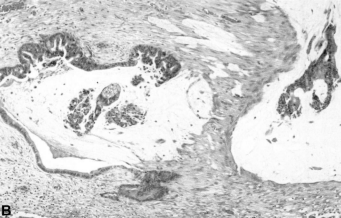

Fig. 6.06 Mucinous adenocarcinoma of the ileum arising in a patient with Crohn disease. **A** Large mucin-filled lakes. **B** More mucin than neoplastic epithelium.

in 65% of patients with small-intestinal adenomas {2534}. More recent studies, however, demonstrate a lower incidence, which is most likely related to the now commonplace practice of performing upper endoscopy in patients with non-specific symptoms. In a recent study by Catalano et al., invasive adenocarcinoma was found in only 6 out of 103 patients (5.8%) with duodenal adenomas {456}. As a result of the widespread use of endoscopy, the earliest stages of neoplastic change have been identified and characterized in adenomas of the duodenum and peri-ampullary region. In patients with FAP, random biopsy specimens of ileal mucosa show foci of abnormal, dysplastic crypts resembling dysplastic aberrant crypt foci of the colon in some patients, supporting the concept that, at least in patients with FAP, oligocryptal adenomas are a step in the development of epithelial neoplasms of the small intestine {247}. Similarly, biopsy of the proximal small-intestine in a group of FAP patients showed frequent microadenomas similar to those observed in *APC*-knockout (Min) mice {2588}. In patients with FAP and in patients with sporadic adenomas, increasing grades of dysplasia are identifiable adjacent to foci of early invasive adenocarcinoma {1457}.

Although adenomas can occur throughout the small intestine, the commonest site is the ampullary and peri-ampullary region {2854}. Adenomas can be multiple, a finding that should prompt evaluation of the patient for a polyposis syndrome.

Histologically, adenomas in the small intestine are similar to those in the colon, but with a propensity to be more villous or tubulovillous in architecture {2271, 3536}. The adenomatous cells resemble those of colonic adenomas, with varying degrees of dysplasia. Goblet cells are prevalent in most adenomas, and some lesions contain Paneth and endocrine cells {846, 2087}.

Intraepithelial neoplasia (dysplasia)

The incidence of small-intestinal adenocarcinoma is increased in patients with chronic inflammatory conditions affecting the small bowel, such as Crohn disease and coeliac disease {1058, 1422, 2038, 2061, 2626}. In patients with Crohn disease, invasive adenocarcinoma is preceded by intraepithelial neoplasia or dysplasia, which may appear either flat or polypoid endoscopically. In one study, dysplasia was identified adjacent to 75% of Crohn disease-associated small-intestinal adenocarcinomas {2966}. Histologically, the dysplasia seen in the small bowel appears similar to inflammatory bowel disease-associated colonic dysplasia.

Genetic susceptibility

Patients with FAP, *MUTYH* polyposis, Lynch syndrome, Peutz-Jeghers syndrome and juvenile polyposis all have an increased risk of developing small-intestinal carcinoma.

Molecular pathology

The relative rarity of small-intestinal adenocarcinoma means that the molecular pathology is poorly understood and the genetic abnormalities only partly characterized. There is uncertainty as to the similarities with large-intestinal carcinoma and the importance of the adenoma–carcinoma sequence, and the molecular abnormalities that underpin that sequence, in small-bowel carcinoma {277, 2871}. *APC* mutations are infrequent in small-bowel carcinoma {134, 3494} but over-expression of p53 is common {3494} and there is good evidence for the involvement of the Wnt signalling pathway {277}. Typical of adenocarcinomas in the gut, there is loss of E-cadherin expression, β-catenin gene (*CTNNB1*) mutation and β-catenin nuclear localization {2190, 3494}. Mutations of *SMAD4* and *KRAS* and activation of the RAS–RAF–MAPK pathway have all been described {134, 277}.

Between 10% and 25% of small-bowel carcinomas show a high level of microsatellite instability (MSI-H) and patients with these tumours have a better prognosis than do those with microsatellite-stable tumours {22, 351, 724, 1184, 2563, 2582, 2635, 3494}. Hypermethylation or loss of *MLH1* and *APC* has also been demonstrated {350, 3142}.

Prognosis and predictive factors

In a review of 4995 patients with small-bowel adenocarcinoma reported to the National Cancer Database (USA) between 1985 and 1995, the overall 5-year survival was 30.5% and median survival was 19.7 months. For stage I lesions, 5-year survival was 65% (median, > 60 months); stage II, 48% (median, 54.5 months); stage III, 35% (median, 29.8 months) and stage IV 4% (median, 9 months). Independent risk factors that significantly correlated with improved survival based upon multivariate analysis were age < 75 years, jejunal or ileal site (versus duodenal), well- or moderately differentiated tumours (relative to poorly differentiated), whether cancer-directed surgery was performed, and tumour stage (local vs regional, regional vs metastatic) {1256}. A study from the Swedish Cancer Registry of 926 patients with small-bowel adenocarcinoma between 1960 and 1988 found an overall 5-year survival of 24% for those with duodenal tumours and 28% for patients with jejunal and ileal tumours. Multivariate analysis revealed that female sex and treatment in the later years of the study (1985–1988) were significantly correlated with improved survival {3678}. In the SEER database for 1988–2001, in 1852 patients diagnosed with small-bowel adenocarcinoma, the median survival was 13.9 months and overall 5-year survival was 27%. For those with localized tumours, the 5-year survival rate was 57% (median, 50 months), regional disease was 34% (median, 22 months), and metastatic disease was 3% (median, 5 months) {1529}.

Neuroendocrine neoplasms of the small intestine

C. Capella
R. Arnold
D.S. Klimstra
G. Klöppel
P. Komminoth
E. Solcia
G. Rindi

Definition
Neoplasms with neuroendocrine differentiation including neuroendocrine tumours (NET) and neuroendocrine carcinomas (NEC) arising in the small intestine. Mixed adenoneuroendocrine carcinomas (MANEC) have an exocrine and an endocrine component, one of which exceeds 30%.

ICD-O codes
Neuroendocrine tumours (NET)
    NET G1 (carcinoid)   8240/3
    NET G2   8249/3
Neuroendocrine carcinoma (NEC) 8246/3
    Large cell NEC   8013/3
    Small cell NEC   8041/3
Mixed adenoneuroendocrine
  carcinoma (MANEC)   8244/3
Enterochromaffin cell (EC cell),
  serotonin-producing NET   8241/3
Gangliocytic paraganglioma   8683/0
Gastrinoma   8153/3
L cell, Glucagon-like peptide-producing
  and PP/PYY-producing NETs   8152/1
Somatostatin-producing NET   8156/3

Synonyms
Synonyms for intestinal NET include: carcinoid, well-differentiated endocrine tumour/carcinoma {3013}. Synonyms for NEC include: poorly differentiated endocrine carcinomas, high-grade neuroendocrine carcinoma, small cell and large cell endocrine carcinomas.

Classification
Intestinal NETs and NECs are classified on the basis of criteria common to all gastrointestinal and pancreatic neuroendocrine

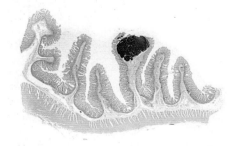

Fig. 6.07 Gastrinoma (gastrin-producing NET) displaying immunoreactivity to gastrin.

neoplasms (see Chapter 1). Neuroendocrine neoplasms of the small intestine exhibit site-related differences, depending on their location in the duodenum and proximal jejunum when compared with distal jejunum, ileum and Meckel diverticulum. For this reason, this chapter is divided into three parts. For details on tumours of the ampullary region, see Chapter 5.

Neuroendocrine neoplasms of the duodenum and proximal jejunum

Neuroendocrine neoplasms of the duodenum comprise NETs, including mainly somatostatin-producing and rare serotonin-producing (EC cell) NETs, rare NECs and MANECs, and the functional ("syndromic") gastrinoma.

Epidemiology
Incidence and time trends
Neuroendocrine neoplasms of the duodenum are rare, accounting for 5.7–7.9% of neuroendocrine neoplasms of the digestive system {1002, 3407}. The number of duodenal endocrine neoplasms showed a gradual and steady increase (57%) between 1986 and 2000 {2998}, which may partly reflect increased diagnosis of incidentally identified lesions as a result of the increased availability of advanced endoscopic and radiological imaging. Jejunal neoplasms account for about 1% of all gut neuroendocrine neoplasms {1002, 3407}. Of NETs, gastrinomas represent the largest group (62%) in reported series of neuroendocrine neoplasms arising in the upper small intestine, followed by somatostatin-producing NETs (18–21%), gangliocytic paragangliomas (9%), undefined neoplasms (5.6%) and pancreatic polypeptide (PP)-producing NETs (1.8%) {3011}. Approximately 50% of sporadic (non-inherited) gastrin-producing NETs (G cell NETs) are functioning (gastrinomas) and are associated with Zollinger-Ellison syndrome (ZES). Of all patients with a sporadic gastrinoma, about 60–75% of neoplasms are located in the duodenum, while in the remaining

patients the gastrinomas are found in the pancreas {1616}. In multiple endocrine neoplasia type 1 (MEN1)-associated ZES, the gastrinomas of most, if not all patients, are in the duodenum {119, 735, 2554}.

Age and sex distribution
Males are more frequently affected (male-to-female ratio, 1.5 : 1), with a mean age at presentation of 59 years {370}. Gastrin-producing NETs associated with ZES (gastrinomas) arise earlier in life than non-functioning NETs (mean age at diagnosis, 39 vs 66 years) {3011}. Somatostatin-producing NETs and gangliocytic paragangliomas are both almost equally distributed between the sexes and are usually diagnosed in the fourth or fifth decade of life {943, 3011}. Poorly differentiated neuroendocrine carcinomas (NECs) of the ampullary region (Chapter 5) are more common in men than women and present at a mean age of 70 years. The few non-ampullary NECs recorded in the literature occurred in males aged 57–69 years {2099, 2817}.

Etiology
For nonfamilial cases, little is known about possible etiological factors. A history of gastritis caused by *Helicobacter pylori* and long-term treatment with proton pump-inhibitors is significantly associated with an increased risk of sporadic duodenal gastrin-producing NETs (G cell NETs) and an increased density of G cells {2052}.

Localization
Most duodenal neuroendocrine neoplasms {370}, are located in the first and the second part, they are rare in the third and fourth part of the duodenum. Nonfunctioning gastrin-producing NETs are located in the duodenal bulb, while the site of gastrinomas associated with ZES is in the first, second or third part of the duodenum or in the upper jejunum {3011}. The preferential location of somatostatin-producing NETs, gangliocytic paragangliomas and NECs is at, or very close to, the ampulla of Vater (Chapter 5) {369, 372, 413, 1960, 3011, 3143, 3670}.

Very few cases of extra-ampullary somato-statin-producing NETs, gangliocytic para-gangliomas or poorly differentiated NEC in the duodenum have been reported {413, 943, 2099, 2817}.

Clinical features

Most neoplasms, especially those located in the duodenal bulb, are asymptomatic and are discovered incidentally, e.g. by imaging, endoscopy or pathological ex-amination of gastrectomy and duodeno-pancreatectomy specimens removed for gastric and pancreatic cancers. Neuro-endocrine neoplasms of the duodenum produce symptoms either by virtue of local infiltration causing haemorrhage, intestinal obstruction and obstructive jaundice (nonfunctioning neoplasms) or, less frequently, by secreted peptide hormones (functioning neoplasms). The localization of somatostatin-producing NETs, gangliocytic paragangliomas, and poorly differentiated neuroendocrine car-cinomas in the ampullary region explains their frequent association with obstructive biliary disease.

ZES with hypergastrinaemia, gastric hyper-secretion, and refractory peptic-ulcer disease, is the only syndrome of neuro-endocrine hyperfunction consistently observed in association with neuroendo-crine neoplasms of the duodenum and upper jejunum {370, 735, 1225, 3011, 3477}.

The association with ZES is found in about 40–50% of duodenal gastrin-producing NETs {1616, 3011}. Neoplasms associ-ated with overt ZES (gastrinomas) differ from their apparently nonfunctioning counterparts in arising earlier in life and having a higher incidence of metastatic and non-bulbar cases {3011}.

Well-differentiated serotonin-producing tumours (carcinoids) are unusual in the upper small intestine. It follows that duo-denal carcinoids only exceptionally give rise to the classical carcinoid syndrome, associated with liver metastases of the neoplasm {413, 3055}. In none of the cases of somatostatin-producing NETs so far reported did the patients develop "somatostatinoma" syndrome (diabetes mellitus, diarrhoea, steatorrhoea, hypo- or achlorhydria, anaemia and gallstones) that has been described in association with some pancreatic somatostatin-producing NETs {943, 3011}.

Macroscopy
NETs

NETs of the duodenum and upper jejunum usually form small (< 2 cm in diameter), grey, polypoid lesions within the submucosa with an intact or focally ulcerated overlying mucosa. However, some examples appear as infiltrative intramural nodules of rather large size (up to 5 cm in diameter). The neoplasms are multiple in about 13% of cases {370}. Gastrin-producing NETs tend to be smaller (0.8 cm) {413}, 1.8 cm for somato-statin-producing NETs {943, 3011, 3055} and 1.7 cm for gangliocytic paragan-gliomas {413}. The gastrinomas in MEN1 are multiple and tiny (sometimes < 1 mm in size) in contrast to sporadic gastrino-mas {118}.

NECs

NECs measure 2–4 cm and present as focally ulcerated, or protuberant lesions {3143, 3670} (Chapter 5).

Histopathology
NETs
Gastrin-producing NETs (G cell NETs). These neoplasms are formed by uniform cells with scant, lightly eosinophilic cytoplasm, arranged in broad gyriform trabeculae and vascular pseudorosettes. Tumour cells have uniform round nuclei containing stippled chromatin and incon-spicuous nucleoli. Necrosis is virtually never seen. Their proliferative index (Ki67) is usually between 2% and 10% {119} and thus G2 (Chapter 1). Angioinvasion is found in some cases. Immunohistochemi-cally, chromogranin A and gastrin are widely expressed. Other peptides detected in tumour-cell subpopulations are chole-cystokinin, PP, neurotensin, somatostatin, insulin, and the α chain of human chorionic gonadotropin {413}. Caudal-related home-obox 2 (CDX2) is positive in three quarters of cases {1706}. G cell NETs also express somatostatin receptors {2450}. Interest-ingly, somatostatin, which is known to inhibit the release of gastrin from gastrino-mas, is detected more frequently in non-functioning G cell NETs than in tumours associated with ZES {413}. MEN1-associ-ated gastrinomas display a multifocal G-cell and somatostatin-cell hyperplasia in the adjacent mucosa and/or Brunner glands, while sporadic G cell NETs lack such lesions {119}. Recently, it has been shown that, in addition to gastrinomas, multiple tiny somatostatin-producing NETs

can also arise in the duodenum of patients with MEN1 {119}. Electron microscopy reveals typical G cells with vesicular granules {413}.
Somatostatin-producing NETs. These neoplasms usually exhibit a predominant tubulo-glandular component admixed with a variable proportion of insular and trabecular areas {943}.
EC cell, serotonin-producing NETs. The classic "midgut EC cell carcinoid" is very rare both in the duodenum and upper jejunum {413}.
Gangliocytic paragangliomas. These neo-plasms appear as an infiltrative lesion composed of an admixture of three cell types: spindle cells, epithelial cells, and ganglion cells (see Chapter 5).

NECs

These aggressive neoplasms may assume the features of either small cell carcinoma or large cell carcinoma.

MANECs

MANECs are most frequently observed in the ampullary–periampullary region (Chapter 5).

Genetic susceptibility
MEN1

This inherited tumour syndrome is signifi-cantly associated with functioning gastrino-mas, but not with other types of NET of the duodenum and upper jejunum. Approxi-mately 25–33% of patients with gastrinomas develop these neoplasms in the setting of MEN1 {413}. The vast majority of these gastrinomas are located in the duodenum {2555}. Loss of heterozygosity (LOH) at the *MEN1* gene locus has been found in 4 out of 19 (21%) duodenal MEN1 gastrinomas {1908}, while a slightly higher rate of LOH on 11q13 for MEN1 gastrinomas (41%; 14 out of 34 neoplasms) was reported in an extended study of MEN1 and sporadic gastrinomas {684}. A low incidence of LOH on 11q13 in MEN1-associated gastrinomas suggests that these neoplasms could arise due to inactivation of the wild-type allele via point mutations or small deletions rather than via loss of a large segment of chromo-some 11 {1908}. Molecular analyses now enable a distinction to be made between hyperplastic G cell lesions and neoplastic lesions in the duodenum of patients with ZES–MEN1. LOH at the *MEN1* locus has been detected in about 50% of MEN1-associated gastrinomas {120}. Allelic loss was found in tiny (300 μm diameter)

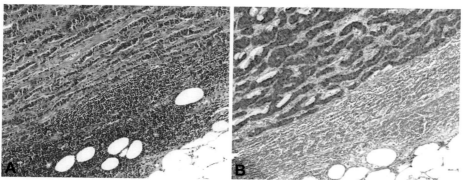

Fig. 6.08 Lymph-node metastasis from duodenal gastrinoma. The tumour cells form trabeculae (**A**) and are intensely immunoreactive for gastrin (**B**).

gastrinomas and (400 μm diameter) somatostatin-producing NETs, which therefore represented true neoplasms. On the contrary, LOH at 11q3 was not found in hyperplastic gastrin and somatostatin cells.

Neurofibromatosis type 1 (NF1)
Patients with von Recklinghausen disease are at significant risk of developing ampullary and periampullary NETs {372, 413, 1586, 3011} (Chapter 5).

Von Hippel-Lindau (VHL) disease
A very rare case in which VHL disease was associated with a duodenal functioning somatostatin-producing NET with a high level of plasma somatostatin has been reported, indicating that VHL-associated NETs of the digestive system occur not only in the pancreas {1480}.

Molecular pathology
In addition to MEN1-associated gastrinomas, the *MEN1* tumour suppressor gene is also involved in the pathogenesis of sporadic duodenal gastrinomas. LOH at the *MEN1* locus was found in 60% of sporadic duodenal gastrinomas {3662} and *MEN1* mutations were detected in 10–25% (40%) of sporadic duodenal gastrinomas {1003}. Mutations were clustered between amino acids 66–166, unlike in patients with familial MEN1.

TP53 mutations are a rare event in sporadic neuroendocrine neoplasms of the digestive system {3221}. β-Catenin mutations were reported in 8 out of 13 (61.5%) duodenal neuroendocrine neoplasms, with cytoplasmic and nuclear accumulation of β-catenin and overexpression of cyclin D1 (*CCND1*), in the absence of *APC* gene mutation. These results suggest that the Wnt pathway is involved in the development of duodenal

neuroendocrine neoplasms {913}, contrary to gastrointestinal NETs at other sites {3108}. Also, *APC* promoter methylation suggests a role for *APC* in Wnt activation {2561}. Methylation of the 5' region of the *CDKN2A* (*p16*) tumour-suppressor gene on chromosome 9p21 has been observed in 52% of gastrinomas, including duodenal ones {2881}. Interestingly, promoter methylation of *CDKN2A*, *APC*, *MEN1*, *HIC1* and *RASSF1A* genes occurs more frequently in gastrointestinal neuroendocrine neoplasms than in pancreatic neuroendocrine neoplasms {471}, indicating that the CpG island methylator phenotype (CIMP) is common among gastrointestinal neuroendocrine neoplasms {146}. Microsatellite instability did not occur in any of the gastrointestinal neuroendocrine neoplasms investigated {146}.

Incidental gastrin-producing (G cell) NETs do not overexpress either basic fibroblast growth factor (bFGF), acidic fibroblast growth factor (aFGF), transforming growth factor-α (TGFα), or their respective receptors FGFR4 and EGFR {1709}. On the contrary, these tumours overexpress the β-subunit of activin, which may be involved in regulating the proliferation of tumour cells {1708}.

Prognosis and predictive factors
The issue of TNM/Staging classification of neuroendocrine neoplasms is as yet unsettled. The classification recently proposed by the American Joint Committee on Cancer (AJCC) and the International Union Against Cancer (UICC) and embraced by WHO is for "carcinoid", i.e. well-differentiated lesions only. Conversely, the classification proposed by the European Neuroendocrine Tumor Society (ENETS) is also meant for high-grade neoplasms {2685}. In addition, it is divided for the upper and

lower intestine. Overall for the small intestine both classifications are substancially in agreement.

Recent studies have demonstrated the prognostic relevance of the newly proposed TNM classification system for foregut neuroendocrine neoplasms with statistical significance for stage and grade {2449}.

NETs
Gastrin-producing NETs (G cell NETs).
NETs with a low-grade malignant potential are those that invade beyond the submucosa or show lymph-node or distant (liver) metastases. Low-grade malignant NETs have been reported to comprise 10% of all G cell duodenal-upper jejunal NETs {413}, 58% of sporadic ZES cases {735} and 45% of ZES–MEN1 cases {735}. Gastrinomas associated with overt ZES are prognostically less favourable than their nonfunctioning counterparts, having a higher frequency of metastases, and being deeply infiltrative {3011}. These findings suggest that the natural history of G cell NETs is different for the two conditions. Nonfunctioning neoplasms represent a generally benign condition, while ZES neoplasms have a low-grade malignancy, especially when arising in sites where G cells are not normally present, such as in the jejunum or pancreas {413}. Metastases in regional lymph nodes have been reported in 4 out of 8 cases of duodenal gastrinomas with ZES–MEN1 syndrome {2555}, in 2 out of 3 cases of jejunal gastrinomas {413} and in 25% of 103 cases of duodenal neoplasms with ZES, 24% of which also had MEN1 syndrome {1225}.

Lymph-node metastases of gastrinomas may be much larger than the primary, which may be < 1 mm in size, and may erroneously be considered to be pancreatic

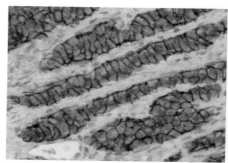

Fig. 6.09 Duodenal gastrinoma revealing immunoreactivity for somatostatin receptor 2A (SSTR2A); expression of SSTR2A is relevant for imaging and therapy.

neoplasms (especially if located at the upper margin of the head of the pancreas {735}), or as primary lymph-node gastrinomas {118}. Local lymph-node metastases seem to have little influence on survival of patients with ZES {689, 3477}. In a study focusing on metastatic rate and survival in patients with ZES, no difference was found in the frequency of metastases to lymph nodes {735}, when comparing primary pancreatic (48%) and duodenal (49%) neoplasms. In contrast, the same study found a significantly higher frequency of metastases to the liver in patients with pancreatic gastrinomas than in patients with duodenal gastrinomas (52% vs 5%). The 10-year survival rate of patients with duodenal gastrinomas (59%) is significantly better than for patients with pancreatic gastrinomas (9%) {3477}. The more favourable prognosis for patients with duodenal NETs is mainly linked to their smaller size and less frequent association with liver metastases.

Somatostatin-producing NETs. About two thirds of these neoplasms were reported as low-grade malignant in one study, despite their rather bland histological appearance {372, 666, 3011}.

Gangliocytic paragangliomas. Gangliocytic paragangliomas are usually benign, in contrast to G cell and somatostatin-producing NETs that arise in the same area. However, occasional large neoplasms (size, > 2 cm) may spread to local lymph nodes, mainly attributable to the endocrine component of the lesion {358, 1327} (see Chapter 5).

NECs

NECs are high-grade malignant, poorly differentiated carcinomas that display a high mitotic rate, tumour necrosis and usually deep mural invasion, angioinvasion, neuroinvasion, and poor survival {2099, 2254, 2817, 3670} (see Chapter 5).

Neuroendocrine neoplasms of the distal jejunum and ileum

Neuroendocrine neoplasms of this segment of the small intestine are only NETs (carcinoids), mainly EC cell, serotonin-producing NETs and, less frequently, L cell, glucagon-like peptide and PP/PYY (peptide YY)-producing NETs. NECs, poorly differentiated endocrine carcinomas, have not been reported.

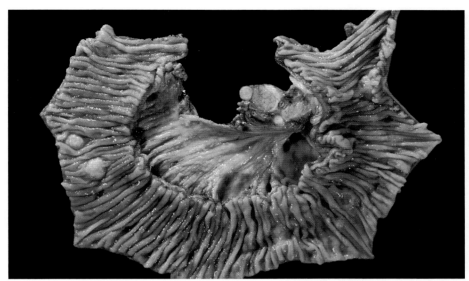

Fig. 6.10 Multiple enterochromaffin cell (EC cell, serotonin-producing) NET of the ileum with mesenteric lymph-node metastases.

Epidemiology
Incidence and time trends
The age-adjusted incidence of jejunum-ileum NETs is 0.4 and 3.2, respectively per 1 000 000 population {2854}. In the gastrointestinal tract, NETs occur predominantly in the small intestine (44.7%) followed in descending frequency by the rectum (19.6%), appendix (16.7%), colon (10.6%), and stomach (7.2%) {1951}. Most small-intestinal NETs occur in the ileum (49.9%). The incidence of ileal NETs increased from 52% in 1973–1977 to 63.6% in 1998–2002), while the incidence of adenocarcinomas has decreased from 18.6% in 1973–1977 to 12.2% in 1998–2002 {2111}.

Age and sex distribution
NETs of the distal jejunum and ileum are almost equally distributed between males and females. NETs are diagnosed between the third and the tenth decades of life, with a peak in the sixth and seventh decades {373, 1002, 2119, 3011}.

Etiology
Although neuroendocrine neoplasms of lower jejunum and ileum are not generally preceded by precursor lesions, there have been reports of focal microproliferations of EC cells in cases of multiple ileal neoplasms {2928} and of intraepithelial neuroendocrine cell hyperplasia in the mucosa adjacent to jejuno-ileal carcinoids {2172}.

Localization
In a series of 167 jejuno-ileal NETs, 70% were located in the ileum, 11% in the jejunum, 3% in Meckel diverticulum {373}. Most of these neoplasms are located in the distal ileum near the ileocaecal valve.

Clinical features
Patients with jejuno-ileal NETs present most commonly with intermittent crampy abdominal pain, suggestive of intermittent intestinal obstruction {2119}. Patients frequently have vague abdominal symptoms for several years before diagnosis, reflecting the slow growth rate of these neoplasms {2119}. Pre-operative diagnosis is difficult since standard imaging techniques rarely identify the primary tumour. Scintigraphic imaging with radiolabelled somatostatin analogues (octreotide) is widely used to localize previously undetected primary or metastatic lesions {1701}. The "carcinoid syndrome" is found in 5–7.7% of patients with EC cell serotonin-producing NETs {1002, 2119} that typically arise in the distal ileum and have already metastasized to the lymph nodes and the liver. Symptoms include cutaneous flushing, diarrhoea, and fibrous thickening of the endocardium and valves of the right heart.

Macroscopy
Jejuno-ileal NETs are multiple (2–100 neoplasms) in about 25–30% of cases {373, 2119, 3099}. Size is < 1 cm in 13% and < 2 cm in 47% of cases {373}. these neoplasms usually appear as mucosal–submucosal nodules with intact or slightly

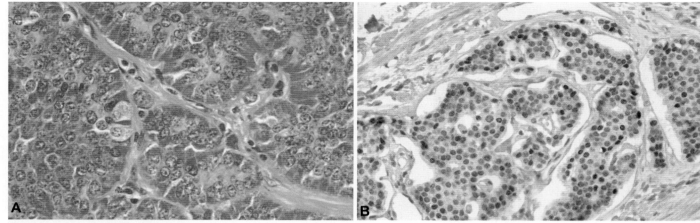

Fig. 6.11 Ileal enterochromaffin cell (EC cell) serotonin-producing NET. **A** The tumour is composed of cells with intense eosinophilic cytoplasm forming rounded nests with peripheral palisading. **B** Note the nuclear immunoreactivity for CDX2.

eroded overlying mucosa. Deep infiltration of the muscular wall and peritoneum is frequent. Extensive involvement of the mesentery associates with considerable fibroblastic or desmoplastic reaction, with consequent angulation and kinking of the bowel and obstruction of the lumen. Infarction of the involved loop of the small intestine may occur as a consequence of fibrous adhesions, volvulus, or occlusion of the mesenteric blood vessels.

Histopathology

Serotonin-producing (EC) cell NETs are composed of rounded nests of closely packed tumour cells that often show a typical peripheral palisading (Type A according to Soga & Tazawa) {3001}. Within the solid nests, rosette type, cribriform and glandular-like structures are frequently detected. The tumour cells are uniform, with little or no pleomorphism or mitotic activity. The proliferative index (Ki67-expressing cells) is very low at

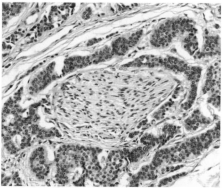

Fig. 6.12 Ileal enterochromaffin cell (EC cell), serotonin-producing NET. Note the invasion of the perineural space.

0–2% {405} and these neoplasms are thus G1 (see Chapter 1). In areas of deep invasion with abundant desmoplastic reaction, the cell nests may be oriented into cords and files. Mesenteric arteries and veins located near the neoplasm, or away from it, may be thickened and their lumen narrowed or even occluded by a peculiar elastic sclerosis, which may lead to ischaemic lesions in the intestine {127}. Most tumour cells are strongly positive with Masson Fontana argentaffin stain and strongly immunoreactive for chromogranin A and B and synaptophysin. In about 30% of cases, a variable number of cells is also reactive for prostatic acid phosphatase {373}.

In the majority of cases, most tumour cells express serotonin. A variety of other neurohormonal peptides or amines have been detected in these neoplasms {267, 1005, 1105, 1986, 3615}. Ileal serotonin-producing (EC) cell NETs and their metastases are positive for the transcription factor protein CDX2 {119} and > 90% of the neoplasms show membranous labelling for somatostatin receptor 2A {2450}. The tumour cells may also express galectin 4 {2757} and cyclooxygenase-2 (COX2) {1706}. In addition, carcinoembryonic antigen (CEA) is found in approximately 70% of neoplasms. Scattered between the tumour cells, S100-positive sustentacular cells may be observed {373}.

The rare jejuno-ileal NETs composed of glucagon-like peptide and PP/PYY-producing L cells feature a typical trabecular structure and an immunoprofile similar to the corresponding colorectal and appendiceal NETs (see Chapters 7 and 8).

Genetic susceptibility

Unlike gastric ECL cell tumours and duodenal G cell NETs, jejuno–ileal carcinoids are only occasionally associated with MEN1 {2431}. Rare examples of familial occurrence of ileal EC cell carcinoids have been reported {2117}.

Molecular pathology

In a microarray analysis performed to identify differentially expressed genes in pancreatic neuroendocrine neoplasms and gastrointestinal NETs (mainly represented by ileal invasive NETs), ileal neoplasms exhibited a gene-expression profile that was significantly different from that of pancreatic neuroendocrine neoplasms {1799}.

Comparative genomic hybridization (CGH) studies of ileal NETs have demonstrated losses of chromosome 9p, 18p, and 18q in 21%, 38%, and 33% of case respectively {3268, 3704}, gains of chromosome 17q and 19p in 57% of cases {3268} and LOH of chromosome 18 has been detected in 88% of ileal NETs {1888}. Furthermore, 22% of ileal NETs showed losses of 16q21 and an accumulation of genetic abnormalities mainly involving a loss of chromosome 16q and gain of chromosome 4p was found in metastases. High-resolution analysis of genetic alterations by single nucleotide polymorphism confirmed that loss of all or most of chromosome 18 was the most frequent aberration in ileal NETs {1546}; this strongly suggests that important candidate genes are located on this chromosome. In addition, losses of chromosome 18 are rare in bronchial and pancreatic neuroendocrine neoplasms, suggesting a different genetic background for these group of neoplasms {1888, 3221, 3704}.

In contrast to foregut (gastric, duodenal and pancreatic) NETs, which show frequent deletions and mutations of the *MEN1* gene, midgut (mainly ileal) NETs rarely show involvement of *MEN1* {683, 3253}. Mutations in *APC* but not in the β-catenin gene (*CTNNB1*) were found in ileal NETs showing nuclear translocation of β-catenin {2561}. Homeobox gene *HOXC6* is upregulated in ileal NETs {912}. Interestingly, *HOXC6* has been reported as target of the *MEN1* gene and also upregulates *CTGF*, which encodes an important growth factor in ileal NETs {912, 1537}.

Accumulation of p53 has not been detected in EC cell NETs examined immunohistochemically, suggesting that this tumour-suppressor gene is not implicated in the pathogenesis of these neoplasms {3011, 3441, 3478}.

Several growth factors, such as TGFα and IGF1, exert a proliferative effect reflected by an increased mitotic index and significantly increased DNA levels in primary cell cultures of ileal NETs, suggesting the involvement of an autocrine loop {44}. PDGF, TGFα, bFGF, and aFGF seem to be mainly involved in tumour stromal reaction, including stromal desmoplasia {44, 1703, 1709}, by acting on receptors expressed on fibroblasts or stimulating the promotion of new vasculature and tumour progression {44, 1703, 1709}. In particular, EC cell NETs overexpress CTGF and TGFβ mRNA and synthesize CTGF and TGFβ proteins that are significantly elevated in patients with clinically documented fibrosis {1537}.

Neural adhesion molecule (NCAM/CNTN6), a member of the immunoglobulin superfamily of cell-adhesion molecules, is highly expressed in ileal NETs {44}. Because NCAM has not been shown in normal gut neuroendocrine cells, the novel expression of this adhesion molecule in carcinoids may be of importance for growth and metastases. Overexpression of snail and sonic hedgehog in NETs of the ileum has been related to their metastatic spread, by a mechanism that leads to downregulation of E-cadherin {833}.

Prognosis and predictive factors

The main criteria for considering a jejuno-ileal carcinoid to have malignant behaviour are deep invasion of the wall (muscularis propria or beyond) and/or presence of metastases. According to these criteria, 141 out of 159 cases (89%) of jejuno-ileal carcinoids in a large series were considered malignant {373}. The mortality rate was 21% for jejuno-ileal EC cell, serotonin-producing NETs (carcinoids) compared with 4% for duodenal, 6% for gastric, and 3% for rectal carcinoids {373}. The overall 5-year survival rate for patients with jejuno–ileal NETs is about 60% and the 10-year survival rate is 43% {373, 3099}. In patients without liver metastases, the 5- and 10-year survival rates are about 72% and 60%, respectively, as opposed to 35% and 15% for patients with liver metastases {3099}, demonstrating the relatively slow rate of growth of some EC cell, serotonin-producing NETs. SEER data for 1973–2002 show that 5-year survival rates for small-intestinal NETs have remained unchanged over 30 years in the USA {2111}. Metastases are generally confined to regional lymph nodes and liver. Extra-abdominal metastases are very rare {2119}.

Tumour stage is the most important predictor of survival. Patients with NETs and a low Ki67 index live longer than those with a high Ki67 index {149}, indicating the importance of a proliferation-based grading system (see Chapter 1). Jejuno-ileal NETs that are clinically nonfunctioning, 1 cm or less in diameter and confined to the mucosa/submucosa are generally cured by complete local excision, but invasion beyond the submucosa or metastatic spread indicates that the lesion is malignant. The malignant potential is retained for ileal NETs > 1 cm but confined to the mucosa/submucosa.

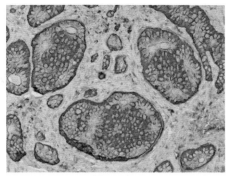

Fig. 6.13 Ileal enterochromaffin cell (EC cell), serotonin-producing NET displaying diffuse immunoreactivity for chromogranin A.

Neuroendocrine tumours of Meckel diverticulum

EC cell, serotonin-producing NETs occur rarely in Meckel diverticulum; 174 cases have been reported {2116}. Meckel NETs prevail in males (three quarters of cases), with a reported age ranging from 14 months to 82 years. About half of the patients present with symptoms such as abdominal pain, nausea, diarrhoea, vomiting and haematochezia and already have metastases {2289}. Because of their considerable metastatic capacity, symptomatic NETs of Meckel diverticulum have been equated to jejuno-ileal carcinoids {2171}. In contrast, tumours detected incidentally in asymptomatic patients are usually not metastatic and are small in size (< 1.7 cm). Histologically, Meckel NETs, like ileal NETs, show a characteristic type A pattern of growth, strong and diffuse expression of neuroendocrine markers and serotonin.

B-cell lymphoma of the small intestine

S. Nakamura
H.K. Müller-Hermelink
J. Delabie
Y.H. Ko
E.S. Jaffe

Definition

Primary small-intestinal B-cell lymphoma is defined as an extranodal B-cell lymphoma arising in the small bowel with the bulk of disease localized to this site. Contiguous lymph-node involvement and distal spread may be seen, but the primary clinical presentation is the small or large intestine, with therapy directed to this site.

ICD-O codes

Burkitt lymphoma	9687/3
B-cell lymphoma, unclassifiable, with features intermediate between diffuse large B-cell lymphoma and Burkitt lymphoma	9680/3
Diffuse large B-cell lymphoma (DLBCL)	9680/3
Immunoproliferative small-intestinal disease (IPSID)	9764/3
Follicular lymphoma	9690/3
Marginal zone lymphoma of mucosa-associated lymphoid tissue (MALT lymphoma)	9699/3
Mantle cell lymphoma	9673/3

Epidemiology

In contrast to lymphomas involving the stomach, primary small-intestinal B-cell lymphomas are uncommon in North America, European and Asian countries {1622, 2219}. However, since epithelial and mesenchymal tumours are uncommon in the small bowel, lymphomas constitute a significant proportion (30–50%) of all malignant tumours at this site. The most frequent histological type among intestinal B-cell lymphomas is diffuse large B-cell lymphoma (DLBCL), which accounts for 40–60% of cases in North America, European and Asian countries {733, 1622, 2219}. Extranodal marginal-zone lymphomas of mucosa-associated lymphoid tissue (MALT lymphomas) are also common lymphomas in the small intestine and colorectum (3–28%).

Immunoproliferative small-intestinal disease (IPSID) is a unique form of intestinal MALT lymphoma that occurs predominantly in the Middle East and Mediterranean. This entity represents part of a spectrum of small-intestinal lymphoproliferations, including α heavy-chain disease (αHCD) and may represent different manifestations or phases of the same disease. IPSID or αHCD occurs predominantly in the Mediterranean area, but may be seen outside this region. It typically affects young adults, while small-intestinal lymphomas in North America and Europe increase in frequency with age, with peak incidence in the seventh decade of life. Most studies have shown a slight predominance in males and an association with lower socioeconomic status {733}.

Burkitt lymphoma occurs in two major forms, defined as endemic and sporadic. Endemic Burkitt is found primarily in Africa and typically presents in the jaw, orbit or paraspinal region, and is strongly associated with infection with Epstein-Barr virus (EBV). In other endemic regions, however, it is relatively common for Burkitt lymphoma to present in the small intestine, usually involving the ileum, with preferential localization to the ileocaecal region. In parts of the Middle East, primary gastrointestinal Burkitt lymphoma is a common disease of children. Sporadic or non-endemic Burkitt lymphoma is a rare disease, not associated with EBV infection, which frequently presents as primary intestinal lymphoma. Burkitt lymphoma is also seen in the setting of infection with human immunodeficiency virus (HIV), where it often involves the gastrointestinal tract {420}.

Etiology

Infection by *Campylobacter jejuni* has shown to be associated with IPSID {1776}. Response to treatment with antibiotics is typical of the early phases of this disease. Chronic inflammatory bowel disease, including Crohn disease and ulcerative colitis, are also risk factors for intestinal B-cell lymphomas, some of which may be associated with iatrogenic immunosuppression and EBV {3350}. Some of these cases may resemble classical Hodgkin lymphoma {1677}. However, the risk for development of lymphoma is much less than that associated with coeliac disease and the development of primary T-cell lymphomas of the small bowel. An increased incidence of lymphoma has also been associated with both acquired and congenital immunodeficiency states,

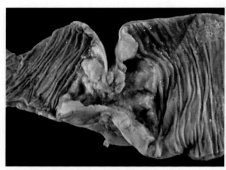

Fig. 6.14 DLBCL of the small intestine. The gross specimen shows a large ulcerating tumour with luminal stricture.

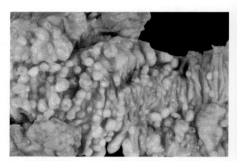

Fig. 6.15 Multiple lymphomatous polyposis with typical polypoid mucosa.

including congenital immune deficiency, iatrogenic immunodeficiency associated with solid-organ transplantation, and acquired immuno-deficiency syndrome (AIDS) {626}. In general, lymphomas associated with immunodeficiency show a predilection for extranodal sites, particularly the gastrointestinal tract, irrespective of the cause of the immunodeficiency {1337, 1817}.

Clinical features

Symptoms produced by small-intestinal lymphomas depend upon the specific histological type. Indolent lymphomas of B-cell lineage typically present with abdominal pain, weight loss and bowel obstruction {733}. Occasional cases present with nausea and vomiting; rarely, cases are discovered incidentally. More aggressive tumours, such as Burkitt lymphoma, may present as a large intra-abdominal mass or acutely with intestinal perforation. IPSID often manifests as abdominal pain, chronic severe intermittent diarrhoea and weight loss. The diarrhoea is mainly the result of steatorrhoea, and a protein-losing enteropathy can be seen. Peripheral oedema, tetany and clubbing are observed in as many as 50% of patients. Rectal bleeding is uncommon in small-bowel lymphoma, but is a common presenting sign in primary colonic lymphoma. Burkitt lymphoma is most frequently seen in the terminal ileum or ileocaecal region, and may cause intussusception.

Imaging and endoscopy

Radiological studies are useful adjuncts to the diagnosis of small-intestinal lymphomas, including computed tomography (CT) and positron emission tomography (PET) scans. Most B-cell lymphomas manifest as exophytic or annular tumour masses in the ileum. Follicular lymphoma, mantle cell lymphoma, and MALT lymphoma may produce nodules or polyps that can be seen both endoscopically and by imaging. Most small-intestinal lymphomas are localized to one anatomic site, but multifocal tumours are detected in approximately 8% of cases.

Multiple lymphomatous polyposis (MLP) consists of numerous polypoid lesions throughout the gastrointestinal tract. Most often, the jejunum and terminal ileum are involved, but lesions can appear in the stomach, duodenum, colon, and rectum. This entity produces a characteristic radiological picture that is virtually diagnostic. Most such cases have been considered to be caused by mantle-cell lymphoma, but other subtypes of lymphoma, such as follicular lymphoma and MALT lymphoma, may produce a similar radiological or endoscopic pattern {1626}.

The macroscopic appearance of IPSID depends on the stage of disease. Early on, the bowel may appear endoscopically normal, with infiltration apparent only on intestinal biopsy. The disease may then progress to thickening of the upper jejunum together with enlargement of the mesenteric lymph nodes and the development of lymphomatous masses. Typically, the spleen is not involved and may even be small and fibrotic, as described for coeliac disease. Distal spread beyond the abdomen is uncommon {1342}.

Histopathology
DLBCL

DLBCL, with or without a MALT lymphoma component, is the dominant type of non-Hodgkin lymphoma of the small intestine. The histological features of small intestinal DLBCL are similar to those of gastric DLBCL. In contrast to gastric lymphomas, DLBCLs arising in the small bowel are much commoner than low-grade B-cell lymphomas of MALT type. Some intestinal DLBCLs may be associated with follicular lymphoma, which most often can be seen in mesenteric lymph nodes. Focal areas of follicular lymphoma may also be present in the intestine, but such cases are considered as nodal lymphomas with spread to the intestine.

MALT lymphoma

The relative frequency of MALT lymphoma (other than IPSID) is much lower in the small intestine than the stomach. The histological features of small-intestinal MALT lymphoma are similar to those of gastric MALT lymphoma, except that lymphoepithelial lesions are less prominent.

IPSID/αHCD

IPSID and αHCD are synonyms for a subtype of small-intestinal MALT lymphoma The histology of this subtype is characteristic of MALT lymphoma with marked plasma-cell differentiation. Three stages of IPSID are recognized.

In stage A, the lymphoplasmacytic infiltrate is confined to the mucosa and mesenteric lymph nodes, and cytological atypia is not present. Although the infiltrate may obliterate the villous architecture, the endoscopic examination appears normal. This phase of the disease is typically responsive to antibiotic therapy.

In stage B, nodular mucosal infiltrates develop and there is extension below the muscularis mucosae. The characteristic features of MALT lymphoma are evident and follicular colonization may be marked. A minimal degree of cytological atypia is apparent. This stage appears to represent a transitional phase. Thickening of mucosal folds can be seen macroscopically, and at this stage, the disease is typically not curable with antibiotics.

Stage C is characterized by the presence of large masses and transformation to DLBCL. Numerous immunoblasts and plasmablasts are present. Marked cytological atypia is found, including Reed-Sternberg-like cells. Mitotic activity is increased. Mesenteric lymph-node involvement occurs early in the course of disease, with infiltration of nodal sinuses and marginal-zone areas. Immunohistochemical studies demonstrate the production of α heavy chain without light-chain synthesis {1342}. IgA produced is almost always of the IgA1 type, with intact carboxy-terminal regions and deletion of most of the V and all of the CH1 domains.

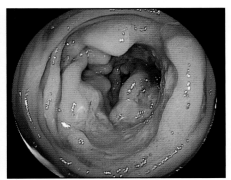

Fig. 6.16 DLBCL of the small intestine. Double-balloon endoscopy reveals a large ulcerating tumour without epithelial irregularity or luminal stricture.

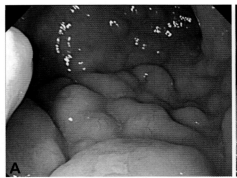
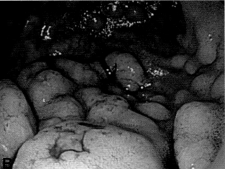

Fig. 6.17 Mantle cell lymphoma of the duodenum with multiple lymphomatous polyposis. **A** Endoscopic appearance. **B** The spraying of indigo carmine highlights the presence of multiple lymphomatous polyposis.

The molecular characterization of individual cases is variable. The small lymphoma cells express CD19 and CD20, but fail to express CD5, CD10 and CD23, while the plasmacytic-cell component may only express plasma-cell markers such as CD138.

Mantle cell lymphoma

Mantle cell lymphoma typically involves both spleen and intestines and may present as an isolated mass or as multiple polyps throughout the gastrointestinal tract where it is referred to as multiple lymphomatous polyposis (MLP) {733, 2174}. Mantle cell lymphoma frequently expresses α-4-β-7 integrin that facilitates homing to the gut. Importantly, other histological subtypes of non-Hodgkin lymphoma, such as follicular lymphoma and MALT lymphoma, can also produce MLP. The polyps range in size from 0.5 cm to 2 cm, with much larger polyps found in the ileocaecal region.

The histology of mantle cell lymphoma involving the small bowel is identical to that involving nodal sites {188}. The architecture is most frequently diffuse, but a nodular pattern and a less common true mantle-zone pattern are also observed. Reactive germinal centres may be found and are usually compressed by the surrounding lymphoma cells, thereby appearing to replace the normal mantle zones. Intestinal glands may be destroyed by the lymphoma, but typical lymphoepithelial lesions are not seen. The low-power appearance is monotonous, with frequent epithelioid histiocytes, mitotic figures and fine sclerosis surrounding small blood vessels. The lymphoma cells are small to medium sized with irregular nuclear outlines, indistinct nucleoli and scant amounts of cytoplasm. Large transformed cells are typically not present. The lymphoma cells are mature

B cells and express both CD19 and CD20. Characteristically the cells weakly co-express CD5 and CD43. Surface immunoglobulins found include both IgM and IgD. Light-chain restriction is present in most cases, with some studies demonstrating a predominance of λ. CD10 and CD11c are virtually always negative. Cyclin D1 is found in virtually all cases and can be demonstrated within the nuclei of the neoplastic lymphocytes in paraffin sections. Rare cases of mantle cell lymphoma that are cyclin D1-negative may be identified by *SOX11* overexpression {2175}.

Follicular lymphoma

Follicular lymphoma occurs in the small intestine, and involvement of the duodenum is a frequent feature {2824, 2838}. Intestinal follicular lymphoma is predominantly found in the second portion of the duodenum, presenting as multiple small polyps, often as an incidental finding on endoscopy performed for other reasons. Recent developments in small-intestinal endoscopies, such as double-balloon or capsule endoscopy, have revealed that the jejunum and ileum are also frequently affected by follicular lymphoma, usually presenting as MLP {1625, 2221}. Morphology is sometimes characterized by glove balloon-like villous hypertrophy caused by extrafollicular infiltration of lymphoma cells. The immunophenotype and genetic features are similar to those of nodal follicular lymphomas. The lymphoma cells co-express CD10, BCL2, and BCL6, but not CD5 or CD43. The expression of BCL2 in conjunction with strong CD10 is useful for distinction from reactive follicles and primary follicles, or marginal zone hyperplasia. MIB1 shows a low proliferation rate. Immunostaining to highlight follicular dendritic cells (antibodies to CD21, CD23 or CD35) help to reveal the unusually

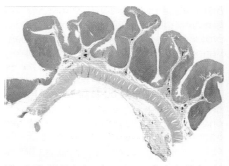

Fig. 6.18 Multiple lymphomatous polyposis. Polypoid mantle cell lymphoma.

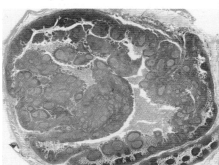

Fig. 6.19 Primary intestinal follicular lymphoma arising in the jejunum.

diminished distribution of follicular dendritic-cell networks, in contrast to nodal counterparts {3162}. Most patients have localized disease (stage IE or IIE), and survival appears to be excellent, even without treatment. This localized polypoid form of follicular lymphoma appears to have a very low risk of extra-intestinal disease.

In contrast to the very localized and limited involvement shown by some intestinal follicular lymphomas, more extensive involvement by primary nodal follicular lymphoma also can be seen, associated with mesenteric lymph-node involvement. These more typical cases of follicular lymphoma present with bulky disease. All cytological grades may be seen: grades 1–2, and grade 3A, or grade 3B. Progression to DLBCL is present in some cases.

Burkitt lymphoma

The histology in all cases is identical and is characterized by a diffuse infiltrate of medium-sized cells with round to oval nuclear outlines, two to five small but distinct nucleoli and a small amount of intensely basophilic cytoplasm. Numerous mitotic figures and apoptotic cells are present. The prominent "starry-sky" appearance is caused by benign phagocytic histiocytes engulfing the nuclear debris resulting from apoptosis. Unusually for

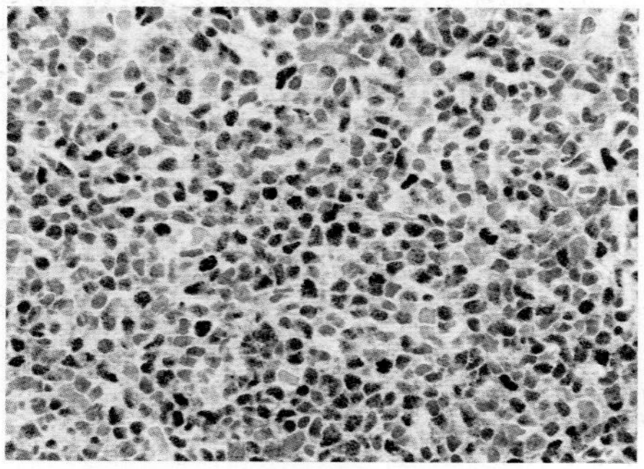

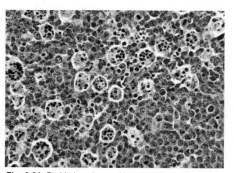

Fig. 6.20 Mantle cell lymphoma. Immunostaining for cyclin D1 shows nuclear positivity.

Fig. 6.21 Burkitt lymphoma. Note the "starry-sky" effect caused by phagocytic histiocytes.

lymphomas, thin sections often show that the cytoplasmic borders of individual cells "square off" against each other; this indicates a mature B-cell lymphoma and the neoplastic cells express pan-B-cell antigens CD19, CD20, CD22, and CD79a. The neoplastic cells co-express CD10, but fail to express CD5 or CD23. Expression of surface immunoglobulins is moderately intense and is nearly always IgM with either κ or λ light-chain restriction. The growth fraction, as assessed by Ki67 or MIB1, is nearly 100% of tumour cells. Burkitt lymphoma cells show positivity for BCL6, but uniformly fail to express BCL2.

B-cell lymphoma, unclassifiable, with features intermediate between DLBCL and Burkitt lymphoma

Most tumours in this group have morphological features that are intermediate between Burkitt lymphoma and DLBCL. Some of these cases were previously classified as Burkitt-like lymphoma. Other cases may be morphologically more typical of Burkitt lymphoma, but have an atypical immunophenotype or genetic features that preclude a diagnosis of Burkitt lymphoma. Unlike Burkitt lymphoma, these lymphomas do not have a predilection for the gastrointestinal tract of adults. They also occur in the setting of HIV infection.

Other B-cell lymphomas

Although rare, any type of B-cell lymphoma other than those described can present as a primary small-intestinal lymphoma.
Indolent lymphomas such as small lymphocytic lymphoma and lymphoplasmacytic lymphoma can present as primary small-intestinal disease.
Lymphoblastic lymphoma in rare cases may present as a mass in the ileocaecal region. Characteristic nuclear features and the expression of terminal nucleotidyl transferase may aid in establishing the diagnosis.

Molecular pathology
DLBCL

In primary intestinal DLBCL, translocations involving *IGH@*, *BCL6*, *BCL2*, and *MYC* are detected in 27%, 23–35%, 0–21%, and 7% of cases, respectively {3649}. *BIRC3-MALT1* translocation has been reported only a single case {3649}.

MALT lymphoma

t(11;18)(q21;q21)/*BIRC3-MALT1* is found in one third of patients, with different frequencies found in primary and secondary intestinal MALT lymphomas (12.5% vs 57%) {3095}. t(1;14)(p22;q32)/*BCL10-IGH@* and trisomy 3 or 18 are detected in 12.5% and 81% of primary intestinal MALT lymphomas, respectively, these frequencies being higher than those for gastric and secondary intestinal MALT lymphomas {3095}.

IPSID

No cytogenetic abnormalities have been consistently described in IPSID. Southern-blot analysis reveals clonal immunoglobulin heavy-chain (*IGH@*) gene rearrangements.

Mantle cell lymphoma

Mantle cell lymphoma is cytogenetically characterized by a t(11;14)(q13;q32) translocation that deregulates expression of the cyclin D1 (*CCND1*) oncogene on chromosome 11.

Follicular lymphoma

Follicular lymphoma is cytogenetically characterized by the t(14;18)(q34;q21) translocation and *BCL2* gene rearrangement. Primary intestinal follicular lymphoma also features a high load of (ongoing) somatic mutations and a biased use of *VH* genes, in particular *VH4*, suggesting a similar etiology to that of MALT lymphoma {2824, 3162}.

Burkitt lymphoma

In most cases, Burkitt lymphoma demonstrates a consistent cytogenetic abnormality that causes rearrangement of the *MYC* oncogene. The characteristic translocation is t(8;14)(q24;q32), in which *MYC* is translocated from chromosome 8 to the *IGH@* locus on chromosome 14.
The remaining cases show variant translocations including the immunoglobulin light-chain loci, t(2;8)(p12;q24) or t(8;22)-(q24;q11), involving κ and λ light-chain genes, respectively. Thus part of the light-chain constant region is translocated to chromosome 8, distal to the *MYC* gene. *MYC* is deregulated by virtue of its juxtaposition to the immunoglobulin light-chain genes.
The molecular characteristics of the *MYC* translocation also differ between endemic and sporadic cases. In endemic Burkitt lymphoma, the (variable) chromosome 8

break-points are usually far 5' of *MYC*, while their chromosome 14 break-points most often occur in the location of the joining segments (*IGHJ@*); it is thus impossible in most cases to demonstrate such rearrangements by Southern-blot analysis. In contrast, sporadic cases frequently have *MYC* break-points within noncoding introns and exons of the gene itself (typically the first exon or intron, or the 5' flanking regions); such rearrangements can be usually be detected by Southern blot {1126}. Fluorescence *in situ* hybridization (FISH) using break-apart probes for *MYC* detects most translocations. In cases lacking *MYC* rearrangements, aberrations in *MYC*-regulating miRNAs have been found {1808A}.

B-cell lymphoma, unclassifiable, with features intermediate between DLBCL and Burkitt lymphoma

This category is cytogenetically heterogeneous and may contain three or more biological groups {2342}. Cases may be double- or triple-hit lymphomas having translocations involving *MYC*, *BCL2*, and/or less frequently *BCL6*, and often show a complex karyotype with multiple abnormalities, in contrast to classical Burkitt lymphoma {3260}.

Prognosis and predictive factors
The main determinant of clinical outcome for small-intestinal lymphomas is histological type {733}. Advanced age at diagnosis, an acute presentation with perforation, and the presence of multifocal tumours have an adverse impact on survival. The prognostic impact of concomitant MALT lymphoma for the behaviour of DLBCL is controversial {733, 2220}.
Mantle cell lymphoma is an aggressive neoplasm. A blastoid cytology, increased mitotic index and peripheral-blood involvement are recognized as adverse factors {144}. Mutations in *TP53* and homozygous deletions of *CDKN2A* have recently been shown to be associated with poor prognosis {1177, 1899}. Patients with intermediate lymphoma between DLBCL and Burkitt lymphoma, which show dual translocations of both *BCL2* and *MYC*, have markedly shortened overall survival {1942, 3260}.

T-cell lymphoma of the small intestine

H.K. Müller-Hermelink
J. Delabie
Y.H. Ko
E.S. Jaffe
S. Nakamura

Definition

An intestinal lymphoma, most often derived from intraepithelial T lymphocytes, occurring as one of two subtypes: enteropathy-associated T-cell lymphoma (EATL) (about 80–90% of cases) and monomorphic CD56+ (NCAM1) intestinal T-cell lymphoma (about 10–20% of cases). Adjacent small intestinal mucosa may show villous atrophy with crypt hyperplasia, as well as increase of intra-epithelial lymphocytes and/or lymphoma cells {540, 542}.

ICD-O codes

T-cell lymphoma   9702/3
Enteropathy-associated T-cell
  lymphoma (EATL)   9717/3

Synonyms

Intestinal T-cell lymphoma (with and without enteropathy). Since different T-cell lymphoma subtypes can present with intestinal disease – extranodal natural killer/T-cell (NK/T-cell) lymphoma, γ-δ T-cell lymphoma, anaplastic large cell lymphoma, peripheral T-cell lymphoma unspecified – this term can be used only descriptively in the setting of incomplete information and does not imply a disease entity.

Enteropathy-associated intestinal T-cell lymphoma (EATL)

Definition

EATL is an intestinal tumour of intra-epithelial T-lymphocytes composed of large, often polymorphic lymphoid cells, which are negative for CD56. It is also referred to as Type I EATL

Epidemiology

The disease is uncommon in most parts of the world, but is seen with increasing frequency in areas with a high prevalence of coeliac disease, e.g. Northern Europe. Conversely, EATL is extremely rare in the oriental population where coeliac disease is also rare. The relative risk of EATL in the small intestine is increased approximately

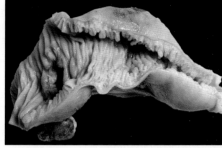

Fig. 6.22 Intestinal T-cell lymphoma. Surgical specimen showing intestinal perforation and severe acute peritonitis.

1020-fold in patients with protracted clinical coeliac disease {2536, 2854}. In a population-based registry of the Netherlands, the annual incidence of EATL of the small intestine is estimated at 0.1 per 100 000 overall and 2.08 per 100 000 in persons aged > 50 years, with a male-to-female ratio of almost 3 : 1 in this age group. The mean age at presentation is 64 years {3392}.

Etiology

This neoplasm is usually manifest in patients with human leukocyte antigen (HLA) haplotypes predisposing to coeliac disease. Histopathological findings suggest an association with coeliac disease that is confirmed by positive serological tests with anti-gliadin and anti-transglutaminase antibodies, HLA-DQ2 or HLA-DQ8 expression and associated clinical findings such as dermatitis herpetiformis and hyposplenism {720, 2785, 3368}. Overexpression of interleukin 15 by enterocytes in coeliac disease may play a role in the continuous stimulation of intraepithelial lymphocytes {2047}.

Localization

The lymphoma occurs most commonly in the jejunum or proximal ileum. Presentation in the duodenum, stomach and colon or outside the gastrointestinal tract may occur but is rare {540}.

Clinical features

A small proportion of patients with EATL have a history of childhood-onset coeliac disease. Most show adult-onset disease

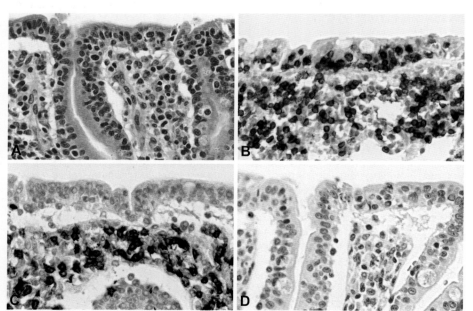

Fig. 6.23 Uninvolved mucosa adjacent to enteropathy-associated T-cell lymphoma (type I EATL). The intraepithelial lymphocytes (**A**) may show an abnormal immunophenotype, with increased numbers being: **B** Positive for CD3; **C** Negative for CD8; and **D** Negative for CD56 (NCAM).

or are diagnosed as having coeliac disease in the same clinical episode in which the lymphoma is diagnosed. Undetected coeliac disease has a higher prevalence in the elderly population than in the population in general (2.45% vs < 1%) {3406}. Patients present with abdominal pain, most often as emergencies associated with intestinal perforation and/or obstruction. In a proportion of patients there is a prodromal period of refractory coeliac disease that is sometimes accompanied by intestinal ulceration (ulcerative jejunitis).

Macroscopy
In the affected bowel segment, the tumour usually presents with a multifocal involvement with multiple ulcerating raised mucosal masses, but may present as one or more ulcers with or without perforation or as a large exophytic mass. The intact mucosa between the lesions may contain thickened folds or appear normal.

Histopathology
The tumour forms an ulcerating mucosal mass that invades the wall of the intestine. There is a wide range of cytological patterns {1344, 3554}. Most commonly, the tumour cells are medium- to large-sized transformed lymphoid cells with roundish or angulated vesicular nuclei, prominent nucleoli and moderate to abundant, pale-staining cytoplasm. Less commonly, the tumour exhibits marked pleomorphism with multinucleated cells bearing a resemblance to anaplastic large cell lymphoma. Most tumours show infiltration by inflammatory cells, including large numbers of histiocytes and eosinophils, and in some cases these may be so abundant that they obscure the relatively small number of tumour cells present. Infiltration of the epithelium of individual crypts is present in many cases. Infiltration of the surface epithelium usually accompanies the destruction of enterocytes and ulceration. However, adjacent to the tumours, especially to those in the jejunum, the intestinal mucosa usually shows enteropathy comprising villous atrophy, crypt hyperplasia, increased lamina propria lymphocytes and plasma cells and intraepithelial lymphocytosis. Intraepithelial lymphocytes may be mixed with transformed lymphoid cells resembling the invasive part of the tumour. The degree of enteropathy is highly variable and may consist only of an increase in intraepithelial lymphocytes without overt villous atrophy.

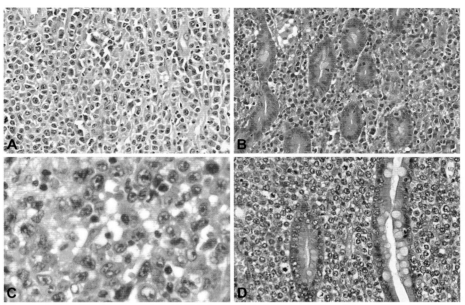

Fig. 6.24 Intestinal T-cell lymphoma (type I EATL). Cytomorphological polymorphism: **A** Immunoblastic morphology; **B** Pleomorphic morphology; and **C** Anaplastic morphology. **D** Intestinal T-cell lymphoma (type II EATL), monomorphic.

Immunohistochemistry
In EATL, the tumour cells are CD3+, CD5–, CD7+, CD8–/+, CD4–, CD103+, TCRß+/– and contain cytotoxic granule-associated proteins (TIA1; granzyme B; perforin). In almost all cases, a varying proportion of the tumour cells express CD30 {3040, 3554}. CD30+ cells are usually CD3–, CD4–,CD8– and predominate in the anaplastic variants of EATL. The intraepithelial lymphocytes in the adjacent enteropathic mucosa may show an abnormal immunophenotype, usually CD3+, CD5–, CD8–, CD4– identical to that of the lymphoma. EATL is usually CD56–.

Precursor lesions
EATL may be preceded by refractory coeliac disease with or without ulceration. This disease is divided into two variants, RCD I and RCD II, according to the absence or presence of intraepithelial lymphocytes with an aberrant phenotype.
RCD II. In RCD II, intraepithelial lymphocytes phenotypically show downregulation of CD8, as in mucosa adjacent to EATL {175, 461}. The intraepithelial lymphocytes also frequently show monoclonal T-cell rearrangement similar to the clonal rearrangements that may be found in the enteropathic mucosa adjacent to EATL {1263}, suggesting that the immunophenotypically aberrant intraepithelial lymphocytes constitute a neoplastic population. In cases of RCD that subsequently develop into EATL, the intraepithelial lymphocytes have the same monoclonal *TCR* gene rearrangement and also gains of chromosome 1q as the subsequent T-cell lymphomas {154, 460, 461, 656, 3396}. Thus, RCD II in which the intraepithelial lymphocytes show these immunophenotypical and genetic features can be considered as examples of intraepithelial T-cell lymphoma or, alternatively, EATL *in situ*. These atypical lymphoid cells are also not strictly confined to the intraepithelial component and may even spread to distant locations, e.g. the skin {3393}. In retrospective analyses, about 40% of RCD II develop overt EATL in a 5-year follow-up period {657, 1965}.
RCD I. In RCD I patients {1690}, intraepithelial lymphocytes express a normal immunophenotype and are polyclonal. These cases only rarely progress to EATL. However, RCD I can also rarely progress to RCD II {657}. Whether this is a necessary intermediate in the multistep

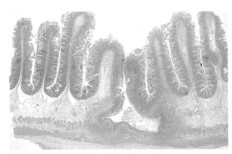

Fig. 6.25 Intestinal T-cell lymphoma. Low-power survey showing deep fissural ulceration and invasion of adjacent mucosa and deep intestinal wall layers.

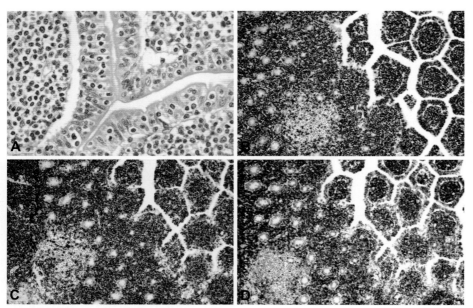

Fig. 6.26 Cytomorphology and immunohistochemistry of type II EATL (monomorphic CD56+) primary intestinal T-cell lymphoma. **A** Monomorphic blastoid cytology. Note intraepithelial invasion of the mucosal surface. The tumours cells are positive for CD3 (**B**), positive for CD8 (**C**) and positive for CD56 (**D**).

transformation process is presently not known.

Molecular pathology

TCRβ and *TCRγ* genes are clonally rearranged {1345, 2193}. Patients with EATL frequently show a HLA-DQ8 and HLA-DQ2, or HLA-DQB1 tumour genotype pattern, which is associated with coeliac disease {1263}. EATL frequently displays chromosomal gains in 1q32.2–q41 and 5q34–q35.2 that may be found also in the intraepithelial lymphocytes of refractory coeliac disease {690, 3697, 3698}. In contrast to primary nodal peripheral T-cell lymphoma (PTCL), most EATL (58–70%) harbour segmental gains of chromosome 9q31.3–qter or deletions of 16q12.1 (23%). These features are prevalent in both subtypes of primary intestinal T-cell lymphoma (EATL and monomorphic CD56+ intestinal T-cell lymphoma) and form a common genetic link between the two types.

Prognosis and predictive factors

Prognosis is usually poor, with death frequently resulting from abdominal complications in patients already weakened by uncontrolled malabsorption. Long-term survivals are recorded. Recurrences are most frequent in the small intestine.

Monomorphic CD56+ intestinal T-cell lymphoma

Definition

An intestinal tumour of intraepithelial T-lymphocytes composed of small- to medium-sized monomorphic cytotoxic T-lymphocytes commonly expressing CD56. This lymphoma also has been referred to as Type II EATL.

Epidemiology

This group comprises 10–20% of gastrointestinal T-cell lymphomas {540, 690}. This type of lymphoma is also seen in populations that are not exposed to nutritional gluten and that have a very low prevalence of coeliac disease, e.g. Taiwan (China) {3319} or Japan {57}.

Etiology

The etiology of this disease is unknown. Although the mucosa adjacent to the invasive tumour may show enteropathy-like changes, the phenotype of intraepithelial lymphocytes may be distinctly different from that for refractory coeliac disease {556}. There is also no clear genetic link with coeliac disease; only 30–40% of Caucasian patients have coeliac disease-associated HLA-DQ2/HLA-DQ8, corresponding to the normal prevalence of these HLA haplotypes in the Caucasian population {690}. Thus, in contrast to Type I EATL, at least a substantial

proportion of cases of this lymphoma arises outside the setting of coeliac disease, confirming the original clinical observation of a lack of any anamnestic link {540}.

Localization

No significant differences from Type I EATL have been reported, but monomorphic CD56+ intestinal T-cell lymphoma more often involves the deeper segments of the small intestine, the ileocaecal region and even the colon.

Histopathology

The neoplastic cells are small, round and monomorphic with darkly staining nuclei and a narrow rim of cytoplasm. There is usually florid infiltration of intestinal crypt epithelium and transmural spread. The adjacent intestinal mucosa may show villous atrophy and crypt hyperplasia with striking intraepithelial lymphocytosis involving both crypt and surface epithelium.

Immunohistochemistry

In monomorphic CD56+ intestinal T-cell lymphoma, the tumour cells are CD3+, CD4–, CD8+, NCAM1/CD56+ and TCRαβ+ {540} and the intraepithelial lymphocytes in the adjacent mucosa are immunophenotypically identical {175}. EBV-related antigen detection and EBV-encoded RNA (EBER) *in situ* hybridization are negative, in contrast to nasal-type NK/T-cell lymphoma involving the small intestine.

Precursor lesions

No precursor lesions have yet been characterized.

Molecular pathology

TCRβ and *TCRγ* genes are clonally rearranged {1345, 2193}. Like EATL, most monomorphic CD56+ intestinal T-cell lymphomas (58–70%) harbour segmental gains of chromosome 9q31.3–qter or show deletions of 16q12.1. In contrast to EATL, this lymphoma is more often characterized by 8q24 (*MYC*) gains and lacks the segmental gains at 1q and 5q found in EATL and RCD II {690, 3697, 3698}.

Prognosis and predictive factors

The clinical course of this disease is similar to that for Type I EATL; the prognosis for overt lymphoma is very bad owing to intestinal complications (perforation, peritonitis) or early spread with lung involvement.

Mesenchymal tumours of the small intestine

M. Miettinen
C.D.M. Fletcher
L.-G. Kindblom
W.M.S. Tsui

ICD-O codes

Leiomyoma	8890/0
Lipoma	8850/0
Angiosarcoma	9120/3
Gastrointestinal stromal tumour	8936/3
Kaposi sarcoma	9140/3
Leiomyosarcoma	8890/3

Gastrointestinal stromal tumour (GIST)

This category includes most smooth-muscle tumours of the small intestine defined before current concepts of GIST. Small-intestinal and duodenal GISTs comprise about 30% and 5%, respectively, of all GISTs.

Clinical features

Duodenal and small-intestinal GISTs occur almost exclusively in adults, usually aged > 50 years. Clinical presentation resembles that of gastric GISTs, but acute complications more commonly include intestinal obstruction and tumour rupture. Smaller GISTs are detected incidentally during endoscopy, surgery, or computed tomography (CT). The frequency of clinical malignancy of small-intestinal GISTs is approximately 35–40%, twice that of gastric GISTs; moreover, most intra-abdominally disseminated GISTs appear to originate in the small intestine. The metastatic pattern resembles that of gastric GISTs. Although most localized intestinal GISTs can be managed by segmental resection, pancreaticoduo-denectomy may be necessary for duodenal tumours abutting or involving the pancreatic head.

Macroscopy

Occurring anywhere in the duodenum or small intestine, GISTs vary from minimal mural nodules to large complex masses, usually with predominant external extension, which may be pedunculated. Some form dumb-bell shaped masses, typically with minor intraluminal and major extra-luminal components. Large tumours are often cystic and haemorrhagic. Advanced tumours involve multiple loops of bowel and develop diffuse or multifocal peritoneal spread, often obscuring the primary site of origin.

Histopathology

Duodenal and small-intestinal GISTs are usually spindle cell tumours with diffuse sheets or vague storiform arrangements of tumour cells. Tumours with low biological potential often contain extracellular collagen globules ("skeinoid fibres"). Anuclear areas are formed that resemble neuropil material in neuroblastoma. Nuclear palisading may occur, but perinuclear vacuolization is rare. Regressive vascular changes (e.g. dilated and thrombosed vessels, haemosiderin deposition, and fibrosis) are common. Nuclear pleomorphism is rare, and mitotic rate is often low. Epithelioid morphology may be associated with higher mitotic activity, reflecting malignancy.

Small-intestinal GISTS generally resemble gastric GISTs, except that immuno-labelling for KIT is almost uniformly positive. DOG1-positivity is nearly consistent. Immunolabelling for α-smooth muscle actin (SMA) and S100 is positive in 50% and 10–15% of cases, respectively. Positive immunolabelling for CD34 is less common (50%) than in gastric GISTs.

Genetic susceptibility

Multiple, often indolent, independent primary tumours occur in patients with neuro-fibromatosis type 1 (NF1). Patients with familial GIST syndrome can develop multiple or diffuse GISTs {323, 1011, 2068, 3324}.

Molecular pathology

KIT-activating mutations are typical of small-intestinal GISTs. Substitutions and deletions in KIT exon 11 mirror those reported in gastric GISTs, while insertions are rare. Duplication of AY502–503 in KIT exon 9 is virtually specific for small-intestinal (vs gastric) GISTs, and occurs in up to 10% of cases. Although not confirmed in one large study cohort, patients with these mutations respond less well to imatinib, prompting dose escalation or use of alternative kinase inhibitors. Monosomy of chromosomes 14 and 22 also occurs {597, 1750}. PDGFRA mutations occur only in duodenal GISTs.

Prognostic factors, grade and stage

The most useful and best studied prognostic factors are tumour size and mitotic activity, typically expressed as number of mitotic figures per 50 high power fields, (total area, 5 mm^2). There is no formal grading system for GISTs; grading for soft-tissue sarcoma is not applicable because relatively low levels of mitotic activity may confer high malignant potential. Staging is based on size and mitotic activity.

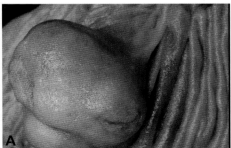
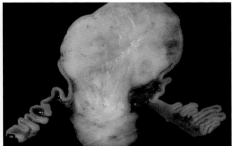
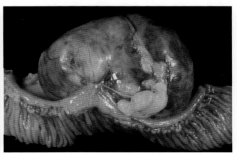

Fig. 6.27 Small-intestinal GISTs often form dumb-bell shaped masses with internal and external components (**A, B**). In larger GISTs, the external component usually predominates (**C**).

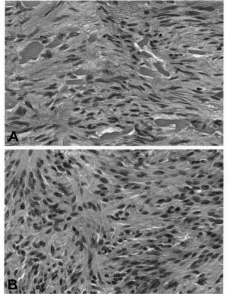

Fig. 6.28 Small-intestinal GIST. **A** Note the distinctive extracellular collagen globules ("skeinoid fibres"). **B** More cellular examples contain uniform spindle cells and often anuclear areas of cell processes, resembling neuropil.

Smooth-muscle tumours

Intramural leiomyomas similar to those seen in the stomach are very rare (about 1 per 100 GISTs). Muscularis mucosae leiomyoma, like that found more commonly in the colon and rectum, has also been reported. Leiomyosarcomas are also rare. Prognosis is better when grade and mitotic rate are low {2078}.

Angiosarcoma

In rare instances, angiosarcoma can involve the small intestine or other parts of the gastrointestinal tract, particularly in older adults with uterine or urinary bladder cancer previously treated by irradiation. Grossly, angiosarcoma forms a haemorrhagic, transmural, often ulcerated mass that often extends into mesentery. The lesions

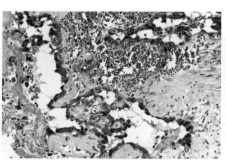

Fig. 6.30 Small-intestinal angiosarcoma contains irregularly shaped vascular lumina lined by highly atypical endothelial cells with mitotic activity.

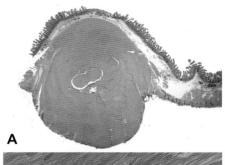

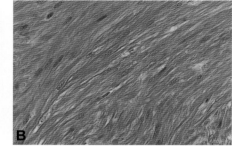

Fig. 6.29 Intramural leiomyoma. **A** The neoplasm forms a well-demarcated transmural mass. **B** It is composed of well-differentiated smooth-muscle cells with abundant eosinophilic cytoplasm and collagenous matrix.

may be multifocal and/or metastases, e.g. from soft tissues of the head and neck.

Histologically, the irregular anastomosing vascular channels are lined by atypical spindled to epithelioid endothelial cells with variable mitotic activity. Although most are high-grade, isolated examples are well-differentiated and low-grade. Immunolabelling is positive in nearly all cases for CD31 (membrane pattern), but more variable for CD34 and FVIII-related antigen. Keratins can be present, especially in epithelioid variants {95, 3207}.

Gastrointestinal clear cell sarcoma

Most cases of this rare, recently recognized tumour occur in the intestine, although it is also reported in the stomach and colon. Clinical presentation resembles

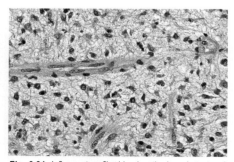

Fig. 6.31 Inflammatory fibroid polyp: the loosely textured tissue contains oval to epithelioid tumour cells, eosinophilic granulocytes, small capillaries, and fibromyxoid matrix.

that for GIST. Often arising in young adults, this sarcoma forms a mural mass of 2–5 cm or larger that may be ulcerated. Metastases to mesenteric lymph nodes and liver are common and often detected at presentation. Histologically, there are sheets of rounded to mildly spindled cells, and packeting to pseudoorganoid clusters is not prominent (unlike peripheral clear cell sarcoma). The presence of multinucleated osteoclast-like histiocytic giant cells is a common although not universal feature {3675}. Immunohistochemically, the tumour cells are positive for S100, but usually negative for HMB45 (gp100), and Melan A (MART1), in contrast to peripheral clear cell sarcomas. Unlike GISTs, this tumour is negative for KIT. The typical tumour translocation is a *EWSR1-CREB1* fusion corresponding to t(2;22)(q32;q12) (unlike peripheral clear cell sarcoma) {130}.

Inflammatory fibroid polyp (IFP)

This lesion occurs throughout the gastrointestinal tract in adults of all ages, but in the small intestine (most frequently in the terminal ileum) more commonly forms a symptomatic mass causing obstruction by intussusception. The polyps usually measure 1–5 cm and are often pedunculated and project intraluminally, appearing greywhite and glistening on sectioning. Mucosal ulceration is possible. The histologically typical appearance is oedematous with spindled to epithelioid tumour cells admixed with eosinophilic granulocytes and histiocytes and a prominent capillary network. In a minority of cases, the tumour cells are (focally) positive for CD34 and SMA. They are negative for KIT and DOG1, but positive for PDGFRA. *PDGFRA*-activating mutations (especially in exon 12) resembling those seen in GISTs are present in > 50% of cases {1751, 2944}. Similar mutations also occur in gastric IFPs {2838}.

Other mesenchymal tumours

Desmoid can form an apparently intestinal mass, despite originating in the mesentery, and can arise in patients with Gardner syndrome. Schwannomas of the small intestine are very rare and resemble those of the stomach. Calcifying fibrous (pseudo)tumour can form a small intestinal mass, but more often shows external serosal involvement only. Inflammatory myofibroblastic tumours may involve the small intestine. Undifferentiated sarcomas are very rare; some may be related to dedifferentiated liposarcoma.

Secondary tumours of the small intestine

C. Iacobuzio-Donahue
G.M. Groisman

Definition

Tumours of the small intestine that originate from an extra-intestinal neoplasm or that are discontinuous with a primary tumour elsewhere in the gastrointestinal tract.

Epidemiology

In autopsy studies, secondary tumours of the small intestine are 2.5 times more common than primary small-bowel carcinoma {725}. Metastatic spread to the small intestine from either an intra- or extra-abdominal primary site is more frequent than to any other site in the tubular gastrointestinal tract {988, 1306}.

Origin

The routes by which secondary neoplasms reach the small bowel include direct extension (i.e. colonic, pancreatic and gastric cancers), intraperitoneal spread (i.e. ovarian cancer) and lymphohaematogenous embolization (i.e. melanoma, lung and breast cancer). Melanoma is the most common malignancy to metastasize to the

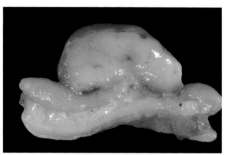

Fig. 6.32 High-grade retroperitoneal sarcoma metastatic to the small intestine, gross micrograph. The metastasis forms an intraluminal mass with a smooth contoured surface.

small intestine, although testis, lung, breast and ovarian cancers also frequently involve the small intestine by metastatic spread {725, 1306}. Melanoma, lung, breast and ovarian cancers also more frequently metastasize to the small intestine than to the stomach or colorectum {3461}. Primary melanomas of the intestine are very rare. Although most melanomas found in the small bowel have

no history of a primary tumour, the general consensus is that they are virtually all metastases from a misdiagnosed or regressed primary melanoma {786, 1802}.

Clinical features

Small intestinal metastases can cause obstruction, perforation, intussusception, malabsorption and/or gastrointestinal bleeding {563, 949, 1239, 1306, 2725, 3413}. Obstruction is more commonly seen in association with metastatic lobular breast carcinoma {1306}. Nonspecific symptoms associated with metastasis to the small intestine include abdominal discomfort, gas distension, and diarrhoea {987}.

Macroscopy

Typical features of intestinal metastases include intestinal-wall thickening, submucosal spread, and ulcers {1306}. Melanomas and sarcomas may appear as nodules or polyps {2444}.

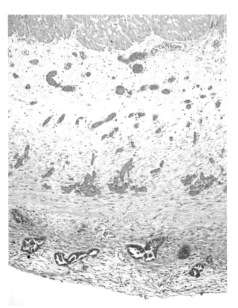

Fig. 6.33 Metastatic high-grade serous ovarian carcinoma within the serosa of the small intestine secondary to intraperitoneal spread. The muscularis propria is present at the top of the image.

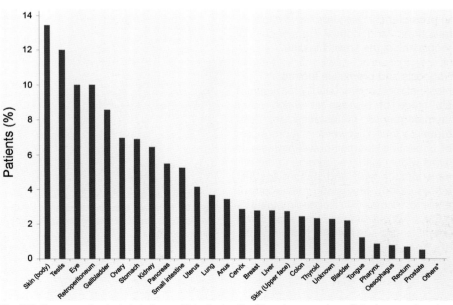

Fig. 6.34 Frequency of metastasis to the small intestine by site of the primary neoplasm. Data shown are based on findings of 3827 autopsies {735}. * Appendix, bile duct, bone, branchial cyst, duodenum, larynx, lip, penis, pleura, salivary gland, skin lower face, tonsil, vagina, vulva.

Histopathology

Metastases are typically located deep within the submucosa or the muscularis propria of the small bowel, with little involvement of the mucosa. The lack of an *in situ* component within the mucosa may also serve as also a clue that the neoplasm is a metastasis, although metastatic carcinoma may grow on the lumenal surface and mimic an *in situ* neoplasm. Obtaining appropriate clinical information about possible primary sites should be the first step in the evaluation of a metastasis. When a possible primary tumour site has been identified, histological, immunohistochemical and molecular comparision of the metastasis with the primary tumour may help to confirm the origin of the metastasis. In difficult cases, immunohistochemistry may help to differentiate between primary small-bowel cancer (positive for keratin 20 and CDX2), metastatic melanoma (positive for Melan A and S100 protein), metastases from ovary and breast (typically positive for keratin 7 and estrogen/progesterone receptors), lung (typically positive for keratin 7 and thyroid transcription factor 1/TTF1) and those from liver, kidney and prostate (typically negative for keratins 7 and 20 and positive for hepatocyte-paraffin-1 antibody/HepPar1, PAX8 and prostate-specific antigen [PSA], respectively) {551, 2380, 3267}. In contrast, the distinction between multiple primary small-bowel carcinoids and their metastases may not be possible. This also applies to leiomyosarcomas and other mesenchymal neoplasms of the small intestine.

Prognosis and predictive factors

Intestinal metastases usually represent a late stage of disease at which other haematogenous metastases are also frequently found. However, the prognosis for patients with small-bowel metastasis varies widely, partly according to the primary tumour type and patient-specific factors {1306}. Metastatic melanoma or renal carcinomas with isolated metastasis to the small intestine may be associated with prolonged survival after resection {62}.

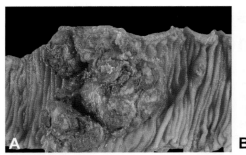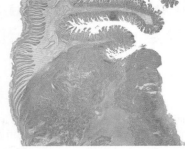

Fig. 6.35 Metastatic malignant melanoma in the small intestine. **A** Gross specimen. **B** Microscopic view.

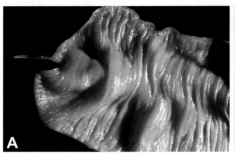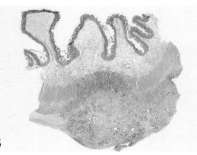

Fig. 6.36 Metastatic adenocarcinoma in the small intestine. **A** The tumour lies beneath swollen mucosa. **B** The tumour is situated in the muscularis propria. Submucosa is oedematous.

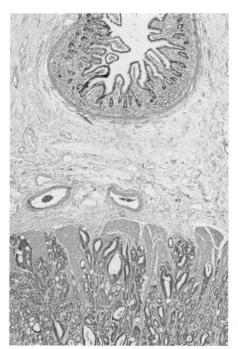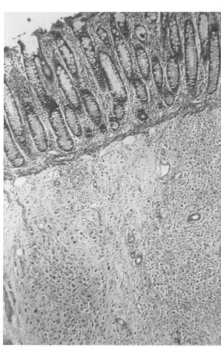

Fig. 6.37 Metastatic adenocarcinoma, small intestine. The muscularis propria contains the tumour. The mucosa is free of neoplasia

Fig. 6.38 Metastatic breast carcinoma in the colon. The tumour cells expand the submucosa.

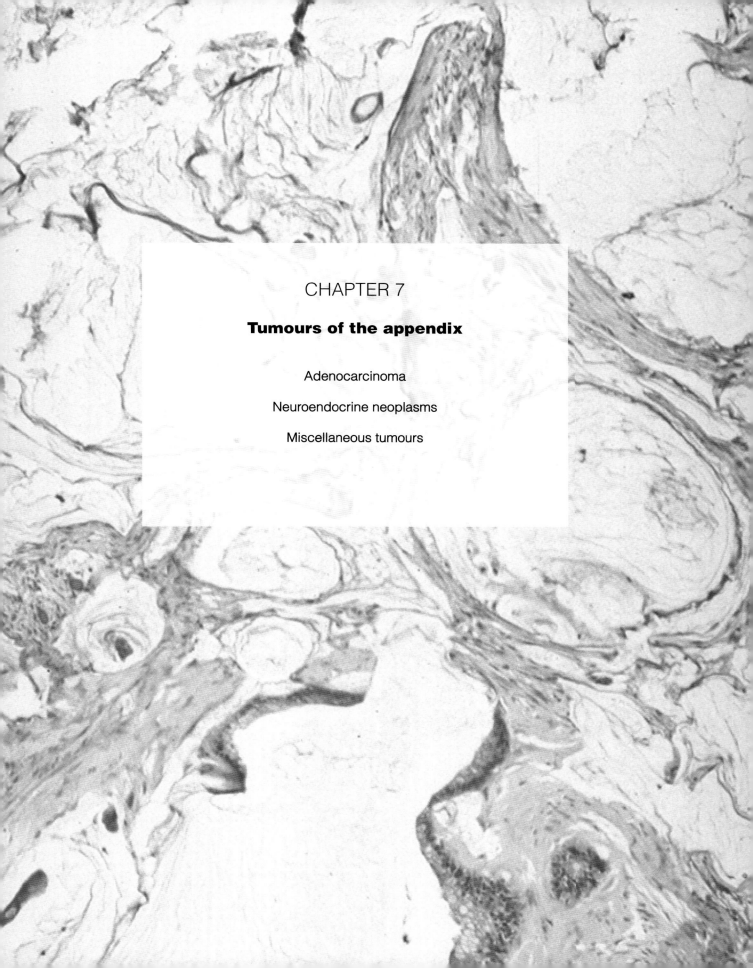

CHAPTER 7

Tumours of the appendix

Adenocarcinoma

Neuroendocrine neoplasms

Miscellaneous tumours

WHO classification[a] of tumours of the appendix

Epithelial tumours

Premalignant lesions

Adenoma	8140/0
Tubular	8211/0
Villous	8261/0
Tubulovillous	8263/0
Dysplasia (intraepithelial neoplasia), low grade	8148/0*
Dysplasia (intraepithelial neoplasia), high grade	8148/2

Serrated lesions	
Hyperplastic polyp	
Sessile serrated adenoma/polyp	8213/0*
Traditional serrated adenoma	8213/0

Carcinoma

Adenocarcinoma	8140/3
Mucinous adenocarcinoma	8480/3
Low-grade appendiceal mucinous neoplasm	8480/1*
Signet ring cell carcinoma	8490/3
Undifferentiated carcinoma	8020/3

Neuroendocrine neoplasms[b]

Neuroendocrine tumour (NET)	
NET G1 (carcinoid)	8240/3
NET G2	8249/3

Neuroendocrine carcinoma (NEC)	8246/3
Large cell NEC	8013/3
Small cell NEC	8041/3
Mixed adenoneuroendocrine carcinoma	8244/3
EC cell, serotonin-producing NET	8241/3
Goblet cell carcinoid	8243/3
L cell, Glucagon-like peptide-producing and PP/PYY-producing NETs	8152/1*
Tubular carcinoid	8245/1

Mesenchymal tumours

Leiomyoma	8890/0
Lipoma	8850/0
Neuroma	9570/0
Kaposi sarcoma	9140/3
Leiomyosarcoma	8890/3

Lymphomas

Secondary tumours

EC, enterochromaffin

[a] The morphology codes are from the International Classification of Diseases for Oncology (ICD-O) {904A} and the Systematized Nomenclature of Medicine (SNOMED). Behaviour is coded /0 for benign tumours, /1 for unspecified, borderline or uncertain behaviour, /2 for carcinoma *in situ* and grade III intraepithelial neoplasia, and /3 for malignant tumours.

[b] The classification is modified from the previous (third) edition of the WHO histological classification of tumours {691} taking into account changes in our understanding of these lesions. In the case of neuroendocrine neoplasms, the classification has been simplified to be of more practical utility in morphological classification.

* These new codes were approved by the IARC/WHO Committee for ICD-O at its meeting in March 2010.

TNM classification[a] of tumours of the appendix

Carcinoma of the appendix

T – Primary tumour
TX   Primary tumour cannot be assessed
T0   No evidence of primary tumour
Tis   Carcinoma *in situ*: intraepithelial or invasion of lamina propria
T1   Tumour invades submucosa
T2   Tumour invades muscularis propria
T3   Tumour invades subserosa or mesoappendix
T4   Tumour perforates visceral peritoneum, including mucinous peritoneal tumour within the right lower quadrant and/or directly invades other organs or structures
   T4a   Tumour perforates visceral peritoneum, including mucinous peritoneal tumour within the right lower quadrant
   T4b   Tumour directly invades other organs or structures

N – Regional lymph nodes
NX   Regional lymph nodes cannot be assessed
N0   No regional lymph node metastasis
N1   Metastasis in 1 to 3 regional lymph nodes
N2   Metastasis in 4 or more regional lymph nodes

M – Distant metastasis
M0   No distant metastasis
M1   Distant metastasis
   M1a   Intraperitoneal metastasis beyond the right lower quadrant, including pseudomyxoma peritonei
   M1b   Nonperitoneal metastasis

G – Histopathological grading

GX	Grade of differentiation cannot be assessed	
G1	Well differentiated	Mucinous low grade
G2	Moderately differentiated	Mucinous high grade
G3	Poorly differentiated	Mucinous high grade
G4	Undifferentiated	

Stage grouping

Stage	T	N	M	G
Stage 0	Tis	N0	M0	
Stage I	T1, T2	N0	M0	
Stage IIA	T3	N0	M0	
Stage IIB	T4a	N0	M0	
Stage IIC	T4b	N0	M0	
Stage IIIA	T1, T2	N1	M0	
Stage IIIB	T3, T4	N1	M0	
Stage IIIC	Any T	N2	M0	
Stage IVA	Any T	N0	M1a	G1
Stage IVB	Any T	N0	M1a	G2–G4
	Any T	N1, N2	M1a	Any G
Stage IVC	Any T	Any N	M1b	Any G

Carcinoid of the appendix[b]

T – Primary tumour
TX   Primary tumour cannot be assessed
T0   No evidence of primary tumour
T1   Tumour 2 cm or less in greatest dimension
   T1a   Tumour 1 cm or less in greatest dimension
   T1b   Tumour more than 1 cm but not more than 2 cm
T2   Tumour more than 2 cm but not more than 4 cm or with extension to the caecum
T3   Tumour more than 4 cm or with extension to the ileum
T4   Tumour perforates peritoneum or invades other adjacent organs or structures, e.g. abdominal wall and skeletal muscle

N – Regional lymph nodes
NX   Regional lymph nodes cannot be assessed
N0   No regional lymph-node metastasis
N1   Regional lymph-node metastasis

M – Distant metastasis
M0   No distant metastasis
M1   Distant metastasis

Stage grouping

Stage	T	N	M
Stage I	T1	N0	M0
Stage II	T2, T3	N0	M0
Stage III	T4	N0	M0
	Any T	N1	M0
Stage IV	Any T	Any N	M1

---

[a] {762, 2996}
[b] Neuroendocrine tumour (NET); well-differentiated neuroendocrine tumour/carcinoma. Goblet cell carcinoid is classified according to the scheme for carcinoma.

A help desk for specific questions about the TNM classification is available at http://www.uicc.org.

Adenocarcinoma of the appendix

N.J. Carr
L.H. Sobin

Definition
A malignant epithelial neoplasm of the appendix with invasion beyond the muscularis mucosae.

ICD-O codes
Adenocarcinoma	8140/3
Mucinous adenocarcinoma	8480/3
Low-grade appendiceal mucinous neoplasm	8480/1
Signet ring cell carcinoma	8490/3
Undifferentiated carcinoma	8020/3

Epidemiology
Adenocarcinoma of the appendix occurs in 0.1–0.2% of appendicectomies, corresponding to an estimated incidence of 0.2 per 100 000 per year {2282, 2985, 3237}. The median age at presentation is in the sixth or seventh decade of life {440, 2092, 3237}. Adenocarcinomas accounted for 58% of malignant appendiceal tumours in the United States Surveillance, Epidemiology and End-Results (SEER) database, the remainder being mostly carcinoids. The incidence rates for the carcinomas stayed constant during 1973–1987 {3237}. Males were more commonly affected than females, but a population study in the Netherlands showed a predominance in females {2985, 3237}.

Etiology
The causes of appendiceal adenocarcinoma are unclear. However, there is an association with neoplasia elsewhere in the large intestine {1530, 2985}. Chronic ulcerative colitis (UC) may also be a risk factor; adenoma and adenocarcinoma of the appendix have been described in patients affected by long-standing UC {2355}.

Clinical features
Many patients with appendiceal adenocarcinoma have clinical features that are indistinguishable from those of acute appendicitis. Others present with an abdominal or pelvic mass. If spread to the peritoneal cavity, appendiceal adenocarcinoma often produces pseudomyxoma peritonei, and the large volumes of mucus can cause abdominal distension or present within a hernia sac {440, 806, 2092, 3658}.

Imaging
Adenomas and adenocarcinomas of the appendix can be demonstrated reliably by computed tomography (CT). They typically show cystic dilatation or a soft-tissue mass. An appendix with a diameter of > 15 mm on CT is suspicious for the presence of a neoplasm {2547}. Pseudomyxoma peritonei is characterized by low-attenuation mucinous ascites on CT, although areas of high attenuation develop in large-volume disease {3127}. Scalloping of the outline of the liver and other viscera is characteristic.

Macroscopy
In cases of primary adenocarcinoma, the appendix may be enlarged, deformed or completely destroyed {440, 441, 2092, 2722}. A cystic swelling of the appendix due to the accumulation of mucus within the lumen can be termed mucocoele, but this is a purely descriptive term, not a pathological diagnosis {440, 441, 2435}. Rarely, the mucin forms small spheres, a condition named myxoglobulosis {2814}.

Tumour spread and staging
Low-grade appendiceal mucinous neoplasms (LAMN) generally grow slowly, and tend to produce the clinical picture of low-grade pseudomyxoma peritonei in which spread beyond the peritoneum or nodal metastasis is unusual. High-grade mucinous adenocarcinomas can also produce pseudomyxoma peritonei, but are more likely to invade the underlying organs and exhibit haematogenous and lymphatic metastasis. On very rare occasions, tumour growth in the retroperitoneum may produce "pseudomyxoma retroperitonei" {393}. The behaviour of nonmucinous carcinomas resembles that of their colonic equivalents.

A distinctive feature of pseudomyxoma peritonei, especially when produced by low-grade neoplasms, is its distribution in the abdomen. There is a tendency to spare the peritoneal surfaces of the

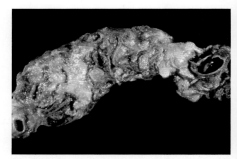

Fig. 7.01 Pseudomyxoma peritonei. Several loops of bowel are encased in a multilocular mucinous mass.

bowel, while large-volume disease is found in the greater omentum, beneath the right hemidiaphragm, in the right retrohepatic space, at the ligament of Treitz, in the left abdominal gutter and in the pelvis {3117}.

In patients with both ovarian mucinous neoplasm and appendiceal mucinous adenocarcinoma, the appendix is almost invariably the primary tumour and the ovarian tumour is secondary, on the basis of molecular analysis {3149, 3632}.

Carcinoma of the appendix was included with colorectal carcinoma in the sixth edition of the TNM classification, but is staged separately in the seventh edition. The basic T, N, and M categories are essentially similar to those of the colon. The separation of mucinous from non-mucinous carcinomas is required, and T4 and M1 are modified to address the particular nature of mucinous carcinomas. Grading was introduced to distinguish between low-grade and high-grade mucinous adenocarcinomas because of differences in behaviour and management. The stage grouping is dependent on these grades. A distinction is made between mucinous peritoneal tumours within the right lower quadrant (T4a) and intraperitoneal metastasis beyond the right lower quadrant, including pseudomyxoma peritonei (M1a) because of the favourable nature of the former compared with the latter {440}. The carcinoma staging scheme also applies to goblet cell carcinoids, but not to typical carcinoids.

Pseudomyxoma peritonei (mucinous carcinoma peritonei). The term "pseudomyxoma peritonei" applies to the clinical picture in which the growth of neoplastic mucin-secreting cells within the peritoneal cavity produces a slow but relentless accumulation of mucin causing gelatinous ascites. In LAMNs, cells may be very scanty within this mucinous material. The appendix is the primary site in the great majority of cases. However, pseudomyxoma can occasionally arise from mucinous adenocarcinomas of other organs, such as colorectum, gallbladder, stomach, pancreas, fallopian tube, urachus, lung, and breast {607, 1686, 2017, 3676}. Evidence now suggests that the ovary is only the primary source on the very rare occasions when a well-differentiated mucinous adenocarcinoma of intestinal type arises in a mature cystic teratoma {1970, 2587, 2722, 3149, 3657}.

Using the criteria in Table 7.01, the lesion causing the pseudomyxoma can be classified as low-grade or high-grade {321, 2092}. The terms "low-grade" and "high-grade mucinous carcinoma peritonei" can be used as alternatives {321}. In general, low-grade pseudomyxoma peritonei is associated with LAMNs, while high-grade disease is associated with mucinous adenocarcinoma, but discordant cases can occur {2092}.

The term "disseminated peritoneal adenomucinosis" (DPAM) has been used for low-grade pseudomyxoma peritonei arising from LAMNs {2722}. The term DPAM should be avoided, since low-grade and high-grade lesions represent a continuous spectrum, and the concept of "ruptured adenoma" does not adequately reflect the clinical course that frequently causes death through obstruction of abdominal viscera {321, 2092, 2435}. Likewise, the term "borderline" is best not applied to appendiceal LAMNs, since similar-appearing borderline tumours of the ovary have a more favourable prognosis {441, 2092}.

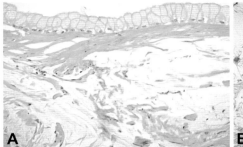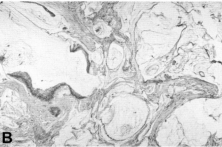

Fig. 7.02 Low-grade pseudomyxoma peritonei (low-grade mucinous carcinoma peritonei). **A** In some cases, the malignant epithelium appears very bland. **B** Many lakes of mucin seem to lack epithelium.

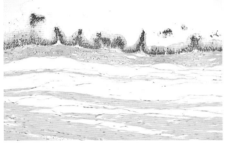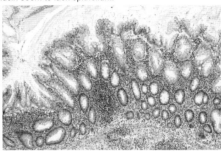

Fig. 7.03 Low-grade appendiceal mucinous neoplasm (LAMN). This undulating morphology can also be seen in adenomas, but there is no lamina propria and the neoplastic epithelium rests on fibrous stroma.

Fig. 7.04 Hyperplastic polyp of the appendix. There is no architectural or cytological atypia.

Histopathology

Appendiceal adenocarcinomas are designated as mucinous if > 50% of the lesion consists of extracellular mucin. The nomenclature of appendiceal mucinous neoplasms is controversial, because low-grade neoplasms that morphologically resemble adenomas can proliferate outside the appendix in a malignant fashion, producing pseudomyxoma peritonei and even distant metastases {441, 957, 2092, 2435}. It is best to diagnose these well-differentiated lesions as LAMNs, a term that avoids the use of "adenoma", an inappropriate designation for a lesion that may produce widespread disease {441}. The classification of mucinous appendiceal neoplasms is shown in Table 7.02. Lesions designated as "mucinous tumours of uncertain malignant potential" are included in the LAMN category. LAMNs may have villous, serrated or undulating morphology but, unlike adenomas, they rest on fibrous tissue rather than lamina propria. Most non-carcinoid appendiceal neoplasms are LAMNs or mucinous adenocarcinomas {440}. They tend to involve the appendix in a circumferential fashion with atrophy of the underlying lymphoid tissue {440, 2092}. The appendix may show widespread epithelial denudation, especially in well differentiated lesions, so that multiple blocks may be required to demonstrate tumour cells {441}. Non-mucinous adenocarcinomas of the appendix resemble their colorectal counterparts. The term "mucinous cystadenocarcinoma" has been used for well-differentiated

Table 7.01 Classification of pseudomyxoma peritonei.

Grade	TNM classification	Architecture	Cellular features	Intracytoplasmic mucin	Mitoses
Low grade	Mucinous, low grade	Cells form strips or small islands. Cells may be very scanty; the mucin may appear acellular.	Neoplastic cells in single layers, sometimes with papillary tufting. Nuclei small and regular. Low-grade dysplasia. Cells may be deceptively bland in appearance.	Variable	Rare
High grade	Mucinous, high grade	Cells form strips, small islands or cribriform structures. Cells numerous. Extensive invasion of underlying organs.	High-grade dysplasia, at least focally.	Variable. Signet-ring cells may be seen.	More common. May be atypical.

a Use of the terms "low-grade dysplasia" and "high-grade dysplasia" is as for the large intestine.

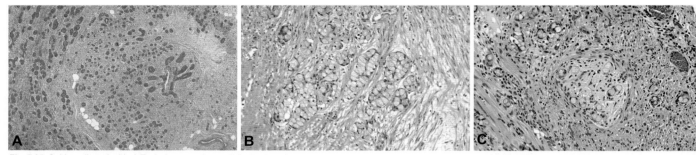

Fig. 7.05 Goblet cell carcinoid. **A** Typical concentric mural distribution of tumour with preservation of the appendiceal lumen. Mucin-positive tumour nests (green) are seen with Movat staining. The lumen is compressed, but intact. **B** Typical clusters of goblet cells. **C** The neoplasm consists of small clusters of cells and single cells, some infiltrating a nerve in the centre of the field.

mucinous tumours with cystic structures; however, such a diagnosis should be avoided because this neoplasm does not constitute a separate disease entity {441}. Appendiceal adenocarcinomas regularly express keratin 20 and CDX2; many express keratin 7 {2317}. They also express MUC2, a gel-forming mucin normally secreted by intestinal goblet cells {2317, 2337}. Comparison of well-differentiated adenocarcinomas of the appendix and colorectum shows similar expression of p53 and CD44s, although the apoptotic count is lower in appendiceal lesions {438}.

Signet ring cell carcinoma

If signet-ring cells account for more than 50% of the neoplasm, the term "signet-ring cell carcinoma" is appropriate. Such lesions should be included in the high-grade category.

Undifferentiated carcinoma

Undifferentiated carcinomas occur in the appendix but are rare. Their histology corresponds to that of undifferentiated carcinomas of the colorectum.

Goblet cell carcinoid

This tumour is characterized by predominantly submucosal growth. It typically infiltrates the appendiceal wall in a concentric manner, thus producing an ill-defined tumour mass {371}. The mucosa is characteristically spared, with the exception of areas of connection of tumour nests with the base of the crypts. The tumour is composed of small, rounded nests of signet-ring-like cells resembling normal intestinal goblet cells, except for the nuclear compression. Glandular lumina are infrequently observed. The cells display mild-to-moderate atypia, low mitotic activity with a Ki67 proliferation index < 20% {3193}. Lysozyme-positive Paneth cells as well as foci resembling Brunner glands may be present {1340}. Mucin staining is intensely positive within goblet cells and extracellular mucin pools. Immunohistochemically, the endocrine-cell component is positive for chromogranin A, synaptophysin, CD56 (NCAM1), serotonin, enteroglucagon, somatostatin, and/or PP {1222, 1340, 3362}. The goblet cells express CEA, keratins 19 and 20 and MUC2 {3193, 3362}. Ultrastructurally, dense-core endocrine granules and mucin droplets are both found {763, 1222}, occasionally within the cytoplasm of the same cell {1340}.

Mixed adenoneuroendocrine carcinoma (see Neuroendocrine neoplasms of the appendix)

This term has been proposed to designate carcinomas of the appendix that arise by progression from a pre-existing goblet cell carcinoid {3193}. Either a signet-ring cell type or poorly differentiated adenocarcinoma type may be encountered {3193, 3446}. The latter type typically exhibits immunohistochemical expression of p53 and MUC1 together with loss of MUC2 {3193}. These carcinomas usually occur in the apparent absence of neoplastic change in the mucosal epithelium {371}.

Grading

Mucinous tumours are classified as low-grade (corresponding to a diagnosis of LAMN or low-grade pseudomyxoma peritonei), or as high-grade (corresponding to a diagnosis of mucinous adenocarcinoma or high-grade pseudomyxoma peritonei). The criteria for these diagnoses are discussed elsewhere in this chapter and are shown in Tables 7.01 and 7.02. Non-mucinous adenocarcinomas of the appendix can be graded using the criteria for colorectal lesions (see Chapter 8). These designations are incorporated into the grading scheme of the TNM classification.

Precursor lesions

By analogy with the rest of the large intestine, an adenoma–carcinoma sequence is assumed to occur in the appendix; the

Table 7.02 Classification of mucinous appendiceal neoplasms.

Neoplasm	TNM classification	Architecture	Cellular features	Intracytoplasmic mucin	Mitoses
Low-grade appendiceal mucinous neoplasm (LAMN)	Mucinous, low-grade	Villous, serrated or undulating architecture, often resembling adenoma. "Broad front invasion" characterized by atrophy and fibrosis of underlying submucosa and muscularis propria, but no desmoplasia.	Neoplastic cells in a single layer; they may be columnar, cuboidal or flattened. Nuclei small and regular. Low-grade dysplasia. Cells may be deceptively bland in appearance.	Large mucin vacuoles common in columnar cells; may compress the nuclei to the cell base. Less mucin in cuboidal cells.	Rare
Mucinous adenocarcinoma	Mucinous, high-grade	Invasive pattern with desmoplastic stroma. Residual luminal mucinous tumour resembling LAMN may be present.	High-grade dysplasia, at least focally.	Variable. Signet-ring cells may be seen.	More common. May be atypical.

^a Use of the terms "low-grade dysplasia" and "high-grade dysplasia" is as for the large intestine.

finding of a residual adenoma in some cases of adenocarcinoma supports this contention. A few adenocarcinomas appear to arise from goblet cell carcinoid tumours {371, 440}.

Adenomas are defined as lesions that are confined to the appendix with no evidence of invasion {2434}. Most appendiceal adenomas are low-grade; high-grade cytology and architectural complexity are only compatible with a diagnosis of adenoma if the lesion resembles an adenoma of the colon and the muscularis mucosae is clearly intact. The designation of adenoma should imply that the lesion is curable by complete excision {441, 2435}. An alternative diagnosis, such as LAMN, is appropriate if there is any doubt. In particular, the presence of any mucin outside the appendix (even if the mucin is acellular) is incompatible with a diagnosis of adenoma {2434}.

The classification of appendiceal adenomas is the same as that in the colon (tubular, tubulovillous, villous). The commonest premalignant lesion of the appendix is the sessile serrated adenoma/polyp {2547}, probably reported in the past as hyperplastic polyps or diffuse hyperplasia. In fact, although hyperplastic polyps of the appendix do occur, they are relatively unusual. A lesion that has villous structures, irregularly branched crypts or dilation at the base of the crypts is probably a sessile serrated adenoma/polyp, not a hyperplastic polyp. Traditional serrated adenomas and mixed hyperplastic-adenomatous polyps form a significant proportion of lesions; the diagnostic criteria are the same as elsewhere in the large intestine {439, 3620}. We no longer recommend the use of "cystadenoma" as a diagnostic term at this site, since cystic change does not indicate a separate disease category.

Genetic susceptibility

Several cases of adenocarcinoma of the appendix have been reported in familial adenomatous polyposis, including one with appendiceal adenocarcinoma as the presenting feature {2481}.

Molecular pathology

Some hyperplastic polyps and sessile serrated adenomas of the appendix show decreased expression of MLH1 and MGMT together with *BRAF* mutations {3620}. However, *KRAS* mutations (mostly in codon 12 and a few in codon 13) are also common and are found in the majority of appendiceal adenomas {1453, 3149}. Appendiceal adenomas frequently show loss of heterozygosity (LOH). In particular, LOH at the 5q locus linked to the *APC* tumour suppressor gene is common {3149}. A study of appendiceal adenocarcinomas showed frequent LOH of chromosome 18q21 and 18q22, mutation of *SMAD4/-DPC4* in a minority of cases, and no mutations of the β-catenin gene (*CTNNB1*) {1992}. Whether mucinous or non-mucinous, appendiceal adenocarcinomas appear to be microsatellite-stable {1453}. Of the reported cases to date, only two lesions showed microsatellite instability; one showed loss of *MSH2* and *MSH6* that was ascribed to a germline defect {2090}, the other showed loss of *MLH1* even though the adjacent serrated polyp was microsatellite-stable {3620}. Thus, the available evidence suggests that appendiceal adenocarcinomas rarely develop via the microsatellite-instability pathway.

Unlike colonic adenocarcinomas, *KRAS* mutations are rarely found in carcinoids or goblet cell carcinoids, while p53 expression at immunohistochemistry or *TP53* mutations were detected in a fraction (25–31%) of goblet cell carcinoids {2624, 3362}. No mutations of *CTNNB1* or *DPC4/SMAD4* were detected in goblet cell carcinoids {3056}. Finally, decreased expression of NLRP1 was identified in goblet cell carcinoids {2112}.

Prognosis and predictive factors

Features that have been associated with a poor prognosis in appendiceal adenocarcinoma include advanced stage, high grade, and nonmucinous histology {606, 2308, 2434, 2989}.

When pseudomyxoma peritonei is present, the distinction between low-grade and high-grade pseudomyxoma has prognostic significance {192, 321, 2092, 2722}. The spread of mucus beyond the right lower quadrant of the abdomen is an independent prognostic variable {440, 2434}. If the mucin deposits appear acellular, the prognosis may be improved {440, 2092, 2434, 3621}.

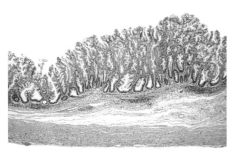

Fig. 7.06 Sessile serrated adenoma/polyp of the appendix. There is architectural complexity and serrations extend into the crypt bases, which are dilated.

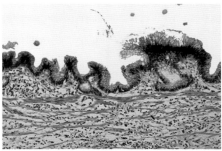

Fig. 7.07 Serrated adenoma of the appendix with undulating morphology. Note the intact muscularis mucosae beneath the lesion. More typical serrated features were present elsewhere.

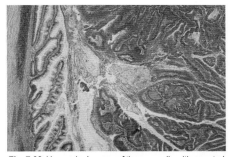

Fig. 7.08 Unusual adenoma of the appendix with serrated features. High-grade morphology is evident (right).

In terms of aggressiveness, goblet cell carcinoids are more aggressive than conventional carcinoids, but less than adenocarcinomas of the appendix.

Metastases to the ovaries are not infrequently seen and may be confused with primary ovarian tumours {1265, 3193}. The 5-year survival of patients with goblet cell carcinoids is 86% for localized disease, 74% for regional disease, and 18% when distant metastases are present {2023}.

Neuroendocrine neoplasms of the appendix

P. Komminoth
R. Arnold
C. Capella
D.S. Klimstra
G. Klöppel
E. Solcia
G. Rindi

Definition

Neoplasms with neuroendocrine differentiation, including neuroendocrine tumours (NET) and neuroendocrine carcinomas (NEC) arising in the appendix. Mixed adenoneuroendocrine carcinomas (MANEC) have an exocrine and an endocrine component, with one component exceeding 30%.

ICD-O codes

Neuroendocrine tumour (NET)
NET G1 (carcinoid)	8240/3
NET G2	8249/3
Neuroendocrine carcinoma (NEC)	8246/3
Large cell NEC	8013/3
Small cell NEC	8041/3
Mixed adenoneuroendocrine carcinoma (MANEC)	8244/3
EC cell, serotonin-producing NET	8241/3
Goblet cell carcinoid	8243/3
L cell, Glucagon-like peptide and PP/PYY-producing NETs	8152/1
Tubular carcinoid	8245/1

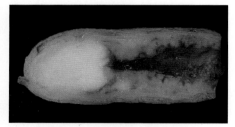

Fig. 7.09 Neuroendocrine tumour (NET) G1 (carcinoid) of the appendix, with typical yellow coloration.

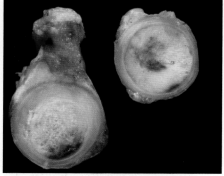

Fig. 7.10 NET G1 (carcinoid) of the appendix infiltrating the mesoappendix.

Synonyms

Synonyms for NET of the appendix include: carcinoid, well-differentiated endocrine tumour/carcinoma {3013}. Synonyms for NEC include: poorly differentiated endocrine carcinomas, high-grade neuroendocrine carcinoma, small cell and large cell endocrine carcinomas. MANECs develop from goblet cell carcinoids.

Epidemiology

Incidence and time trends

NETs account for 50–77% of all appendiceal neoplasms {1934, 2118} and for 19% of all gastrointestinal NETs. They are found in 0.3–0.9% of patients undergoing appendectomy {1324, 1995, 2023, 3209}. The annual incidence rate is 0.15 new cases per 100 000 population {3624}. However, this figure may be an underestimate, since not all cases are reported and some registries do not record "benign" neoplasms (e.g. NETs of < 1 cm). NECs are exceedingly rare {2339, 2732}.

Age and sex distribution

The mean age at presentation is 32–43 years (range, 6–80 years) {2115, 2118, 2713}. Tubular NETs occur at a significantly younger age than goblet cell carcinoids (average, 29 vs 53 years) {371}. Appendiceal NETs occur more frequently in females than in males {1161}, which may reflect the greater number of incidental appendicectomies performed in women; however, in the Surveillance, Epidemiology and End Results (SEER) database, the frequency of non-endocrine appendiceal neoplasms is similar in males and females, suggesting that the higher rate of appendiceal NETs in women may not be due solely to higher rates of appendectomy {2115, 2118}. Furthermore, the prevalence of girls among children with appendiceal NETs cannot be explained by differences in rates of appendectomy {1447, 2121}.

Clinical features

Most appendiceal NETs are found incidentally in appendectomy specimens, detection depending on careful histological examination. Most appendiceal NETs are asymptomatic and located in the distal end of the appendix {1004}. In a small number of cases, NETs involving the remaining portions of the appendix may obstruct the lumen and produce appendicitis {371, 1004}. A carcinoid syndrome is extremely rare and almost always related to widespread metastases, usually to the liver and retroperitoneum {2118, 3236}.

Macroscopy

NETs

For routine cases, it is recommended that the entire tip of the appendix (two longitudinal pieces) be examined together with the resection margin in one block and several diametrical cuts through the rest of the appendix in a second block. Appendiceal NETs are firm, greyish-white (yellow after formalin fixation), and fairly well-circumscribed, but not encapsulated. In 80%, 14% and 6% of cases, the diameter is < 1 cm, 1–2 cm and > 2 cm, respectively {681, 3081}. Most neoplasms (75%) are located at the tip of the appendix, followed by the middle appendix (15%) and the base (10%) {681, 3081}.

MANECs

MANECs (e.g. goblet cell carcinoids) of the appendix may be found in any portion of the appendix and appear as an area of whitish, sometimes mucoid induration, without dilatation of the lumen. They range in size from 1 to 5 cm, with a mean of 2 cm {100}, but may occasionally not be assessed accurately because of their diffuse infiltrative growth {371}. They are discussed under *Adenocarcinoma of the appendix*.

Histopathology

Most NETs of the appendix are enterochromaffin (EC) cell, serotonin-producing tumours (see Table 7.03). Only a minority are glucagon-like peptide, PP/PYY-producing or L cell NETs. Also relatively rare are goblet cell carcinoids. Primary NECs, either pure endocrine or MANEC, are exceedingly rare in the appendix {2339, 2732}.

NETs

EC cell NET. The tumour cells are arranged in rounded solid nests that sometimes show peripheral-cell palisading. Occasionally, there may also be glandular formations, forming a tubular or acinar pattern. Tumour cells are uniform, with little or no pleomorphism or mitotic activity and a Ki67 proliferative index of < 2% {3362}, thus mostly belonging to the G1 class (for grading, see Chapter 1). NET with a predominantly clear cell phenotype may rarely be encountered and can easily be confused with goblet cell carcinoids. Most EC cell NETs display invasion of the muscular wall and also lymphatic and perineural invasion. Subserosal/meso-appendiceal fatty tissue is infiltrated in 10–40% of cases {681, 3081}. Despite such aggressive growth patterns, appendiceal NETs, in contrast to ileal NETs, infrequently present with lymph-node or distant metastases {2023}. Like ileal EC cell NETs, they stain for both serotonin and substance P and may also exhibit S100-positive sustentacular cells. However, in contrast to ileal and colonic EC cell NETs, which seem to develop from EC cells of the mucosal crypts {1914, 2172}, the S100-positive cells in appendiceal EC cell NETs may surround some nests of neoplastic cells, forming subepithelial neuroendocrine complexes {1001, 1914}. No other relevant histological, cytological, or immunohistochemical differences between ileal and appendiceal NETs have been detected, despite their rather different clinical behaviour. Thus, the tumour cells are positive for chromogranin A, synaptophysin, keratins 8 and 19, CD56 (NCAM1), CDX2 and usually negative for keratins 7 and 20, CEA and TTF1 {100, 3052, 3362}.

L cell NET. These rare NETs produce glucagon-like peptides (GLP1, GLP2, and the enteroglucagons glicentin and oxyntomodulin) and PP/PYY. They feature a characteristic trabecular pattern {1366, 2911}. These neoplasms generally measure only 2–3 mm in diameter and are the appendiceal counterpart of L cell NETs in the rectum, showing a similar immunoprofile (see Chapter 8).

Tubular carcinoid. This neoplasm is often misdiagnosed as a metastatic adenocarcinoma, because it does not resemble the typical EC cell NET and shows little contact with the mucosa. It is composed of small, discrete tubules, some with inspissated mucin in their lumen. Short trabecular structures are frequent, but solid nests are generally absent. Useful criteria for diagnosing this neoplasm are origin from the base of the crypts, integrity of the luminal mucosa, orderly arrangements, and absence of cytological abnormalities and mitoses. Immunohistochemically, the tumour cells are often positive for chromogranin A, glucagon and serotonin, but negative for S100 protein {371, 1001}.

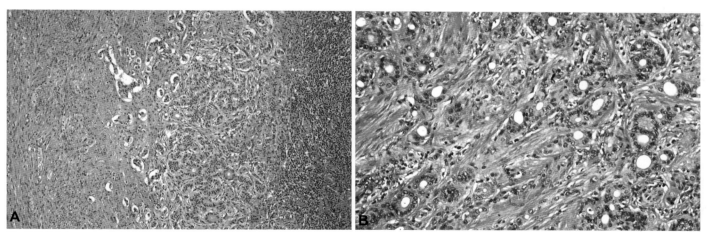

Fig. 7.11 Tubular carcinoid of the appendix. Typical tubular pattern (**A**) with gland-like structures (**B**) arising at the tip of the appendix.

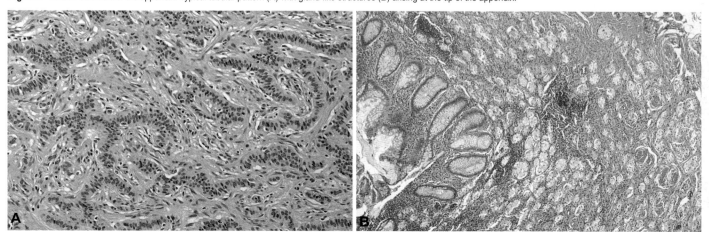

Fig. 7.12 Neuroendocrine tumours (NETs) of the appendix. **A** L cell NET, low power. **B** Clear cell carcinoid.

Table 7.03 Types and characteristics of neuroendocrine neoplasms of the appendix.

Type	Subtype	Characteristics
Neuroendocrine tumour (NET)	Enterochromaffin cell (EC cell) NET	Majority of tumours Produce serotonin, substance P; S100-positive May show muscular invasion, lymphatic or perineural invasion and invasion of peritoneum
	L cell NET	Minority of tumours Produce glucagon-like peptides, PP/PYY Tubular and trabecular pattern Mostly 2–3 mm in size
	Tubular carcinoid	Affect younger patients (average age, 29 years) Little contact with the mucosa Small tubules with mucin in lumina; no cell nests Originate from base of the crypts Produce glucagons, serotonin; no S100-positive cells
Mixed adenoneuroendocrine carcinoma (MANEC)	Goblet cell carcinoid	Affect older patients (average age, 52 years) Submucosal concentric growth Positive staining for mucin Produce serotonin, somatostatin, carcinoembryonic antigen (CEA)
Neuroendocrine carcinoma (NEC)	Small cell NEC	Extremely rare Mostly associated with adenocarcinoma

NECs

NECs (poorly differentiated endocrine carcinomas) are exceedingly rare in the appendix {2339, 2732}. Both the histology and the immunoprofile are consistent with those reported for NECs at other sites of the gastrointestinal tract (see Chapters 2, 4, 6, 8).

Goblet cell carcinoid.

See *Adenocarcinoma of the appendix.*

Molecular pathology

In contrast to other NETs of the gastrointestinal tract, loss of heterozygosity (LOH) at the *MEN1* gene locus appears to be rare {2528, 3056, 3253}. A gene-expression study identified overexpression of *NAP1L1*, *MAGED2* and *MTA1* in appendiceal NETs with lymph-node or liver metastases as well as in goblet cell carcinoids, but not in incidentally detected small NETs.

Prognosis and predictive factors

The issue of TNM/staging classification of neuroendocrine neoplasms is as yet unsettled. The classification presented in Chapter 1 is for "carcinoid", i.e. well-differentiated lesions only. Conversely, the classification proposed by the European Neuroendocrine Tumor Society (ENETS) is also intended for high-grade neoplasms {2684, 2685}. In the appendix, the American Joint Committee on Cancer/International Union Against Cancer (AJCC/UICC) classification for T (tumour) is based on size only, while the ENETS proposal considers invasion of subserosa/-mesoappendix, an issue that requires data confirmation.

The vast majority of patients with NETs of the appendix have a favourable prognosis. Neoplasms of < 1 cm hardly ever metastasize. Nonfunctioning, non-angioinvasive neoplasms confined to the appendiceal wall and of < 2 cm in diameter are generally cured by complete local excision, the risk for developing lymph-node metastases being 1% or less. A risk of 21–44% {2120} for metastatic spread to the lymph nodes {1936} has to be taken into account if the neoplasm exceeds 2 cm in size or invades deeply into the meso-appendiceal/subserosal fatty tissue or shows angioinvasion {109, 183, 1936, 2120, 2773, 3147}. The significance of several other parameters, such as invasion of peritoneum, an elevated proliferation index, expression of additional immunohistochemical markers such as p53 {2173}, localization of the neoplasm in the basis of the appendix, the distance from the meso-appendiceal resection margin are still unclear and remain to be investigated in larger series.

While there is agreement that a right-sided hemicolectomy (including lymphadenectomy) should be performed in patients with neoplasms of > 2 cm in diameter, there is still significant uncertainty as to appropriate therapy in cases where one of the aforementioned adverse prognostic factors is present in a patient with a neoplasm of < 2 cm in diameter. For example, while some claim that meso-appendiceal invasion in neoplasms of < 2 cm has no prognostic impact and simple appendectomy is sufficient {2733}, others perform right-sided hemicolectomy and lymphadenectomy in such cases, since lymph-node metastases may be found in about 1% of patients {355, 681, 2191, 2566}. Location of neoplasms at the base of the appendix with involvement of the surgical margin or of the caecum is prognostically unfavourable, requiring at least a partial caecal resection to avoid residual tumour or subsequent recurrence.

The 5-year survival of patients with appendiceal NETs is 88–94% for localized disease, 78–83% for regional disease, and 25–31% when distant metastases are present {2023, 3624}.

Tubular NETs behave in a clinically benign manner {371}.

Of the two cases of NECs in the appendix so far reported, one was associated with an adenocarcinoma and the patient was alive 65 months after diagnosis, while the other patient only survived 2 months after surgery, which is consistent with the overall poor prognosis of pure NECs of other gastrointestinal sites.

Several studies have shown that patients with appendiceal NETs exhibit an increased risk for other gastrointestinal malignancies, which warrants follow-up of all patients via colonoscopic screening {356}.

Miscellaneous tumours of the appendix

N.J. Carr
L.H. Sobin

Neural proliferations

Neural proliferations are common in the appendix. By far the most frequent is the neuroma, also called neurogenic appendicopathy or neurogenous hyperplasia {441, 2401}. This lesion causes obliteration of the appendiceal lumen by replacing the normal mucosa and lymphoid tissue with a proliferation of spindle cells that immunoexpress S100 protein, together with nerve fibres, neuroendocrine cells, mast cells and eosinophils within a variably myxoid and collagenous stroma. These lesions were previously diagnosed as fibrous obliteration. Occasionally, neuromas may be found in the mucosa or submucosa without luminal obliteration. Neuromas of the appendix can be encountered in any age group, but their prevalence increases with age; one study found that 58% of appendices removed at autopsy exhibited luminal obliteration by this process {2401}.

Other neural proliferations, such as neurofibroma, ganglioneuroma, schwannoma and gangliocytic paraganglioma are rare in the appendix {2076, 2400, 3363, 3679}. Gastrointestinal stromal tumours are probably the most frequent mesenchymal neoplasm at this site {2076}. One reported case had ganglion cells and nerve fibres within the tumour {38}.

Lymphomas

Lymphomas involve the appendix usually as part of more general intestinal spread. Lymphomas presenting as primary disease of the appendix are rare; some

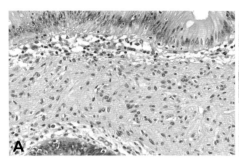 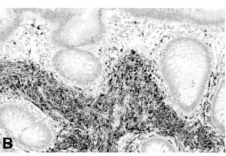

Fig. 7.13 Neuroma of the appendix. **A** The tumour occupies part of the lamina propria mucosae and comprises an eosinophilic bundle composed of fibroblastic cells with eosinophilic cytoplasm and spindle- or oval-shaped nuclei. **B** Immunohistochemical staining for S100 protein is positive.

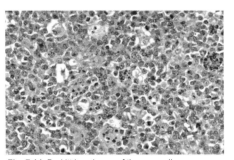

Fig. 7.14 Burkitt lymphoma of the appendix.

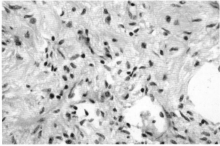

Fig. 7.15 Neuroma of the appendix. This lesion caused luminal obliteration. Spindle cells positive for S100 are intermingled with eosinophils.

are of Burkitt type {2180}.

Other rare primary appendiceal neoplasms that have been described are Kaposi sarcoma and small cell carcinoma {710, 2339}.

Secondary tumours

Secondary tumours are unusual in the appendix. Primary sites include carcinomas of the gastrointestinal and urogenital tract, breast, lung, and gallbladder. Metastatic thymoma and melanoma have also been reported {170, 959, 1032, 2727, 3066, 3537}. A common pattern is serosal involvement, presumably due to transcoelomic spread. Endometriosis involving the appendix wall may mimic metastatic adenocarcinoma.

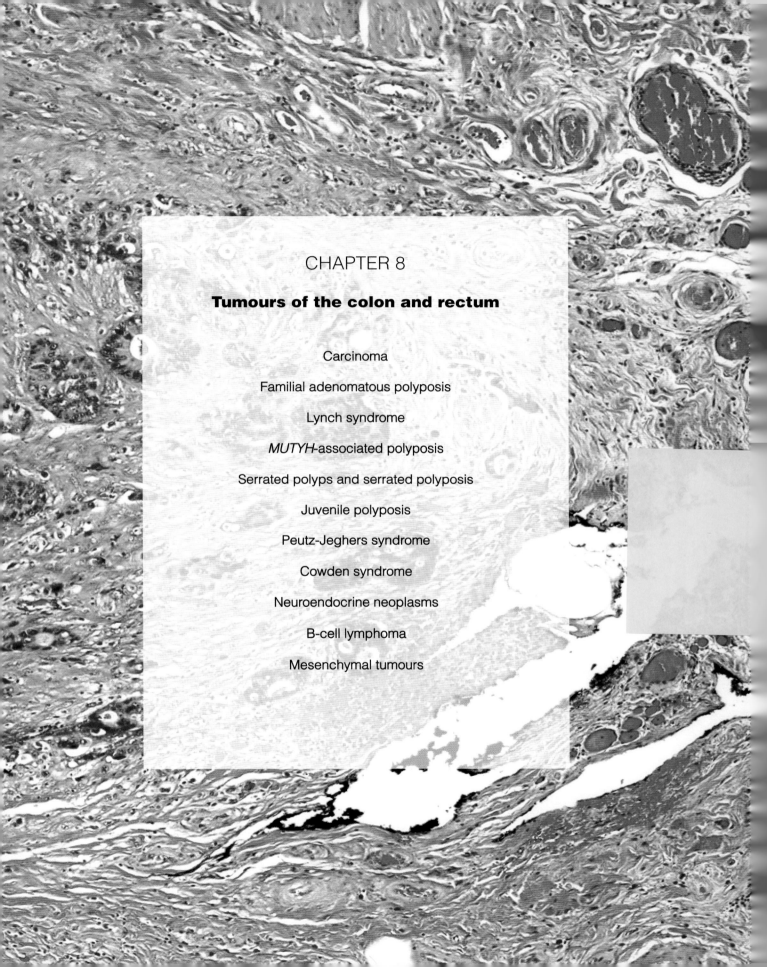

CHAPTER 8

Tumours of the colon and rectum

Carcinoma

Familial adenomatous polyposis

Lynch syndrome

MUTYH-associated polyposis

Serrated polyps and serrated polyposis

Juvenile polyposis

Peutz-Jeghers syndrome

Cowden syndrome

Neuroendocrine neoplasms

B-cell lymphoma

Mesenchymal tumours

WHO classification[a] of tumours of the colon and rectum

Epithelial tumours

Premalignant lesions

Adenoma	8140/0
Tubular	8211/0
Villous	8261/0
Tubulovillous	8263/0
Dysplasia (intraepithelial neoplasia), low grade	8148/0*
Dysplasia (intraepithelial neoplasia), high grade	8148/2
Serrated lesions	
Hyperplastic polyp	
Sessile serrated adenoma/polyp	8213/0*
Traditional serrated adenoma	8213/0*

Hamartomas

Cowden-associated polyp
Juvenile polyp
Peutz-Jeghers polyp

Carcinomas

Adenocarcinoma	8140/3
Cribriform comedo-type adenocarcinoma	8201/3*
Medullary carcinoma	8510/3
Micropapillary carcinoma	8265/3*
Mucinous adenocarcinoma	8480/3
Serrated adenocarcinoma	8213/3*
Signet ring cell carcinoma	8490/3
Adenosquamous carcinoma	8560/3
Spindle cell carcinoma	8032/3
Squamous cell carcinoma	8070/3
Undifferentiated carcinoma	8020/3

Neuroendocrine neoplasms[b]

Neuroendocrine tumour (NET)	
NET G1 (carcinoid)	8240/3
NET G2	8249/3
Neuroendocrine carcinoma (NEC)	8246/3
Large cell NEC	8013/3
Small cell NEC	8041/3
Mixed adenoneuroendocrine carcinoma	8244/3
EC cell, serotonin-producing NET	8241/3
L cell, Glucagon-like peptide-producing and PP/PYY-producing NETs	8152/1*

Mesenchymal tumours

Leiomyoma	8890/0
Lipoma	8850/0
Angiosarcoma	9120/3
Gastrointestinal stromal tumour	8936/3
Kaposi sarcoma	9140/3
Leiomyosarcoma	8890/3

Lymphomas

Secondary tumours

EC, enterochromaffin.

[a] The morphology codes are from the International Classification of Diseases for Oncology (ICD-O) {904A}. Behaviour is coded /0 for benign tumours, /1 for unspecified, borderline or uncertain behaviour, /2 for carcinoma *in situ* and grade III intraepithelial neoplasia, and /3 for malignant tumours.

[b] The classification is modified from the previous (third) edition of the WHO histological classification of tumours {691} taking into account changes in our understanding of these lesions. In the case of neuroendocrine neoplasms, the classification has been simplified to be of more practical utility in morphological classification.

* These new codes were approved by the IARC/WHO Committee for ICD-O at its meeting in March 2010.

TNM classification[a] of tumours of the colon and rectum[b]

Carcinoma of the colon and rectum

T – Primary tumour
TX   Primary tumour cannot be assessed
T0   No evidence of primary tumour
Tis   Carcinoma *in situ*: intraepithelial or invasion of lamina propria
T1   Tumour invades submucosa
T2   Tumour invades muscularis propria
T3   Tumour invades subserosa or into non-peritonealized pericolic or perirectal tissues
T4   Tumour perforates visceral peritoneum and/or directly invades other organs or structures
   T4a   Tumour perforates visceral peritoneum
   T4b   Tumour directly invades other organ or structures

N – Regional lymph nodes
NX   Regional lymph nodes cannot be assessed
N0   No regional lymph-node metastasis
N1   Metastasis in 1 to 3 regional lymph nodes
   N1a   Metastasis in 1 regional lymph node
   N1b   Metastasis in 2 to 3 regional lymph nodes
   N1c   Tumour deposit(s), i.e. satellites, in the subserosa, or in non-peritonealized pericolic or perirectal soft tissue without regional lymph-node metastasis
N2   Metastasis in 4 or more regional lymph nodes
   N2a   Metastasis in 4 to 6 regional lymph nodes
   N2b   Metastasis in 7 or more regional lymph nodes

M – Distant metastasis
M0   No distant metastasis
M1   Distant metastasis
   M1a   Metastasis confined to one organ
   M1b   Metastases in more than one organ or the peritoneum

Stage grouping

Stage	T	N	M
Stage 0	Tis	N0	M0
Stage I	T1, T2	N0	M0
Stage II	T3, T4	N0	M0
Stage IIA	T3	N0	M0
Stage IIB	T4a	N0	M0
Stage IIC	T4b	N0	M0
Stage III	Any T	N1, N2	M0
Stage IIIA	T1, T2	N1	M0
	T1	N2a	M0
Stage IIIB	T3, T4a	N1	M0
	T2,T3	N2a	M0
	T1,T2	N2b	M0
Stage IIIC	T4a	N2a	M0
	T3, T4a	N2b	M0
	T4b	N1,N2	M0
Stage IVA	Any T	Any N	M1a
Stage IVB	Any T	Any N	M1b

Carcinoid of the colon and rectum[c]

T – Primary tumour
TX   Primary tumour cannot be assessed
T0   No evidence of primary tumour
T1   Tumour invades lamina propria or submucosa and is no greater than 2 cm in size
   T1a Tumour less than 1 cm in size
   T1b Tumour 1 to 2 cm in size
T2   Tumour invades muscularis propria or is greater than 2 cm in size
T3   Tumour invades subserosa, or non-peritonealized pericolic or perirectal tissues
T4   Tumour perforates peritoneum or invades other organs

N – Regional lymph nodes
NX   Regional lymph nodes cannot be assessed
N0   No regional lymph-node metastasis
N1   Regional lymph-node metastasis

M – Distant metastasis
M0   No distant metastasis
M1   Distant metastasis

Stage grouping

Stage	T	N	M
Stage I	T1	N0	M0
Stage IIA	T2	N0	M0
Stage IIB	T3	N0	M0
Stage IIIA	T4	N0	M0
Stage IIIB	Any T	N1	M0
Stage IV	Any T	Any N	M1

---

[a] {762, 2996}
[b] The TNM classification and stage grouping for GISTs of the colon and rectum can be found on page 47.
[c] NET; well-differentiated endocrine tumour/carcinoma.
[d] The term "carcinoma *in situ*" is not consistently used in diagnostic practice. The intraepithelial lesions are comprised in the dysplasia/intraepithelial neoplasia, high-grade, category; when intramucosal invasive growth is encountered, the term used is "intramucosal carcinoma."

A help desk for specific questions about the TNM classification is available at http://www.uicc.org.

Carcinoma of the colon and rectum

S.R. Hamilton
F.T. Bosman
P. Boffetta
M. Ilyas
H. Morreau

S.-I. Nakamura
P. Quirke
E. Riboli
L.H. Sobin

Definition

A malignant epithelial tumour originating in the large bowel. Metastasis, and therefore the use of the term "carcinoma" for tumours of the colon and rectum, requires invasion through the muscularis mucosae into the submucosa. More than 90% of colorectal carcinomas (CRC) are adenocarcinomas {319}.

ICD-O codes

Adenocarcinoma	8140/3
Cribriform comedo-type adenocarcinoma	8201/3
Medullary carcinoma	8510/3
Micropapillary carcinoma	8265/3
Mucinous adenocarcinoma	8480/3
Serrated adenocarcinoma	8213/3
Signet ring cell carcinoma	8490/3
Adenosquamous carcinoma	8560/3
Spindle cell carcinoma	8032/3
Squamous cell carcinoma	8070/3
Undifferentiated carcinoma	8020/3

Epidemiology

An estimated 1.23 million new cases of CRC occurred worldwide in 2008, representing about 9.7% of all new cancers. CRC ranks as the fourth most frequent cancer in men (after lung, prostate and stomach cancer), and third in women (after cancers of the breast and uterine cervix) {319, 842}. However, the age-standardized incidence of this cancer varies by at least 25-fold around the world.

Higher rates occur in industrialized, high-resource countries of Europe, Australia, New Zealand, North America and Japan (about 40–60 per 100 000), and much lower rates in other countries in Asia (e.g. India) and Africa. The incidence, and therefore the impact of CRC on the burden of cancer, are changing in many areas of the world and will affect priorities for cancer control and cancer services. Incidence rates are rising in many countries where rates were previously low, but falling (e.g. North America), stabilizing (e.g. northern and western Europe), or increasing only gradually in countries where rates were previously high. Among immigrants and their descendants, incidence rates rapidly approach those of their adopted countries, indicating that lifestyle, dietary and perhaps other environmental factors are important risk factors {319}.

Incidence increases with age {1816}, and carcinomas are rare before the age of 40 years, except in individuals with genetic predisposition or predisposing conditions such as chronic inflammatory bowel diseases in high-incidence countries. However, age-standardized incidence rates among young patients are often higher in low-incidence than in high-incidence populations {1650, 3016}. Rates of rectal cancer are about 50% higher and colon cancer rates about 20% higher in men than in women. The ratio of colon to rectal cancer is higher in populations with a high incidence than in populations with a low incidence {3697}.

The worldwide mortality rate is about half the incidence rate (about 608 000 deaths from CRC in 2002), but there is wide variation in mortality rates according to available treatment options, with lower rates in countries with high incidences and high resources {319, 842}. Nonetheless, CRC is the most common cause of deaths from cancer that is not directly attributable to tobacco usage in some of these countries.

Etiology

Diet, lifestyle, and other exposures

A high incidence of CRC is observed consistently in populations with a "Western-type" diet (highly caloric food rich in animal fat) combined with a sedentary lifestyle. Epidemiological studies have indicated that obesity, meat consumption, smoking and alcohol consumption are important modifiable risk factors. "Westernization" of previously low-incidence populations is followed by increased incidence rates. Inverse associations in populations include dietary consumption of fruits, vegetables, whole grains, calcium and vitamin D; prolonged use of nonsteroidal anti-inflammatory drugs (NSAIDs); estrogen replacement therapy in women; and physical activity. Numerous other putative protective and predisposing dietary components and exposures have been reported {319, 882A, 1984A, 3360A}.

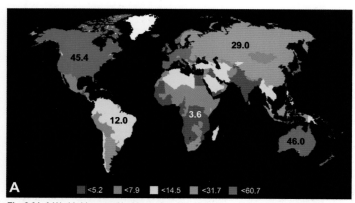

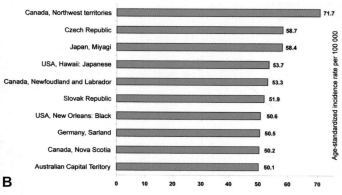

Fig. 8.01 A Worldwide annual incidence (per 100 000) of cancer of the colon and rectum in men {842A}. Numbers on the map indicate regional average values and are higher in developed countries {842A}. **B** Age-standardized incidence (per 100 000) of colorectal cancer in men in selected countries {842}.

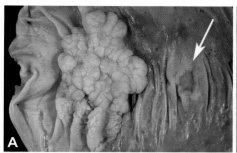 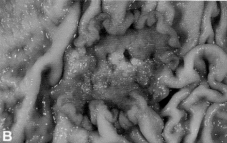 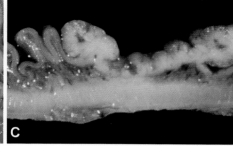

Fig. 8.02 Advanced colorectal carcinomas. **A** Small depressed invasive carcinoma with a nearby protruding adenoma. **B** Advanced colorectal carcinoma, depressed type. **C** Cross-section of adenocarcinoma with extension into the submucosa (pT1).

The molecular pathways underlying the epidemiological associations are poorly understood because of complex interactions that probably involve dietary patterns, macro- and micronutrient composition of foodstuffs, food preparation techniques, hormonal effects, genetic characteristics, and gene–diet and gene–gene effects. Research methodologies are inadequate to characterize precisely the various etiological components and their interactions, contributing to the insufficient levels of evidence upon which interventions could be based with confidence. Patients with colorectal adenomas, known to be precursors to CRC, have been studied in clinical trials of prevention strategies. Dietary modifications, e.g. fibre supplementation and reduction in fat, have been minimally effective {63, 2701} and supplemental folate that was expected to be protective may promote neoplasia {579, 854}. In contrast, NSAIDs {1102, 1736}, especially when combined with an inhibitor of the polyamine pathway {2058}, and dietary calcium supplementation {1052} have shown evidence of chemopreventive activity.

Chronic inflammation
Chronic inflammatory bowel diseases are etiological factors for CRC {1639, 3292} These diseases include ulcerative colitis (UC), Crohn disease (CD), and *Schistosoma mansoni* infection {3653}. Despite recurrent episodes of inflammation in diverticular disease, diverticulitis is not a specific risk factor for carcinoma {2054}.

Other risk factors
Rare but well-recognized etiological factors include therapeutic pelvic irradiation {2632} and ureterosigmoidostomy {1000}.

Localization
Most CRCs are located in the sigmoid colon and rectum, but the proportion of carcinomas that are more proximally located increases with age {3057}. Molecular pathology has site differences: tumours with high levels of microsatellite instability (MSI-H) and CpG-island methylation microsatellite-stable tumours are frequently located in the caecum, ascending colon and transverse colon; CpG-island methylation microsatellite-stable tumours in both the right and left colon; and microsatellite-stable tumours without CpG-island methylation mainly in the left colon {227, 1317}.

Clinical features
Signs and symptoms
Some patients are asymptomatic and the neoplasm is identified by screening or surveillance. Haematochezia and anaemia are common presenting features attributable to bleeding from the tumour. Many patients experience change in bowel habits, especially constipation, because the solid faeces in the left colon are often impeded by the mass. There may be associated abdominal distension, bowel obstruction or perforation. Rectosigmoid lesions can produce tenesmus and rectal bleeding. Other nonspecific symptoms include fever, malaise, weight loss, and abdominal pain.

Imaging
Imaging techniques permit noninvasive detection and clinical staging. Barium enema has been replaced by computer assisted tomography (CT) that may be useful for screening (CT colonography). Cross-sectional imaging by CT, magnetic resonance imaging (MRI), and transrectal ultrasonography are used to estimate depth of tumour invasion and the possibility of regional and distant metastases {722, 2546}. Scintigraphy and positron emission tomography (PET) are also used to assess the spread of disease {1174, 1477}.

Endoscopy
Colonoscopy allows observation of the mucosal surface of the entire large bowel. In addition, biopsy or therapeutic removal of identified lesions can be done by snare polypectomy, endoscopic mucosal resection or submucosal dissection, especially for adenomas and superficial carcinomas {416, 3187}. Improved magnification, chromoendoscopy employing dyes, and confocal endoscopy improve visualization of non-protruding lesions. Other innovations such as narrow band imaging with different wavelengths of light, Raman spectroscopy

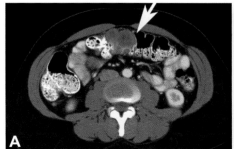 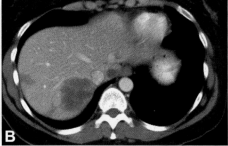

Fig. 8.03 CT scan of carcinoma of the colon and rectum. **A** Primary tumour (arrow) in the transverse colon. **B** Metastases in the liver.

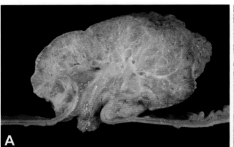
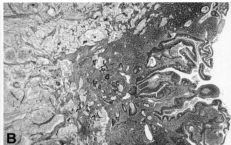
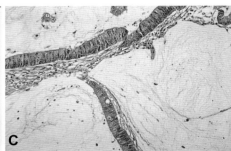

Fig. 8.04 Mucinous adenocarcinoma. **A** Cut surface with gelatinous appearance. **B** Mucinous adenocarcinoma beneath high-grade dysplasia in ulcerative colitis. **C** Multilocular mucin deposits with malignant epithelium.

and optical coherence tomography are of unproven value {2433}.

Macroscopy

Carcinomas have variable macroscopic appearances: exophytic/fungating with predominantly intraluminal growth, endophytic/ulcerative with predominantly intramural growth, annular with circumferential involvement of the colorectal wall and luminal stenosis, and, least commonly, diffusely infiltrative/linitis plastica pattern. Overlap among these types and ulceration are common. Some cancers, usually arising in a pedunculated adenoma, occur on a stalk of uninvolved mucosa and submucosa and are amenable to colonoscopic polypectomy. Carcinomas proximal to the splenic flexure tend to grow as exophytic masses while those in the descending colon and rectum are more often endophytic and annular. On cut section, most CRCs have a relatively homogeneous grey/white appearance, although a gelatinous cut surface can be seen in mucinous tumours.

Tumour spread and staging

Following transmural direct extension through the muscularis propria into pericolic or perirectal soft tissue, carcinomas may involve contiguous structures. The consequences depend on the anatomic site. Advanced rectal carcinomas may extend into pelvic structures such as the vagina and urinary bladder, but cannot gain direct access to the peritoneal cavity when located distal to the peritoneal reflection. In contrast, colonic carcinomas can extend directly to the serosal surface with transcoelomic spread in the peritoneal cavity (peritoneal carcinomatosis) and/or perforation. Since the peritoneal surface infiltrated by tumour cells may become adherent to adjacent structures, direct extension into adjoining organs can also occur. Implantation attributable to surgical manipulation, including laparoscopic resection, occurs only occasionally {103}. Spread via lymphatic or blood vessels can occur early in the natural history and lead to lymph node involvement and systemic disease. Despite the presence of lymphatic vessels in the colorectal mucosa, lymphatic spread does not occur unless the muscularis mucosae is

breached and the submucosa is invaded. Involvement of veins and venules that are portal vein tributaries in the colon and vena cava tributaries in the rectum contribute to haematogenous dissemination.

Staging

The classifications proposed by Cuthbert Dukes in 1929–1935 for rectal cancer are the basis for many staging systems for CRC, including the current TNM {89, 671}. This family of classifications for patients who underwent resection of their primary with curative intent takes into account two histopathological features: depth of penetration relative to the muscularis propria and presence or absence of metastasis in regional lymph nodes.

The TNM classification has now largely replaced other classifications thanks to its greater utility and standardization. The classification has undergone relatively few major modifications between the sixth (2002) and seventh (2009) editions, such that the main T, N, and M categories and stages I to IV can be compared easily.

In the T categories, the designations of the subdivisions of T4 are reversed. The N1 and N2 categories separating tumours

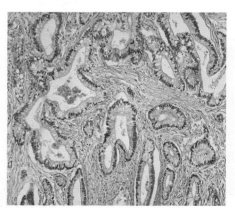

Fig. 8.05 Well-differentiated adenocarcinoma of the colon.

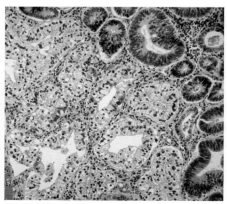

Fig. 8.06 Clear cell carcinoma of the colon.

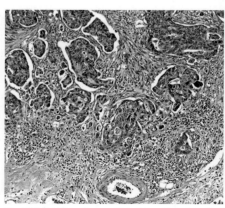

Fig. 8.07 Rectal carcinoma with budding at invasive edge.

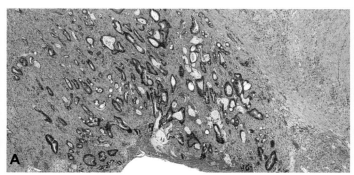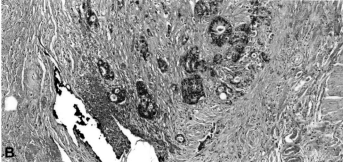

Fig. 8.08 Adenocarcinoma in a pT4 stage category. **A** The tumour extends through the muscularis propria and subserosa and penetrates the serosa, accessing the peritoneal cavity. The obliterated serosal surface does not represent a surgical margin of resection. **B** The tumour extends through the subserosa, which shows active inflammation and mesothelial reaction on the serosal surface. Black ink was applied to the gross specimen to assist in histopathological identification of the serosa.

involving three or fewer lymph nodes and four or more are retained, but further subdivision by number of involved nodes is added for finer distinction. The categorization of mesenteric tumour deposits or satellites without identifiable residual lymph node is clarified. These may represent discontinuous spread, venous invasion with extravascular spread, or a totally replaced lymph node. Such a deposit, regardless of size or configuration (used as criteria in the fifth and sixth editions, respectively), is changed to equivalency to a lymph-node metastasis, and in the absence of lymph-node involvement is designated N1c in the seventh edition to favour treatment with postoperative adjuvant chemotherapy. This categorization leads to the paradoxical situation in which in the presence of a single lymph-node metastasis changes the category from N1c to N1a and therefore underestimates the prognostic influence of the mesenteric deposit {2600, 2601, 3336}.

The M category is subdivided into a category with distant metastasis confined to one organ and potentially amenable to surgical resection (although extent of single-organ involvement, e.g. unilobar vs bilobar liver metastases, is not incorporated, and preoperative neoadjuvant chemotherapy may convert some tumours from unresectable to resectable) and a second category with more widely disseminated metastases in more than one organ or the peritoneum. The prefix "p" is used to indicate pathological, as contrasted with clinical or imaging, assessment.

All the subdivisions of the T, N, and M categories are expressed in subdivisions of the stage groupings, generating three subdivisions each for stages II and III and two subdivisions of stage IV, with comparability to previous TNM staging systems

over the last 30 years. Molecular characteristics and other histological features such as extramural vascular invasion and depth of invasion in T1 carcinoma that are not included in the TNM classification but influence outcome and treatment are discussed below.

Histopathology

The defining feature of CRC is invasion through the muscularis mucosae into the submucosa. More than 90% of CRCs are adenocarcinomas {319}. Lesions with the histopathological characteristics of adenocarcinoma that are confined within the mucosa and completely removed have no risk of metastasis even when intramucosal invasion is present. Because these lesions are cured when removed completely, the terms "high-grade dysplasia" or "intramucosal carcinoma" are often used to avoid inappropriate overtreatment for carcinoma, e.g. surgical resection {3024}. However, "intramucosal adenocarcinoma" is used routinely with associated treatment recommendations in the *Guidelines for Treatment of Colorectal Carcinoma* edited by the Japanese Society for Cancer of the Colon and Rectum {1391, 1392}.

Most colorectal adenocarcinomas are negative for keratin 7 and positive for keratin 20 by immunohistochemistry and also express CDX2 transcription factor. A proportion of tumours is negative for keratin 20, and these tend to be MSI-H {2024}. Expression of CDX2 is not associated with MSI status {172, 2387}.

Other variants

Several histopathological variants can be distinguished, some associated with specific molecular characteristics.

Mucinous adenocarcinoma

This designation is used if > 50% of the lesion is composed of pools of extracellular mucin that contain malignant epithelium as acinar structures, layers of tumour cells, or individual tumour cells including signet-ring cells. The level of maturation of the epithelium determines differentiation, but many mucinous adenocarcinomas are MSI-H {1061, 1804} and therefore low-grade. Mucinous adenocarcinomas that are microsatellite-stable (MSS) or have low levels of instability (MSI-L) behave as high-grade lesions. Carcinomas with mucinous areas of < 50% are categorized as having a mucinous component.

Signet ring cell carcinoma

This variant of adenocarcinoma is defined by the presence of > 50% of tumour cells with prominent intracytoplasmic mucin, typically with displacement and moulding of the nucleus. Signet-ring cells can occur within the pools of mucinous adenocarcinoma or in a diffusely infiltrative process with minimal extracellular mucin in a linitis-plastica pattern. Large signet-ring cells can be termed "globoid cells". Some signet ring cell carcinomas are MSI-H and

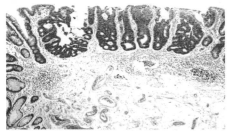

Fig. 8.09 Intramucosal adenocarcinoma. Criteria of the Japanese Society for Cancer of the Colon and Rectum {1391, 1392}.

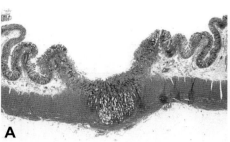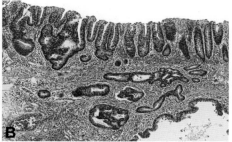

Fig. 8.10 A Small adenocarcinoma arising in a depressed adenoma and invading the muscularis propria. **B** Early adenocarcinoma arising in a flat adenoma and invading the submucosa.

are low-grade, but those that lack MSI-H are usually highly aggressive {2442}. Carcinomas with signet-ring cell areas of < 50% are categorized as adenocarcinoma with a signet-ring cell component (signet ring cell carcinoma).

Medullary carcinoma

This rare variant is characterized by sheets of malignant cells with vesicular nuclei, prominent nucleoli and abundant eosinophilic cytoplasm exhibiting prominent infiltration by intraepithelial lymphocytes. It almost invariably has MSI-H and usually a favourable prognosis {1573, 2872}.

Serrated adenocarcinoma

This rare variant has architectural similarity to a sessile serrated polyp with glandular serration that may be accompanied by mucinous, cribriform, lacy and trabecular areas and a low nucleus-to-cytoplasm ratio. These tumours can have MSI-L or MSI-H, BRAF mutations, and CpG island hypermethylation {1400, 1404, 1963}.

Cribriform comedo-type adenocarcinoma

This rare tumour has extensive large cribriform glands with central necrosis analogous to breast adenocarcinomas and is usually microsatellite-stable with CpG island hypermethylation {528}.

Micropapillary adenocarcinoma

This rare variant has small clusters of tumour cells within stromal spaces mimicking vascular channels and has also been described in breast and bladder cancer. The pattern can be seen as a component of conventional CRC. Immunohistochemistry shows a characteristic MUC1 staining pattern {1211, 1687, 2780, 3283}.

Adenosquamous carcinoma

This unusual tumour has features of both squamous cell carcinoma and adenocarcinoma, either as separate areas within the tumour or admixed. This variant has more than just occasional small foci of squamous differentiation. Pure squamous cell carcinoma is very rare.

Spindle cell carcinoma

This is a biphasic carcinoma with a spindle-cell sarcomatoid component in which the tumour cells are at least focally immunoreactive for keratins {135, 1421, 1553}.

Undifferentiated carcinoma

These rare tumours lack morphological, immunohistochemical, and molecular biological evidence of differentiation beyond that of an epithelial tumour and have variable histological features. Some of these tumours have MSI-H.

Rare variants

There is an additional heterogeneous group of very rare CRC variants, e.g. clear cell carcinoma, that often have a component of conventional adenocarcinoma or mimic other types of cancers, e.g. choriocarcinoma {1050}, Paneth cell-rich papillary adenocarcinomas {2959}. The differential diagnosis includes metastasis from elsewhere or rare primary colorectal tumours, e.g. primary melanoma or nonepithelial cell types such as gastrointestinal stromal tumours (GISTs).

Grading

Colorectal adenocarcinoma was graded traditionally as well-, moderately, poorly, and undifferentiated on the basis of the percentage of gland formation. "Undifferentiated adenocarcinoma" is an oxymoron, and "undifferentiated carcinoma" (grade 4) is now a term of exclusion reserved for malignant epithelial tumours that show no gland formation, mucin production, or neuroendocrine, squamous or sarcomatoid differentiation. The terms "low-grade" and "high-grade" are now favoured for clinical usage owing to the similar behaviour of well- and moderately differentiated carcinomas and greater reproducibility. Morphological grading of tumours applies only to "Adenocarcinoma, NOS". Other morphological variants carry their own prognostic significance and grading does not apply. Adenocarcinomas and undifferentiated carcinomas that have MSI-H behave as low-grade.

Carcinomas are sometimes heterogeneous, and grading is then based upon the least differentiated component. The invading edge of CRC is regarded as suboptimal to evaluate tumour grade, but the presence of "tumour budding" with poorly differentiated foci characterized by rudimentary gland formation and individual invasive carcinoma cells has been associated with aggressive behaviour {2360, 3452}. Classification of morphologic variants and carcinomas other than adenocarcinomas, e.g. NEC, as low- or high-grade requires consideration of specific criteria other than those for adenocarcinoma.

Precursor lesions
Aberrant crypt foci (ACF)

ACF are clusters of abnormal crypts seen on staining colorectal mucosa in resection specimens with methylene blue or mucosal examination with a magnifying endoscope or chromoendoscopy. Increased numbers

Table 8.01 Criteria for histological grading of colorectal adenocarcinomas.

Criterion	Differentiation category	Numerical grade[a]	Descriptive grade
> 95% with gland formation	Well-differentiated	1	Low
50–95% with gland formation	Moderately differentiated	2	Low
> 0–49% with gland formation	Poorly differentiated	3	High
High level of microsatellite instability[b]	Variable	Variable	Low

[a] The category "undifferentiated carcinoma" (grade 4) is reserved for carcinomas with no gland formation, mucin production, or neuroendocrine, squamous or sarcomatoid differentiation; [b] MSI-H.

of ACF are seen in association with neoplasia. Histopathology shows two main types: those resembling hyperplastic polyps that are common, and those with dysplasia (microadenomas) that are rare, except in familial adenomatous polyposis (FAP) {531, 2326}. The clinical importance of sporadic ACFs is uncertain {1088, 1737}.

Adenomas

Adenomas are defined by the presence of dysplastic epithelium. This is characterized histopathologically by enlarged, hyperchromatic nuclei, varying degrees of nuclear spindling and stratification, and loss of polarity. Dysplasia can be low-grade or high-grade, depending on the degree of architectural complexity, extent of nuclear stratification, and severity of abnormal nuclear morphology. Foci in invasive growth can be encountered in an adenoma with high-grade dysplasia. For such lesions, the terms high-grade dysplasia as well as intramucosal carcinomas are used. Paneth cells, neuroendocrine cells and squamous-cell aggregates may be seen in adenomas {189, 1370, 3426}.

Macroscopically, most adenomas are polypoid with protrusion into the colorectal lumen, either sessile with broad attachment or on a stalk. A smaller number are flat or depressed {1734, 2469} and often recognizable macroscopically by mucosal reddening, subtle changes in texture, or highlighting by specialized endoscopic techniques.

Most adenomas are < 1 cm in size and have tubular architecture. Villous architecture is defined as leaf- or finger-like projections of epithelium overlying a small amount of lamina propria. Tubulovillous adenomas are defined by a mixture of tubular and villous structures with arbitrary percentages in different studies, typically between 25% and 75% villous component. Unusual histopathological patterns such as microtubular adenoma occur.

The characteristics of adenomas are associated with the occurrence of synchronous and metachronous carcinoma. Adenomas of larger size (1 cm), more extensive villous architecture, and high-grade intraepithelial neoplasia/dysplasia, termed "advanced adenomas" {1155}, and flat depressed adenomas {1734} have a higher frequency of malignancy, although depressed adenomas have a lower frequency of KRAS mutation than do polypoid adenomas {2158}. Patients who have an adenoma of 20 mm or more with tubulovillous or villous architecture in a proximal location in the

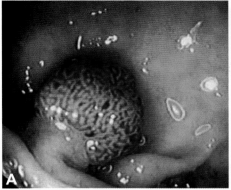 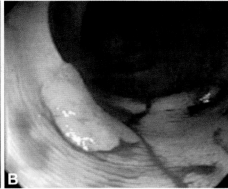

Fig. 8.11 Endoscopic features of adenoma. **A** Polypoid. **B** Flat, slightly elevated.

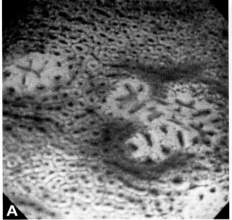 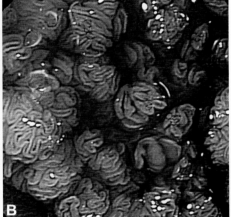

Fig. 8.12 Endoscopic features of adenomas highlighted with indigo carmine. **A** Two small flat adenomas; note the abnormal tubular pit pattern. **B** Tubulovillous adenoma seen by magnifying video endoscopy; the cerebriform pattern is highlighted.

colon, multiplicity of adenomas (five or more) or are male have more frequent development of a metachronous advanced adenoma or carcinoma {1991}. The clinical implications of serration in adenomas and of sessile serrated adenomas/polyps are not yet well-defined.

Serrated lesions

This is a heterogeneous group of lesions characterized morphologically by a serrated (sawtooth or stellate) architecture of the epithelial compartment, and includes the hyperplastic polyp, sessile serrated adenoma/polyp and traditional serrated adenoma.

Juvenile polyp

Sporadic juvenile polyps occur most commonly in children {3451}. This lesion contains abundant stroma composed of inflamed, often oedematous, granulation tissue that surrounds cystically dilated glands containing mucin. The glands are lined by cuboidal to columnar epithelial

cells with reactive changes.

The juvenile polyps in patients with juvenile polyposis syndrome often have a frond-like growth pattern with less stroma, fewer dilated glands and more proliferated small glands (microtubular pattern) than the sporadic type. Dysplasia is rare in sporadic juvenile polyps, but there is an increased risk of colorectal carcinoma in patients with juvenile polyposis syndrome {1280}.

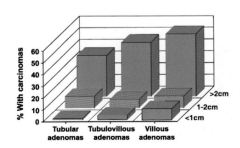

Fig. 8.13 Frequency of colorectal adenocarcinoma in adenomas relative to size and architecture.

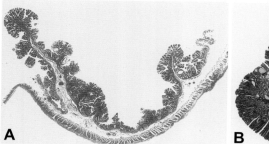
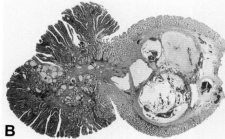

Fig. 8.14 Tubulovillous adenoma. **A** Partly sessile, partly pedunculated. **B** With pseudoinvasion. Small clusters of adenomatous cells produce multilocular, large mucin deposits that expand the stalk of the adenoma. This growth pattern can be mistaken for mucinous adenocarcinoma.

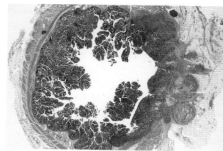

Fig. 8.15 Villous adenoma of the rectum and invasive adenocarcinoma.

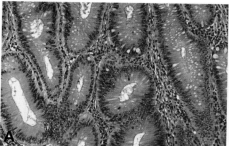
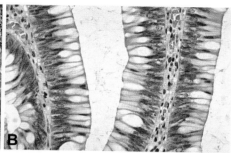

Fig. 8.16 A Adenoma with low-grade dysplasia and well-maintained glandular architecture. **B** Low-grade dysplasia with regular but slightly elongated, hyperchromatic nuclei. Cytoplasmic mucin is retained.

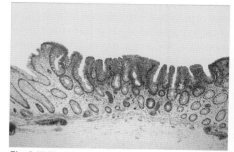

Fig. 8.17 Flat "elevated" tubular adenoma showing low-grade dysplasia.

Peutz-Jeghers polyp

These are hamartomatous gastrointestinal polyps that preferentially affect the small intestine and that, together with muco-cutaneous melanin pigmentation, are a component of the inherited predisposition syndrome, Peutz-Jeghers syndrome (PJS).

Other lesions
Reactive lesions/mimics of carcinoma
Inflammatory polyp/"pseudopolyp." These are composed of varying proportions of reactive epithelium, inflamed granulation tissue and fibrous tissue, often with morphological similarity to juvenile polyps. Inflammatory polyps are seen in a variety of chronic inflammatory diseases including ulcerative colitis, Crohn colitis, diverticulitis, and schistosomiasis {3574, 3653}. Mucosal prolapse changes/solitary rectal ulcer syndrome/colitis cystica profunda. Polyps, masses, erosions and ulcers characterized histopathologically by elongated, distorted regenerative glands surrounded by proliferated smooth-muscle fibres from the muscularis mucosae can occur together with inflamed granulation tissue and fibrosis in prolapsing mucosa and entrapped glands in deeper layers {761, 2410, 2974}. When located in the rectum, the lesion is termed solitary rectal ulcer syndrome, but these findings can occur with prolapse in other sites, e.g. colostomy stomas. The features can be confused with inflamed adenoma or invasive adenocarcinomas and are an important cause of misdiagnosis of neoplasia. On the other hand, mucosal prolapse changes can occur due to an underlying neoplasm {1836}.

In addition to mucosal prolapse changes/solitary rectal ulcer syndrome/colitis cystica profunda, misplacement of epithelium in the submucosa of adenomas ("pseudoinvasion") {3198} and muciphages may be misdiagnosed as carcinoma.

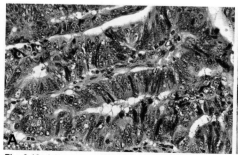
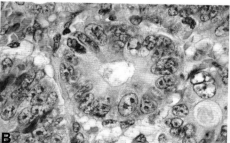
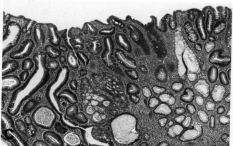

Fig. 8.18 Adenomas with high-grade dysplasia. **A** Loss of normal glandular architecture, hyperchromatic cells with multi-layered irregular nuclei and loss of mucin, and a high nucleus-to-cytoplasm ratio. According to Japanese criteria, this would be an intramucosal carcinoma. **B** Loss of polarity with little nuclear stratification; marked nuclear atypia with prominent nucleoli (Japanese criteria: intramucosal adenocarcinoma). **C** Adenoma with focal cribriform pattern (Japanese criteria: adenocarcinoma in adenoma).

Neoplasia in chronic inflammatory bowel diseases

The natural history and morphology of CRC associated with chronic colitis differ from those of sporadic carcinomas {45, 1164, 3723}. The risk in ulcerative colitis and Crohn disease increases after 8–10 years and is highest in patients with early-onset and extensive involvement of the colorectum, especially pancolitis.

Ulcerative colitis (UC)

This chronic inflammatory disorder of unknown etiology affects children and adults, with a peak incidence in the early third decade of life. A risk of CRC of 30% after 30 years is reported in patients with pancolitis in whom the inflammatory disease began before the age of 15 years. Population-based studies show a 4.4-fold increase in mortality from CRC {771, 2039, 2532, 3078}, but in clinical studies, the increase in incidence is usually higher, up to 20-fold {1095, 1698}. Involvement of more than half of the colorectum by UC is associated with a risk of developing carcinoma of approximately 15%, whereas less extensive left-sided disease has a lower risk of malignancy of about 5% {1801, 2915}, and ulcerative proctitis is not associated with increased risk.

UC-associated CRCs are often multiple, flat, infiltrative, and mucinous or signet-ring cell type. Low-grade tubuloglandular adenocarcinoma occurs almost exclusively in UC or Crohn disease and is particularly problematic to diagnose because of its well-differentiated nature {1815, 3341}. The carcinomas evolve through low-grade and high-grade dysplasia that have heterogeneous macroscopic appearances and may be difficult to distinguish histopathologically from inflammation-induced reactive epithelium. Flat lesions may be difficult to recognize endoscopically without chromoendoscopy {469}. Raised dysplastic lesions ("dysplasia-associated lesion or mass", DALM) may present as polyps, plaques or subtle velvety patches in inflamed areas. Extensive biopsy sampling is therefore essential. DALM is strongly associated with carcinoma and considered an indication for colectomy {1880}, but distinction of colitis-associated dysplasia from a sporadic adenoma that can be adequately treated by polypectomy may be very difficult {1880, 1882, 3370}.

Although the molecular alterations in sporadic and UC-related cancer are

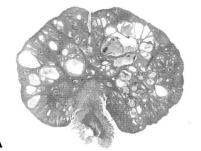
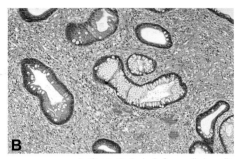

Fig. 8.19 Juvenile polyp. **A** Smooth eroded surface with numerous mucus retention cysts, typical of sporadic juvenile polyps. **B** Expanded inflamed stroma with distorted glands showing reactive changes.

similar {3443}, they seem to differ in frequency and sequence: *APC* mutation occurs late and *TP53* mutation occurs early in UC-associated CRC {3568}, and MSI-H CRC is frequent {915}. Multiple heterogeneous molecular alterations may be found in the surrounding mucosa {582, 2476, 2693}, indicating field abnormalities that explain the multiplicity. Use of molecular markers, including transcriptome analysis, to allow early detection of intraepithelial neoplasia/dysplasia in UC has been extensively investigated, but to date no markers have achieved a level of evidence to be included in follow-up surveillance.

Crohn disease

This disease is associated with an increased risk of carcinoma in the small and the large intestine. The risk of CRC appears to be about threefold that in individuals without chronic inflammatory bowel disease {890, 989}. Long duration and early onset of disease are risk factors, as in UC. The characteristics of CRC in Crohn disease are similar to those in UC {2966}, but there is also an increased frequency of adenocarcinoma within perianal fistulae and of squamous cell carcinoma of the anus {1702}.

Genetic susceptibility

Twin studies suggest that up to 35% of all CRCs can be ascribed to inherited susceptibility {637}. Approximately 10–35% of all CRC cases show familial clustering, and only a proportion can be explained by known syndromes. The currently known CRC-predisposition syndromes with high-risk germline mutations account for < 6% of all cases {1}.

The high-risk genetic diseases are classified morphologically into polyposis syndromes characterized by large numbers of polyps (e.g. FAP) and nonpolyposis syndromes characterized by a small number of or absence of polyps, e.g. Lynch syndrome. Although most of these syndromes show autosomal dominant inheritance, recessive inheritance is evident in *MUTYH*-associated polyposis (MAP) due to mutation of the base excision-repair gene inherited from each parent {1906}.

For individuals from unexplained family clusters, the lifetime risk for CRC is more than twice that of the general population when these individuals have an affected first-degree relative, and more than threefold when the first-degree relative is younger than 50 years {177, 388, 1435}. Some of the currently unexplained familial risk could be attributable to as yet

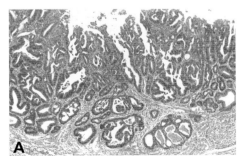
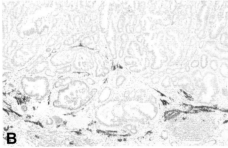

Fig. 8.20 Moderately differentiated adenocarcinoma with tubular adenoma, excised by endoscopic mucosal resection. **A** Part of the adenocarcinoma invaded the lamina muscularis mucosae. **B** Immunohistochemical staining for desmin reveals entanglement of the tissues of the invading adenocarcinoma with muscle fibres of the muscularis mucosae.

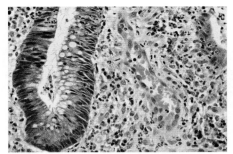

Fig. 8.21 Reactive epithelial changes in ulcerative colitis.

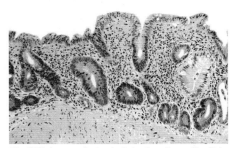

Fig. 8.22 Low-grade dysplasia in ulcerative colitis. Note the haphazardly arranged dysplastic glands.

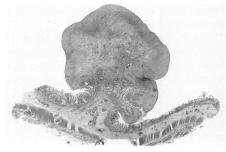

Fig. 8.23 Inflammatory polyp in ulcerative colitis.

unidentified highly penetrant genetic risk factors. Another explanation could be the combination of several cancer-susceptibility alleles of low or moderate penetrance {1251}.

Unexplained high- or moderate-risk genetic predisposition

Evidence for additional high- or moderate-risk alleles comes from the 30–40% of large families with CRC who fulfil the so-called "Amsterdam" clinical criteria for Lynch syndrome but lack a deficiency in mismatch repair and germline mutations in mismatch-repair genes {669, 1863, 1864}. Such families have been termed "familial colorectal cancer type X" {1862} or mismatch repair-proficient hereditary nonpolyposis colorectal cancer (HNPCC). {2794}. Linkages with chromosomes 3q22 and 9q22 have been reported {1517, 1519, 2447, 2545, 2983, 3502}.

Low-penetrance cancer-susceptibility alleles

Numerous genome-wide polymorphic genetic variations that may determine individual susceptibility to cancer have been studied in candidate-gene approaches and genome-wide association studies (GWAS) {670, 2768, 3265}. Loci identified by GWAS collectively account for about 6% of the risk of developing CRC. Low-penetrance alleles can act as modifiers in highly penetrant diseases {3505}. Functional causal variants and genes and the mechanisms of their actions are only partly known. The novel variants may act as regulatory elements of gene expression.

Genetic risk of CRC associated with other cancer syndromes or diseases

Risk of CRC may be influenced by germline defects that lead to cancer syndromes not typically involving the colorectum, e.g. Li-Fraumeni syndrome, characterized by germline mutation of *TP53* {2367, 3544}, and *BRCA1* hereditary breast and ovarian cancer syndrome {648, 881}. Genetic polymorphisms or alterations in inflammatory-response genes are related to the occurrence of UC and Crohn disease that in turn predispose to CRC. Alterations in *TNF* and *NOD2/-CARD15* may influence the risk of CRC at older ages and with no relationship to inflammatory bowel disease {1691, 3111}.

Molecular pathology

Cancer-associated genes and biomarkers can be grouped into categories based upon the types of information they provide:

Predisposition: germline (i.e. inherited) variants that result in increased risk.
Profile: somatically mutated or altered in expression within tumours.
Prognostic: associated with natural history and clinical outcome.
Predictive: associated with responsiveness or resistance of a tumour to specific therapies.
Pharmacogenomic: associated with metabolism and may affect levels and effectiveness of specific therapies

These five categories overlap, and many genes and biomarkers are in more than one category.

Profile genes and biomarkers in the adenoma–adenocarcinoma sequence

CRC is a paradigm for multistep carcinogenesis with morphological–genomic associations in the adenoma–adenocarcinoma sequence, as introduced by Fearon and Vogelstein in 1990 {829, 2199}. The body of evidence indicates that: (1) some alterations segregate together or inversely as part of a "genetic pathway" {1316}; and (2) functional pathways can be disrupted at different points so that different alterations may have functional "equivalence" in the same pathway {2493}.

Chromosomal instability pathway

Around 75% of sporadic CRCs in developed countries, a higher percentage in low-incidence populations, and most syndromic CRCs other than Lynch syndrome develop along the chromosomal-instability pathway {1046, 1486}. These cancers are characterized by gross chromosomal abnormalities, such as aneuploid karyotype, large chromosome-segment deletions and duplications, and increased nuclear DNA content. The tumours almost always have an *APC* mutation (> 90%) while *KRAS* mutations occur in about 50%,

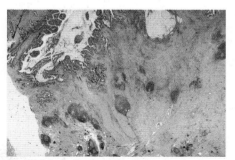

Fig. 8.24 Crohn-like lymphoid reaction associated with a colonic adenocarcinoma.

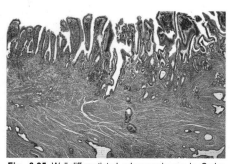

Fig. 8.25 Well-differentiated adenocarcinoma in Crohn disease, invading the wall beneath high-grade dysplasia with villous architecture.

TP53 mutations in about 70%, and 18q allelic loss in about 80%. Some tumours have a BRAF mutation as an alternative to KRAS mutation {2887}. The molecular characteristics of individual CRCs associate with DNA methylation status owing to epigenetic and genomic interactions. Mutations in PIK3CA are reported to occur in about 25% of tumours and are considered to be late events {2362}. Mutations in FBXW7/CDC4 are also reported as late occurrences, and it is claimed these are responsible for aneuploidy {1518, 2618}, since adenomas are rarely aneuploid. Low-frequency mutations are reported in mitotic checkpoint genes such as CHEK2 {3519} and BUB1 {391} that also may contribute to aneuploidy.

Microsatellite instability (MSI) pathway

Approximately 15% of sporadic CRCs in developed countries, a lower percentage in low-incidence populations, and almost all CRCs in HNPCC patients develop along the MSI pathway {472, 1104}. These tumours have lost the mismatch-repair function. Microsatellites are nucleotide repeat sequences that are prone to formation of insertion/deletion loops during DNA replication. Mismatch repair usually corrects insertion/deletion loops and keeps microsatellites at germline length, whereas deficient repair allows insertion/deletion loops to persist. After additional rounds of replication without mismatch repair, multiple alleles of varying lengths develop, now termed MSI-H {227, 1317} and previously reported as ubiquitous somatic mutations (USM) and DNA replication errors (RER).

In sporadic tumours, MSI-H and loss of mismatch repair occur mainly due to methylation of the MLH1 gene promoter with resultant epigenetic loss of protein expression of MLH1 and its binding partner PMS2. Sporadic MSI-H cancers usually have global hypermethylation (i.e. CpG island methylator phenotype, CIMP). In Lynch syndrome, loss of mismatch repair usually occurs because of germline mutation of one of four mismatch-repair genes (MSH2, MLH1, MSH6, or PMS2) or the TACSTD1 regulatory gene {1851}. Usually, but not invariably, there is loss of expression of the corresponding gene product in the case of MSH2 or MLH1 and their binding partners (MSH6 and PMS2, respectively). MSH6 can also be lost as a result of defective mismatch repair because the MSH6 gene itself contains a

microsatellite, or as a result of germline mutation.

Classification of MSI status is based on altered size of various mononucleotide and dinucleotide repeat sequences (e.g. BAT25, BAT26, D5S346, D2S123, D17S250, known as the Bethesda panel) {296, 2977, 3342}. MSI-H is defined by altered size of at least two of the five (40%) microsatellite markers. Sporadic MSI-H CRCs have more extensive alteration of microsatellites than Lynch syndrome CRCs. Most MSI-H cancers are diploid or near diploid, and the frequency of loss of heterozygosity (LOH) is low, including chromosome 5q (962,841). Microsatellite-stable tumours have no instability identified in the panel. Tumours with one abnormal marker among the five in the panel (or more than one and < 40% of markers in larger sets) are termed MSI-L. The classification, and therefore the clinical significance, of MSI-L is controversial owing in part to lack of standardization of the number and type of markers used, and this small subset of tumours is

often grouped with microsatellite-stable tumours. Indirect diagnosis of MSI-H can also be made using immunohistochemistry for loss of mismatch-repair proteins, with greater accuracy for sporadic than for inherited cases {2420}.

Many genes contain small runs of nucleotide repeats in exonic coding regions, and consequently MSI-H tumours frequently have frameshift mutations in these genes, e.g. TGFBR2, IGF2R, BAX, TCF7L2, E2F4, PTEN, MSH6, MSH3, and CASP5 {916, 1434, 1978, 2627, 2862, 3027, 3592}. Instability in 3' untranslated regions can lead to loss of expression, exemplified by BMPR2 {1623}. Numerous single-nucleotide mismatches also persist. The mutational profile of sporadic MSI-H tumours includes APC, BRAF (approximately 50%), but rarely KRAS. Lynch syndrome-associated cancers may contain CTNNB1 mutations {1437} as an alternative to APC, and never contain BRAF mutation {732}, providing a useful marker to identify sporadic cases among those that have lost MLH1. MSI-H tumours have a

Table 8.02 Genetic syndromes associated with a possible risk of colorectal carcinoma.

Syndrome	Gene (chromosome)	MIM No.
Autosomal dominant inheritable colorectal carcinoma		
No or few adenomatous polyps		
Lynch syndrome[a,b]	MLH1 (3p21–p23), MSH2 (2p21), MSH6 (2p21), PMS2 (7p22)	120435
Adenomatous polyps		
Familial adenomatous polyposis (FAP)[a] and attenuated FAP (AFAP)	APC (5q21–q22)	175100
Hamartomatous / mixed / hyperplastic polyps		
Peutz-Jeghers syndrome (PJS)	LKB1/STK11 (19p13.3)	175200
Juvenile polyposis syndrome (JPS)	SMAD4 (18q21.1) BMPR1A (10q22.3)	174900
Hereditary haemorrhagic telangiectasia syndrome (HHT)[c]	ENG (9q33–q34.1), ACVRL1 (12q11–q14)	187300
Hyperplastic polyposis syndrome (HPS)[c]	MUTYH (1p34.1; autosomal recessive), MBD4 (3q21.3)	Unassigned
Hereditary mixed polyposis syndrome (HMPS)[c]	CRAC1 (15q13–q21)	601228
PTEN hamartoma syndrome (Cowden syndrome/ Bannayan-Ruvalcaba-Riley syndromes)[c]	PTEN (10q23)	158350/153480
Birt-Hogg-Dube syndrome[c]	FLCN (17p11.2)	135150
Autosomal recessive inheritable colorectal carcinoma		
Adenomatous, serrated adenomas and hyperplastic polyps		
MUTYH-associated polyposis (MAP)[b]	MUTYH (1p34.1)	608456

[a] Turcot syndrome is a variant of Lynch syndrome, or FAP with brain tumours.
[b] Muir-Torre syndrome is a variant of Lynch syndrome, or MAP with sebaceous gland tumours.
[c] Risk of colorectal carcinoma is not clear.

Table 8.03 Genes harbouring alleles that confer susceptibility to colorectal cancer, identified from candidate screens.

Genetic pathway	Gene variants	References
Carcinogen pathway	NAT2, GSTT1	{670}
Folate pathway	MTHFR	{670, 1251A, 3473A}
Alcohol detoxification	ALDH2	{670}
Oncogene	HRAS1	{670, 1251A}
Tumour-suppressor genes	APC, TCF7L2, TP53, CHEK2, BRCA1	{670, 877A, 1251A}
Others	CaSR, AKAP9, PTGS1, TNFα, NOD2/CARD15	{1691, 2536A, 3111, 3473A}

Table 8.04 Loci conferring susceptibility to colorectal cancer, identified from genome-wide association studies (GWAS).

Single nucleotide polymorphism (SNP)	Chromosome	Tagging gene	Reference
rsl6892766	8q23.3	EIF3F	{3265A}
rs6983267/rs10505477	8q24.21	MYC	{3265B, 3677A}
rs719725	9p24		{2583A}
rsl075668	10p14		{3265A}
rs3802842	11q23.3		{2555B, 3212A}
rs4444235	14q22.2	BMP4	{1251B}
rs4779584	15q13.3	CRAC1 (HMPS)	{1376A}
rs9929218	16q22.1	CDH1	{1251B}
rs4939827/rs12953717/rs4464148/Novel1'	18q21.1	SMAD7	{336A, 2555A, 3212A}
rs10411210	19q13.1	RHPN2	{1251B}
rs961253	20p12.3		{1251B}

distinguishable gene-expression transcriptome and microRNAome {1743}. Tumours with MSI-H, whether sporadic or Lynch-associated, have morphological differences from tumours with chromosomal instability. They are frequently right-sided, mucinous or occasionally medullary type, associated with a Crohn-like peritumoral lymphocyte infiltrate and an intratumoral lymphocyte infiltrate, devoid of "dirty" necrosis, and at lower stage and with expansile growth and better stage-specific prognosis {952, 1416, 1548}. MSI-H tumours may be less responsive to certain chemotherapies, such as 5-fluorouracil {698, 2975}, but more responsive to irinotecan {244}.

Microsatellite-stable and chromosome-stable tumours

Up to 15% of tumours do not show the classical pathways of genome instability i.e. they will show neither MSI nor chromosomal instability. These tumours are little studied since demonstration of chromosomal stability requires specialized techniques such as flow cytometry or image analysis for total DNA content {476, 1526}, evaluation of LOH at multiple loci, or array comparative genomic hybridization.

CpG island methylator phenotype (CIMP)

Many genes contain areas rich in cytosine and guanine dinucleotides, termed CpG islands, within their promoter regions. Methylation of the cytosine residues in these CpG islands changes chromosomal structure and inhibits gene expression, including that of tumour-suppressor genes, thereby allowing epigenetic loss of function without mutation. Methylation of gene promoters can occur as an age-related phenomenon (called Type A methylation) but also occurs as a specific widespread phenomenon in certain cancers (called Type C methylation) {2361, 3282, 3724}. Tumours with CIMP often have MSI-H because of methylation of the MLH1 mismatch-repair gene; however, > 50% of CIMP carcinomas are microsatellite-stable. CIMP status clusters with MSI status and mutations in KRAS, BRAF, and TP53. Tumours with frequent MSI-H and BRAF

mutation are referred to as CIMP1, whereas CIMP tumours that are microsatellite-stable with a high frequency of KRAS mutations are referred to as CIMP2, and CIMP-negative tumours are microsatellite-stable with frequent TP53 mutations {2918, 3115}.

Noncoding RNAs

Small noncoding RNAs termed "microRNAs" regulate gene expression, resulting in loss of expression of tumour-suppressors and expression of oncogenes. {2734}.

Stem-cell markers

The cancer stem-cell hypothesis states that a small number of stem cells undergo asymmetric division and are responsible for the generation of the bulk of the tumour cells {92, 297}. Cancer stem cells may be the counterparts of normal tissue stem cells and are proposed to be the source of tumour recurrence and resistance to chemotherapy, leading to therapeutic strategies to attempt to specifically target cancer stem cells. However, identification of these cells is problematic since they usually represent only a small fraction of the tumour cell population. In addition, cancer stem cells may be in a state of plasticity, rather than representing a fixed tumour-cell subtype.

Several potential stem-cell markers that have been proposed for CRC include CD133, CD166, CD24, LGR5, DCAM kinase-like II, Bmi, Musashi-1, and aldehyde dehydrogenase-1 {647, 2013, 2331, 2671, 3133, 3204, 3397}.

Prognosis and predictive factors

Anatomic extent of disease, i.e. tumour stage, is the strongest prognostic factor for CRC. Additional factors are summarized in Table 8.05 {675, 1022, 3462, 3725}:

Morphology

In addition to deeper invasion, especially serosal-surface involvement, greater extent of involvement of a particular layer of the wall, an infiltrative pattern of the invasive edge and tumour budding as contrasted with an expansile pattern, a microacinar pattern with discrete small and relatively regular tubules {3499}, poor differentiation including signet ring cell and mucinous adenocarcinomas in the absence of MSI-H, and other histopathological types of carcinoma (i.e. adenosquamous carcinoma and small cell carcinoma) are associated with poorer prognosis {3437, 3438}.

Additional lymph-node characteristics

Metastasis to numerous or a high proportion of nodes, to those near the mesenteric margin and/or at great distance from the primary tumour, or to retrograde lymph nodes, and pathological examination of a smaller number of negative nodes (e.g. 12–18) have been associated with poorer prognosis {1043}. The prognostic value of identification of isolated tumour cells or micrometastasis in lymph nodes by immunohistochemical or molecular techniques remains controversial {2474}.

Extent of resection

The term "margin" refers to the areas of a resection or excision specimen that have been cut by the surgeon or gastroenterologist. Margins are not natural structures such as the serosal surface. A short longitudinal surgical resection margin (2–5 cm) reflecting the surgical technique employed and anatomical considerations has been associated with poor outcome. In rectal cancer, distance from the circumferential margin representing the adventitial soft tissue margin closest to the deepest penetration of the tumour is important owing to the anatomical proximity of pelvic structures {2866}. For all segments of the large intestine that are either incompletely or not enveloped by peritoneum, the circumferential margin created by blunt or sharp dissection at operation is also important, as is the mesocolic margin in colon cancer. The distance of the carcinoma from the margins in specimens from polypectomy, endoscopic mucosal resection, submucosal excision, and transanal excision also has prognostic importance.

Extramural venous invasion

Carcinomas sometimes invade muscular veins. Many studies have shown that invasion of extramural (i.e. beyond the muscularis propria) muscular veins is a poor prognostic feature {2599}.

Other prognostic features

Angiolymphatic invasion and involvement of perineural spaces and nerves are adverse features, whereas peritumoral lymphocytic response and tumour-infiltrating lymphocytes are favourable and often associated with MSI-H {939}.

Prognostic genes and biomarkers

The published literature is awash with studies reporting molecular or immunohistochemical prognostic factors in CRC, but none has been adopted into routine clinical practice. Tumour stage continues to be the mainstay for patient-management decisions affected by prognostic considerations. This situation is attributable to lack of the necessary levels of evidence to support the use of potential markers, as a consequence of lack of cross-validation. The complexity of CRC with the recognition of molecular subtypes that often share markers despite very different biological behaviour contributes to the lack of marker utility. In studies of markers, variability in quality of pathology, in protocols and methodologies used, and in scoring or assessing markers, under-powering due to sample size, tendency to study single markers rather than complete pathways, and the retrospective nature of the studies are problematic {2031}. The marker with the highest level of evidence is MSI-H for improved stage-specific survival, with a hazard ratio of about 0.65 {2578}. Good prognosis is also reported where there is infiltration of tumours by cytotoxic T cells {3432}, a feature of MSI-H. Reported markers for poor prognosis include mutations of *BRAF* {2788}, allelic imbalance at 18q {2577}, mutation of *PIK3CA* {2362}, or high expression of CD133 stem-cell marker {297}, osteopontin {2703}, or CXCL12 {55}.

Predictive genes and biomarkers

These genes or biomarkers that indicate likelihood of tumour response or resistance to specific therapies and of their toxicities must be used within the context of the pathway that is being targeted, the combination of agents administered, and the clinical setting. Between 1995 and 2005, the number of efficacious therapeutic agents for CRC increased from one (i.e. 5-fluorouracil) to seven (i.e. 5-fluorouracil, capecitabine, oxaliplatin, irinotecan, bevacizumab, cetuximab, and panitumumab), including the latter three targeted antibodies {2270}. Some of the best examples of predictive tumour markers are described below.

KRAS *mutation and epidermal growth factor receptor (EGFR) inhibitors*

EGFR is expressed in most CRCs and, because it is located on the cell surface, it is an attractive target. The anti-EGFR monoclonal antibodies cetuximab and panitumumab block ligand binding and produce a dramatic response in some CRC patients, whereas small-molecule tyrosine

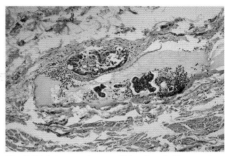

Fig. 8.26 Adenocarcinoma within a lymphatic vessel.

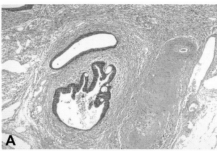

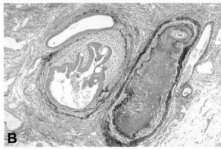

Fig. 8.27 Well-differentiated adenocarcinoma that was excised by endoscopical mucosal resection. **A** Veinous invasion in a well-differentiated adenocarcinoma. **B** Elastic (Van Gieson) stain reveals an artery that runs parallel to the vein; the vein is invaded by adenocarcinoma.

kinase inhibitors are inactive against CRC. However, EGFR signals through the RAS/RAF pathway, and mutation in downstream *KRAS,* leading to constitutive activation, renders tumours unresponsive to upstream inhibition by anti-EGFR antibodies {1847, 2321, 2810, 3025}. Testing for *KRAS* mutation is therefore required before the antibodies are used. *KRAS* may be mutated at any of three potential hotspots (i.e. codons 12/13, 61 and 146) that should be tested. The role of *BRAF* mutation is less certain. *EGFR* also signals through *PIK3CA*, and mutation of that gene and loss of *PTEN* expression may be adverse predictive markers. Expression of epi- and amphiregulin ligands and *EGFR* amplification are potential favourable predictive markers.

Table 8.05 Prognostic factors not included in the TNM staging of carcinoma of the colon and rectum.

Adverse features of primary tumour	Adverse vessel invasion	Favourable host response	Adverse surgical technique
Greater extent of circumferential involvement Bowel obstruction Bowel perforation Poor differentiation[a] Infiltrative pattern of invasion/budding Selected molecular characteristics	Muscular veins Lymphatic vessels Perineural spaces	Intratumoral inflammation Peritumoral inflammation Desmoplasia Reactive lymph nodes	Short distance between resection margin and tumour Incomplete excision with residual tumour
[a] See Table 8.02 for exceptions related to high levels of microsatellite instability (MSI-H).			

MSI-H and 5-fluorouracil, oxaliplatin and irinotecan

MSI-H predicts poor response to 5-fluorouracil and oxaliplatin. Mismatch repair detects mutations produced by the insertion of 5-fluorouracil into DNA and the formation of oxaliplatin adducts, and then induces apoptosis if these alterations cannot be repaired. In the absence of mismatch repair, apoptosis may not occur, resulting in resistance to these agents {3667}. Cell lines with MSI-H are usually sensitive to irinotecan {325}, and the survival of patients with MSI-H colon cancers may be better survival after adjuvant therapy that includes this agent {244}.

Other markers with mechanistic plausibility have been reported, including expression of thymidylate synthase (TYMS/TS), the target of 5-fluorouracil and of the fluoropyrimidine catabolizing enzymes dihydropyrimidine dehydrogenase (DPD) and thymidine phosphorylase (TP). The reported data are conflicting on the relationship of expression to response to this drug, which is the most commonly used therapeutic agent for CRC {328, 1917}.

Tumour topoisomerase I (Topo 1) expression may predict a good response to irinotecan and oxaliplatin. This enzyme unwinds DNA during replication and repair, and irinotecan is a Topo I inhibitor, but the mechanistic link to oxaliplatin is uncertain {1741}.

Germline gene characteristics have the potential to provide pharmacogenetic predictive biomarkers {2796}. Exposures including lifestyle factors such as diet {2056}, physical activity {2055} and other drugs {2663} may also affect outcome after therapy. A large number of additional agents directed at targets in CRC, e.g. *MET* and insulin-like growth factor 1 receptor (*IGF1R*), are in the drug-development pipeline {474}. Research on genes and biomarkers for current and emerging therapeutic agents is targeted to providing personalized cancer therapy with optimal efficacy, toxicity and cost-effectiveness.

Familial adenomatous polyposis

F.M. Giardiello
R.W. Burt
H.J. Järvinen
G.J.A. Offerhaus

Definition

Familial adenomatous polyposis (FAP) is an autosomal dominant disorder characterized by the development of hundreds to thousands of colorectal adenomatous polyps and the inevitable occurrence of colorectal adenocarcinoma if the colon is not removed {384, 936, 3385}. Fundic gland polyps of the stomach and duodenal and small-bowel adenomas are also common. FAP is caused by germline mutations in the adenomatous polyposis coli (*APC*) gene, which is located on the long arm of chromosome 5 (5q21–22) {378}.

Gardner syndrome is a variant of FAP that includes epidermoid cysts, osteomas, dental anomalies and desmoid tumours, in addition to the expected gastrointestinal polyps {947}. It is now more of historical interest, as these extra-intestinal growths are known to correlate more with mutation location in the *APC* gene, rather than occurring together in specific families. Nonetheless, the name persists and is often applied to families in which the extra-intestinal manifestations of the disease are particularly obvious and common.

The name "Turcot syndrome" is applied to a variant of FAP with typical intestinal polyps but also brain tumours, almost always medulloblastoma in type {1108, 3321}, although the original Turcot family had Lynch syndrome (658).

An attenuated form of FAP, called attenuated FAP or attenuated APC, has been distinguished from classic FAP {380, 1178, 1619}. The number of colorectal adenomas in attenuated FAP averages approximately 30, while the number of polyps is extremely variable; the upper gastrointestinal polyps are similar to those arising in typical FAP. Extra-intestinal growths may occur in attenuated FAP, but are far less common than in the classical form.

MIM No.

FAP (including Gardner syndrome
 and attenuated FAP)   175100
Turcot syndrome   276300

Synonyms

Adenomatous polyposis coli, familial polyposis coli, Bussey-Gardner polyposis, Gardner syndrome, familial multiple polyposis, multiple adenomatosis, familial polyposis of the colon and rectum, familial polyposis of the gastrointestinal tract, familial adenomatous polyposis coli, etc.

Incidence

Estimates of the incidence of FAP vary between 1 per 7000 and 1 per 30 000 newborns. In general, FAP underlies < 1% of all new cases of colorectal cancer. Between 30% and 50% of new FAP patients are *de novo* cases, representing new mutations of the *APC* gene or *APC*-gene mosaicism in one of the parents (much less common) {1179}.

Diagnostic criteria

Classical FAP is defined clinically by the finding of at least 100 colorectal adenomatous polyps in a patient in whom the syndrome is fully developed {384, 3385}. The finding of fewer adenomas in a first-degree relative of an affected person is likewise diagnostic, especially in younger individuals. Histological confirmation of polyps as adenomas is required to distinguish FAP from other forms of polyposis, including hamartomatous polyposes, lymphoid hyperplasia and lymphomatous polyposis. In cases in which the number of synchronous adenomas is < 100, the possibility of MUTYH polyposis should also be considered.

A conclusive diagnosis of FAP is achieved by demonstration of a disease-causing germline mutation in the *APC* gene {378}. The rate of detection of such mutations in an index case with the expected phenotype is 60–80%, but much lower for attenuated FAP. Once the disease-causing mutation is known in a family, genetic testing of family members for the presence or absence of that specific mutation is diagnostic with near 100% accuracy. The presence of the mutation confirms the diagnosis, while its absence rules out FAP. In patients for whom the fulfilment of the clinical criteria remains doubtful and genetic diagnosis is not achieved, the finding of extracolonic features of FAP (e.g. epidermoid cysts, osteomas, desmoid tumour, gastric fundic-gland polyps, duodenal adenomas) may give additional diagnostic support. The following diagnostic criteria have been established: (1) 100 or more colorectal adenomas; or (2) a germline disease-causing mutation of the

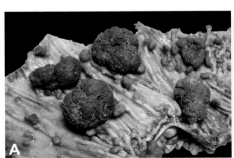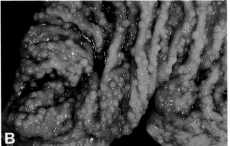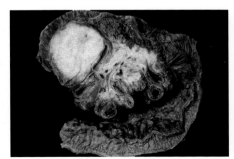

Fig. 8.28 Colectomy specimens from patients with familial adenomatous polyposis. **A** Multiple adenomas at different stages of development. **B** Numerous small early (sessile) adenomas.

Fig. 8.29 Mesenteric fibromatosis (desmoid tumour) in a patient with familial adenomatous polyposis. The lesion entraps loops of small intestine.

APC gene; or (3) family history of FAP and any number of adenomas at a young age. Diagnostic criteria for attenuated FAP are more difficult to establish. An autosomal dominant pattern of a smaller number of adenomatous polyps is very suggestive and best confirmed by genetic testing for mutations in expected areas of the APC gene. As noted previously, the number of adenomas averages 30, but is extremely variable, making clinical diagnosis in a specific individual difficult. "Rectal sparing" is common in patients with attenuated FAP.

Localization

Colorectal adenomas in FAP occur throughout the colon, but follow the general distribution of sporadic adenomas, often with a slight excess of polyps in the left colon {384}. The distribution of cancers follows that of the adenomas. This colonic distribution is reversed in attenuated FAP, with both adenomas and cancers exhibiting a more proximal colonic distribution with frequent "rectal sparing" {380}.

Clinical features

Age at clinical manifestation

Colorectal adenomas become detectable at endoscopic examination in the second or third decade of life, occurring at an average age of 15.9 years (range, 8–34 years) {2537}. Polyps increase in number and size with age. The most important clinical feature of FAP is the almost invariable progression of one or more colorectal adenomas to cancer. The mean age at which cancer develops is about 40 years, but the risk of cancer is already 1–6% by the age of 21 years {384}. By age 50 years, > 90% of untreated patients will have colorectal cancer. Rare cases of colorectal cancer have been reported in children with FAP. Extracolonic manifestations such as epidermoid cysts, mandibular osteomas, desmoid tumours or congenital hypertrophy of the retinal pigment epithelium (CHRPE) may present in children and can serve as markers of FAP.

Symptoms and signs

In the early phase of FAP, adenomas do not cause any symptoms. Specific symptoms attributable to colorectal adenomas do not usually occur until late in the second or early in the third decade of life and include rectal bleeding and diarrhoea, often accompanied by mucous discharge and abdominal pain. Such symptoms appear gradually and may be easily overlooked;

the mean age at which symptoms appear is 33 years and the mean age of diagnosis is 36 years in unscreened/untreated FAP patients. Two thirds of patients diagnosed with FAP on the basis of symptoms already have colorectal cancer, whereas cancer in asymptomatic members of known FAP families is very rare, if regular surveillance and appropriate therapy have been undertaken. The symptoms and signs of extra-intestinal manifestations may sometimes precede those of the colorectum. Symptoms from benign polyps of the upper gastrointestinal tract are rare. Symptoms occur with gastric and duodenal cancers, but these virtually never precede symptoms or cancer of the colon.

Macroscopy

Most polyps in FAP are small (usually < 5 mm), sessile, and spherical, but may be lobulated. Scattered larger pedunculated polyps are much less common {979}. In the completely expressed disease, polyps often number hundreds or thousands and may "carpet" the lining of the whole large bowel. The number of adenomas per patient varies between families, in some families being little more than 100 even in adults, whereas most families are affected by profuse polyps, numbering hundreds or thousands {979}.

Histopathology

Adenomas in FAP begin as dysplastic aberrant crypt foci, so-called "single-crypt adenomas" {1414}. In practice, to find more than one of these in a colon is considered virtually pathognomic for FAP. By excessive and asymmetrical crypt fission {3459} subsequent to loss of APC-controlled growth and tissue organization, these aberrant crypt foci develop into oligocryptal adenomas, which may not be visible as polyps before further growth into grossly visible adenomatous polyps. FAP adenomas have the same architecture as their sporadic counterparts; most are tubular adenomas or, less frequently, tubulovillous or villous. Nonpolypoid "flat" adenomas account for approximately 5% of colon adenomas in affected family members {1997}. Adenomas and carcinomas in FAP are histologically identical to sporadic lesions. As for sporadic adenomas and colorectal carcinomas, the incidence of malignancy depends on size and frequency. Adenomas in attenuated FAP show the same cytological features as adenomatous epithelium, but more often appear flat or depressed {598}.

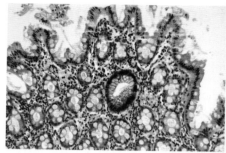

Fig. 8.30 A single crypt adenoma (aberrant crypt focus), the earliest microscopically recognizable adenoma in a person affected by familial adenomatous polyposis.

Proliferation

The histologically normal intestinal mucosa in FAP shows no increase in the rate of epithelial-cell proliferation {3459}. Mitotic activity is not increased {2218}, except in the adenomatous epithelium in which cell proliferation is identical to that in sporadic adenomas. Interestingly, in multiple intestinal neoplasia (Min) mice, a model for the development of FAP, the histologically normal-looking mucosa has an extended proliferative compartment and decreased rate of cellular crypt–villus migration {1954}. Mutation of APC is associated with a dominant-negative effect upon intestinal-cell migration {1954}. Studies on the cellular kinetics of proliferative patterns in the normal-looking colonic mucosa of humans with FAP have also shown expansion of the proliferative compartment {699}. Moreover, the stem-cell dynamics of normal-appearing crypts in the colon of FAP patients indicate that stem-cell survival is enhanced compared with unaffected individuals {1554}.

These observations show that before somatic loss of the wild-type APC allele, haploinsufficiency has apparently already lead to microscopically occult alterations in cell growth, differentiation and migration in the colonic crypts of FAP patients, a phenomenon considered as pre-tumour progression {394}.

Small-intestinal polyps

Small-bowel polyps, particularly duodenal polyps, are also adenomas. They develop preferentially in the periampullary region of the duodenum, probably due to a co-carcinogenic effect of bile {3043}. They become evident 10 years later than colorectal polyps. Using side-viewing endoscopy, adenomas have been found in 92% of patients with FAP at routine screening {3047}. The severity of duodenal polyposis can be classified according to Spigelman by the number, size, structure, and degree of dysplasia of adenomas {3047}. These adenomas increase in size and number with time and carry a lifetime risk of duodenal or periampullary cancer of 4–10% {272, 1805}. Ampullary and peri-ampullary adenocarcinoma is one of the principal causes of death in patients who have undergone prophylactic proctocolectomy {3047}. Adenomas develop rarely in the jejunum or ileum, but after prophylactic proctocolectomy with ileoanal pouch, the prevalence of ileal adenomas may exceed 50% {252}.

Extraintestinal manifestations

Several other organs are involved in FAP, but extra-intestinal manifestations rarely determine the clinical course of the disease, except for desmoid tumours.

Stomach. Gastric adenomas do occur with increased frequency {734}, but the most common abnormality is the fundic-gland polyp. This is a non-neoplastic mucus-retention type of polyp, grossly visible as a smooth dome-shaped nodule in the gastric body and fundus, and is usually multiple. Histologically, the lesion is characteristically undramatic, consisting of gastric-body mucosa that is often normal apart from cystic dilatation of glands. There is evidence for increased cell proliferation and dysplasia developing in these polyps {3561}, but progression to adenocarcinoma is a rare occurrence {3728}.

Liver and biliary tract. There is an increased incidence of hepatoblastoma in male infants of families with FAP {980}. Dysplasia has been demonstrated in the bile-duct and gallbladder epithelium in patients with FAP {2328}, and these patients are at risk of developing adenocarcinoma of the biliary tree {3044}.

Extra-gastrointestinal manifestations

Soft tissues. Tissues derived from all three germ layers are affected in FAP. As well as the endodermal lesions so far described, mesodermal lesions in the form of a fibromatosis unique to FAP, usually referred to as desmoid tumour, develop in a substantial proportion of patients (10–25%) {245, 1752}. Desmoid tumours arise in either the retroperitoneal tissues, mesenterium or in the abdominal or thoracic wall. Trauma, previous surgery (at an early age), female sex, family history of desmoids, and the site of the *APC* mutation beyond codon 1399 or 1444 are associated with an increased risk of desmoids {753}.

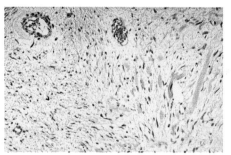

Fig. 8.31 Mesenteric fibromatosis (desmoid tumour) in a patient with familial adenomatous polyposis. Note the collagen bands and small vessels.

A desmoid is a mass of firm pale tissue, characteristically growing by expansion, usually rounded in shape. Desmoids begin as small scar-like foci of fibrosis in the retroperitoneal fat and, when large, typically extend around and between other structures such as the small or large bowel, ureters, and major blood vessels. Histologically, these lesions are composed of sheets of elongated myofibroblasts, arranged in fascicles and whorls. The lesions have a dense, tough, consistency, and there is a variable amount of collagen. They are well-vascularized and contain numerous small blood vessels that bleed profusely when incised. Desmoid tumours may grow rapidly, but can resolve spontaneously; some show cycles of growth and regression, while others remain stable {569}. Mesenteric and retroperitoneal desmoids may cause bowel or ureteric obstruction or other life-threatening complications.

Bones. Bone lesions include exostoses and endostoses. Endostoses of the mandible are found in the majority of patients {365}. They are almost always small and symptomless. Exostoses may be solitary or multiple and tend to arise in the long bones.

Teeth. Dental abnormalities have been described in 11–80% of individuals with FAP {3503}. The abnormalities may be impaction, supernumerary or absent teeth, fused roots of first and second molars or unusually long and tapered roots of posterior teeth.

Eye. In 75–80% of patients, ophthalmoscopy reveals multiple patches CHRPE {487}. Ultrastructurally, they are freckle-like plaques of enlarged melanin-containing retinal epithelial cells {2482}. Their value for diagnosis is limited by inconsistency and variation between families.

Skin. Epidermal cysts, usually of the face and often multiple, were first described in FAP by Gardner {948}.

Endocrine system. There is a definite but relatively slight increase in the incidence of neuroendocrine neoplasms in FAP, including neoplasia of the pituitary, pancreatic islets and adrenal cortex {1975}, as well as multiple endocrine neoplasia syndrome (MEN), type 2b {2527}, but these are of insufficient frequency or gravity to form part of a routine screening protocol. The best documented endocrine association is papillary carcinoma of the thyroid {464}, which is largely restricted to women {364}.

Nervous system. The concurrent presence of a brain tumour and multiple colorectal polyps constitutes Turcot syndrome. Some individuals affected in this way have FAP and carry a germline defect in the *APC* gene. These are infants or young children who present with medulloblastoma and colorectal polyps {1108}. Other individuals present later in life with a glioma, usually an astrocytoma or glioblastoma multiforme that is usually associated with Lynch syndrome rather than FAP {1900}.

Genetic susceptibility
Genetics

FAP is an autosomal dominant disease with almost complete penetrance by age 40 years. In 1991, germline mutations in the *APC* gene were identified as the cause of FAP by several investigators, including Kinzler, Groden, and Nishisho {1069, 1572, 2305}.

Gene structure and expression

The *APC* gene was localized to chromosome 5q21–22 by Bodmer et al. {291} and Leppert et al. {1806}. It was isolated by the group of White {1069} and by the laboratories of Nakamura and Vogelstein {2305}. It spans a region of 120 kb and is composed of at least 21 exons, 7 of which are alternatively expressed {2798}. Sixteen APC transcripts that differ in their most 5' regions and arise by the alternative inclusion of six of these exons have been identified.

The *APC* gene is ubiquitously expressed in normal tissues, with highest levels in the central nervous system. Tissue-specific differences have been observed in the expression of *APC* transcripts without exon 1, a coding region for a heptad repeat that supports homodimerization of the APC protein.

Gene product and function

The *APC* gene encodes a 2843 amino-acid protein with a relative molecular mass of 309 000. The protein has several

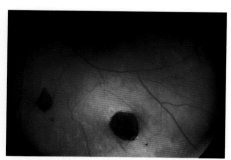

Fig. 8.32 Congenital hypertrophy of the retinal pigment epithelium (CHRPE) in a 41-year-old man with familial adenomatous polyposis attributable to an *APC* gene mutation in exon 15, codon 1157.

important structural areas {131}, including the oligomerization domain, armadillo region, 15 amino-acid repeat area, 20 amino-acid repeat area, basic domain, end-binding protein 1 (EB1) binding site and the HDLG (homologue of the Drosophila, discs large tumour-suppressor protein) binding site. The oligomerization domain is essential for the formation of dimers with wild-type and truncated mutant APC proteins. The armadillo region binds the regulatory B56 subunit of protein phosphatase 2A, the enzyme that also binds axin via its catalytic subunit. The 15 amino-acid and 20 amino-acid repeat areas are essential for binding axin and β-catenin, respectively. The basic domains and EB1 binding-site complex with microtubules. The HDLG binding site is involved in the inhibition of cell-cycle progression. The APC protein functions in tumour suppression and is considered important in cell adhesion, signal transduction, and activation. The APC protein is a negative regulator in the Wnt signalling pathway. The domains described above act as binding and degradation sites for β-catenin and control the intracellular concentration of β-catenin {2742}. In the normal situation, glycogen synthase kinase 3β (GSK3β) promotes phosphorylation of the protein conductin/axin that is added to the APC–GSK3β complex {224}. Phosphorylated axin recruits β-catenin, which is in turn phosphorylated and targeted for degradation through an APC-dependent ubiquitin–proteasome pathway {7}. When this system is perturbed, β-catenin is not degraded. This can occur when Wnt signalling inhibits GSK3β activity and dephosphorylates axin. As a result, β-catenin is released from the complex. Free β-catenin shuttles to the nucleus where it binds to the transcription factors of the TCF/LEF

family. The resulting complexes activate *MYC* {1145} and transcription of the cyclin D1 gene {3224}. Lack of functional APC can also cause unregulated intracellular accumulation of β-catenin, and, thereby, constitutive expression of *MYC* and of the cyclin D1 gene (CCND1) {3513}. In the cytoplasm, β-catenin is involved in cytoskeletal organization with binding to microtubules. It also interacts with E-cadherin, a membrane protein involved in cell adhesion. Unregulated concentrations of β-catenin also perturb these processes.

Gene mutations

A deleterious germline mutation in *APC* is found in up to 95% of individuals with classic FAP {1727}. Mutations in the base-pair excision gene *MYH* account for some of the remaining individuals {2961}. The majority (95%) of *APC* mutations are nonsense or frameshift mutations producing a truncated protein with abnormal function. About 10% of *APC* mutations are large interstitial deletions that may involve the entire gene. Rare missense mutations, most with uncertain functional consequences, have been described. Also, germline mutation in the *APC* promoter region has been identified as a cause of FAP {489}. More than 700 different deleterious *APC* gene mutations have been identified (primarily in the 5' region of the gene), but those at codons 1061 and 1309 account for 33% of all reported. The rate of germline mutation leading to a new deleterious *APC* allele is estimated to be five to nine mutations per million gametes. Consequently, individuals with no previous family history of FAP (*de novo* cases) are not uncommon, representing up to one quarter of *propositi* {266}. In addition to spontaneous mutation, gonadal mosaicism has been reported to account for about 10% of new cases of FAP {140, 2861}.

Application of genetic testing in the clinical setting

Genetic testing is the standard of care for screening at-risk members of families affected by FAP {975}. The indications for *APC*-gene testing include confirming the diagnosis of FAP and pre-symptomatic diagnosis of individuals aged 10 years or older at risk for this condition. Currently, commercial laboratories generally use sequencing for mutation analysis and some additionally test for large-segment rearrangement. The strategy for testing an at-risk individual begins with first testing

an affected member of the family to determine whether a detectable mutation exists in the pedigree {622}. If a deleterious mutation is found in an affected family member, then at-risk relatives can obtain true positive or negative test results. If a mutation is not identified, testing at-risk relatives should not be conducted because the results will be inconclusive {976} (in this situation, a negative test result for an at-risk individual could be a false negative since the laboratory technology may not be of sufficient sensitivity to detect a mutation, if one is present). When an affected family member is not available for evaluation, testing of at-risk family members can provide only positive or inconclusive results. In this case, a true negative test result for an at-risk individual can only be given if another at-risk family member tests positive for a deleterious mutation. In patients with classic or the attenuated FAP phenotype, in which no mutation in the *APC* gene has been found, *MYH* gene testing should be considered.

Molecular pathology

In accordance with the two-hit model of carcinogenesis, the wild-type *APC* allele is lost or mutated in most FAP-associated tumours, including colorectal adenoma and carcinoma, desmoid tumours {2102}, medulloblastoma {364}, gastroduodenal tumours {3281}, thyroid carcinoma {1368}, and hepatoblastoma {1683}. Each colorectal adenomatous polyp is a premalignant lesion that may progress to carcinoma in an unpredictable fashion. In addition to *APC* mutations, colon carcinomas in FAP patients contain somatic mutations similar to those found in sporadic colon cancers not associated with replication errors. *TP53* mutation and 17p allele loss are observed in 40% of invasive carcinomas {1541}. However, *TP53* may not be involved in some families {58}. Loss of alleles on chromosome 18 and 22 were observed in 46% and 33% of cases, respectively. The frequency of mutation of *KRAS* increases from 11% in moderately to 36% in severely dysplastic adenomas {58}. *KRAS* mutations may potentiate the transcription of cyclin D1 {1145}. Interestingly, the type of *APC* germline mutation may influence the mode of inactivation of the second *APC* allele {58}.

Animal model

The first mouse model of *APC* mutation was developed via random mutagenesis {2164}.

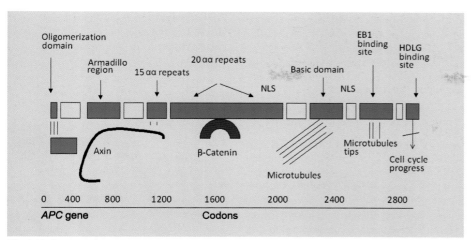

Fig. 8.33 Structure of the protein encoded by the *APC* gene. αα, amino acid; EB1, end-binding protein 1; HDLG, homologue of Drosophila, discs large tumour-suppressor protein; NLS, nuclear localization signal.

This Min mouse, designated APCmin, has a heterozygous truncating mutation at codon 850 of the *APC* gene and develops approximately 30 small intestinal adenomas. Homozygous mutant embryos die before gastrulation {2164}. Other murine APC models were subsequently constructed using gene-knockout technology to create mutations in codons 716, 1638, and 14; such mice have varying numbers of small-bowel adenomas {3165}. Investigators have also created *APC*-mutant mice carrying additional mutations that modify the number of intestinal polyps and induce progression of adenomas to cancer {2164, 3165}.

Genotype–phenotype relationships
Several definitive associations exist between specific *APC*-gene mutations and colorectal and extracolorectal FAP phenotype {3048}. Attenuated FAP, characterized by patients with colorectal oligopolyposis (< 100 colorectal adenomas) and later age of colorectal-cancer development is caused by mutations before codon 158 (5' end of the gene), after codon 1595 (3' end of the gene) or in the alternatively spliced region of exon 9 (codons 312–412) {332, 974}. Severe colorectal polyposis (> 1000 adenomas) correlates with mutations between codons 1250 and 1464 {2207}. CHRPE is associated with mutations between codons 311 and 1444, and desmoid tumours may be more prevalent in persons with mutations after codon 1444 {450, 2290}. Multiplicity of extracolonic manifestations appears to occur more frequently in mutations that are 3' to codon 1445 {981}. No consistent associations with tumours of the upper gastrointestinal tract have been found.

Prognosis and management
Colorectal screening and surveillance
Screening for FAP includes sigmoidoscopy or colonoscopy beginning at age 10–15 years in individuals known to have a disease-causing mutation or in all children of an affected parent, if genetic testing is not available or not informative {3385}. If a mutation in *APC* has been detected in a family member, genetic testing should be offered to determine which relatives require screening. Once adenomas are detected, annual or biannual colonoscopy should be continued until an appropriately timed colectomy is completed.

When genetic diagnosis is not possible, endoscopic surveillance should be continued at 1–2 year intervals up to the age of 40 years. If FAP is not apparent by that age, screening as per persons with an average risk of colon cancer can then be performed. In persons at risk or with a genetic diagnosis of attenuated FAP, colonoscopy should always be used in view of the more proximal distribution of polyps {380}. Colonoscopy should start late in the second decade of life and be repeated every 1–2 years, depending on the presence and number of adenomas. More intensive screening should probably continue until age 50 or 60 years for persons with this condition.

Colorectal therapy
Surgery can be anticipated once colonic adenomas appear in a person with FAP {1395, 1488, 2461}. In most cases, surgery is delayed until the patient has completed his/her secondary education, for psychosocial reasons; however, annual surveillance should be performed in these persons to determine whether earlier surgery is necessary. If colectomy has not already been performed, it should certainly be undertaken when approximately 100 adenomas occur, when multiple adenomas of more than 1 cm in diameter are found, or if advanced histology appears in any adenoma. Surgical options include: (1) restorative proctocolectomy; (2) colectomy with mucosal proctectomy, ileal pouch construction and ileo-anal pouch anastomosis; and (3) colectomy with ileorectal anastamosis. Restorative proctocolectomy has the advantage that about 1 cm of low rectal tissue is left in place, allowing the patient to distinguish air, liquid and solid material. It has the disadvantage, however, that residual rectal tissue may form adenomas. Colectomy with ileo-anal pouch anastomosis is necessary if adenomas are found at or near the dentate line at the anus before surgery. Colectomy with ileorectal anastomosis can be done with rectal sparing and is almost always the procedure of choice for persons with attenuated FAP.

Surveillance is always necessary after surgery, as adenomatous polyps may develop in the ileal pouch or rectal tissue of any patient. The incidence of ileal cancer is low, but that of rectal cancer (when rectal tissue remains) is substantial if continued surveillance is not performed. Annual or 6-monthly flexible sigmoidoscopy can be done, depending on the number of polyps observed. Polyps should be removed or ablated. Some patients with a remaining rectum or rectal cuff will eventually need completion surgery because of adenomas or advanced adenomas that are not well-controlled endoscopically.

Lynch syndrome

P. Peltomaki
G.J.A. Offerhaus
H.F.A. Vasen

Definition

Lynch syndrome (previously "hereditary nonpolyposis colorectal cancer", HNPCC) is an autosomal dominant disorder caused by a defect in a DNA mismatch repair (MMR) gene. The syndrome is characterized by the development of colorectal carcinoma, endometrial carcinoma and other cancers.

MIM No.

120435-6

Diagnostic criteria

Before the discovery of the DNA MMR-gene defects responsible for Lynch syndrome in the 1990s, clinical diagnostic criteria (the "Amsterdam criteria") were used to identify families with a presumably inherited form of colorectal carcinoma {3384, 3388}. Families that met these criteria were referred to as having HNPCC. Further molecular genetic analysis, however, showed that HNPCC constitutes a heterogeneous group of families. In about half of the families with HNPCC, neither microsatellite instability (MSI) in tumours nor a germline defect in an MMR gene could be identified {1864, 3506}. Such families are referred to as having "familial colorectal cancer type X" {1864}, "non-Lynch syndrome colorectal cancer predisposition" {738} or just "familial colorectal cancer" {3386}. The genetic basis for this disease is still unknown {3383}.

Currently, the term "Lynch syndrome" is reserved for families with an identified pathogenic germline mutation in one of the DNA MMR genes {295}. In addition, patients with inactivation of MutS homologue 2 (MSH2) due to a deletion of the 3' exons of the TACSTD1 gene (tumour-associated calcium signal transducer 1) are considered to have Lynch syndrome {1851}. Recently, patients with methylation

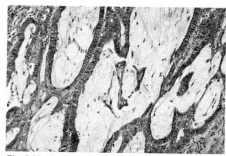

Fig. 8.34 Mucinous adenocarcinoma from a patient with Lynch syndrome.

of the MutL homologue 1 (MLH1) promotor in the germline have also been reported {1213, 2143} and may be designated as having Lynch syndrome, although segregation and penetrance in subsequent generations remain unclear. Patients without an identified germline defect in a DNA MMR gene but with a tumour showing MSI and absence of immunohistochemical expression of the MMR proteins are very likely to have Lynch syndrome if other causes of MSI, such as methylation of the MLH1 promoter, are excluded.

In 2004, a set of clinical guidelines (the revised Bethesda guidelines) was proposed that can be used to select individuals for MSI analysis {3342}. Individuals that meet one of these criteria are suspected to have Lynch syndrome.

Clinical features

Carriers of a pathogenic mutation in a DNA MMR gene have a high lifetime risk of developing colorectal carcinoma (10–53%), endometrial carcinoma (15–44%), and certain other cancers (< 15%) {178, 509, 2877, 3471}. The risk of developing cancer depends on sex, type of gene involved and environmental factors. Colorectal carcinomas are often diagnosed at an early age (mean, 45–50 years), and are located in the proximal part of the colon in about two thirds of patients. Synchronous or metachronous colorectal carcinoma is present in 18% of patients {3382}. In almost all cases, MSI is evident. The adenomas that occur in Lynch syndrome tend to develop at an early age, have villous components and are more dysplastic than

Table 8.06 Overview of clinical criteria for Lynch syndrome: Amsterdam I and II and revised Bethesda criteria.

Amsterdam criteria I
There should be at least three relatives with CRC; all the following criteria should be present:
1. One should be a first-degree relative of the other two
2. At least two successive generations should be affected
3. At least one CRC should be diagnosed before the age of 50 years
4. Familial adenomatous polyposis should be excluded
5. Tumours should be verified by pathological examination

Amsterdam criteria II
There should be at least three relatives with a Lynch syndrome-associated cancer (CRC, cancer of the endometrium, small bowel, ureter or renal pelvis); all of the following criteria should be present:
1. One should be a first-degree relative of the other two
2. At least two successive generations should be affected
3. At least one should be diagnosed before the age of 50 years
4. Familial adenomatous polyposis should be excluded in the CRC case(s) if any
5. Tumours should be verified by pathological examination

Revised Bethesda criteria
1. CRC diagnosed in a patient of less than 50 years of age
2. Presence of synchronous, metachronous colorectal, or other Lynch syndrome-related tumours,[a] regardless of age
3. CRC with MSI-H phenotype diagnosed at less than 60 years of age
4. Patient with CRC and a first-degree relative with a Lynch syndrome-related tumour, with one of the cancers diagnosed before the age of 50 years
5. Patient with CRC with two or more first-degree or second-degree relatives with a Lynch syndrome-related tumour, regardless of age.

CRC, colorectal cancer.
[a] Lynch syndrome-related tumours include colorectal, endometrial, stomach, ovarian, pancreas, ureter, renal pelvis, biliary-tract and brain tumours, sebaceous gland adenomas, keratoacanthomas and carcinoma of the small bowel. [b] MSI-H, high level of microsatellite instability.

Table 8.07 Current terminology for families with inherited colorectal cancer without polyposis.

Terminology	Clinical definition	Molecular genetic analysis
Hereditary nonpolyposis colorectal cancer (HNPCC)	Amsterdam criteria I and II	*Defined solely by clinical criteria[a]*
Familial colorectal cancer (type X) Non-Lynch syndrome colorectal cancer predisposition	Amsterdam criteria I	Genetic basis unknown; no evidence for defects in DNA MMR genes
Lynch syndrome	Familial clustering of colorectal cancer and/or other cancers	Presence of pathogenic germline defects in DNA MMR genes Germline methylation of the *MLH1* promoter Inactivation of *MSH2* due to deletion of 3' exons of the *EPCAM (TACSTD1)* gene
Probable Lynch syndrome	Familial clustering of colorectal cancer and/or other cancers	Presence of microsatellite instability and absence of expression of DNA MMR proteins in tumours Additionally, no evidence for methylation of the *MLH1* promoter
Suspected Lynch syndrome	Revised Bethesda criteria, Amsterdam criteria I and II	*Defined solely by clinical criteria[a]*

MMR, mismatch repair, [a] This terminology is used if no molecular genetic data are available.

adenomas detected in the general population {668, 2678}. Although multiple adenomas may be observed in Lynch syndrome, florid polyposis is not a feature. Patients with mutations of *MSH6* and *PMS2* may present at an older age with more left sided tumours than those with mutations of the other genes.

Extracolonic lesions include cancer of the endometrium, renal pelvis/ureter, stomach, small bowel, ovary, brain, hepatobiliary tract, and also sebaceous tumours. Of these, the relative risk of carcinoma of the endometrium, ovaries, ureter, renal pelvis, and small bowel is highest, and these tumours are therefore the most specific for Lynch syndrome {3471}. The occurrence of sebaceous gland tumours together with Lynch syndrome-type internal malignancy is referred to as the Muir-Torre syndrome {577}. The association of primary brain tumours (usually glioblastomas) with multiple colorectal adenomas is referred to as Turcot syndrome {3321}. The latter has a shared genetic basis with Lynch syndrome

on the one hand and familial adenomatous polyposis (FAP) on the other {1108}.

Pathology

Although the pathogenesis and also certain morphological features differ between Lynch tumours and sporadic colorectal cancers with a high frequency of MSI (MSI-H) {1398}, the pathology of Lynch tumours is very similar to that of sporadic colorectal carcinoma with MSI-H. Many studies make no distinction between familial and non-familial carcinomas with MSI-H. Therefore, the following descriptions apply to all carcinomas with MSI-H, but highlight subtle differences between cancers from the Lynch syndrome and their sporadic counterparts, where these are known.

Macroscopy

Lynch syndrome-associated cancers show a predilection for the proximal colon, including the caecum, ascending colon, hepatic flexure and transverse colon {1933}. At least 60% of such cancers

occur in the proximal colon. Gross appearances have not been studied in detail. However, since HNPCC and MSI-H colorectal carcinomas show a consistent trend towards good circumscription {1402, 2909}, they are more likely to present as polypoid growths, plaques, ulcers or bulky masses and less likely to present as diffuse growths or tight strictures. Adenomas are not numerous, but are likely to be more frequent in subjects with Lynch syndrome than in age-matched controls {1405}. Colonoscopic studies indicate that the distribution of adenomas in Lynch syndrome may not mirror the proximal colonic predilection of carcinoma {1405}. This could be due to the occurrence of sporadic distal adenomas in older subjects with Lynch syndrome or because proximal adenomas are more likely to progress to cancer. It is considered that colorectal carcinomas in Lynch syndrome arise from conventional adenomas, while the precursors of sporadic MSI-H tumours are serrated polyps {1398}

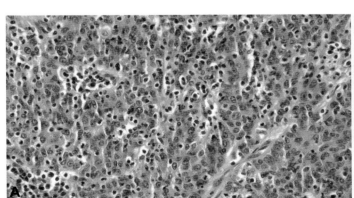 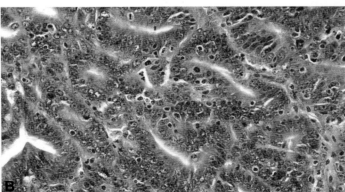

Fig. 8.35 Abundant lymphocytes infiltrate the neoplastic epithelium in poorly differentiated (**A**) and moderately differentiated (**B**) adenocarcinomas from patients with Lynch syndrome.

Histopathology

No individual microscopic feature is specific to Lynch syndrome, but particular groups of features are diagnostically useful {1416, 2909, 3297}. Similar features are found in the 10–15% of sporadic colorectal cancers that show MSI-H {1402}. However, sporadic MSI-H cancers present in older subjects lacking a family history of bowel cancer. Colorectal cancers from Lynch syndrome fall into different groups on the basis of site and microscopic criteria.

Proximally located mucinous adenocarcinomas

These are usually well circumscribed and well- or moderately differentiated. Lymphocytic infiltration is not prominent, but tumour-infiltrating (intraepithelial) lymphocytes (TIL) may be evident in nonmucinous areas. There may be tubulo-villous or villous adenomatous remnants adjacent to the cancer. Mucin production may be more common in subjects with a germline mutation in *MSH2* {2909}. Sporadic MSI-H tumours more often show a mucinous appearance than their Lynch-syndrome counterparts {1061}.

Proximally located, poorly differentiated adenocarcinomas

Poor differentiation indicates failure of gland formation, the malignant epithelium being arranged in small clusters, irregular trabeculae or large aggregates. These tumours are well-circumscribed and lack an abundant desmoplastic stroma. Some are peppered with TIL. A Crohn-like lymphocytic

reaction may be present. This subtype has been described as medullary or "undifferentiated", although most of these tumours contain subclones in which glandular differentiation is evident. This subtype may be more common in subjects with a mutation in *MSH2* {2909}. In general, colorectal cancers showing TIL and/or a Crohn-like lymphocytic reaction appear to be more common in subjects with a germline mutation in *MLH1* {2909}. Poor differentiation is another microscopic feature that is more frequent in sporadic MSI-H tumours than in their Lynch-syndrome counterparts {1061, 1398}.

Adenomas in Lynch syndrome

These are more likely to show features indicative of increased risk of cancer, including villosity and high-grade intraepithelial neoplasia {1405}. Immunohistochemical staining to demonstrate loss of expression of MMR proteins (MLH1, MSH2, postmeiotic segregation 2 [PMS2], MutS homologue 6 [MSH6]) may assist in pinpointing the underlying germline mutation. However, immunoreactivity may be retained in the case of MLH1, even if genetic changes result in the production of a nonfunctioning protein {3233}. Virtually all sporadic MSI-H carcinomas lose *MLH1* through methylation; *BRAF* mutations are also largely restricted to the sporadic MSI-H tumours and are not found in Lynch-syndrome tumours {1398}. Immunohistochemical staining of MSI-H colorectal cancers confirms that most TIL are CD3-positive T cells and most are cytotoxic (CD8-positive) {731}. In sections stained

with haematoxylin and eosin, lymphocytes are difficult to discern when the percentage of CD3-positive lymphocytes (out of all epithelial nuclei) is less than about 5%. CD3 counts in excess of 5% occur in about 70% of MSI-H cancers. CD3 counts in excess of 10% are highly specific for MSI-H cancers, and are the best predictors. The feature of TIL does not, however, distinguish between Lynch tumours and their sporadic MSI-H counterparts {1061, 1416, 3297}. The nodular arrangements of lymphocytes occurring peri-tumourally or within the serosa (Crohn-like reaction) are B-lymphocytes surrounded by T-lymphocytes.

Molecular pathology
Acquired genetic changes in Lynch-syndrome cancers

The demonstration of MSI serves as an important biomarker for cancers associated with Lynch syndrome. Lynch-syndrome cancers and sporadic MSI-H cancers share the mutator pathway.

Mode of inheritance, chromosomal location, and structure

Lynch syndrome is transmitted as an autosomal dominant trait. It is associated with heterozygous germline mutations in one of five genes with a verified or putative function in DNA MMR, namely *MLH1*, *MSH2*, *MSH6*, *PMS2*, and *MLH3* (MutL homologue 3). Biallelic mutations cause a syndrome of constitutional deficiency in MMR, which is characterized by childhood cancers of the haematological system and brain, in addition to early-onset colorectal cancer {3524}. Furthermore, most patients with biallelic mutations show signs of neurofibromatosis type 1 (NF1).

Gene product

Lynch-syndrome-associated DNA MMR genes are ubiquitously expressed in adult human tissues; the expression pattern therefore does not seem to explain the selective organ involvement observed in this syndrome. Expression is particularly prominent in the epithelium of the digestive tract as well as in testis and ovary {862, 1774, 3523}. In the intestine, expression is confined to the replicating compartment, i.e. the bottom half of the crypts. Immunohistochemical staining of MMR proteins shows nuclear localization. Mutations typically lead to the absence of the respective MMR protein (and occasionally, other MMR proteins, in a defined pattern {1166}).

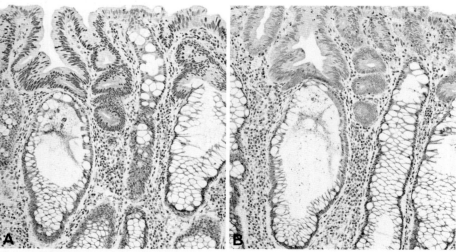

Fig. 8.36 Tubular adenoma from a patient with Lynch syndrome. **A** Immunostaining for MLH1. **B** Immunostaining for MSH2; the neoplastic epithelium shows loss of MSH2 expression (upper portion).

Function

The protein products of genes involved in Lynch syndrome are key players in the correction of mismatches that arise during DNA replication {1831}. Two different MutS-related heterodimeric complexes are responsible for mismatch recognition: MSH2–MSH3 and MSH2–MSH6. While the presence of MSH2 in the complex is mandatory, MSH3 can replace MSH6 in the correction of insertion–deletion mismatches, but not single-base mispairs. Following mismatch binding, a heterodimeric complex of MutL-related proteins, MLH1–PMS2 (and possibly another alternative complex formed by MLH1–MLH3) is recruited, and this larger complex, together with numerous other proteins, accomplishes MMR. The observed functional redundancy in the DNA MMR protein family may help explain why mutations in MSH2 and MLH1 are prevalent in families with Lynch syndrome, while mutations in MSH6, PMS2, and MLH3 are less frequent, and no Lynch-syndrome-associated germline mutations in MSH3 have been reported. MMR deficiency gives rise to MSI, and as such may aid in the diagnosis of this syndrome {2}. However, MSI is not specific to Lynch syndrome since it also occurs in 10–15% of apparently sporadic colorectal and other tumours {296}. Correction of biosynthetic errors in the newly synthesized DNA is not the only function of the DNA MMR system. In particular, it is also able to recognize lesions caused by exogenous mutagens and mediate DNA-damage signalling {1831}.

Gene mutations

The International Society for Gastrointestinal Hereditary Tumours (InSiGHT) maintains a central database for Lynch syndrome-associated mutations and polymorphisms (http://www.insight-group.org). Most are found in MLH1 and MSH2, with fewer mutations in MSH6, PMS2 and MLH3. More than a thousand mutations are

Table 8.08. Characteristics of Lynch syndrome-associated human DNA mismatch repair genes.

Gene	Chromosomal location	Length of cDNA (kb)	No. of exons	Genomic size (kb)	References
MLH1	3p21–p23	2.3	19	58–100	{339, 1112, 1635, 1861, 1869, 2446}
MSH2	2p21	2.8	16	73	{869, 1636, 1773, 1871, 2515, 2847}
MSH6	2p21	4.2	10	20	{21, 2847, 2441, 2280}
PMS2	7p22	2.6	15	16	{2279, 2281}
MLH3	14q24	4.4	12	36	{1866}

presently known that are likely to be pathogenic {2517, 3547}. While > 80% of mutations are specific to each family, prevalent founding mutations occur in certain populations {2517}. As a rule, the mutations are scattered throughout the genes. Most mutations in MSH2 and MLH1 are truncating {2517, 3547}. However, one third of the mutations in MLH1 are missense, which constitutes a diagnostic problem concerning their pathogenicity. Commonly used theoretical criteria in support of pathogenicity include the following: the mutation leads to a nonconservative amino-acid change, the involved codon is evolutionarily conserved, the change is absent in the normal population, and it segregates with the disease phenotype. However, functional testing is often mandatory for the proper assignment of pathogenicity to unclassified variants. Characteristics of variants with reported results of functional and/or in silico testing can be viewed in a database (http://www.mmruv.info; {2419}). Functional studies have shown that Lynch syndrome-associated mutations in DNA MMR genes can be pathogenic in multiple ways {2398, 2615}. Furthermore, the mechanism behind constitutional inactivation of a DNA MMR gene is not always genetic (point mutation or large rearrangement) but may be epigenetic (germline epimutation) {1212, 1851}.

Mutations in DNA MMR genes account for two thirds of all families with classical Lynch syndrome that meet the Amsterdam criteria and show MSI in tumours {1870}. The occurrence of these mutations is clearly lower (< 30%) in kindreds not meeting the Amsterdam criteria {2329, 3504}.

Prognosis and predictive factors

MLH1 and MSH2 mutations have a high penetrance, with > 80% of carriers developing some form of cancer during their lifetime {3387}. There is no clear-cut correlation between the involved gene, mutation site within the gene, or mutation type vs clinical features. MSH2 mutations may confer a higher risk of extracolonic cancer than do MLH1 mutations, while MSH6 mutations may be associated with atypical clinical features, including an elevated occurrence of endometrial cancer relative to colorectal cancer as well as late age of onset {1166}. PMS2 mutations are associated with a lower penetrance and variable clinical phenotypes ranging from early- or late-onset, apparently sporadic colorectal cancer (heterozygosity for germline mutations {2877, 3296}) to Turcot syndrome or a distinct childhood-cancer syndrome (homozygosity or compound heterozygosity for germline mutation {3524}). Kindreds with the Muir-Torre phenotype {1666} as well as a subset of those with Turcot syndrome {1108} show predisposing mutations similar to those observed in classical Lynch syndrome (with the distinction that in Turcot syndrome the mutations are often biallelic).

MUTYH-associated polyposis

H. Morreau
R.H. Riddell
S. Aretz

Definition

MUTYH-associated polyposis (MAP) is an autosomal recessive disorder characterized by a variable number of colorectal polyps with different histological phenotypes, that have a tendency to progress to malignancy. Since the disorder was not recognized until 2002 {60}, the full spectrum of *MUTYH*-associated phenotypes and the prediction of risk associated with *MUTYH* mutations are still being elucidated and are the subject of ongoing debate.

Characteristically, > 10 polyps are found, although in population-based series of colorectal cancer (CRC) up to one third of patients with biallelic *MUTYH* mutations have no or < 10 polyps at presentation {142, 163, 180, 571, 621, 822, 1075, 2284, 2583, 2790, 2961, 3369, 3448}. Small-intestinal (mostly duodenal) and stomach polyposis is part of the MAP spectrum and extra-intestinal manifestations of MAP might occur {3408}.

MIM No.

MAP	608456
MUTYH	604933

Synonyms

The approved abbreviation of the syndrome is MAP, the approved gene symbol is *MUTYH*. The terms *MYH* and *MYH*-associated polyposis should no longer be used.

Diagnostic criteria

MAP is suspected in patients with multiple (> 10) synchronous colorectal adenomas of rather late onset in the absence of a germline mutation in the adenomatous polyposis coli (*APC*) gene and a pedigree suggestive of autosomal recessive inheritance. However, since most MAP patients present as seemingly sporadic cases and pseudo-dominant families have also been reported, genetic testing by screening for *MUTYH* mutation is imperative to guarantee a confident diagnosis {2790}.

The most important differential diagnosis is the *APC*-related attenuated or atypical form of familial adenomatous polyposis (AFAP). In cases where there are few adenomas, Lynch syndrome (hereditary nonpolyposis colorectal cancer, HNPCC) should be considered {1166}. Since hyperplastic polyps and sessile serrated adenomas are a common finding in MAP {302, 2340} and the occurrence of colorectal cancer in the absence of colorectal polyps has been reported {571, 1906}, the clinical presentation could be misdiagnosed as hyperplastic polyposis or sporadic colorectal cancer in some patients. In patients of any age with few adenomas, without an overt family history (and no carcinoma), the likelihood of identifying MAP, AFAP or Lynch syndrome is very small.

Epidemiology

The prevalence of MAP is yet unknown. Assuming that the frequency of carriers of a heterozygous *MUTYH* mutation is approximately 2% in Caucasian populations, the incidence of biallelic mutations is about 1:10 000 in Europe and North America. According to studies on large population-based cohorts of patients with colorectal cancer (CRC), biallelic carriers account for < 1% of cases of CRC {571, 1906}, but can be identified in 3–42% of patients with colorectal adenomatous polyposis who are negative for *APC* mutations, depending on the inclusion criteria applied, the methods used for mutation screening, and the patient's ethnic background {1863}.

Localization

MAP polyps are located throughout the colon, but also in the small intestine (mostly duodenum) and stomach. Similarly, MAP carcinomas can be found throughout the colorectum; however, when all reported cases are compiled, MAP carcinomas are more often found in the right side of the colon compared with sporadic CRCs {142, 1867, 2283, 2340}. MAP carcinomas can also be found in the duodenum {360, 2286, 3408}.

Clinical features

Colorectal manifestations

Most clinical information on carriers of biallelic *MUTYH* mutations has come from studies of polyposis cohorts, which are biased in favour of description of a more severe phenotype. According to this clinic-based approach, MAP is characterized by the occurrence of tens to a few hundreds of

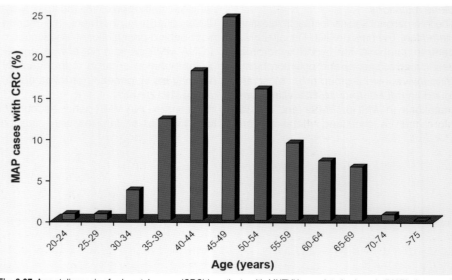

Fig. 8.37 Age at diagnosis of colorectal cancer (CRC) in patients with *MUTYH*-associated polyposis (MAP); the age at diagnosis ranged from 21 to 70 years. Modified from Sampson & Jones {2790}.

colorectal polyps throughout the colorectum; around two thirds of patients have < 100 polyps at diagnosis {2790}. However, a proportion of patients have > 100, sometimes even up to 1000 polyps, but do not have the carpets seen in some variants of FAP in which some folds are studded with polyps.

About 60% of MAP patients are diagnosed with CRC at first presentation; in large population-based series, the penetrance of biallelic mutations has been estimated to be around 70% at age 70 years {1906}. Colorectal polyps and CRC usually manifest between the fourth and seventh decades of life, with a mean age at diagnosis of 45 years {2285}. Even in patients with > 100 polyps, the mean age at diagnosis is significantly older than that for classic FAP {142}.

According to recent studies on large population-based cohorts of persons with CRC, up to one third of carriers of biallelic MUTYH mutations exhibit CRC in the absence of multiple adenomas {571}, suggesting that a substantial number of patients are not identified by current screening strategies. Considerable inter- and intra-familial variability in phenotype expression was recognized, even between patients carrying the same mutations.

Extracolonic manifestations

Extracolonic manifestations have been described only in several case reports and small sample series suggesting coincidence with limited clinical relevance {2583}. A systematic retrospective evaluation in a large cohort of MAP patients (n = 276) recruited from a European multicentre study identified a moderate but significant over-representation of several extracolonic tumours {3408}. Gastric lesions occurred in 11% of examined MAP cases. The majority had fundic gland polyps only, but a few gastric adenomas were described. The incidence of gastric cancer was not significantly increased. Duodenal polyposis was seen in 17% of cases and the relative risk of duodenal cancer was high. The incidence of extraintestinal malignancies was almost twice that of the general population and the lifetime risk was almost 40%, although no predominant tumour and no shift towards early onset was observed. The tumour spectrum is wide and points to a certain phenotypic overlap with Lynch syndrome that may reflect shared aspects of pathophysiology. In particular, sebaceous gland tumours do not seem to be restricted to germline mutations of mismatch repair genes (Muir-Torre syndrome) but might also serve as marker lesions in a small subset of MAP patients.

Implications of heterozygous MUTYH mutations

The clinical relevance of monoallelic MUTYH mutations is still controversial. According to studies on large (partly population-based) series using different approaches, carriers of heterozygous mutations have a modest and late-onset increase in the risk of CRC (odds ratio, 1.5–2.1) comparable to that of first-degree relatives of individuals with apparently sporadic CRC {571, 822, 1442}. In contrast, another large population-based study and a meta-analysis of 11 case–control series failed to identify a significantly increased risk of CRC {1906}. In the latter, however, screening for MUTYH mutations was restricted to the c.536A>G;p.Tyr179Cys (Y179C) and c.1187G>A;p.Gly396Asp (G396D) mutations.

Macroscopy
Polyps and carcinomas
The gross appearance of MAP adenomas usually resembles attenuated FAP (< 100 polyps); indeed, up to 40% of cases of AFAP have been attributed to MAP. For reporting, it is thus important to count the number of polyps as accurately as possible. Apart from the greater tendency of MAP cancers to be located in the proximal colon, no characteristic macroscopic features have yet been described.

Histopathology
Colon polyps
Conventional adenomas (mostly of low grade) are the predominant type of polyps found in MAP {1863, 1867, 2961}. The unexpected feature of MAP is their association with serrated polyps of all kinds, which also resemble their non-MAP counterparts. While hyperplastic polyps (usually less than five) are usually only found occasionally, some MAP patients have an excess of hyperplastic polyps and, to a much lesser extent, sessile serrated adenoma/polyps (SSA/P), some of which fulfil the criteria for serrated polyposis (see *Serrated polyps of the colon and rectum and serrated polyposis*) {302, 2340}.

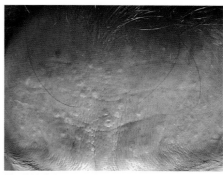

Fig. 8.38 Sebaceous gland adenomas of the forehead in a patient with proven biallelic *MUTYH* mutations (a patient with *MUTYH*-associated polyposis). Reprinted from Ponti et al. {2575A}.

Colon carcinomas
So far, there are no established histological features that differentiate MAP carcinomas from FAP or sporadic carcinomas {2340}. However, it has been suggested that MAP CRCs can show similarities to microsatellite-unstable cancers (such as predilection for the proximal colon, a more often mucinous histotype, presence of tumour-infiltrating lymphocytes or intraepithelial lymphocytes) and a Crohn-like infiltrate {2283}). A small proportion of MAP carcinomas also has a high level of microsatellite instability (MSI-H) owing to sporadic promoter hypermethylation of *MLH1* {580, 1795}. Although initially reported, there is no consensus that immunohistochemical staining of MUTYH is helpful in the diagnosis of MAP {714, 2340, 3360}. Aberrant immunohistochemical staining of other molecules such as p53 or β-catenin (*CTNNB1*), differs in frequency in MAP carcinomas in comparison to sporadic CRC, but is not helpful in the identification of MAP carcinomas.

Duodenal carcinomas
To date six duodenal carcinomas have been described in MAP patients in the context of duodenal polyposis {360, 2286, 3408}. In two of those that were analysed further, a typical c.34G>T *KRAS* tranversion mutation was found, providing evidence that the duodenal lesions were indeed induced by a *MUTYH* deficiency. Duodenal carcinomas were also observed in the absence of duodenal adenomas.

Stomach polyps
Fundic-gland polyps and adenomas can be found {2583, 3408}.

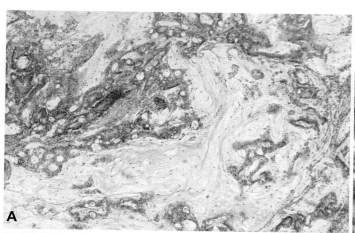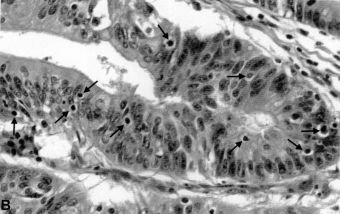

Fig. 8.39 Histology of colorectal cancer in patients with *MUTYH*-associated polyposis (MAP). **A** Mucinous carcinoma in the ascending colon of a MAP patient with a p.G396D/p.P405L mutation in *MUTYH*. Reprinted from Nielsen *et al.*, 2009 {2283} . **B** Adenocarcinoma in the ascending colon with tumour-infiltrating lymphocytes (arrows) in a patient with p.Y179C/p.Y179C mutation in *MUTYH*.

Genetic susceptibility

MUTYH gene

MAP is caused by biallelic germline mutations of the base excision repair (BER) gene *MUTYH* on chromosome 1p34.1, the human homologue of the *Escherichia coli* mutY gene {60}. *MUTYH* consists of 16 exons encompassing 1650 bp and encodes a highly conserved DNA glycosylase that is responsible for removing adenine residues mismatched with 8-oxo-7,8-dihydro-2'-deoxyguanosine (8-oxoG), the most stable product of DNA damage caused by reactive oxygen species.

Mutation spectrum

By 2009, > 100 different *MUTYH* mutations had been reported in a variety of biallelic combinations in MAP patients worldwide (Human gene mutation database, www.hgmd.org; Leiden open variation database, www.lovd.nl/MUTYH, {877}). The current annotation for the description of *MUTYH* mutations (GenBank: NM_001128425) extends the numbering after nucleotide position c.157 by 42 nucleotides (14 amino acids) compared to the originally introduced reference sequence (GenBank: U63329.1). The predominant mutation type (about 50% of cases) is missense changes followed by protein-truncating mutations that span the whole gene, except the most 3′and 5′ends {2583, 2790}. Large genomic deletions do not seem to contribute substantially to the mutation spectrum. In Caucasian populations, the two missense mutations c.536A>G;p.Tyr179Cys (Y179C) in exon 7 and c.1187G>A;p.Gly396Asp (G396D) in exon 13 (previously designated c.494A>G;p.Tyr165Cys and c.1145G>A;p.-Gly382Asp, respectively) account for around 70% of all mutant alleles. However, ethnic and geographic differences in the pattern of *MUTYH* mutations are evident and point to founder events. To date, few missense changes have been characterized by functional assays.

Recurrence risk and predictive testing

Genetic counselling should be offered to all patients with suspected or proven monogenic disease and to their relatives, in particular in a setting of predictive genetic testing. Siblings of MAP patients have a recurrence risk of 25%, thus, predictive testing is reasonable once the mutations are identified in the index case. Due to a heterogeneous carrier frequency of *MUTYH* mutations of around 2% in the Caucasian general population, children of a MAP patient have a low but not negligible risk (approximately 1%) of carrying two mutations; screening of the spouses of MAP patients and MUTYH heterozygotes for *MUTYH* mutation should thus be considered {2790}.

Molecular pathology

Oxidative DNA damage (especially with 8-oxoG) is not readily repaired in the absence of functional *MUTYH* base-excision repair {2583}. A defect in the latter leads to increased misincorporation of adenine opposite 8-oxo-guanine and is thereby associated with increased frequency of G:C > T:A transversions in tumour-suppressor genes and oncogenes in daughter cells, leading to the formation of intestinal adenoma. For unknown reasons, there is a high occurrence of these transversions at GAA sites, especially in the *APC* gene, leading to selection of the stop codon TAA. The finding of such somatic *APC* mutations in adenomas has led to the elucidation of the underlying cause of MAP in humans {60}. The requirement for two rather than a single somatic *APC* mutation for initiation of adenoma might be the reason for the more attenuated colorectal phenotype in MAP compared with classic FAP {142, 2790}. In MAP adenomas and carcinomas (in the latter with a frequency of up to 64%), but also in SSA/P/Ls and hyperplastic polyps of MAP patients, a characteristic c.34G>T;p.Gly12Cys *KRAS* tranversion mutation in codon 12 is found {60, 302, 1867, 2961}. This mutation is infrequent in consecutive series of sporadic CRC {115} and thus can be used to identify (atypical) MAP patients {3369}. The c.35G>T; p. Gly>Val *KRAS* transversion is not typically associated with MAP and occasionally c.39G>A; p. Gly>Asp is found in adenomas. In other genes often implicated in colorectal tumorigenesis, such as *TP53* and *SMAD4*, G>T transversions are found but to a lesser extent than other types of mutations, which might indicate a predominant *MUTYH* effect in early carcinogenesis {1867, 2283}.

As the *APC* gene is a preferred target of somatic mutations caused by insufficient *MUTYH* activity, consequently MAP-associated adenomas and carcinomas are expected to use the chromosomal-instability pathway associated with the Wnt signalling pathway, and therefore should resemble typical sporadic adenomas and carcinomas. However, in contrast to most sporadic forms of CRC, about half of MAP carcinomas are close to diploid. Although MAP CRCs are without alterations that are detectable with array comparative genomic hybridization, loss of heterozygosity (LOH) is present at different loci, owing to widespread copy-neutral LOH {1867, 2062}.

For MAP adenomas, the picture is less clear as near diploid and aneuploid adenomas have been identified using different technical platforms {422, 1439}. Loss of human leukocyte antigen (HLA) class I is a frequent event in MAP carcinomas, similarly to mismatch repair-deficient tumours {673}. This can be explained by the loss of caretaker functions leading to abundance of somatic mutations in the genome and resulting in presentation of aberrant peptides at the cell surface in the context of HLA. The latter most likely triggers a strong selective pressure by the immune system favouring outgrowth of cells with an immune evasive phenotype.

Surveillance and predictive testing

The gastrointestinal surveillance protocol applied in AFAP has been suggested for MAP by a European expert panel {3385}. It includes complete colonoscopy at biannual intervals starting from age 18–20 years and gastroduodenoscopy starting at age 25–30 years. Accordingly, predictive genetic testing should be performed at these ages. However, these recommendations might be modified as the full clinical spectrum becomes better understood. A significant

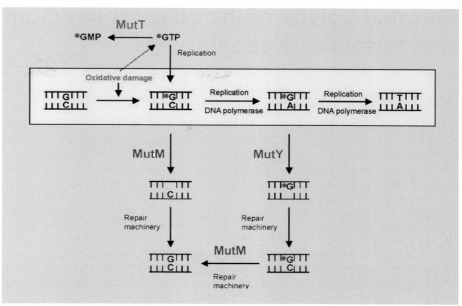

Fig. 8.40 The 8-oxoG repair system of *Escherichia coli*. The 8-oxoG is denoted by a red dot next to the G. The human homologues of the three *E. coli* DNA glycosylases MutY, Mut and MutM are termed *MUTYH*, *MTH1* and *OGG1*, respectively. GMP, guanine monophosphate; GTP, guanine triphosphate. From Cheadle & Sampson {499A}.

genotype–phenotype correlation has been established: Y179C homozygotes present earlier and have a higher risk of developing CRC than do Y179C/G396D compound heterozygotes and G396D homozygotes {2285}. In the light of current data, intense surveillance for extra-intestinal tumours is unlikely to offer great benefit {3408}. In heterozygous relatives of MAP patients, CRC screening measures similar to those offered to first-degree relatives of patients with sporadic CRC seem to be appropriate {1442}. Prognostic and predictive factors for MAP-associated CRC are under study. The timing and procedure for colorectal surgery are similar to those for FAP and must be determined on an individual basis {2790}.

Serrated polyps of the colon and rectum and serrated polyposis

D.C. Snover
D.J. Ahnen
R.W. Burt
R.D. Odze

Sporadic serrated polyps

Definition
This is a heterogeneous group of lesions characterized morphologically by a serrated (sawtooth or stellate) architecture of the epithelial compartment. The lesions include hyperplastic polyps (HPs), sessile serrated adenoma/polyp (SSA/P) and traditional serrated adenomas (TSA). Definitions of the subtypes of serrated polyps of the large intestine and of serrated polyposis are summarized in Table 8.09.

ICD-O codes
Sessile serrated adenoma/polyp   8213/0
Traditional serrated adenoma   8213/0

Synonyms
At the present time, "hyperplastic polyp" without a modifier (i.e. microvesicular) is acceptable since there is no known clinical utility to distinguishing subtypes. Sessile serrated adenoma (SSA) and sessile serrated polyp (SSP) are currently considered synonyms and both are acceptable diagnostic terms. Filiform serrated adenoma may be a subset of TSA. It is recommended that giant hyperplastic polyp, variant hyperplastic polyp and serrated adenoma (without a modifier) should not be used since they are potentially misleading and evolving concepts have led to new nomenclature.

Clinical features
Hyperplastic polyps (HPs)
HPs are most frequent in the distal colon and rarely cause symptoms {198}. Histologically, several subtypes have been recognized that differ slightly in terms of morphology, distribution and molecular characteristics, but without clinical relevance as yet. Goblet-cell rich hyperplastic polyps (GCHP) are almost exclusively seen in the left colon, whereas microvesicular hyperplastic polyps (MVHP) are more widely distributed.

HPs are typically sessile lesions of 1–5 mm in size and rarely > 1 cm. It is not uncommon for distal HPs to be multiple (10–20). They are generally described as looking like pearl-coloured dew drops, tend to flatten and are more difficult to see when the lumen is fully distended. Using newer high-definition endoscopes and chromoendoscopy, the polyp surface has been described as having crypt openings that are larger than the surrounding normal crypts, with lumens that are rounded in GCHP and stellate in MVHP {2333, 3109}. These techniques may make endoscopic diagnosis of HPs and other serrated polyps feasible, but the current standard for diagnosis is polypectomy and histology. HPs in the proximal colon are larger, on average, than those in the distal colon. Large proximal HPs may be difficult to visualize because they tend to be flat and are often covered with yellowish mucus.

Sessile serrated adenomas/polyps (SSA/P)
SSA/Ps rarely cause clinical symptoms. They are more likely to be located in the proximal colon. Their average size is larger than that of hyperplastic polyps; more than half of SSA/Ps measure > 5 mm and 15–20% are > 10 mm {3049}. They appear flat to sessile, with a soft, smooth-appearing surface. They are often covered with mucus, giving them an initial yellow appearance {2332}. When the mucus is washed off, the underlying polyp may be similar in colour to the adjacent mucosa or may be reddish. When viewed by chromoendoscopy or narrow-band imaging, the surface characteristics of SSA/Ps are similar to those of MVHPs {1394}.

Traditional serrated adenoma (TSA)
TSAs are much less common than other serrated polyps, are usually found in the distal colon and rarely cause clinical symptoms. Although there are limited endoscopic data, TSAs have been described as having an endoscopic appearance that resembles that of conventional colonic adenomas, which are more commonly reddish and protuberant than SSA/Ps {1192, 1277, 2006}. The endoscopic surface appearance of TSAs is not well characterized.

Histopathology
The distinction of HP from SSA/P and TSA is based mainly on architectural criteria, although cytological features play a more important role in TSA {757, 2994, 2993, 3274}. SSA/P and TSA can develop additional cytological features indicative of progression toward the development of carcinoma. It is recognized that not all serrated lesions are easily classified, often because of sampling issues or poor orientation of the specimen. In such cases, the term "serrated polyp, unclassified" may be used.

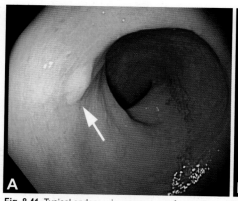
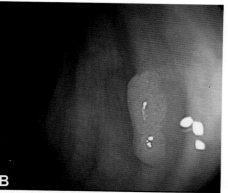

Fig. 8.41 Typical endoscopic appearance of sporadic serrated polyps in the sigmid colon. **A** Hyperplastic polyp (HP). The lesion (arrow) is sessile and pearly white. **B** Sessile serrated adenoma/polyp (SSA/P). The lesion is somewhat larger than a typical hyperplastic polyp, sessile and has a yellow mucus cap.

Hyperplastic polyps (HP)

HPs are the most common serrated lesions, accounting for > 75% of all serrated polyps. Three types have been described: the microvesicular (MVHP), goblet-cell rich (GCHP) and mucin-poor types (MPHP) {3274}. The subtypes have demographic and molecular differences {2333}. All three types are characterized by elongation of the crypts with variable degrees of serration. The crypts are straight and proliferation is located in the lower third of the crypts, with serration developing in the more luminal aspects {3276}. The bases of the crypts are narrow and lined with undifferentiated cells with interspersed neuroendocrine cells. MVHPs are characterized by epithelial cells with microvesicular (small-droplet)

mucin with or without interspersed goblet cells and tend to show more prominent serrations. GCHPs are mostly composed of goblet cells and show much more subtle serrations. Both MVHP and GCHP have bland nuclei without atypia. MPHPs are mucin-depleted, may show prominent serration and may show reactive-appearing nuclear atypia. MVHP is the most common, followed by GCHP. MPHP is very rare and little is currently known about this variant.

SSA/P

SSA/P constitutes about 15–25% of all serrated polyps and in one prospective study was found in 9% of all patients undergoing screening colonoscopy {1021, 3049, 3274}. This lesion is thought to be

the precursor to sporadic carcinomas with microsatellite instability (MSI) and is probably also the precursor for CpG island-methylated microsatellite-stable carcinomas {1399}. Like HP, SSA/P has bland cytology and elongation of crypts with prominent serration. The distinguishing feature of SSA/P is an overall distortion of the normal architecture resulting from alterations of the proliferative zone {3276}. The proliferative zone is often not located in the base of the crypts but rather on one or the other side of the crypts and is often asymmetrical. Ki67 staining emphasizes this abnormal proliferation and reveals cells with goblet-cell or gastric-foveolar differentiation at the base of the crypts. The crypts are often dilated and assume abnormal shapes including L-shaped and

Table 8.09 Histological and genetic features distinguishing different types of sporadic serrated polyps and serrated polyposis.

Type	Synonyms	Histological features[a]				Genetic features[b]			
		Crypts	Proliferation	Cytological dysplasia	Mucin type	BRAF mutation	KRAS mutation	CIMP	MLH1 methylation
MVHP	Hyperplastic polyp; metaplastic polyp	Straight with serrations toward lumen	Located uniformly in basal portion of crypts	No	Microvesicular or mixed goblet cell & microvesicular	+++	–	+	–
GCHP	Hyperplastic polyp; metaplastic polyp	Straight, serrations may be minimal	Located uniformly in the basal portion of crypts	No	Pure goblet cells	–	+++	U	–
MP/HP	Hyperplastic polyp; metaplastic polyp	Straight, serration toward lumen	Located uniformly in the basal portion of crypts	Atypia present but appears reactive	None	U	U	U	U
SSA/P	Serrated polyp with abnormal proliferation; giant hyperplastic polyp; variant hyperplastic polyp	Crypts distorted, often dilated near base, excess serration near base	Proliferation abnormally located often away from the base of the crypts, variable from crypt to crypt	No	Usually microvesicular, sometimes with goblet cells or gastric foveolar differentiation	+++	–	+++	–
SSA/P with cytological dysplasia	Mixed hyperplastic-adenomatous polyp; advanced SSA/P	As for SSA/P	As for SSA/P but with more proliferation in cytologically dysplastic areas	Present	As for SSA/P	+++	–	+++	++
TSA	Serrated adenoma; filiform serrated adenoma	Hyperserrated in part owing to formation of ectopic crypts	Proliferation present at base of ectopic crypts	May be present, usually in the form of cells with eosinophilic cytoplasm	None or goblet cells	+[c]	+[c]	++	–
Serrated polyposis	Hyperplastic polyposis; giant hyperplastic polyposis	Mostly SSA/P with some MVHP	As per polyp subtype	Present as disease advances	As per polyp subtype	++[c]	+[c]	+++	+

CIMP, CpG island methylator phenotype; GCHP, goblet cell-rich hyperplastic polyp; MPHP, mucin-poor hyperplastic polyp; MVHP, microvesicular hyperplastic polyp; SSA/P, Sessile serrated adenoma/polyp; TSA, traditional serrated adenoma.
[a] Please see text for details of histology. [b] –, not present; +, present often to a limited extent or in some cases; ++ and +++, present extensively; U, unknown. [c] KRAS and BRAF mutations are mutually exclusive. Individuals only carry a mutation in one of these two genes.

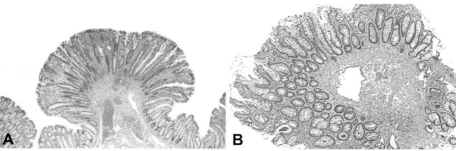

Fig. 8.42 Hyperplastic polyps. **A** Microvesicular hyperplastic polyp (MVHP). The crypts are elongated but relatively straight, with serrations that are visible mainly near the luminal end of the crypts. **B** Goblet cell-rich hyperplastic polyp (GCHP). The crypts are elongated and slightly serpiginous, but generally straight. Serrations are minimal in most cases.

inverted T-shaped. Serration may be very prominent and is often seen at the base of the crypts, rather than superficially, as for HPs. There is often subtle nuclear atypia, usually in the form of vesicular nuclei with prominent nuclei, and mitoses may be seen anywhere in the crypts, including in the upper third. Some areas of SSA/P may have straight crypts similar to those of MVHP; however, usually the straight crypts account for less than half of the lesion and if more than two or three contiguous crypts demonstrate features of SSA/P, the lesion should be classified as SSA/P.

Cytological dysplasia is not present in uncomplicated SSA/P, but develops with progression toward carcinoma, often in conjunction with methylation of the *MLH1* gene and with the development of MSI {1019, 2927}. In addition to dysplasia resembling that of conventional adenomas (with narrow elongated hyperchromatic nuclei and basophilic cytoplasm) more cuboidal cells with eosinophilic cytoplasia and more vesicular nuclei with prominent nucleoli may occur, referred to as "serrated dysplasia". These advanced lesions have been referred to as "mixed SSA/P-tubular adenomas" (or mixed HP-TA) in the older

literature; however, the term "SSA/P with cytological dysplasia" is preferred since biologically the cytologically dysplastic part of these lesions is not the same as conventional adenoma, essentially never with mutation of the *APC* gene but rather with MSI resulting from methylation of *MLH1*. The behaviour of these lesions may be more aggressive than that of conventional adenoma.

TSA

The term "serrated adenoma" was initially coined for any lesion showing serration and cytological dysplasia {1891}. As it turns out, several disparate lesions fulfil this definition, including the lesions now known as TSA, SSA/P with cytological dysplasia and some conventional adenomas with an overall serrated architecture. Because of this potentially confusing ambiguity, it is recommended that the term "serrated adenoma" never be used without a qualifier. The most unique lesion falling under this category, TSA, is a lesion characterized by an overall complex and villiform growth pattern, often with cells showing cytological features characterized as "dysplasia", but

quite different from the dysplasia of conventional adenomas or of SSA/P with cytological dysplasia {2994, 3274}. The lesion reported as "filiform" serrated adenoma may represent a subset of TSA {3619}. TSAs are uncommon, making up < 1% of all polyps.

The original definition of TSA referred to a lesion with a protuberant although sessile growth pattern with an overall complex, often villiform configuration. In many examples, the villi are lined with a very characteristic cell – a tall columnar cell with a narrow pencillate nucleus and eosinophilic cytoplasm, often refered to as a "dysplastic" cell. Mitoses are very rare in these cells, unlike the dysplastic cells of conventional adenoma, and there is no proliferation according to Ki67 staining. These cells are, therefore, not "dysplastic" in the same sense as the "dysplastic" cells of conventional adenoma or SSA/P with cytological dysplasia, and appear to be senescent. Conventional or serrated dysplasia can occur in TSA, probably reflecting progression toward carcinoma. Recent studies have suggested that the cytological features of the individual cells of TSA may not be the best defining feature, but rather that TSA differs from HP and SSA/P in that the crypts have lost their anchoring to the underlying muscularis mucosae, leading to the formation of "ectopic" crypts {3276}. If the presence of ectopic crypts is considered to be the defining feature of TSA, lesions having the overall growth pattern of TSA but with a predominance of goblet cells may also be categorized as TSA.

TSA has some features in common with SSA/P, but the lesions have more differences than similarities, including considerable differences in histology, location, progression and molecular pathology.

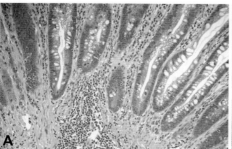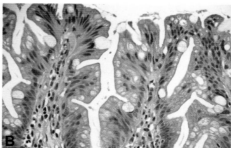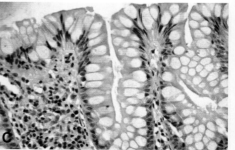

Fig. 8.43 Hyperplastic polyps: all types have crypts with narrow bases and a component of undifferentiated small proliferating cells as well as a variable number of interspersed goblet cells. **A** Microvesicular hyperplastic polyp (MVHP) generally has a higher proportion of proliferating cells than goblet cell-rich hyperplastic polyps (GCHP). **B** In MVHP, the maturing cells near the lumen contain very small droplets of mucin. **C** In GCHP, the primary maturing cell is the goblet cell and there are no microvesicular cells.

TSA is generally not associated with carcinoma with high MSI but may be associated with low MSI {757}.

Molecular pathology

The serrated pathway involves a sequence of genetic and epigenetic alterations that lead to the development of sporadic carcinomas with MSI and probably also microsatellite stable CpG island-methylated carcinomas (CIMP+ MSS). An early event in the pathway involves activating mutations of the *BRAF* gene, a pro-proliferative, anti-apoptotic serine-threonine kinase. Mutations of *BRAF* are present in the majority of SSA/Ps and are also common in MVHP. This explains why some sporadic MSI-H adenocarcinomas (but not Lynch syndrome-associated MSI carcinomas) contain *BRAF* mutatations. GCHPs tend to carry *KRAS* mutations. The serration of both SSA/P and MVHP is thought to be attributable to failure of apoptosis, which leads to the accumulation of mature cells that pile up into serrations. Although it has been speculated that MVHP may be a precursor lesion to SSA/P, there are several arguments against this possibility, including the marked difference in distribution of the lesions and the fact that SSA/Ps can occasionally be only two or three crypts in size. Therefore, this possibility remains to be clarified.

It is clear that SSA/P acts as a more immediate precursor to carcinoma. SSA/Ps are prone to methylation of the promoter regions of a number of genes, the most important of which is *MLH1*, a DNA mismatch repair gene. SSA/Ps without cytological dysplasia are generally not methylated at *MLH1*, and hence are not MSI. When methylation of *MLH1* occurs, the polyp becomes MSI, and at this point has a propensity to develop into carcinoma, probably at a rate similar to

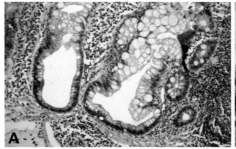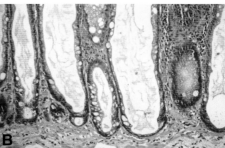

Fig. 8.44 Sessile serrated adenoma/polyp (SSA/P), high-power view. **A** Mature cells are often seen at the base of the crypts; in this case, they mainly resemble gastric foveolar cells. Note the dilated, distorted appearance of the crypt, sometime referred to as "anchor-shaped". **B** In this case, the crypts are uniformly dilated and there are goblet cells at the crypt bases.

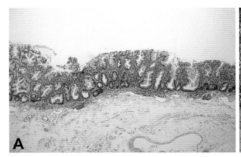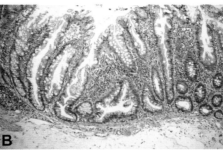

Fig. 8.45 Sessile serrated adenoma/polyp (SSA/P), low-power view. **A** Note that although the crypts still reach the muscularis mucosae, they are generally distorted and dilated, L-shaped, inverted T-shaped or anchor-shaped. **B** SSA/P with excess serration at the base of a crypt.

that of adenomas in patients with Lynch syndrome. The *MLH1* gene is not methylated in CIMP-H microsatellite-stable carcinomas and the specific genes and sequence of events that drive the progression from SSA/P to CIMP-H microsatellite-stable carcinomas is unknown.

TSA shows considerable differences from SSA/P in terms of mutation and methylation status {757}. Although many TSAs are reported to have *BRAF* mutations, at least 25% of TSAs have mutations of *KRAS,* not *BRAF*. Since such mutation studies have not always used the current definition of TSA,

it is likely that many of the cases in which *BRAF* is mutant are SSA/P with cytological dysplasia, rather than TSA. TSA does show increased methylation, but essentially never shows methylation of *MLH1*, and is never associated with CIMP-H MSI carcinomas. It has been suggested that TSA may be the precursor to MSI-L carcinoma by way of methylation of the *MGMT* promoter. Much remains to be learned about TSA, which has only recently been distinguished from the other serrated lesions.

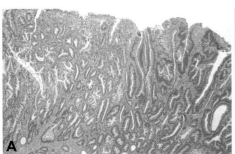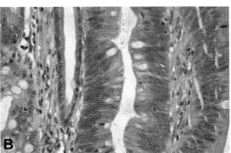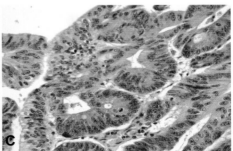

Fig. 8.46 Sessile serrated adenoma/ polyp (SSA/P) with cytological dysplasia. **A** At low power, the SSA/P on the left is sharply demarcated from the cytologically dysplastic area on the right. **B** Here the cytological dysplasia resembles that of a conventional adenoma, although the molecular profile of this lesion is likely to be very different. **C** The cytological dysplasia in this example is slightly different from that of a conventional adenoma; the cells are shorter, and the nuclei have more open chromatin and prominent nucleoli. The cytoplasm tends to be more eosinophilic (less amphophilic) than that found in conventional adenomas. This is sometimes referred to as "serrated" dysplasia.

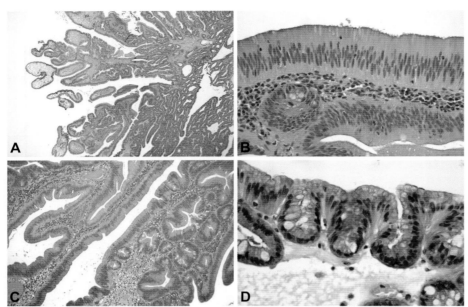

Fig. 8.47 Traditional serrated adenoma (TSA). **A** At low power, TSA often appears very complex with a prominent "villiform" or "filiform" configuration. **B** In many cases, the cells lining the villi are predominantly tall and columnar with eosinophilic cytoplasm and oval nuclei, which are typically minimally pseudostratified and generally show little if any mitotic activity (and are usually negative for the proliferation marker Ki67). **C** Note the presence of small abortive or "ectopic" crypts (seen protruding from the surface) that do not extend to the muscularis mucosae. This detachment of crypts from the muscularis mucosae may allow these lesions to become villiform. **D** At higher power, the cells of these ectopic crypts are differentiated near the surface, but proliferating and undifferentiated at the base.

Prognosis and predictive factors

The current recommendation is to remove all polyps when technically possible {2664}, except where there are many diminutive (< 5 mm) distal HP-appearing polyps that can be sampled (six to eight polyps biopsied) to confirm that they are HPs). Diminutive distal HPs are thought to have little or no malignant potential and their presence does not otherwise affect screening for colorectal cancer and intervals for colonoscopic surveillance.

Follow-up recommendations for individuals with large (> 1 cm) HPs are not clearly defined but, given that many SSA/Ps will have areas that are histologically indistinguishable from HPs, complete excision is important, if possible, to assure accurate diagnosis. Surveillance recommendations for SSA/Ps and TSAs are not standardized nor validated. Two groups have published similar recommendations based on current terminology and predicted behaviour, but they have not been tested {757, 2994}. Recommended surveillance intervals may be partly based on the number and size of the polyps (5-year surveillance for one or two small [< 1 cm] polyps; 3-year surveillance for any large [> 1 cm] lesion or for three or more of any size). Some authors recommend that any SSA/P with cytological dysplasia be considered as a histologically advanced lesion, given the likelihood that it is MSI, and that a 1-year post-intervention examination should be considered to guarantee complete removal of the lesion, with a subsequent surveillance interval of 3 years, but this approach has not been rigorously tested.

Serrated polyposis

Synonyms

Historically, serrated polyposis has been called hyperplastic polyposis; however, the term "serrated polyposis" is preferred, given the common presence of SSA/P in this process {3275}.

Diagnostic criteria

Differing criteria to define serrated polyposis have been suggested, although all are empirical and the described categories may represent different diseases. Definitions include: (1) at least five serrated polyps proximal to the sigmoid colon with two or more of these being > 10 mm; (2) any number of serrated polyps proximal to the sigmoid colon in an individual who has a first-degree relative with serrated polyposis; or (3) > 20 serrated polyps of any size, but distributed throughout the colon {1106, 2636, 1401}.

Clinical features

Serrated polyposis occurs in males and females and at any age, although it is more often reported in middle and later life {845, 1296, 2636, 2658, 2744}. It is generally asymptomatic, but larger polyps may bleed. The condition is most often identified unexpectedly at screening colonoscopy. The polyps are most often sessile and < 1 cm in diameter, with rare larger pedunculated lesions. Small polyps are often distributed throughout the colon while larger polyps are usually found in the proximal colon. One or several cytologically dysplastic lesions are often found in this condition during surveillance. Serrated polyps have been observed to progress to high-grade dysplasia. Extracolonic or extraintestinal manifestations have not been observed. Two clinical variants are recognized, although overlap may be present {381, 1401}. In type 2, numerous small (usually 5 mm or smaller) classical hyperplastic polyps are present throughout the colon and the risk of cancer is modestly increased, if at all {1401}. In type 1, multiple SSA/Ps occur that can be larger and often more proximal {1401}. The risk of cancer is substantial for type 1. Ultimately, molecular genetic alterations may define these two and possibly other variants.

Histopathology

The lesions of serrated polyposis are predominately SSA/P, with fewer MVHPs, which may be larger than typical HPs {3275, 757, 1401}. With progression, SSA/Ps with cytological dysplasia appear, at which point carcinoma may develop quickly. Lesions that are indistinguishable from conventional adenoma are sometimes present, and may represent SSA/P

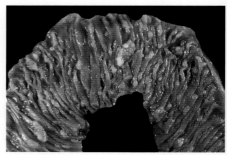

Fig. 8.48 Serrated polyposis in a colectomy specimen.

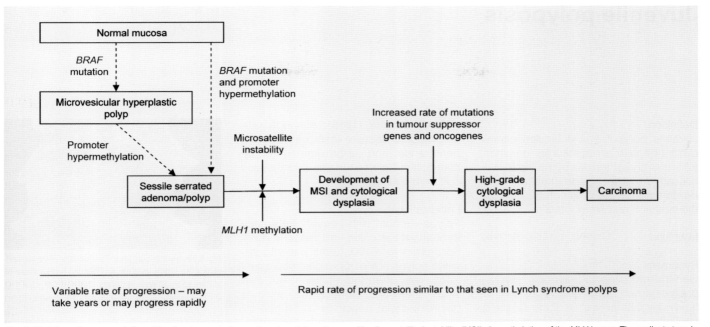

Fig. 8.49 Schematic representation of the development of sporadic colorectal carcinoma with microsatellite instability (MSI) via methylation of the *MLH1* gene. The earliest steps in the progression from normal mucosa to sessile serrated adenoma/polyp (SSA/P) are currently under debate (dotted lines).

that has been overtaken by cytologically dysplastic cells and hence are not technically conventional adenomas.

Genetic suscepibility

Relatives have not generally been examined for polyposis. Few cases of familial serrated polyposis have been described {1401}.

Molecular pathology

The genetic etiology and pathogenesis of serrated polyposis is not known. The serrated pathway, described for sporadic polyps, is certainly one possibility {1406, 1465, 3656}. Additional pathways have been postulated, suggesting that the disease may be heterogeneous {1401, 2636}. *MUTYH* gene-associated polyposis has occasionally been reported to include multiple serrated polyps as part

of the phenotype {544}. It has been suggested that the lesions in type 2 serrated polyposis generally have *KRAS* mutations while lesions in type 1 serrated polyposis tend to have mutant *BRAF* {1401}.

Prognosis and predictive factors

Untreated serrated polyposis is thought to be associated with a substantial (although undetermined) increased risk of developing colon cancer {3275, 845, 1138, 1296, 1403, 1401, 1796, 2658, 2744}. Suggested management is colonoscopy for polyp removal every 1–3 years, depending on the number of polyps present {845, 1719, 2744, 3635}. Polyps of < 3–4 mm can probably safely be observed with annual examination, although larger polyps should be removed. If colonoscopic management becomes technically difficult or ineffective, or if any progression to cytological

dysplasia is observed, then colectomy with ileo-rectal anastamosis should be recommended, followed by regular rectal clearing of new polyps. The presence of multiple, large proximal colonic serrated polyps, which can be difficult and risky to remove by colonoscopy, is a common reason to move to surgery, although large numbers of polyps may also lead to this decision. Screening colonoscopy should probably also be offered to first-degree relatives, particularly those aged > 40 years, in view of the possible familial risk {1719, 3635}. Properly managed patients with serrated polyposis appear to have a very good prognosis. Some cases of *MUTYH*-associated polyposis are also reported to have SSA/P.

Juvenile polyposis

G.J.A. Offerhaus
J.R. Howe

Definition
Juvenile polyposis is a familial cancer syndrome with an autosomal dominant trait. It is characterized by multiple juvenile polyps of the gastrointestinal tract, predominantly the colorectum, but also the stomach and small intestine.

MIM Nos   174900, 175050, 612242

Synonyms
Generalized juvenile polyposis; juvenile polyposis coli; juvenile polyposis of infancy; juvenile polyposis of the stomach; familial juvenile polyposis; hamartomatous gastrointestinal polyposis; combined juvenile polyposis/hereditary haemorrhagic telangiectasia (Osler-Weber-Rendu) syndrome.

Diagnostic criteria
After the initial report by McColl in 1964 {2020}, the following diagnostic criteria were established: (1) more than three to five juvenile polyps of the colorectum; or (2) juvenile polyps throughout the gastrointestinal tract; or (3) any number of juvenile polyps with a family history of juvenile polyposis {978, 1407}. Other syndromes involving hamartomatous gastrointestinal polyps should be ruled out clinically or by pathological examination.

Epidemiology
Incidence
Juvenile polyposis is ten times less common than familial adenomatous polyposis (FAP) {1397}, with an incidence of 0.6–1 case per 100 000 population in European countries and North America {379}. In less developed countries, however, juvenile polyposis may be the most common gastrointestinal polyposis syndrome {2662, 3515}. About half of cases arise in patients with no family history {572}.

Age and sex distribution
Two thirds of patients with juvenile polyposis present within the first two decades of life, with a mean age at diagnosis of 18.5 years {572}, although some present in infancy, and others not until their seventh decade {1258}. Although epidemiological data are limited, incomplete penetrance and approximately equal distribution between males and females can be presumed.

Localization
Polyps occur with equal frequency throughout the colon and range in number from 1 to > 100. Some patients develop polyps of the upper gastrointestinal tract, most often the stomach, but also small intestine. Generalized juvenile gastrointestinal polyposis is defined by the presence of polyps in the stomach, small intestine and colon {2770}.

Clinical features
Signs and symptoms
Patients usually present with gastrointestinal bleeding, manifesting as haematochezia. Melaena, prolapsed rectal polyps, passage of tissue *per rectum*, intussusception, abdominal pain, and anaemia are also common.

Imaging
Air-contrast barium enema and upper gastrointestinal series may reveal filling defects, but are non-diagnostic for juvenile polyps.

Endoscopy. Small juvenile polyps may resemble hyperplastic polyps, while larger polyps generally have a well-defined stalk with a bright red, rounded head, which may be eroded. In the stomach, polyps are less often pedunculated and are more

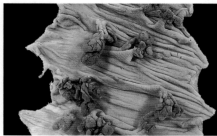

Fig. 8.50 Juvenile polyposis. The contours of the multiple polyps are highly irregular and fronded, unlike those of solitary sporadic juvenile polyps.

commonly diffuse. Biopsy or excision of polyps by colonoscopy can be both diagnostic and therapeutic. Endoscopic screening of the colorectum and upper gastrointestinal tract is recommended at age 15 years or at the time of first symptoms {344, 1259} and should be repeated every 2–3 years.

Extraintestinal manifestations
Congenital anomalies have been reported in 11–15% of patients with juvenile polyposis {572, 1226}, mostly in sporadic cases {385}. These anomalies most commonly involve the heart, central nervous system, soft tissues, gastrointestinal tract and genitourinary system {572, 2020}. Several patients have been reported with ganglioneuromatous proliferation within juvenile polyps {2042, 2539, 3483}. An association exists between juvenile polyposis and hereditary haemorrhagic telangiectasia, characterized by vascular malformations affecting many organs {938}, and various

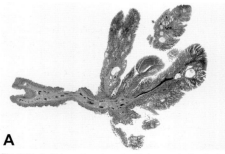
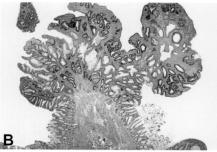

Fig. 8.51 A, B Juvenile polyposis with low-grade dysplasia: the bizarre architecture is unlike the round, uniform structure of sporadic juvenile polyps.

reports of patients with juvenile polyposis who have pulmonary arteriovenous malformations and hypertrophic osteoarthropathy have been published {174, 611, 2972}.

Macroscopy

Most subjects with juvenile polyposis have 3–200 polyps throughout the colorectum. The rare and often lethal form occurring in infancy may be associated with diffuse gastrointestinal polyposis {2770}. In cases presenting in later childhood to adulthood, completely unaffected mucosa separates the lesions. This is unlike the dense mucosal carpeting that is characteristic of FAP. The polyps are usually pedunculated, but can be sessile in the stomach. Smaller examples have the spherical head of a typical solitary juvenile polyp. They may grow up to 5 cm in diameter, with a multilobulated head. The individual lobes are relatively smooth and separated by deep, well-defined clefts. The multilobulated polyp therefore appears as a cluster of smaller juvenile polyps attached to a common stalk. Such multilobulated or atypical juvenile polyps account for about 20% of the total number of polyps {1407}.

Histopathology

Smaller polyps are indistinguishable from their sporadic counterparts, i.e. they have an eroded surface, abundant oedematous stroma with inflammatory cells and cystically dilated glands with reactive epithelium. In the multilobulated or atypical variety, the lobes may be either rounded or finger-like. There is a relative increase in the amount of epithelium vs stroma. Glands show more budding and branching but less cystic change than the classical solitary polyp {1407}.

Neoplastic potential. There are two histogenetic explanations for the well-documented association between juvenile polyposis and colorectal cancer, which could (1) arise in co-existing adenomas; or (2) develop via neoplastic change within a juvenile polyp. While both mechanisms may apply, pure adenomas appear to be uncommon in juvenile polyposis. In contrast, foci of dysplasia are regularly seen, particularly in atypical or multilobulated juvenile polyps {1407, 3546}. Additional support for the second mechanism comes from a transgenic-mouse model of juvenile polyposis in which

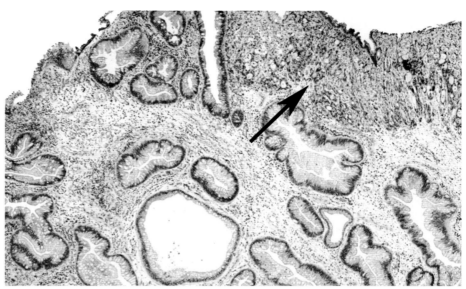

Fig. 8.52 Juvenile polyp with low-grade dysplasia and an area of early adenocarcinoma (arrow).

disruption of signalling by intestinal bone morphogenetic protein (BMP) leads to the development of neoplasia in the polyps {1122}.

Molecular pathology

Germline mutations in *SMAD4* or *BMPR1A* are identified causes of juvenile polyposis in 50–60% of patients {893, 1254, 1261, 2736}. Most such alterations are point mutations or small base-pair deletions that can be detected by conventional sequence analysis; however, about 5–15% are deletions of one or more exons, or the entire *SMAD4* or *BMPR1A* gene. To analyse such large genomic deletions, techniques such as multiplex ligation-dependent probe amplification (MPLA) are necessary {141, 401, 3365}.

Since the molecular cause of juvenile polyposis remains unknown in about half of cases, other candidate genes, mostly those involved in the TGFβ/BMP pathway, have been investigated. Germline mutation of the TGFβ coreceptor endoglin (*ENG*) has been reported in two patients with juvenile polyposis {3144}, but since no *ENG* mutations were found in an additional 65 patients, the role of this gene in susceptibility is under debate {1255}. No germline mutations have been found in *SMAD1–3*, *SMAD5*, *SMAD7*, *BMPR2*, *BMPR1B*, *ACVRL1*, *TGFBR2* or *CDX2* {345, 3365}. Although one unconfirmed report has suggested a role for *PTEN* {2399}, the present notion is that individuals with *PTEN* mutations should be considered as having Cowden syndrome {795}.

Prognosis and predictive factors

The most severe form of juvenile polypsis presents in infancy, with diarrhoea, anaemia, and hypoalbuminaemia; these patients rarely survive past age 2 years. Although polyps in patients with juvenile polypsis are considered to be hamartomas, they do have malignant potential. A recent analysis found a cumulative lifetime risk of colorectal cancer of 39% and a relative risk of 34 for patients with juvenile polyposis {343}. The lifetime risk of other cancers of the stomach, small bowel and pancreas has been reported as 10–15% {1258}. The typical age at diagnosis is between 35 and 45 years (range, 15–68 years) for colon carcinoma and 58 years (range, 21–73 years) for upper gastrointestinal carcinoma {1258, 1407}. Most cases occur in patients who have not been screened radiologically or endoscopically, suggesting that cancers may be preventable by close surveillance. Prophylactic surgery should be considered for patients who cannot be managed endoscopically and have polyps with dysplasia or who have a strong family history of colorectal cancer. Mutations in *SMAD4* and *BMPR1A* may be associated with phenotypic differences in severity {1116}. In general, carriers of *SMAD4* mutations are more likely to develop polyps and cancers of the upper gastrointestinal tract {894, 2831} and hereditary haemorrhagic telangiectasia {938}, while carriers of *BMPR1A* mutations are more likely to have cardiac defects.

Peutz-Jeghers syndrome

G.J.A. Offerhaus
M. Billaud
S.B. Gruber

Definition
Peutz-Jeghers syndrome (PJS) is an inherited cancer syndrome characterized by mucocutaneous melanin pigmentation and hamartomatous gastrointestinal polyposis, which preferentially affects the small intestine. PJS patients also have an increased risk of extraintestinal cancer, including tumours of the ovary, uterine cervix, testis, pancreas and breast.

MIM No.   175200

Synonyms and historical annotation
The syndrome was first described by Peutz in 1921 {2538} and later by Jeghers in 1949 {1411}. The pedigree of the Dutch family described by Peutz continues to be followed {3492}. Several designations have been used synonymously, including Peutz-Jeghers polyposis, periorificial lentiginosis, and polyps-and-spots syndrome.

Incidence
As this condition is rare, well-documented incidence data are not available. Based on numbers of families registered in the Finnish Polyposis Registry, the incidence of PJS is roughly one tenth that of familial adenomatous polyposis (FAP), with an estimated prevalence of 1 per 50 000 to 1 per 200 000 births.

Diagnostic criteria
The following diagnostic criteria are recommended: (1) three or more histologically confirmed Peutz-Jeghers polyps;

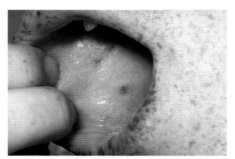

Fig. 8.53 Peutz-Jeghers syndrome. Note the pigmentation of the lips, peri-oral skin, tongue and fingers.

or (2) any number of Peutz-Jeghers polyps with a family history of PJS; or (3) characteristic, prominent, mucocutaneous pigmentation with a family history of PJS; or (4) any number of Peutz-Jeghers polyps and characteristic, prominent, mucocutaneous pigmentation. Some melanin pigmentation is also regularly seen in unaffected individuals, hence the emphasis on the prominence of the pigmentation. Moreover, the pigmentation in PJS patients may disappear with time or can, in rare cases, be absent altogether.

Intestinal neoplasms
Penetrance appears to be high and males and females are equally affected {1160}. Polyps are most common in the small intestine, but may occur anywhere in the gastrointestinal tract. Polyps in PJS have also been described at locations outside the gastrointestinal tract, such as the gallbladder, bladder and nasopharynx {1515}. Note that counting only the number

of polyps that come to clinical attention (e.g. upon intussusception) might misrepresent the true number and distribution of polyps {3331}.

Clinical features
Signs and symptoms. These include abdominal pain, intestinal bleeding, anaemia, and intussusception, which typically manifest in the first two decades of life {344}. The characteristic pigmentation, if present, allows diagnosis of asymptomatic patients in familial cases, but the hamartomatous PJS polyps constitute the main clinical hallmark.

Imaging. The presence of polyps may be detected by upper-gastrointestinal and small-bowel contrast radiography, and by air-contrast barium enema. Periodic small-bowel X-ray examination is advisable in the follow-up of affected patients. Endoscopy is superior to radiological imaging since simultaneous polypectomy can be used for diagnostic and therapeutic purposes. Current recommendations include biannual endoscopy of the upper gastrointestinal tract and colonoscopy with polypectomy, and small-bowel X-ray series {982}. Since the enteroscope is rarely able to view the full length of the bowel, imaging remains an integral component of clinical management, although solid evidence on the impact of surveillance strategies in these patients is lacking.

Macroscopy
On gross inspection, the surface of Peutz-Jeghers polyps shows coarse lobulation somewhat resembling that of an adenoma but with larger lobules and in marked contrast to the smooth surface of a juvenile polyp. The stalk is generally short and broad or absent. Polyp size can vary from 5–50 mm.

Histopathology
A typical Peutz-Jeghers polyp has a diagnostically useful central core of smooth muscle that shows tree-like branching. This is covered by the mucosa native to

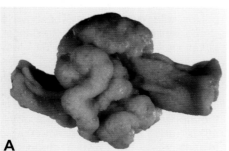

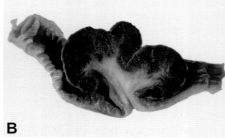

Fig. 8.54 A Lobulated Peutz-Jeghers polyp of the small intestine, gross specimen. **B** Small-intestinal Peutz-Jeghers polyp with haemorrhagic infarction caused by intussusception.

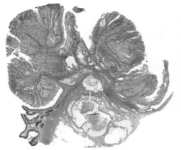
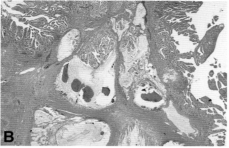
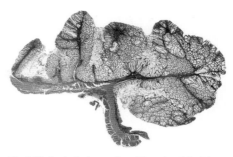

Fig. 8.55 Peutz-Jeghers polyp of the small intestine. **A** Whole mount. **B** Pseudoinvasion characterized by benign mucinous cysts extending through the bowel wall into mesentery. The patient was well 10 years after removal of the polyp.

Fig. 8.56 Peutz-Jeghers polyp of the colon. Arborizing smooth muscle separates colonic glands into lobules (Masson trichrome stain).

the region, heaped into folds producing a villous pattern {1385}. Diagnosis may be complicated when there is secondary ischaemic necrosis, which can arise when a polyp has caused intussusception, a common form of presentation. Occasionally, polyps (especially smaller ones) lack diagnostic features. Epithelial misplacement involving all layers of the bowel wall ("pseudoinvasion") has been described in up to 10% of intestinal PJS polyps {2923}. Mechanical forces associated with intussusception and episodes of mucosal prolapse {1385} is the likely explanation for this observation. Epithelial misplacement may be florid and extend into the serosa, thereby mimicking a well-differentiated adenocarcinoma. Useful discriminatory features are the lack of cytological atypia, presence of all the normal cell types, mucinous cysts and haemosiderin deposition {2923}.

Intraepithelial neoplasia (dysplasia) and cancer in Peutz-Jeghers polyps.
While PJS is associated with a 10- to 18-fold excess of gastrointestinal and non-gastrointestinal cancers {977, 3045}, the

question of whether or not the hamartomatous Peutz-Jeghers polyp is itself precancerous has proved difficult to resolve. Epithelial misplacement has apparently been overdiagnosed as cancer in the past {2923}, and it is questionable whether the increased risk of malignancy in the stomach, small bowel and colon is attributable to malignant progression from hamartoma to adenocarcinoma. Intraepithelial neoplasia (dysplasia) is very uncommon in PJS polyps {1865, 2923}, although it has been described occasionally {573, 2534}. Human PJS polyps appear to be polyclonal {672}, while murine PJS models have demonstrated that loss of the wildtype *LKB1/STK11* allele, the gene responsible for PJS, is not a prerequisite for polyp formation {2731}. The incidence of adenomas in PJS patients remains ill-defined, although an increased risk of developing adenoma has been reported {2021}. It is conceivable that prolapse of a well-formed adenoma may mimic the histopathology of dysplasia in a hypothetically pre-existing hamartomatous PJS polyp.

Extraintestinal manifestations
Predisposition to cancer of multiple organ systems is an important feature of PJS {977}. The most well-documented extraintestinal neoplasms include sex-cord tumours with annular tubules (SCTAT) of the ovary {3659}, adenoma malignum of the uterine cervix {3659}, Sertoli cell tumours of the testis {3521}, carcinoma of the pancreas {980}, and carcinoma of the breast {2680}. The risk of breast cancer in female PJS patients is comparable to that of carriers of *BRCA1* or *BRCA2* mutations {1146}. Cutaneous melanin pigmentation occurs typically around the mouth as freckle-like spots. Other sites commonly affected are the digits, palms and feet, buccal mucosa, and anal region. While dramatic pigmentation is a helpful sign, it may fade with time, and some affected individuals never display pigmentation.

Genetic susceptibility
PJS is an autosomal dominant trait with nearly complete penetrance. The PJS gene, *LKB1/STK11*, maps to 19p13.3. Although some initial evidence suggested

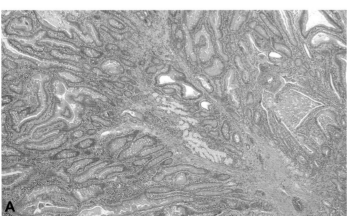
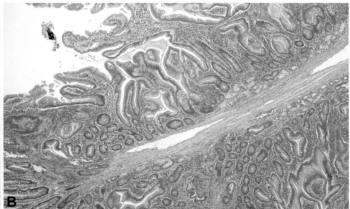

Fig. 8.57 Peutz-Jegher polyp of the small intestine. **A** Note the branching muscularis mucosae with overlying small-intestinal mucosa. **B** The small-intestinal mucosa is essentially normal and overlies an arborized muscularis mucosae.

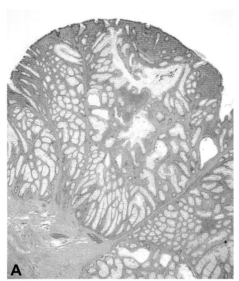
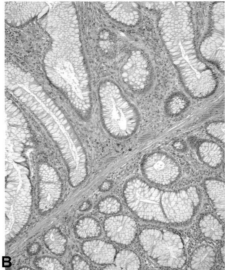

Fig. 8.58 Peutz-Jeghers polyp of the large intestine. **A** Note the arborizing muscularis mucosae with overlying relatively normal colonic mucosa. **B** At high power, the appearance of the mucosa is nearly normal.

locus heterogeneity {2034}, the advent of novel molecular techniques for the analysis of large genomic deletions (e.g. multiplex ligation probe amplification), PJS in most families can now be linked to pathogenic germline mutations in *LKB1/STK11* {671, 1147}. However, the identification of a germline mutation in the gene encoding smooth-muscle myosin (*MYH11*) in a PJS patient suggests that alterations in genes other than *LKB1/STK11* may also be involved in this disease {89}.

Gene structure

The *LKB1* gene spans 23 kb and comprises 11 exons, 9 of which are coding. It is transcribed in the telomere-to-centromere direction. The open reading frame consists of 1302 base pairs, corresponding to 433 amino acids. Codons 50–337 encode the catalytic kinase domain of the protein, which is most similar to the SNF1-/AMP-activated protein kinase (AMPK) family. Two alternatively spliced forms of *LKB1* exist: in *LKB1* long (*LKB1L*), the C-terminal sequence is encoded by exon 9B, while in the recently described *LKB1* short (*LKB1S*) this sequence is encoded by exon 9A {3280}. In *LKB1S*, the 63 residues of *LKB1L* are substituted by a 39-residue unique sequence.

Germline mutations

Germline mutations are usually truncating, but missense mutations have also been described {1159, 1417}. Since wildtype LKB1 is capable of autophosphorylation {2034, 3642}, the effect of missense mutations occurring in the kinase domain can be evaluated in assays for autophosphorylation. Interestingly, inactivating mutations in PJS patients and in sporadic cases are not restricted to the kinase domain {86, 1494} and functional analyses have revealed that such mutations interfere with LKB1-mediated regulation of AMPK and cell polarity {880}. Recent research shows that LKB1/STK11 is frequently targeted for inactivation in pulmonary cancers in patients with sporadic tumours, particularly the most frequent subtype, adenocarcinoma {1424, 2793}.

Gene product

The human *LKB1* gene is ubiquitously expressed in fetal and adult tissues {1159, 1417}. LKB1L is a 50 kDa protein that possesses a serine/threonine kinase domain framed by a short *N*-terminus sequence (48 residues) and a more extended *C*-terminus region of 122 amino acids that contains five phosphorylation sites and a farnesylation motif {1159, 1417}. LKB1S lacks two phosphorylation sites and the prenylation motif; it is mostly expressed in the testis where it is required

during spermiogenesis {3280}. Homologues of LKB1 have been identified in several species, including mouse, *Xenopus*, *Drosophila* and *Caenorhabditis elegans* {2987, 3106, 3472}. Unlike most kinases, LKB1 is not activated by phosphorylation of its activation loop by an upstream kinase, but by binding to the adapter proteins STRAD and MO25. Formation of this trimeric complex stabilizes and activates LKB1. LKB1 is a master kinase that regulates cell polarity and energetic metabolism {879}. Although the crucial downstream target of LKB1 remains to be defined, it has been shown that LKB1 can effectively phosphorylate AMPK, a key sensor of cellular energy status that relays LKB1 tumour-suppressor activity in invertebate models {879}. Furthermore, the LKB1–AMPK signalling cascade negatively regulates the mTOR pathway, which is a major regulator of cell growth and is constantly hyperactivated in hamartomatous polyposis syndromes, including PJS {1329}. These findings suggest that topical inhibition of mTOR with rapamycin analogues may prove beneficial in the treatment of PJS-associated tumours {2889}. In humans, the AMPK family includes 14 kinases that are involved in a wide array of functions ranging from control of cell metabolism to the regulation of cellular polarity {1386}. The LKB1 protein behaves as a tumour suppressor in various model systems and, curiously, hemi-allelic inactivation has been shown to accelerate tumour formation in murine models {1424}, suggesting that LKB1 may be haplo-insufficient for suppression of neoplastic transformation under certain conditions.

Prognosis and predictive factors

While intussusception has been a major source of mortality in PJS kindreds {3492}, surgery constitutes an effective treatment. The prognosis for individuals affected by PJS is thus mainly determined by the risk of malignancy {977}. Although little information on prognosis is available, one report suggests that PJS-associated cancers are particularly aggressive {3045}. Research shows that a diagnosis of PJS has great psychosocial impact {3545}, although the physical impact on the patient is not greater than that in the general population.

Cowden syndrome

Ch. Eng
C. Eng
R.W. Burt

Definition

Cowden syndrome (CS), also known as PTEN hamartoma syndrome, is an autosomal dominant disorder characterized by multiple hamartomas involving organs derived from all three germ-cell layers. The classical hamartoma associated with CS is trichilemmoma. Affected family members have a high risk of developing breast and epithelial thyroid carcinomas. Other clinical manifestations include mucocutaneous lesions, nonmalignant thyroid abnormalities, fibrocystic disease of the breast, gastrointestinal hamartomas, early-onset uterine leiomyomas, macrocephaly, mental retardation and dysplastic gangliocytoma of the cerebellum (Lhermitte-Duclos disease). The syndrome is caused by germline mutations of the phosphatase and tensin homologue (*PTEN*) gene. A subset of individuals with CS and CS-like symptoms without germline *PTEN* mutations have been found to habour germline variants of dehydrogenase complex subunits B (*SDHB*) or D (*SDHD*).

MIM No.   158350

Synonyms

Cowden disease; multiple hamartoma syndrome.

Diagnostic criteria

Because of the variable and broad expression of CS and the lack of uniform diagnostic criteria prior to 1996, the International Cowden Consortium {2263} compiled operational diagnostic criteria for CS on the basis of the published literature and their own clinical experience {793, 3683}. Trichilemmomas and papillomatous papules are particularly important to recognize. CS usually presents within the third decade of life. It has variable and broad expression and an age-related penetrance. By the third decade of life, 99% of affected individuals have developed mucocutaneous stigmata, although any of the other features could already be present. Because the clinical literature on CS consists mostly of reports of the most

florid and unusual families or case reports by subspecialists interested in their respective organ systems, the spectrum of component signs is unknown. Despite this, the most commonly reported manifestations are mucocutaneous lesions, thyroid abnormalities, fibrocystic disease and carcinoma of the breast, gastrointestinal hamartomas, multiple, early-onset uterine leiomyoma, macrocephaly (specifically, megencephaly) and mental retardation {1119, 1895, 3058, 3683}.

Epidemiology

The single most comprehensive clinical epidemiological study estimated the prevalence to be 1 per million population {3058}. After identification of the gene for CS {1842}, a molecular-based estimate of prevalence in the same population was 1 : 200 000 {2262}. Because of difficulty in recognizing this syndrome, prevalence figures are likely to be underestimates.

Intestinal neoplasms

Hamartomatous polyps

In a small but systematic study comprising nine well-documented individuals with CS, seven of whom had a germline mutation in *PTEN*, all nine had hamartomatous polyps {3476}. Several varieties of hamartomatous polyps are seen in this syndrome, including hamartomas most similar to juvenile polyps composed of a mixture of connective tissues normally present in the mucosa, principally smooth muscle in continuity with the muscularis mucosae, along with lipomatous and ganglioneuromatous lesions and lymphoid

hyperplasia {424, 3476}. These polyps are found in the stomach, duodenum, small bowel and colon. Those in the colon and rectum usually measure 3–10 mm in diameter, but can reach 2 cm or more. Some of the polyps are no more than tags of mucosa, but others have a more definite structure. Examples containing adipose tissue have been described. The mucosal glands within the lesion are normal or elongated and irregularly formed, but the overlying epithelium is normal and includes goblet cells and columnar cells {424}. Some ganglion tissue is not unusual in the juvenile-like polyps, but lesions in which autonomic nerves are predominant, giving a ganglioneuroma-like appearance, have been described but seem to be exceptional {1749}.

The vast majority of CS hamartomatous polyps are asymptomatic, although anecdotally, adenomatous polyps and colon cancers have been observed in young patients with this condition {3684}. The association and risk of gastrointestinal malignancy with CS is unknown, but appears to be likely. In a study of nine CS individuals, glycogenic acanthosis of the oesophagus was found in six out of seven individuals with *PTEN* mutation {3476}. It is likely that many more CS patients will be identified in the future with ongoing screening for colon cancer, which should allow a more precise characterization of the phenotypic gastrointestinal features of this disease and possible risk of gastrointestinal cancer.

In order to determine the prevalence of *PTEN* germline mutations in an unselected series of individuals with hamartomatous

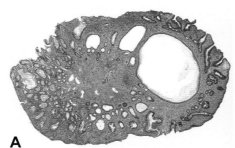
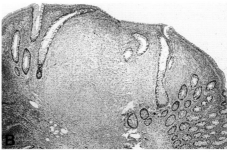

Fig. 8.59 A, B Colonic polyps in Cowden syndrome. Distorted glands and fibrous proliferation in the lamina propria.

Table 8.10 International Cowden Consortium diagnostic criteria for Cowden syndrome and operational diagnosis.

Diagnostic criteria
Pathognomonic criteria
Mucocutaneous lesions:
Trichilemmomas, facial
Acral keratoses
Papillomatous papules
Mucosal lesions
Major criteria
Breast cancer
Thyroid cancer, especially follicular carcinoma
Macrocephaly (megencephaly) (≥ 97th percentile)
Lhermitte-Duclos disease
Minor criteria
Other thyroid lesions (e.g. adenoma or multinodular goitre)
Mental retardation (IQ ≤ 75)
Gastrointestinal hamartomas
Fibrocystic disease of the breast
Lipomas
Fibromas
Genitourinary tumours (e.g. uterine fibroids) or malformation

Operational diagnosis in an individual
1. Mucocutaneous lesions alone if:
(a) there are six or more facial papules, of which three or more must be trichilemmoma; or
(b) cutaneous facial papules and oral mucosal papillomatosis; or
(c) oral mucosal papillomatosis and acral keratoses; or
(d) palmoplantar keratoses, six or more.
2. Two major criteria but one must include macrocephaly or Lhermitte-Duclos disease
3. One major and three minor criteria.
4. Four minor criteria.

Operational diagnosis in a family where one individual is diagnostic for Cowden
1. At least one pathognomonic criterion.
2. Any one major criterion with or without minor criteria.
3. Two minor criteria.

polyps, a prospective pilot series of 49 individuals who had five or more colonic polyps, at least one of which was hamartomatous or hyperplastic, were accrued irrespective of age or family history {3144}. Of these 49 individuals, approximately 20% were found to have germline mutations in *PTEN*, *SMAD4*, *BMPR1A* or *STK11*. Of these eleven germline mutations, four involved *PTEN* – two intragenic mutations and two large deletions {3144}. In a child with juvenile polyposis of infancy, this deletion also involved *BMPR1A* upstream of *PTEN*. Subsequently, germline deletion involving both *PTEN* and *BMPR1A* was shown to characterize at least a subset of juvenile polyposis of infancy {692}.

Extraintestinal manifestations
Breast cancer
The two most commonly recognized cancers in CS are carcinoma of the breast and thyroid {3058, 3683}. In the general population, lifetime risks of breast and thyroid cancers are approximately 11% (in women), and 1%, respectively. Breast cancer has been observed rarely in men with CS {1979}. In women with CS, estimates of lifetime risk of breast cancer range from 25% to 50% {793, 1119, 1895, 3058, 3683}. The mean age at diagnosis is likely to be 10 years earlier than for breast cancer occurring in the general population {1895, 3058}. Although Rachel Cowden died of breast cancer at the age of 31 years {349, 1875} and the earliest recorded age at diagnosis of breast cancer is 14 {3058}, the great majority of breast cancers are diagnosed after the age of 30–35 years (range, 14–65 years) {1895}. The predominant histology is ductal adenocarcinoma. Most CS breast carcinomas occur in the context of ductal carcinoma *in situ* (DCIS), atypical ductal hyperplasia, adenosis and sclerosis {2856}.

Thyroid cancer
The lifetime risk of epithelial thyroid cancer can be as high as 10% in males and females with CS. Because of small numbers of cases, it is unclear whether the age of onset is truly earlier than that of the general population. Histologically, thyroid cancer is predominantly follicular carcinoma, although papillary histology has also been rarely observed {1119, 1968, 3058, 3683}. Medullary thyroid carcinoma has not been observed in patients with CS.

Benign tumours
The most important benign tumours are trichilemmomas and papillomatous papules of the skin. Apart from those of the skin, benign tumours or disorders of breast and thyroid are most frequently noted and probably represent true component features of this syndrome. Fibroadenomas and fibrocystic disease of the breast are common signs of CS, as are follicular adenomas and multinodular goitre of the thyroid. An unusual tumour of the central nervous system, cerebellar dysplastic gangliocytoma or Lhermitte-Duclos disease, has recently been associated with CS {794, 1900, 2432}. Interestingly, adult-onset Lhermitte-Duclos disease, even in the absence of other features or family history, is highly predictive of finding a germline mutation in *PTEN* {3713}. Other malignancies and benign tumours have been reported in patients or families with CS. Some authors believe that endometrial carcinoma could also be a component tumour of CS. It remains to be shown whether other tumours (sarcomas, lymphomas, leukaemia, meningiomas) are true components of CS.

Genetic susceptibility
Chromosomal location and mode of transmission
CS is an autosomal dominant disorder, with age-related penetrance and variable expression {794}. The CS susceptibility gene, *PTEN*, resides on 10q23.3 {1834, 1842, 2263}.
Pilot data suggest that a subset of individuals with CS and CS-like features, who are negative for *PTEN* mutations, harbour germline variants of *SDHB* (on 1p35–p36) or *SDHD* (on 11q23), both of which have been shown to affect the same downstream signalling pathways as PTEN (AKT and MAPK) {2277}.

Gene structure
PTEN/MMAC1/TEP1 consists of nine exons spanning 120–150 kb {1834, 1979, 3063}. It is believed that intron 1 occupies much of this genomic distance (approximately 100 kb). *PTEN* is predicted to encode a 403 amino-acid phosphatase. Similar to other phosphatase genes, *PTEN* exon 5 specifically encodes a phosphatase core motif. Exons 1 to 6 encode amino acid sequence that is homologous to tensin and auxilin {1830, 1834, 3063}.

Gene product
PTEN is virtually ubiquitously expressed {3063}. Detailed studies of expression in human development have not been performed. Only a single study has examined expression of PTEN protein during human embryogenesis using a monoclonal antibody against the terminal 100 amino acids of PTEN {992}. This study revealed high levels of expression of PTEN protein in the skin, thyroid and

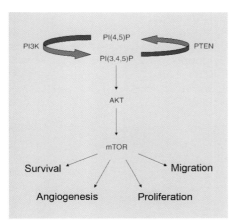

Fig. 8.60 Schematic representation of the PI3K-Akt-mTOR signalling pathway. When PTEN is downregulated, Akt is upregulated, leading to upregulation of mTOR. Reprinted by permission from Macmillan Publishers Ltd: *European Journal of Human Genetics*, Blumenthal GM et al. {287A}, Copyright 2008.

central nervous system, organs that are affected by the component neoplasias of CS. It also revealed prominent expression in the developing autonomic nervous system and gastrointestinal tract. Moreover, early embryonic death in pten -/- mice also imply a crucial role for PTEN in early development {713, 2569, 3138}. PTEN is a tumour suppressor and a dual-specificity lipid phosphatase that plays multiple roles in the cell cycle, apoptosis, cell polarity, cell migration and even genomic stability {2200, 2919, 3683}. The major substrate of PTEN is phosphatidylinositol-3,4,5-triphosphate (PIP3) which lies in the PI3 kinase pathway {643, 926, 1833, 1949, 3053}. When PTEN is ample and functional, PIP3 is converted to 4,5-PIP2, which results in hypophosphorylated AKT/PKB, a known cell-survival factor. Hypophosphorylated AKT is apoptotic. When PTEN is in the cytoplasm, it predominantly signals via its lipid phosphatase activity down the PI3K-AKT pathways {2082}. In contrast, when PTEN is in the nucleus, it predominantly signals via protein phosphatase activity down the cyclin D1/MAPK pathway, eliciting G1 arrest at least in breast and glioma cells {926, 927, 1833, 2082}. It is also believed that PTEN can dephosphorylate focal adhesion kinase (FAK; PTK2B) and inhibit integrin and mitogen-activated protein (MAP) kinase signalling {1078, 3179}.

Gene mutations
Approximately 85% of CS cases, as strictly defined by the Consortium criteria, have a germline mutation in *PTEN*, including intragenic mutations, promoter mutations and large deletions/rearrangements {1842, 1979, 3714}. If the diagnostic criteria are relaxed, then mutation frequencies drop to 10–50% {1925, 2264, 3303}. A formal study that ascertained 64 unrelated CS-like cases revealed a mutation frequency of 2% if the criteria were not met, even if the diagnosis were made short of one criterion {1980}. However, it should be noted that this study only looked at the nine exons of *PTEN*, and it would be predicted that further mutations would have been identified in the promoter or in *SDHB/SDHD*. A single research-centre study involving 37 unrelated CS families, ascertained according to the strict diagnostic criteria of the Consortium, revealed a mutation frequency of 80% {1979}. Exploratory genotype–phenotype analyses revealed that the presence of a germline mutation was associated with a familial risk of developing malignant breast disease {1979}. Further, missense mutations and/-or mutations 5` of the phosphatase core motif seem to be associated with a surrogate for disease severity (multi-organ involvement). A small study comprising 13 families with 8 *PTEN* mutation-positive members could not find any genotype–phenotype associations {2262}, but this may be due to the small sample size.

Bannayan-Riley-Ruvalcaba syndrome (BRRS)
Previously thought to be clinically distinct, BRRS (MIM 153480), characterized by macrocephaly, lipomatosis, haemangiomatosis and speckled penis, is likely to be allelic to CS {1981}. Approximately 60% of BRRS families and isolated cases combined carry a germline mutation in *PTEN* {1982}. There were 11 cases classified as true CS–BRRS overlap families in this cohort, and 10 of these had a *PTEN* mutation. Another 10% of BRRS individuals were subsequently shown to harbour larger germline deletions of *PTEN* {3714}. The overlapping mutation spectrum, the existence of true overlap families and the genotype–phenotype associations suggest that the presence of germline mutation of

PTEN is associated with cancer strongly suggest that CS and BRRS are allelic and part of a single spectrum at the molecular level. The aggregate term of PTEN hamartoma tumour syndrome (PHTS) has been suggested {1982}, and has become more germane when germline mutations in *PTEN* were subsequently identified in autism spectrum disorder with macrocephaly, Proteus syndrome and VATER (association of birth defects) with macrocephaly {386, 2643, 3712}. The identification of a germline intragenic mutation in *PTEN* in a patient previously thought to have juvenile polyposis {2399} excludes that specific clinical diagnosis, and points to the correct molecular designation of PHTS {795, 1260, 1261, 1689, 1983, 2408}. This has been further borne out by finding germline mutations/deletions of *PTEN* in individuals with juvenile polyps and of large deletions involving both *PTEN* and *BMPR1A* in juvenile polyposis of infancy {692, 3144}. A significant finding of the polyp-ascertainment study was that the reasons for referral based on original pathology readings were often incorrect, suggesting that re-review of all polyp histologies by gastrointestinal pathologists based in major academic medical centres is vital for focusing on the correct genetic etiology {3144}.

Prognosis and predictive factors
There have been no systematic studies to indicate whether the prognosis for CS patients who have cancer is different from that of their counterparts with sporadic cancer.

When activated mTOR signalling was uncovered as an important downstream response to PTEN dysfunction or deficiency, mTOR inhibition was shown to be effective *in vitro* and in animal models {3051}. In fact, rapamycin was shown to be effective in a child with Proteus syndrome who also carried a germline mutation in *PTEN* {1984}. An open label phase II trial of mTOR inhibitor is currently underway for human CS with demonstrated germline *PTEN* mutation (NCI-08-C-0151).

Neuroendocrine neoplasms of the colon and rectum

D.S. Klimstra
R. Arnold
C. Capella
G. Klöppel
P. Komminoth
E. Solcia
G. Rindi

Definition

Neoplasms with neuroendocrine differentiation including neuroendocrine tumours (NET) and neuroendocrine carcinomas (NEC) arising in the large intestine and presacral region; mixed adeno-neuroendocrine carcinomas (MANEC) have an exocrine and a neuroendocrine component, with one component exceeding 30% (see Chapter 1).

Synonyms

Synonyms for colon and rectum NET include: carcinoid, well differentiated endocrine tumour/carcinoma {3013}. Synonyms for NEC include: poorly differentiated endocrine carcinomas, high grade neuroendocrine carcinoma, small cell and large cell endocrine carcinomas.

ICD-O codes

Neuroendocrine tumour (NET)
    NET G1 (carcinoid)   8240/3
    NET G2   8249/3
Neuroendocrine carcinoma (NEC) 8246/3
    Large cell NEC   8013/3
    Small cell NEC   8041/3
Mixed adenoneuroendocrine
    carcinoma (MANEC)   8244/3
EC cell, serotonin-producing NET 8241/3
L cell, Glucagon-like peptide
    and PP/PYY-producing NETs   8152/1

Epidemiology

Incidence and time trends

The annual incidence of NETs of the colon is 0.11 to 0.21 cases per 100 000 population {2115} and NETs make up 0.4% of colorectal neoplasms {1648}. NETs of the caecum to transverse colon (midgut) represent about 8% of all gastrointestinal NETs, while NETS of the descending colon and rectosigmoid (hindgut) represent about 27% {2113, 2115}. Rectal NETs have an annual incidence of 0.14–0.76 cases per 100 000 population. In the 40 years between 1950 and 1991, the proportion of caecal NETs, among NETs of all sites, nearly doubled, as did the proportion of rectosigmoid lesions {2115, 3440}. It has been suggested that rectal NETs are particularly prevalent in Asian/Pacific Islanders, Native Americans, and African Americans {3624}.

NECs are rare in the large bowel, but more common in this location than elsewhere in the intestines. NECs comprise approximately 0.6% of all carcinomas of the large bowel {243}.

Age and sex distribution

The reported average age at diagnosis is 56 years for rectal NETs, and 66 years for colonic NETs, and the male-to-female ratio is 1.02 and 0.66, for rectal and colonic NETs, respectively {620, 815, 1738, 2115}. Although colorectal NETs are rare in childhood, they make up 34% of solid colorectal neoplasms in patients aged < 20 years {3617}.

The average age of patients with NECs of the large bowel is 61.5 years, and the male-to-female ratio is essentially 1 : 1, similar to the values for large-bowel adenocarcinomas {243, 3071}.

Etiology

Some colorectal neuroendocrine neoplasms, including both NETs and NECs, have been reported in the large bowel of patients with ulcerative colitis {995, 1062} or Crohn disease {1062, 1188, 1220, 2965}. In association with these conditions, the neoplasms tend to be multiple {2029}. However, there appears to be no evidence to substantiate a direct association between inflammatory bowel disease and neuroendocrine oncogenesis, because almost all cases are found incidentally after surgery for inflammatory bowel disease {1062}. A case of rectal NET in a patient with Peutz-Jeghers syndrome has also been reported {3425}. Multiple rectal NETs have been reported in diffuse ganglioneuromatosis {1121}.

Rarely, NETs or so-called "microcarcinoids" (microscopic NET cell nests) are found associated with adenomatous polyps of the large bowel {1924, 2598}, but there is no evidence that the majority of colorectal NETs are etiologically related to adenomas or adenocarcinomas of the large bowel. In contrast, high-grade NECs commonly arise in association with adenomas

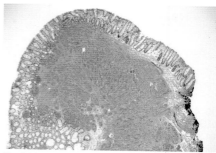

Fig. 8.61 Endoscopically resected rectal neuroendocrine tumour (NET) invading the mucosa–submucosa, but not the muscularis propria.

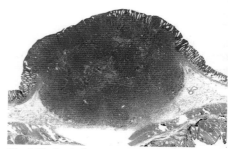

Fig. 8.62 Surgically resected neuroendocrine tumour (NET) invading the mucosa–submucosa, but not the muscularis propria.

or adenocarcinomas and presumably share some molecular alterations and etiological associations with conventional colorectal adenocarcinomas.

Patients with colorectal NETs are reported to have an increased risk of other malignancies, including carcinomas of the gastrointestinal tract, lung, and prostate {3246}, and metachronous or synchronous non-NET neoplasms are found in 13% of cases {2115}.

Localization

NETs are more common in the rectum (54% of cases), followed by the caecum (20%), sigmoid colon (7.5%), rectosigmoid colon (5.5%) and ascending colon (5%) {2115, 3013}. A NET arising in a caecal duplication cyst has been reported {1379}. NECs can arise in either the right colon or the rectosigmoid {3071}. Most NECs of the anal canal are small cell carcinomas, whereas those of the colon and rectum may be small cell, large cell, or have mixed features {2932}.

Clinical features

Symptomatic patients with colonic NETs most commonly present in the seventh decade of life with symptoms of abdominal pain and weight loss, although some present at a late stage with liver metastases {2730}. Less than 5% of patients present with the carcinoid syndrome {234, 2730}.

Half of rectal NETs are asymptomatic and are discovered at routine rectal examination or endoscopy {1699}, while the other half give rise to symptoms, typically rectal bleeding, pain or constipation {1423, 3080}. Rectal NETs are practically never associated with the carcinoid syndrome {1423, 3080}.

NECs are aggressive neoplasms and can present with symptoms attributable to local disease or to widespread metastases.

Macroscopy
NETs

The majority of colonic NETs are detected in the right colon {234, 2730} and are larger than their counterparts in the small intestine, appendix, and rectum. The average size has been reported as 4.9 cm {234}.

Rectal NETs appear as solitary submucosal nodules, sometimes polypoid, often with intact overlying epithelium {2936}. Larger neoplasms may be ulcerated {2936}. Up to half of rectal NETs are < 1.0 cm in diameter, perhaps because they are more readily detected on physical examination or endoscopy than those that are more proximally located {396, 1699}. Reviewing 356 cases reported in the literature, Caldarola *et al.* {396} found that only 13% of rectal NETs measured > 2 cm in diameter. Larger lesions tend to

be fixed to the rectal wall. In the majority of cases, the neoplasm is found 4–13 cm above the dentate line and on the anterior or lateral rectal walls {396}.

NECs

NECs of the colorectum are grossly similar to conventional adenocarcinomas. If an associated adenoma is present, they may be polypoid; if not, they are typically ulcerated neoplasms with a raised border, and on cut section they are infiltrative.

Histopathology
NETs

Since the large bowel is derived from both the embryonic midgut and hindgut, NETs of the colon can be either midgut-type serotonin (enterochromaffin, EC) cell NETs (in the caecum and ascending colon) or hindgut-type NETs that arise in the more distal colon and rectum and are L cell (glucagon-like peptide-producing and PP/PYY-producing) NETs {864}.

Colonic EC cell serotonin-producing NETs show histological, cytological, cytochemical, and ultrastructural features that are identical to those of jejuno–ileal EC cell serotonin-producing NETs {3013}. L cell, glucagon-like peptide and PP/PYY-producing NETs are characterized histologically by the predominance of a trabecular pattern, often admixed with tubuloacini or broad, irregular trabeculae with rosettes, and only occasionally with solid nests {3001}. These patterns are different from those of EC cell serotonin-producing NETs, in which solid nests prevail. The cytological features resemble those of other gastrointestinal NETs, with uniform round to oval nuclei having indistinct nucleoli and a coarsely granular

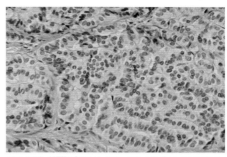

Fig. 8.63 NET of the rectum, with a trabecular pattern, typical of L cell NET.

chromatin pattern. Most colorectal NETs have minimal if any necrosis. The mitotic rate is, by definition, < 20 per 10 high power fields (HPF), but most cases have very few mitoses (< 2 per 10 HPF), corresponding to grade G1 {2685}. Typically (but not always), a slightly higher mitotic rate is found in larger (> 2.0 cm) colorectal NETs.

Immunohistochemically, colorectal NETs stain for the neuroendocrine markers chromogranin A and synaptophysin, keratins (especially Cam5.2, low-molecular-mass keratins 8–18), NCAM1/CD56 and for a variety of peptide hormones {831}. About 80% of rectal NETs display more or less abundant glucagon-like peptides (GLP-1, GLP-2, glicentin) and/or PP/PYY immunoreactivity typical of intestinal L cells, whereas only 30% show serotonin immunoreactivity and 20% somatostatin immunoreactivity, usually in only a few cells {864, 3011}. Although there is a prevalence of L cells in these neoplasms, minority populations of substance P, insulin, enkephalin, β-endorphin, neurotensin, and motilin immunoreactive cells have also been identified {831, 3011}. The vast majority (82%) of colorectal NETs tested

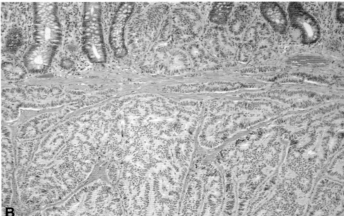

Fig. 8.64 Neuroendocrine tumour (NET) of the rectum. **A** Note the trabecular arrangement of cells in the submucosa. **B** High-power view of the trabecular growth pattern.

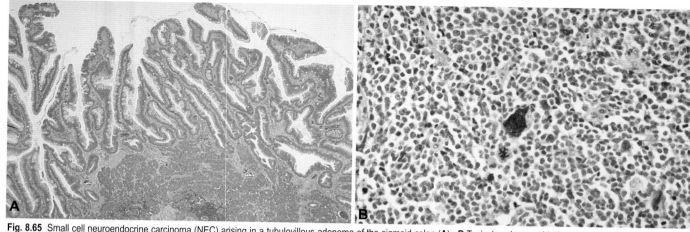

Fig. 8.65 Small cell neuroendocrine carcinoma (NEC) arising in a tubulovillous adenoma of the sigmoid colon (**A**). **B** Typical oval or moulded nuclei with diffuse chromatin, scant cytoplasm and little stroma.

in one series of 84 cases showed immunoreactivity for prostatic acid phosphatase, a finding that is unusual in other gut NETs and is possibly related to the common origin of the rectum and prostate from cloacal hindgut {831}. Most midgut NETs are positive for CDX2, whereas hindgut NETs are rarely positive {193, 801, 3052}. TTF1 is negative in colorectal NETs and keratin 20 may be positive in 24% of cases {392}. The Ki67-labelling index, like the mitotic rate, is defined as < 20% {2685}, and most cases a Ki67 index of 1–2%, corresponding to G1.

NECs

These are morphologically similar to small cell carcinoma and large cell NEC of the lung, and correspond to class G3 {2682, 2685}. They are usually found in the right colon, and are frequently associated with an overlying adenoma or adenocarcinoma {2081, 2932}, but not associated with NETs (carcinoid tumours) {368, 2932}. In the colon and rectum, 75% of NECs are large-cell type, whereas in the anus most are small cell carcinomas {2932}. Primary NECs in the colon without an associated adenoma component must be distinguished from metastases of pulmonary neuroendocrine carcinomas or cutaneous Merkel cell carcinomas {1281, 1755}.

Small cell NEC. Small cell carcinomas have a diffuse or nesting growth pattern and are composed of small to medium sized cells with minimal cytoplasm and have fusiform nuclei with granular chromatin and inconspicuous nucleoli. Some larger cells or occasional cells with nucleoli (< 25% of the neoplastic population) are acceptable findings. Necrosis is common.

The mitotic rate is very high, averaging 65 per 10 HPF {2932}. One quarter of cases have a minor component (< 30%) of adenocarcinoma or (in the anal canal) squamous cell carcinoma {2932}. Small cell carcinomas typically express chromogranin A, synaptophysin and CD56, although less consistently or diffusely than NETs {1045}. Seventy-five percent express either chromogranin A or synaptophysin and 95% express at least one of the above three markers {2932}. Keratins are also expressed, often dot-like {933}. The Ki67-labelling index is usually > 50% and may be nearly 100%. One out of five colorectal small cell carcinomas stains for CDX2 {801}. Keratin 20 may also be expressed {1498}. TTF1 is also expressed in some colorectal small cell carcinomas, limiting its use to define the site of origin {523}.

Large cell NEC. These neoplasms show organoid, nesting, trabecular, rosette-like and palisading patterns that suggest neuroendocrine differentiation, which must be confirmed by immunohistochemistry or electron microscopy {613}. In contrast to small cell carcinoma, the neoplastic cells have more abundant cytoplasm, more vesicular nuclei, and often prominent nucleoli {2932, 3289}. A component of adenocarcinoma is relatively common (61%), and in some cases this component exceeds 30% of the neoplasm, qualifying for a diagnosis of MANEC {2932}. The Ki67 labelling index is usually very high (30–80%) {2103}. At immunohistochemistry, pure neuroendocrine areas are diffusely positive for synaptophysin and usually for chromogranin A, although to a lesser extent {243, 2932}. At least two neuroendocrine markers (synaptophysin,

chromogranin A, or CD56) must be diffusely positive to establish a diagnosis of large cell NEC. CDX2 may also be expressed, but TTF1 usually is not {1498}.

MANECs

Although examples have been reported of NETs or neuroendocrine micronests arising in adenomatous polyps {1924, 2598}, NETs arising in association with adenocarcinomas are exceedingly rare {107, 1220, 1429, 1618}. Thus, most *bona fide* MANECs of the large bowel consist of components of adenocarcinoma (or, in the anal canal, squamous cell carcinoma) mixed with high-grade NEC, which can be either small cell or large cell {1964, 2932}. In fact, as mentioned above, many high-grade NECs have minor exocrine components, and an origin in association with adenomatous polyps is frequent {2081}. Conversely, immunohistochemically detectable neuroendocrine cells are found in up to 41% of colorectal adenocarcinomas, most of which have no morphological suggestion of a discrete neuroendocrine component {1328, 3130, 3623}.

A neoplasm with morphologically recognizable adeno- and neuroendocrine phenotypes is defined as carcinoma since both components are malignant and should be graded. The identification of scattered neuroendocrine cells by immunohistochemistry in adenocarcinoma does not qualify for this definition. A squamous cell carcinoma component is rare.

Molecular pathology

Loss of heterozygosity at the *MEN1* gene locus is rare {683, 1380, 3253} and colorectal NETs do not represent an integral part of the MEN1 syndrome {2431}. Colorectal NECs, like NECs developing at other gastrointestinal sites, display higher frequency of allelic imbalances than NETs, the most frequent abnormality involving the p53 and CDKN2/Rb pathways, *FHIT* (3p), *DCC/SMAD4* (18q) and *MEN1* {924, 2560}. NECs may share some molecular features with adenocarcinomas of the colorectum, with which they may be associated, suggesting a common origin {3325, 3422}. In contrast to colorectal adenocarcinoma, however, they often demonstrate loss of expression of the Rb gene product (especially small cell carcinomas), a feature they share with their pulmonary counterparts {1583, 1754}. DNA mismatch repair proteins are intact in most NECs {3071}.

Staging, prognosis and predictive factors

The issue of TNM/staging classification of neuroendocrine neoplasms is as yet unsettled. The classification presented in this book is for "carcinoid", i.e. well-differentiated, lesions only. Conversely, the classification proposed by the European Neuroendocrine Tumor Society (ENETS) is also meant for high-grade neoplasms {2684, 2685}. In the large intestine, both classifications are largely concordant.

Colonic EC cell serotonin-producing NETs frequently show malignant behaviour; local spread is found in 36–44% of patients and distant metastases in 38% {2115, 2730}. The reported 5-year and 10-year survival rates are 25–42% and 10%, respectively {2115, 2730}. Modlin found that metastatic neoplasms represent 82% of caecal NETs, but only 11–18% of rectal NET patients develop metastases {815, 831, 1699, 2113, 2115}. Patients with rectal NETs generally have a good prognosis, with a 5-year survival rate of 72–89% {2113, 2115}, which is better than the 5-year survival rate of 60% for patients with jejuno–ileal NETs {373}.

Recognized risk factors for malignant behaviour include: size > 2 cm {1423, 1585, 2256}, invasion of the muscularis propria {1423, 2256}, lymphatic invasion {815, 1648}, atypical histology {1659},

presence of > 2 mitoses per 10 HPF (and thus fitting the G2 class), and DNA aneuploidy {3301}. A scoring system based on size, depth of invasion, lymph-node metastases, and distant metastases that accurately stratifies prognosis has been developed for rectal NETs {1738}. Some authors suggest that rectal NETs measuring < 1.0 cm with no lymphatic invasion have a low enough rate of metastasis to justify endoscopic local resection as definitive therapy {1648, 519}, although one case of a rectal NET of < 0.5 cm with liver metastases has been reported {3304}.

Although rectal NETs limited to the mucosa and submucosa generally do not metastasize, the size of the neoplasm remains important, since those measuring > 1.0 cm have a greater metastatic rate than stage-equivalent adenocarcinomas {3000}. Immunoexpression of peripherin, a type-III neuronal intermediate filament, had been reported to be more consistent in rectal NETs without metastases than in those with metastases {1353}.

NECs of the large bowel are highly aggressive, and 70% of patients have metastases at presentation; median survival is 10.4 months, 2-year survival is 25%, and 5-year survival is 13% {243, 329, 933, 2932}. Mixed adenoneuroendocrine neoplasms are so rare that generalizations about behaviour are not possible. Those cases with a high-grade NEC component are aggressive, similar to the pure high-grade NECs, one case being reported with liver metastases in the presence of invasion limited to mucosa-submucosa {3325}.

Neuroendocrine neoplasms of the presacral region

Neuroendocrine neoplasms of the presacral region are rare, with only 25 cases reported in the English literature {746, 1561, 1840, 1916, 3017}. An origin from hindgut remnants in the region has been proposed, 12 of the reported cases being associated with teratoma or tailgut cysts, one case being associated with imperforate anus {1561}. Patients are more often female, age ranging from 18 to 72 years,

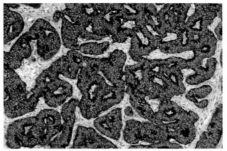

Fig. 8.66 Rectal neuroendocrine tumour (NET) showing diffuse and intense immunoreactivity for prostatic acid phosphatase.

presenting with mass-related symptoms and often pain. Neuroendocrine neoplasms of the presacral region are NETs displaying histological and immunohistochemical features similar to those of rectal NETs, with trabecular-gyriform structure, bland cytology and immunoreactivity for chromogranin A and synaptophysin {746}. One case also showed positive nuclear immunohistochemistry for estrogen and progesterone receptors {1840}. The low mitotic rate, the absence of necrosis and the low Ki67 index reported qualify most presacral region NETS as G1 (for grading, see Chapter 1) {746, 1561, 1840}. Malignant NETs with proven metastatic capacity also displayed foci of necrosis, angioinvasion and increased Ki67 index, qualifying these NETs as G2 {1916, 3017}. Patients with sacrococcigeal NETs in general have a good prognosis, largely depending on appropriate management with either surgery or local radiation therapy, one patient being alive and well after 28 years of evolution {746}. A poor outcome is reported for G2 cases {1840, 1916, 3017}.

B-cell lymphoma
of the colon and rectum

H.K. Müller-Hermelink
J. Delabie
Y.H. Ko
E.S. Jaffe
J.H. van Krieken
S. Nakamura

Definition
Primary B-cell lymphoma of the colorectum is defined as an extranodal lymphoma arising in either the colon or rectum with the bulk of disease localized to this site {1341}. Locoregional lymph-node involvement and distal spread may be seen, but the primary clinical site of presentation is the colon and/or rectum.

ICD-O codes
B-cell lymphoma, unclassifiable, with
  features intermediate between
  diffuse large B-cell lymphoma and
  Burkitt lymphoma   9680/3
Burkitt lymphoma   9687/3
Diffuse large B-cell lymphoma 9680/3
Mantle cell lymphoma   9673/3
Marginal zone lymphoma of
  mucosa-associated lymphoid
  tissue (MALT lymphoma)   9699/3

Epidemiology
Primary lymphomas arising in the large intestine are less frequent than either gastric or small bowel lymphomas {1344}. They account for < 10% of gastrointestinal lymphomas and most commonly (73%) occur in the caecum. The incidence of colonic lymphoma is increasing owing to increased numbers of cases associated with acquired or iatrogenic immunodeficiency {1093}. Most colorectal malignant lymphomas are B-cell lymphomas, but a higher prevalence of T-/NK-cell lymphomas of the colon and rectum may also account for a slightly higher incidence in Asian countries {1472}. Primary lymphomas account only for about 0.2–0.4% of all malignant neoplasms at this site. There is a male predominance with a male :female ratio of 2 : 1.
The mean age at presentation of colonic B-cell lymphomas is between 50 and 70 years, presentation at a younger age is common in immunodeficient individuals. The majority (54.7%) of these neoplasms are diffuse large B-cell lymphoma (DLBCL), which includes immunodeficiency-associated cases, followed by marginal zone B-cell lymphoma of mucosa-associated lymphoid tissue (MALT) type, follicular lymphoma, mantle cell lymphoma and Burkitt lymphoma {1093}. The frequencies in Asia are similar {1629}. In mantle cell lymphoma, colonic involvement by systemic lymphoma is frequent and detected by colonoscopy in 88% of cases {2718}.

Etiology
The main risk factors are medical immunosuppression, e.g. long-term treatment with corticosteroids and inhibitors of tumour necrosis factor α (TNFα), and immunodeficiency associated with human immunodeficiency virus (HIV). The standardized incidence rate of malignant non-Hodgkin lymphoma in HIV-seropositive individuals has declined considerably as a result of the use of highly active antiretroviral therapy (HAART). Colorectal lymphomas in HIV-infected patients were more common in the pre-HAART era {2498}.
Inflammatory bowel disease, Crohn disease and ulcerative colitis in their natural course are not thought to be associated with increased frequency of lymphoma; however, the incidence of treatment-related lymphomas has increased. Recent reports suggest that patients receiving anti-TNFα therapy might have a higher chance of developing non-Hodgkin lymphoma, but this remains to be firmly established {1726}. Colonic B-cell lymphomas associated with inflammatory bowel disease frequently harbour Epstein-Barr virus (EBV) {3542}. EBV-associated colonic large B-cell lymphomas and primary Hodgkin lymphoma may also occur in age-related immunodeficiency, long-term medical immunosuppression or HIV-associated acquired immunodeficiency.

Localization
Most colorectal lymphomas involve the caecum or ascending colon, followed by the rectum. There is a preference for rectal lymphoma in heavily immunodeficient patients infected with HIV {1337, 1817}. Multifocal involvement is uncommon, with the exception of multiple lymphomatous polyposis {2925}.

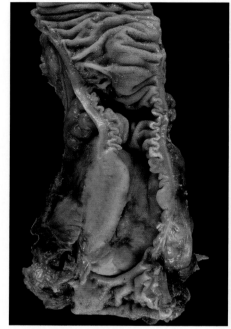

Fig. 8.67 Malignant lymphoma of the rectum.

Clinical features
The presenting features are very similar to those of epithelial neoplasms at this site. The most frequent clinical signs are abdominal pain, palpable mass, anaemia, weight loss, rectal bleeding, diarrhoea or constipation, irregular bowel habit and worsening of the symptoms of ulcerative colitis. Occasional cases are found incidentally, while an acute presentation with rupture of the colon is distinctly uncommon {1042, 1563, 2925}. Colorectal lymphomas are usually diagnosed using endoscopy and biopsy. Computerized tomography (CT) and barium enema have a role in diagnosis and determining the extent of disease and staging. Multiple lymphomatous polyposis has a characteristic radiological picture with numerous polyps of variable size throughout the colon. Transrectal ultrasonography may also be a useful adjunct for diagnosis.

Macroscopy
Most low-grade lymphomas present as well-defined protuberant growths that

deeply invade the bowel wall. DLBCL and Burkitt lymphoma tend to form larger masses with stricture and ulcer formation involving long segments of the colorectum. Low-grade and aggressive MALT lymphomas typically remain localized for prolonged periods, but may spread to involve locoregional lymph nodes. Mantle cell lymphoma may present as an isolated mass or as multiple polyps producing the clinical picture of multiple lymphomatous polyposis {3485}. In most cases, the colon is more significantly involved than the small bowel. The polyps range in size from 0.5 cm to 2 cm, with much larger polyps found in the ileocaecal region {1343, 2174}. Although multiple lymphomatous polyposis is characteristic of mantle cell lymphoma, it may also be found in other lymphoma entities, and more than half of patients with mantle cell lymphoma show subclinical involvement of the colonic mucosa without any visible abnormality {2718}.

Histopathology and immunohistochemistry
Diffuse large B-cell lymphoma (DLBCL)
DLBCL is the most frequent malignant lymphoma found in the colon. In contrast to gastric DLBCL, low-grade components are rarely seen and if present may represent a follicular lymphoma component. The lymphoma forms large ulcerating tumours with transmural infiltration by tumour cells. Sporadic DLBCL of the colon shows often centroblastic morphology and its variants (multilobulated, monomorphic, polymorphic). In the setting of immunodeficiency-associated DLBCL, the lymphoma cells are more often immunoblastic or even plasmablastic. Association with EBV is frequent and is investigated by EBV-encoded RNA (EBER) hybridization. These DLBCLs also show an inflammatory component consisting of activated T cells, macrophages, polytypic plasma cells and eosinophils. The phenotype is that of a mature B cell, being positive for CD20 and CD79a.

MALT lymphoma
Marginal zone B-cell lymphoma of MALT-type (MALT lymphoma) may occur as solitary mass or nodular lesion in the caecum or rectum {1341}. The histological and immunophenotypical features are discussed in detail with tumours of the stomach (Chapter 4). Low-grade colorectal MALT lymphomas resemble those of the small intestine in that lymphoepithelial

lesions are less prominent than in the stomach. Multiple gastrointestinal involvement of more than one anatomical site is frequent {1622}.

The immunophenotype is positive for CD20, negative for CD10 and BCL6; CD5 is usually negative but may be weakly expressed in rare cases; CD21 is often expressed, but CD23 is usually negative. Plasma-cell differentiation may be detected by immunoglobulin light-chain restriction.

Mantle cell lymphoma
The morphology of mantle cell lymphoma involving the large bowel is identical to that of mantle cell lymphoma at nodal sites {188}. The architecture is most frequently diffuse, but a nodular pattern and a less common true mantle-zone pattern are also seen. Intestinal glands may be destroyed by the lymphoma, but typical lymphoepithelial lesions are not seen. The low-power appearance is monotonous with dispersed histiocytes, while mitotic figures may be more frequent than in MALT lymphomas. The lymphoma cells are small- to medium-sized with irregular nuclear outlines, indistinct nucleoli and scant amounts of cytoplasm. Large transformed cells are typically not present.

The lymphoma cells are mature B cells expressing both CD79a and CD20. Characteristically the cells weakly co-express CD5 and CD43. Surface immunoglobulin is found, including both IgM and IgD. Light-chain restriction is present in most cases, with a predominance of lambda. CD10 and CD11c are virtually always negative. Cyclin D1 is found in almost all cases and can be seen within the nuclei of the neoplastic lymphocytes in paraffin sections. The Ki67-defined proliferation rate is an important predictive marker {1584}, since the proliferation-signature gene score has been shown to be the most important prognostic factor on gene-expression profiling {1128}. Rare cases of mantle cell lymphoma that are negative for cyclin D1 may be identified by *SOX11* overexpression {2175}.

Burkitt lymphoma
Typical Burkitt lymphoma as primary colorectal lymphoma is rare. The caecum and ascending colon may be involved {1629}. Sporadic cases of childhood Burkitt lymphoma in the rectum have been described {827, 960}. Burkitt lymphoma in HIV-infected individuals may still present as a

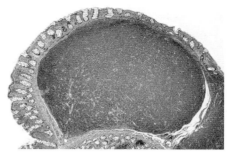

Fig. 8.68 Mantle cell lymphoma predominantly infiltrating the submucosa, thereby causing a polypoid lesion.

colorectal tumour in the HAART era, as these lymphomas have also been observed in immunocompetent patients in the past {419, 3032}. The details of the histology, immunophenotype, cytogenetics and molecular genetics of these tumours are described in detail for the small intestine (Chapter 6).

B-cell lymphoma, unclassifiable, with features intermediate between DLBCL and Burkitt lymphoma
B-cell lymphomas with morphological and genetic features intermediate between DLBCL and Burkitt lymphoma for clinical and biological reasons should be diagnosed separately and not included in one of these categories {3145}. The so-called "double-hit" lymphomas showing a *BCL2* translocation with a *MYC* translocation, as well as cases with *MYC* translocations involving partners other than immunoglobulin genes. Cases are often found at extranodal sites and are resistant to current therapies.

Other B-cell lymphomas
Most subtypes of B-cell lymphoma {3349} can present primarily as colorectal tumour and may mimic the clinical appearance of lymphomas or other neoplasms that are more frequent in this site. Chronic lymphocytic leukaemia involving the colonic mucosa may mimic mantle cell lymphoma or MALT lymphoma. Rectal involvement of plasmablastic lymphoma is difficult to distinguish from undifferentiated carcinoma or malignant melanoma. Intestinal T-cell lymphoma may present as multiple lymphomatous polyposis. Therefore biopsies that are suspicious for a lymphoproliferative disease should be thoroughly investigated by immunophenotyping. In the diagnostic work-up of large cell lymphoma also EBER *in situ* hybridization and genetic studies by fluorescent *in situ*

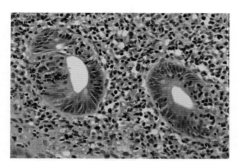

Fig. 8.69 MALT lymphoma of the rectum with lymphoepithelial lesions.

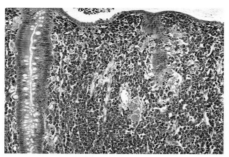

Fig. 8.70 Burkitt lymphoma of the colon. Malignant cells infiltrate the lamina propria and produce lymphoepithelial lesions.

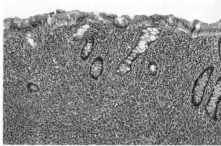

Fig. 8.71 Mantle cell lymphoma of the colon.

hybridization (FISH) techniques for *MYC* rearrangement and/or other breakpoints (*BCL2*, *BCL6*) are often necessary for definitive classification.

Genetic susceptibility

Lymphomas have been considered to be part of the Lynch syndrome-associated tumour spectrum, described earlier in this chapter, as a childhood cancer syndrome with biallelic homozygous or compound heterozygous mutations in DNA mismatch repair genes. Rarely, these lymphomas may arise within the gastrointestinal tract and show the underlying genetic defect in DNA mismatch repair {1199, 2551}.

Molecular pathology

Genetic information is included in the definition of lymphoma entities and found in the WHO classification of haematopoietic and lymphoid tumours, fourth edition {3145}.

MALT lymphoma

Genetic alterations and the frequencies of distinct types of balanced translocation show a site specific variation in MALT lymphomas. The cytogenetic and molecular features of low-grade colorectal MALT

lymphomas are incompletely investigated. The presence of t(11;18)(q21;q21) and the corresponding molecular abnormalities, rearrangement of *BCL10* or *BIRC3-MALT*, have been seen rarely at this site, sometimes together with a gastric tumour and multiple intestinal involvement. Trisomy of chromosome 3 has also been seen in colonic MALT lymphoma.

Mantle cell lymphoma

MCL is characterized by a recurrent cytogenetic abnormality, t(11;14)(q13;q32). This translocation deregulates expression of the cyclin D1 oncogene on chromosome 11.

Burkitt lymphoma

Burkitt lymphoma demonstrates a consistent cytogenetic abnormality in most cases, with rearrangement of the *MYC* oncogene on chromosome 8. The characteristic translocation, t(8;14)(q24;q32), is seen in most cases; the remainder shows variant translocations including the immunoglobulin light-chain loci, t(2;8)(p12;q24) or t(8;22)(q24;q11), involving kappa and lambda light-chain genes, respectively. In the classical t(8;14), *MYC* is translocated from chromosome 8 to the

heavy-chain locus on chromosome 14. In the variant translocations, a part of the light-chain constant region is translocated to chromosome 8, distal to the *MYC* gene. Thus, in the variant translocations, *MYC* remains on chromosome 8 and is deregulated by virtue of its juxtaposition to the immunoglobulin light-chain genes.

The molecular characteristics of the *MYC* translocation also differ between endemic and sporadic cases. In endemic Burkitt lymphoma, the chromosome 8 breakpoints are variable and usually far 5' of *MYC*, while the chromosome 14 breakpoints most often occur in the location of the *IGHJ@* gene joining segments. FISH analysis using break-apart probes for *MYC* detects most translocations. In cases without *MYC* rearrangements, aberrations in miRNA regulating *MYC* have been found {1808A}.

Prognosis and predictive factors

Prognostic factors for colorectal lymphoma are similar to those for lymphoma of the small intestine (Chapter 6).

Mesenchymal tumours of the colon and rectum

M. Miettinen
C.D.M. Fletcher
L.-G. Kindblom
W.M.S. Tsui

ICD-O codes

Leiomyoma	8890/0
Lipoma	8850/0
Gastrointestinal stromal tumour	8936/3
Angiosarcoma	9120/3
Kaposi sarcoma	9140/3
Leiomyosarcoma	8890/3

Definition

Gastrointestinal stromal tumour (GIST)
For definition, terminology and incidence, we refer to the chapters on gastric and small-intestinal GISTs (Chapter 4 and 6). GISTs are very rare in the colon (about 1% of all GISTs) and have a predilection for the sigmoid. However, microscopic GISTs have been detected in 0.2% of retrospectively examined sigmoid-colon resections. Rectal GISTs comprise 4% of all GISTs and occur in any segment. These tumours vary from incidentally detected small mural nodules to large, complex pelvic masses that can cause intestinal obstruction or gastrointestinal bleeding. Those with anterior extension can abut the prostate gland and clinically simulate prostate cancer {39, 1131, 2064, 2074}.

The histological features of colonic GISTs are generally similar to those of small-intestinal GISTs. While most have spindle-cell morphology, some are epithelioid. Skeinoid fibres may occur. Nuclear palisading is a common feature, whereas perinuclear vacuolization is not usually prominent. Rectal GISTs are usually highly cellular spindle cell tumours, and many contain nuclear palisades, whereas perinuclear vacuolization and skeinoid fibres do not occur. Occasional epithelioid examples have been reported.

Immunohistochemically, colonic GISTs are similar to small-intestinal ones, whereas rectal GISTs resemble gastric GISTs by being consistently positive for KIT, DOG1, and CD34 and usually negative for smooth-muscle antigen (SMA).

The *KIT* mutation spectrum of colorectal GISTs is similar to that of small-intestinal GISTs, with a majority of cases showing mutations in exon 11 and a minority showing mutations in exons 9, 13 or 17 {1131, 2064, 2074}.

Most colonic GISTs are advanced tumours when detected, and have a poor prognosis. The behaviour of rectal GISTs is often aggressive, and even small tumours of < 2 cm in size with mitotic activity can recur and metastasize. Pelvic extension and liver metastasis is common, and bone metastases may develop more often than in gastric and small-intestinal GISTs.

Smooth muscle tumours

A distinctive type of leiomyoma that usually occurs in the colon and rectum is that of the muscularis mucosae. These tumours are roundish nodules that usually measure < 1 cm and not more than 2 cm. They are usually incidental endoscopic findings in older adults and are clinically indolent.

Histologically, these tumours are composed of bundles of well-differentiated smooth muscle that merge into the muscularis mucosae. Although focal nuclear atypia may be present, mitotic activity is not detectable.

Immunohistochemical features are typical of well-differentiated smooth muscle tumours: positive for SMA and desmin, and negative for CD34, S100 protein, KIT, and DOG1 {2072}.

Intramural leiomyomas are rare. They usually measure 1–3 cm, and are composed of well-differentiated smooth muscle cells with limited, if any, atypia and virtually no mitotic activity, although tumours with both atypia and mitotic activity are more appropriately designated as leiomyosarcomas.

Leiomyosarcomas occur both in the colon and rectum. They are often obstructing polypoid intraluminal masses. Prognosis varies, but may be good after complete excision, despite high-grade histology. Histological and immunohistochemical features are similar to those of leiomyosarcomas at other sites {2064}.

Schwannoma

Schwannomas similar to those in the stomach occur in the colon and rectum, usually in older adults. Presentations include gastrointestinal bleeding and a polypoid, obstructing, intraluminal mass. The histological features of these tumours are similar to those in the stomach, with the

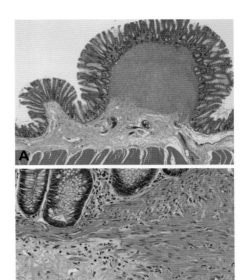

Fig. 8.72 Leiomyoma of muscularis mucosae. **A** The tumours forms a sharply demarcated mucosal mass that merges with muscularis mucosae layer. **B** It is composed of well-differentiated smooth muscle cells.

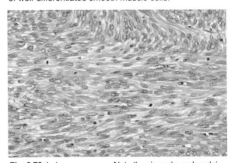

Fig. 8.73 Leiomyosarcoma. Note the cigar-shaped nuclei.

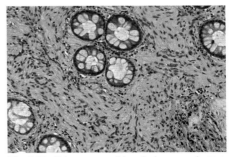

Fig. 8.74 Schwannoma: this colonic mucosal nerve sheath tumour contains mildly palisaded spindle-cell infiltration between crypts. The inset shows positivity for S100 protein.

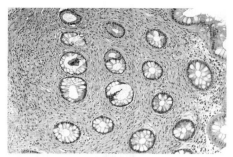

Fig. 8.75 Colonic perineurioma contains uniform spindle cells spaced between crypts. This tumour was positive for epithelial membrane antigen (EMA).

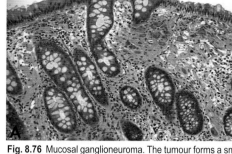

Fig. 8.76 Mucosal ganglioneuroma. The tumour forms a small polyp (**A**) that contains spindled Schwann cells, ganglion cells, and often also eosinophilic granulocytes (**B**). The inset shows positivity for S100 protein.

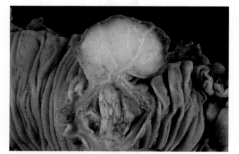

Fig. 8.77 Colonic lipoma.

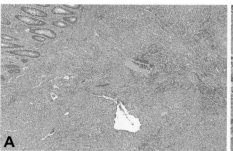

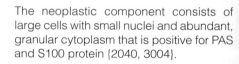

Fig. 8.78 Kaposi sarcoma. **A** Submucosal infiltrate. **B** Vascular slit pattern.

typical features including peritumoral lymphoid cuff and microtrabecular architecture. Small mucosal nerve sheath tumours occur in the colon and rectum. The designation "mucosal Schwann cell hamartoma" has also been used for apparently similar lesions. These tumours are clinically indolent and are not associated with neurofibromatosis type 1 (NF1) {985, 2075}.

Perineurioma

Perineuriomas in the gastrointestinal tract usually occur in the colon and are most often identified by chance as a small sessile polyp in adults. Most measure < 0.5 cm, rarely being larger. Histologically, these are typically intramucosal lesions, which fill and expand the lamina propria, entrapping crypts. They are composed of uniform spindle cells with short tapering nuclei and indistinct eosinophilic cytoplasm, often arranged in a whorled fashion within a delicate collagenous stroma. Perineuriomas are consistently immunopositive for EMA and less often claudin-positive. They show no evident tendency to recur {1241}. Lesions formerly known as fibroblastic polyps of the colon appear to represent intramucosal perineuriomas {1071}.

Ganglioneuroma

Most gastrointestinal ganglioneuromas occur in the colon with a predilection to the left side and the rectum, and a few are seen in the appendix. They are seen at a wide range of ages and equally in men and women. The usual presentation is a small mucosal polyp of < 1–2 cm, or sometimes multiple polyps. They are usually sporadic and indolent. However, diffuse murally extending ganglioneuromas (ganglioneuromatosis) have a high association with NF1 and multiple endocrine neoplasia type 2b (MEN2B) syndromes {436, 2914}.

Histologically, there are large numbers of mucosal ganglion cells and spindled Schwann cells, often with numerous eosinophilic granulocytes. Cystic glands can be present, imparting a resemblance to juvenile polyp in some cases. Immunohistochemically, the ganglion cells are positive for neuron-specific enolase (NSE), neurofilaments, and synaptophysin, whereas the Schwannian components are positive for S100 protein and often also for glial fibrillary acidic protein (GFAP).

Granular cell tumour

These tumours usually present as small mucosal nodules incidentally detected at endoscopy. Multiple lesions can be present, and occurrence together with peripheral granular cell tumours is also possible. The neoplastic component consists of large cells with small nuclei and abundant, granular cytoplasm that is positive for PAS and S100 protein {2040, 3004}.

Lipoma

Submucosal lipomas occur especially in the colon, usually detected in older adults as an incidental finding. Larger tumours may cause obstruction, ulcerate and undergo necrosis resulting in gastrointestinal haemorrhage. Histologically, there is mature adipose tissue without significant atypia. Thick-walled dilated blood vessels are often present in these lipomas, although they differ from peripheral angiolipomas.

Other mesenchymal tumours

A wide spectrum of vascular tumours such as haemangiomas, lymphangiomas, angiosarcoma and Kaposi sarcoma may occur in the colon and rectum. Mesenteric desmoid can involve the colonic wall, potentially simulating a GIST. Rare undifferentiated, phenotypically nonspecific sarcomas occur in the colon, and these should be separated from GISTs. Variably HMB45-positive PEComas (spindle cell and epithelioid variants, related to angiomyolipoma family) may occur in the colon. The pathology of these neoplasms is discussed in Chapter 10.

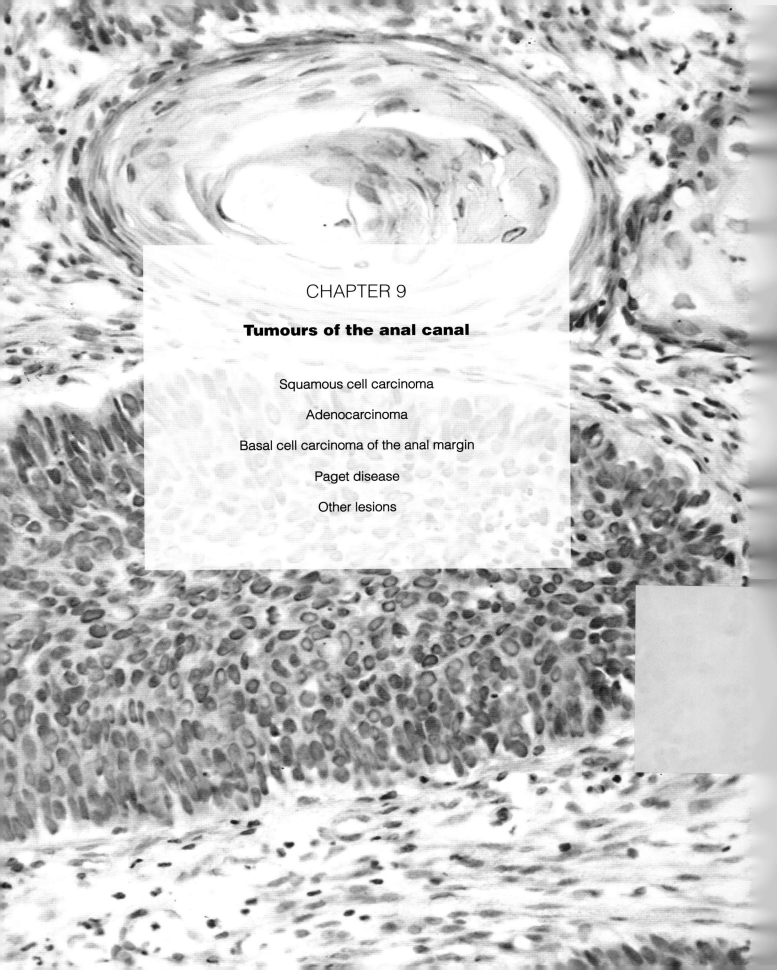

CHAPTER 9

Tumours of the anal canal

Squamous cell carcinoma

Adenocarcinoma

Basal cell carcinoma of the anal margin

Paget disease

Other lesions

WHO classification[a] of tumours of the anal canal

Epithelial tumours

Premalignant lesions

Anal intraepithelial neoplasia (dysplasia), low grade   8077/0*
Anal intraepithelial neoplasia (dysplasia), high grade   8077/2

Bowen disease
Perianal squamous intraepithelial neoplasia
Paget disease   8542/3

Carcinoma

Squamous cell carcinoma	8070/3
Verrucous carcinoma	8051/3
Undifferentiated carcinoma	8020/3
Adenocarcinoma	8140/3
Mucinous adenocarcinoma	8480/3

Neuroendocrine neoplasms[b]

Neuroendocrine tumour (NET)	
NET G1 (carcinoid)	8240/3
NET G2	8249/3
Neuroendocrine carcinoma (NEC)	8246/3
Large cell NEC	8013/3
Small cell NEC	8041/3
Mixed adenoneuroendocrine carcinoma	8244/3

Mesenchymal tumours

Secondary tumours

---

[a] Morphology code of the International Classification of Diseases for Oncology (ICD-O) {904A}. Behaviour is coded /0 for benign tumours, /1 for unspecified, borderline or uncertain behaviour, /2 for carcinoma *in situ* and grade III intraepithelial neoplasia, and /3 for malignant tumours.
[b] The classification is modified from the previous (third) edition of the WHO histological classification of tumours {691} taking into account changes in our understanding of these lesions. In the case of neuroendocrine neoplasms, the classification has been simplified to be of more practical utility in morphological classification.
* These new codes were approved by the IARC/WHO Committee for ICD-O at its meeting in March 2010.

TNM classification[a] of carcinoma of the anal canal

T – Primary tumour
TX   Primary tumour cannot be assessed
T0   No evidence of primary tumour
Tis   Carcinoma *in situ*, Bowen disease, high-grade squamous
        intraepithelial lesion (HSIL), anal intraepithelial neoplasia
        II–III (AIN II–III)
T1   Tumour 2 cm or less in greatest dimension
T2   Tumour more than 2 cm but not more than 5 cm in greatest
        dimension
T3   Tumour more than 5 cm in greatest dimension
T4   Tumour of any size invades adjacent organ(s), e.g. vagina,
        urethra, bladder (direct invasion of rectal wall, perianal skin,
        subcutaneous tissue or the sphincter muscle(s) alone is not
        classified as T4)

N – Regional lymph nodes
NX   Regional lymph nodes cannot be assessed
N0   No regional lymph-node metastasis
N1   Metastasis in perirectal lymph node(s)
N2   Metastasis in unilateral internal iliac and/or inguinal lymph
        node(s)
N3   Metastasis in perirectal and inguinal lymph nodes and/or
        bilateral internal iliac and/or bilateral inguinal lymph nodes

M – Distant metastasis
M0   No distant metastasis
M1   Distant metastasis

Stage grouping

Stage	T	N	M
Stage 0	Tis	N0	M0
Stage I	T1	N0	M0
Stage II	T2, T3	N0	M0
Stage IIIA	T1, T2, T3	N1	M0
	T4	N0	M0
Stage IIIB	T4	N1	M0
	Any T	N2, N3	M0
Stage IV	Any T	Any N	M1

---

[a] {762, 2996}
A helpdesk for specific questions about the TNM classification is available at http://www.uicc.org.

Tumours of the anal canal

M.L. Welton
R. Lambert
F.T. Bosman

Topographic definition of the anal canal, anal margin and perianal region

The anal canal is defined as the terminal part of the large intestine. The uppermost boundary of the anal canal is defined by the passage of the rectum through the proximal portion of the anorectal ring, usually 1–2 cm above the dentate line. The large bowel passes through the muscular diaphragm of the sphincter mechanism and terminates at the intersphincteric groove, which is created by the termination of the circular muscle of the large bowel. This anatomic landmark correlates roughly with the transition from the highly specialized squamous mucosa of the anal canal to the perianal skin. The dentate (pectinate) line denotes the mucosal transition from rectum to anus that occurs on average 1–2 cm proximal to the termination of the anal canal. The proximal anal canal is lined with colorectal mucosa. This colorectal mucosa may be involved with squamous metaplasia resulting in a "transformation zone" blurring the original dentate line.

This transformation zone is particularly susceptible to involvement with human papillomavirus (HPV). Immediately proximal to the dentate line and extending by 0–12 mm is a variably present anal transitional zone (ATZ) of specialized epithelium that is similar to urothelium {835, 3240}. The distal anal canal extends from the dentate line downwards to the mucocutaneous junction with the perianal skin, the anal verge. It is lined with a highly specialized nonkeratinizing squamous mucosa, formerly termed pectin, lacking

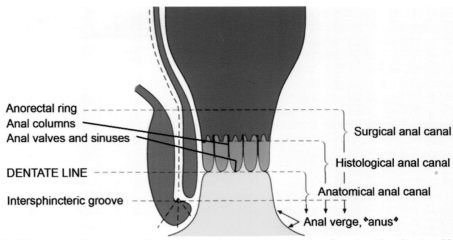

Fig. 9.01 Anatomy of the anal canal. The light blue area is the anal transitional zone. Reproduced from Sternberg SS, *Histology for pathologists*, 2nd edition {835}, with permission.

hair follicles, apocrine glands and sweat glands. The perianal skin is denoted by the appearance of these skin appendages. These landmarks, the dentate line and the anal verge, have historically been used to define cancers of the anal canal and anal margin. Unfortunately, much confusion has persisted, leading to miscategorization of tumours and quite possibly overtreatment.

Recently, new definitions have been proposed to simplify classification: anal canal, perianal and transformation zone. A tumour of the anal canal is defined as a tumour that cannot be seen in its entirety, or at all, when gentle traction is placed on the buttocks. A perianal cancer is found within a 5 cm radius of the anus and is seen completely when gentle traction is placed on the anus. The rectal transformation zone represents the area of distal rectal mucosa proximal to the dentate line involved with squamous metaplasia.

Squamous cell carcinoma

Definition

Squamous cell carcinoma (SCC) of the anal canal is a malignant epithelial neoplasm that is frequently associated with chronic infection with HPV.

ICD-O code   8070/3

Epidemiology

The age-standardized rate of incidence of anal SCC is < 1 per 100 000. Most anal cancers occur among patients in the sixth or seventh decade of life {903}. However, in individuals with cellular immune incompetence, anal cancer may occur at a young age {2036}.

The incidence of anal cancer is higher in females than in males {592, 903, 2037}, with a male-to-female ratio of 0.81. Anal cancer is more common in females of all ages and basaloid tumours in particular are more frequent in women. The evolution of sexuality, HPV infection and sex hormones play a causal role in the increasing predominance of females {901}; the latter as estrogen and androgen receptors are present in the supportive tissue of anal mucosa {2358}.

Anal cancer has increased in incidence during recent decades by about 2.5-fold in men and 5-fold in women {903, 1240, 1436, 2037, 3487}. The risk is higher in urban than in rural areas {903, 2037}. The overall incidence of invasive and *in situ* anal carcinoma increased to about 2.5 per 100 000 {1436}.

Racial differences exist: the age-standardized incidence in the USA is 1.4 and

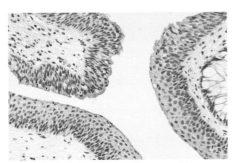

Fig. 9.02 Normal histology of the anal transition zone.

1.9 per 100 000 for white men and women, respectively, and 1.6 per 100 000 for African-American men and women {1240}.

Geographic variations in the respective proportion of SCC and adenocarcinoma exist: for SCC, the age-standardized rate of incidence is < 0.5 per 100 000 men but > 0.5 per 100 000 women {634}.

The age-standardized rate of incidence for adenocarcinoma varies from 0.1 to 0.5 per 100 000 men and from 0.1 to 0.2 per 100 000 women. The proportion of adenocarcinoma is particularly low in Northern Europe, constituting < 15% of all cases {634}. Adenocarcinoma is more frequent in some African or Asiatic countries and represents the majority of anal cancers in Japan.

Mortality

The rate of mortality is significantly lower than the rate of incidence. In the USA in 2002–2006, the age-standardized rate of mortality was 0.2 per 100 000. In 1980–2006 in the USA, a significant annual increase in mortality occurred in females {1240}.

Survival

The prognosis for patients with anal cancer varies according to the stage of the tumour at detection. In the USA, the SEER survival monograph {1943} reports a relative 5-year survival rate of 60.2 for Caucasian men and 47.0 for African-

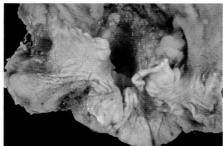

Fig. 9.03 Squamous cell carcinoma arising at the dentate line of the anal canal.

American men and of 69.5 and 58.5 for Caucasian women and African-American women, respectively. The 5-year relative survival for localized anal cancer (48% and 42% of the registered cases for white and African-American people, respectively) was slightly more than 81% for Caucasian people and 67% for African American people. The 5-year relative survival with extensive disease is around 15%.

Etiology

Several recent studies have identified risk factors for anal SCC, including infection with HPV, immunodeficiency with human immunodeficiency virus (HIV) seropositivity, a low CD4-T-cell count, immunosuppression following solid-organ transplantion, anoreceptive sexual intercourse, and tobacco-smoking {3346}.

HPV infection

The association between HPV infection and anal cancer has been extensively analysed and included in the burden of HPV-related cancers {2484}. HPV infection is also associated with development of anal squamous intraepithelial neoplasia in persons with immunodeficiency. Sexually transmissible HPV can be detected in the majority of anal SCCs in more developed countries {900, 1180, 1230, 2784, 3151}. Different results have been reported in Asia; in China, only a single case involving HPV type 16 DNA was detected among 72 anal cancers {1724}. HPV was detected in 90% of women and 63% of men with invasive anal cancer {898}. In women, HPV-associated gynaecological (cervical, vulvar, vaginal) cancer has been reported to be strongly associated with anal cancer {1431, 3079}. While many HPV types can infect the genital mucosa, their potential to induce malignancy differs. The prevalence of HPV16 and HPV18 DNA was 72% in invasive cancer, 69% in high-grade squamous intraepithelial neoplasia and 27% in low-grade intraepithelial neoplasia {1237}. Low-risk HPV types are identified in anal lesions with low-grade dysplasia and high-risk types (HPV types 16, 18, 31, 33, 35, 39, 45, 50, 51, 53, 56, 58, 59 and 68) occur in high-grade anal intraepithelial neoplasia (AIN) or invasive cancer {3682}. HPV-16 is detected in around 70% of cases {649, 900}. Involvement of high-risk HPV is less frequent in lesions confined to the perianal skin {898}.

HIV and immunosuppression

Homosexual men who are infected with HIV appear to be at a particularly high risk of developing anal cancer {1015, 2036, 2438}. Development of squamous intraepithelial lesions is inversely related to CD4-T-cell count. The risk of HPV-related cancers was analysed in the USA in nearly 500 000 individuals diagnosed with acquired immunodeficiency syndrome (AIDS); the incidence of invasive anal cancer was increased in men with a CD4-T-cell count of < 100 per mm³. Incidence was also higher during 1996–2004 than in 1990–2005, suggesting that prolonged survival attributable to antiretroviral treatment may be associated with an increased risk of developing HPV-associated cancer {498}. Antiretroviral treatments do not seem to decrease the risk of anal cancer, suggesting that a vaccine against HPV (now available) could prove

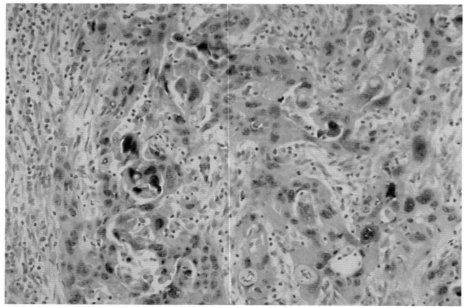

Fig. 9.04 *In situ* hybridization for human papilloma virus HPV16/18 is positive in this anal carcinoma.

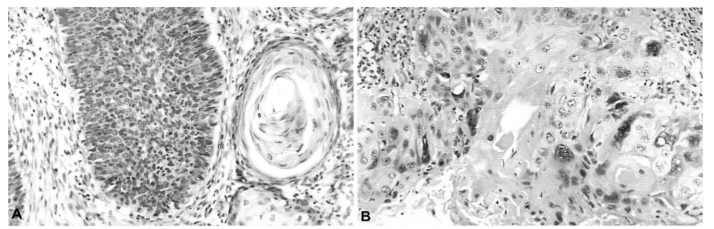

Fig. 9.05 Squamous cell carcinoma of the anus. **A** The tumour shows a combination of basaloid features and keratinization. **B** Note the large cells that are poorly differentiated.

to be protective {886}. The association between HIV infection and anal cancer is subject to confounding factors because HIV-positive patients are often infected with more than one HPV type {2438}. The role of HIV infection in the development of malignancy is proposed to be through HPV infection {902}.

Patients receiving long-term immunosuppressive therapy after solid-organ transplantion are at a higher risk of developing SCC {2519}, with a increased risk of 100-fold after renal transplantation {568}. An increased risk of anal cancer has also been reported in patients receiving immunosuppressive therapy with corticoids for other indications {649}.

Sexual practices

The risk of anal cancer is linked to sexual practice. Homosexual men constitute a high-risk group {900, 903, 2037}. In the USA, the incidence of anal SCC has been estimated to be 11–34 times higher in homosexual men than in the general male population and approximately as high as the incidence of cervical cancer before the introduction of cervical cytology screening {2437}.

A population-based study {650} has shown an increased risk in men who are not exclusively heterosexual and in those practicing anal intercourse. A further study of the same group {649} has shown that the odds ratio for anal cancer in men who are not exclusively heterosexual was 17.3. The risk is also increased when there is a history of genital warts, with an odds ratio of 7.4. Other factors include number of sexual partners, receptive anal intercourse, and coinfection with other sexually transmitted diseases {900}.

Anal cancer was also found to be more common in women practising anal intercourse.

Other factors

Several studies have identified smoking as a risk factor for the development of anal cancer {901, 1231}. Case–control studies estimate the relative risk of anal cancer in smokers at 3.0–7.7 for women and 3.9–9.4 for men {649}. Haemorrhoids and fissures, fistulae and abcesses in the anal region had been considered as predisposing factors, but at the present time three case–control studies {650, 899, 1231} and two cohort studies {904, 1857} have failed to support this association. Crohn disease of long duration has also been implicated in the etiology of anal SCC according to some case reports {1702}. The association was not confirmed in a controlled study addressing this issue {899}. An increased risk of anal cancer is reported in persons with longstanding perianal Crohn disease {707}, but the majority of cases concern adenocarcinoma. In addition, the occurrence of an adenocarcinoma is not an unusual complication at the ileo-anal anastomosis after establishment of an ileal pouch.

Clinical features

Symptoms and signs

AIN is often an unexpected finding in minor surgical specimens. Clinical manifestations of anal cancer are often late and nonspecific and are mainly related to tumour size and extent of infiltration. They include anal pruritus, discomfort in the sitting position, sensation of a pelvic mass, pain, change in bowel habit, incontinence caused by sphincter infiltration, discharge,

bleeding, fissure, or fistula. The initial nonspecificity of clinical features combined with physician and patient reluctance to examine and discuss anal diseases contribute to a delay in diagnosis {2139A}. The clinical diagnosis of an anal tumour should always be confirmed by histological examination. A forceps or needle biopsy is usually sufficient to establish the diagnosis. The biopsy should be accompanied by an exact description of the location and appearance of the biopsy site. An excisional biopsy may be inadvisable, because delay in wound-healing may postpone optimal chemoradiotherapeutic treatment. However, small lesions may lend themselves to local excision more readily and the wound is often small enough to be of little clinical impact. Enlarged lymph nodes, if symptomatic, may be excised, but are generally included in the planned radiation fields. If lymph-node biopsy is necessary for planning, needle aspiration under radiological guidance is often useful.

Imaging

Computed tomography (CT) scan, magnetic resonance imaging (MRI), and fine-needle aspiration may be used to establish inguinal and pararectal node involvement. Endo-anal ultrasound is useful in the follow-up of irradiated carcinomas {1985}. CT scan and MRI allow detection of involved lymph nodes and distant metastases {3078}.

Exfoliative cytology

In patients with an increased risk, such as those with HIV, those who are immunocompromised (kidney transplant patients), or women with SCC of the genital tract,

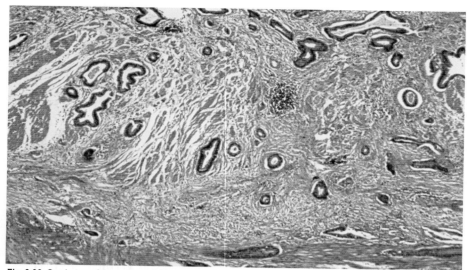

Fig. 9.06 Carcinoma of the anal canal. Note the small neoplastic glands that resemble anal glands.

the use of anal smears taken with a cyto-logy brush from the area above the dentate line is recommended {895, 2851}.

Macroscopy

The entire anal canal and distal rectum must be considered at risk. A digital rectal exam may detect a tiny lump, or ulceration in the distal rectal mucosa or a fissure with slightly exophytic and indurated margins. Inspection may reveal an irregular thickening of the anoderm and anal mar-gin with chronic dermatitis. The lesion in the anal mucosa and perianal skin may have a different colour from the surrounding tissue and the lesion in the distal rectal

mucosa may appear somewhat granular and friable or may be completely invisible and only detected upon palpation or with the aid of high-resolution anoscopy (HRA). In HRA, a magnified view of the anus is augmented by the painting of the anal canal and distal rectal mucosa with acetic acid. Ulceration and infiltration result in bleeding and fixation.

Tumour spread and staging

Anal SCC should be staged according to the TNM (tumour, node, metastasis) system {1107}. Treatment for anal SCC has now changed from surgery alone to sphincter-preserving procedures, including radiation

and chemotherapy, sometimes in combi-nation with local excision. Large surgical specimens are therefore rare. The exami-nation should include resection lines in all directions and a careful search for lymph nodes. Clinical results for the combined treatment regimes are comparable or better than those for surgery alone, but detection of residual disease can be more difficult using imaging techniques owing to local fibrosis. The question of persistent versus recurrent disease often arises in the first months after combined modality therapy has been completed. Serial digital rectal examination with anoscopy and ultrasound is recommended for mon-itoring. Routine biopsy is discouraged as non-healing painful ulcers often result, requiring abdominal–perineal resection for "benign" disease {2737}. Larger lesions may take 6–8 months to resolve and patience is encouraged as long as the lesion continues to decrease in size.
In 15–20% of cases, the lesion may infil-trate the lower rectum and the neighbour-ing organs, including the rectovaginal septum, bladder, prostate and posterior urethra, sometimes with suppuration and fistulas. The vulva is usually spared. Lymphatic spread occurs in up to 40% of cases {2472}. Tumours proximal to the pectinate line drain into the pelvis along the middle rectal vessels to the pelvic side walls and internal iliac chains and superiorly via the superior rectal vessels to the periaortic nodes. Tumours distal to the dentate line drain along cutaneous pathways to the inguinal and the femoral nodal chains. Inguinal nodes are involved in about 10–20% of cases {966, 2472}. Inguinal lymph nodes can be involved bilaterally in a small number of cases at time of presentation. Retrograde lym-phatic drainage occurs in advanced cases when the lymphatics are obstructed by malignant spread {2472}.

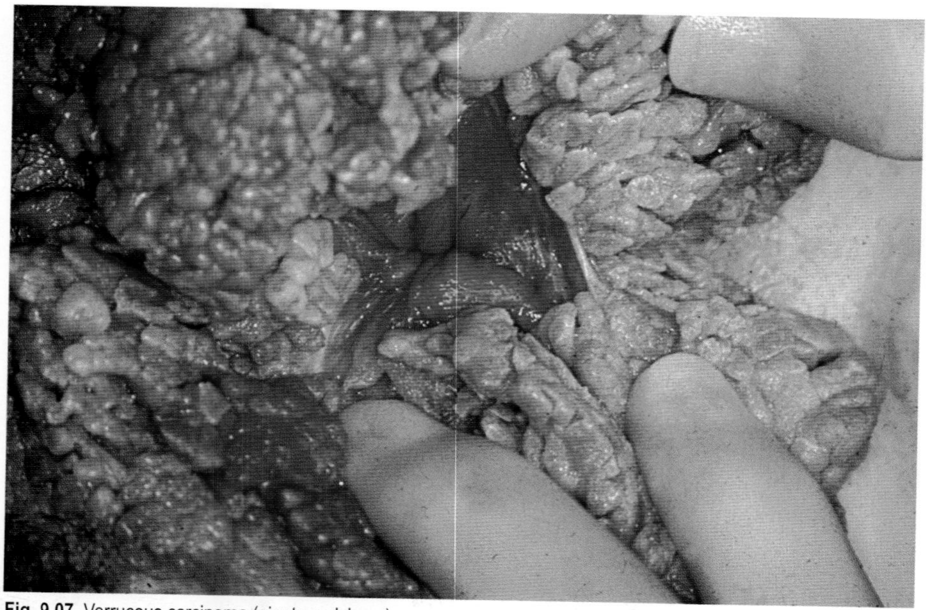

Histopathology
SCC of the anal canal

Anal SCC may show homogeneous histo-logical characteristics, but most tumours exhibit a mixture of areas with different histological features. One pattern is that of large, pale eosinophilic cells and keratinization of either lamellar or single-cell type. Another is that of small cells with palisading of the nuclei in the periphery of tumour-cell islands. The latter often contain necrotic eosinophilic centres. Intermediate stages between these two

Fig. 9.07 Verrucous carcinoma (giant condyloma).

extremes are often present. Tubular architecture or spindle-cell transformation may be found. The invasive margin can vary from well-circumscribed to irregular, and a lymphocytic infiltrate may be pronounced or absent. None of these features have been shown to have any prognostic significance; histological features do not consistently correlate with HPV type {1892, 3151}. The usual patterns of immunoexpression are summarized in Table 9.01 {2210}.

The second edition of the WHO classification of SCC of the anal canal included the large cell keratinizing subtype, the large cell nonkeratinizing subtype, and the basaloid subtype, often referred to as cloacogenic carcinoma. The value of this classification of anal SCC has been questioned in recent years. Many tumours show more than one subtype. Thus in a study of 100 cases of anal carcinomas, 99 showed some features of squamous differentiation (keratinization, stratification and prickles), 65 showed basaloid features (small cell change, palisading, retraction artefact and central eosinophilic necrosis) and 26 showed focal evidence of ductal proliferation and occasionally positive staining for periodic acid–Schiff (PAS) after diastase digestion {3517}. Furthermore, the diagnostic reproducibility of these subtypes is low {837}. This is probably the reason that the proportion of basaloid carcinoma in larger series has varied from 10% to almost 70%, and that no significant correlation between histological subtype and prognosis has been established. In addition, histological diagnosis is nowadays nearly always performed on small biopsies, that may not be representative of the whole tumour, and therapy is not influenced by histological subtype {837}. Therefore, it is recommended that the generic term "squamous cell carcinoma" be used for these tumours, accompanied by a comment describing those histopathological features that may possibly affect the prognosis, i.e. size of predominant neoplastic cell, basaloid features, degree of keratinization, adjacent squamous intraepithelial neoplasia, presence of mucinous microcysts or degree of differentiaton {258}.

Apart from the verrucous carcinoma mentioned below, the only rare histological subtype that seems to have a different biological course, having a less favourable prognosis, is characterized by a rather uniform pattern of small tumour cells with nuclear moulding, high mitotic rate, extensive apoptosis and diffuse infiltration in the surrounding stroma. This has been called small cell (anaplastic) carcinoma {2922}, but should not be confused with small cell carcinoma (poorly differentiated neuroendocrine carcinoma).

Perianal SCC

The distinction between anal canal and perianal SCC may be difficult, as tumours often involve both areas at the time of diagnosis. This may account for the varying data on prognosis; however, prognosis is generally better for patients with perianal SCC than with anal-canal SCC, in particular if local resection is possible {2510}. Perianal SCC is often the large cell variant {898, 2510}.

Verrucous carcinoma

In the anogenital area, this tumour is also called giant (malignant) condyloma or Buschke-Löwenstein tumour {1077}. It has a cauliflower-like appearance, is larger than the usual condyloma (with a diameter of up to 12 cm), and fails to respond to conservative treatment. In contrast to an ordinary condyloma, it is characterized by a combination of exophytic and endophytic growth. Histologically, it shows acanthosis and papillomatosis with orderly arrangement of the epithelial layers and an intact but often irregular base with blunt downward projections and keratin-filled cysts. The endophytic growth may represent invasive activity, but convincing evidence of invasive growth is rare.

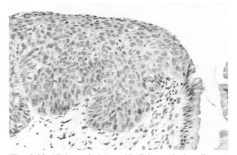

Fig. 9.08 High-grade intraepithelial neoplasia adjacent to normal rectal epithelium.

Cytologically, the epithelial cells appear benign. Large nuclei with prominent nucleoli may be present, but cytonuclear atypia is usually minimal and mitoses are restricted to the basal layers {1892}.

Some verrucous carcinomas contain HPV, the most common types being HPV6 and HPV11. They are regarded as an intermediate state between the ordinary condyloma and SCC, and the clinical course is typically that of local destructive invasion without metastases {248, 1892}. The presence of severe cytological changes, unequivocal invasion or metastases should lead to the diagnosis of SCC and to the appropriate therapy.

Grading

Poor prognosis has been related to poor differentiation {298}, especially if this was defined only by the degree of dissociation of tumour cells {1016}. However, such differences may be related to tumour stage in multivariate analysis {2926}.

Table 9.01. Immunoreactivity profiles for anal tumours.[a]

Tumour	Keratins			Mucin	CEA	Vimentin	Others
	8 + 18	7 / 20	5 + 14				
Colorectal adenocarcinoma	+	– / +	–	+	+	–	—
Squamous cell variants	–	– / –	+	–	–	–	Keratin 13 / 19
Basal cell carcinoma	–	– / –	+	–	–	–	Ber-EP4[b]
Neuroendocrine tumour (NET)	+	– / –	–	–	–	–	Chrom / Synap
Malignant melanoma	–	– / –	–	–	–	+	S100, HMB45[c]
Bowen (also pigmented)	–	– / –	+	–	–	–	
Paget cells (local)	+	+ / –	–	+	+	–	GCDFP-15
Paget cells (from colorectal carcinoma)	+	+ / +	–	+	+	–	
Prostatic carcinoma	+	– / –	–	–	–	–	PSA, PSAP
Malignant lymphoma	–	– / –	-	-	-	+	LCA and others

CEA, carcinoembryonic antigen; Chrom, chromogranin A; GCDFP, gross cystic disease fluid protein, a marker for apocrine cells; LCA, leukocyte common antigen; PSA, prostate-specific antigen; PSAP, prostate-specific acid phosphatase; Synap, synaptophysin. [a] Exceptions occur, especially among keratins and mucin; [b] Antibody to epithelial cell-adhesion molecule; [c] Melanocyte-specific antibody.

Grading on the basis of biopsies is not recommended, as these may not be representative of the tumour as a whole.

Precursor lesions
Chronic HPV infection
Warts in the perianal skin and lower anal canal (condyloma acuminatum) show the same histology as their genital counterparts. Flat koilocytic lesions also occur. They should always be totally embedded and examined histologically for possible presence of intraepithelial neoplasia.

Intraepithelial neoplasia
Precancerous AIN in the ATZ and the squamous zone has also been termed dysplasia, carcinoma *in situ* and anal squamous intraepithelial lesion (ASIL) {839, 2438}. The corresponding lesions in the perianal skin are commonly referred to as Bowen disease. This terminology is complicated by the fact that the precancerous changes are not always restricted to one area.

Given the confusion engendered by multiple terms referring to the same pathology, the American Joint Committee on Cancer (AJCC) has recommended using simply "low-grade squamous intraepithelial lesion" (LSIL) and "high-grade squamous intraepithelial lesion" (HSIL). The term preferred by WHO is AIN (see Chapter 1). "Leukoplakia" is a clinical term and should not be used as a histological diagnosis.

Anal squamous intraepithelial neoplasia (ASIN)
Most cases of ASIN are incidental findings in specimens taken during minor surgery for benign conditions. When detected macroscopically, ASIN may present as an eczematoid or papillomatous area, or as papules or plaques. The latter may be irregular, raised, scaly, white, pigmented or erythematous and occasionally fissured. Induration or ulceration may indicate invasion.

Histologically, ASIN is characterized by varying degrees of loss of stratification and nuclear polarity, nuclear pleomorphism and hyperchromatism, and increased mitotic activity with presence of mitoses high in the epithelium. The surface may or may not be keratinized, and koilocytic changes may be present. ASIN should be graded as either ASIN-L (low-grade) or ASIN-H (high-grade) and the terminology of dysplasia and the grading

in mild, moderate and severe should be abandoned because reproducibility studies have shown considerable variation between observers {446}. Expression of *CDKN2A* (*p16*) and assessment of proliferative activity according to the Ki67-labelling index can assist in grading {3439}.

Perianal squamous intraepithelial neoplasia (PSIN, previously known as Bowen disease)
Clinically, this presents as a white or red area in the perianal skin that may be in continuity with dysplastic lesions in the anal canal. HPV DNA is sometimes detected, including HPV types 16 and 18, among others. Histologically, it shows full-thickness dysplasia of the squamous and sometimes the pilosebaceous epithelium, with disorderly maturation, mitoses at all levels and dyskeratosis. Occasionally, atypical keratinocytes may resemble Paget cells, but are negative for low relative-molecular-mass keratins and for mucin. In pigmented PSIN, the neoplastic cells are invariably negative for S100 protein and HMB45. PSIN has a strong tendency to recur after local treatment, but only a few percent of cases will progress to SCC. This tendency is higher in immunocompromised patients who develop PSIN {2850}

Genetic susceptibility
Human leukocyte antigens (HLAs) are involved in the presentation of viral antigens to the immune system. Since the etiology of most anal SCCs involves HPV infection {898}, susceptibility to cancer development might be HLA type-dependent. However, no study has addressed the association between specific HLA class I or II alleles and risk, and attempts to identify other genetic susceptibility markers for anal SCC have so far been unsuccessful {501, 502}.

Molecular pathology
HPV DNA is detectable in most anal SCCs; in a large population-based series of anal SCCs in Denmark and Sweden, 84% contained HPV DNA, with higher proportions of HPV DNA-positive cancers among women and homosexual men than among non-homosexual men {898}. Loss of functional tumour-suppressor protein p53 appears to play a central role in the development of anal and anogenital SCCs {623, 624, 1180, 1793}. Inactivation of p53 (*TP53*) may occur at the gene level through point mutations leading to the

production of inactive p53 or, less frequently, by means of deletions in the relevant area of chromosome 17p {1180}. More typically, p53 inactivation occurs at the protein level through formation of a complex between the viral protein E6 (expressed by "high-risk" HPV types) and a cellular protein, the E6-associated protein, which when bound to p53 leads to rapid proteolytic degradation of p53 {3491}. The level of p53 expression does not correlate with HPV status {1180}. The E7 protein of high-risk HPV types binds to the retinoblastoma protein, pRb {755}, disrupting signals that normally restrict proliferation to the basal epithelial layer. The resulting increased proliferation increases the risk of malignant transformation on exposure to DNA-damaging stimuli. The combination of increased cell proliferation (pRb inactivation) and impaired ability to induce cell-cycle arrest or apoptosis following DNA damage (p53 inactivation) are two central mechanisms through which high-risk types of HPV increase the risk of anogenital cancer. Additional gene alterations appear to be involved in malignant progression and invasion. Amplification of the *MYC* gene was found in 30% of anal SCCs {623}. Furthermore, gains in chromosomes 3q, 17, and 19 as well as losses in chromosomes 4p, 11q, 13q, and 18q, loss of heterozygosity at the *APC*, *DCC/SMAD4* and *D2S123* gene loci and epigenetic alterations such as inactivation of the *TSLC1* tumour-suppressor gene occur with increased frequency in SCC {969, 1180, 2179, 3064}.

Prognosis and predictive factors
The most important prognostic factors reported in recent larger series of SCC of the anal canal are tumour stage and nodal status {258, 892, 2511, 2926}. Perianal SCC has a slightly better prognosis, which depends only on inguinal-node involvement {2510}. DNA ploidy status has only been shown to be of independent prognostic significance in one of three larger series {1016, 2867, 2926}. Expression of p53, cyclin A, tumour-budding and tumour-infiltrating T-cells have been found to be of prognostic significance {1044, 2292, 2293}.

Adenocarcinoma

Definition
Adenocarcinoma of the anal canal is an adenocarcinoma arising in the epithelium of the anal canal, including the mucosal surface, the anal glands and the lining of fistulous tracts.

ICD-O code   8140/3

Clinical features
The clinical features of anal adenocarcinoma of colorectal type do not differ from those of anal squamous cell carcinoma (SCC). Perianal adenocarcinomas may present as submucosal tumours, sometimes in combination with fistulae. Occasionally, there may be associated Paget disease of the anus. Tumour spread and staging largely correspond to that for anal SCC.

Histopathology
Adenocarcinoma arising in anal mucosa
Most adenocarcinomas found in the anal canal represent downward spread from an adenocarcinoma in the rectum or arise in colorectal-type mucosa above the dentate line. Macroscopically and histologically, they are indistinguishable from ordinary colorectal-type adenocarcinoma, and do not seem to represent a special entity, except for their low location. Adenocarcinoma in the ATZ may develop after restorative proctocolectomy for ulcerative colitis {2878}.

Extramucosal (perianal) adenocarcinoma
Approximately 200 cases of extramucosal adenocarcinoma have been reported, the largest series unfortunately with insufficient histological data {5}. A minimum criterion for diagnosis is an overlying non-neoplastic mucosa, which may be ulcerated. Recent reports indicate that about two thirds of these tumours manifest in men with a mean age of about 60 years. Reliable data for the prognosis for such patients have not been identified. Difficulties in establishing the correct diagnosis may delay proper treatment. Extramucosal adenocarcinomas seem to fall into two groups on the basis of their association with either fistulae or remnants of anal glands. At present, no laboratory methods can distinguish between these two groups. The epithelium of persistent anal fistulae is most often of the same type as that found in the anal glands and ATZ {1915}, and the epithelia in these two locations show the same profile with regard to mucin composition {836} and keratin expression {1217, 3518}.

Adenocarcinoma within anorectal fistulae
These tumours develop in pre-existing anal sinuses or in fistulae {129}. Some are associated with Crohn disease {707, 1702}. Others may contain epithelioid granulomas, often related to foci of inflammation or extravasated mucin, but without other signs of inflammatory bowel disease {1440}. Rarely, the tumours may be related to fistulae lined by normal rectal mucosa, including muscularis mucosae, most likely representing adenocarcinomas arising in congenital duplications {1440}. Histologically, carcinomas arising in fistulae usually are of the mucinous type, but tubular adenocarcinomas and squamous neoplasia can also be found {1702, 3636}.

Adenocarcinoma of anal glands
Only a few cases have been reported in which convincing evidence for origin in an anal gland has been demonstrated by continuity between anal-gland epithelium and tumour {209, 1099, 2490, 3486, 3540}. With a single exception {1099}, these patients have had no history of previous or concomitant fistula. The tumours were all characterized by a ductular architecture with scant production of mucin. Pagetoid spread was present in at least one case {3540}. Carcinomas of the anal gland express keratin 7 as well as keratin 5/6 and show a loss of p63 expression, which may be helpful in diagnosis {1217, 1868}.

Grading
Anal adenocarcinomas are graded in the same way as colorectal adenocarcinomas.

Precursor lesions
Anal adenocarcinomas without predisposing conditions as described above are rare. They can arise from adenomas {584A}, which can be graded as for the colorectum.

Prognosis and predictive factors
The prognosis for anal adenocarcinoma seems to be related only to stage at diagnosis and is poorer than that for SCC {209, 481, 513, 1585, 2201}.

Basal cell carcinoma of the anal margin

Basal cell carcinoma, the most common skin cancer, is primarily found on areas of the skin that are exposed to the sun, and little more than 100 cases have been reported to occur in the anal area {984, 2287}. The etiology is unknown and there is no evidence for a role of infection by HPV {2261}. The tumour commonly presents as an indurated area with raised edges and central ulceration, located in the perianal skin, but occasionally involves the squamous zone below the dentate line. Histologically, it can show the same variability in morphology as basal cell carcinoma elsewhere, most reported cases having had a solid or adenoid pattern.

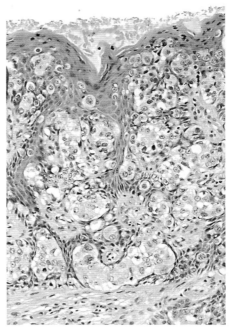

Fig. 9.09 Paget disease of the anal canal. Large Paget cells are distributed throughout the non-neoplastic squamous epithelium.

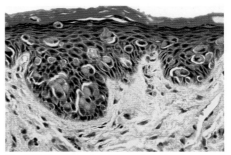

Fig. 9.10 Paget disease of the anal canal.

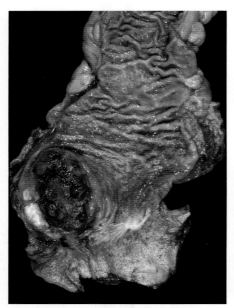

Fig. 9.11 Malignant melanoma of the anus with typical polypoid appearance.

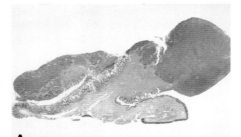

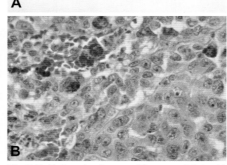

Fig. 9.12 Malignant melanoma of the anus. **A** Polypoid growth is frequent. **B** Epitheloid melanoma cells with prominent nucleoli.

Other lesions

Squamous cell papilloma, papillary hidradenoma, keratoacanthoma, mesenchymal tumours, neurogenic tumours and lymphomas rarely involve the anal canal and perianal region. Patients with AIDS have an increased risk of developing lymphoma and Kaposi sarcoma. Neuroendocrine neoplasms of the anal canal are conventionally classified as rectal and are discussed in Chapter 8.

Squamous cell papilloma of the anal canal

Rarely, papillomatous processes covered by normal, more or less keratinized squamous epithelium can be found in the anus. Such lesions should be tested for the presence of HPV. Lesions that are negative for HPV are commonly regarded as "burned-out" condylomas.

Papillary hidradenoma

This rare tumour arises in the perianal apocrine glands, typically in middle-aged women and only exceedingly rarely in men {1877}. It presents as a circumscribed nodule approximately 1 cm in diameter and may resemble a haemorrhoid. Histologically, it consists of a papillary mass with a cyst-like capsule. The papillae are lined by a double layer of epithelial cells, the outer layer being composed of cells containing mucin. The tumour does not express the eccrine marker IKH4, but it must be remembered that adenocarcinoma metastases are also negative for this marker {1357}. Convincing examples of anal apocrine adenocarcinoma have not been published.

Keratoacanthoma

There are a few reports on keratoacanthoma arising in the perianal skin {783}.

Neuroendocrine tumours

Neuroendocrine tumours may arise in the anus {838, 1243}. They are, however, conventionally classified as rectal. An immunohistochemical study of 17 rectal neuroendocrine tumours showed that most were of L cell type {519} (see Chapter 5).

Malignant melanoma

Anal melanoma is rare, representing 1–3% of all anal tumours. Patients most commonly present in the fifth or sixth decades of life with pain, rectal bleeding or a mass.

Basal cell carcinoma is treated adequately by local excision and metastases are extremely rare. It is therefore important to distinguish basal cell from squamous cell carcinoma; this may be particularly difficult when relying solely on small biopsies. Both types of tumours can be found in the squamous zone, and both can show a combination of basaloid, squamous and adenoid features and an inflammatory infiltrate in the stroma {101}. Numerous and even atypical mitoses may be present in basal cell carcinomas {2593}. However, basaloid areas in squamous carcinoma usually show less conspicuous peripheral palisading, more cellular pleomorphism, and often large, eosinophilic necrotic areas. Immunohistochemistry may be helpful in establishing the diagnosis. Basal cell carcinoma is positive for Ber-EP4 and negative for keratins 13, 19 and 22, and for carcinoembryonic antigen (CEA), epithelial membrane antigen (EMA), erythroid band 3 (AE1) and *Ulex europaeus* agglutinin 1 (UEA1), while basaloid variants SCC usually show the opposite pattern {101}.

Paget disease

Extramammary Paget disease usually affects sites with a high density of apocrine glands, such as the anogenital region, where it presents as a slowly spreading, erythematous eczematoid plaque that may extend up to the dentate line {2808}. Histologically, the basal part or whole thickness of the squamous epithelium is infiltrated by large cells with abundant pale cytoplasm and large nuclei. Occasional cells have the appearance of signet rings. Paget cells invariably react positively for mucin stains and nearly always for keratin 7, but Merkel cells and Toker cells may also be positive for the latter.

Paget disease of the anus appears to represent two entities. About half of the cases are associated with a synchronous or metachronous malignancy, most often a colorectal adenocarcinoma. Such cases can be regarded as a pagetoid extension of the tumour. They usually react positively for keratin 20 and negatively for gross cystic-disease fluid protein-15 (GCDFP-15), a marker for apocrine cells. This is in contrast to the other half of the cases, which are not associated with internal malignancies but have a high rate of local recurrence and may become invasive {1976}. Only the latter entity can be regarded as a true epidermotrophic apocrine neoplasm {145, 215, 1012, 2325}. Recently, it has been proposed that this disease arises from adnexal stem cells residing in the infundibulo-sebaceous unit of hair follicles and adnexal structures, on the basis of expression of keratins 15 and 19 {2652}.

Macroscopy. Lesions may be polypoid or sessile and infiltrating. Pigmentation of the lesion is often apparent. Satellite nodules may occur.

Histopathology. The features are similar to those of cutaneous melanomas that express S100 protein. Most cases show a junctional component adjacent to the invasive tumour, and this finding is evidence that the lesion is primary rather than metastatic.

Prognosis. Anal melanomas spread by lymphatics to regional nodes, and haematogenously to the liver and thence to other organs. Metastases are frequent at time of presentation, and the prognosis is poor; 5-year survival is < 20% {3087}. Outcomes do not support radical surgery, except for the purposes of palliation in the unusual cases that present at an early stage {292, 322}.

Mesenchymal and neurogenic tumours

These are all rare and the exact point of origin may be difficult to establish. Reports on tumours in the anorectal and perianal area include haemangioma, lymphangioma {653}, haemangiopericytoma {804}, leiomyoma, malignant fibrous histiocytoma and leiomyosarcoma {1913}, rhabdomyoma in a newborn {1744}, and rhabdomyosarcoma in childhood {2631} and adulthood {1524}, fibrosarcoma, neurilemmoma and neurofibroma {961}, granular cell tumour (myoblastoma) {1438}, spindle cell lipoma and aggressive angiomyxoma {852} and extraspinal ependymoma in a newborn {3475}. Persons infected with HIV may, in addition to the increased risk of squamous neoplasia, develop Kaposi sarcoma in the perianal area {202}.

Lymphoma

Primary lymphomas of the anorectal region are rare in the general population, but much more common in patients with AIDS, particularly homosexual men. All are of B-cell type, the most common types being large cell immunoblastic or pleomorphic {1154, 1336}. Langerhans-cell histiocytosis has been described in children {1051, 1454} and in an adult {587}.

Secondary tumours

Metastases to the anal canal and perineum are rare and present as any other lesion involving this region with pain, bleeding, a mass, or altered bowel control. Most primaries are found in the rectum or colon, but occasionally also in the respiratory tract, breast and pancreas {662, 834, 1474, 2986}. There are few reports of metastatic squamous cell carcinoma {965}. Malignant lymphoma, leukaemia and myeloma may infiltrate the anal canal, and eosinophilic granuloma has also been described {834}.

Neoplasia-like lesions / Fibroepithelial polyp

Also called fibrous polyp or anal tag, this is one of the most frequent anal lesions and is found at the dentate line, anal mucosa or in the perianal skin {3501}. Fibroepithelial polyps may be associated with local inflammation such as fissure or fistula {1879}. Granulomas can be found in about one third of skin tags in cases of Crohn disease {3208}. Others may represent the end stage of a thrombosed haemorrhoid, but remnants of haemorrhoidal vessels or signs of previous bleeding are rarely found. Most are probably of idiopathic nature as the incidence is rather similar in patients with or without anal diseases {3501}.

Grossly, the polyp is spherical or elongated with a greater diameter ranging from a few millimetres up to 4 cm. The surface is white or grey and may show superficial ulceration. Histologically, it consists of a fibrous stroma covered by squamous epithelium, which usually is a

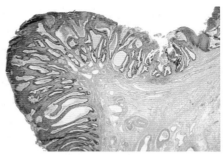

Fig. 9.13 Inflammatory cloacogenic polyp. Dilated elongated hyperplastic glands showing regenerative atypia. Surface erosion is a constant feature.

slightly hyperplastic and may be keratinized. The stroma may be more or less dense and often contains fibroblastic cells with two or more nuclei and a considerable number of mast cells {1070}. Neuronal hyperplasia is a common feature {840}.

Inflammatory cloacagenic polyp

Inflammatory cloacagenic polyps, first described in 1981 {1878}, are commonly associated with mucosal prolapse and sometimes with haemorrhoids {520, 1812}. These polyps arise in the ATZ and form a rounded or irregular mass measuring 1–5 cm in diameter. Histologically, the polyp consists of hyperplastic rectal mucosa, partly covered with ATZ-type or squamous epithelium. The surface is typically eroded and the stroma shows oedema, vascular ectasia, inflammatory cells and granulation tissue. Vertically oriented smooth-muscle fibres are found between the elongated and tortuous crypts. It can be confused with a prolapsed rectal adenoma {2464}.

Malacoplakia

Cutaneous malacoplakia may arise in immunocompromised patients and present as perianal nodules {1903}.

CHAPTER 10

Tumours of the liver and intrahepatic bile ducts

Focal nodular hyperplasia and hepatocellular adenoma

Hepatocellular carcinoma

Intrahepatic cholangiocarcinoma

Combined hepatocellular-cholangiocarcinoma

Hepatoblastoma

Mucinous cystic neoplasms

Lymphoma

Mesenchymal tumours

Secondary tumours

Diagnostic algorithms

WHO classification[a] of tumours of the liver and intrahepatic bile ducts

Epithelial tumours: hepatocellular

Benign

Hepatocellular adenoma	8170/0
Focal nodular hyperplasia	

Malignancy-associated and premalignant lesions

Large cell change (formerly "dysplasia")
Small cell change (formerly "dysplasia")
Dysplastic nodules
    Low grade
    High grade

Malignant

Hepatocellular carcinoma	8170/3
Hepatocellular carcinoma, fibrolamellar variant	8171/3
Hepatoblastoma, epithelial variants	8970/3
Undifferentiated carcinoma	8020/3

Epithelial tumours: biliary

Benign

Bile duct adenoma (peribiliary gland hamartoma and others)	8160/0
Microcystic adenoma	8202/0
Biliary adenofibroma	9013/0

Premalignant lesions

Biliary intraepithelial neoplasia, grade 3 (BilIN-3)	8148/2*
Intraductal papillary neoplasm with low- or intermediate-grade intraepithelial neoplasia	8503/0
Intraductal papillary neoplasm with high-grade intraepithelial neoplasia	8503/2*
Mucinous cystic neoplasm with low- or intermediate-grade intraepithelial neoplasia	8470/0
Mucinous cystic neoplasm with high-grade intraepithelial neoplasia	8470/2

Malignant

Intrahepatic cholangiocarcinoma	8160/3
Intraductal papillary neoplasm with an associated invasive carcinoma	8503/3*
Mucinous cystic neoplasm with an associated invasive carcinoma	8470/3

Malignancies of mixed or uncertain origin

Calcifying nested epithelial stromal tumour	8975/1*
Carcinosarcoma	8980/3
Combined hepatocellular-cholangiocarcinoma	8180/3
Hepatoblastoma, mixed epithelial-mesenchymal	8970/3
Malignant rhabdoid tumour	8963/3

Mesenchymal tumours

Benign

Angiomyolipoma (PEComa)	8860/0
Cavernous haemangioma	9121/0
Infantile haemangioma	9131/0
Inflammatory pseudotumour	
Lymphangioma	9170/0
Lymphangiomatosis	
Mesenchymal hamartoma	
Solitary fibrous tumour	8815/0

Malignant

Angiosarcoma	9120/3
Embryonal sarcoma (undifferentiated sarcoma)	8991/3
Epithelioid haemangioendothelioma	9133/3
Kaposi sarcoma	9140/3
Leiomyosarcoma	8890/3
Rhabdomyosarcoma	8900/3
Synovial sarcoma	9040/3

Germ cell tumours

Teratoma	9080/1
Yolk sac tumour (endodermal sinus tumour)	9071/3

Lymphomas

Secondary tumours

PEComa, perivascular epithelioid cell tumour.
[a] The morphology codes are from the International Classification of Diseases for Oncology (ICD-O) {904A} and the Systematized Nomenclature of Medicine (SNOMED). Behaviour is coded /0 for benign tumours, /1 for unspecified, borderline or uncertain behaviour, /2 for carcinoma in situ and grade III intraepithelial neoplasia, and /3 for malignant tumours.
* These new codes were approved by the IARC/WHO Committee for ICD-O at its meeting in March 2010.

TNM classification[a] of tumours of the liver and intrahepatic bile ducts

Hepatocellular carcinoma

T – Primary tumour
TX   Primary tumour cannot be assessed
T0   No evidence of primary tumour
T1   Solitary tumour without vascular invasion
T2   Solitary tumour with vascular invasion or multiple tumours, none more than 5 cm in greatest dimension
T3   Multiple tumours any more than 5 cm or tumour involving a major branch of the portal or hepatic vein(s)
     T3a   Multiple tumours any more than 5 cm
     T3b   Tumour involving a major branch of the portal or hepatic vein(s)
T4   Tumour(s) with direct invasion of adjacent organs other than the gall bladder or with perforation of visceral peritoneum

N – Regional lymph nodes
NX   Regional lymph nodes cannot be assessed
N0   No regional lymph-node metastasis
N1   Regional lymph-node metastasis

M – Distant metastasis
M0   No distant metastasis
M1   Distant metastasis

Stage grouping

Stage	T	N	M
Stage I	T1	N0	M0
Stage II	T2	N0	M0
Stage IIIA	T3a	N0	M0
Stage IIIB	T3b	N0	M0
Stage IIIC	T4	N0	M0
Stage IVA	Any T	N1	M0
Stage IVB	Any T	Any N	M1

Carcinoma of the intrahepatic bile ducts[b]

T – Primary tumour
TX   Primary tumour cannot be assessed
T0   No evidence of primary tumour
Tis   Carcinoma *in situ* (intraductal tumour)
T1   Solitary tumour without vascular invasion
     T2a   Solitary tumour with vascular invasion
     T2b   Multiple tumours, with or without vascular invasion
T3   Tumour perforates the visceral peritoneum or directly invades adjacent extrahepatic structures
T4   Tumour with periductal invasion (periductal growth pattern)

N – Regional lymph nodes
NX   Regional lymph nodes cannot be assessed
N0   No regional lymph-node metastasis
N1   Regional lymph-node metastasis

M – Distant metastasis
M0   No distant metastasis
M1   Distant metastasis

Stage grouping

Stage	T	N	M
Stage I	T1	N0	M0
Stage II	T2	N0	M0
Stage III	T3	N0	M0
Stage IVA	T4	N0	M0
	Any T	N1	M0
Stage IVB	Any T	Any N	M1

---

[a] {762, 2996}

[b] The classification applies to intrahepatic cholangiocarcinoma, cholangiocellular carcinoma, and combined hepatocellular and cholangiocarcinoma (mixed hepatocellular-cholangiocellular carcinoma).

A helpdesk for specific questions about the TNM classification is available at http://www.uicc.org.

Focal nodular hyperplasia and hepatocellular adenoma

P. Bioulac-Sage
C. Balabaud
I. Wanless

Focal nodular hyperplasia

Definition
Focal nodular hyperplasia (FNH) is not a true neoplasm, but a regenerative hyperplastic response of hepatocytes, secondary to localized vascular abnormalities {3456}.

Epidemiology
FNH is the second most frequent benign liver nodule (after haemangioma) and has been reported to occur in 0.8% of an adult autopsy population {3455}. In 80–90% of cases, FNH is discovered in women in their third or fourth decade of life. Three quarters of women with FNH have been long-term users of oral contraceptives (OC) suggesting that female hormones play a role in the pathogenesis of FNH {973}, although use of OC did not correlate with the size or number of lesions, making it unlikely that this is an important risk factor {2000}. In countries where OC use is less prevalent (e.g. China), FNH tends to be a lesion found in men or children of either sex {1860}.

Etiology
Pathogenesis
While the pathogenesis of FNH is not fully established, the association with conditions in which there are vascular anomalies (e.g. hereditary haemorrhagic telangiectasia) and the presence of unusually large vessels within the lesions has led to the belief that FNH is a response to focally increased blood flow {3456}. The presence of focal hepatic vein obstruction and association with Budd-Chiari syndrome suggest a role for outflow obstruction. A current hypothesis is that the primary lesion is outflow obstruction and the secondary congestive injury results in parenchymal collapse and fibrosis, arteriovenous shunting, and loss of portal veins and ducts. The sequential loss of portal veins and ducts and the replacement of congested tissue with fibrosis explain the spectrum of histological findings (Table 10.01). Since all histological features are local events in or adjacent to individual, lesional portal tracts, mixed forms occur within this spectrum.

Clinical features
In two thirds of cases, FNH is solitary {3455}. Most lesions are asymptomatic and discovered incidentally during surgery, autopsy, or imaging for unrelated symptoms. Large lesions can present with abdominal pain or compression of adjacent organs. Rare reports of haemorrhage or malignant transformation still require confirmation. FNH lesions may regress with age, as documented by serial imaging {1681, 2373}, although histological proof is absent.

The background liver is usually normal; however, classical FNH, and especially FNH variants, can occur in abnormal livers with vascular alterations (Table 10.01) {1843, 3186, 3454, 3455}.

FNH is associated with hepatic haemangioma in 20% of cases. Coexistence with hepatocellular adenoma (HCA) is rare. Associated vascular lesions outside the liver have also been reported.

Macroscopy
On cut section, classical FNH is a pale, firm mass, ranging from a few millimetres to > 10 cm in diameter. The margin is well-delimited, lobulated, and non-encapsulated. The lesion is composed of component nodules each measuring 2–3 mm, separated by zones of atrophy giving a multinodular appearance. The lesion characteristically has a central or excentric stellate scar with radiating

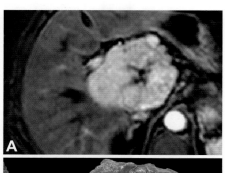

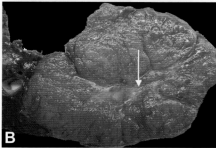

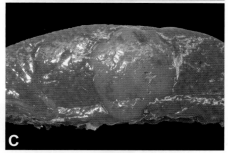

Fig. 10.01 Focal nodular hyperplasia. **A** MRI: fat-suppressed gadolinium-enhanced T1-weighted sequence (arterial phase). **B** Fresh specimen: note the multinodularity and central stellate scar (arrow). **C** Small lesion without stellate scar, but with focal areas of congestion.

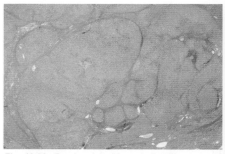

Fig. 10.02 Focal nodular hyperplasia. Fibrous septa separate hepatocellular nodules of different sizes that resemble cirrhosis (Masson trichrome).

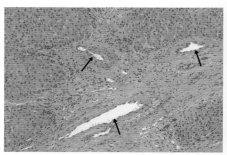

Fig. 10.03 Focal nodular hyperplasia. The arteries in the central scar are variably thick-walled (arrows).

extensions that partially surround some component nodules. FNH variants, incomplete or early forms may lack a central scar and have variably prominent regions of congestion.

Histopathology

Classical FNH lesions are composed of benign hepatocellular nodules arranged in plates no more than two cells thick. Steatosis, usually focal, may occur. The central scar contains one or more large dystrophic vessels and numerous small arterioles. The large vessels have irregular, fibrous, intimal thickening with focal medial attenuation. The internal elastic lamina is poorly formed and duplicated. Portal veins are absent. The radiating branches of scar contain portal tract-like structures with arteries unaccompanied by portal veins or ducts. When fibrous septation is prominent, the appearance may be indistinguishable from cirrhosis, especially in biopsy specimens. Stromal inflammatory infiltrates, lymphocytic or mixed, are frequent. At the stromal-parenchymal interface, cholate stasis and/or ductular reactions are often present. Sinusoids adjacent to arterial sources are lined by CD34-positive endothelium. Immunostaining reveals broad, anastomosing ("map-like") areas of (hepatocellular) expression of glutamine synthetase, often adjacent to hepatic veins {263}.

In addition to classical FNH, other nodules thought to be regenerative in nature have been reported under many different names {1335, 2274, 3455}. The existing literature concerning these rare FNH variants is confusing because diagnostic criteria have not been standardized; a

Table 10.01 Histological criteria for classical focal nodular hyperplasia (FNH) and its variants.

Criterion	Classical FNH[a]	FNH variants[b]
Fibrosis	+++	– to ++
Duct loss and ductular reaction (keratin 19+)	+++	– to +
Sinusoidal dilatation	+/– to +	– to ++
Glutamine synthetase immunostaining	Large positive anastomosing areas, often around central veins	Few data available
Background liver	Normal[c]	Normal or abnormal[d]

+ , positive; –, negative.
[a] Fibrous scar or ductular reaction may be absent, particularly in a biopsy.
[b] These variants are rare compared with classical FNH and include a variety of benign nodules considered to be regenerative in nature and containing portal tracts. These have been classified over the years under a variety of names that are not yet universally accepted, including early FNH, pre-FNH, subtle FNH, FNH-like nodules, telangiectatic FNH, large regenerative nodules, or partial nodular transformation. These lesions may have a focal component of classical FNH.
[c] Steatosis may be seen in the otherwise normal liver.
[d] In addition to possible steatosis, livers may show vascular disorders, including portal thrombosis or atresia, patent ductus venosus, hepatic vein thrombosis, hereditary haemorrhagic telangiectasia, or cirrhosis.

universally accepted terminology awaits further characterization of the FNH variants using modern techniques of imaging, immunohistochemistry and molecular analysis {264, 2456, 3608}.

Molecular pathology

Clonal analysis using the human androgen receptor (HUMARA) test demonstrates the reactive, polyclonal nature of FNH liver cells in 50–100% of cases {264, 2459}. Recent studies have shown that mRNA expression of the angiopoietin genes (ANGPT1 and ANGPT2) involved in vessel maturation is altered, with the ratio of ANGPT1 to ANGPT2 being increased compared with normal liver, cirrhosis, and other liver tumours {2457, 2645}, supporting the importance of vascular alterations in the pathogenesis of FNH.

In FNH lesions, the β-catenin pathway is activated, including the downstream target, glutamine synthetase {2646}, which explains the expansion of hepatocytes expressing glutamine synthetase that is so useful for histological diagnosis. While the molecular mechanisms of this activation are uncertain, they do not involve demonstrable mutations in β-catenin (CTNNB1) or axin 1 (AXIN1).

Prognosis and predictive factors

In centres with experience in this field, an accurate diagnosis can be made using imaging techniques in 90% of cases. Contrast-enhanced ultrasonography (CEUS) is the modality of choice {376, 1562}. Magnetic resonance imaging (MRI) and triple-phase computed tomography (CT) are useful when CEUS is not available. In < 10% of cases, the differential

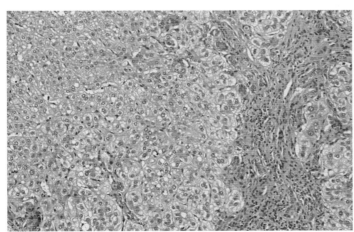

Fig. 10.04 Focal nodular hyperplasia displaying cholate stasis in periseptal hepatocytes, ductular reaction at stromal–parenchymal interface, and septal inflammation.

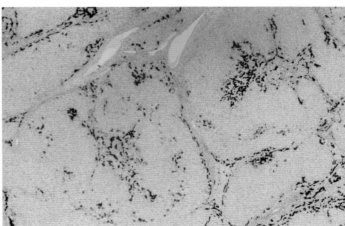

Fig. 10.05 Focal nodular hyperplasia. Immunostaining for keratin 7 highlights the prominent ductular reaction at the septal–parenchymal interface.

Table 10.02 Typical features of focal nodular hyperplasia (FNH) with various imaging modalities.

Imaging modality	Main nodule	Central scar region
Magnetic resonance imaging (MRI)		
T1-weighted	Iso- or slightly hypointense	Hypointense
Chemical shift sequences	No signal dropout	
T2-weighted	Iso- or slightly hyperintense	Hyperintense
Gadolinium-enhanced imaging		
Arterial phase	Hyperintense	Hypointense
Portal venous phase	Isointense	Hypo-, iso-, or hyperintense
Delayed phase	Isointense	Hyperintense
Baseline grey-scale ultrasonography	Slightly hypoechoic, isoechoic, or hyperechoic	Slightly hyperechoic[a]
Colour Doppler		
Vascularity	Hypervascular	
Arteries	Feeding artery[a]	Central stellate vasculature[a]
Veins	Peripheral draining veins[a]	
Contrast-enhanced ultrasonography (CEUS)		
Arterial phase	Hypervascular	Central scar not visualized
Filling pattern	Centrifugal	
Portal venous phase	Iso- or hyperechoic	Hypoechoic[a]
Delayed phase	Isoechoic	Hypoechoic[a]
[a] Inconsistent		

diagnosis of FNH, hepatocellular adenoma (HCA), and hepatocellular carcinoma (HCC) cannot be solved by imaging alone. A biopsy with standard and/or immunohistochemical stainings, interpreted by an experienced liver pathologist, can resolve most of these problem cases. Differential diagnosis may be impossible on the basis of biopsy only; if the result is not definitive, surgery may be advocated.

The histological diagnosis of FNH requires two main criteria: the lesion must be composed of benign-appearing hepatocytes and must be supplied by altered portal tracts. Ensuring that the biopsy includes the lesion may be difficult, since cirrhosis attributable to any cause may closely resemble FNH. It is therefore recommended that a biopsy be accompanied by a sample of nonlesional liver.

HCA is the most frequent lesion to be distinguished from FNH. In most cases this is straightforward because adenomas are supplied by isolated arteries, not portal tracts. A source of difficulty in this regard is the presence of ductular elements that are positive for keratin 7 in HCA of the inflammatory type. The key feature is that expression of glutamine synthetase shows a distinctive map-like distribution adjacent to hepatic veins in FNH, while expression is diffusely positive in β-catenin-activated HCA and mostly negative in other types of HCA.

HCC may mimic FNH by the presence of focal scarring, arterialized sinusoids, and residual portal-tract remnants. Warning signs of malignancy include nuclear pleomorphism, wide plates, a high nucleus-to-cytoplasm ratio, mitotic figures in the lesion and often cirrhosis in the background liver.

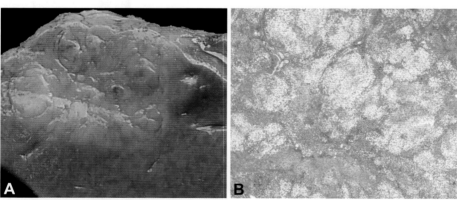

Fig. 10.06 Small steatotic focal nodular hyperplasia. **A** Surgical specimen. **B** Masson trichrome staining.

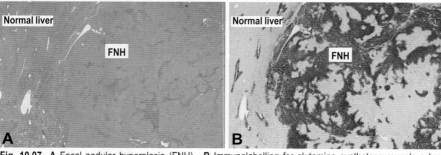

Fig. 10.07 A Focal nodular hyperplasia (FNH). **B** Immunolabelling for glutamine synthetase reveals a broad, anastomosing "map-like" pattern of staining within the lesion and the normal, perivenular pattern outside.

Hepatocellular adenoma

Definition
Hepatocellular adenoma (HCA) is a benign liver neoplasm composed of hepatocytes.

ICD-O code
8170/0

Epidemiology
The incidence of HCA is about 3–4 per 100 000 population in Europe and North America {2723} but lower in Asia. Eighty-five percent of cases occur in young women; HCA is rare in children, men, and the elderly.

Etiology
The major risk factor for HCA is exposure to estrogenic or androgenic steroids. In young women with HCA, 80% have been users of oral contraceptives (OC) and risk increases with duration of use. The prevalence appears to be declining as low-estrogen preparations become more widespread. The lesions usually shrink after stopping OC or after menopause. Most men developing HCA have been

users of anabolic steroids for the purpose of bodybuilding. Patients taking androgens for Fanconi anaemia or acquired aplastic anaemia are also at risk {3389}. Nonhormonal risk factors include glycogenosis type 1 (von Gierke disease) or 3 (Forbes disease), galactosaemia, tyrosinaemia, familial polyposis coli, and hepatic iron overload with β-thalassemia {2960}. Obesity has recently been shown to be a risk factor for a particular HCA subtype.

Clinical features

Clinical presentation may include abdominal pain, abdominal mass, intraperitoneal haemorrhage, abnormal liver tests, or a liver mass found incidentally during an imaging study. HCA can be single or multiple. When 10 or more adenomas occur, the condition is known as "adenomatosis" {873, 3400}. Clinically significant haemorrhage is observed in 20–25% of cases; the risk being highest when the tumours are > 5 cm. Malignant transformation to hepatocellular carcinoma (HCC) is rare but well-documented, occurring in up to 7% of cases reported from referral centres {260, 730, 2059}. The risk of transformation varies with HCA subtype and with clinical association, being higher in patients with glycogenosis or androgenic–anabolic steroid use.

Macroscopy

HCAs are typically large, globular tumours with prominent vessels in the overlying hepatic capsule. On cut section, the parenchyma is soft and relatively uniform, although congestion, necrosis, haemorrhage, or fibrosis are frequent. The margins of the lesion are ill-defined, grossly and microscopically, with little or no fibrous capsule. Size varies from microscopic to 20 cm in diameter. In livers with adenomatosis, hundreds of lesions may be visible grossly as minute ill-defined nodules or only microscopically. HCA may be similar in colour and texture to the background liver, but steatosis, major congestion and haemorrhage or degenerative changes can make it distinct. The background liver is usually normal or altered in colour related to associated fatty-liver disease, glycogen-storage disease, or iron overload.

Histopathology

HCA is typically composed of benign hepatocytes arranged in regular plates, usu-

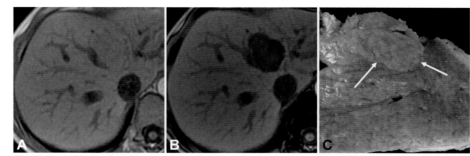

Fig. 10.08 HNF1α-inactivated hepatocellular adenoma. MRI: Homogeneous segment IV lesion displaying isointensity on T1W image (**A**) and critical homogenous signal drop-out on phased opposed T1W image (**B**) due to massive fat component. **C** Fresh specimen: yellowish tumour (arrows).

ally one or at most two cells thick. There may be very focal pseudogland formation. Tumour hepatocytes have cytoplasm that may be normal, clear (glycogen-rich), steatotic, or contain pigment in lysosomes. Nuclear atypia and mitoses are unusual. The tumour parenchyma is supplied by isolated arteries unaccompanied by bile ducts. Variations in this typical pattern are frequently seen in some of the subtypes.

As the deviation from normal liver histology may be minimal, it is very important to obtain a simultaneous biopsy of nontumoral liver, to confirm the presence or absence of cirrhosis in particular.

Differential diagnosis

Fibrosis or the presence of ductules within the lesion, particularly in inflammatory HCA, may hinder differential diagnosis with FNH. In such cases, the identification of FNH or HCA by immunostaining for glutamine synthetase is very useful.

Mitoses are extremely rare in HCA and their presence indicates that HCC should be considered. Arterialized sinusoids (CD34+) are almost always found in HCCs, but may also be found in some HCAs. Cytoplasmic pigment, when present, suggests that the lesion is slow-growing and thus favours HCA over HCC. Angiomyolipoma may also resemble HCA, but can be differentiated by immunohistochemistry.

Molecular pathology

HCA represents a heterogeneous entity, recently subclassified into several groups according to genotype and phenotype. These subtypes vary greatly in their clinical, pathological, and radiological features {265, 1757, 3727}.

HNF1α-inactivated HCA

The *HNF1A* gene encodes hepatocyte nuclear factor 1 (HNF1α), a transcription factor that is involved in hepatocyte

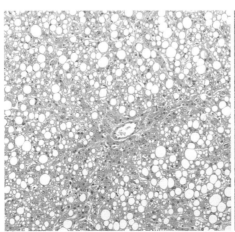

Fig. 10.09 HNF1α-inactivated hepatocellular adenoma. Benign, steatotic hepatocytes are intermingled with isolated thin-walled arteries.

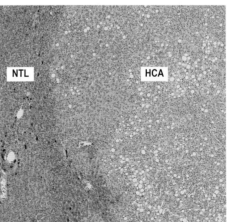

Fig 10.10 HNF1α-inactivated hepatocellular adenoma. In contrast to the adjacent nontumoral liver (NTL), the steatotic and nonsteatotic tumoral hepatocytes lack normal expression of L-FABP.

Table 10.03 Histological features of subtypes of hepatocellular adenoma (HCA).

Histological feature	HNF1α–inactivated HCA	β-Catenin-activated HCA	Inflammatory HCA[a]	Unclassified HCA
Steatosis	Usually +++ Rarely + Extremely rarely –	–	– to ++ (heterogeneous) rarely +++	+/–
Sinusoidal dilatation and peliosis	– to +	– to +/–	– to +++	– to ++
Ductular reaction	–	–	+/– to +++	–
Abnormal thick arteries	–	–	+ to ++	– to +/–
Inflammatory reaction	– to +/–	–	+ to +++	–/+
Cytological abnormalities	–	+	–[b]	–
Remodelling (necrosis, haemorrhage, fibrotic bands)	– to +/–	– to +/–	– to ++	– to +/–
Immunohistochemistry				
L-FABP[c]	–	+	+	+
Glutamine synthetase[d]	–	+	–[b]	–
β-Catenin (aberrant nuclear expression)	–	+	–[b]	–
SAA/CRP[e]	–	–	+ to +++	–

L-FABP, liver fatty acid-binding protein; HNF1α, hepatocyte nuclear factor 1 α; SAA/CRP, Serum amyloid A/C reactive protein. Grading: +, mild; ++, moderate; +++, severe; –, absent.

[a] Can also have mutant β-catenin; [b] Except if β-catenin is mutated; [c] Normally expressed in nontumoral liver; [d] Glutamine synthetase is occasionally expressed at the periphery and around veins of any HCA without β-catenin mutation; [e] Rarely, only one is expressed; occasionally, both can be overexpressed in nontumoral liver as a general inflammatory reaction (i.e. in response to bleeding).

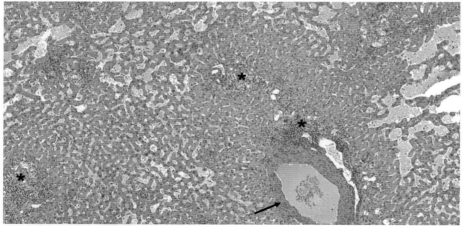

Fig. 10.11 Inflammatory hepatocellular adenoma. Note the sinusoidal dilatation, inflammatory infiltrates (asterisks) and thick-walled artery (arrow).

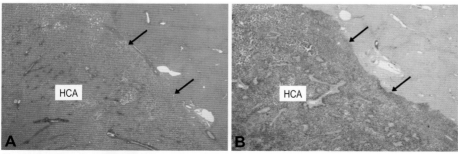

Fig. 10.12 Inflammatory hepatocellular adenoma (HCA). **A** The limits of the tumour (arrows) are ill-defined on haematoxylin & eosin staining. **B** Amyloid A is strongly overexpressed by adenomatous hepatocytes, clearly demarcated from the nontumoral liver (arrows).

differentiation. Biallelic inactivating mutations of this gene are found in approximately 35–40% of HCA; 90% of *HNF1A* mutations are somatic, while the remaining 10%, are constitutional (germline) {288}. Heterozygous germline mutations in *HNF1A* are responsible for an autosomal dominant form of diabetes, MODY3 (maturity-onset diabetes of the young type 3). Patients with MODY3 and HCA carry an additional somatic mutation of the second allele. In rare cases, germline mutations of *HNF1A* could cause genetic predisposition to the development of HCA via a carcinogenic pathway other than the complete inactivation of HNF1α. Germline heterozygous mutations in *CYP1B1* could also participate in genetic predisposition to the development of HNF1α-inactivated HCA {1410}.

HNF1α-inactivated HCAs represent a homogeneous group of tumours with lobulated contours, showing typically marked and diffuse steatosis, and absence of significant inflammation or nuclear atypia. *FABP1*, encoding L-FABP (liver fatty-acid binding protein), a gene that is positively regulated by *HNF1A*, is expressed in normal liver tissue and clearly downregulated in this HCA subtype. Immunohistochemically, there is nearly complete absence of L-FABP staining, in contrast to the nontumoral surrounding liver, which appears homogeneously, although faintly stained. Therefore, lack of L-FABP expression is an excellent diagnostic argument for HNF1α-inactivated HCA. Furthermore, the downregulation of L-FABP may contribute to the fatty phenotype through impaired fatty-acid trafficking {2647}. HCA associated with mutant *HNF1A* occurs almost exclusively in women. Nodules can be solitary or multiple. Most adenomatosis contains mutant *HNF1A*. Constitutional mutations can affect both sexes, and can be discovered in children, sometimes in a familial form or in association with MODY3 {173}.

β-Catenin-activated HCA

An activating mutation in β-catenin is found in 10–15% of HCA cases. *GLUL*, which encodes glutamine synthetase, a target of β-catenin, is also upregulated. This HCA subtype is often associated with specific conditions (i.e. glycogenosis, administration of male hormones) and male sex. The lesions are usually solitary (except in glycogenosis) and have an increased risk of malignant transformation,

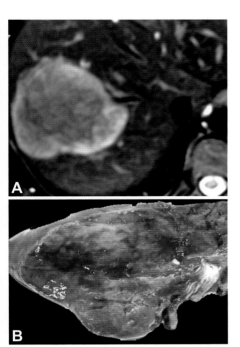

Fig. 10.13 Inflammatory hepatocellular adenoma. **A** On the fat-suppressed T2-weighted MRI sequence, the tumour displays a high signal intensity, especially at the periphery. **B** The resected specimen shows an ill-defined tumour with congested areas.

compared with the other subtypes. Steatosis and inflammation are usually absent. Since nuclear atypia and a pseudoglandular growth pattern are frequent in this subtype, distinguishing β-catenin-activated HCA from well-differentiated HCC may be very difficult. By immunohistochemistry, glutamine synthetase is usually strongly expressed in a diffuse pattern, associated with aberrant cytoplasmic and nuclear β-catenin. When glutamine synthetase staining is heterogeneous and β-catenin staining is non-conclusive, molecular techniques can identify the presence of mutations in β-catenin.

Inflammatory HCA

Inflammatory HCA, also known as telangiectatic adenoma {2458}, represents more than half of HCA cases. IHCA is characterized by increased expression of inflammation-associated proteins such as amyloid A (SAA) and C-reactive protein (CRP), at both the mRNA and protein levels. About 60% of these adenomas have mutations in gp130 {2644}; β-catenin mutations coexist with gp130 mutations in

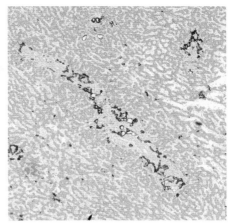

Fig. 10.15 Inflammatory hepatocellular adenoma. Immunostaining for keratin 7 highlights ductular reaction.

10% of inflammatory HCAs.

Most patients with this subtype are women. Obesity and fatty-liver disease are frequent {260, 2458}. In 50% of cases, serum levels of CRP are elevated and erythrocyte sedimentation rate is increased, in rare cases, in association with fever and anaemia; these features can regress after resection. Nodules can be solitary or multiple.

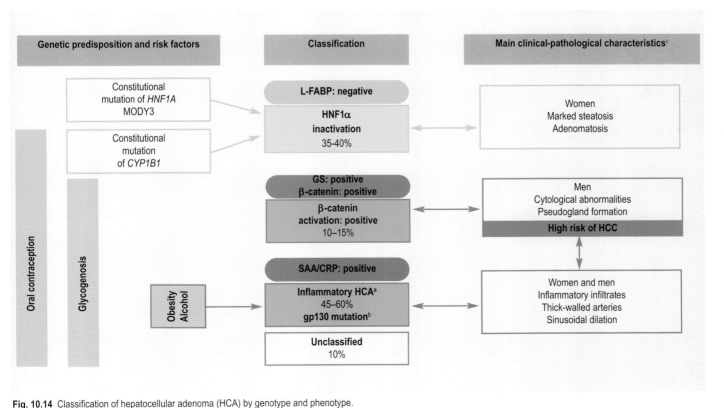

Fig. 10.14 Classification of hepatocellular adenoma (HCA) by genotype and phenotype.
GS, glutamine synthetase; HCC, hepatocellular carcinoma; SAA/CRP, serum amyloid A/C-reactive protein.
[a] 10% of HCAs also have mutant β-catenin; [b] Mutations in the gene encoding gp130 are found in 60% of inflammatory HCAs; [c] These characteristics are frequent, but not exclusive.

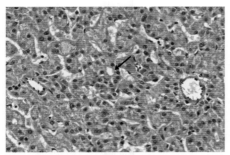

Fig. 10.16 Hepatocellular adenoma with mutant β-catenin in a young boy treated with androgens for anaplastic anaemia. There are mild cytological and architectural abnormalities, including rare pseudoglands (arrow).

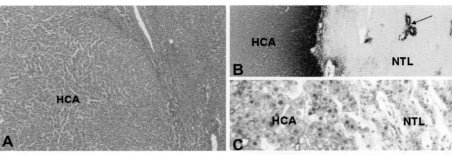

Fig. 10.17 Hepatocellular adenoma (HCA) with mutant β-catenin (**A**). **B** Note the strong and diffuse overexpression of glutamine synthetase, contrasting with normal expression in centrilobular hepatocytes (arrow) of nontumoral liver (NTL). **C** There is aberrant cytoplasmic and nuclear expression of β-catenin in the tumoral hepatocytes.

Histologically, inflammatory HCA typically exhibits focal or diffuse inflammation, sinusoidal dilatation, congestion and peliotic areas, numerous thick-walled arteries often in association with ductular reaction, lying in small amounts of connective tissue. There may be focal steatosis. Immunohistochemistry reveals strong expression of SAA and CRP in tumour hepatocytes. Micronodules can also be detected by immunostaining for SAA and CRP in the liver parenchyma, outside the main tumours {261}. There is a risk of malignant transformation, particularly for cases in which β-catenin is also mutant.

Unclassified HCA
HCAs without distinguishing histological features and without known mutations represent < 10% of all cases.

Prognosis and predictive factors
Radiological diagnosis can be difficult owing to the variable and nonspecific features of HCA. However, the two major HCA subtypes (i.e. HNF1α-inactivated and inflammatory) can now be identified using magnetic resonance imaging (MRI), which has greatly helped the diagnosis of HCA {324, 1757, 1824}.
Clinical or biological context, including absence of cirrhosis and history of hormone exposure is often helpful, but cannot be definitive. Biopsy fulfils two goals: to make the differential diagnosis between HCA, FNH, and well-differentiated HCC, and to classify HCA subtypes. Recognition of β-catenin-activated HCA is important for patient management {260}. Patients with large (> 5 cm) nodules, either HCA or unclassified, should be treated (surgery, radiofrequency, embolization); but tissue should be taken for confirmation of diagnosis {260, 730}.

Hepatocellular carcinoma

N.D. Theise
M.P. Curado
S. Franceschi
P. Hytiroglou
M. Kudo

Y.N. Park
M. Sakamoto
M. Torbenson
A. Wee

Definition
A malignant tumour with hepatocellular differentiation.

ICD-O codes
Hepatocellular carcinoma   8170/3
   Fibrolamellar variant   8171/3
   Undifferentiated carcinoma   8020/3

Epidemiology
Primary liver cancer is the second most common cancer in Asia and the fourth most common in Africa. In 2002, the global number of new cases in males was estimated at 442 119; there were 416 882 deaths, 94% of which occurred in the first year after diagnosis. For females, there were an estimated 184 043 new cases globally, most of which occurred in eastern regions of Asia {634, 842}.

Hepatocellular carcinoma (HCC) is the most common histological type of primary liver cancer. Population-based cancer registries show that the incidence of HCC, as a percentage of histologically specified tumours, is higher in North America and Europe than in Asia. Regions where the incidence of HCC is < 30% of histo-logically specified tumours are exceptional, e.g. Lampang, Thailand, where intrahepatic cholangiocarcinoma is predominant owing to infection by endemic liver fluke (*Opisthorchis viverrini*) {2487}.

Geographical distribution
Rates of HCC are highest in East Asia (China, Japan), but are also moderately high in Italy. With annual age-standardized incidence rates (ASIR, standardized to world population) of < 7 per 100 000, low-risk areas include North and South America, South–Central Asia, Northern Europe, Australia and New Zealand. With > 80% of reported global cases, less developed countries carry the greatest burden of disease.

Geographical variations in HCC incidence and mortality are ascribed to different levels of exposure to HCC-associated risk factors: chronic infection with hepatitis B virus (HBV) or hepatitis C virus (HCV) and exposure to aflatoxin in developing countries, smoking and alcohol abuse in developed countries {2389, 2509, 2605}. In Japan, local differences in the age-standardized mortality rate (ASMR, standardized to world

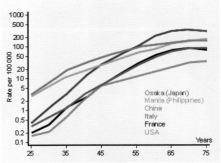

Fig. 10.19 Age-specific incidence of liver cancer in men in selected countries {842A}.

population) reflect the sero-prevalence of antibodies to HCV among blood donors {122, 2488, 3183, 3314}.

Time trends
The overall incidence of HCC remains high in developing countries and is steadily rising in most industrialized countries {2903}. In Asia, incidence rates are highest in China, but a slight decrease has been reported for the period 1998–2002 {3701}. A decrease in incidence rates has also been observed in other regions of Asia {2489}.

In the United States of America (USA), there has been an increase of about 80% in the annual incidence of HCC, and this has been more marked in African Americans. Similar increases have been reported in the United Kingdom (UK), Canada and Australia. These changes may, at least in part, be ascribed to increases in chronic infection with HCV.

Age and sex distribution
Age-specific incidence rates differ significantly between countries. In males aged 25–49 years, liver cancer is the second most common tumour in Asia and the third most common in Africa, while in males aged 50–69 years, liver cancer ranks as the second most common tumour in Africa and the third in Asia. In females, liver cancer is the fifth most common in Africa in those aged 50–69 years and the third most common cancer at age 70 years. The geographical distribution

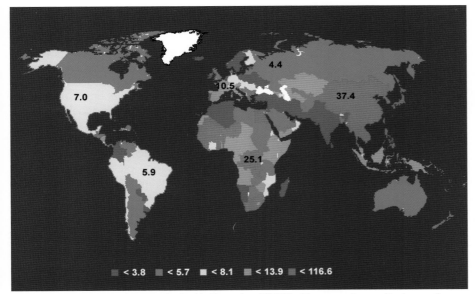

Fig. 10.18 Worldwide annual age-standardized incidence (per 100 000) of liver cancer in men. Numbers on the map indicate regional average values {842A}.

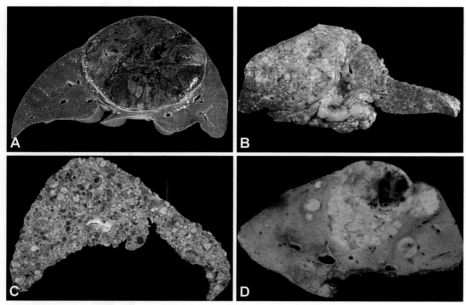

Fig. 10.20 Hepatocellular carcinoma. **A** Nodular type. **B** Massive type. **C** Diffuse type. **D** With multiple ("satellite") nodules of intrahepatic metastases.

of HCC is similar for males and females, although males have a considerably higher risk of developing HCC. Data for 2002 show that ASIR reaches 50–25 per 100 000 males in East Asia (China, Japan), while rates in Europe reach about 25 per 100 000 in some regions of Italy.

A similar pattern is found for females in the same regions; however, the highest rates are about 14 per 100 000 {634, 842}.

Etiology

Chronic viral infection (HBV or HCV or coinfection) is the most important cause

of HCC, accounting for approximately 85% of cases {2483, 2641}. Alcohol-induced liver injury constitutes the most important nonviral risk factor {887}. Tobacco-smoking has also been recently recognized as a risk factor for HCC {1333}. In southern China and sub-Saharan Africa, high dietary ingestion of aflatoxin is an environmental hazard, particularly in individuals infected with HBV {1331}. Iron overload, particularly in the context of hereditary haemochromatosis, is also an exogenous risk factor {1528}. α-1-Antitrypsin deficiency greatly increases the risk of developing HCC. It has become apparent that obesity, with its accompanying problems of diabetes mellitus and nonalcoholic steato-hepatitis, can increase the risk of HCC, even without viral infection {781, 2570}. The risk of acquiring HCC increases if multiple risk factors are present {887, 3131}.

Liver cirrhosis

The major clinical risk factor for HCC is liver cirrhosis, largely independently of its etiology, though cirrhosis itself is now not considered premalignant, but rather a parallel process to malignant transformation in the setting of chronic liver disease {3229}.

HBV

HBV is a DNA virus belonging to the hepadnavirus group. The virus consists of an outer envelope, composed mainly of hepatitis B surface antigen (HBsAg), and an internal core (nucleocapsid), which contains hepatitis B core antigen (HBcAg), a DNA polymerase/reverse transcriptase, and the viral genome. The genome comprises a well-characterized, partly double-stranded, circular DNA molecule of about 3200 base pairs. Sequencing of HBV genomes and the S gene has revealed eight genotypes (A–H) and several subgenotypes {2320}; the distribution of the different types and subtypes differs according to geographical location and the predominant transmission modality and can affect response to antiviral treatment with lamivudine.

The World Health Organization (WHO) estimates that about 350 million people are chronically infected with HBV worldwide. HBV is the predominant cause of HCC in most Asian, African, and Latin American countries {2641}. Epidemiological studies show a convincing link between chronic HBV infection and HCC development.

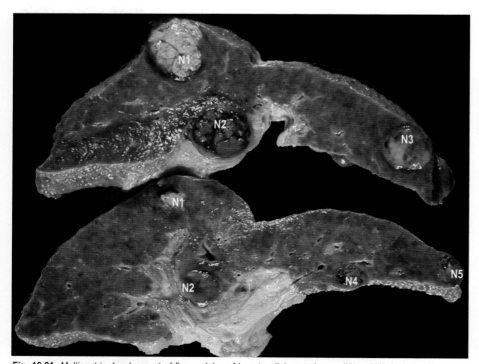

Fig. 10.21 Multicentric development of five nodules of hepatocellular carcinoma (N1 to N5), including two early hepatocellular carcinomas (N4 and N5).

The incidence of HCC in individuals who are chronically infected with HBV is approximately 100 times higher than in the uninfected population, and the lifetime risk of HCC in males infected at birth approaches 50%. Several lines of evidence support a direct oncogenic role for HBV in the development of HCC: (1) the integration of HBV DNA into the chromosomal DNA of HCCs; (2) the role of the HBV X gene in the pathogenesis of HBV-associated HCCs, in particular, binding to and inactivation of p53; (3) the development of HCC in animal models of chronic he-

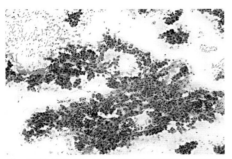

Fig. 10.22 Well-differentiated hepatocellular carcinoma: the cohesive clusters of malignant hepatocytes appear as slender arborizing cords (Papanicolaou).

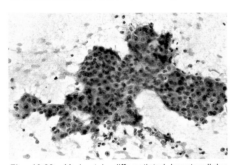

Fig. 10.23 Moderately differentiated hepatocellular carcinoma: the cohesive clusters of malignant hepatocytes with broad cords (more than five cells thick) are wrapped by endothelium. Note the granular cytoplasm, increased nucleus:cytoplasm ratio, centrally placed round nuclei with well-delineated nuclear membrane, granular chromatin and distinct nucleolus (Papanicolaou).

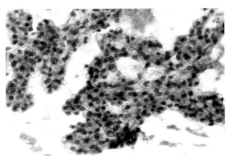

Fig. 10.24 Hepatocellular carcinoma with trabecular arrangement and clear cell change (Papanicolaou).

padnavirus infection; and (4) the declining incidence of HCC after mass HBV vaccination {484}.

HCV
HCV has a single-stranded RNA genome that codes for a single polyprotein consisting of 3010–3033 amino acids. Post-translational processing yields the structural protein C (RNA-binding nucleocapsid protein), E1 and E2 envelope proteins, and nonstructural proteins NS1–NS5, including RNA-dependent RNA polymerase {3241}. HCV isolated from various geographical regions shows marked genetic heterogeneity, with at least six different genotypes in distinct patterns of geographical distribution. The HCV genome readily mutates, with the genes for the envelope proteins E1 and E2 appearing to be particularly variable. Rapid replication and lack of proofreading function – characteristics that are typical of RNA viruses – explain the enormous genetic variability of HCV and the difficulties encountered in eradicating HCV infection, even with multidrug therapy. There is no prophylactic vaccine against HCV. WHO estimates that about 180 million people are infected with HCV worldwide, but there is evidence that the prevalence of HCV is greatly underestimated and is still increasing in some less developed countries {2641}.

HCV is more commonly found than HBV in patients with HCCs in Europe, Japan and the USA, but also in a few less developed countries (e.g. Egypt, Mongolia and Pakistan) {2641} where HCV is spread through unscreened blood and non-sterile injections {2586}.

HCV-associated HCCs typically develop 20–30 years after infection and are usually, but not always, preceded by cirrhosis. Thus far, there is no evidence to suggest a direct, molecular role for HCV in the pathogenesis of HCC. Rather, HCC develops via HCV-induced chronic liver injury in parallel with progression to fibrosis and cirrhosis. The average time from infection to onset of cirrhosis in published studies was 13–25 years and time to onset of liver cancer 17–31 years {1841}. The risk of liver cancer among individuals with HCV-related cirrhosis ranged between 1% and 7% per year.

Hepatitis D virus (HDV)
HDV ("delta") is an RNA-defective virus requiring HBV for infection {2695}. It is un-

clear whether chronic HDV infection increases the risk of developing HCC over that for HBV infection alone {825}.

Alcohol
In the USA and northern Europe, alcohol-induced liver injury is a leading cause of chronic liver disease and liver cirrhosis {2641}. Heavy alcohol consumption in men {3681} and even moderate consumption (two or more drinks per day) in women {93} are associated with a two-fold increased risk of acquiring HCC. Patients who drink heavily and have coexisting liver disease from other causes have the highest risk of developing HCC {887}.

Tobacco
An association between tobacco-smoking and HCC has been established recently {1333}. Independently of alcohol use or viral infection, the risk of acquiring HCC has been shown to increase with duration of smoking and number of cigarettes smoked per day.

Aflatoxin B1 (AFB1)
AFB1 is a potent liver carcinogen {2485} produced by the moulds *Aspergillus parasiticus* and *A. flavus*. Under hot and humid tropical conditions, these moulds can contaminate grain, particularly ground nuts (peanuts). Dietary ingestion

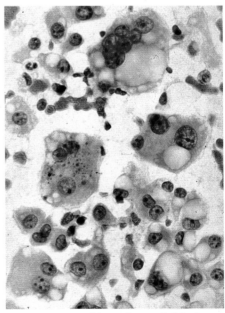

Fig. 10.25 Hepatocellular carcinoma with fatty change, bile and giant cells. Dissociated malignant hepatocytes show pleomorphism and multinucleation (Papanicolaou).

of high levels of aflatoxins, particularly in the context of coexisting chronic HBV infection {2133, 3131}, increases the risk of HCC by more than 50-fold. AFB1 is metabolized by cytochrome P450 enzymes to its reactive form, AFB1-5,9-oxide. Binding to DNA at the N7 position of guanine preferentially causes a G:C > T:A mutation in codon 249 of the *TP53* tumour-suppressor gene, resulting in the substitution of arginine for serine {333}, which is most often found in areas of the world with the highest levels of food contamination with AFB1 {2133}. Use of low-technology approaches at the subsistence-farm level in sub-Saharan Africa reduces exposure to aflatoxins {3323}.

Clinical features

Symptoms and signs

The presenting signs and symptoms in patients with HCC may be caused by the tumour itself or by an advanced stage of chronic liver disease predisposing to malignancy. Thus, symptoms include abdominal pain, general malaise, anorexia or weight loss, and nausea or vomiting. Common clinical signs include hepatomegaly, ascites, fever, jaundice, and splenomegaly.

The laboratory findings are partly determined by the underlying liver disease and may be reflected in changes in the results of blood tests for liver enzymes, which are not, however, HCC-specific. A significantly raised serum level of α-fetoprotein (AFP) of > 400 ng/ml, or a continuous rise even if < 100 ng/ml, strongly suggests HCC. However, most HCCs are not associated with elevated AFP levels, particularly as HCC lesions are detected at earlier stages, and mildly raised AFP lev-

els may also be found in liver disease without HCC. AFP levels, therefore, have to be interpreted individually in the context of other clinical symptoms and signs, as well as imaging studies.

There are also uncommon paraneoplastic syndromes, such as erythrocytosis, hypoglycaemia or hypercalcaemia.

Imaging

Imaging studies are important in patient management for the identification and localization of HCC. Useful techniques include ultrasonography (US), colour Doppler US, contrast-enhanced US, computed tomography (CT), lipiodol CT, magnetic resonance imaging (MRI), angiography, CT during hepatic arteriography (CTHA), and CT during arterial portography (CTAP). The standard imaging techniques are US, CT and MRI. In most cases, these allow detection and staging of HCC. Typical findings associated with HCCs that have progressed are arterial hypervascularity with venous wash-out on dynamic CT, dynamic MRI or contrast-enhanced US {352, 1672}.

However, early HCC (vaguely-nodular type HCC) presents a different dynamic imaging pattern: isovascular, hypovascular, or rarely hypervascular arterial supply on dynamic CT, dynamic MRI, or CTHA associated with preserved portal supply on CTAP. A problematic issue in the diagnosis of early HCC via imaging is that these findings are frequently shared by dysplastic nodules (DN) {125, 1672}. Of the existing imaging modalities, gadolinium-ethoxybenzyl DTPA (Gd-EOB-DTPA) MRI seems to be the most sensitive imaging tool for the differentiation of early HCC from DN {1671A}.

Macroscopy

Most HCCs are nodular lesions. The macroscopic features vary according to tumour size and the presence or absence of liver cirrhosis. In the presence of cirrhosis, HCC often has a fibrous pseudocapsule, while in livers without cirrhosis HCC tends to be unencapsulated. HCCs are typically softer than the background liver and may be unifocal or multifocal. Multifocality is defined as tumour nodules clearly separated by intervening non-neoplastic liver. Multifocal tumours may represent either independent HCCs arising simultaneously (i.e. multicentric HCC), or intrahepatic metastases from a primary tumour. Unifocal tumours may grow as single nodules or as clusters of closely approximated and contiguous individual nodules.

The term "massive type" has been used for HCC growing as a large dominant mass, with or without smaller satellite nodules. Another subtype, pedunculated HCC, is defined as a tumour mass protruding outside of the liver, with or without a pedicle. Pedunculated HCC was initially reported to have a good prognosis, although this has not been confirmed in all studies. HCC metastatic to the right adrenal gland can mimic and should be distinguished from pedunculated HCC. Diffuse or cirrhotomimetic HCC is a rare HCC growth pattern in which numerous small tumour nodules are distributed throughout the liver in a diffuse pattern that closely mimics the regenerative nodules of liver cirrhosis. The macroscopic appearance of HCC can be further modified by varying degrees of necrosis and tumour involvement of portal and hepatic veins.

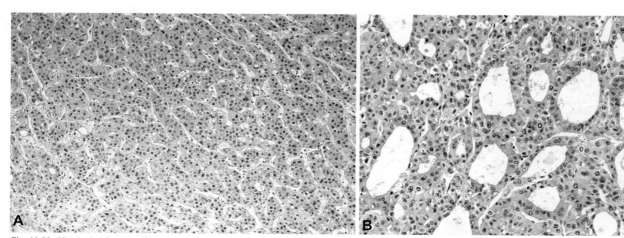

Fig. 10.26 Histological features of hepatocellular carcinomas. **A** Trabecular pattern. **B** Pseudoglandular or acinar pattern.

In addition, the production of bile or fat and the accumulation of cytoplasmic material such as glycogen can affect the macroscopic findings.

Tumour spread

HCC may spread by lymphatic and haematogenous routes. Intrahepatic spread via the portal veins is common and its frequency increases with tumour size. Tumour invasion into the major bile ducts is infrequent clinically, but found in about 5% of autopsy cases. In clinical follow-up studies, the lungs are the most common target for extrahepatic metastasis (47% of metastatic HCCs), followed closely by the lymph nodes (45%), bone (37%), and the adrenal glands (12%) {3338}.

Histopathology
Classical HCC

HCCs consist of tumour cells that usually resemble hepatocytes. The stroma is composed of sinusoid-like blood spaces lined by a single layer of endothelial cells. Unlike the sinusoidal endothelial cells in normal liver tissue, those of HCC show changes of "capillarization", i.e. they resemble normal capillaries, including immunohistochemically demonstrable CD34, factor-VIII-related antigen and subendothelial laminin and type IV collagen. Ultrastructural observation confirms a basement-membrane-like structure between the endothelial cells and tumour-cell trabeculae {797, 1565, 1569}. The blood supply of HCCs is derived from newly formed arteries, which are termed "unpaired" or "nontriadal" arteries because they are not part of portal tracts. Portal tracts are not present in HCC tissue; however, at the tumour periphery, entrapped portal tracts may be seen among invasive neoplastic cells.

HCCs vary architecturally and cytologically. The different architectural patterns and cytological variants frequently occur in combination. Immunohistochemically, HCC is characterized by cytoplasmic positivity with antibodies to carbamoyl phosphate synthetase-1 (HepPar1). It has been reported that about 90% of all HCCs are positive for HepPar1; positivity is less frequent in poorly differentiated or scirrhous HCCs {552}. Canalicular patterns may be seen with immunohistochemical staining with polyclonal antibodies to carcinoembryonic antigen(CEA) or antibodies to CD10 or ABCB1/MDR1. HCC is also often positive for AFP, fibrinogen, and keratins 8 and18, but usually negative for keratins 19 and 20 and epithelial membrane antigen.

Architectural patterns
Trabecular (plate-like) pattern. This pattern is the most common in well- and moderately differentiated HCCs. Tumour cells grow in cords of variable thickness that are separated by sinusoid-like blood spaces. Well-differentiated tumours have a thin trabecular pattern and trabeculae become thicker with de-differentiation. Sinusoid-like blood spaces sometimes show varying degrees of dilatation, or may be difficult to recognize owing to compression by tumour cells. Reticulin staining or CD34 immunostaining is helpful in the recognition of a trabecular pattern.

Pseudoglandular or acinar pattern. HCC frequently has a gland-like pattern, usually admixed with the trabecular pattern.

The gland-like structures are referred to as "pseudoglands" or "pseudoacini" because they are not true glands but actually modified, abnormal bile canaliculi formed between tumour cells. The structure is formed mostly by a single layer of tumour cells. Pseudoglands frequently contain proteinaceous fluids, which often stain with periodic acid–Schiff (PAS), but not with mucicarmine or Alcian blue. Bile may be present. Cystic dilatation of the pseudoglands sometimes occurs and may occasionally be formed by the degeneration of thick trabeculae. Generally, the pseudoglandular structures are smaller in well-differentiated tumours than in moderately differentiated tumours.

Compact pattern. Sinusoid-like blood spaces are inconspicuous and slit-like, giving the tumour a solid appearance. The compact pattern is common in poorly differentiated tumours.

Cytological variants
Pleomorphic cells. Tumour cells show marked variation in cellular and nuclear size, shape, and staining. Bizarre multinucleated or mononuclear giant cells are often present, and osteoclast-like giant cells are rarely seen. Generally, pleomorphic tumour cells lack cohesiveness, do not show a distinct trabecular pattern and are common in poorly differentiated tumours.

Clear cells. Tumour cells have clear cytoplasm owing to the presence of abundant glycogen. If the tumour consists predominantly of this type, it is sometimes difficult to distinguish from metastatic renal cell carcinoma of clear-cell type. Clinical information and immunohistochemical

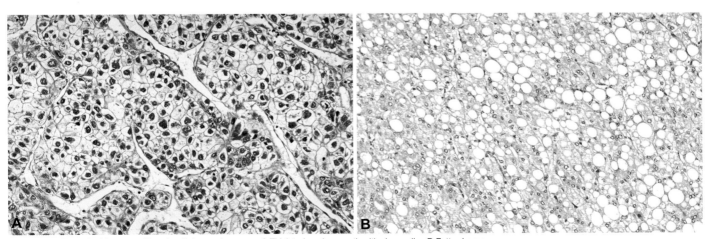

Fig. 10.27 Histological features of hepatocellular carcinomas. **A** Thick trabecular growth with clear cells. **B** Fatty change.

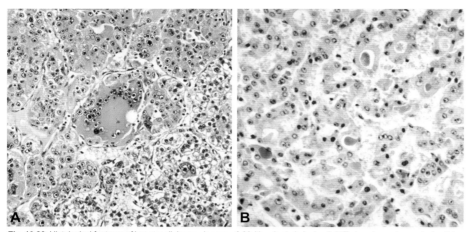

Fig. 10.28 Histological features of hepatocellular carcinomas. **A** Multinucleated giant cell. **B** Trabecular and pseudoglandular pattern with bile plugs.

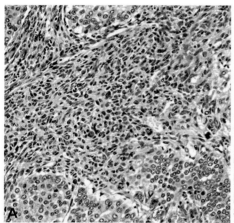
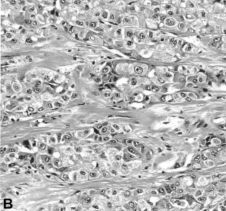

Fig. 10.29 Special types of hepatocellular carcinomas. **A** Sarcomatoid hepatocellular carcinoma. **B** Scirrhous hepatocellular carcinoma.

stains can be helpful in this regard.

Spindle cells. Spindle cells are observed in sarcomatoid HCC, which is discussed in the section on special types.

Fatty change. Diffuse fatty change is most frequent in small, early-stage tumours (< 2 cm in diameter). Its frequency declines as tumour size increases and it is

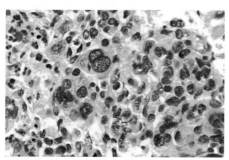

Fig. 10.30 Poorly differentiated hepatocellular carcinoma with no evidence of trabecular arrangement.

infrequent in advanced tumours. Metabolic disorders related to hepatocarcinogenesis and insufficient blood supply in the early neoplastic stages have been suggested as possible mechanisms underlying fatty change in small tumours.

Bile production. Bile is occasionally observed, usually as plugs in dilated canaliculi or pseudoglands. When bile production is prominent, the tumour is yellowish in colour and turns green after formalin fixation.

Hyaline bodies. Mallory-Denk bodies (reticular hyaline bodies) are intracytoplasmic, irregular in shape, eosinophilic and PAS-negative. Some take a globular shape and are called globular hyaline bodies. They consist of aggregated intermediate filaments and show immunohistochemical positivity with antibodies to ubiquitin and keratins. However, another type of globular hyaline body is small,

round, homogeneous, strongly acidophilic, PAS-positive and stains orange to red with Masson trichrome stain. Immunohistochemically, they are often positive for α-1-antitrypsin.

Pale bodies. These are intracytoplasmic, round to ovoid, amorphous, and lightly eosinophilic. They consist of amorphous material accumulated in cystically dilated endoplasmic reticulum, and often contain immunostainable fibrinogen {3100}. They are commonly seen in the fibrolamellar variant of HCC but are also found in the common types of HCC and in scirrhous HCC.

Ground glass inclusions. Like those of HBsAg-positive hepatocytes, these are rarely also observed in neoplastic cells of HCC arising in HBsAg-positive patients. They stain with modified orcein, Victoria blue, aldehyde fuchsin, and with immunohistochemistry.

Special types of carcinoma

Fibrolamellar carcinoma. Fibrolamellar carcinomas (FLC) are distinctive liver cancers of children and young adults that differ from classical HCC at the clinical, histological, and molecular levels {3270}. FLC account for 0.5–9.0% of primary liver cancers in various case series, with reported frequency being influenced by country and study design. Overall, FLC appears to be less common in Asia and in Africa than in North America and European countries. FLC arises in non-cirrhotic livers; etiology and risk factors are not known. There is no strong gender predilection. The age at presentation shows a unimodal distribution peaking at age 25 years and 85% of all FLC occur in individuals aged 35 years or younger. Two-thirds of cases involve the left lobe of the liver. Grossly, FLC tend to be yellow to pale tan and are firm to hard. A central scar may be found in about 75% of cases, but FLC do not appear to be etiologically related to focal nodular hyperplasia.

Histologically, FLC typically grow with broad pushing borders and benign portal tracts can occasionally be found entrapped within the growing tumour front. FLC are made up of large polygonal cells with abundant eosinophilic (oncocytic) cytoplasm, large vesicular nuclei, and large nucleoli. These distinctive cytological findings in conjunction with the lamellar fibrosis are the defining features of FLC. The eosinophilic cytoplasm is rich in mitochondria. In a subset of FLC, areas of gland-like formation are present, with tumour cells lining circular or ovoid spaces, some of which may contain mucicarmine and/or alcian blue-positive secretions. Such cases can be misclassified as combined hepatocellular-cholangiocarcinoma in the absence of careful attention to the complete histological findings. Other findings include calcifications, either in stroma or as luminal calcification of pseudogland secretions. "Pale bodies" and/or "hyaline bodies" may be found, as in classical HCC. The prognosis for FLC is better than for typical HCC that arises in cirrhotic livers, but similar to typical HCC that arises in non-cirrhotic livers.

Scirrhous HCC. About 5% of HCCs show a scirrhous growth pattern characterized by marked fibrosis along the sinusoid-like blood spaces with varying degrees of atrophy of tumour trabeculae {1688}. Most of these tumours arise immediately below the liver capsule. In cases of multifocal carcinoma, some tumour foci may show a scirrhous growth pattern while others show a classical HCC pattern. A better prognosis has been reported in some, but not all studies. The scirrhous type of HCC should not be confused with cholangiocarcinoma or FLC. In addition, similar fibrotic changes can occur following chemotherapy, radiation, and transarterial chemoembolization. Such post-therapeutic fibrosis should be distinguished from the scirrhous variant. The term "sclerosing hepatic carcinoma", has been used to designate a variety of tumours arising in non-cirrhotic livers that can be associated with hypercalcaemia, but does not constitute a distinct histopathological entity {1349}; some of these tumours appear to be hepatocellular, but others are intrahepatic (peripheral) cholangiocarcinomas.

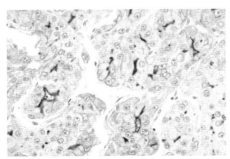

Fig. 10.31 Hepatocellular carcinoma: immunostaining with polyclonal antibodies to carcinoembryonic antigen (CEA) shows a characteristic canalicular pattern.

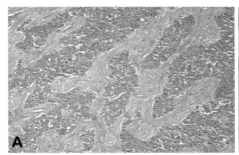 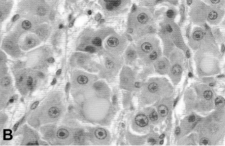

Fig. 10.32 Fibrolamellar carcinoma (FLC). **A** Intratumoral fibrosis often runs in parallel bands separating nests of oncocytic hepatocytes. **B** The diagnosis depends on the diffuse presence of oncocytic hepatocytes, as well as fibrous bands. The vesicular nuclei and large nucleoli are important diagnostic features. Pale bodies are also present in this field.

Undifferentiated carcinoma. Undifferentiated carcinomas are tumours that are primary to the liver and can be diagnosed as carcinomas based on immunohistochemistry, but cannot be further classified. Undifferentiated carcinoma is rare, accounting for < 2% of epithelial liver tumours. There is a male preponderance, but data on geographical distribution are not available. Localization, clinical features, symptoms and signs, and diagnostic procedures display no differences compared with hepatocellular carcinoma. Undifferentiated carcinomas are postulated to have a worse prognosis (compared with HCC), although greater case numbers to support this are not available {614, 1349}.

Lymphoepithelioma-like carcinoma. Lymphoepithelioma-like carcinoma is a rare type of HCC with pleomorphic tumour cells intermixed with numerous lymphocytes {2265}. The tumour cells tend to be small with focal syncytial growth. In some but not all cases, the tumour cells are positive for Epstein-Barr virus (EBV). Because of the rarity of this tumour type, information regarding histological findings, clinical features and prognosis is limited.

Sarcomatoid hepatocellular carcinoma. Occasionally, HCC is partially or fully comprised of malignant spindle cells, and may be difficult to distinguish from various sarcomas. When such sarcomatoid features are prominent, the tumour is called sarcomatoid HCC. Most sarcomatoid HCCs have areas of more typical HCC identified by sufficient sampling; however, immunohistochemical stains and clinicopathological correlation are also of value in correctly classifying such tumours, especially when the histological material is limited. Sarcomatoid change is more frequent in HCC with repeated chemotherapy or transarterial chemoembolization {1634}.

Grading

Histological grading of HCC is based on tumour differentiation: well-differentiated, moderately differentiated, poorly differentiated, and undifferentiated types are recognized.

Well-differentiated HCC

Well-differentiated HCC is most common in small, early-stage tumours of < 2 cm, and is rare in advanced tumours. The lesions are composed of cells with mild atypia and increased nucleus-to-cytoplasm ratio in a thin trabecular pattern, often with pseudoglandular structures. Fatty change is frequent. In most tumours of > 3 cm in diameter, well-differentiated carcinoma is observed only in the periphery, if at all.

Moderately differentiated HCC

Moderately differentiated HCC is most common in tumours of > 3 cm in diameter and is characterized by trabecular growth of three or more cells in thickness. Tumour cells have abundant eosinophilic cytoplasm and round nuclei with distinct

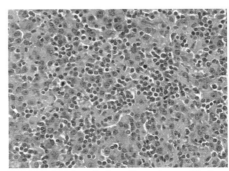

Fig. 10.33 Lymphoepithelioma-like carcinoma of the liver.

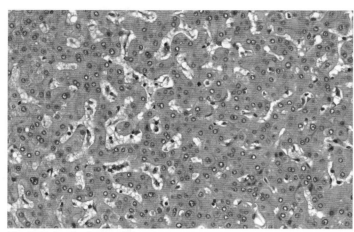

Fig. 10.34 Small cell change in hepatocytes.

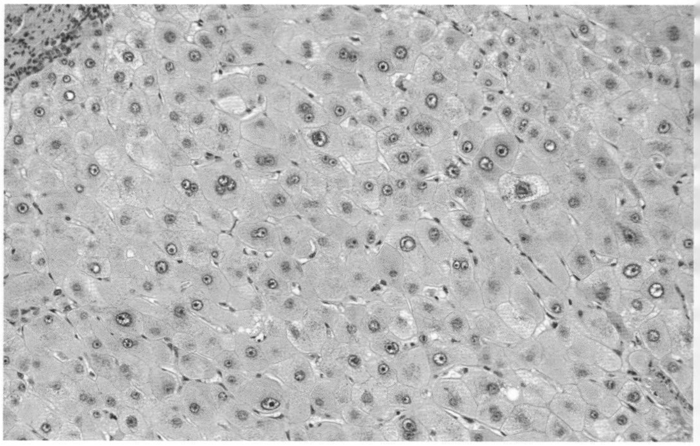

Fig. 10.35 Large cell change in hepatocytes.

nucleoli. A pseudoglandular pattern is also frequent, and pseudoglands often contain bile or proteinaceous fluid.

Poorly differentiated HCC

Poorly differentiated HCC, which is extremely rare in small, early-stage tumours, grows in a solid pattern without distinct sinusoid-like blood spaces; only slit-like blood vessels are observed in large tumour nests. The neoplastic cells show an increased nucleus : cytoplasm ratio and frequently moderate to marked pleomorphism.

Undifferentiated HCC

Undifferentiated tumour cells contain little cytoplasm, are spindle or round-shaped, and exhibit solid growth.
Edmondson and Steiner classified HCCs on a scale ranging from grade 1 to grade 4, on the basis of nuclear and cellular atypia. However, approaches using nuclear/cytological grading and/or proliferative index are not widely used in routine diagnostic practice for HCC.
It should be kept in mind that HCC often varies histologically even within a single nodule. In terms of histological grade, most primary cancer nodules of < 1 cm in diameter are uniformly well-differentiated, while approximately 40% of nodules of 1.0–3.0 cm in diameter consist of different types of neoplastic tissue with different histological grades {1520}. Less differentiated tissues are always located inside, surrounded by well-differentiated tumour on the outside; these less differentiated areas come to predominate as tumours enlarge to 3 cm {2153, 2381}. Stromal changes during tumour progression include increasing frequency of unpaired

arteries and capillarization of sinusoids, in parallel with increased arterial supply on radiological imaging.

Precursor and early lesions

Precancerous lesions of HCC include: (1) cytological changes indicative of hepatocellular dysplasia, often occurring as expansile foci (seen on microscopic, but not on gross examination), termed "dysplastic foci"; and (2) nodular lesions detectable on gross and, often, on radiological examination, characterized by cytological or structural atypia and termed "dysplastic nodules" (DN). Recently, international consensus has been reached regarding the histological features of early HCC, which is a low-grade, early-stage tumour.

Hepatocellular changes and dysplastic foci

Hepatocellular changes that have mostly

been associated with carcinogenesis in chronic liver disease include small cell change, large cell change, and iron-free foci.
Small cell change, originally described as small cell dysplasia {3466}, is defined as hepatocytes showing decreased cell volume, increased nucleus : cytoplasm ratio, mild nuclear pleomorphism and hyperchromasia, and cytoplasmic basophilia, giving the impression of nuclear crowding. Small cell change is characterized by higher proliferative activity than surrounding hepatocytes, chromosomal gains and losses, telomere shortening with p21-check-point inactivation, a morphological resemblance to early HCC, and a histological continuum to HCC {24, 1298, 1977, 2565, 3466}. These data support the precancerous nature of small cell change.
Large cell change, originally termed "liver

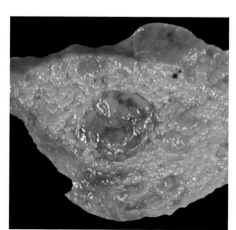

Fig. 10.36 Dysplastic nodule in a cirrhotic liver.

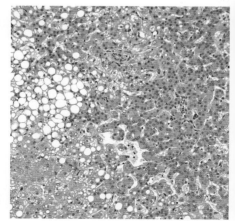

Fig. 10.37 High-grade dysplastic nodule with cytological and structural atypia, including high cell density, two-to-three-cell thick plates, small cell change and focal fatty change.

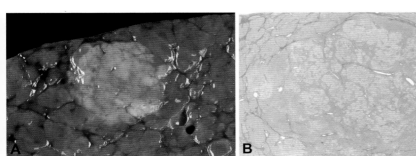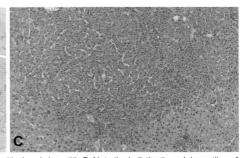

Fig. 10.38 Early hepatocellular carcinoma (HCC). **A** An early HCC with fatty change arising in a cirrhotic liver affected with chronic hepatitis B. Note the indistinctly nodular outline of the lesion. **B** Low-power view of an early HCC. **C** At high power, the cell plates at the border of early HCCs can be seen to be composed both of hepatocytes and neoplastic cells.

cell dysplasia" {128}, is defined as hepatocytes with both nuclear and cellular enlargement (therefore, a preserved nucleus : cytoplasm ratio), nuclear pleomorphism, frequent nuclear hyperchromasia, and multinucleation. The data for the nature of such change have been conflicting and suggest that large cell change may be a heterogeneous entity {311, 1299, 1787, 1977, 2479, 2565, 3220}. This change has been linked to cellular senescence {1787} and cholestasis {2255}; however, large cell change in chronic hepatitis B appears to be a tumour-related lesion {1549}. Actually, the presence of large cell change in cirrhosis associated with chronic hepatitis B or C has been reported to be an important independent risk factor for subsequent development of HCC {310, 941}. Thus, there is consensus that large cell change is at least an indication of chronic injury that predisposes to hepatocarcinogenesis; whether there are subtypes of large cell change that are directly premalignant remains uncertain.

The term "dysplastic focus" was introduced by an international consensus article published in 1995 {1335}, and has been subsequently used to describe groups of hepatocytes with features suggestive of precancerous change, which are incidentally discovered on histological examination. According to the original definition, dysplastic foci measure < 1 mm in diameter; this arbitrary size criterion is related to the fact that these microscopic lesions are usually contained within a single hepatic lobule or cirrhotic nodule. Dysplastic foci are mostly identified in livers with cirrhosis, and are often multiple.

Histologically, most recognizable dysplastic foci consist of expansile groups of hepatocytes with small cell change {1298}. At least a subset of iron-free foci arising in livers with hereditary haemochromatosis are precancerous, i.e. dysplastic foci {705}. Other cytological changes that may be seen in dysplastic foci of humans almost certainly exist, but are still under investigation; as discussed above, a subset of large cell change may represent such lesions. The efforts to study the biological nature of dysplastic foci have been limited by the inability to follow these lesions over time. However, from a practical point of view, identification of small or large cell change, or iron-free foci in liver biopsy specimens signifies an increased risk of HCC.

Dysplastic nodules (DN)

DNs are usually detected in cirrhotic livers, but are occasionally found with chronic liver disease without developed cirrhosis {125, 1298, 1335, 1633}. They may be single or multiple, and may have distinct or indistinct margins on gross examination. Their size varies from few millimetres to few centimetres, but most are < 15 mm in diameter. On the cut surface of the liver, DNs differ from the surrounding cirrhotic nodules because of their size, colour, texture, or degree of bulging. Nevertheless, identification of these lesions relies on histological examination. According to international consensus {1335}, DNs are classified as low-grade (LGDN) or high-grade (HGDN), depending on degree of atypia.

On microscopic examination, DNs often appear hypercellular when compared with the adjacent hepatic parenchyma;

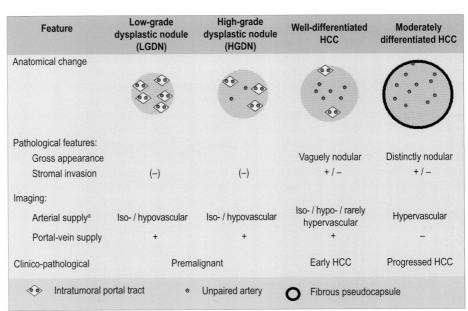

Feature	Low-grade dysplastic nodule (LGDN)	High-grade dysplastic nodule (HGDN)	Well-differentiated HCC	Moderately differentiated HCC
Anatomical change				
Pathological features:				
Gross appearance			Vaguely nodular	Distinctly nodular
Stromal invasion	(–)	(–)	+ / –	+ / –
Imaging:				
Arterial supply[a]	Iso- / hypovascular	Iso- / hypovascular	Iso- / hypo- / rarely hypervascular	Hypervascular
Portal-vein supply	+	+	+	–
Clinico-pathological	Premalignant		Early HCC	Progressed HCC

⬙ Intratumoral portal tract   • Unpaired artery   ◯ Fibrous pseudocapsule

Fig. 10.39 International consensus on the classification of small nodular lesions in cirrhotic liver: clinical and pathological correlations. The diagnosis must also consider the context of the lesion, especially the presence of cirrhosis, imaging findings, and growth rate.
HCC, hepatocellular carcinoma. [a] Hypovascularity, hypervascularity, and isovascularity refer to density or signal intensity in the arterial phase of contrast-enhanced imaging relative to the nontumoral liver {125}.

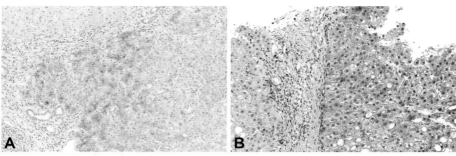

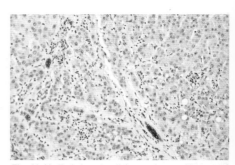

Fig. 10.40 Early hepatocellular carcinoma. **A** Immunostaining for glypican-3 (GPC3) reveals pericanalicular and cytoplasmic patterns of expression. **B** Immunostaining for heat-shock protein-70 (HSP70) is positive in tumour cells, including nuclei, and in biliary epithelium, but negative in non-lesional hepatocytes.

Fig. 10.41 Early hepatocellular carcinoma. Absence of ductular reaction in an area of stromal invasion (immunostaining for keratin 19).

such increase in cell density can be marked in HGDN {125}. Both LGDN and HGDN may exhibit features suggesting the presence of a clonal cell population, such as iron or copper accumulation, or steatosis in a liver without significant fatty change. DNs may derive their blood supply both from portal vessels and from newly formed arteries (termed "unpaired" or "nontriadal" arteries) {2480, 2721, 3332}. Portal tracts are commonly seen, but may be few and scarred. Unpaired arteries of DN are least prominent in LGDN, both in number and in size, and increase through HGDN and early HCC developmental stages. Therefore, in the arterial phase of contrast-enhanced hepatic imaging, DNs usually appear isovascular or hypovascular, as compared to the surrounding parenchyma.

Diffuse or focal small cell change is commonly found in HGDN. Other cytological changes that are indicative of atypia, distinguishing HGDN from LGDN, include clear cell change, focal fatty change with Mallory-Denk bodies and resistance to iron accumulation. HGDN may also demonstrate evidence of structural atypia, such as thick cell plates (up to three cells in thickness), occasional pseudoglandular structures, and expansile subnodules (foci), often differing from the remaining nodule in degree of cytological atypia or cell proliferation rate. In order to make a diagnosis of HGDN, the atypia observed in the lesion should be insufficient for a confident diagnosis of HCC. Sometimes, a subnodule with features diagnostic for HCC may be seen in a DN; the most appropriate term for such lesions is "HCC arising in DN". On other occasions, definite distinction between HGDN and well-differentiated HCC may be difficult or impossible, especially on needle biopsy material. Recently developed immunohistochemical markers may be of assistance in this regard.

At the other end of the spectrum, there is currently consensus that distinction between LGDN and large regenerative nodules of cirrhotic livers cannot be made confidently by morphology alone, remaining a task for future resolution {125}. However, presence of unpaired arteries or evidence of a clone-like cell population in a large nodule indicate that the nodule is dysplastic rather than regenerative. The practical implication of this diagnosis is that the patient is at increased risk of developing HCC. Useful histological features for the differential diagnosis among large regenerative nodule, FNH-like nodule, LGDN, HGDN, early HCC and classical HCC are presented in the section on *Algorithmic approach to diagnosis of liver tumours*.

Early hepatocellular carcinoma

Early HCC is a low-grade, early-stage tumour that may be difficult to recognize both grossly and microscopically. Although the pathological features of early HCC have been well described by Japanese authors during the last two decades {1642, 2242, 2781, 2782}, international consensus regarding the biological nature of this lesion and its distinction from HGDN has only recently been achieved {125}. Grossly, early HCC usually is a poorly defined nodular lesion measuring < 2 cm in diameter (hence the terms "vaguely nodular small HCC" and "small HCC with indistinct margins" that have been used for this tumour in the literature).

On microscopic examination, early HCC is a well-differentiated neoplasm, commonly composed of small hepatocyte-like cells that merge imperceptibly with the surrounding hepatic parenchyma. Char-acteristic features, often seen in combination, include: (1) increased cell density, more than twice that of the surrounding liver, with increased nucleus : cytoplasm ratio; (2) irregular thin trabecular pattern of growth; (3) pseudoglandular structures; (4) fatty change; (5) unpaired arteries; and (6) intratumoral portal tracts {125, 1633}. Any of these features may be present diffusely in the tumour, or may be seen in an expansile subnodule. Because the histological features listed above may be observed both in early HCC and in HGDN, distinction between the two types of lesion may sometimes be impossible, especially in biopsy material {1641}. However, detection of stromal invasion qualifies a lesion as HCC {125}. If the presence of invasion is questionable, detection of a ductular reaction by immunohistochemical stains for keratins 7 or 19 will favour pseudoinvasion rather than true invasion {2478}.

It should be emphasized that not all small HCCs (defined by the international consensus article of 1995 as HCCs measuring < 2 cm {1335}) represent early HCC. As a rule, distinctly nodular small HCCs have similar histological features to those of larger examples of classical HCC, including: variably differentiated neoplastic cell populations; well-developed trabecular architecture, pseudoglandular structures and unpaired arteries; absence of portal tracts; and presence of fibrous pseudocapsule at the tumour margin. Thus, distinctly nodular small HCCs are biologically progressed lesions, as evidenced by the presence of portal vein branch invasion and intrahepatic metastases in a significant proportion of cases {125, 1633}. Although early HCC is considered to be an earlier stage of tumour than distinctly nodular HCC, it should also be noted that the characteristic histologi-

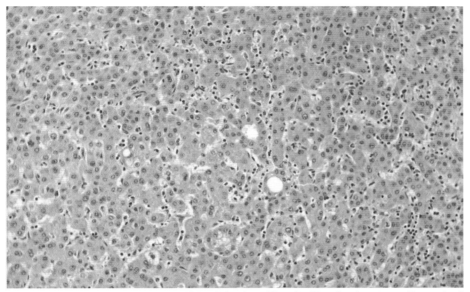

Fig. 10.42 Early hepatocellular carcinoma. High cell density and irregular thin trabecular pattern with occasional pseudoglands are typical features.

cal features of early HCC may sometimes be seen in tumours measuring > 2 cm in diameter, suggesting that some HCCs have a slow biological evolution.

The differences in vascular supply between early HCC (portal vessels, variable number of unpaired arteries) and distinctly nodular HCC (no portal vessels, well-developed unpaired arteries) are reflected in their imaging findings: early HCCs usually appear iso- or hypovasular when compared with the surrounding parenchyma, while distinctly nodular HCCs appear hypervascular on the arterial phase and hypovascular on the venous phase. Consequently, an early HCC with a subnodule of classical HCC may provide a nodule-in-nodule pattern on imaging studies {765, 1142}.

Hepatocellular adenoma

Transformation of hepatocellular adenoma to HCC has been considered rare. However, recent molecular studies have identified a subset of adenomas with an increased risk of malignant transformation, which are characterized by activating mutations in the gene encoding β-catenin {265}.

Molecular pathology

The great majority of HCCs develop in patients with chronic liver disease as a result of accumulating genetic and epigenetic changes in concert with clonal expansion of hepatocytes and/or hepatic

progenitor cells. When cirrhosis develops, the likelihood of HCC is increased, reflecting an increase in cell proliferation (owing to architectural remodelling and vascular alterations) and, possibly, replicative senescence. Nevertheless, the early molecular alterations leading to hepatocarcinogenesis appear before cirrhosis is established and are epigenetic in nature, including overexpression of growth factors, such as TGFα and IGF-2, as well as gene inactivation by promoter methylation {1645, 3242}. In addition, in chronic hepatitis B, viral X protein acts as an oncoprotein, while HBV DNA integration in the host genome induces genomic instability and deregulates genes involved in cell signalling and replication, such as the gene encoding cyclin A and the human telomerase reverse transcriptase (*TERT*) gene {712, 1759}. Other structural DNA changes, such as allelic deletions, also occur in livers with chronic hepatitis, with or without cirrhosis. However, the incidence of genomic changes escalates rapidly from chronic hepatitis and cirrhosis to dysplastic lesions and HCC {3242}.

Clonal expansion is enhanced by telomerase activation with diminished apoptosis. Active telomerase has been detected in cirrhotic nodules, DN and HCC {1297, 1658}. A large variety of genetic and epigenetic changes have been identified in precancerous hepatic lesions and HCC, including chromosomal amplifications,

mutations, loss of heterozygosity, global DNA hypomethylation and promoter hypermethylation {1759, 2089, 3242}. These changes derange several signal transduction pathways, each with a relatively low frequency; therefore, HCC is characterized by remarkable molecular heterogeneity. The Wnt/β-catenin pathway is commonly disrupted in HCC, mostly as a result of mutations in *CTNNB1* or *AXIN1*, epigenetic silencing of *CDH1*, or changes in the expression of Frizzle receptors {1759, 2089}. Activation of this pathway causes accumulation of nuclear β-catenin, where it regulates specific oncogenes, including *CCND1*, *MYC* and *BIRC5*. The p53 and Rb1 pathways are also often disturbed in HCC, p53 particularly by aflatoxin exposure (although also by other mechanisms) {2427}, and Rb1 by mutation, loss or silencing of *RB1* or *CDKN2A*, or due to reduced expression of other genes, such as *CDKN1A* {137}. The PI3K/Akt/mTOR pathway is also commonly disrupted {3404}, sometimes due to abnormal activation of tyrosine kinase receptors, or to constitutive activation of PI3K following loss of function of the tumour-suppressor gene *PTEN*. Derangements of other signal transduction pathways, such as the MAPK pathway and the TGFβ pathway, also play roles in hepatocarcinogenesis {137, 2427}. Finally, mutations of the *KRAS* oncogene in HCC are associated with exposure to vinyl chloride {3484}.

Molecular diagnosis of early HCC

Most early HCCs are negative for serum markers (AFP and PIVKA-II), lack typical radiological findings and show relatively mild histological atypia. The lack of typical features of classical HCC causes difficulty in the detection and accurate diagnosis of early HCC. Therefore, large-scale methods of gene expression have been employed to identify easily applicable immunomarkers to aid the diagnosis of carcinoma in these tumours.

The mRNA and protein expression of heat-shock protein 70 (HSP70) is upregulated in early HCC, increasing in a stepwise manner in the multistage process of hepatocarcinogenesis. Normal HSP70 immunoreactivity of biliary epithelium serves as an internal positive control (nontumorous hepatocytes are negative). Positive expression (defined as immunopositivity of at least 10% of tumour cells) was reported in about 80% of early HCC and

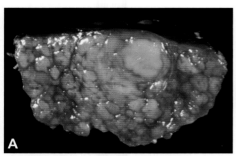 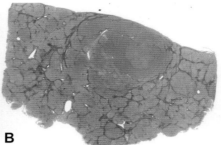 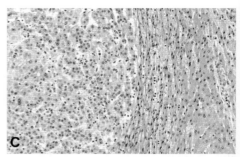

Fig. 10.43 Nodule-in-nodule type of hepatocellular carcinoma. **A** Macroscopy. **B** Low-power view. **C** Note the border between the early (right side) and advanced (left side) components.

only exceptionally in DNs or other non-cancerous nodules {557, 718}. Glypican-3 (GPC3), an oncofetal protein, is expressed abundantly in fetal liver, is inactive in the normal adult liver, and is frequently reactivated in HCC {418}. Immunohistochemical expression of GPC3 is much higher in small HCCs than in cirrhosis and DNs. GPC3 has a reported sensitivity of 77% and specificity of 96% in the diagnosis of small HCC. The expression of glutamine synthetase, a target of β-catenin signalling, also increases in a stepwise fashion from precancerous lesions to advanced HCC, as seen by immunohistochemistry {2412}. Glutamine synthetase is expressed in hepatocytes surrounding the terminal hepatic venules in normal livers, while positive areas comprise < 10% of the parenchyma in cirrhotic livers; therefore, staining in 10% of cells or more is considered suggestive of malignancy.

Applying the above markers (HSP70, GPC3, glutamine synthetase) as a panel can raise the diagnostic accuracy in tumour biopsy specimens, particularly when definite stromal invasion is not seen {717, 2478}. Investigation of additional markers holds promise for the future.

Molecular diagnosis of multicentric HCC
HCCs frequently occur as multiple intrahepatic nodules, synchronously or metachronously. Genetic analysis of the HBV integration pattern, chromosomal allele loss, and mutational inactivation of tumour-suppressor genes has often indicated multicentric, independent development of these nodules {2349, 2783}. These studies have shown that nodules apparently growing from portal-vein tumour thrombi or satellite nodules surrounding a large main tumour represent intrahepatic metastases, whereas other nodules can be considered to be multicentric HCCs. The following histological criteria are proposed to recognize multicentric HCC in routine practice: (1) multiple early HCCs or concurrent early HCCs and classical HCCs; (2) presence of peripheral areas of well-differentiated HCC in the smaller lesions; and (3) multiple HCCs of obviously different histology. Multicentric HCC appears to be most frequent with HCV infection {2381}.

Prognosis and predictive factors
The prognosis for patients with classical HCC is generally very poor, particularly for cases in which AFP levels are > 100 ng/ml at the time of diagnosis, partial or complete portal vein thrombosis,

and presence of a *TP53* gene mutation {94, 3126}. Cases of morphologically pure HCC (i.e. without the morphological features of combined hepatocellular cholangiocarcinoma), but which demonstrate significant (5% of tumour cells or greater) immunostaining for keratin 19 have been found to have a poorer prognosis and higher rates of recurrence and lymphnode metastasis than keratin 19-negative HCC {3335}. Spontaneous regression has been reported rarely. Most studies report a 5-year survival rate of < 5% in patients with symptomatic HCC.

Established HCCs are largely resistant to radio- and chemotherapy, although a subset of patients have shown a response to sorafenib, a new agent that inhibits several tyrosine protein kinases, a success that gives hope that novel efficacious agents will be developed based on better knowledge of the molecular mechanisms responsible for HCC development {314}. Currently, however, long-term survival is likely only in patients with small, asymptomatic HCCs that can be treated by resection, including liver transplantation, or by nonsurgical methods, including percutaneous ethanol or acetic acid injection and percutaneous radiofrequency thermal ablation.

Intrahepatic cholangiocarcinoma

Y. Nakanuma
M.-P. Curado
S. Franceschi
G. Gores
V. Paradis
B. Sripa

W.M.S. Tsui
A. Wee

Definition

Intrahepatic cholangiocarcinoma (ICC) is an intrahepatic malignancy with biliary epithelial differentiation. ICC can arise in any portion of the intrahepatic biliary tree, from the segmental and area ducts and their major branches to the smallest bile ducts and ductules {1106, 2390, 2499}. ICC arising from the intrahepatic small bile ducts is often called "peripheral ICC", but use of this term is discouraged.

Cholangiocarcinoma arising from the right and left hepatic ducts at or near their junction is referred to as "hilar CC" (often called "Klatskin tumour") and is considered to be an extrahepatic lesion {3489}, although the differentiation of hilar cholangiocarcinoma from ICC arising from the intrahepatic large bile ducts (perihilar ICC) is usually controversial at advanced stages, and such cases could be included in the definition of perihilar ICC {1106, 2248}. Likewise, it should be kept in mind that the distinction of hilar from perihilar depends on the pathological examination of resected specimens. The uses and meanings of the terms "hilar" and "perihilar" therefore may differ between pathologists, surgeons and radiologists.

ICD-O codes

Biliary intraepithelial neoplasia,
grade 3 (BilIN-3)   8148/2
Intraductal papillary neoplasm with:
   Low- or intermediate-grade
     intraepithelial neoplasia 8503/0
   High-grade intraepithelial
     neoplasia   8503/2
An associated invasive carcinoma
     8503/3
Intrahepatic cholangiocarcinoma 8160/3

Epidemiology

Incidence and geographical distribution

ICC is a relatively infrequent tumour in most populations, but is the second most common primary hepatic malignancy after hepatocellular carcinoma (HCC); about 5–15% of primary liver cancers are estimated to be ICCs {1967, 3489, 3602}. ICC is sometimes coded by cancer registries together with liver cancer, and this can lead to an underestimation of the true incidence of this tumour. The technological requirements for morphological sampling of ICC means that verification is low in areas where incidence is high {634}.

The prevalence of ICC shows a wide geographic variation, and the highest incidence is reported in areas of Asia where *Opisthorchis viverrini* (Thailand and Laos {1855}) and *Clonorchis sinensis* (southern China and the Republic of Korea {3468}) are endemic. The age-standardized incidence of ICC in Khon Kaen (Thailand) was 88 per 100 000 in males and 37 per 100 000 in females {2486}.

In the United States of America (USA), considered to be a low-risk population, the incidence of ICC from 1976 to 2000 was greatest in men of African descent.

Age distribution

Patients with ICC are usually elderly, with a slight male dominance, in areas where liver flukes are or are not endemic {532, 1855, 3468}. The age-specific incidence of this tumour is consistent with a linear increase with age, being highest in the oldest age group (≥ 85 years) {2022}.

Time trends

The incidence of ICC is increasing in many regions, including non-endemic areas {1531, 1621, 2499, 2898, 3489}. In the USA, a nearly three-fold increase was reported in the diagnosis of ICC between 1975 and 1999.

Etiology

Although the etiology of most cases of ICC remains obscure, some cases are associated with prior biliary or hepatic disease and a number of other risk factors {488}. For example, case–control studies in the USA have shown that several risk factors, including nonspecific cirrhosis, alcoholic liver disease, hepatitis C virus (HCV) infection, human immunodeficiency virus (HIV) infection, diabetes mellitus, and inflammatory bowel diseases are significantly more prevalent among patients with ICC {2899}.

Chronic inflammatory biliary disease

Some cases of ICC are preceded by a chronic inflammatory process of the bile ducts. Carcinogenesis is probably related to the duration and severity of bile-duct inflammation, and ICC tends to proliferate and spread along the affected intrahepatic bile ducts.

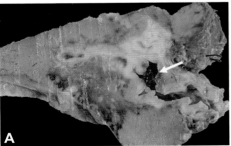 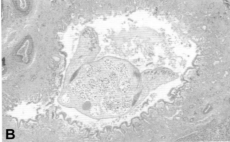 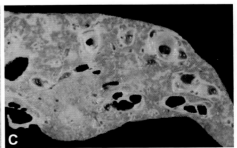

Fig. 10.44 Predisposing conditions for intrahepatic cholangiocarcinoma. **A** Hepatolithiasis with intrahepatic cholangiocarcinoma (arrow, stone). **B** *Opisthorchis viverrini* (liver fluke) in an intrahepatic bile duct. **C** Fibropolycystic disease of the liver with features of Caroli disease and of congenital hepatic fibrosis.

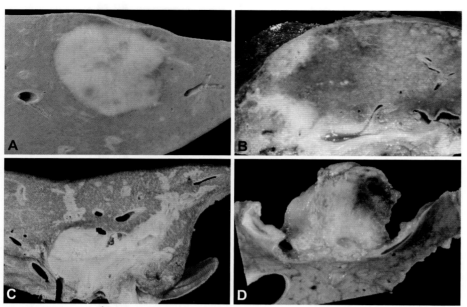

Fig. 10.45 Macroscopic features of intrahepatic cholangiocarcinoma. **A** Mass-forming type. **B** Periductal infiltrating type. **C** Periductal-infiltrating and mass-forming type. **D** Intraductal growth type.

Primary sclerosing cholangitis (PSC)
PSC with or without inflammatory bowel disease, usually ulcerative colitis, is a common risk factor for ICC in North America and European countries, and the prevalence of ICC in PSC is 5–15% with a cumulative risk of 1.5% per year {238, 289}. This risk is higher in northern European countries. Clinically undetected ICC or precursor lesions are occasionally encountered in explanted livers at liver transplantation.

Hepatolithiasis
Hepatolithiasis, which is not rare in the Far East, is the primary independent risk factor for ICC {1778}; about 7% of patients with hepatolithiasis eventually develop ICC {526} and 27–65% of ICCs are associated with hepatolithiasis {507, 508}. Calcium bilirubinate stones predominate, but some ICCs are associated with cholesterol stones {526}. The hepatic lobe or segments containing calculi involved by ICC are sometimes atrophic. The calculi-containing bile ducts have a proliferative epithelial lining and, not infrequently, dysplasia {3694}.

Parasitic biliary infestation
Epidemiological studies, such as a case-control study in an endemic area (Pusan) in the Republic of Korea and Hong Kong (China), have shown that the relative risk of ICC in persons infected with *C. sinen-*sis ranges from 2.7 to 6.5 {634, 3468}. Liver flukes, especially *O. viverrini* and *C. sinensis*, are risk factors for ICC {532, 1855, 3468}. The presence of parasites in the biliary tree leads to a chronic inflammatory response and bile-duct epithelial hyperplasia with an increased risk of ICC {2818}.

Biliary malformations and other lesions
ICC may arise in fibropolycystic disease of the liver, including congenital segmental or multiple dilatation of the intrahepatic bile ducts (Caroli disease), choledochal cysts, solitary unilocular or multiple liver cysts, and congenital hepatic fibrosis {3606}.

Non-biliary cirrhosis
Non-biliary cirrhosis, particularly hepatitis virus-related cirrhosis, is known as a background lesion of ICC {2899, 3597}. HCV infection may play a role in the development of ICC {1621, 3488}. In Japan, patients with cirrhosis attributable to HCV have a 1000-fold risk of ICC compared with the general population {1621}. In areas where both HBV and ICC are endemic, the two may also be related {1778, 1791}. Such ICCs are usually smaller, mass-forming types, when clinically detectable, and are frequently associated with neutrophilic infiltration {2237}.

Other risk factors
Deposition of thorotrast, Epstein-Barr virus (EBV) infection and genetic haemochromatosis are rare risk factors {511}.

Clinical features
ICC is an aggressive cancer, with high mortality and poor survival rates {1080}. The site of the tumour in the liver, its growth pattern and the presence or absence of strictures of the biliary tree relate to the clinical features of ICC.

Symptoms and signs
Clinical features are dependent on the anatomical location, growth pattern and stage of disease {762, 1967, 2996}. ICC without central bile-duct obstruction and presenting as mass(es) often go unnoticed until attaining a large size. General malaise, night sweats, right upper-quadrant abdominal pain and weight loss are frequent clinical symptoms. The liver itself is enlarged to a lesser extent, ascites is uncommon, and signs of portal hypertension are absent or minimal. Perihilar ICC usually presents with cholestasis {758}. Other symptoms that may coexist are related to hepatitis viral infection, cirrhosis, and prior biliary diseases such as PSC, or systemic metastases.

Imaging
Imaging is essential for diagnosis. The mass-forming type of ICC is expansile, and the borders between the cancer and non-neoplastic tissues are relatively clear {1106, 3604}. On arterial dominant phase of dynamic enhanced computed tomography (CT) or magnetic resonance imaging (MRI), usually only the periphery of the tumour enhances; the centre of the tumour (with few cells and abundant stroma) remains poorly enhanced. The centre of the tumour gradually enhances on equilibrium phase (late phase, delayed enhancement). This progressive contrast enhancement from early to late phase differs from that commonly seen in HCC (which shows early enhancement and a delayed contrast washout) {2681}. The periductal-infiltrating type of ICC develops along the intrahepatic bile ducts and appears as a solid mass extending along portal tracts, showing delayed enhancement on contrast-enhanced CT or MRI. Endoscopic retrograde cholangiopancreatography (ERCP) reveals secondary dilatation of the upstream ducts as a result of tumoral obstruction, and the anatomical location of the involved ducts

can be evaluated by calibre changes or duct rigidity.

Intraductal tumours are confined within the dilated part of an intrahepatic large bile duct, commonly showing contrast-enhanced papillary mural nodules with no or mild extension beyond the bile-duct walls. Marked, localized dilatation of affected ducts caused by mucin hypersecretion is identifiable by all imaging modalities, especially ultrasound and MR cholangiography (MRCP). Cholangiography reveals filling defects in the biliary tract, which are caused by polypoid tumours and/or hypersecreted mucin.

Advanced cases of ICC often have a mixed pattern of growth with central necrosis and/or intrahepatic metastases. Secondary dilated bile ducts around the tumour are more frequently detectable by CT, MRI and ultrasonography.

Macroscopy

ICC often develops in a non-cirrhotic liver. ICC is grossly classifiable into three types: mass-forming (MF) type, periductal infiltrating (PI) type and intraductal-growth (IG) type {1106, 3604}. The MF type presents a nodular or mass lesion in the hepatic parenchyma, and the carcinoma is grey to grey-white, firm and solid. The PI type spreads along the portal tracts with narrowing of the involved ducts. Peripheral bile ducts show obstructive dilatation and cholangitis. The IG type is a polypoid or papillary tumour within the dilated bile-duct lumen, and this type represents malignant progression of intraductal papillary neoplasm (IPN) of the bile duct. These three types may overlap in the same case. According to recent experience in North America and European countries, the MF type was present in 34 patients (65%), the MF + PI type in 13 patients (25%), the PI type in 3 patients (6%), and the IG type in 2 patients (4%) {1080}. Fibrous encapsulation is not seen in any type.

ICC arising in the intrahepatic small bile ducts or ductules usually presents as MF type {2237}, while ICC arising in the intrahepatic large bile ducts (perihilar ICC) presents as any of the three types. ICC cases involving the hepatic hilum are associated with cholestasis, biliary fibrosis, and cholangitis of the intrahepatic bile ducts. At more advanced stages, ICCs consist of variably sized nodules, usually coalescent. The MF type can be quite large. Central necrosis or scarring are

common, and mucin may be visible on the cut surfaces.

Tumour spread and staging

ICC directly invades the surrounding hepatic parenchyma and may spread along the portal pedicles. The IG type often spreads intraluminally along the ducts. Intrahepatic metastases develop in nearly all advanced cases. The incidence of metastases to regional lymph nodes is higher than in HCC. Blood-borne metastases occur later, particularly to the lungs; other sites of metastasis include bone, adrenals, kidneys, spleen, and pancreas. The TNM (tumour, node, metastasis) classification of extrahepatic bile-duct carcinoma (sixth edition) has divided these carcinomas into perihilar and distal bile-duct types. The perihilar classification applies to carcinomas of the right, left, and common hepatic ducts, i.e. those proximal to the origin of the cystic duct (Klatskin tumour).

Histopathology

Most ICCs are adenocarcinomas with variable differentiation and fibroplasia, resembling adenocarcinoma of the hilar and extrahepatic bile ducts or pancreas. There is no dominant histological type in cases associated with preceding biliary disease, while ICC arising in non-biliary cirrhosis frequently presents with bile-ductule differentiation, possibly arising

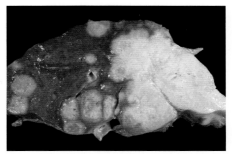

Fig. 10.46 Macroscopic features of intrahepatic cholangiocarcinoma, advanced stage.

from the hepatic progenitor cells {1778, 2237}.

Adenocarcinoma

Most ICCs have a tubular pattern of growth with variable-sized lumina, though micropapillary, acinar or cord-like patterns also occur. The neoplastic cells are usually small or medium-sized, cuboidal or columnar, and can be pleomorphic. They have small nuclei and nucleoli, and most have pale, slightly eosinophilic or vacuolated cytoplasm. The neoplastic cells may sometimes have clear and abundant cytoplasm or resemble goblet cells. These features resemble cholangiocytes (lining epithelium of the bile ducts), while some cases resemble bile ductules.

A variable and occasionally abundant fibrous stroma is an important characteristic

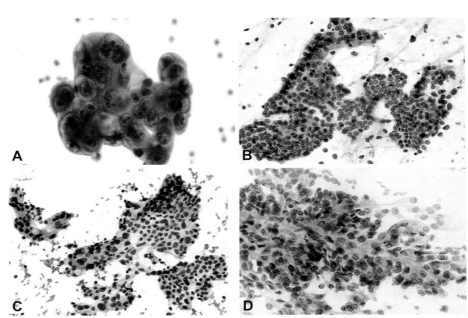

Fig. 10.47 Cytology of intrahepatic cholangiocarcinoma according to fine-needle aspiration. **A** Malignant epithelial cells. **B** Differentiated carcinoma. **C** Less well-differentiated carcinoma. **D** Intraductal papillary neoplasm.

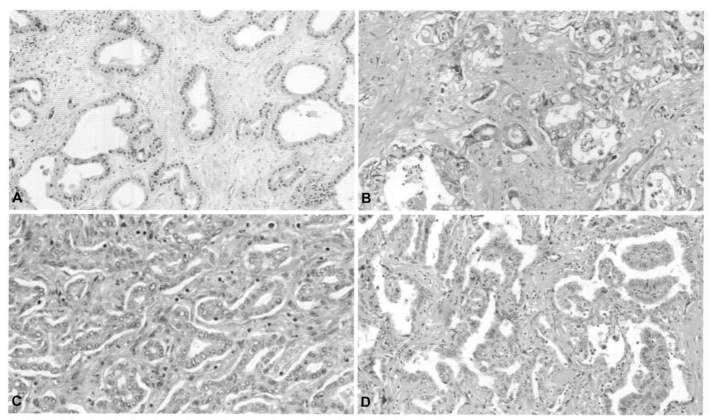

Fig. 10.48 Intrahepatic cholangiocarcinoma. **A** Well-differentiated adenocarcinoma. **B** Moderately differentiated adenocarcinoma. **C** Well-differentiated tubular cholangiocarcinoma. **D** Well-differentiated papillotubular adenocarcinoma.

of ICC. Usually, the centre of the tumour is more sclerotic and hypocellular, the neoplastic cells appearing lost in the dense, hyaline stroma. There may be focal calcifications in these areas. The periphery of the tumours contains more abundant, proliferating cells. ICC often extends by compressing hepatocytes, by infiltrating along sinusoids, or directly replacing adjoining hepatocytes in their trabeculae. As a result, portal tracts may be incorporated within the tumour and appear as tracts of elastic fibre-rich connective tissue. ICC also frequently infiltrates the portal tracts, and invades portal vessels (lymphatics and portal venules). This pattern of invasion is a frequent and relatively early histological finding, suggesting the development of early metastasis. Infiltrating, well-differentiated tubular carcinoma must be differentiated from the non-neoplastic pre-existing small bile ducts and ductules. ICC also often infiltrates intrahepatic nerves, frequently forming variably-sized glands surrounding the nerve.

ICCs arising from the large intrahepatic bile ducts are often associated with a noninvasive IPN. Once there is invasion of the ductal wall, the lesion may be well- to moderately differentiated adenocarcinoma, with considerable desmoplasia and stenosis of the bile-duct lumen. In the IG type of invasive carcinoma, a grossly visible papillary tumour growing in the duct lumen is supported by fine fibrovascular cores, and the surrounding mucosa is frequently replaced by superficial spreading carcinoma.

ICC arising from the intrahepatic peribiliary glands is also recognized and mainly involves these glands, sparing the lining epithelial cells at an early stage. The tumour cells can also infiltrate the peribiliary glands of the intrahepatic large bile ducts and their conduits, and this lesion should be differentiated from invasion of carcinoma in the portal connective tissue. Occasionally it may be difficult to distinguish this lesion from reactive proliferated peribiliary glands.

Grading

ICCs can be graded as well-, moderately,

and poorly differentiated adenocarcinoma according to their morphology. Most ICCs are well-differentiated tubular adenocarcinoma with or without micropapillary structures. Moderately differentiated carcinomas are composed of moderately distorted tubular glands with cribriform formations and/or a cord-like pattern, while the poorly differentiated cancers are recognized by distorted tubular or cord-like structures with marked cellular pleomorphism.

Histological variants

The following rare variants of ICC are recognized: adenosquamous and squamous carcinoma, mucinous carcinoma, signet-ring cell carcinoma, clear cell carcinoma, mucoepidermoid carcinoma, lymphoepithelioma-like carcinoma, and sarcomatous ICC. Adenosquamous and squamous carcinoma are occasionally seen at advanced stages of ICC. Mucinous carcinoma is not infrequently associated with the IG type of ICC, particularly cases with intestinal differentiation. EBV-encoded nuclear RNAs have been demonstrated in lymphoepithelioma-like carcinoma {511, 1272, 3420}. Sarcomatous ICC shows spindle-cell areas resembling spindle cell sarcoma or fibrosarcoma or with features of malignant fibrous histiocytoma. Carcinomatous foci, including squamous cell carcinoma, are scattered focally.

Immunohistochemistry

The production of mucin can be demonstrated in most ICCs by staining with mucicarmine, diastase-PAS or Alcian blue, though the amount of mucin is usually small and especially negligible in carcinoma resembling bile ductules. Mucin core (MUC) proteins 1, 2, and 3 are detectable in the carcinoma cells {2811, 2812}. ICC cells are often immunoreactive for keratins 7 and 19, carcinoembryonic antigen (CEA), epithelial membrane antigen (EMA), and blood group antigens. EMA is expressed on the luminal surface of carcinoma cells with ductular features. A keratin profile is useful for the differentiation of ICC from metastatic carcinoma: Keratin 7 is constantly expressed in ICC, while keratin 20 is constantly expressed in metastatic colon carcinoma {2756}.

Cytopathology

Bile and suspicious lesions encountered during biliary instrumentation can be sampled for cytology. In routine cytology, epithelial cells with prominent nucleoli, thickening of the nuclear membrane and increased chromatin are diagnostic for malignancy, with sensitivity varying from 9% to 24% and specificity from 61% to 100% {1125}. Advanced cytological techniques such as fluorescent *in situ* hybridization (FISH), for evaluation of aneuploidy, increases both sensitivity (up to 34%) and specificity (up to 98%) {200, 1572A}. Percutaneous or endoscopic ultrasound-guided fine-needle aspiration (FNA) cytology can be used to sample ICCs, especially the MF type {499, 625, 785}. Cellularity varies with degree of desmoplasia. In well-differentiated ICCs, sheets of cuboidal or columnar epithelial cells show a honeycomb appearance with round to eccentric nuclei, fine chromatin, small to inconspicuous nucleoli and ample, lacy or vacuolated cytoplasm. However, there is disorderly growth with crowding, piling up and loss of nuclear polarity. Characteristically, cell and nuclear enlargement can be abrupt, with an increased nucleus-to-cytoplasm ratio, irregular nuclear contour, hyperchromasia and distinct nucleolus. Less differentiated ICCs exhibit greater pleomorphism. Squamous features with dense cytoplasm and distinct cell borders may be seen. In IPN of the bile ducts, the hypercellular aspirates are composed of broad and often double-cell layered sheets of ductal columnar epithelium with distinctive, three-dimensional, complex and branching papillary configurations {3310}.

Differential diagnosis

Bile duct adenoma (BDA) is usually single, usually < 1 cm in size, and is sub-

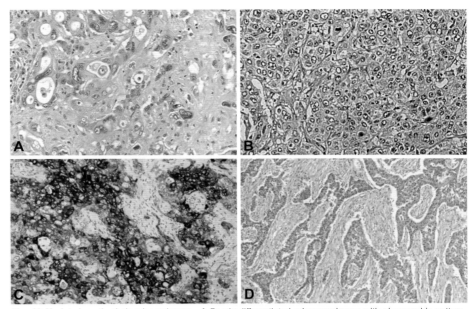

Fig. 10.49 Intrahepatic cholangiocarcinoma. **A** Poorly differentiated adenocarcinoma with pleomorphic pattern. **B** Poorly differentiated adenocarcinoma with solid growth pattern. **C** Cells of poorly differentiated adenocarcinoma in B are positive for epithelial membrane antigen (EMA). **D** Adenocarcinoma with cord-like and solid pattern.

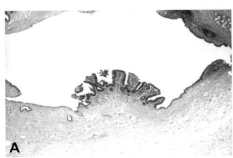
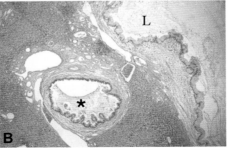

Fig. 10.50 A Intraductal papillary biliary neoplasm (IPBN) showing a multilocular pattern; this growth pattern, which can be mistaken for mucinous cystic neoplasm (cystadenocarcinoma), can be distinguished histologically by the absence of ovarian-like stroma. **B** IPBN showing a unilocular cystic pattern and filled with carcinoma and mucin.

Fig. 10.51 Intraductal papillary biliary neoplasm of the bile duct (IPBN). **A** Microscopic papillary lesion remote from the main lesion (multifocal occurrence). **B** Intraductal *in situ*-like spread of the small bile duct (*) and also large bile duct (L).

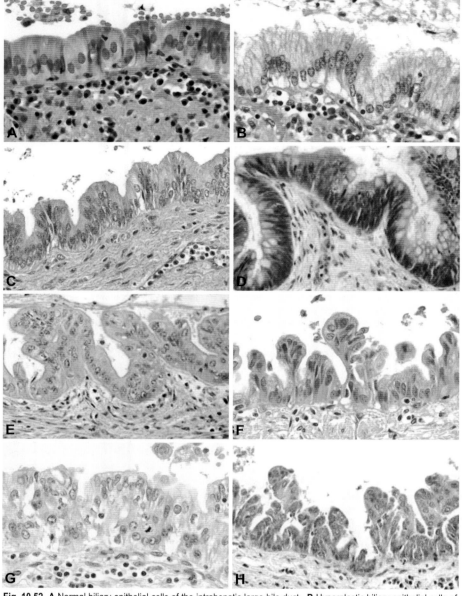

Fig. 10.52 A Normal biliary epithelial cells of the intrahepatic large bile duct. **B** Hyperplastic biliary epithelial cells of the intrahepatic large bile duct. **C, D** Biliary intraepithelial neoplasia 1 (BilIN-1). **E, F** Biliary intraepithelial neoplasia 2 (BilIN-2). **G, H** Biliary intraepithelial neoplasia 3 (BilIN 3).

premalignant neoplasm.

Von Meyenburg complex (biliary microhamartoma) is small, up to several millimetres in diameter. These lesions are usually multiple and are adjacent to a portal tract and, if widespread, may be an indication of fibropolycystic disease of the liver. Within a fibrous or hyalinized stroma, they present as irregular or round ductal structures that appear somewhat dilated and have a flattened or cuboidal epithelium. The lumina contain proteinaceous or bile-stained secretions.

Intrahepatic peribiliary cysts are usually found in chronic advanced liver disease, in syndromes with biliary anomalies, and also in normal livers. Multiple cysts may be seen around the intrahepatic large bile ducts {2236}. They are visible by ultrasound or CT and are thought to derived from peribiliary glands and should be differentiated from ICC clinically and histologically. Multicystic biliary hamartoma consists of ductal structures, periductal glands, and fibrous connective tissues containing blood vessels {3695}. Smooth muscle bundles focally surrounded ductal structures. Ductal epithelium and periductal glands resemble biliary epithelium and peribiliary glands, respectively.

Multifocal hyperplasia of peribiliary glands comprises macroscopically recognizable dilatation and hyperplasia of the peribiliary glands of intrahepatic and extrahepatic bile ducts in apparently normal livers and also in acquired liver diseases {748}. Some ducts may be cystically dilated. Lack of familiarity with this lesion could lead to an erroneous diagnosis of a well-differentiated cholangiocarcinoma.

Precursor and early lesions

Two types of precursor lesions are proposed for the development and progression of ICC arising from the intrahepatic large bile ducts: flat biliary intraepithelial neoplasia (BilIN) and papillary intraductal papillary neoplasm (IPN) of the bile duct. Molecular and genetic alterations related to cholangiocarcinogenesis have been described in these lesions {2235, 3689, 3691, 3694}.

Biliary intraepithelial neoplasia

BilIN is not infrequently encountered in the intrahepatic large bile ducts in chronic biliary diseases such as hepatolithiasis {3689}. BilINs are characterized by atypical

capsular and well-circumscribed but nonencapsulated. BDA is composed of a proliferation of small, uniform small-sized ducts with cuboidal cells that have regular nuclei. These ducts have no or little lumen and can elaborate mucin. Their associated fibrous stroma shows varying degrees of chronic inflammation and collagenization. Enclosed in the lesion are normally spaced portal tracts. BDA and peribiliary glands share common antigens, suggesting a common line of differentiation and leading some to consider it

a peribiliary gland hamartoma {253}.
Biliary adenofibroma is characterized by a complex tubulocystic biliary epithelium without mucin production, together with abundant fibroblastic stromal components. There is evidence that this might be related to Von Meyenburg complex on the basis of similar morphological architecture and epithelial expression of D10, but not 1F6 {3380}. Because of its size, proliferative activity and immunopositivity for p53, biliary adenofibroma is believed to be a potentially

epithelial cells with multilayering of nuclei and micropapillary projections into the duct lumen {3688, 3689}. The atypical cells have an increased nucleus-to-cytoplasm ratio, partial loss of nuclear polarity, and nuclear hyperchromasia. They are divisible into BilIN-1, BilIN-2 and BilIN-3 according to degree of atypia: BilIN-1 and BilIN-2 correspond to low- and intermediate-grade lesions (ICD-O code, 8148/0), and BilIN-3 to high-grade lesions (ICD-O code, 8148/2) {3688}. Some peribiliary glands in chronic hepatobiliary diseases may show BilIN lesions. BilINs are also seen in the hilar and extrahepatic bile ducts. Interestingly, similar intraepithelial biliary lesions are also encountered in the small intrahepatic bile ducts in livers with chronic hepatis C, alcoholic cirrhosis, thorotrast deposition, and PSC, suggesting that they may be precursor and early lesions of ICC arising from small bile ducts and ductules {876, 3273}. Extensive intraductal spread of BilINs along the intrahepatic bile ducts without grossly visible tumour lesions has been reported {48}.

Intraductal papillary neoplasms
IPN of the bile ducts includes the previous categories of biliary papilloma and papillomatosis, and is characterized by dilated intrahepatic bile ducts filled with a noninvasive papillary or villous biliary neoplasm covering delicate fibrovascular stalks {11, 12, 510, 1364, 3690, 3691, 3694}. Dilated bile ducts are fusiform or cystic (unilocular or multilocular). The papillary lesions are soft and white, red or tan. Similar neoplasia can develop in the hilar and extrahepatic bile ducts, and synchronous and metachronous IPNs can develop in the intrahepatic and extrahepatic biliary tree. About one third of IPNs secrete mucin in the duct lumen (mucin secreting biliary tumour) {2933, 3691}.
Although IPN of the bile ducts is usually not so mucinous, there are a number of parallels between IPN of the bile ducts and intraductal papillary mucinous neoplasm (IPMN) of the pancreas {1611, 2933, 3690, 3691}. Both lesions are papillary and intraductal, both show similar range of possible differentiation of the neoplastic cells (pancreatobiliary type, intestinal type, oncocytic type, and gastric type), and both have similar types of associated invasive carcinomas {3691}. The pancreatobiliary type is the most common type of IPN of the bile ducts. As

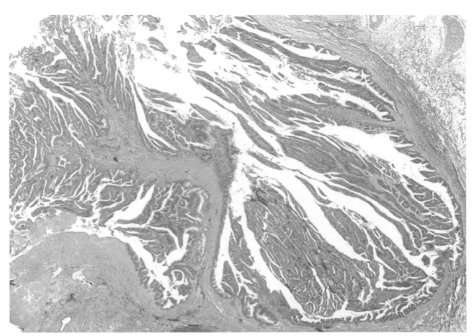

Fig. 10.53 Intraductal papillary biliary neoplasm (IPBN) showing papillary-villous growth in the cystically dilated bile duct.

in the pancreas, when associated with an invasive carcinoma, the pancreatobiliary type of bile-duct IPN is usually associated with a tubular adenocarcinoma, while the intestinal type of bile-duct IPN is usually associated with a colloid type of invasive carcinoma {1611, 2933}.
IPN with cystic luminal dilatation can be distinguished from biliary mucinous cystic neoplasm (biliary cystadenoma/cystadenocarcinoma) applying the criteria used in the differentiation of IPMN of pancreas from pancreatic mucinous cystic neoplasm, namely the presence of ovarian-type stroma and female sex are supportive of biliary mucinous cystic neoplasm, while luminal communication with the bile ducts and absence of

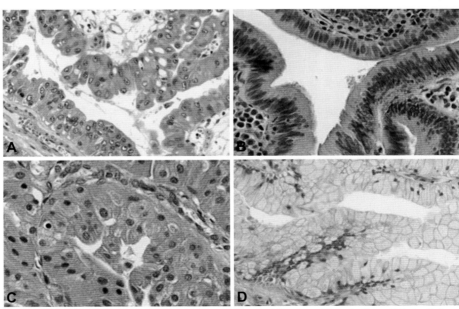

Fig. 10.54 Phenotype of intraductal papillary neoplasia. **A** Pancreatobiliary type. **B** Intestinal type. **C** Oncocytic type. **D** Gastric type.

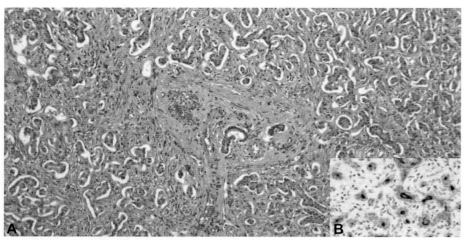

Fig. 10.55 Bile duct adenoma. **A** A proliferation of normal-appearing, small bile ducts is surrounded by connective tissue with an entrapped portal tract. **B** Bile-duct cells stain positively for epithelial membrane antigen.

ovarian-type stroma support the diagnosis of IPN {3690, 3691}.

IPN of the bile ducts is classifiable as low, intermediate or high grade on the basis of degree of cellular and nuclear atypia {2235, 3690, 3691}. IPNs are not infrequently associated with invasive carcinoma (IPN with an associated invasive ICC). IPN with an associated invasive ICC in the intrahepatic bile ducts corresponds to the IG type of ICC. When an invasive carcinoma is present, it should be separately designated and staged.

Molecular pathology

Cholangiocytes are continuously exposed to genotoxic insults such as chronic inflammation, oxidative stress and hydrophobic bile acids, predisposing them to genetic and epigenetic alterations {2167}. There are also accompanying increases of inflammatory mediators {1967}. Decreased membranous expression of E-cadherin, α-catenin, and β-catenin leads to weaker intercellular adhesion {790}, correlating with high-grade ICC and related to invasiveness {153, 1364}.

IL6 appears to play an important role in cholangiocarcinogenesis; tumour cells constitutively secrete IL6, which activates cell survival pathways and enhances tumour growth via autocrine mechanisms

{2045, 3120}. IL6 can also regulate the activity of DNA methyltransferases, and overexpression results in methylation of the promoters of several genes, including the epidermal growth factor receptor (*EGFR*) {2045}. Telomerase activity is detectable in carcinoma cells of almost all ICC cases {2423}. *EGFR* expression is a significant prognostic factor and also a risk factor for tumour recurrence {3650}. Increased gene signals of proto-oncogene *ERRB2* (human epidermal growth factor receptor-2, HER2) have been reported in ICC and may relate to progression {3339}. Promoter mutations leading to loss of transcriptional activity of *CDKN2A/p16INK4a* occur in PSC-associated cholangiocarcinoma {3194}, while overexpression of polycomb group protein *EZH2* may induce methylation of the *CDKN2A* promoter followed by decreased expression of *CDKN2A* in hepatolithiasis-associated ICC {2813}.

Prognosis and predictive factors

ICC is associated with a high rate of fatality because of early invasion, widespread metastasis, and lack of effective therapeutic modalities. Few patients are candidates for surgical resection as many patients present with advanced disease {2390, 2499, 3489}. The postoperative prognosis for patients with ICC depends

on growth type: the 5-year survival rate is 39% in patients with the MF type and 69% for the IG type, while the PI type shows a poor prognosis; no patients with the MF + PI type survived more than 5 years {1426, 3141, 3599}. Patients with mucinous carcinoma of the IG type have a better prognosis after surgical resection, when compared with conventional adenocarcinoma {2933, 3691}. These growth types reflect different biological behaviours: the MF + PI tumours had a positive lymph-node metastasis rate of 50% and a macroscopic vascular involvement rate of 61%, and perineural infiltration was higher in MF + PI types (80%) than in the MF group (33%). ICC arising in non-biliary cirrhosis is usually detectable as a small nodule during follow-up of hepatitis virus-related cirrhosis, and is treatable with hepatectomy {3597}. Concomitant hepatolithiasis prevents precise diagnosis preoperatively, with a poor prognosis {1426}. Lymph-node spread, macroscopic vascular invasion, positive surgical margins and bilobar distribution are associated with a high recurrence rate and a poor prognosis {1426, 3598}. In addition, intrahepatic metastasis, macroscopic vascular invasion, noncurative resection and advanced TNM stage are associated with a poor prognosis {1426}. Poor histological differentiation and squamous-cell or sarcomatous elements confer a poor prognosis. The mucin phenotype is also of prognostic significance: MUC2 expression is relatively frequent in well differentiated ICC, suggesting a favourable prognosis {1189}, while MUC5AC was more often associated with aggressive tumour development. In a single-centre experience, liver transplantation for highly selected patients with perihilar CC with neoadjuvant chemoirradiation has a 5-year disease-free survival of > 80% {1424}.

Combined hepatocellular-cholangiocarcinoma

N.D. Theise
O. Nakashima
Y.N. Park
Y. Nakanuma

Definition

A tumour containing unequivocal, intimately mixed elements of both hepatocellular carcinoma (HCC) and cholangiocarcinoma (ChC). This tumour should be distinguished from separate HCC and ChC arising in the same liver {1030}. Such tumours may be separated or intermixed ("collision tumour").

ICD-O code   8180/3

Epidemiology

This tumour type comprises < 1% of all liver carcinomas. Age- and sex-specific incidence and variations in geographical distribution of this tumour are similar to those for HCC.

Macroscopy

The gross morphology of this tumour is not significantly different from that of HCC. In tumours with a major component of ChC with fibrous stroma, the cut surface is firm and fibrotic.

Histopathology

Combined hepatocellular-cholangiocarcinoma, classical type

The most typical form of combined hepatocellular-cholangiocarcioma contains areas of typical HCC and areas of typical ChC. The hepatocellular component may be well-, moderately or poorly differentiated. Confirmation of hepatocellular differentiation is easily provided by immunohistochemical staining, e.g. with HepPar1 (granular cytoplasmic staining) or specific canalicular staining with anti-CD10 and/or rabbit polyclonal antibody to carcinoembryonic antigen (CEA) {309, 1123, 1803, 2455, 3244, 3567}. α-Fetoprotein may or may not be present. Bile may be produced, highlighted if necessary by Prussian blue stain or histochemical staining.

The biliary component is usually a typical adenocarcinoma, well-, moderately, or poorly differentiated, often accompanied by abundant stroma. Mucin may be demonstrated histochemically (periodic acid–Schiff stain after diastase digestion, mucicarmine). Keratins 7 and 19 are usually highlighted by immunostains; these do not however confirm biliary differentiation, as hepatocellular components may also be positive for these antigens {723, 3335}.

In many of these mixed hepatobiliary carcinomas, there are foci of intermediate morphology at the interface of the HCC and ChC components; immunohistochemistry often provides confirmatory evidence of mixed phenotypes in these regions. Cells that have phenotypical or

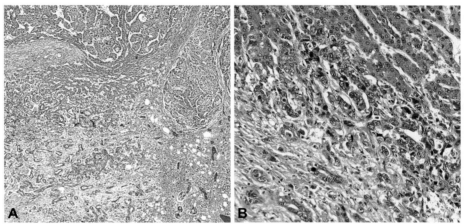

Fig. 10.56 Combined hepatocellular-cholangiocarcinoma. **A** The classical type shows a border zone between an hepatocellular carcinoma component with thick trabeculae (upper right) and a cholangiocarcinoma component with malignant glands in an abundant fibrous stroma (lower left). **B** The transitional area between the two components often shows mixed features with intermediate morphology.

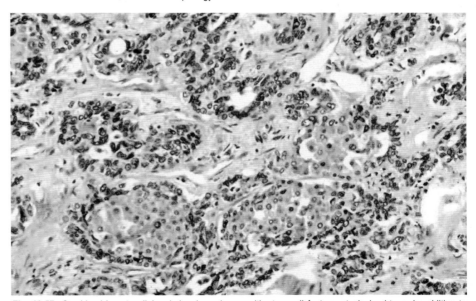

Fig. 10.57 Combined hepatocellular-cholangiocarcinoma with stem-cell features, typical subtype. In addition to components of hepatocellular and cholangiocarcinoma (not shown), these tumours have nests of mature appearing hepatocytes with peripheral, small, stem/progenitor-like cells, which may be positive for keratin 19, neural cell adhesion molecule (NCAM1/CD56), KIT and/or EpCAM.

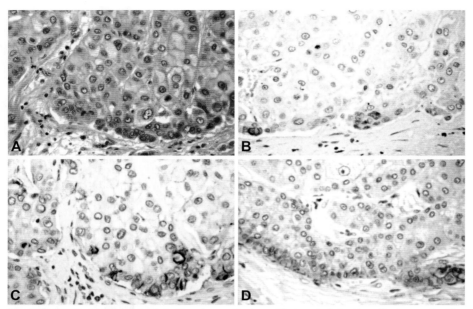

Fig. 10.58 Combined hepatocellular-cholangiocarcinoma with stem-cell features, typical subtype. Carcinoma cells at the periphery of tumour cell nests are small, dark-stained and face the fibrous septa (**A**). These cells are immunopositive for keratin 19 (**B**), neural cell adhesion molecule (NCAM1/CD56) (**C**), and epithelial cell adhesion molecule (EpCAM) (**D**).

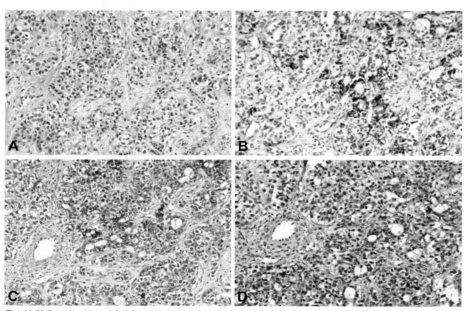

Fig. 10.59 Combined hepatocellular-cholangiocarcinoma with stem-cell features, intermediate-cell type. **A** Tumour cells are small and oval-shaped with scant cytoplasm and arranged in solid nests and strands within fibrotic stroma. There is simultaneous expression of HepPar-1 (**B**), α-fetoprotein (**C**), and keratin 19 (**D**).

immunophenotypical features of stem/-progenitor cells may also be present; if these predominate, classification as one of the subtypes "combined hepatocellular-cholangiocarcinoma with stem-cell features" should be considered.

Subtypes with stem-cell features
Three specific forms of stem-cell features have been highlighted in the literature, although they are not at this time considered to be distinctive clinicopathological entities, since it is as yet uncertain whether there are biological differences between them. Therefore, the clinical term "combined hepatocellular-cholangiocarcinoma with stem-cell features" includes all these subtypes and any other as yet unidentified variants.

Combined hepatocellular-cholangiocellular carcinoma with stem-cell features, typical subtype demonstrates nests of mature appearing hepatocytes with peripheral clusters of small cells which have high nucleus : cytoplasm ratio and hyperchromatic nuclei {910, 3231}. These cells are positive for keratins 7 and 19, nuclear cell adhesion molecule (NCAM1/CD56), KIT and/or epithelial cell adhesion molecule (EpCAM), thus recapitulating the morphological features and immunohistochemical profile of stem/progenitor cells. These nests may be separated by sufficient stroma to impart a schirrous appearance. In some cases, the hepatocytes in the centre of the nests show clear cell change.

Combined hepatocellular-cholangiocarcinoma with stem-cell features, intermediate-cell subtype consists of tumour cells with features intermediate between hepatocytes and cholangiocytes {1550}. These tumour cells are small and oval-shaped with hyperchromatic nuclei and scant cytoplasm. They are arranged in trabeculae, solid nests or strands and set within a background of marked desmoplasia. Elongated, ill-defined gland-like structures may be present, but well-defined glands are not seen. Cellular atypia is not marked and mucin production is not present. The tumour cells show simultaneous cytoplasmic expression of hepatocytic (HepPar1 or α-fetoprotein) and cholangiocytic markers (keratin 19 or CEA), much like ductular reactions in non-neoplastic, diseased liver; KIT expression is common.

Combined hepatocellular-cholangiocarcinoma with stem-cell features, cholangiolocellular type has populations of small cells with high nuclear:cytoplasmic ratio and hyperchromatic, oval nuclei, growing in a tubular, cord-like, anastomosing pattern, the so-called "antler-like" pattern {1638, 2953}. They are embedded in a fibrous stroma, and appear to recapitulate the canals of Hering or cholangioles. These tumour cells may be immunohistochemically positive for keratin 19, KIT, NCAM and EpCAM. Cellular atypia is usually mild and mucin production is absent. HCC-like and/or ChC-like areas are frequently present at the periphery of the tumours, where the tumour cords are continuous with the nontumoral liver-cell cords in a replacing pattern of growth. This tumour has traditionally been classified as a special type of cholangio-

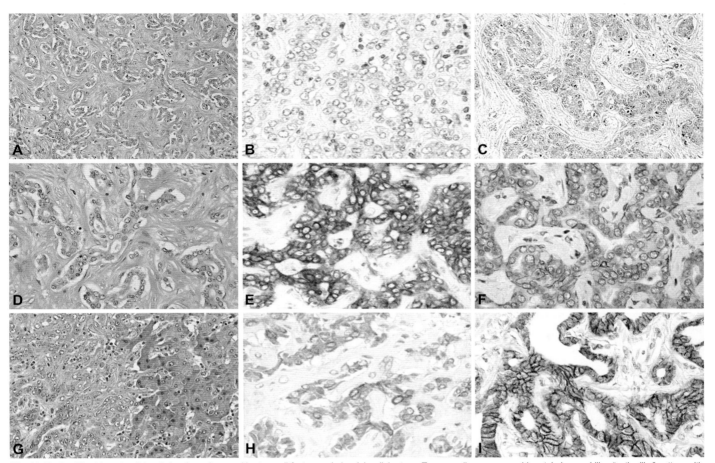

Fig. 10.60 Combined hepatocellular-cholangiocarcinoma with stem-cell features, cholangiolocellular type. Tumour cells are arranged in a tubular, cord-like, "antler-like" pattern with marked fibrous stroma (**A**, **D**). The tumour cords are continuous with the nontumoral liver-cell cords in a replacing growth pattern (**G**). There is no mucin production (**B**) and tumour cells are usually immunohistochemically positive for keratin 7 (**E**) and keratin 19 (**H**), and also frequently show a positive but variable reaction for KIT (**C**), NCAM1/CD56 (**F**) and EpCAM (**I**).

carcinoma, but is now considered a stem-cell subtype of combined hepatocellular-cholangiocarcinoma.

Prognosis and predictive factors
The prognosis for patients with combined hepatocellular-cholangiocarcinoma with-out stem cell features is thought to be worse than for pure HCC {1489}. Prognosis for combined hepatocellular-cholangiocarcinoma with stem-cell features is unknown, with conflicting evidence based on small series and numbers of patients {723, 1550, 1638, 2386, 2606, 3231, 3335, 3605}. Long-term follow-up of larger cohorts of strictly categorized tumours is needed to adequately define the clinical and biological behaviour of all the combined variants.

Hepatoblastoma

A. Zimmermann
R. Saxena

Definition

A primary malignant blastomatous tumour of the liver characterized by various combinations of several epithelial and mesenchymal cell lineages. The epithelial lineages recapitulate early hepatic ontogenesis and include immature cells, embryonal and fetal hepatoblasts, and more mature hepatocyte-like cells.

ICD-O codes

Hepatoblastoma
    Epithelial variants   8970/3
    Mixed epithelial-mesenchymal   8970/3
Calcifying nested epithelial
    stromal tumour   8975/1

Epidemiology

A rare tumour with 1 case per 1–1.5 million population, hepatoblastoma is the most frequent liver tumour in children; 80–90% of hepatoblastomas present before the age of 5 years, 70% present in the first 2 years of life, and 4% are present at birth. Prenatal presentation with placental metastasis has been reported. There is a slight male predominance (1.5–2 : 1).

Etiology

The strong association of hepatoblastoma with prematurity and low birth weight {2026, 2667, 2984, 3037} was first reported in a study from Japan {3197}, which found that hepatoblastomas accounted for 58% of all malignancies in children with birth weights of < 1000 g. The underlying etiopathogenesis is not

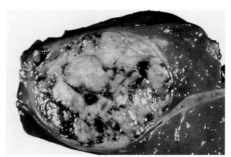

Fig. 10.61 Epithelial hepatoblastoma presenting as a large, well-demarcated lesion with central haemorrhage.

clear; therapeutic agents used to maintain low-birth-weight infants possibly play a role.

Localization

Hepatoblastomas occur as a single mass in 80–85% of cases, involving the right lobe in 55–60% of cases, the left lobe in 15% of cases, and both lobes in the remaining cases. Multiple masses may occur in either or both liver lobes.

Clinical features

Hepatoblastomas are often noted by a parent or physician as an enlarging abdomen in the infant or small child, often accompanied by anorexia or weight loss. Nausea, vomiting and abdominal discomfort or pain may be present. Jaundice is seen in < 5% of patients. Hepatoblastoma is often associated with haematological paraneoplastic syndromes, including anaemia and thrombocytosis {2891}. Very rarely, hepatoblastomas may produce chorionic gonado-

tropin, causing precocious puberty.
A marked elevation of serum α-fetoprotein (AFP) is noted in up to 90% of cases; a subgroup of hepatoblastomas show low or normal levels of serum AFP. The latter are associated with an aggressive course {680} and high-risk histologies such as small cell undifferentiated (SCUD) hepatoblastoma and tumours with rhabdoid features. AFP levels markedly decrease or fall to normal after chemotherapy-induced regression or complete removal of the tumour and rise with recurrence of disease. It should be borne in mind that "adult" levels of AFP (< 25 ng/mL) are not normally reached until approximately 6 months of age.

Imaging

Ultrasonographically, most hepatoblastomas present as hyperechoic masses. Computed tomography (CT) shows well-delineated single or multiple masses that are hypoattenuated compared with the surrounding liver. Up to 50% of tumours appear calcified or ossified. Magnetic resonance imaging (MRI) in combination with CT can help to differentiate hepatoblastoma from infantile haemangioendothelioma, mesenchymal hamartoma, undifferentiated (embryonal) sarcoma, and hepatocellular carcinoma by demonstrating cystic or vascular features peculiar to each lesion {3372}. MRI may also be used to characterize epithelial and mesenchymal components of hepatoblastoma.

Macroscopy

Hepatoblastomas often present as well-circumscribed, single or multiple lesions varying from 5 cm to > 20 cm in size, and from 150 to about 1500 g in weight. Hepatoblastomas are often nodular and bulge from the cut surface. An irregular, usually thin pseudocapsule formed by compressed liver may be present. The texture and colour of the cut surface depends on the tumour components; and presence or absence of necrosis and haemorrhage. Fetal hepatoblastomas display a tan-brown colour similar to that of

Table 10.04 Histopathological patterns in hepatoblastoma.

Histological type	Subtype
Wholly epithelial type	Fetal
	Mixed fetal and embryonal
	Macrotrabecular
	Small cell undifferentiated (SCUD)
Mixed epithelial and mesenchymal (MEM) type[a]	Without teratoid features
	With teratoid features
Hepatoblastoma, not otherwise specified	

[a] The epithelial component should be specified according to the category listed under wholly epithelial type.

normal liver. In the other subtypes, the cut surface is often variegated, with soft or gelatinous, brown to red areas {3082}. When osteoid is present, the tumour is typically gritty and the cut surface exhibits multiple whitish and slightly transparent speckles which may be clustered in a focal area. A standardized protocol for the examination of surgically resected hepatoblastoma specimens has been published {861}.

Histopathology

Hepatoblastomas and related tumours display a distinct variety of histological patterns that may be present in varying proportions {6, 2739}. These tumours are classified as wholly epithelial or mixed epithelial and mesenchymal types; the most widely-used classfication is given in Table 10.04. A more extended classification, based on the concept of a hepatoblastoma family of tumours and containing variants of hepatoblastoma and hepatoblastoma-related neoplasms, has been published {3720}.

Wholly epithelial types of hepatoblastoma
Fetal subtype

Accounting for nearly one third of hepatoblastomas, the fetal subtype presents as thin plates or nests of small- to medium-sized cells resembling hepatocytes of the developing fetal liver. The cytoplasm is either finely granular and eosinophilic or clear, reflecting variable amounts of glycogen and lipids, which impart a characteristic "light and dark" pattern at low magnification. The cells contain a small round nucleus with fine nuclear chromatin and an indistinct nucleolus. They are arranged in trabecula, and canalicular domains may develop, with visible bile droplets. The intervening thin-walled sinusoid-like vascular channels are lined by endothelial cells that demonstrate diffuse CD34 immunostaining in contrast to the focal staining of sinusoidal endothelium in normal liver {2746}. The tumours may contain vascular areas that may be mistaken for portal tracts, especially in needle biopsies, but that lack bile ducts. Foci of extramedullary haematopoiesis composed mainly of clusters of erythroid precursors are seen, more often in pretreatment biopsies {3417}.

In the typical fetal subtype, mitotic figures are commonly < 2 per 10 high power fields, the PCNA proliferative index is low

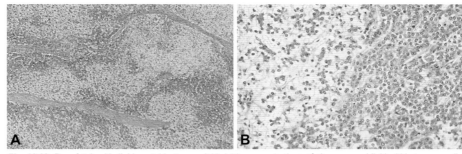

Fig. 10.62 Pure fetal epithelial hepatoblastoma. **A** Variable concentrations of glycogen and lipid within tumour cells sreate dark and light areas. **B** At higher magnification, the marked difference between the glycogen-rich clear cells (left) and the glycogen-poor dark cells (right) is evident.

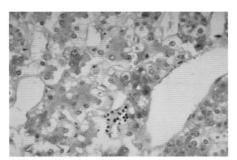

Fig. 10.63 Pure fetal epithelial hepatoblastoma. Cuboidal cells form trabeculae. Immunoreactivity for α-fetoprotein is present in most tumour cells. A cluster of haematopoietic cells is present, lower centre.

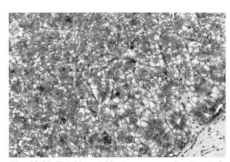

Fig. 10.64 Fetal hepatoblastoma expressing β-catenin on the cell surface, as on normal hepatocytes.

and the DNA content is diploid {2755}. A subset of fetal hepatoblastomas shows significant mitotic activity (> 2 per 10 high power fields) and is associated with larger, more pleomorphic nuclei and decreased cytoplasmic glycogen, creating a crowded, cellular appearance. This variant is termed "crowded fetal". Hepatoblastomas with an exclusively fetal morphology and absence of crowding have been termed "pure fetal hepatoblastoma".

Immunohistochemically, fetal hepatoblastomas may express AFP and show membranous expression of β-catenin.

Mixed fetal and embryonal subtype

This subtype of hepatoblastoma accounts for about 20% of cases. Apart from a few tumours post-chemotherapy, embryonal components do not usually occur alone, but develop in combination with the fetal phenotype. The morphology of embryonal hepatoblastoma resembles that of the liver at 6–8 weeks of gestation. Embryonal hepatoblasts have scant, dark granular cytoplasm devoid of visible glycogen (no periodic acid–Schiff, PAS, staining) and lipid droplets; and contain enlarged nu-

clei with coarse chromatin, thus resembling blastemal cells found in other blastomatous tumours, such as nephroblastoma. The cells are arranged as solid nests or glandular/acinar structures, sometimes with papillary profiles and formation of pseudorosettes. The mitotic activity is more pronounced than in the embryonal areas. Foci of extramedullary haematopoiesis are rarely present {1575}. Immunohistochemistry for β-catenin shows normal membranous staining of the fetal cells while the less mature cells often show nuclear staining.

A subset of fetal and fetal/embryonal hepatoblastomas contain (sometimes numerous) roughly spherical foci of pale, small cells. These foci may be surrounded by a rim of embryonal-looking cells, followed by fetal-type cells. It has been shown that these foci consist of poorly differentiated cells with marked nuclear expression of β-catenin and very low proliferative activity. In contrast, the embryonal cells surrounding these pale foci have very high proliferative activity, are rich in mitochondria, and exhibit a mixed nuclear and cytoplasmic/membranous pattern of β-catenin staining. The

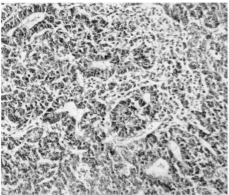

Fig. 10.65 Mixed fetal and embryonal hepatoblastoma. Embryonal epithelial cells occur singly and in glandlike structures.

Fig. 10.66 Macrotrabecular hepatoblastoma. The tumour consists of macrotrabeculae (left).

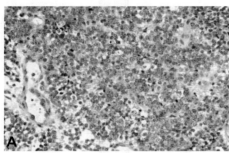
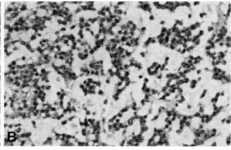

Fig. 10.67 Hepatoblastoma, small cell undifferentiated subtype (SCUD). **A** Small immature cells with increased nucleus : cytoplasm ratio form a diffuse growth pattern. **B** Clusters of small cells are embedded in a myxoid matrix (myxoid/mucoid variant).

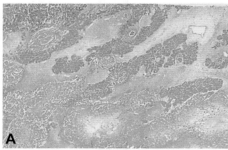
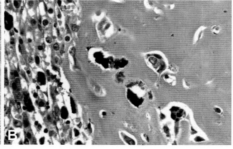

Fig. 10.68 Mixed epithelial and mesenchymal (MEM) hepatoblastoma. **A** Areas showing mesenchymal tissue and foci of osteoid-like material are present, together with areas of epithelial hepatoblastoma. **B** MEM type with teratoid features. There are numerous dark-brown melanin granules within the mesenchyme and in osteoblast-like cells.

peripheral rim of fetal-type cells demonstrate low proliferation and membranous β-catenin staining {3720}. These findings suggest microheterogeneity in some epithelial hepatoblastomas, with formation of distinct proliferation and differentiation "pacemakers" possibly driven by clones of mutated progenitor cells.

Macrotrabecular subtype

Macrotrabecular hepatoblastomas account for 3% of tumours and display trabecula that are 6–12 or more cells in thickness; the pattern is best appreciated on a reticulin stain. This subtype therefore denotes a growth pattern and not a distinct differentiation pathway. The term "macrotrabecular" is applied only to those tumours in which the pattern is a prominent feature of the lesion. When present focally, the tumour is classified according to its predominant components.

The trabeculae are composed of fetal and embryonal epithelial cells and a third, larger cell type resembling hepatocytes. Fetal and embryonal cells show the same morphological and proliferative features as described above, while the hepatocyte-like cells with vesicular nuclei and prominent nucleoli may resemble hepato-

cellular carcinoma. It has been proposed that macrotrabecular hepatoblastoma be divided into MT-1, consisting exclusively of hepatocyte-like cells and suspected to have a more aggressive course; and MT-2, consisting of fetal/embryonal cells assumed to have biologically standard risk. The MT-1 phenotype may be difficult to distinguish from hepatocellular carcinoma occurring in older children {3720}.

Small cell undifferentiated (SCUD) subtype

Approximately 2–3% of epithelial hepatoblastomas are composed entirely of non-cohesive sheets of small cells resembling the cells of neuroblastoma or other so-called small cell blue tumours. Formerly termed anaplastic hepatoblastoma, this variant is now called SCUD hepatoblastoma {1026}. In contrast to other epithelial hepatoblastomas, this subtype shows low or normal levels of serum AFP and is regarded as the least differentiated form of hepatoblastoma. Tumours consisting exclusively of small undifferentiated cells are very rare (2% or less) but foci of SCUD are common in other subtypes of hepatoblastoma. The SCUD phenotype, is an adverse prognostic factor, even when present focally {1096}.

This tumour grows diffusely and is highly invasive. The cells are arranged as solid sheets with abundant apoptosis, necrosis and numerous mitotic figures. Sinusoids are present but decreased in amount compared with fetal-type tumours, and there is pronounced expression of distinct extracellular matrix proteins {2745}. Immunostaining shows reactivity for keratin 8, sometimes for vimentin, and rarely for CD99, but not for AFP. In the Ki67 immunostain, the proliferation fraction usually exceeds 80%.

Similiar to certain subsets of neuroblastoma and medulloblastoma, some SCUD hepatoblastomas contain tumour cells of intermediate or even large size (intermediate cell and large cell undifferentiated hepatoblastoma; ICUD and LCUD) {3720}. In addition, SCUD hepatoblastoma sometimes exhibits rhabdoid features, histologically resembling malignant extrarenal rhabdoid tumour. A pathogenic connection between these two lesions is suspected, since some liver neoplasms that histologically qualify as SCUD are immunohistochemically SMARCB1(INI1)-negative, a *bone fide* feature of rhabdoid tumours {3294, 3294, 3427}.

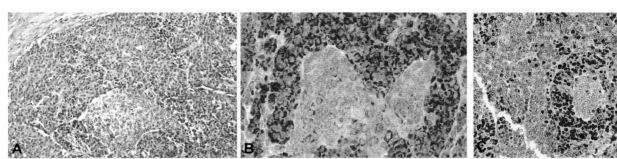

Fig. 10.69 Microheterogeneity in some fetal and mixed fetal/embryonal hepatoblastomas. **A** Foci of immature-looking cells, but with inconspicuous nuclei, are seen embedded in fetal or mixed fetal and embryonal tissue. **B** Mitochondrial immunostain: the cells of the nests have a poor organelle complement, whereas the surrounding, rapidly proliferating cells are rich in mitochondria. **C** Ki67 immunostain: the nest of progenitor cells exhibits very low proliferative activity, the surrounding rim of cells shows marked proliferation and the hepatoblastoma tissue shows low proliferation.

Mixed epithelial and mesenchymal (MEM) type

MEM type without teratoid features. MEM hepatoblastomas account for 45% of hepatoblastomas and consist of epithelial (usually fetal or mixed fetal/embryonal) elements admixed with neoplastic mesenchymal components, i.e. not tumour-induced stroma. Most of these tumours (about 80%) contain mature and immature fibrous tissue, osteoid or osteoid-like tissue, and rarely hyaline cartilage. The other 20% display more complex heterologous tissues of all germ layers, and are termed MEM hepatoblastomas with teratoid features. The fibrous mesenchyme may be rich in glycosaminoglycans, producing a myxoid appearance, but it also contains myofibroblast-like cells and bundles of collagen fibres. Islands of osteoid-like tissue composed of a hyaline matrix containing lacunae filled with one or more cells are the hallmark of MEM hepatoblastoma. Rarely, they are the only mesenchymal component noted in a predominantly fetal hepatoblastoma. There is strong evidence that the cells located within lacunae and osteoblast-like cells at the border of osteoid are derived from epithelial cells, because: (1) they may blend with adjacent fetal/embryonal hepatoblastoma cells; (2) they show immunostaining for keratin 8 and epithelial membrane antigen, in addition to AFP and vimentin {6, 3457}; and (3) the osteoid cells share molecular abnormalities of the β-catenin gene and expression/signalling pathways with epithelial hepatoblastoma cells.

Mixed epithelial and mesenchymal (MEM) type with teratoid features. This subtype, so-named owing to the variable presence of diverse heterologous components, is not related to teratomas, which are germ cell tumours. There is, however, a report of a discrete cystic teratoma contiguous to a hepatoblastoma. Between 3% and 20% of MEM hepatoblastomas display endodermal, neuroectodermal (melanin-producing cells, glial elements and neuronal cells), and complex mesenchymal tissues, including striated muscle cells {3084}. Melanin granules may be seen in osteoblast-like cells situated in osteoid, but the mere presence of osteoid does not qualify a tumour as teratoid. Similarly, stratified squamous epithelium, seen in tumours subsequent to chemotherapy, is not a teratoid feature. The pathogenesis of teratoid MEM is not established, but a role for pluripotent stem/precursor cells is hypothesized. The prognostic significance of teratoid features is not clear.

Pathology of hepatoblastoma subsequent to chemotherapy

Pre-surgical or pre-transplantation chemotherapy, a common therapeutic strategy in the treatment of hepatoblastomas {2525}, induces shrinkage of the tumour which aquires a more spherical configuration with more clearly delineated borders. The cut surface of such tumours is typically nodular; most of the nodules consist of firm fibrotic tissue intermingled with necrosis and/or haemorrhage. Microscopically, small foci of residual tumour may be detectable; the amount of detectable residual tumour depends upon the extent of sampling {2830}. Adequate sampling may be guided by careful inspection of the cut surfaces; viable epithelial tumour appears as pale friable foci located within fibrotic nodules, whereas MEM tumour remnants may be seen as white specks of osteoid. Histologically, residual embryonal, macrotrabecular and small cell components can be identified without difficulty, but the small nests of clear and dark cells of fetal hepatoblastoma embedded in fibrous tissue may be difficult to distinguish from entrapped and damaged benign hepatocytes.

Chemotherapy causes complex secondary changes in tumour cells, including cell enlargement with or without ballooning, fatty change and marked nuclear anomalies precluding proper identification of cell types. In some treated hepatoblastomas, only crowded foci of osteoid may remain without any epithelial tumour

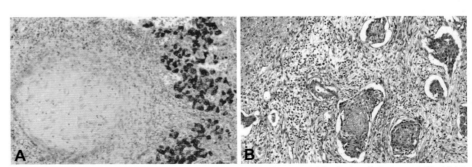

Fig. 10.70 A Hepatoblastoma with post-chemotherapy alterations. Immunostaining for keratin 8 shows residual fetal-type tumour cells adjacent to a scar. There is admixed inflammation. **B** Several typical foci of partly keratinized squamous epithelium in an inflammatory tissue.

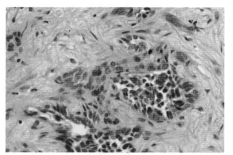

Fig. 10.71 Cholangioblastic hepatoblastoma.

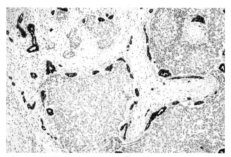

Fig. 10.72 "Ductal-plate tumour." In this hepatoblastoma variant, nests of nodules of hepatoid epithelial cells encircled by keratin 7-positive cholangiocytes often form duplicated profiles with slits, mimicking the ductal plate.

elements. Keratinized squamous epithelium is a typical post-chemotherapy feature, and is often accompanied by a foreign-body giant-cell reaction. Completely regressed tumour often shows fibrous spheres containing scarred vessels, necroses, old blood and haemosiderin granules.

Differential diagnosis

Hepatoblastoma must be differentiated from other liver tumours and pseudotumours that occur in the same age group. Modern imaging techniques, especially MRI, allow distinction from infantile haemangioendothelioma, which presents almost exclusively in the first year of life as an asymptomatic liver mass or masses with or without shunting phenomena and heart failure {2870}.

Mesenchymal hamartoma, a benign but sometimes very large lesion, occurs during the first 2–3 years of life and presents as a rapidly enlarging mass owing to cyst formation {3086}, a feature not encountered in hepatoblastoma. Rapid enlargement may also be seen in undifferentiated embryonal sarcoma, which however occurs in older children than for mesenchymal hamartoma and hepatoblastoma.

Focal nodular hyperplasia (FNH) may be seen in the first few years of life, but is more common in older children; the radiological features of this lesion are distinctive.

Hepatocellular adenoma is rarely found in the first 5–10 years of life, but may be difficult to differentiate from a pure fetal hepatoblastoma on the basis of imaging. Mesenchymal neoplasms such as hepatic angiomyolipomas or other perivascular epithelioid cell tumours (PEComas) occurring in children are, owing to their imaging morphology and anatomical localization, relatively easy to differentiate from malignant liver-cell tumours.

Variants of hepatoblastoma and tumours related to hepatoblastoma
Hepatoblastomas and related tumours with cholangiocellular components

A proportion of hepatoblastomas are characterized by the presence of cholangiocellular elements with or without formation of bile duct-like structures (hepatoblastoma with cholangioblastic features; cholangioblastic hepatoblastoma) {3719}. Duct-like profiles may be seen on staining with haematoxylin and eosin, while cholangiocellular elements may be revealed by immunostaining for keratins 7 and 19. In rare instances, slit-like ductular structures surround nodules of immature hepatoblasts or hepatocytes, mimicking an abortive ductal plate ("ductal plate tumours") {1035}.

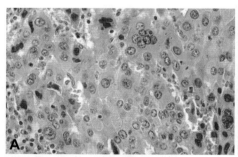
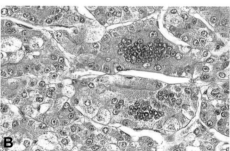
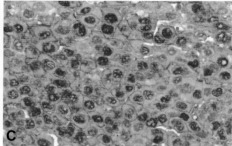

Fig. 10.73 Transitional liver cell tumour (TLCT). **A** Tumour composed of large hepatoid cells, few giant cells and smaller cells growing in a trabecular to diffuse pattern. **B** Note the very large multinuclear tumour giant cells and a few hepatoblastoma-like cells. **C** After immunostaining for β-catenin, TLCTs often show a mixed pattern, i.e. nuclear, cytoplasmic, and membranous staining.

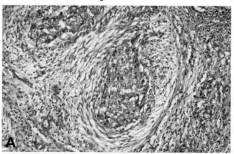
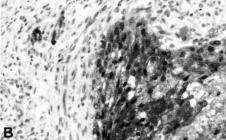
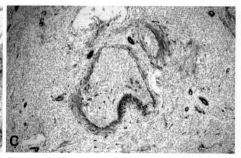

Fig. 10.74 Calcifying nested stromal epithelial tumour. **A** A nest of epithelial cells, reminiscent of immature hepatoid cells, is surrounded by a mantle of spindle cells. **B** The epithelial cells show prominent nuclear immunostaining for β-catenin. **C** The mesenchymal elements of the tumour are positive for smooth muscle actin.

Transitional liver cell tumour

Transitional liver cell tumour

Transitional liver cell tumour (TLCT) is a recently characterized malignant hepatocellular neoplasm {2595} that occurs in older children and young adolescents, and is distinct in regard to clinical presentation, histopathology, immunohistochemistry and treatment response. The term "transitional" implies a putative intermediate position of the neoplastic cells between hepatoblasts and hepatocytes. Clinically, TLCT presents as large or very large, expanding masses commonly located in the right liver lobe. These masses are hypo-dense and non homogeneous in CT scans and may demonstrate extensive central necroses. Very high levels of serum AFP are typical. Histologically, the growth pattern is more often diffuse than trabecular, lacking a prominent sinusoidal vascular network or prominent stroma. The tumour cells represent a mixture of cells resembling those of hepatocellular carcinoma, hepatoblastoma-like cells (mainly with a fetal morphology), and multinucleated giant cells. Acinar structures staining for keratins 7 and 19 may also be encountered. The tumour cells express β-catenin, in a mixed nuclear and cytoplasmic pattern.

TLCT are very aggressive neoplasms that pursue a rapid course and do not respond to chemotherapy.

Calcifying nested stromal epithelial tumour of the liver

This neoplasm is an unusual, probably favourable hepatic tumour in children of young to older age {1149, 1194}. It is characterized histologically by nested spindle and epithelioid cells and sometimes marked desmoplasia. The nests of epithelioid cells resemble immature, keratin 8- and epithelial membrane antigen-positive hepatoid cells with eosinophilic cytoplasm. These nests are surrounded by spindle cells that stain for vimentin and α-smooth muscle actin. Calcifications and bone formation may occur. An possible relationship to mixed blastomatous tumours of the paediatric liver is uncertain, but, like hepatoblastomas, the epithelioid cells in nested tumours have nuclear positivity for β-catenin, suggesting a pathogenic role for mutations in the β-catenin gene.

Tumour spread and staging

Some 40–60% of hepatoblastomas are either very large or involve both liver lobes

Table 10.05 The Pretreatment Extent of Disease (PRETEXT) staging system {2706}.

PRETEXT I	One section[a] is involved and three adjoining sections are free.
PRETEXT II	One or two sections are involved, but two adjoining sections are free
PRETEXT III	Two or three sections are involved, and no two adjoining sections are free.
PRETEXT IV	All four sections are involved.

Additional criteria for liver tumour

Caudate lobe involvement (C)

C0	Caudate lobe not involved
C1	Tumour involving the caudate lobe

Tumour focality (F)

F0	Patient with solitary tumour
F1	Patient with two or more discrete tumours

Additional criteria for venous involvement

Portal-vein involvement (P)

P0	No involvement of the main portal vein or its left or right branches
P1	Involvement of either the left or the right branch of the portal vein
P2	Involvement of the main portal vein
a	Suffix "a" if intravascular tumour is present (e.g. P1a)

Involvement of the inferior vena cava (IVC) and/or hepatic veins (V)

V0	No involvement of the hepatic veins or IVC
V1	Involvement of one hepatic vein but not IVC
V2	Involvement of two hepatic veins but not the IVC
V3	Involvement of all three hepatic veins and/or the IVC
a	Suffix "a" if intravascular tumour is present (e.g. V1a)

Additional criteria for abdominal involvement

Tumour rupture or intraperitoneal haemorrhage (H)

H0	No evidence of tumour rupture or intraperitoneal haemorrhage
H1	Imaging and clinical findings of intraperitoneal haemorrhage

Extrahepatic abdominal disease (E)

E0	No evidence of abdominal involvement (except M1 or N1)
E1	Direct extension of tumour into adjacent organs or diaphragm
E2	Peritoneal nodules
a	Suffix "a" if intravascular tumour is present (e.g. E1a)

Additional criteria for metastases

Distant metastases (M)

M0	No metastases
M1	Any metastases except E and N

Lymph-node metastases (N)

N0	No nodal metastases
N1	Metastases in abdominal lymph nodes only
N2	Metastases in extra-abdominal lymph nodes (with or without abdominal lymph-node metastases)

[a] PRETEXT groups the liver into four sections: left lateral section (segments 2 and 3); left medial section (segments 4a and 4b); right anterior section (segments 5 and 8); right posterior section (segments 6 and 7). The term "section" is synonymous with the previously used term "sector."

Table 10.06 Children's Oncology Group (COG) staging of hepatoblastoma {2666}.

Stage	Criterion
Stage I	Tumour completely resected with no microscopic residual disease
Stage II	Microscopic residual disease present
	Preoperative or intraoperative rupture
Stage III	Tumour unresectable
	Tumour resected with grossly visible residual disease
	Nodal involvement
Stage IV	Distant metastases

Table 10.07 Molecular findings in hepatoblastoma.

Gene or genetic pathway	Alteration	References
Chromosomal changes	Gain or loss of 1q, 2q, 4q, 8, 11q, 17q and 20	
Microsatellite instability		{635}
TGFB1 (TGFβ)	Upregulation	{25}
PPARA	Upregulation	{25}
Adipocytokine signalling	Upregulation	{25}
Extracellular matrix-receptor interaction	Upregulation	{25}
Apoptopic pathways	Downregulation	{25}
Upregulation of the WNT β-catenin signalling pathway[a]		{25}
CTNNB1	Mutation; deletions in exons 3 and 4	{1897, 635}
AXIN1 and *AXIN2*	Mutations	{3427}
APC	Mutations (found in hepatoblastoma associated with familial adenomatous polyposis	{1208}
Upregulation of cell-cycle pathways and loss of check-point control		
PLK1 (polo-like kinase-1)	Upregulation	{3579}
CDKN2A (p16)	Promoter methylation	{2936A}
CDKN1B (p27/KIP1)	Loss of expression	{345A}
DLK1, the NOTCH ligand	Upregulation	{1897}
Dysregulation of insulin-like growth factor (IGF) signalling		{1053, 3414, 3264}
PLAG1	Overexpression	{3681A}
11p15 gene cluster	Imprinting errors (found in hepatoblastoma associated with Beckwith-Wiedemann syndrome)	{595}
Molecular markers with prognostic significance		
PLK1	Expression is an indicator of poor prognosis	{3579}
RASSF1A	Methylation suggests that tumour is less likely to respond to preoperative chemotherapy	{1232}

[a] Seen on immunohistochemistry as nuclear localization of β-catenin.

at presentation, rendering them unresectable {3084}. However, preoperative chemotherapy, such as employed in trials by the International Childhood Liver Tumor Strategy Group (SIOPEL), reduces the size of the tumour masses in > 80% of patients, allowing complete resection. {860, 2057, 2525, 2707}. Tumour spread includes local extension into the hepatic veins and the inferior vena cava. The lung is the most frequent site of remote metastases; approximately 10–20% of patients have pulmonary metastases at diagnosis. Hepatoblastomas also metastasize to the skeleton, brain, ovaries, and the eye. Prenatally developing hepatoblastomas may metastasize to the placenta {318, 789, 2698}.

There are two main systems for staging of hepatoblastoma; the first is the PRETEXT (pretreatment extent of disease) system formulated by SIOPEL and the second is the COG (Children's Oncology Group) system adopted by the American Children's Oncology Group. The PRETEXT system is used for staging tumours before the initiation of any therapy and has been shown to correlate with overall and event-free survival. It is also useful in assessing the efficacy of neoadjuvant chemotherapy and predicting surgical resectability. The COG system assesses completeness of resection, which is the single most important prognostic factor in hepatoblastoma. It is therefore designed for post-surgical staging of the tumour and is more appropriate for use in treatment protocols that favour surgery immediately after diagnosis.

The PRETEXT stage consists of a number from 1 to 4, which indicates the extent of liver involvement by tumour, plus several additional criteria {2706}. The PRETEXT number is derived by subtracting the number of contiguous sections not involved by tumour from 4 (Table 10.05). When assigning this number, it is important to distinguish actual involvement of the section from mere compression by an adjacent tumour. The COG staging system is shown in Table 10.06 {2666}.

Genetic susceptibility

Congenital anomalies are noted in approximately 5% of patients and include renal malformations such as horseshoe kidney, renal dysplasia and duplicated ureters, gastrointestinal malformations such as Meckel diverticulum, inguinal hernia and diaphragmatic hernia, and other disparate malformations such as absent adrenal gland, heterotopic lung tissue and hemihypertrophy. Other syndromes with an increased incidence of hepatoblastoma include Beckwith-Wiedemann syndrome, trisomy 18, trisomy 21, Acardia syndrome, Goldenhar syndrome, Prader Willi syndrome, type-1a glycogen storage disease {2677} and familial adenomatous polyposis (FAP). FAP kindreds include patients with hepatoblastoma who have a mutation at the 5' end of the *APC* gene {463, 983}. Alterations in *APC* have also been noted in cases of hepatoblastoma in patients with nonfamilial adenomatous polyposis {2347}.

Molecular pathology

Genetic and molecular studies of hepatoblastoma have identified gains or losses of several chromosomes as well as alterations in pathways affecting cell fate, growth, apoptosis, signalling and differentiation (Table 10.07) {1054}. Of these, the two most commonly implicated pathways are the Wnt/β-catenin and the insulin growth factor signalling pathways. Approximately 70% of sporadic hepatoblastomas show accumulation of β-catenin {635} and a common deletion in exon 4 of the *CTNNB1* gene was demonstrated in 86% of hepatoblastomas {1897}. There appears to be some correlation between molecular patterns and histological subtypes, with the most significant differences being observed at the two ends of the differentiation spectrum of hepatoblastoma, namely the fetal subtype and SCUD subtype (Table 10.08). In general, fetal hepatoblastomas show more molecular evidence of differentiation than SCUD hepatoblastomas.

Prognosis and predictive factors

Prognosis is directly affected by the ability to completely resect the lesion {591, 1097, 3418}. Modern treatment strategies developed and tested in large international trials during the past years have impressively improved the prognosis and outcome of hepatoblastoma, primarily by shrinking the tumour, thereby downstag-ing and rendering it resectable {1244, 2525}. High initial (PRETEXT) tumour stage, low serum AFP, vascular invasion and certain histological subtypes (SCUD; rhabdoid features; TLCT) are powerful predictors of aggressive biology (high-risk tumours), whereas low stage and purely fetal morphology are favourable prognostic factors (standard risk) {3416}. Serum AFP levels are useful in predicting outcome by monitoring the response of AFP-producing tumours to surgery and chemotherapy {3371}.

Of all the molecular markers studied, only Polo-kinase 1 expression has been reported to have prognostic value independent of β-catenin mutation, age, stage or histology {3579}. This protein is crucial for various events in mitotic progression. In one study, higher mRNA levels correlated with poor outcome: the 5-year survival rate was 56% for high expression versus 87% for low expression {3579}. A separate study showed that hepatoblastomas with *RASSF1A* methylation (RAS association domain family protein 1) are less likely to respond to preoperative chemotherapy than those without *RASSF1A* methylation {1232}.

Table 10.08 Correlation of molecular changes with histological subtypes of hepatoblastoma.

Histological subtype	Molecular change	References
Small cell undifferentiated (SCUD) hepatoblastoma[a]	Differential overexpression of MAPK pathway genes	{25}
	Loss of *CDKN1B* (*p27/KIP1*)	
	Overexpression of *FOXG1*	{26}
	Decreased expression of *HES1* (a NOTCH target gene)	{1897}
	Decreased expression of *GLUL* (encoding glutamine synthetase)	{1897}
Fetal hepatoblastoma[a]	Large deletions in exons 3 and 4 of the β-catenin gene (*CTNNB1*)	{1897}
Mesenchymal hepatoblastoma	Upregulation of genes involved in extracellular matrix-receptor interaction pathways	{25}

MAPK, mitogen-activated protein kinase.
[a] Molecular changes for SCUD are compared to those for fetal hepatoblastoma and *vice versa*.

Mucinous cystic neoplasms of the liver

W.M.S. Tsui
N.V. Adsay
J.M. Crawford
R. Hruban
G. Klöppel
A. Wee

Definition

A cyst-forming epithelial neoplasm, usually showing no communication with the bile ducts, composed of cuboidal to columnar, variably mucin-producing epithelium, associated with ovarian-type subepithelial stroma. This neoplasm occurs almost exclusively in women. Noninvasive mucinous cystic neoplasms (MCN) are categorized on the basis of the highest degree of cytoarchitectural atypia into MCN with low-grade dysplasia, MCN with intermediate-grade dysplasia, and MCN with high-grade dysplasia. If there is a component of invasive carcinoma, the lesion should be designated as MCN with an associated invasive carcinoma. MCNs occur principally in the liver and occasionally in the extrahepatic biliary system (including the gallbladder).

ICD-O codes

MCN with low- or intermediate-grade
  intraepithelial neoplasia   8470/0
MCN with high-grade
  intraepithelial neoplasia   8470/2
MCN with an associated invasive carcinoma
                                     8470/3

Synonyms

These lesions have previously been referred to as cystadenoma and cystadenocarcinoma.

Epidemiology

MCNs are rare {706}. Without an associated invasive carcinoma they are seen almost exclusively in women. Cases of "cystadenocarcinoma" have been reported in males and females with equal frequency; however, based on the current requirement for the presence of ovarian-type stroma, it is likely that many of these neoplasms would now be classified as intraductal papillary neoplasms (IPN) of the bile ducts with marked cystic changes. Patients who present with MCN with an associated invasive carcinoma tend to be older (mean age, 59 years) than patients with noninvasive MCN (mean age, 45 years).

Clinical features

MCNs nearly always cause symptoms at

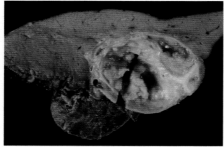

Fig. 10.75 Mucinous cystic neoplasm, high grade, with invasive carcinoma (biliary cystadenocarcinoma). Multiloculated cystic tumour with solid fleshy nodules arising in the wall.

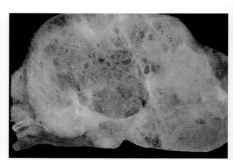

Fig. 10.76 Biliary adenofibroma. Circumscribed tumour with solid and spongy areas formed by microcysts.

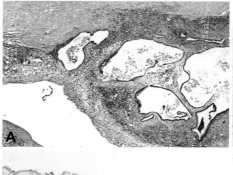
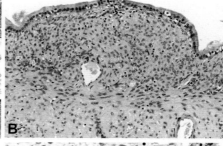
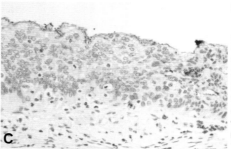
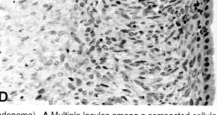

Fig. 10.77 Mucinous cystic neoplasm, low grade (biliary cystadenoma). **A** Multiple locules among a compacted cellular stroma with an outer fibrous capsule. **B** The columnar lining epithelium is mucin-secreting and lies on an ovarian-like stroma. **C** Carcinoembryonic antigen (CEA) is focally expressed on the luminal border of dysplastic epithelium. **D** The ovarian-like stroma is immunoreactive for estrogen receptors.

the time of presentation, typically abdominal pain and swelling. Biliary obstruction with resultant jaundice and ascending infection, haemorrhage, rupture, venacaval obstruction and biliary calculi formation have also been reported. Serum levels of the tumour marker CA19-9 may be elevated, particularly if there is an associated invasive carcinoma. Imaging techniques show a multilocular cystic mass, with irregular thickness of the wall, internal septation, and papillary projections observed in the malignant tumours.

Macroscopy

Most MCNs are multilocular and range in size from 2.5 to 28 cm {706}. The fluid content of locules is usually thin and watery, but it can also be haemorrhagic or composed of a mucinous semi-solid material. The cysts typically do not directly communicate with the larger bile ducts. When an associated invasive carcinoma is present, there may be a large papillary mass as well as solid areas of grey-white tumour in a thickened wall.

Tumour spread and staging

MCNs are slow-growing, frequently reaching a large size. They can progress to invasive carcinoma over a period of many years. When present, an associated invasive carcinoma is usually limited to within the primary neoplasm so that complete surgical removal is often feasible. However, invasive carcinoma can sometimes spread to the parenchyma of the liver, or metastasize to regional lymph nodes in the hepatoduodenal ligament. Distant metastases most frequently involve the lungs, pleura and peritoneum. Staging follows the protocol of TNM (tumour, node, metastasis) classification for intrahepatic cholangiocarcinoma

Histopathology

These tumours should be extensively sampled for microscopy, especially in areas with papillary projections and mural nodules. By microscopy, noninvasive MCNs are usually multilocular and are well-defined by a fibrous capsule, which may contain smooth muscle fibres. The inner surface of the cysts are lined by columnar, cuboidal, or flattened, mucus-secreting epithelial cells resting on a basement membrane; polypoid or papillary projections may be present. A mucicarmine stain can highlight the mucin, particularly when the neoplastic epithelial cells are columnar. Compared with MCNs of the pancreas, hepatic MCNs more commonly have cuboidal, non mucinous epithelium. However, the presence of ovarian-type stroma defines these neoplasms as MCN. The use of the term "serous cystadenoma" for neoplasms with ovarian-type stroma is inappropriate. The

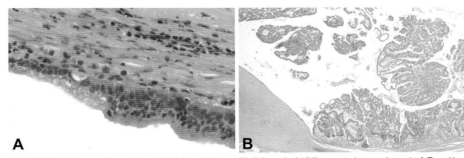

Fig. 10.78 Mucinous cystic neoplasm with high-grade intraepithelial neoplasia (biliary cystadenocarcinoma). **A** Transition from normal to dysplastic epithelium. **B** Complex papillary projections and crypt-like invaginations in the area of high-grade neoplasia.

epithelial cells in most hepatic cases have pale eosinophilic cytoplasm and basally oriented nuclei, and express biliary-type keratins (7, 8, 18, 19), epithelial membrane antigen (EMA), and focally carcinoembryonic antigen (CEA). Gastric and intestinal differentiation and squamous metaplasia may also occur. About half of the tumours contain scattered endocrine cells, as identified by expression of chromogranin and synaptophysin {3213}.

Subjacent to the basement membrane is a cellular, compact, ovarian-like, mesenchymal stroma, which in turn is surrounded by looser fibrous tissue. The stromal cells are spindle-shaped or rarely oval, and may be focally luteinized. They express vimentin, actin and desmin. This mesenchymal component is immunoreactive with estrogen and progesterone receptors, and α-inhibin {3}. A xanthogranulomatous reaction, with foam cells, cholesterol clefts and pigmented lipofuscin-containing macrophages, may be present in the cyst wall.

Foci of epithelial dysplasia comprising micropapillary projections or crypt-like invaginations, nuclear enlargement and hyperchromasia, multilayering, and mitosis may be seen. Severe dysplasia is

characterized by significant architectural atypia, such as exophytic papillae with back-to-back glands, as well as nuclear pleomorphism and numerous mitotic figures. Most associated invasive carcinomas are ductal adenocarcinomas with tubulopapillary or tubular growth patterns. Although often multifocal, malignant foci may be focal, and these neoplasms therefore need to be extensively sampled {706}.

Cytopathology

Diagnostic fine-needle aspiration (FNA) cytology samples are characterized by aggregates of cuboidal to columnar epithelium with occasional papillary arrangement. The background can be watery, or composed of abundant thick mucin containing degenerated cellular debris and macrophages. The neoplastic cells show varying degrees of architectural and nuclear atypia corresponding to heterogeneity of the cyst lining. The ovarian-type stromal component is usually not seen {1884, 3479}. The cytological features overlap with those of IPN, in which papillary clusters with fibrovascular cores and nuclear grooves are abundant {3310}.

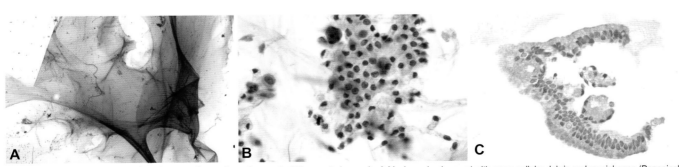

Fig. 10.79 Fine-needle aspirate of mucinous cystic neoplasm, low grade (biliary cystadenoma). **A** Mucinous background with some cellular debris and muciphages (Papanicolaou). **B** A sheet of columnar cells with bland nuclei in basal location (Papanicolaou). **C** Cell block reveals a short strip of columnar cells with basally oriented nuclei and mucin-positive apical cytoplasm (mucicarmine).

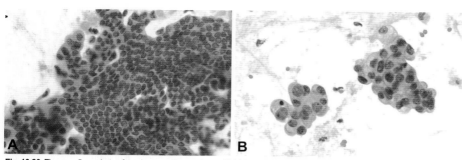

Fig. 10.80 Fine-needle aspirate of mucinous cystic neoplasm with high-grade intraepithelial neoplasia (biliary cystadenocarcinoma). **A** Sheets of moderately dysplastic epithelium with larger nuclei, nuclear crowding, and irregular nuclear membrane. **B** Clusters of malignant cells with much enlarged, pleomorphic hyperchromatic nuclei, prominent nucleoli and pale cytoplasm.

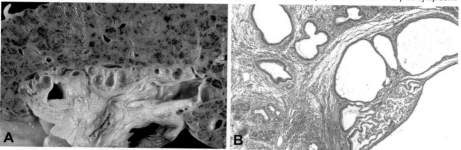

Fig. 10.81 Peribiliary cysts. **A** Large cysts in the connective tissue of the hilus; the background liver shows advanced cirrhosis. **B** Variably sized cysts are intermingled with peribiliary glands.

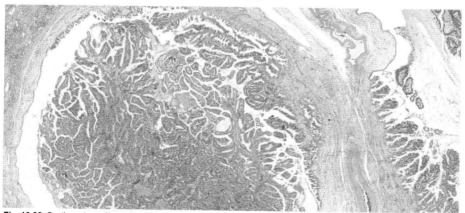

Fig. 10.82 Cystic variant of intraductal papillary neoplasm (IPN) closely mimicking high-grade mucinous cystic neoplasm (right side) but lacking the ovarian-like stroma. Note the intraductal papillary neoplasm (IPN) in the adjacent dilated bile duct (left side).

In practice, FNA lacks sensitivity owing to sampling problems and often cannot differentiate between the various types of hepatobiliary cysts. The findings usually only permit distinction between benign cyst contents or adenocarcinoma. Stains for mucin can help distinguish mucinous from nonmucinous cystic lesions. The cyst fluid can be also assayed for CA19-9 and CEA to distinguish a mucinous neoplasm from non-neoplastic lesions {1627}.

Differential diagnosis
MCN and IPN of the biliary tree can both form mucin-containing cysts lined by a cuboidal to columnar neoplastic epithelium. Communication with the bile ducts and absence of ovarian-like stroma favour a diagnosis of IPN of the bile ducts {3114, 3690}.

Hepatic microcystic serous cystadenoma of pancreatic type is characterized by multiple small locules lined by a single layer of glycogen-rich cuboidal cells with clear cytoplasm and lacking the ovarian-type mesenchymal stroma. This benign tumour is exceedingly rare in the liver {706, 1350, 1564}. Biliary adenofibroma, another rare member of the group of benign bile-duct tumours, is basically a solid tumour with some microcystic spaces, comprising microcystic and tubuloacinar glandular structures lined by non-mucin-secreting biliary epithelium and supported by a fibroblastic stromal scaffolding {3311}.

Endometriosis with its specialized stroma can mimic MCN, as can adult mesenchymal hamartoma with multicystic appearance. In cases where the mesenchymal stroma is lacking, distinction of MCN from non-neoplastic bile duct cysts and other large cystic lesions can be problematic. Bile duct cysts (simple hepatic cysts) are characterized by flat to columnar lining epithelium and absence of mucin-secretion; accompanying von Meyenburg complexes and corpora albicans-like collapsed cysts are common when multiple bile duct cysts are present in the liver.

Intrahepatic cystic carcinomas that communicate with bile ducts and do not contain ovarian-like stroma are most likely to be associated with IPN {132, 2238}. Peribiliary cysts comprising cystically dilated peribiliary mucin-secreting glands may simulate MCN. In fact, it is currently thought likely that MCN originates from peribiliary glands, considering the site of occurrence, histological morphology, close relationship with these glands, and frequent presence of endocrine cells.

Prognosis and predictive factors
The prognosis for patients with a noninvasive biliary MCN is excellent if complete resection is possible. The prognosis for patients with an invasive adenocarcinoma arising in association with MCN is much harder to predict. In the past, a variety of different carcinomas were lumped together under this designation, including carcinomas arising in association with MCN with ovarian stroma, carcinomas arising in the context of fibropolycystic disease, carcinomas arising in congenital liver cysts, and carcinomas in the hepatoduodenal ligament {706, 3230}.

Additional data are needed to define more precisely the prognosis for patients with MCN with an associated invasive carcinoma when current definitions, specifically inclusive of the requirement for ovarian-like stroma, are rigorously applied. At present, it appears that invasive adenocarcinomas arising in association with biliary MCN have a better prognosis than do pure cholangiocarcinomas, highlighting the importance of this distinction.

Lymphoma of the liver

E.S. Jaffe
H.K. Müller-Hermelink
J. Delabie
Y.H. Ko
S. Nakamura

Definition
Primary hepatic lymphoma is defined as an extranodal lymphoma arising in the liver, with the bulk of the disease localized to this site. More often, the liver is a secondary site of involvement by lymphoma. Some rare lymphomas, such as hepatosplenic T-cell lymphoma, may present with dominant manifestations in the liver, but the disease is in reality systemic.

Epidemiology
Primary lymphoma of the liver is rare {1341} and mainly a disease of middle-aged men {2041}, although occasional paediatric cases are reported. Most are diffuse large B-cell lymphomas (DLBCL), mucosa-associated lymphoid tissue (MALT) lymphomas are second most common. Hepatosplenic T-cell lymphoma is a disease that mainly affects young adult males (male : female ratio, approximately 5 : 1) {593}. Predominantly paediatric lymphomas, such as Epstein-Barr virus (EBV)-positive T-cell lymphoproliferative disease of childhood, are also recognized {2610}.

Etiology
A proportion of cases are associated with infection with hepatitis C virus, with or without mixed cryoglobulinaemia {114, 152, 652, 677, 2122, 2197, 2741}. Other lymphomas have been reported arising within a background of infection with hepatitis B virus {1999, 2424}, HIV {2544, 2835} or primary biliary cirrhosis {2584}. Hepatosplenic T-cell lymphomas have been linked to iatrogenic immunosuppression, especially in children with Crohn disease {2257, 3228, 3394}. EBV infection of T cells is found in systemic EBV-positive T-cell lymphoproliferative disease of childhood, and may follow chronic active EBV infection in some cases {576, 2375}.

Clinical features
The most frequent presenting symptoms are right upper-abdominal/epigastric pain or discomfort, weight loss and fever {2041}, although some patients (e.g. those with EBV-postiive T-cell lymphoproliferative disease of childhood) may present with abnormal results for serum liver enzyme tests {2610}. Most cases are solitary or multiple masses within the liver, sometimes misdiagnosed as primary hepatocellular or metastatic cancer {2041}. Some cases have been reported with diffuse infiltration of the liver associated with hepatomegaly, but without a discrete mass, simulating hepatic inflammation. T-cell/histiocyte-rich large B-cell lymphomas often present with marked hepatomegaly, but the disease is usually disseminated with splenic and bone-marrow involvement {455}.

In contrast to primary lymphoma, secondary liver infiltration is a frequent occurrence in many low-grade B-cell malignancies, including chronic lymphocytic leukaemia and follicular lymphoma, and is an indication of stage IV disease. Hepatosplenic T-cell lymphomas present with hepatosplenomegaly, usually without peripheral lymphadenopathy or lymphocytosis. There is almost always thrombocytopenia and most patients are anaemic. The results of tests of liver function are usually abnormal, with moderate elevation of levels of transaminases and alkaline phosphatase. Serum lactate dehydrogenase levels may be very high {593}. Evidence of hepatic failure is common in lymphomas associated with a haemophagocytic syndrome, most often EBV-positive T-cell or natural-killer cell (NK) malignancies {1323, 1383}.

Histopathology
B-cell lymphoma
The majority of primary hepatic lymphomas are DLBCLs and are composed of a monotonous proliferation of large cells expressing CD20 and other B-cell-associated antigens, with formation of a destructive mass lesion. T-cell/histiocyte-rich large B-cell lymphomas involve the liver more diffusely, usually with infiltration of portal triads. Occasional cases of Burkitt lymphoma have been described {1276}, usually presenting as a solitary mass. Low-grade B-cell lymphomas of MALT type are characterized by a dense

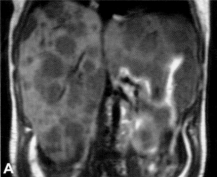
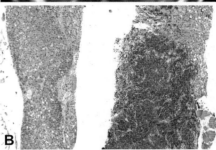

Fig. 10.83 Diffuse large B-cell lymphoma (DLBCL). **A** MRI for the patient shown in B. Multiple filling defects are seen in the liver. **B** HIV-associated. Sheets of abnormal lymphoid cells diffusely infiltrate the hepatic parenchyma.

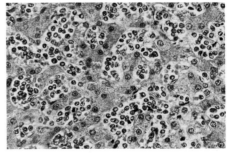

Fig. 10.84 Hepatosplenic T-cell lymphoma. Abnormal lymphoid cells with abundant pale cytoplasm infiltrate hepatic sinusoids.

lymphoid infiltrate within the portal tracts. The atypical lymphoid cells have centrocyte-like cell morphology and surround reactive germinal centres. Lymphoepithelial lesions may involve the bile-duct epithelium, and these may be highlighted by staining with antibodies to keratins {1574, 1950}. IgG4-associated sclerosing cholangitis should be considered in the differential diagnosis of hepatic MALT lymphoma and is usually associated with autoimmune pancreatitis {702}.

Secondary involvement of the liver by low-grade B-cell malignancies shows preferential involvement of the portal triads, with the morphology and phenotype related to the specific entity.

T-cell lymphoma

Hepatosplenic T-cell lymphoma is characterized by infiltration of the sinusoids by a monomorphic population of medium sized cells with a moderate amount of eosinophilic cytoplasm. The nuclei are round or slightly indented with moderately dispersed chromatin and contain small, usually basophilic, nucleoli. Portal infiltration is variable, but generally not prominent. A similar sinusoidal pattern of infiltration is seen in the spleen and bone marrow, both of which are usually involved by the lymphoma at diagnosis {593, 819}. The cells are most often of γ δ T-cell derivation with a minority derived from α β T-cells. They are cytotoxic, but with an immature or inactivated phenotype {225, 593, 819}.

Systemic T-cell malignancies, including T-cell large granular lymphocytic leukaemia, and adult T-cell leukaemia/ lymphoma usually involve the sinuses more prominently

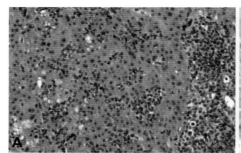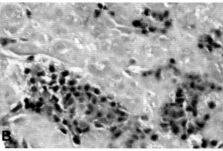

Fig. 10.85 Aggressive NK-cell leukaemia with prominent sinusoidal infiltration. **A** Neoplastic cells infiltrate the sinuses. **B** *In situ* hybridization shows that tumour cells are positive for Epstein-Barr virus-encoded RNA (EBER).

than portal tracts. Systemic EBV-positive T-cell lymphoproliferative disease of childhood and aggressive NK-cell leukaemia are both sinusoidal in distribution and often associated with haemophagocytic syndrome. In haemophagocytic syndrome, Kupffer cells show erythrophagocytosis and bile stasis is usually evident. Extranodal NK/T-cell lymphoma also has a high frequency of hepatic infiltration, with or without haemophagocytic syndrome.

Molecular pathology

Hepatic MALT lymphomas have been associated with a translocation involving *IGHα* and *MALT1* {3094}. Hepatosplenic T-cell lymphomas are associated with isochromosome 7q and trisomy 8 in most

cases {98}. For other lymphoma subtypes, the genetics are specific to the particular diagnosis, with no features specific for cases with hepatic involvement.

Prognosis and predictive factors

The prognosis for patients with primary hepatic lymphoma relates to the specific disease entity. DLBCL is an aggressive disease, with the international prognostic index providing guidance for expected treatment response and outcome {2041, 2954}. Liver involvement is indicative of stage IV disease. Hepatosplenic T-cell lymphomas are very aggressive, with a mean patient survival time of 1 year {225, 593}.

Mesenchymal tumours of the liver

M. Miettinen
C.D.M. Fletcher
L.G. Kindblom
A. Zimmermann
W.M.S. Tsui

Definition
A group of benign or malignant tumours with specific mesenchymal cell differentiation or lack of specific differentiation (undifferentiated sarcoma).

ICD-O codes

Angiomyolipoma (PEComa)	8860/0
Cavernous haemangioma	9121/0
Infantile haemangioma	9131/0
Lymphangioma	9170/0
Solitary fibrous tumour	8815/0
Angiosarcoma	9120/3
Carcinosarcoma	8980/3
Embryonal sarcoma (undifferentiated sarcoma)	8991/3
Epithelioid haemangioendothelioma	9133/3
Kaposi sarcoma	9140/3
Leiomyosarcoma	8890/3
Malignant rhabdoid tumour	8963/3
Rhabdomyosarcoma	8900/3
Synovial sarcoma	9040/3

Mesenchymal hamartoma

Mesenchymal hamartoma (MH) of the liver is a benign tumour-like lesion that develops before birth and is characterized by a commonly multicystic and well-delineated hepatic mass {600, 686, 1712, 3083, 3086, 3098}. It accounts for 8% of

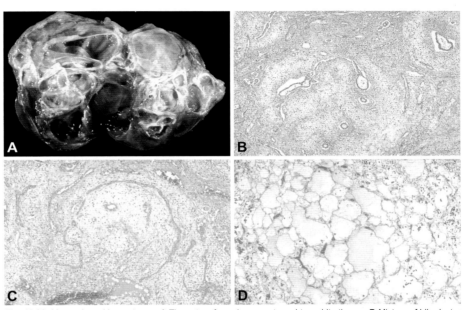

Fig. 10.86 Mesenchymal hamartoma. **A** The cut surface shows cysts and tan-white tissue. **B** Mixture of bile ducts, mesenchymal tissue and blood vessels. **C** Bile ducts display a ductal plate malformation; the primitive mesenchymal tissue consists of loosely arranged stellate cells. The tumour contains liver cells (top) in addition to blood vessels. **D** Fluid accumulation in the mesenchyme mimics lymphangioma, but the spaces lack an endothelial lining.

all liver tumours and pseudotumours from birth to age 21 years, but represents 12% of all liver tumours and pseudotumours arising during the first 2 years of life, and 22% of all benign liver neoplasms. About 85% of affected children present before the age of 3 years, and < 5% of MHs are diagnosed after the age of 5 years {693}. About 15% of cases have been observed in the neonatal period {2183}. The lesion is slightly more common in boys than in girls. In contrast, the rare MHs occurring in adults are more frequent in women {3637}.

Clinical features
Clinically, MH typically presents with abdominal distension and an upper abdominal mass, although some cases are found incidentally. Pain is rarely a dominant feature, and only few patients show anorexia, vomiting or failure to thrive {693}. Abdominal distension may rapidly progress owing to fluid accumulation in the loose tissues and in cysts and may cause respiratory distress. Large MH in neonates and infants may compromise blood circulation and evolve into life-threatening lesions. Specifically, tumoral

Table 10.09 Mesenchymal tumours of the liver.

Mode of presentation	Examples
Asymptomatic (incidental finding)	Any
Upper abdominal mass +/- hepatomegaly	Any
Sudden increase in size of tumour	Mesenchymal hamartoma, cavernous haemangioma
Febrile illness with weight loss	Inflammatory pseudotumour, embryonal sarcoma, angiosarcoma
Acute abdominal crisis from rupture	Cavernous haemangioma, infantile haemangioma, angiomyolipoma, angiosarcoma, epithelioid haemangioendothelioma
Budd-Chiari syndrome	Epithelioid haemangioendothelioma
Congestive heart failure	Infantile haemangioma
Cardiac tumour syndrome	Embryonal sarcoma
Consumption coagulopathy	Cavernous haemangioma, infantile haemangioma
Hypoglycaemia	Solitary fibrous tumour
Portal hypertension	Epithelioid haemangioendothelioma, inflammatory pseudotumour
Liver failure	Epitheliod haemangioendothelioma, angiosarcoma
Obstructive jaundice	Inflammatory pseudotumour
Lung metastases	Epithelioid haemangioendothelioma, angiosarcoma

arteriovenous shunts may induce heart failure. A complication of macrocystic MH is cyst rupture followed by neonatal ascites {964}. MH is sometimes associated with malformations, including defects in the common mesentery and mesenchymation, such as protrusion through the chest wall. It may also sometimes be associated with mesenchymal stem villus hyperplasia/dysplasia of the placenta {444, 1711}. A subset of MHs is already detectable prenatally (fetal mesenchymal hamartoma), usually diagnosed by fetal ultrasonography and/or computed tomography (CT) in the last trimester of pregnancy. The results of liver-function tests are usually normal, but serum levels of α-fetoprotein (AFP) may be slightly elevated owing to AFP production by regenerating hepatocytes located around the tumour mass {299}; in exceptional cases, MH is associated with high levels of serum AFP, a phenomenon that poses differential diagnostic problems in regard to hepatoblastoma {891, 1084, 3344}.

Ultrasonography and CT reflect the main gross components of MH, ranging from a predominantly cystic lesion or multicystic mass to a complex solid mass, which is usually hypodense and hypovascular and often multiloculated {1559}. Calcification (usually peripheral) may occur {3069}. Cysts are commonly septated, with mobile septa. These features are, together with parietal solid and nodular components, very suggestive of MH {1464, 2820, 3633}.

Macroscopy

Grossly, MH occur in the right liver lobe in 75% of cases, the left lobe in 22% of cases, and both lobes in 3% of cases. Most present as expanding, well-delimited masses without a capsule, but with perifocal liver atrophy. Very large tumours may involve both lobes or even most of the organ. Few to multiple cystic spaces lacking a communication with bile ducts are noted on cut surfaces (85% of cases). Very young patients show fewer cysts and a more solid phenotype, suggesting that cysts develop in parallel with progressive tumour growth; in some cases cysts may reach > 10 cm in size and contain an amber fluid or a gelatinous mass. In one series, 41% of tumours were solid and 59% were cystic {483}. Similar to other hepatic tumours, a subset of MH shows a pedunculated growth pattern, usually situated at the inferior surface of the liver.

Histopathology

The lesion is composed of loose connective tissue and epithelial bile duct- or ductule-like in varying proportions. The mesenchyme is typically loose and myxoid, or collagenous and arranged concentrically around the the ductules. The latter may be tortuous and occasionally dilated. These biliary cell profiles are often arranged in a ductal-plate malformation pattern. Islets of liver cells without an acinar architecture may be present. MH usually contains foci of extramedullary haematopiesis (in > 85% of cases).

Molecular pathology

On the basis of analyses of cytogenetics and DNA, there is some evidence that a neoplastic process may be involved. This has received some support from the observation of evolution of undifferentiated sarcoma from MH. Chromosomal aberrations in MH include balanced translocations between chromosomes 15 and 19 {3038} and chromosomes 11 and 19 with a break-point at 19q13.4 {1998}, interstitial deletion involving chromosome band 19q13.4 {3175}, and a complex translocation between chromosomes 11, 17 and 19 {2196} termed "MHLB1" (mesenchymal hamartoma of the liver breakpoint 1) {2619}, suggesting that the break-point

19q13.4 might be a common clonal abnormality in MH {2902}.

Prognosis

As a rule, MH has a benign course in the absence of complications, with good prognosis if the mass is resected {3633}. Exceptions are patients with severe cardiopulmonary complications and the rare instances of evolution into undifferentiated (embryonal) sarcoma {1487, 2622}.

Infantile haemangioma

Infantile haemangioma (formerly often designated as infantile haemangioendothelioma) is a benign vascular tumour similar to capillary haemangioma of the skin in infancy. It is the most common mesenchymal tumour of the liver in infants and children, accounting for about 20% of all liver tumours arising between birth and age 21 years. The clinically significant cases usually present in the first 2 years of life, when infantile haemangioma represents 40% of all tumours and 70% of benign tumours {3084}. It occurs more frequently in females (63%) than in males. Patients usually present with an enlarging abdomen, some may develop congestive heart failure or consumption coagulopathy {687, 2870}, and about 10% have haemangiomas in the skin or other sites. There may be a variety of associated con-

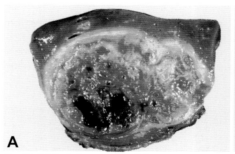 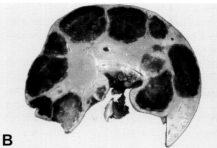

Fig. 10.87 Infantile haemangioma (infantile haemangioendothelioma). **A** A red and brown tumour with focal haemorrhage. **B** Multiple brown cavitary lesions.

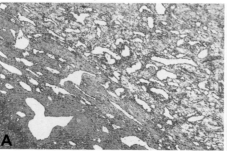 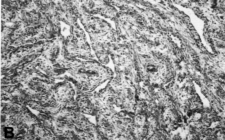

Fig. 10.88 Infantile haemangioma (infantile haemangioendothelioma). **A** The tumour is well-circumscribed but not encapsulated, and consists of small vessels. **B** Vessels are lined by a single layer of plump endothelial cells surrounded by a scant fibrous stroma; note the scattered bile ducts (Masson trichrome stain).

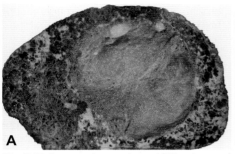 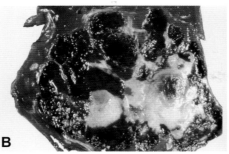 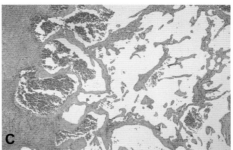

Fig. 10.89 Cavernous haemangioma. **A** Diffuse haemangiomatosis showing numerous dark blood-filled vessels extending beyond the central spongy mass and involving the whole liver lobe. **B** Multilocular blood-filled structures with pale solid areas. **C** Note the large thin-walled vascular spaces.

genital anomalies, including hemihypertrophy and Cornelia de Lange syndrome.

Macroscopy

The tumours are single in 55% and multiple in 45% of cases. Single tumours are as large as 15 cm and located equally in both lobes. Multiple lesions are often < 1 cm in size and frequently involve large portions of the liver. The large, single lesions are red-brown or red-tan, often with haemorrhagic or fibre-optic centres and focal calcification. The small lesions appear spongy and red-brown on sectioning.

Histopathology

The tumour, especially the peripheral portion, is composed of numerous small vascular channels (capillary-like) lined by plump endothelial cells usually arranged in a single layer. The vessels are supported by a scanty fibrous stroma that may be loose or compact. Larger cavernous vessels lined by flat endothelium and increased stromal fibrosis are often present in the centre of the larger lesions, corresponding to tumour regression. These vessels may undergo thrombosis with infarction, haemorrhage and calcification. Other characteristic features are small bile ducts and hepatocytes trapped

within the advancing edges, and foci of extramedullary haematopoiesis. Endothelial cells in the tumour express factor VIII-related antigen, CD31 and CD34. Distinction from congenital vascular malformation with capillary proliferation has been advocated, using GLUT1 as an immunomarker that is only positive in haemangioma {2110}.

Prognosis

This benign tumour exhibits rapid postnatal proliferation, and then maturation, followed by slow involution during childhood. Yet deaths are not uncommon, with an overall survival of 70%; adverse risk factors include congestive heart failure, jaundice, multiple tumours and absence of cavernous differentiation {2870}. Clinical management takes account of possible spontaneous regression and the severity of associated complications. The first line of treatment is with drugs, followed in the nonresponders by surgical resection, hepatic-artery ligation or transarterial embolization, with liver transplantation being the last resort {548}.
"Infantile haemangioendothelioma" was classified into two histological types {687}. The histologically more aggressive type 2 was characterized by nuclear atypia, multilayered and papillary projec-

tions of the endothelial lining; and solid cellular masses with whorls of spindle cells and Kaposiform features: this is now classified as angiosarcoma. There are also occasional reports of transformation of infantile haemangioendothelioma to angiosarcoma {2870}.

Cavernous haemangioma

This is the most common benign tumour of the liver {262}. The reported incidence varies from 0.4% to 20% in autopsy studies, the highest figure being the result of a thorough prospective search {1484}. It occurs at all ages, but is more commonly seen in young adult females. It is known to increase in size or even rupture during pregnancy, and also may enlarge or recur in patients on estrogen therapy. Haemangiomas are symptomatic only when they are > 4 cm in size, leading to pain or a mass syndrome. Rupture or acute thrombosis are exceptional, as well as the severe Kasaback-Merritt syndrome with consumptive coagulopathy.

Macroscopy

Cavernous haemangiomas vary from a few millimetres in size to huge tumours that can replace most of the liver. They are usually single, and soft or fluctuant. When sectioned, they partially collapse owing to the escape of blood and have a spongy appearance. Recent haemorrhages, organized thrombi, fibrosis and calcification may be seen.

Histopathology

Lesions are typically composed of varying sized blood-filled vascular channels lined by a single layer of flat endothelial cells and separated by fibrous septa of various thicknesses. Small arborizing vessels may be present in the fibrous stroma. Although grossly well-circumscribed, microscopic extension of dilated vascular

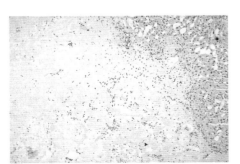

Fig. 10.90 Sclerosed haemangioma. Pale hyalinized nodule with remnants of obliterated vessels.

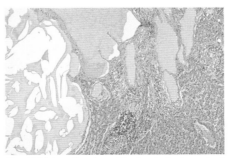

Fig. 10.91 Lymphangioma. The lymphatic channels of variable size contain clear pink-staining fluid.

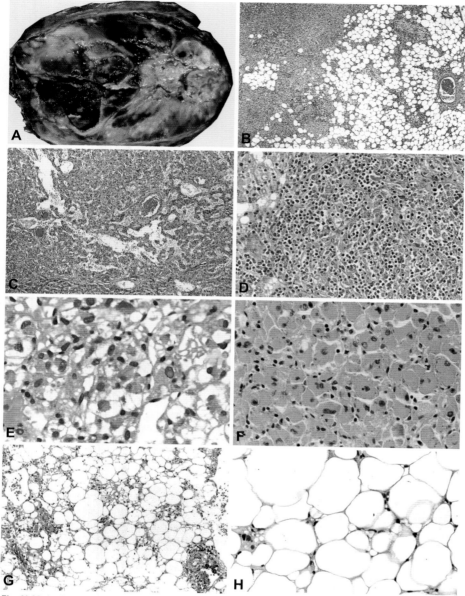

Fig. 10.92 Angiomyolipoma of the liver. **A** Cirumscribed tumour with variegated appearence including yellowish fatty areas. **B** Classic mixed tumour with admixture of myoid and fat cells. **C** Trabecular pattern featuring epitheloid myoid cells arranged in trabeculae separated by sinusoids. **D** Inflammatory infiltrate among spindle-cell stroma resembling inflammatory pseudotumour. **E** Epithelioid clear myoid cells with perinuclear condensation of cytoplasm. **F** Oncocytic myoid cells with abundant eosinophilic granular cytoplasm. **G** Lipomatous tumour with diffuse sheets of adipocytes and scanty myoid cells resembling a tumour originating from adipose tissue. **H** This neoplasm can easily be mistaken for liposarcoma owing to the presence of lipoblast-like cells.

or diffuse lesions must be differentiated from peliosis hepatis and hereditary haemorrhagic telangiectasia.

Lymphangioma and lymphangiomatosis

Lymphangioma is a rare benign tumour that is usually observed in children and adolescents. It may occur as a solitary mass or more commonly as multiple masses composed of multiple endothelial-lined spaces that vary in size from capillary channels to large, cystic spaces containing clear pink-staining lymph. The vascular spaces are lined by a single layer of endothelial cells. The supporting stroma is usually scanty and may contain lymphoid tissue.

Hepatic lymphangiomas extremely rarely occur in isolation; they are often accompanied by lymphangiomatosis of the spleen, skeleton, and other tissues, and may represent a malformation syndrome. Diffuse lymphangiomatosis involving the liver and multiple organs is associated with a poor prognosis {655}. Single lesions have been successfully resected {2897}.

Angiomyolipoma and lipomatous lesions

Angiomyolipoma is defined as a benign tumour composed of variable admixtures of adipose tissue, smooth muscle (spindled or epithelioid), and thick-walled blood vessels {1029}. It is currently regarded as a tumour of perivascular epithelioid cells (PEComa) exhibiting dual myomatous and lipomatous differentiation and melanogenesis {1987, 3309}. This tumour occurs principally in adults, with a wide age range (10–86 years) and female predominance (female-to-male ratio, 2 : 1 to 5 : 1). An association with tuberous sclerosis is recognized (5–10%); these patients have coexisting renal tumours and often multiple liver tumours. Most patients are asymptomatic, and the tumours are found incidentally. Large lesions may cause epigastric pain. Rarely, rupture with haemoperitoneum occurs in large subcapsular tumours.

Macroscopy

Angiomyolipomas are usually single and variable in size (0.8–36 cm). They are sharply demarcated but not encapsulated, fleshy or firm and, when sectioned, with a homogeneous yellow, yellow-tan or tan appearance, depending on their fat content. Larger tumours may have grossly evident necrosis or haemorrhage.

spaces into adjacent hepatic parenchyma may be observed {1547}. Thrombi in various stages of organization with areas of infarction may be present, and older lesions show dense fibrosis and calcification. In sclerosed haemangiomas, most or all of the vessels are occluded and sometimes are only demonstrable by stains for elastic tissue. Capillary-type haemangiomas are only rarely recorded in adult livers. Cavernous haemangiomas are not known to undergo malignant change. Only large symptomatic tumours require surgical excision. Extremely rarely, diffuse and multiple lesions (diffuse hemangiomatosis) with progressive development do occur {1797}; some cases are associated with involvement of multiple organs. Multiple

Histopathology

The components of smooth muscle, adipose tissue and thick-walled, sometimes hyalinized blood vessels occur in varying proportions, and are responsible for the protean morphological appearance {3309}. The smooth muscle is the only specific diagnostic component, comprising mainly epithelioid cells in sheets and, to a lesser extent, spindle-shaped cells arranged in bundles. The epithelioid cells may be clear (sugar cell), oncocytic, or pleomorphic. Unusual growth patterns (trabecular, pelioid, inflammatory) may be seen, especially in myomatous tumours with few or no fat cells. Extramedullary haematopoiesis is a frequent and characteristic feature of hepatic tumours. Immunohistochemically, the defining myoid cells are consistently positive for HMB45 and other melanogenesis markers (e.g. Melan A) {1962}; S100, CD117, actin,

desmin and vimentin expression is variable. The microscopic appearances are extensively varied and may imitate hepatocellular carcinoma, sarcomas or even vascular malformation.

Angiomyolipomas are benign neoplasms, despite their occasional large size, infiltrative margins and pleomorphic appearance. Rare malignant examples are being recognized, with monotypic epithelioid morphology, necrosis, marked nuclear atypia, and high proliferation activity suggested as potentially ominous features {651, 696, 2276, 2463}.

Lipomatous tumours and lesions

Traditionally, the lipomatous tumours of the liver are designated according to the elements present, e.g. lipoma, hibernoma, angiolipoma, myelolipoma, angiomyelolipoma. In fact, some of the lipomatous tumours reported under these

different appellations and even liposarcomas are all basically angiomyolipomas with varying proportions and/or unusual morphology of the different components. The correct terminology should be adopted, as with the soft-tissue tumours in other organs.

Pseudolipoma is believed to represent an appendix epiploica attached to the Glisson capsule after becoming detached from the large bowel. Lesions are usually a small, encapsulated mass of fat located in a concavity on the surface of the liver, the fat typically showing necrosis and calcification {1483}.

Focal fatty change of the liver is not a mesenchymal lesion, but may be mistaken for lipomatous lesions on imaging. It is characterized by multiple, contiguous acini showing macrovesicular steatosis of hepatocytes, with preservation of acinar architecture. About 45% of cases in a series of focal fatty change occurred in patients with diabetes mellitus {1072}. Distinction has to be made from steatotic microadenomas in liver adenomatosis associated with mutations in hepatocyte nuclear factor 1α ($HNF1\alpha$) {1807}.

Solitary fibrous tumour

Solitary fibrous tumour (previously also known as localized fibrous tumour and localized fibrous mesothelioma) originates from the submesothelial tissue of the liver. It occurs in patients aged 16–84 years (mean, 55 years) {2145, 2526} and with a female-to-male predominance of 2:1. Clinical presentation includes mild abdominal discomfort and presence of a solid abdominal mass. Some cases are associated with hypoglycaemia caused by the production of an insulin-like growth factor.

Macroscopy

Lesions vary considerably in size, from 2–32 cm in diameter. They arise in either lobe and are occasionally pedunculated. The external surface is smooth and the consistency firm. They are sharply demarcated but not encapsulated. Cross sections show a light tan to almost white colour with a whorled texture.

Histopathology

Solitary fibrous tumour is composed of bland uniform fibroblast-like spindle cells in a collagenized stroma and often shows alternating hypocellular and hypercellular areas. There are accompanying branching

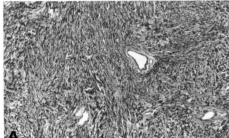
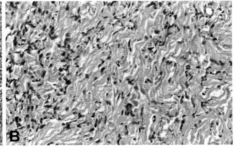

Fig. 10.93 Solitary fibrous tumour of the liver. **A** Cellular area comprising uniform spindle cells in patternless architecture. **B** Spindle cells are separated by keloid-like collagen.

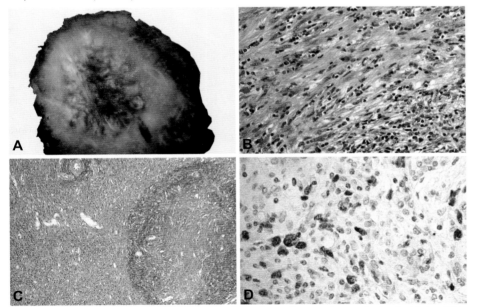

Fig. 10.94 Inflammatory pseudotumour of the liver. **A** The tumour forms a circumscribed yellowish-tan mass. **B** Mononuclear inflammatory cells in a stroma of spindle cells. **C** Note the presence of obliterative phlebitis. **D** There are many IgG4-positive plasma cells among the inflammatory infiltrate.

haemangiopericytoma-like vessels. Nuclei of the spindle cells are uniform and lack pleomorphism, but these tumours may undergo malignant change as evidenced by the presence of infiltrative margins, high cellularity, prominent cellular atypia, tumour necrosis, and increased mitotic activity (> 4 mitoses per 10 HPF) {473, 2145}. The tumour cells characteristically express CD34 and often CD99.

Inflammatory pseudotumour

This lesion is defined as a benign, non-neoplastic, non-metastasizing mass composed of fibrous tissue and proliferated myofibroblasts, with a marked inflammatory infiltration, predominantly plasma cells. It has been described under many other names, such as plasma cell granuloma, pseudolymphoma, fibroxanthoma, and histiocytoma, a reflection of the variability of its appearance. In liver lesions, there is a 3 : 1 predominance in males, and mean age at presentation is 37 years (range, 1–83 years) {2913}. Most patients present with recurrent fever, weight loss and abdominal pain; jaundice develops in a minority.

The etiology of this lesion remains unknown, although the myofibroblastic nature of the spindle cells has been well established. Most probably it is a heterogenous lesion, with various infectious and inflammatory causes being proposed.

Macroscopy
Inflammatory pseudotumours are solitary (about 80% of cases) or less often multiple (about 20% of cases) and usually intrahepatic, but some can involve the hepatic hilum (about 10% of cases). About half of the solitary tumours are located in the right lobe. They vary in size from 1 cm to large masses involving an entire lobe, and are firm, tan, yellow-white or white in colour.

Histopathology
The lesions are composed of inflammatory cells in a stroma of interlaced bundles of myofibroblasts, fibroblasts, and collagen. Most of the inflammatory cells are mature polyclonal plasma cells, but lymphocytes (and occasional lymphoid aggregates or follicles), as well as eosinophils and neutrophils, may be present. Macrophages, sometimes showing xanthomatous changes, occasional granulomas and, rarely, phlebitis involving portal vein branches or outflow veins, may be seen. Lately, IgG4-related disease turns out to be an important subgroup, which features a fibroblastic mass with marked lymphoplasmacytic infiltration, many eosinophils, numerous IgG4-positive plasma cells, dense fibrosis of hilar and extrahepatic bile ducts and obliterative phlebitis, and responds to steroid therapy {3692, 3693}.

Differential diagnosis
The clinical presentation and gross appearance of inflammatory pseudotumour may mimic that of malignant tumours, and the lesion may be mistaken for a sarcoma. On the contrary, other neoplasms with an inflammatory infiltrate are not uncommonly misdiagnosed as inflammatory pseudotumours. Examples include follicular dendritic tumour harbouring Epstein-Barr virus (EBV) {524, 2873}, inflammatory myofibroblastic tumour/low-grade inflammatory fibrosarcoma {3107}, and the inflammatory type of angiomyolipoma {1632, 3309}.

Embryonal sarcoma
Undifferentiated (embryonal) sarcoma of the liver (UES; synonym: malignant mesenchymoma of the liver) is a malignant hepatic tumour that is composed of undifferentiated mesenchymal cells and that chiefly occurs in older children.
More than 75% of cases of UES have been diagnosed in children aged 6–15 years {3082}. Few cases occur in adults. It has been estimated that UES ranks as the third most common primary malignant paediatric liver tumour, after hepato-

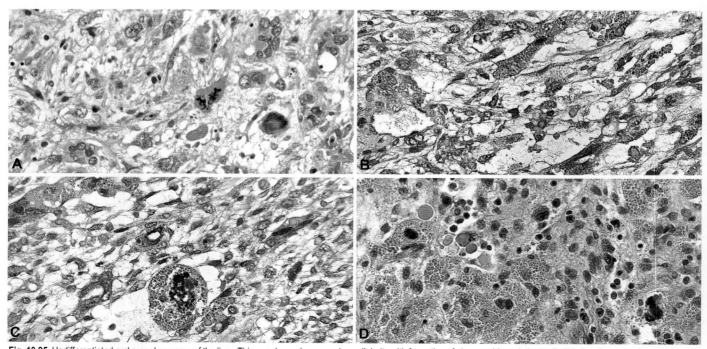

Fig. 10.95 Undifferentiated embryonal sarcoma of the liver. This neoplasm shows varying cellularity with formation of pleomorphic and giant cells (**A**). Focally, a myxoid matrix is seen (**B**). The presence of cytoplasmic (**C**) or extracellular (**D**) hyaline globules is a typical feature of this tumour.

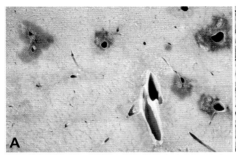
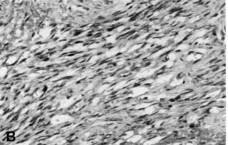

Fig. 10.96 Kaposi sarcoma. **A** Multiple dark-brown lesions are centred in large portal areas. **B** Spindle cells and slit-like vascular spaces.

blastoma and hepatocellular carcinoma, representing 9–15% of hepatic tumours in this age group {3085}. The incidence in males and females is equal. There is no pre-existing liver disease.

Clinically, affected children show abdominal pain and enlargement, weight loss and fever, and may be severely sick at presentation, with systemic signs of malignancy. Levels of serum AFP are not elevated {1715}, or only to a minimal degree owing to hepatocyte regeneration. A few patients exhibit spontaneous tumour rupture followed by haematoperitoneum and haemorrhagic shock {1304, 1715, 3085}. UES may invade the inferior vena cava and grow into the right atrium, producing a cardiac murmur.

Imaging shows that UES is located more frequently in the right liver lobe {1715}. Ultrasonographically, > 80% of these tumours are solid, whereas CT and magnetic resonance imaging (MRI) have shown low-attenuation masses with a cystic appearance {1158, 2138, 2724}. It has been shown that the CT/MR findings for cysts do not correlate well with pathological findings {361}, most of the cystic structures not being true cysts but liquified necroses and blood clots {3085}. However, true cystic spaces may also occur {3663}, sometimes with intracystic septa suggesting echinococcosis at imaging {1449}.

Macroscopy

Macroscopically, UES varies from 10 to 20 cm in diameter. It is typically well-demarcated but not encapsulated. Gross sections reveal a variegated cut surface with glistening, solid, grey-white tumour tissue alternating with fluid-rich and gelatinous areas, necroses and haemorrhage.

Histopathology

UES is chiefly composed of a loose or myxoid tissue containing an immature-looking population of spindle, stellate, polymorphous and giant cells. These cells form a diffuse growth, but cellularity may be higher around blood vessels and entrapped bile ducts. Tumour cells often display prominent anisonucleosis with hyperchromasia. The giant cells are isolated or form small clusters; they may be multinucleated and often contain bizarre nuclei with massively deranged chromatin structure, anomalies resembling those produced by ionizing radiation. A characteristic feature is the presence of sometimes numerous eosinophilic intracytoplasmic globules of variable size, located mainly in large and polymorphous cells and in giant cells. These globules are strongly positive on periodic acid-Schiff (PAS) (diastase-resistant) staining and seem ultrastructurally to represent electron-dense lysosomes with dense precipitates {40}.

Some UES show a storiform pattern resembling malignant fibrous histiocytoma {1511} or haemangiopericytoma-like areas. Spindle cells suggesting a myoid differentiation may occur {3433}, and a subset of UES displays anaplastic components (mainly in adult patients) {2304} or small undifferentiated cells {3433} resembling those in undifferentiated hepatoblastoma or some rhabdoid tumours. Osteoid formation has been reported {1715}. UES contains bile duct-like profiles, sometimes with dilated lumina, and hepatocyte nests, both structures being thought to be entrapped pre-existing structures.

Immunohistochemically, the reaction profile seems to represent an immature phenotype involving putative precursors of both mesenchymal and epithelial lineages and possibly reflecting abnormal mesenchymal–epithelial transition (MET). Positivity for several markers has been detected, including vimentin (the most consistent reaction) {1811}, desmin (highly variable), keratins, α-smooth muscle actin, α-1-antitrypsin and α-1-antichymotrypsin, CD10, CD68 and calponin {1536, 1715, 1811, 2065, 2304, 2465, 3482}. MyoD1 is not detectable in UES, an important feature for distinguishing UES from hepatobiliary rhabdomyosarcoma {2278}. In contrast to many hepatoblastomas, UES does not show nuclear expression of β-catenin {3603}.

Molecular pathology

The etiology and pathogenesis of UES are unknown. Cytogenetically, UES are diploid or aneuploid {543, 1811}, and there is evidence for extensive chromosomal rearrangements {1315}. Comparative genomic hybridization (CGH) has demonstrated several chromosomal gains and deletions, but without a specific pattern {3029}. Together, these findings suggest marked and probably progressive genomic instability. In a few instances, UES evolves in connection with pre-existing MH of the liver {667, 1762}. Cytogenetic analysis of UES secondary to MH showed a translocation at 19q13.4, a potential marker of MH {1762} and termed MHLB1 {2619}, suggesting the involvement of a common pathogenic pathway in these two lesions. In a case of UES arising in mesenchymal hamartoma and showing t(11;19)(q13;q13.4), the breakpoint at 11q13 occurred in the *MALAT1* gene, which is known to be rearrranged in a subset of renal tumours {2619}.

Prognosis

Until recently, the prognosis for patients with UES has been poor, with a median survival of < 1 year after diagnosis. With considerable improvements in recent years, long-term survival has been achieved after combined modality treatments {269, 1545, 2430}. .

Kaposi sarcoma

Disseminated Kaposi sarcoma involving the liver, mostly associated with AIDS, is usually an incidental finding on autopsy detected in 15% of patients with AIDS. In the liver, Kaposi sarcoma typically involves portal and periportal areas, often grossly detectable as red-brownish foci. Histologically, these tumours typically show poorly vasoformative spindle-cell proliferation accompanied by haemorrhage and focal deposition of

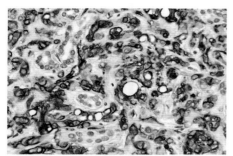

Fig. 10.97 Epithelioid hemangioendothelioma with strong positivity for CD34.

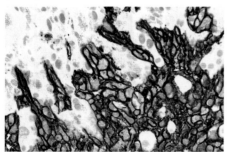

Fig. 10.98 Hepatic angiosarcoma showing strong membrane positivity for CD31.

haemosiderin. Cytoplasmic eosinophilic hyaline globules are a typical finding, and immunohistochemical demonstration of membranous/cytoplasmic CD31 and CD34, and nuclear human herpesvirus 8 (HHV-8) are diagnostic {2310}.

Epithelioid haemangioendothelioma

A tumour of variable malignant potential that is composed of spindle or epithelioid cells growing along preformed vessels or forming new vessels.

Epithelioid haemangioendothelioma (EHE) of the liver acquired its name because of the involvement of a neoplastic cell with an epithelioid morphology, but the neoplasm is clearly not epithelial. It is an uncommon tumour that presents between the ages of 12 and 86 years. The overall incidence of this tumour is unknown, but more hepatic EHEs are reported in females (about 60%) than in males (about 40%), in contrast to EHEs arising in soft tissues. Most patients are adults; of 137 patients with EHE of the liver, only seven patients were aged 20 years or < 20 years {1961}.

Clinical features

Apart from asymptomatic patients (42%), hepatic EHE may present with abdominal pain, jaundice, and ascites {230, 1961}. In rare circumstances, the tumour may be complicated by Budd-Chiari syndrome {1143} or by hepatic-vein invasion with a venoocclusive disease (VOD)-like presentation.

Radiologically, EHE presents as nodular and solitary lesions at early stages, often changing into multiple lesions. On MRI images, the nodules may show a multilayered target appearance with prominent peripheral rim with high signal intensity on T1-weighted and very low signal intensity on T2-weighted images (the bright-dark ring sign), corresponding to thrombosed vascular channels {760}. In the largest published series, 82% of hepatic EHE were manifest as multiple tumours {1961}. About 20% of these lesions exhibit focal calcifications, sometimes resulting in subtotal liver calcification {695}.

Macroscopy

Grossly, hepatic EHE presents as pale or whitish and firm to rubbery nodules with infiltrative borders. Subcapsular tumours may show typical umbilication. Solitary lesions have an average diameter of 5.6 cm, and multiple lesions range in diameter from 0.2 cm to 14 cm {1961}.

Histopathology

The neoplastic cell exhibits epithelioid, dendritic, or intermediate features {1351}. The characteristic, slightly eosinophilic epithelioid cells occur in all cases and may show vacuolated signet ring-cell-like features representing intracytoplasmic lumina sometimes containing erythrocytes. Epithelioid cells typically invade the liver sinusoids, causing marked hepatocyte plate atrophy and destruction. Dendritic cells display a spindle or stellate morphology with interdigitating processes and may also contain intracytoplasmic vacuoles. The third cell type, intermediate cell, is cytologically situated between the other two types {1351}. The mitotic rate varies considerably; no mitoses were found in 58% of tumours {1961}. EHE reveals a sometimes marked desmoplastic stromal reaction, more pronounced in the tumour centre.

Immunohistochemically, EHE cells are reactive for vimentin, factor VIII-associated antigen, CD31 and CD34 {1143, 1351, 1961, 3434}, CD34 reactivity is a particularly useful marker {694}. Some of the tumour cells are positive for keratins, in particular, keratin18 {1961, 2063}, but this observation does not prove an epithelial lineage. Podoplanin (D2-40 antibody) has been shown to be a useful marker for hepatic EHE {911}. An endothelium-related cell seems to be involved, also supported by the finding of Weibel-Palade bodies in the tumour cells {2865}.

Prognosis

EHE of the liver generally behaves as a low-grade malignant neoplasm with slow progression, but appears to be resistant to chemotherapy and may undergo a fatal course {3328}, frankly malignant behaviour also occurring rarely in children and adolescents {1490, 3154}. Tumour-related death has also been reported after EHE recurrence subsequent to liver transplantation {1679}. So far, there is no standardized effective therapy, but the results of surgical resection in cases of localized and monolobar intrahepatic disease {2166} and liver transplantation are encouraging {1808, 2327}.

Angiosarcoma

This is a variably vasoformative malignant neoplasm composed of spindled or epithelioid endothelial cells. The typical occurrence is in patients aged > 60 years and there is a 3 : 1 predominance in men. However, angiosarcomas occur even in children with a very low frequency. Known etiological factors (seen in 20% of hepatic angiosarcomas) include occupational exposure to vinyl chloride monomer, arsenic, and androgenic-anabolic steroids. Iatrogenic thorium oxide (thorotrast), an α particle-radiating substance previously used as a radiological contrast medium, is historically important, but presently a very rare etiological factor.

Clinical features

Patients with angiosarcoma present with abdominal pain, ascites, or sometimes with acute abdomen caused by tumour rupture. Prognosis is poor, and most patients die within 1 year.

Macroscopy

Grossly, hepatic angiosarcomas are typically ill-defined masses that often involve much of the liver. Many also involve the spleen. On sectioning, the tumour varies from greyish-white to haemorrhagic and focally cystic.

Histopathology

Microscopically, angiosarcomas can show solid and pseudopapillary patterns with formation of irregular vascular channels lined by variably atypical endothelial cells that often show multilayering and mitotic activity. The tumour cells frequently line pre-existing vascular channels and hepatic sinusoids. Cases associated with thorothrast often contain portal fibrosis, with granules of thorothrast present in these areas.

Molecular pathology

Mutations in the *TP53* gene have been examined in angiosarcomas that are associated or otherwise with exposure to vinyl chloride. The former were found to have A to T transversion missense mutations in codons 249 and 255 (two out of four cases), whereas the latter lacked such mutations and instead had G to A transitions in codons 141 and 136 (2 out of 21 cases) suggesting that vinyl-chloride associated angiosarcomas may have a distinctive *TP53* mutation profile {1228, 3008}. *KRAS* mutations seem to be common in both sporadic and thorothrast- and vinyl-chloride associated hepatic angiosarcomas {2596}.

Carcinosarcoma

These neoplasms are currently understood to be carcinomas that have undergone sarcoma-like differentiation (sarcomatoid carcinoma). The sarcomatoid component represents clonal evolution from the differentiated component (hepatocellular or cholangiocarcinoma). Morphology varies from spindled to epithelioid and pleomorphic. Mitotic rare is usually high, and atypical mitoses are frequent. These are clinically aggressive tumours with a poor prognosis.

Hepatobiliary rhabdomyosarcoma

Hepatobiliary rhabdomyosarcoma (RMS) is a clinically and pathologically distinct tumour entity characterized by the devel-opment and growth of a usually embryonal-type rhabdomyosarcoma along the biliary tract in children {659, 1714}. Although rare, this neoplasm is the most common tumour of the biliary tract in children, representing 1% of all paediatric rhabdomyosarcomas. The tumour occurs predominantly in infants, with a marked male preponderance, and about 2% of lesions are present at birth.

Clinical features

Clinical presentation is dominated by the sequelae of the tumour's intrabiliary growth, i.e. mainly intermittent obstructive jaundice, but fever and nonspecific abdominal manifestations may also occur. The tumour can involve the extrahepatic and/or the intrahepatic bile ducts. In localized disease, hepatobiliary RMS is classified as stage I according to the Intergroup RMS Study Group/COG {1767}. A novel classification of risk associated with RMS has recently been formulated {1144}.

Ultrasonography shows an intraductal stenosing mass causing biliary dilatation, and CT reveals hypodense and heterogeneous attenuation patterns. The typical cholangiographic finding is that of variegated filling defects representing the intraductal tumour masses {963, 2705, 2708}.

Macroscopy

Grossly, hepatobiliary RMS forms soft and often transparent masses that grow into the biliary lumina, producing polypoid and grape-like masses (botryoid growth pattern).

Histopathology

Hepatobiliary RMS commonly exhibits the morphology of embryonal RMS, charac-terized by a loose and sometimes myxoid tissue with interspersed spindled or stellate neoplastic cells. These cells have a sparse cytoplasm and small and dense nuclei, in the absence of easily recogniz-able mitotic figures, potentially causing misinterpretations in small biopsies. A characteristic feature is the rather low cellularity in deeper parts of the tumour and a band of higher cellularity immediately beneath the biliary epithelium, the so-called "cambium" layer. Diagnosis requires immunohistochemistry, the neoplastic cells being immunoreactive for desmin, myogenin and MyoD.

Prognosis

For treatment, chemotherapy with or without surgery has been performed, leading to complete tumour regression in some patients and avoiding aggressive surgery, but treatment strategies and results are constantly changing owing to improved imaging procedures for staging and novel therapy regimes {619, 1283, 1990, 2573, 2763, 2800, 3050, 3436}

Extrarenal malignant rhabdoid tumour of the liver

Malignant rhabdoid tumour (RT) primary to the liver is a rare and highly aggressive tumour that is characterized by a diffuse growth of undifferentiated cells with so-called rhabdoid features and a distinct molecular change in some cases.

The concept of rhaboid tumour or of tumours with rhabdoid features is based on the observation of intracellular filamentous aggregates manifest as distinct paranuclear spherical inclusions {1027}, rendering the cell asymmetrical and somewhat resembling a rhabdomyoblast. However, the cell lineage involved in RT has nothing to do with rhabdomyosarcoma, and the cell type involved is still unknown.

RT is a well-known entity in the kidney, but primary hepatic RT is a rare high-risk lesion of still unknown frequency {1289, 2466}.

Clinical features

Clinically, hepatic RT presents in a similar fashion to other malignant liver tumours in childhood, but serum AFP levels are consistently normal, an important differential diagnostic feature. RT of the liver can undergo spontaneous rupture {565}. Grossly, RT of the liver are often large or very large tumours predominantly located in the right liver lobe, forming lobulated masses with necrosis and haemorrhage.

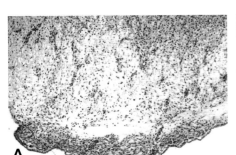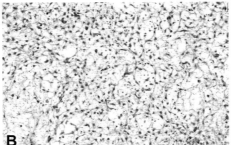

Fig. 10.99 Hepatobiliary rhabdomyosarcoma. **A** This neoplasm is characterized by the typical loose tissue of the embryonal variant. It is covered by atrophic biliary epithelium and forms the mucosal surface of a duct. Note the subepithelial hypercellular band of tumour tissue, the "cambium." **B** Spindle cells and stellate cells show marked positivity for desmin.

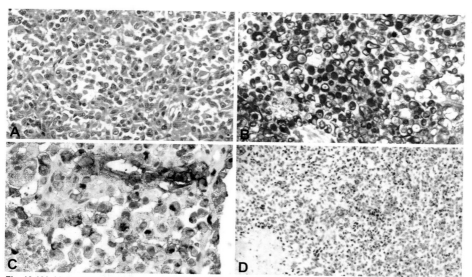

Fig. 10.100 Malignant rhabdoid tumour of the liver. **A** There is a diffuse growth of rather large cells with partly vesicular nuclei. In some (rhabdoid) cells, the nucleus is excentrically placed, caused by a paranuclear inclusion. **B, C** The paranuclear bodies of rhabdoid cells are better visualized after immunostaining for vimentin. **D** Unlike the normal surrounding cells, the nuclei of the neoplastic cells fail to stain for SMARCB1/BAF47.

Histopathology

RT shows a diffuse growth pattern, the lesion being composed of noncohesive small- to medium-sized undifferentiated cells with a generally inconspicuous cytoplasm. Some of the cells display the rhabdoid feature described above. The recognition of these paranuclear bodies seems to depend on a good fixation and high-quality haematoxylin and eosin staining of the tissue. Immunohistochemically, RT are polyantigenic, with immunoreactivity to a wide array of antibodies against mesenchymal, epithelial, neural, glial and myogenic markers {2466, 2837}, but they commonly express vimentin (mainly in the paranuclear inclusion, resulting in a characteristic "dot") and sometimes epithelial markers such as keratins (in particular, keratins 8 and 18, but not keratins 1, 10, 13–17 or 20) {3666} and epithelial membrane antigen. It has been reported that intracytoplasmic inclusion-body formation in RT may be related to mutations in the keratin 8 gene {2955}. Loss of SMARCB1 (caused by truncating mutations) can be detected by immunohistochemistry using the BAF47 antibody {1450}, which shows loss of nuclear immunostaining in the nuclei of RT cells, including those of the liver {3427, 3562}.

A fraction of hepatic RTs consist of small and anaplastic-looking cells, easily confounded with small cell undifferentiated hepatoblastoma; these cells are SMARCB1-negative, suggesting that a subset of undifferentiated hepatoblastomas have rhabdoid features {3294, 3427}.

Molecular pathology

Most RT show a characteristic molecular feature, i.e. loss of the SWI/SNF related, matrix associated, actin-dependent regulator of chromatin *SMARCB1* (*INI1*). In the regulation of gene expression, chromatin organization in nuclei is a crucial mechanism. Complexes of the SWI/SNF (SMARCA1/SMARCB1) family of proteins control or alter chromatin structure via ATP-dependent nucleosome remodelling {2129, 3088}. Most malignant rhabdoid tumours are caused by loss of function of the SMARCB1 component of the SWI/SNF chromatin-remodelling complex {1628}. It is thought that this loss of function affects key regulator proteins of cell-cycle progression and cell-cycle check-point (G1/S transition) control, as this protein regulates the activities of cyclin D1, CDKN2A (p16INK4A) and pRb(f). However, it has been reported that SMARCB1-deficient tumours and rhabdoid tumours are convergent, but not fully overlapping entities {315}.

Prognosis

RT (including primary hepatic RT) are generally highly aggressive lesions. Modern chemotherapy regimes have delivered promising results {1409, 1499}.

Leiomyosarcoma

Conventional leiomyosarcomas are almost always metastatic when involving the liver, and search for a primary tumour in locations such as the retroperitoneum is always necessary. EBV-associated leiomyosarcomas/smooth-muscle tumours can form primary hepatic masses. These tumours occur in patients with immunosuppression, either acquired (HIV/AIDS-associated) or iatrogenic (usually transplant-associated). In liver-transplant patients, occurrence from donor cells has been reported in allografts, and occurrence from recipient cells outside the graft.

Histologically, these tumours are typically less differentiated than typical leiomyosarcomas, composed of oval to spindled mesenchymal cells with immunoreactivity for α smooth muscle actin, but usually not for desmin. Demonstration of nuclear EBER is diagnostic.

Tumour behaviour is unpredictable, and multifocal lesions do not necessarily indicate metastasis, but are a feature of this tumour {3249}. In some cases, antiviral treatment and restoration of immune response have resulted in tumour regression and long-term survival {300}.

Secondary tumours of the liver

C. Iacobuzio-Donahue
L. Ferrell

Definition

Malignant neoplasms that have metastasized to the liver from extrahepatic primary tumours.

Epidemiology

Metastases predominate over primary hepatic tumours in a ratio of 40 : 1 in Europe and North America {235, 2548} and by 2.6 : 1 in Japan {2548}. In contrast, primary hepatic tumours are more common than metastases in south-east Asia and sub-Saharan Africa {2168} owing to the high incidence of hepatocellular carcinoma (HCC), shorter life expectancy (common extrahepatic carcinomas affect older age groups) and the low incidence of certain tumour types (e.g. carcinomas of the lung and colorectum). Autopsy studies in Japan and the USA have shown that up to 40% of patients with an extrahepatic primary tumour have hepatic metastases {614, 725, 2548}.

Etiopathogenesis

The liver has a rich systemic (arterial) and portal (venous) blood supply, providing a fertile environment for entrapping circulating neoplastic cells. The arrest of such cells is controlled by Kupffer cells in the sinusoids {217, 1469} and may be enhanced by growth factors such as transforming growth factor α (TGFα) {3453}, tumour necrosis factor (TNF) {1581}, or insulin-like growth factor-1 (IGF-1) {2215}, chemokines such as CXCR4 {951} and adhesion molecules such as integrin αb6 {3614}. As tumour deposits enlarge, they induce angiogenesis using native sinusoidal endothelium, thus enhancing their chances of survival {970}.

Most metastases from unpaired abdominal organs reach the liver via the portal vein, and from other sites via the systemic arterial circulation. Lymphatic spread is less common and extension to the liver via the peritoneal fluid is rare {614}. Cirrhosis provides a measure of relative protection against seeding by secondary tumours {2522}. In contrast, experimental models suggest that steatohepatitis promotes metastatic formation {3376}, as

does excess consumption of alcohol {1947}. In most patients, metastases to the liver are a manifestation of systemic, disseminated disease. Colorectal carcinoma, neuroendocrine neoplasms, and renal cell carcinoma are exceptions, as these neoplasms sometimes produce isolated, even solitary, deposits {102, 2015}.

Origin of metastases

The most frequent secondary neoplasms of the liver are carcinomas followed by melanomas {725, 2973}. Hepatic involvement by lymphomas or sarcomas is uncommon {1377, 1881, 3062}. In autopsy studies in North America and Europe, the frequency of hepatic metastases per primary site is greatest for testicular, ocular (uveal melanoma) and pancreaticobiliary cancers. Breast, lung and colorectal carcinomas also frequently metastasize to the liver {725}. In terms of absolute numbers, the most common metastases to the liver are derived from breast, colorectal and gastric carcinomas {725}. Hodgkin and non-Hodgkin lymphomas may involve the liver in up to 20% of patients at presentation and 55% at autopsy {1377}. Only 6% of patients with sarcoma may have

hepatic metastases at presentation, but 34% have hepatic metastases at autopsy {1393}.

Clinical features

Signs and symptoms

In many patients, the presence of a hepatic metastasis is asymptomatic. Patients with symptomatic hepatic metastases often present with ascites, hepatomegaly or abdominal fullness, hepatic pain, jaundice, anorexia, and weight loss. There may be constitutional symptoms, such as malaise, fatigue and fever {2893}. On examination, nodules or a mass are felt in up to 50% of cases, and a friction bruit may be heard on auscultation. Symptomatic presentation is associated with bulky, rapidly progressing tumours with a poor prognosis {2893}. Rarely, patients present with fulminant hepatic failure {2620} caused by diffuse infiltration of the liver, most often seen in association with metastatic small cell carcinoma. Patients with functioning neuroendocrine carcinomas that metastasize to the liver may present with carcinoid syndrome {231}. "Carcinomatous cirrhosis" with jaundice, ascites, and bleeding

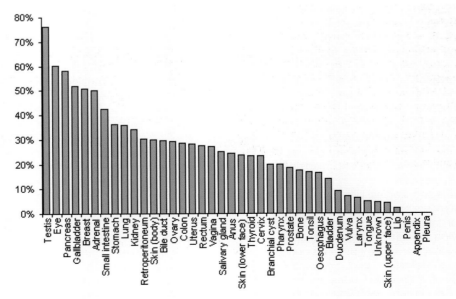

Fig. 10.101 Frequency of metastasis to the liver according to site of the primary neoplasm. Data from 3827 autopsies {725}.

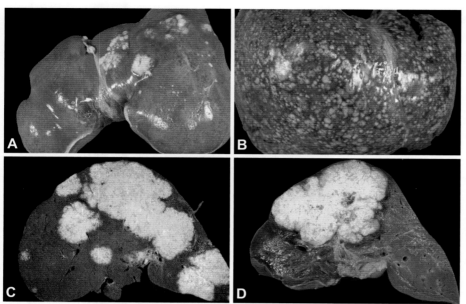

Fig. 10.102 Gross specimens. **A** Metastatic colon carcinoma showing umbilication and hyperaemic borders. **B** Metastatic small cell carcinoma of the lung forming innumerable small nodules. **C,D** Metastatic large-intestinal carcinoma, cut surfaces.

varices due to diffuse infiltration of the liver has also been described {2815}.

Laboratory studies: Levels of alkaline phosphatase and serum transaminase, although nonspecific, are elevated in about 80% and 67% of patients respectively, and probably represent the effects of hepatic parenchymal infiltration by the tumour and of generalized wasting. Elevated levels of lactic dehydrogenase are relatively specific for the presence of metastatic melanoma. Tests of synthetic function, e.g. prothrombin time and levels of serum albumin, may be normal despite extensive metastatic involvement. Levels of α-fetoprotein (AFP) may be slightly to moderately elevated, but very high concentrations are more consistent with a diagnosis of HCC {3710}. Levels of carcinoembryonic antigen (CEA), which are raised in as many as 90% of patients with metastases from colorectal carcinoma, can be useful in monitoring patients after resection of the primary tumour, together with routine clinical and imaging follow-up studies {3181}.

Imaging studies: Ultrasound can identify tumours measuring 1–2 cm in size, differentiate solid from cystic lesions, and provide guidance for percutaneous needle biopsy. However, it provides poor anatomical definition and frequently misses smaller lesions. Computed tomography (CT), using contrasted and non-contrasted images, can also serve as a

screening tool. The administration of intravenous contrast permits the detection of tumours as small as 0.5 cm in diameter {2981}. Most metastases display decreased vascularity in comparison to the surrounding hepatic parenchyma and thus appear as hypodense defects. Tumours that are hypervascular (e.g. melanoma, carcinoids and some breast cancers) or calcified (e.g. colorectal carcinoma) are better delineated by non-contrast views. Magnetic resonance imaging (MRI) is more sensitive than CT in the detection of hepatic tumours and can detect additional lesions, too small to be seen via CT. Positron emission tomography (PET) can detect metastatic disease in the liver and elsewhere. The radiolabelled glucose analogue 2-(18)fluoro-2-deoxy-D-glucose (F-18 FDG) can be used with PET to highlight metabolically active tissues. Through co-registration with anatomical studies like CT or MRI, viable malignant tumours can be differentiated from benign or necrotic lesions {111}. However, a high rate of false-negatives has been shown for PET when evaluating mucinous carcinomas {236}.

Preoperative CT arterial portography or intraoperative ultrasound is associated with the highest sensitivities {3031}. The former is capable of detecting lesions of 15 mm, although a false-positive rate of 17% has been reported {3030}. Its suc-

cess relies on the fact that tumours are not fed by portal-vein blood, so that metastases appear as filling defects. Intraoperative ultrasound, capable of detecting lesions of 2–4 mm in diameter, delineates the anatomical location of tumours in relationship to major vascular and biliary structures and provides guidance for intraoperative needle biopsies. It is the definitive step for determining resectability at the time of exploratory laparotomy or laparoscopy. Although the use of angiography has declined in recent years, it is helpful in defining vascular anatomy for planned hepatic resections, selective chemotherapy, chemo-embolization, or devascularization procedures, for assessing whether there is metastatic involvement of the portal venous system and/or hepatic veins, or for differentiating between benign and malignant vascular lesions when other imaging studies have yielded equivocal results.

Macroscopy

Some studies suggest that right-sided colon cancers predominantly metastasize to the right lobe of the liver, while left-sided colon cancers metastasize to both lobes, supporting the existence of the "streaming" effect in the portal vein {1649}. Metastases may be multinodular, diffusely infiltrative, or solitary. Very large solitary metastases are most often seen in association with metastatic colorectal or renal cell carcinoma. Umbilication (a central depression on the surface of a metastatic deposit) is caused by necrosis or scarring and is typical of metastatic adenocarcinomas from the stomach, pancreas or colorectum. A vascular rim around the periphery of the metastatic lesion is often seen. Mucin-secreting adenocarcinomas appear as glistening, gelatinous masses, while well-differentiated keratinizing squamous cell carcinomas are granular. Metastatic carcinoid tumours are typically solid but can form pseudocysts {697}. Extensive haemorrhage is more frequently seen in metastatic choriocarcinoma, carcinomas of the thyroid or kidney, neuroendocrine neoplasms, or vascular leiomyosarcomas. Diffusely infiltrating neoplasms, such as small cell carcinoma, lymphoma and sarcoma may have a soft, opaque, fleshy appearance. Rarely, metastatic breast carcinoma can produce extensive fibrosis simulating cirrhosis. Calcification of

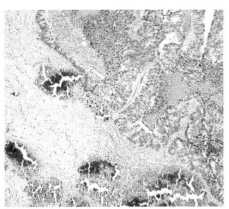

Fig. 10.103 Metastatic colorectal carcinoma. The tumour is necrotic and the cell type is typically columnar.

hepatic metastases may be seen in association with a variety of primary neoplasms. In colon cancer, calcifications within hepatic metastases are associated with a better prognosis {756}.

Histopathology and differential diagnosis

Metastatic neoplasms to the liver are usually histologically similar to their primary tumour of origin and to related metastases at other organ sites.

Metastases arising from renal cell carcinoma, adrenocortical carcinoma or melanoma may mimic HCC, which can usually be distinguished by its trabecular structure and presence of sinusoids, absence of mucin secretion or desmoplastic stroma, bile production, and the demonstration of bile canaliculi by polyclonal CEA antisera (specific for a liver-cell origin). Other useful immunophenotypic features are the presence of liver export proteins (albumin, fibrinogen, α-1-antitrypsin) and expression of hepatocyte-paraffin-1 (HepPar1), AFP and the oncofetal protein glypican-3 {1458}. Of note, AFP and glypican-3 also stain germ cell tumours, and glypican-3 can also be positive in melanoma. Moreover, AFP is expressed in only a minority of HCCs, and glypican-3 is often not positive in well-differentiated HCCs {1849, 2892}. Adrenocortical carcinomas are typically positive for inhibin and melanA {2189, 2659}, and renal cell carcinomas are typically positive for paired box gene 8/PAX8 {3267}. Amelanotic melanoma is easily identified by positive immunolabelling for S100 protein and HMB45 {2380}.

The distinction between cholangiocarcinoma and *metastatic adenocarcinomas* is much more difficult, if not impossible

{1803, 2380}. The presence of high-grade intraepithelial neoplasia within intrahepatic bile ducts near an adenocarcinoma is strong evidence that the neoplasm is a primary cholangiocarcinoma; without this finding, panels of immunohistochemical stains are required.

Cholangiocarcinoma may assume any of the histological patterns of a metastatic adenocarcinoma; it is usually tubular but may be mucinous, signet-ring, papillary, cystic, or undifferentiated. Some metastases form reproducible patterns that may provide clues to their primary origin, e.g. small tubular or tubulo-papillary glands frequently derive from the pancreaticobiliary system, while a signet ring-cell appearance suggests a gastric or breast primary.

Perhaps the easiest pattern to recognize as metastatic in origin is that exhibited by adenocarcinomas of the colon and rectum, which nearly always show glands of variable size and shape, lined by tall columnar cells, with lumina containing abundant necrotic debris. Metastases from the colorectum frequently have well-defined edges whereas those from other glandular sites tend to be more diffuse. Of note, some metastatic colonic adenocarcinomas are associated with prominent intrabiliary ductal growth that mimics high-grade intraepithelial neoplasia of intrahepatic bile ducts {2689}. Cholangiocarcinomas typically express keratins 7 and 19 but not 20, while colorectal carcinomas are typically negative for keratins 7 and 19 and positive for keratin 20 {1948, 2756}. Nuclear positivity for CDX2 is also a marker for gastrointestinal origin {3490}. Metastases from the breast may be identified by immunostains for gross cystic disease fluid protein 15, estrogen and progesterone receptors {2335}. Metastatic adenocarcinoma from the lung is typically positive for TTF1; however, occult breast or lung carcinoma with hepatic metastases as the initial presentation is rare. The same applies to squamous cell carcinomas of the oesophagus and cervix. In patients presenting with hepatic metastasis, the most common primary is a small cell carcinoma of the lung, characteristically producing an enlarged liver caused by diffuse infiltration {2620}.

Neuroendocrine/islet cell/carcinoid tumours are easily identified by their organoid nesting pattern, uniform cytology and vascularity, and positive immunostaining for chromogranin, synap-

tophysin and neuron-specific enolase. Islet cell tumours also produce specific hormones, e.g. insulin, glucagon, gastrin, vasoactive intestinal peptide and somatostatin, which either give rise to clinical syndromes or can be detected in the blood or tumour tissue. In some instances, the site of origin of the neuroendocrine neoplasm (e.g. gastrointestinal vs pulmonary) can be identified by nuclear positivity for CDX2 or TTF1, respectively {2801}.

Although uncommon, most *sarcomas* that metastasize to the liver are gastrointestinal stromal tumours (typically positive for CD34 and KIT) or uterine leiomyosarcomas (that may be positive for desmin or muscle-specific actin) {3062}. Some carcinomas, notably of the kidney, may be sarcomatoid in their morphology. Sarcomatoid renal cell carcinomas nonetheless retain PAX8 expression {3267}.

Leukaemias, myeloproliferative disorders, Hodgkin and non-Hodgkin lymphomas may involve the liver at advanced stages of disease. Leukaemias tend to produce diffuse sinusoidal infiltrates. Hodgkin and high-grade non-Hodgkin lymphomas produce tumour-like masses, while low-grade nonHodgkin lymphomas produce diffuse portal infiltrates {1377}.

Rarely, *carcinomas of the thyroid, prostate and testis* may metastasize to the liver. In these cases, the diagnosis can be confirmed by immunohistochemical detection of thyroglobulin, prostate-specific antigen and AFP and bHCG, respectively. Squamous cell carcinomas of the head and neck seldom involve the liver.

The presence of a characteristic histological triad of features – proliferating bile ducts, leukocytes and focal sinusoidal dilatation – in a core biopsy suggests that a metastatic deposit (a space-occupying lesion) has been missed by the biopsy needle. Three lesions – *bile duct adenoma, sclerosed haemangioma, and larval granuloma* – may resemble metastatic tumours at laparotomy {3573}.

Prognosis

In most patients, the presence of hepatic metastasis indicates an advanced and disseminated stage of disease that precludes surgical intervention. However, for patients with colorectal carcinoma and low-burden metastatic disease, 5-year survival can be as high as 40%. Without surgical therapy, median survivals of < 12 months should be expected.

Diagnostic algorithms for tumours of the liver

R. Saxena
J. Albores-Saavedra
P. Bioulac-Sage
P. Hytiroglou
M. Sakamoto
N.D. Theise
W.M.S. Tsui

Introduction

Hepatocellular carcinoma (HCC) and metastatic tumours constitute the vast majority of clinically significant liver tumours worldwide. The most common liver tumour is cavernous haemangioma, which is most often discovered incidentally during imaging for unrelated conditions.

An important consideration in the differential diagnosis of a liver tumour is whether the background liver is cirrhotic. While exceptions occur, a malignant tumour in a cirrhotic liver in children or adults is HCC, and needs to be differentiated from large regenerative nodules and dysplastic nodules, which also form distinctive nodules in the cirrhotic liver. In contrast, there are major geographic differences in the types of tumours that occur in the non-cirrhotic liver; in adults, HCC is the most common liver tumour in South-East Asia and sub-Saharan Africa, while metastatic tumours and benign hepatocellular lesions (focal nodular hyperplasia and hepatocellular adenoma) outnumber HCC in the USA and Europe. In children, paediatric tumours such as hepatoblastoma, mesenchymal hamartoma and infantile haemangioma account for the majority of tumours arising in non-cirrhotic livers. While HCCs do occur in children, only 20–30% occur in a background of cirrhosis in contrast to 80–90% in adults, at least in European countries and North America. Similarly, the fibrolamellar variant of HCC occurs in non-cirrhotic livers of older children and young adults.

The vast majority of cystic liver lesions are either developmental or infectious in nature, which thus form an important differential diagnostic consideration with cystic liver neoplasms. True primary cystic neoplasms of the liver, i.e. neoplasms with epithelium-lined cysts, are few and include biliary intraductal papillary neoplasm, mucinous cystic neoplasm and cystic cholangiocarcinoma. On the other hand, almost any solid tumour can undergo cystic degeneration; in these tumours, the cystic cavities are not lined by epithelium. Solid neoplasms most likely to appear cystic on radiological or gross examination are mesenchymal hamartoma, undifferentiated embryonal sarcoma, HCC post-embolization and large cavernous haemangioma.

The diagnosis of a liver tumour is facilitated by four vital pieces of clinical and radiological information: the age of the patient; whether the tumour is solid or cystic; whether the tumour is single or multicentric; and whether there is underlying fibrotic chronic liver disease. While imaging studies offer clues about the nature of a liver tumour, they offer a specific diagnosis only in a subset of HCCs arising in the cirrhotic liver. This includes lesions > 2 cm in diameter that demonstrate radiological features specific for HCC by one dynamic imaging modality or lesions < 2 cm in diameter that demonstrate these specific features by two dynamic imaging modalities {352}. Radiological findings considered specific for HCC in a cirrhotic liver are "rapid wash-in" during arterial phase followed by "rapid wash-out" during early-late portal phases. A confirmatory biopsy is not needed in these cases of HCC, representing perhaps the only instance in which diagnosis of malignancy is established by radiology alone. These noninvasive criteria do not apply for the diagnosis of HCC in a non-cirrhotic liver.

Cellular lines of differentiation of liver tumours

The repertoire of primary epithelial liver tumours is largely limited to tumours that display hepatocytic and/ or cholangiocytic phenotypes. This rather small group of primary tumours is matched by an almost indefinite variety of metastatic tumours. Mesenchymal tumours of the liver are similar to those arising elsewhere in the body except for mesenchymal hamartoma, which is specific to the liver. Mesenchymal tumours that occur preferentially in the liver include inflammatory pseudotumour, cavernous haemangioma, angiomyolipoma, infantile haemangioma, epithelioid haemangioendothelioma, undifferentiated embryonal sarcoma and angiosarcoma.

Tumours with predominant hepatocytic phenotype may contain a variety of intracellular inclusions such as ground glass inclusions, pale bodies, eosinophilic globules and Mallory-Denk hyalin. The cells are arranged in trabeculae with intervening endothelium-lined sinusoids, a pattern that recapitulates the architecture of the normal liver. These tumours may also form gland-like structures that do not contain mucin (pseudoglands or acini) but may have bile (biliary rosettes), a pattern recapitulating the biliary canalicular system of the normal liver. The presence of bile is the most convincing evidence of hepatocellular differentiation on an haematoxylin and eosin stain. Immunohistochemical evidence of hepatocyte lineage is provided by cytoplasmic positivity for hepatocyte-specific antigen (carbomyl phosphate synthetase-1, recognized by HepPar1 antibody) and α-fetoprotein (AFP); and by canalicular positivity for CD10 and polyclonal antibody to carcinoembryonic antigen (pCEA). The latter cross-reacts with a biliary glycoprotein present in the canalicular membrane of hepatocytes; cytoplasmic reactivity with either pCEA or monoclonal antibody to CEA (mCEA) is evidence against HCC.

Immunohistochemical evidence for the hepatocellular phenotype is useful in two situations: first, in the distinction of well-differentiated HCC from other tumours that may show large eosinophilic cells with or without a trabecular architecture (Table 10.10); and second, in the distinction of poorly differentiated HCC from other poorly differentiated tumours, including metastatic carcinomas.

Tumours with predominant cholangiocytic phenotype form ductal and/or glandular structures of varying complexity and are usually associated with a fibrous stroma (bile duct adenoma, intrahepatic cholangiocarcinoma). These tumours may contain mucin and demonstrate immunohistochemical positivity for keratins AE1, 8/18, 7, and 19, and for epithelial membrane antigen (EMA), pCEA, MOC31 and MUC1; however, none of these markers

Table 10.10 Differential diagnosis of hepatocellular carcinoma (HCC) and its mimics: useful histological and immunohistochemical features.[a]

Features	HCC	AdCa	RCC	ACC	OCT	NET / NEC	AML	MEL
Histological / histochemical								
Trabecular architecture	●		●	●	●	●	●	●
Pseudoglandular structures	●	●			●	●		
Bile production	●							
Tubuloglandular architecture		●				●		
Desmoplastic reaction		●			●	●		
Organoid pattern					●	●		●
Cytoplasmic fat in tumour cells	●		●	●			●	
Mucin		●						
Immunohistochemical[b]								
α-Fetoprotein	●							
HSA / carbamoyl phosphate synthetase-1	●							
CEA, canalicular staining	●							
CEA, cytoplasmic staining		●						
Glypican-3	●							●
Keratins 8/18	●	●	●		●	●		
Keratins 7/19		●			●	●		
MOC31		●				●		
Epithelial membrane antigen		●	●		●	●		
Vimentin			●	●	●		●	●
PAX2			●					
Inhibin				●				
Melan A				●			●	●
Chromogranin						●		
Synaptophysin				●		●		
Smooth muscle actin							●	
HMB45 antigen							●	●
TTF1 nuclear staining		●[c]			●	●[c]		
Thyroglobulin					●			

ACC, adrenocortical carcinoma; AdCa, adenocarcinoma; AML, angiomyolipoma, epithelioid variant; CEA, carcinoembryonic antigen; HCC, hepatocellular carcinoma; HSA, hepatocyte-specific antigen (HepPar1 antibody); MEL, melanoma; NET/NEC, neuroendocrine tumour/ neuroendocrine carcinoma; OCT, follicular carcinoma of thyroid, oncocytic variant; RCC, renal cell carcinoma.

[a] The selection of features was based on utility, not completeness. Dots indicate features that are commonly present in each tumour. Absence of a dot signifies that the specific feature is either absent or uncommonly present in the specific tumour.

[b] Other immunohistochemical markers may be useful in specific situations (see Table 10.13), e.g. metastatic colorectal adenocarcinomas are usually keratin 20-positive, CDX-2 positive, MUC2-positive, and keratin 7-negative; HCCs arising in patients with chronic infection with hepatitis B virus (HBV) occasionally express hepatitis B surface antigen (HBsAg); CDX-2 may be positive in NET/NEC of the gut.

[c] Positive in adenocarcinoma and NET/NEC of the lung, and in small cell NEC of other organs.

are specific for cholangiocytic differentiation. The diagnosis of intrahepatic cholangiocarcinoma necessitates exclusion of morphologically similar and more frequently occuring metastatic adenocarcinomas; both lesions usually occur in non-cirrhotic livers (Table 10.13).

Clues from the clinical picture
Information on age, sex, multicentricity and the presence or absence of fibrotic chronic liver disease help to significantly narrow the differential diagnosis. Tumours that may present at birth include mesenchymal hamartoma, hepatoblastoma and infantile hemangioma. A large tumour in a child aged < 6 months with a hyperdynamic circulation or consumptive thrombocytopenia (Kassabach-Merritt syndrome) is most likely to be an infantile haemangioma. Other tumours that occur in children aged < 2 years are malignant rhabdoid tumour and rhabdomyosarcoma. Tumours in children aged > 2 years include undifferentiated embryonal sarcoma, calcifying nested epithelial stromal tumour, transitional liver cell tumour and HCC (Table 10.14). In a child with a cirrhotic liver, the differential diagnosis of a distinctive liver nodule is the same as in adults and includes large regenerative nodule, dysplastic nodule and HCC.

Table 10.11 Differential diagnosis of well-differentiated hepatocellular tumours arising in non-cirrhotic liver: useful gross, microscopic and immunohistochemical features.

Tumour	Gross characteristics	Microscopy	Immunohistochemistry	
Focal nodular hyperplasia (FNH)	Firm, multinodular mass, well-limited, non-encapsulated; often central stellate fibrous scar (classical FNH); any size; single (in about two thirds of cases) or multiple	Nodules of benign hepatocytes, separated by fibrous bands radiating from stellate scar; thick, dystrophic arteries, ductular reaction and lymphocytic infiltration in fibrosis (classical FNH)	Overexpression of glutamine synthetase, forming large interconnected areas in a "map-like" pattern; keratin 7 or 19 to highlight ductular reaction	
Hepatocellular adenoma (HCA)[a]	Soft, non-encapsulated mass, often necrotic and haemorrhagic; any size; single (in about two thirds of cases) or multiple	Benign hepatocytes, isolated arteries and arterioles. **Subtypes:**	The following panel is useful in subclassification of HCA: [b]	
		HNF1α-inactivated Steatosis, usually marked	Loss of L-FABP in tumoral hepatocytes	
		β-Catenin-activated Focal, mild to moderate nuclear atypia and pseudoglands	Glutamine synthetase: strong, diffuse overexpression; β-Catenin: aberrant, often focal, nuclear and cytoplasmic expression	
		Inflammatory HCA[c] Inflammatory infiltrate, thick arteries, ductular reaction; often prominent sinusoidal dilatation and peliotic areas	Serum amyloid A, C-reactive protein: diffuse overexpression	
Well-differentiated hepatocellular carcinoma[a]	Soft tumour, often encapsulated, often large	Trabecular architecture (plates often more than two to three cells thick), pseudoglands; variable nuclear atypia; bile production (common); numerous isolated arteries; decreased reticulin network	Glypican-3: for this differential diagnosis, this stain is useful only if positive AFP: useful if positive, but usually negative	
Fibrolamellar hepatocellular carcinoma	Large, firm, variegated tumour with fibrous scar; calcifications (imaging)	Large, eosinophilic (oncocytic) hepatocytes; thick plates separated by thick parallel fibrous lamellae; cytoplasmic inclusions common	Keratin 7: useful, if strongly and diffusely positive	
Hepatoblastoma, fetal type	Large, variegated tumour, often haemorrhagic	Small hepatocytes in two-cell thick plates; little to no pleomorphism; "light" and "dark" areas; extramedullary haematopoiesis	AFP: positive	

AFP, α-fetoprotein; L-FABP, liver fatty acid-binding protein.

[a] The differential diagnosis of HCA and well differentiated HCC may be impossible. Often additional clinical information, radiological examination (including assessment of rapid growth), and/or more extensive sampling are necessary for diagnosis.

[b] This panel may also be used for distinguishing FNH from HCA (in FNH, L-FABP is normally expressed, i.e. diffusely positive, and β-catenin is exclusively membranous, whereas C-reactive protein and serum amyloid A are negative).

[c] 10% of inflammatory HCAs are also β-catenin-activated.

A young woman taking the contraceptive pill who presents with acute abdominal haemorrhage is most likely to have a hepatocellular adenoma. A cystic tumour in a young woman is likely to be a mucinous cystic neoplasm, formerly referred to as "biliary cystadenoma." If the tumour demonstrates areas of invasion, it is called a mucinous cystic neoplasm associated with invasive carcinoma; a term that is preferred to the formerly used " biliary cystadenocarcinoma." These cystic neoplasms are analogous to their counterparts in the pancreas and, as in that organ, their defining feature is the presence of "ovarian-like" stroma. Furthermore, as in the pancreas, a number of cystic, mass-like lesions do not show an "ovarian-like" stroma and are lined by papillary epithelium, which may be biliary, mucinous or oncocytic in nature. Like their pancreatic counterparts, they arise from biliary intraductal papillary lesions (biliary papilloma/biliary papillomatosis) and become cystic as they enlarge and obstruct the ducts of origin. These cystic neoplasms occur with equal frequency in men and women and are distinct from the mucinous cystic neoplasms with "ovarian-like" stroma in both the pancreas and liver {257, 1837, 2250}. Thus, these tumours, originally thought to represent variants of "cystadenoma" and "cystadenocarcinoma" without the typical "ovarian-like" stroma, are more appropriately termed "biliary intraductal papillary neoplasms" (whether cystic or not) in alignment with intraductal papillary tumours of the pancreas. In contrast to intraductal papillary neoplasms of the pancreas, which are most often lined by mucinous epithelium, the vast majority of intraductal papillary neoplasms of the biliary tree are lined by biliary epithelium. Oncocytic variants are rare at both sites.

The new suggested terminology acknowledges the similarities between cystic tumours arising in the pancreas and the liver and their respective ductal systems, and distinguishes the two distinct clinico-pathological groups of cystic tumours in the liver; those that have an intraductal origin and those that do not {2719}.

The presence of underlying chronic liver disease, especially when there is advanced fibrosis or cirrhosis, represents high odds for the presence of HCC. In addition, HCC may arise in the context of haemochromatosis and chronic hepatitis B infection even in the absence of cirrhosis; this is especially true in areas with high incidence of HCC, such as South-East Asia and sub-Saharan Africa, where a male preponderance is noted.

Clues from the radiological and gross appearance of liver tumours

Most liver tumours are solid in appearance but cystic changes may occur in any tumour, including HCC. Cystic changes are rare in cholangiocarcinomas, which usually are white, firm masses without significant necrosis or haemorrhage. The presence of fibrosis in these tumours leads to delayed central enhancement on dynamic computed tomography (CT) and magnetic resonance imaging (MRI); this feature when associated with biliary dilatation is strongly suggestive of cholangiocarcinoma. Almost any tumour can cause compression of the bile ducts, but an abrupt biliary stricture is indicative of cholangiocarcinoma, especially when there are known predisposing factors such as primary sclerosing cholangitis. While both focal nodular hyperplasia and fibrolamellar carcinoma occur in non-cirrhotic livers and show a central stellate scar, focal nodular hyperplasia has a soft appearance while fibrolamellar carcinoma is firm. A yellow colour representing underlying steatosis is more common in focal nodular hyperplasia.

Most primary liver tumours are solitary; HCC may show multiple satellite nodules situated around the main tumour at a distance of 1 cm or less. On the other hand, the presence of multiple tumours, both solid and cystic, is suspicious for metastatic disease, especially when they arise in older individuals without cirrhosis. Bile duct adenomas are often multiple and appear as tiny, subcapsular lesions measuring 1–5 mm. They raise alarm for metastatic disease during abdominal surgery and account for a significant number of intraoperative consultations. Multiple, centrally calcified or ossified tumour masses in a non-cirrhotic liver of an elderly individual are distinctive for epithelioid haemangioendothelioma.

Different types of cysts cannot be reliably distinguished from one another by radiological or gross examination, except in the case of hydatid cysts which have pearly white, slimy walls and characteristic imaging features. Large cavernous haemangiomas with cystic degeneration typically appear spongy and beefy-red on gross examination. The latter also show peripheral puddling of contrast material on imaging studies, the intensity of which is the same as that of the aorta, an important diagnostic feature. When imaging shows multiple liver cysts, developmental cysts or metastatic disease are the major considerations. Liver tumours that are entirely or predominantly intraductal include

Table 10.12 Differential diagnosis of distinctive hepatocellular nodular lesions arising in cirrhotic liver: useful histological and immunohistochemical features.

Histological feature	Hepatocellular lesion					
	LRN	FNH-like	LGDN	HGDN	eHCC	clHCC
Features characteristic of carcinoma						
Cell plates more than three cells in width	–	–	–	–	+/–	+
Moderate nuclear-contour irregularities	–	–	–	–	+	+
Stromal invasion	–	–	–	–	+/–	+/–
Vascular invasion	–	–	–	–	–	+/–
Widespread loss and irregularity of reticulin framework	–	–	–	–	–	+/–
Other features						
Cell density more than twice that of the surrounding parenchyma (reflecting increased nucleus : cytoplasm ratio)	–	–	–	+/–	+	+/–
Pseudogland formation in the absence of cholestasis	–	–	–	+/–	+/–	+/–
Expansile subnodules (foci)	–	–	–	+/–	+/–	+/–
Nuclear hyperchromasia	–	–	–	+	+	+
Mild nuclear-contour irregularities	–	–	–	+	+	+
Cytoplasmic basophilia	–	–	–	+/–	+/–	+/–
Prominent steatosis (more than in the background liver)	–	?	+/–	+/–	+/–	+/–
Prominent hepatocellular siderosis (more than in the background liver)			+/–	+/–	–	–
Resistance to iron accumulation[a]	–	–	–	+/–	+	+
Portal tracts within the nodule	+	+/–	+	+	+/–	–
Unpaired arteries	–	+	+/–	+/–	+/–	+
Immunohistochemical stains						
α-Fetoprotein	–	–	–	–	–[b]	+/–
Three-marker panel:[c]						
Glypican-3	–[b]	?	–[b]	+/–	+/–	+/–
Heat shock protein 70	–	?	–[b]	–[b]	+/–	+/–
Glutamine synthetase (diffuse pattern, not just perivenular)	–	–	–	–	+/–	+/–

FNH-like, focal nodular hyperplasia-like nodule; HGDN, high-grade dysplastic nodule; LGDN, low-grade dysplastic nodule; LRN, large regenerative nodule; eHCC, early hepatocellular carcinoma; clHCC: "classic" hepatocellular carcinoma.

–, absent; +, present; +/–, can be absent or present; ?, not known.

[a] "Resistance to iron accumulation" refers to an iron-free focus in an otherwise siderotic nodule.

[b] Rarely positive.

[c] Currently, positive immunostaining for any two markers of the three-marker panel is considered strong suggestive evidence for hepatocellular carcinoma (either early or classic).

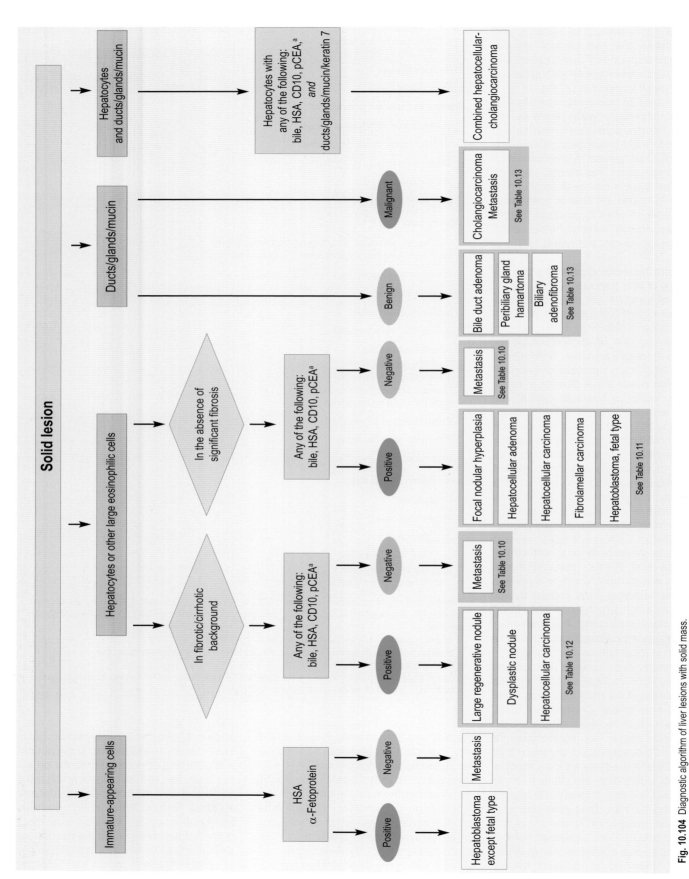

Fig. 10.104 Diagnostic algorithm of liver lesions with solid mass.

[a] Only the canalicular pattern of staining for CD10 and pCEA is specific for the hepatocellular phenotype; this may, however, coexist with a membranous pattern. pCEA, polyclonal antibody to carcinoembryonic antigen; HSA, hepatocyte-specific antigen, recognized by HepPar1 antibody, corresponds to cytoplasmic carbamoyl phosphate synthetase-1.

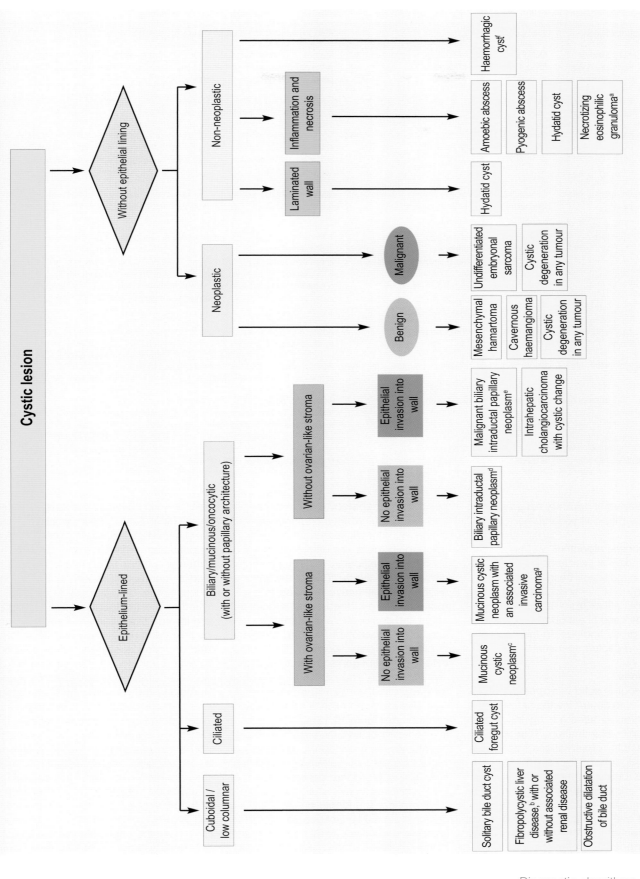

Fig 10.105 Diagnostic algorithm of cystic lesions of the liver.

[a] This does not refer to Langerhans cell histiocytosis, but to an inflammatory lesion, often associated with parasitic infections.

[b] Inclusive of Caroli disease; [c] Biliary cystadenoma; [d] Biliary papilloma or papillomatosis, with low- or high-grade dysplasia; [e] Biliary papillomatosis with invasion; [f] Cystic haematoma; [g] Biliary cystadenocarcinoma.

Table 10.13 Differential diagnosis of solid, benign and malignant, biliary and gland-forming lesions of the liver: useful gross, histological and immunohistochemical features.

Solid glandular lesion	Gross characteristics	Histological and immunohistochemical characteristics
von Meyenburg complex (bile duct microhamartoma)	Multiple discrete nodules, related to portal tracts; may contain bile; usually < 0.5 cm	Irregular or rounded ductal structures lined by flattened or cuboidal epithelium; lumina may contain proteinaceous fluid or bile concretions; dense fibrous stroma; usually portal or periportal; expresses keratins 7 and 19.
Bile duct adenoma (peribiliary gland hamartoma)	Solitary subcapsular, whitish firm discrete nodule; usually < 2 cm	Small, round tubules, lined by cuboidal epithelium,[a] may contain mucin; often contains normal portal tracts; expresses keratins 7 and 19.
Biliary adenofibroma	Circumscribed, whitish tumour; may contain microcystic areas; may be as large as 16 cm.	Complex tubulo-cystic structures with complex branching; single-layered biliary epithelium of variable height, sometimes with mitotic activity; lumina may contain cellular debris or proteineous fluid; abundant fibroblastic stroma and/or areas of hyalinization; expresses keratins 7 and 19.
Serous cystadenoma (microcystic adenoma)	Circumscribed, sponge-like tumour, with microcysts filled with clear, watery fluid; any size.	Multiple small cysts separated by thin fibrous septa, lined by a single layer of clear, glycogen-rich cuboidal cells; expresses keratins 7 and 19, and occasionally CA19-9 and B72.3.
Cholangiocarcinoma	Variable appearances; any size: • Single firm nodule; • Multiple nodules (mimicking metastases); • Diffuse growth; • Irregular periductal thickening; • Intraductal polypoid mass; • Any combination of the above.	Adenocarcinoma, often with abundant desmoplastic stroma, perineural invasion and/or mucin secretion. Immunoprofile: keratins 7 and 19, EMA, and CEA: usually positive; keratin 20: positive in 20% of cases. (Epithelioid hemangioendothelioma may mimic cholangiocarcinoma, but is negative for epithelial immunomarkers and positive for endothelial markers, e.g. CD31 and CD34)
Metastatic pancreatobiliary ductal carcinoma	Single or multiple firm nodules of any size.	Adenocarcinoma indistinguishable from cholangiocarcinoma either by morphology or by immunohistochemistry.
Metastatic colorectal adenocarcinoma	Single or multiple nodules of any size, often with central necrosis.	Adenocarcinoma, often with garland pattern and central "dirty" necrosis. Immunoprofile: keratin 20, CDX2, MUC2 and CEA: positive; keratin 7: negative.
Metastatic adenocarcinoma from other sites	Single or multiple nodules of any size.	Adenocarcinoma with variable appearance. Immunoprofile: first segregate according to pattern of keratins 7 and 20; then apply markers according to the suspected primary site.

CEA, carcinoembryonic antigen; EMA, epithelial membrane antigen.
[a] The rare clear cell variant may be easily confused with metastatic renal cell carcinoma or cholangiocarcinoma, clear cell type.

biliary intraductal papillary neoplasm and embryonal rhabdomyosarcoma.

The diagnostic algorithm

The diagnosis of liver tumours initially requires that the lesion be identified as predominantly cystic or solid; this information is available either from the radiology report, in the case of a biopsy specimen, or from the gross findings, in the case of a surgically resected specimen.

Solid lesions

If the tumour is solid in appearance, the next step is to determine the nature of the cells and/or architecture on low-power microscopic examination. This leads to four possible observations, as noted in the algorithm for solid tumours. When the tumour is composed predominantly of immature-appearing cells, the differential diagnosis includes hepatoblastoma and metastasis; the former can be differentiated from morphologically similar appearing metastatic tumours by positivity for hepatocyte-specific antigen and AFP {824}. When the tumour demonstrates hepatocellular phenotype or large eosinophilic cells, the differential diagnosis differs significantly in cirrhotic versus non-cirrhotic livers. The overwhelming majority of distinctive nodules in a cirrhotic liver are indeed of hepatocellular origin and demonstrate differentiation features of this phenotype, such as presence of bile, cytoplasmic positivity for hepatocyte-specific antigen and canalicular positivity for pCEA and CD10. Such lesions may represent large regenerative nodules, dysplastic nodules or hepatocellular carcinomas (Table 10.12).

In a non-cirrhotic liver, the presence of large hepatocyte-like eosinophilic cells with or without a trabecular pattern may represent true hepatocytic differentiation or be effectively mimicked by metastatic tumours from other organs. The former group of lesions demonstrate markers of hepatocytic differentiation and include focal nodular hyperplasia, hepatocellular adenoma, HCC, fibrolamellar carcinoma and hepatoblastoma (Table 10.11). The differential diagnosis of metastatic lesions with a hepatocytoid appearance is listed in Table 10.10.

When a tumour is composed of ducts and/or glands with or without mucin production, the first step is to determine whether the ductal/glandular structures are benign or malignant. Benign lesions usually demonstrate a biliary phenotype and are often accompanied by a fibrous stromal background. The differential diagnosis of malignant gland-forming and/or mucin-producing lesions in the liver in one of the most difficult in diagnostic surgical pathology. It encompasses the distinction of intrahepatic cholangiocarcinoma from metastatic adenocarcinoma and in the latter case, the identification of the primary site of origin. This can be accomplished in most cases by correlation of the histological features with the staining profile for keratins 7 and 20, combined with the application of site-specific antibodies. In this context, it is pertinent that cholangiocarcinomas may be positive for keratin 20 in about 40%, and for CDX2 in about 20% of cases, making distinction from metastatic colonic adenocarcinoma difficult. However, in contrast to intrahepatic cholangiocarcinoma, the latter usually shows abundant necrosis and no desmoplasia. The morphological and immunohistochemical profile of pancreatic adenocarcinoma is identical to that for intrahepatic cholangiocarcinoma and the two cannot be distinguished without additional clinical and radiological data.

A tumour containing both hepatocytes and ducts/glands is most commonly a combined hepatocellular-cholangiocarcinoma (mixed hepatobiliary carcinoma). These tumours show immunopositivity for hepatocyte markers in the hepatocellular-looking areas and for cholangiocytic markers in the ductal and glandular elements. Cholangiocarcinoma with reported positivity for hepatocellular markers such as hepatocyte-specific antigen, CD10 and AFP (2–5% of cases), probably represent examples of this tumour.

Cystic lesions

The first step in the diagnosis of a liver cyst is to determine whether it is a true cyst, i.e. whether the cystic space is lined by epithelium. When lined by epithelium, the nature of the epithelium is assessed. Cysts lined by cuboidal or low columnar epithelium are common and the vast majority are developmental in origin; a minority are a result of biliary obstruction. If the lining epithelium is ciliated, the cyst represents a ciliated foregut cyst and will usually show smooth muscle in its wall. A benign cyst with a mucinous or biliary lining epithelium and ovarian-like stroma in the wall is a mucinous cystic neoplasm (formerly, biliary cystadenoma). These cysts occur almost exclusively in women and the stroma is immunohistochemically positive for estrogen and progesterone receptors. Uncommonly, these tumours may undergo malignant change manifested by invasive epithelial growth into the cyst wall (mucinous cystic neoplasm with invasive carcinoma; formerly, biliary cystadenocarcinoma).

A cyst lined by biliary or mucinous epithelium in papillary configurations is a biliary intraductal papillary neoplasm, biliary or mucinous type, respectively. Rare cases may be lined by oncocytic cells. The epithelium in these cysts may show low-, intermediate-or high-grade intraepithelial neoplasia. These neoplasms may show epithelial invasion into the cyst walls, giving rise to their malignant counterpart, malignant biliary intraductal papillary neoplasm (biliary papillomatosis with invasion). Uncommonly, intrahepatic cholangiocarcinoma may demonstrate cystic change and may be difficult to differentiate from malignant biliary intraductal papillary neoplasm.

Liver cysts not lined by epithelium may represent cystic change in solid tumours or necrosis in inflammatory lesions; the first step is therefore to distinguish between neoplastic and non-neoplastic lesions. Almost any tumour may be seen but those most prone to appear cystic on radiological and gross examination are mesenchymal hamartoma, undifferentiated embryonal sarcoma and large cavernous haemangioma. Mesenchymal hamartoma occurs at < 2 years of age and contains abundant myxoid tissue, while undifferentiated embryonal sarcoma occurs more commonly at > 2 years of age and shows undifferentiated, obviously malignant cells with eosinophilic intracytoplasmic globules. A cyst showing a laminated wall of acellular eosinophilic material, often lined by a germinal layer, is a hydatid cyst. The presence of inflammation and necrosis should raise suspicion of an infectious process, e.g. a pyogenic abscess, amoebic abscess, hydatid cyst or necrotizing eosinophilic granuloma. The latter term is used to denote inflammatory nodules with central necrosis that are usually associated with parasitic infections and systemic symptoms and should not be confused with Langerhans cell histiocytosis {1475}. It is uncertain whether the solitary necrotic nodule is also related to necrotizing eosinophilic granuloma {3715}. Large haematomas may sometimes appear as cystic tumours and are easily identified by the presence of organizing blood and absence of epithelial lining, neoplastic tissue and inflammatory reaction.

Comments

The diagnostic algorithm focuses on commonly encountered lesions and does not include rare epithelial tumours (microcystic adenoma), rare variants of epithelial tumours (cholangiocellular variants of hepatoblastoma, transitional liver cell tumour), mixed epithelial-mesenchymal tumours (calcifying nested stromal epithelial tumour) and mesenchymal tumours (angiomyolipoma and others). On the other hand, non-neoplastic

Table 10.14 Age at presentation of liver tumours in infants and children.

Age < 2 years
Infantile haemangioma
Mesenchymal hamartoma
Hepatoblastoma
Hepatic malignant rhabdoid tumour
Rhabdomyosarcoma

Age > 2 years
Focal nodular hyperplasia
Hepatocellular adenoma
Fibrolamellar carcinoma
Hepatocellular carcinoma
Transitional liver cell tumour
Calcifying nested epithelial stromal tumour
Undifferentiated embryonal sarcoma

cysts that form mass lesions are included since they outstrip cystic neoplasms in incidence. Similarly, the algorithm outlines the most common pathways of tumour morphology and behaviour; and does not include rare morphological and biological variants.

It is pertinent to note that although immunohistochemical stains form an important part of the diagnostic algorithm, they are neither sensitive nor specific. The sensitivity of hepatocyte-specific antigen for diagnosis of HCC is 70–90% {818, 1735, 1911} and seems to decrease with the degree of differentiation of the tumour {552}. This marker is also positive in gastric, pulmonary, ovarian and pancreatobiliary carcinomas {1735}. AFP is detectable by immunohistochemistry in only 30–40% of HCCs {552, 3271} and approximately 50–60% of hepatoblastomas {2628}. On the other hand, approximately 10–20% of HCCs may be positive for keratins 7 and 20. The issue of immunohistochemical sensitivity and specificity is particularly compounded in poorly differentiated tumours that display aberrant phenotypes as they diverge markedly from normal differentiation pathways. Many of these tumours may morphologically appear as solid sheets of cells, which do not indicate a definite differentiation pathway.

A biopsy aimed at a mass lesion in the liver may miss its target and instead sample adjacent compressed hepatic parenchyma, which shows a characteristic triad of histological findings. These include sinusoidal dilatation, ductular reaction, and portal inflammation and oedema. These features reflect obstruction of bile and blood flow by an adjacent space-occupying lesion, thus suggesting the presence of such a lesion {967}.

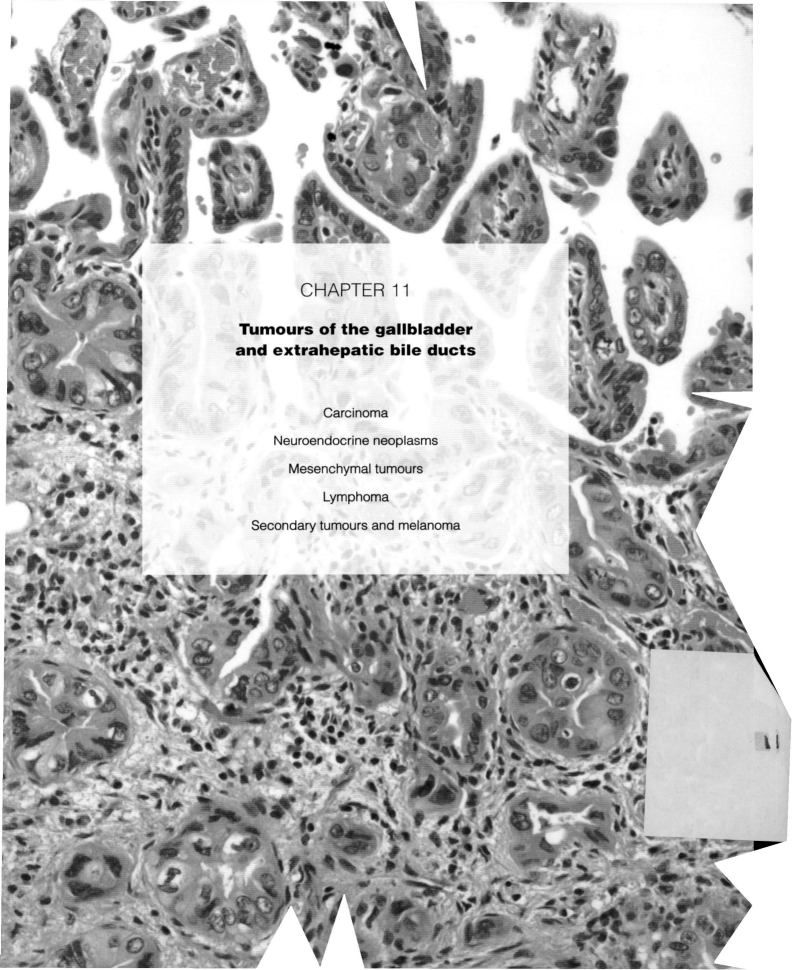

CHAPTER 11

Tumours of the gallbladder and extrahepatic bile ducts

Carcinoma

Neuroendocrine neoplasms

Mesenchymal tumours

Lymphoma

Secondary tumours and melanoma

WHO classification[a] of tumours of the gallbladder and extrahepatic bile ducts

Epithelial tumours

Premalignant lesions

Adenoma	8140/0
Tubular	8211/0
Papillary	8260/0
Tubulopapillary	8263/0
Biliary intraepithelial neoplasia, grade 3 (BilIN-3)	8148/2
Intracystic (gallbladder) or intraductal (bile ducts) papillary neoplasm with low- or intermediate-grade intraepithelial neoplasia	8503/0
Intracystic (gallbladder) or intraductal (bile ducts) papillary neoplasm with high-grade intraepithelial neoplasia	8503/2*
Mucinous cystic neoplasm with low- or intermediate-grade intraepithelial neoplasia	8470/0
Mucinous cystic neoplasm with high-grade intraepithelial neoplasia	8470/2

Carcinoma

Adenocarcinoma	8140/3
Adenocarcinoma, biliary type	8140/3
Adenocarcinoma, gastric foveolar type	8140/3
Adenocarcinoma, intestinal type	8144/3
Clear cell adenocarcinoma	8310/3
Mucinous adenocarcinoma	8480/3
Signet ring cell carcinoma	8490/3
Adenosquamous carcinoma	8560/3
Intracystic (gallbladder) or intraductal (bile ducts) papillary neoplasm with an associated invasive carcinoma	8503/3*
Mucinous cystic neoplasm with an associated invasive carcinoma	8470/3*
Squamous cell carcinoma	8070/3
Undifferentiated carcinoma	8020/3

Neuroendocrine neoplasms[b]

Neuroendocrine tumour (NET)	
NET G1 (carcinoid)	8240/3
NET G2	8249/3
Neuroendocrine carcinoma (NEC)	8246/3
Large cell NEC	8013/3
Small cell NEC	8041/3
Mixed adenoneuroendocrine carcinoma	8244/3
Goblet cell carcinoid	8243/3
Tubular carcinoid	8245/1

Mesenchymal tumours

Granular cell tumour	9580/0
Leiomyoma	8890/0
Kaposi sarcoma	9140/3
Leiomyosarcoma	8890/3
Rhabdomyosarcoma	8900/3

Lymphomas

Secondary tumours

---

[a] The morphology codes are from the International Classification of Diseases for Oncology (ICD-O) {904A}. Behaviour is coded /0 for benign tumours, /1 for unspecified, borderline or uncertain behaviour, /2 for carcinoma *in situ* and grade III intraepithelial neoplasia, and /3 for malignant tumours.

[b] The classification is modified from the previous WHO histological classification of tumours {691} taking into account changes in our understanding of these lesions. In the case of neuroendocrine neoplasms, the classification has been simplified to be of more practical utility in morphological classification.

* These new codes were approved by the IARC/WHO Committee for ICD-O at its meeting in March 2010.

TNM classification[a] of tumours of the gallbladder and extrahepatic bile ducts

Carcinoma of the gallbladder

T – Primary tumour
TX   Primary tumour cannot be assessed
T0   No evidence of primary tumour
Tis Carcinoma *in situ*
T1   Tumour invades lamina propria or muscular layer
   T1a Tumour invades lamina propria
   T1b Tumour invades muscular layer
T2   Tumour invades perimuscular connective tissue; no extension beyond serosa or into liver
T3   Tumour perforates the serosa (visceral peritoneum) and/or directly invades the liver and/or one other adjacent organ or structure, such as stomach, duodenum, colon, pancreas, omentum, extrahepatic bile ducts
T4   Tumour invades main portal vein or hepatic artery or invades two or more extrahepatic organs or structures

N – Regional lymph nodes
NX   Regional lymph nodes cannot be assessed
N0   No regional lymph-node metastasis
N1   Regional lymph-node metastasis (including nodes along the cystic duct, common bile duct, hepatic artery, and portal vein).

M – Distant metastasis
M0   No distant metastasis
M1   Distant metastasis

Stage grouping

Stage 0	Tis	N0	M0
Stage I	T1	N0	M0
Stage II	T2	N0	M0
Stage IIIA	T3	N0	M0
Stage IIIB	T1, T2, T3	N1	M0
Stage IVA	T4	Any N	M0
Stage IVB	Any T	Any N	M1

Carcinoma of the distal extrahepatic bile ducts[b]

T – Primary tumour
TX   Primary tumour cannot be assessed
T0   No evidence of primary tumour
Tis Carcinoma *in situ*
T1   Tumour confined to the bile duct
T2   Tumour invades beyond the wall of the bile duct
T3   Tumour invades the gallbladder, liver, pancreas, duodenum or other adjacent organs
T4   Tumour involves the coeliac axis or the superior mesenteric artery

N – Regional lymph nodes
NX   Regional lymph nodes cannot be assessed
N0   No regional lymph-node metastasis
N1   Regional lymph-node metastasis

M – Distant metastasis
M0   No distant metastasis
M1   Distant metastasis

Stage grouping

Stage 0	Tis	N0	M0
Stage IA	T1	N0	M0
Stage IB	T2	N0	M0
Stage IIA	T3	N0	M0
Stage IIB	T1, T2, T3	N1	M0
Stage III	T4	Any N	M0
Stage IV	Any T	Any N	M1

Carcinoma of the perihilar extrahepatic bile ducts[c]

T – Primary tumour
TX   Primary tumour cannot be assessed
T0   No evidence of primary tumour
Tis Carcinoma *in situ*
T1   Tumour confined to the bile duct, with extension up to the muscle layer or fibrous tissue
T2a Tumour invades beyond the wall of the bile duct to surrounding adipose tissue
T2b Tumour invades adjacent hepatic parenchyma
T3   Tumour invades unilateral branches of the portal vein or hepatic artery
T4   Tumour invades the main portal vein or its branches bilaterally; or the common hepatic artery; or the second-order biliary radicals bilaterally; or unilateral second-order biliary radicals with contralateral portal-vein or hepatic-artery involvement

N – Regional lymph nodes
NX   Regional lymph nodes cannot be assessed
N0   No regional lymph-node metastasis
N1   Regional lymph-node metastasis including nodes along the cystic duct, common bile duct, hepatic artery, and portal vein

M – Distant metastasis
M0   No distant metastasis
M1   Distant metastasis

Stage grouping

Stage 0	Tis	N0	M0
Stage I	T1	N0	M0
Stage II	T2a, T2b	N0	M0
Stage IIIA	T3	N0	M0
Stage IIIB	T1, T2, T3	N1	M0
Stage IVA	T4	N0, N1	M0
Stage IVB	Any T	Any N	M1

---

[a] {762, 2996}; [b] The classification applies to carcinomas of the extrahepatic bile ducts distal to the insertion of the cystic duct. Cystic duct carcinoma is included under gallbladder; [c] The classification applies to carcinomas of the extrahepatic bile ducts of perihilar localization (Klatskin tumour). Included are the right, left, and common hepatic ducts, i.e. those proximal to the origin of the cystic duct.
A helpdesk for specific questions about the TNM classification is available at http://www.uicc.org.

Carcinoma of the gallbladder and extrahepatic bile ducts

J. Albores-Saavedra
N.V. Adsay
J.M. Crawford
D.S. Klimstra

G. Klöppel
B. Sripa
W.M.S. Tsui
V. Paradis

Carcinoma of the gallbladder

Definition
A malignant epithelial neoplasm, usually with biliary, intestinal, foveolar or squamous differentiation, arising in the gallbladder.

ICD-O codes

Adenocarcinoma	8140/3
Biliary type	8140/3
Gastric foveolar type	8140/3
Intestinal type	8144/3
Clear cell adenocarcinoma	8310/3
Mucinous adenocarcinoma	8480/3
Signet ring cell carcinoma	8490/3
Adenosquamous carcinoma	8560/3
Intracystic (gallbladder) or intraductal (bile ducts) papillary neoplasm with an associated invasive carcinoma	8503/3
Mucinous cystic neoplasm with an associated invasive carcinoma	8470/3
Squamous cell carcinoma	8070/3
Undifferentiated carcinoma	8020/3

Epidemiology
Most patients with carcinoma of the gallbladder are in the sixth or seventh decade of life. From 1985 to 2005, the incidence of invasive carcinoma of the gallbladder in the USA was 0.9 per 100 000 males and 1.6 per 100 000 females, accounting for 0.16% and 0.39% of all cancers in males and females, respectively {1240}. The female-to-male ratio is 1.77. Cancer of the gallbladder accounts for 51% of all cancers arising in the biliary tract in women and 28% in men. The incidence of this cancer decreased between 1973 and 2005 {1240}.
The incidence of carcinoma of the gallbladder varies geographically and also in different ethnic groups within the same country. In the USA, it is more common in American Indians and Hispanic Americans than in whites or African Americans {70, 708, 2890}. Recent studies indicate that rates are declining in American Indians, possibly because of the increasing use of cholecystectomy {191}. High rates are also found in certain populations in Mexico, Central and South America, eastern Europe and in parts of Asia {1800, 2630}.

Etiology
The most important risk factors for carcinoma of the gallbladder are genetic background (described later), gallstones and an abnormal choledochopancreatic junction.
Gallstones are present in > 80% of gallbladders harbouring a carcinoma {70}. However, the overall incidence of carcinoma of the gallbladder in patients with cholelithiasis is < 0.2% {70}, so although gallstones are considered to be a contributing risk factor, most individuals with gallstones never develop gallbladder carcinoma. Correlation between gallstone size and the risk of cancer is suspected, but has not been confirmed {70}.
Diffuse calcification of the gallbladder wall ("porcelain gallbladder") is present in < 1% of cholecystectomy specimens and 8–10% of such resected specimens (some estimates reaching 13–62%) harbour a carcinoma {631, 3075, 3279}. Some studies have suggested that selective mucosal calcification poses a significant cancer risk, while diffuse intramural calcification does not {3075}. In studies in which such an association was reported, the carcinomas detected included not only well-differentiated adenocarcinoma but also mucinous and squamous cell carcinomas {70}.
Data reported largely from Japan indicate an association between an abnormal junction between the pancreatic and common bile ducts and cancer of the gallbladder and the extrahepatic bile ducts {2105}. Of patients with gallbladder carcinoma, those with an abnormal choledochopancreatic junction are on average 10 years younger than those with a normal junction {2105}.
A small number of patients with familial adenomatous polyposis (FAP) will develop dysplasia and carcinoma of the gallbladder {1198}.
The inflammatory disorders ulcerative colitis and primary sclerosing cholangitis have also been reported to be associated with carcinoma of the gallbladder, although less frequently than with carcinoma of the extrahepatic bile ducts {1826, 3601}.

Clinical features
Currently, close to 50% of gallbladder carcinomas are diagnosed incidentally in cholecystectomy specimens from patients with symptoms attributed only to the presence of gallstones (cholelithiasis) {745}. Unfortunately, gallbladder carcinoma usually presents at a late stage, even when found incidentally. The signs and symptoms are not specific, often resembling those of chronic cholecystitis. Right upper-quadrant pain is common. Computed tomography (CT) and ultrasonography aid detection of the neoplasm. Less than 1% of patients with carcinomas of the gallbladder present with a paraneoplastic syndrome that may be the first

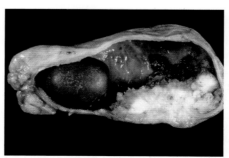

Fig. 11.01 The white, irregular cut surface of an intracystic papillary neoplasm projecting into the gallbladder lumen next to a large gallstone.

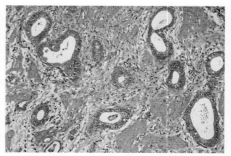

Fig. 11.02 Well-differentiated adenocarcinoma infiltrating the wall of the gallbladder, biliary type.

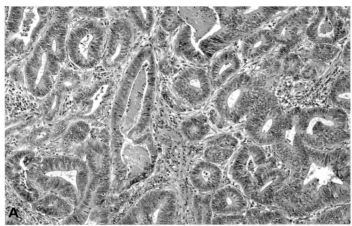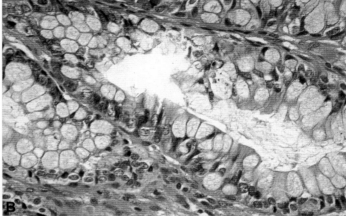

Fig. 11.03 Adenocarcinoma of the gallbladder, intestinal type. **A** Note the tubular glands similar to those seen in colonic adenocarcinoma. **B** Goblet-cell variant.

manifestation of the neoplasm {3345}. Adenocarcinomas of the gallbladder have been reported in association with acanthosis nigricans {2623}, bullous pemphygoid-type lesions {70}, the Leser-Trelat sign {70}, dermatomyositis {3640} and Guillain-Barré syndrome {2540}.

Macroscopy

Carcinoma of the gallbladder usually forms an infiltrating grey-white mass. Some carcinomas cause diffuse thickening and induration of the entire gallbladder wall. The gallbladder may be distended by the tumour, or collapsed owing to obstruction of the neck or cystic duct. It can also assume an hourglass deformity when the neoplasm arises in the body and constricts the lateral walls. Carcinomas arising in association with intracystic papillary neoplasms are usually sessile and exhibit a polypoid or cauliflower-like appearance. Mucinous and signet ring cell carcinomas have a mucoid or gelatinous cut surface.

Tumour staging

The TNM (tumour, node, metastasis) classification for the gallbladder also applies for carcinomas of the cystic duct. Changes in the classification of regional lymph nodes and stage grouping occurred between the sixth and seventh editions of TNM {2996}.

Histopathology

The WHO histological classification of tumours of the gallbladder is based on previous classifications published by WHO {1106} and by the Armed Forces Institute of Pathology (AFIP) in 2000 {70} and has been updated to align the nomenclature

of intracystic papillary neoplasms and biliary intraepithelial neoplasia (BilIN) with those of the intrahepatic biliary tree and the pancreas. Two new histological types, cribriform carcinoma and the benign giant cell tumour, have been added {69, 71}.

Adenocarcinoma, biliary type

Well- to moderately differentiated invasive adenocarcinomas of biliary type are the most common malignant epithelial neoplasms of the gallbladder. They are composed of short or long tubular glands lined by cells that vary in height from cuboidal to tall columnar, superficially resembling biliary epithelium. Cytoplasmic and luminal mucin is frequently present {1745}. Rarely, the extracellular mucin may become calcified. About one third of the well-differentiated adenocarcinomas show focal intestinal differentiation and contain goblet and neuroendocrine cells {76, 3582, 3596}. These sometimes numerous neuroendocrine cells may be immunoreactive for serotonin and peptide hormones, but a diagnosis of neuroendocrine

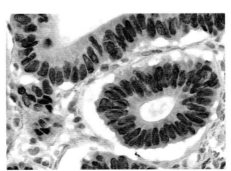

Fig. 11.04 Intestinal-type adenocarcinoma of the common hepatic duct showing diffuse nuclear expression of CDX2.

neoplasm is not warranted. Rarely, Paneth cells may be seen. Adenocarcinomas may contain osteoclast-like giant cells {52} or show focal cribriform or angiosarcomatous patterns {70, 185}. They may also contain cyto- and syncytio-trophoblast cells {20, 70}.

Gallbladder adenocarcinomas tend to be more poorly differentiated and show less desmoplasia than their counterparts in the extrahepatic bile ducts. Most adenocarcinomas of the gallbladder are immunoreactive for carcinoembryonic antigen (CEA), MUC1, MUC2, p53 and keratin 7 {76, 77, 214, 660, 754, 1790, 2011, 2779, 3177, 3530, 3596}.

Adenocarcinoma, intestinal type

Two morphological variants of invasive adenocarcinoma of intestinal type have been described in the gallbladder. The most common is composed of tubular glands closely resembling those of colonic adenocarcinomas. The glands are lined predominantly by columnar cells with pseudostratified ovoid or elongated nuclei. The second variant consists of glands lined predominantly of goblet cells usually with a variable number of neuroendocrine and Paneth cells {70, 75}. Both variants label with antibodies to CDX2, MUC2, CEA and keratin 20.

Adenocarcinoma, gastric foveolar type

This unusual but distinctive, well-differentiated variant is composed of tall columnar cells with basally oriented nuclei and abundant mucin-containing cytoplasm; it usually labels with antibodies to MUC5A. Combined forms (adenocarcinoma or adenosquamous carcinoma with foveolar

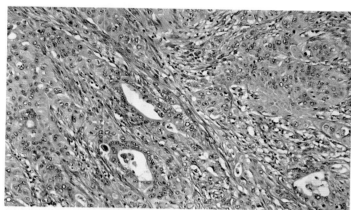

Fig. 11.05 Adenosquamous carcinoma of the gallbladder, composed of gland-forming elements alternating with solid, squamous nests.

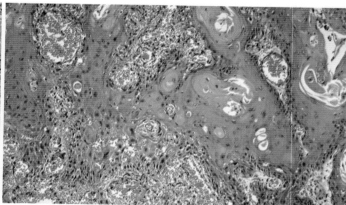

Fig. 11.06 Squamous cell carcinoma of the gallbladder.

differentiation) have been reported in the gallbladder {70}.

Adenosquamous carcinoma

The extent of differentiation of the two malignant components, glandular and squamous, varies, but in general they tend to be moderately differentiated {54, 69, 475, 1856, 2088, 2295}. Keratin pearls are often present in the squamous component, and mucin is usually demonstrable in the neoplastic glands.

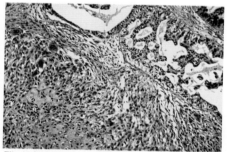

Fig. 11.07 Carcinosarcoma of the gallbladder. The tumour has malignant glandular elements and a sarcomatous component with osteoid formation.

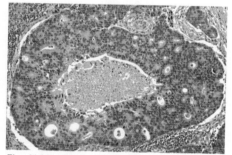

Fig. 11.08 High-grade cribriform carcinoma of the gallbladder with comedo-type necrosis.

Carcinosarcoma

The epithelial (carcinomatous) elements usually predominate in the form of glands, but may be arranged in cords or sheets. Foci of squamous differentiation are reported. The sarcomatous component can include heterologous elements such as chondrosarcoma, osteosarcoma, and rhabdomyosarcoma. Keratin and CEA are absent from the mesenchymal component, helping to distinguish carcinosarcomas from undifferentiated spindle and giant cell carcinomas {70}.

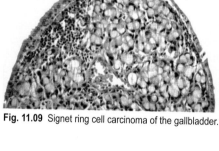

Fig. 11.09 Signet ring cell carcinoma of the gallbladder.

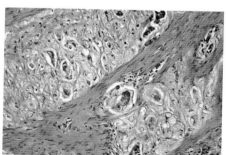

Fig. 11.10 Mucinous adenocarcinoma. Clusters of malignant epithelial cells are surrounded by abundant extracellular mucin.

Cribriform carcinoma

Cribriform carcinoma is a distinctive invasive neoplasm of the gallbladder that resembles cribriform carcinoma of the breast, but accounts for < 1% of all gallbladder carcinomas {71}. Patients are younger than those with conventional adenocarcinoma of the gallbladder and the neoplasms are usually associated with cholelithiasis. In addition to typical cribriform growth, high-grade tumours have large vesicular nuclei with prominent nucleoli and show comedo-type necrosis. In contrast to cribriform carcinomas of the breast, the gallbladder carcinomas are negative for estrogen and progesterone receptors and behave aggressively, like conventional adenocarcinomas of the gallbladder {71}.

Clear cell adenocarcinoma

This rare malignant neoplasm is composed predominantly of glycogen-rich clear cells with well-defined cytoplasmic borders and central hyperchromatic nuclei arranged in glandular or other growth patterns {73, 270, 3139, 3377}. Some cells contain eosinophilic granular cytoplasm. Foci of conventional adenocarcinoma with mucin production are usually found and can distinguish primary carcinomas from metastatic clear cell carcinomas of the kidney. Exclusion of renal cell carcinoma is also accomplished by immunohistochemical labelling for PAX8 and RCC {162}. In some clear cell adenocarcinomas, the columnar cells contain subnuclear and supranuclear vacuoles similar to those seen in secretory endometrium. Production of α-fetoprotein has been documented in clear cell carcinomas with or without hepatoid differentiation {2107, 3465}.

Hepatoid adenocarcinoma

This is an exceedingly rare neoplasm of the gallbladder that closely mimics hepatocellular carcinoma {2779, 3356}. For diagnosis, > 50% of the neoplasm should be composed of hepatoid cells usually arranged in a trabecular pattern. The neoplastic hepatoid cells label with HepPar1 antibody and rarely with α-fetoprotein. A minor component of conventional adenocarcinoma has been reported in all of these carcinomas. The biological behaviour of hepatoid adenocarcinoma appears to be similar to that of conventional adenocarcinoma.

Mucinous adenocarcinoma

These neoplasms are more common in the gallbladder than in the extrahepatic bile ducts, and are similar to those that arise at other anatomical sites. By convention, > 50% of the tumour contains extracellular mucin {70, 72}. Mucinous carcinoma should be distinguished from a benign mucocele. The abundant extracellular mucin present in a mucocele may be recognized grossly in the gallbladder wall as nodules of different sizes. The mucin can extend to the serosa through the Rokitansky-Aschoff sinuses and induce a histiocytic response. The histiocytes may phagocytize mucin and be confused with signet ring cells. Immunolabelling for keratin and CEA is positive in mucinous carcinoma and negative in mucocele. Ruptured, mucin-containing, Rokitansky-Aschoff sinuses with abundant extracellular mucins having small benign glandular and papillary structures should not be confused with mucinous carcinoma {68}.

Signet ring cell carcinoma

Cells containing intracytoplasmic mucin displacing the nuclei toward the periphery predominate in this variant of adenocarcinoma. A variable amount of extracellular mucin is usually present. Lateral spread through the lamina propria is a common feature. A diffusely infiltrating linear pattern resembling linitis plastica (diffuse-type adenocarcinoma) of the stomach has been observed {70}.

Squamous cell carcinoma

This malignant epithelial neoplasm is composed entirely of squamous cells with highly variable degrees of differentiation. Keratinizing and nonkeratinizing types exist {136, 954, 3137}. Spindle cells pre-

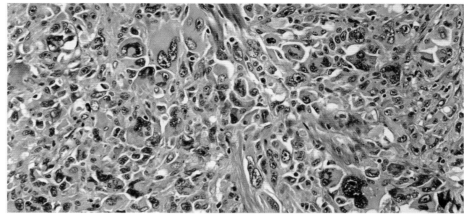

Fig. 11.11 Undifferentiated carcinoma of the gallbladder, spindle cell and giant cell type; note the absence of glandular differentiation.

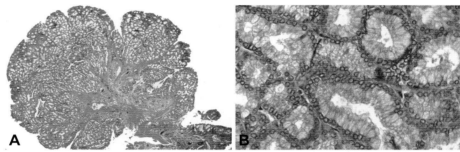

Fig. 11.12 Tubular adenoma, pyloric-gland type, of the gallbladder. **A** A vague lobular patern is seen at low magnification. **B** Tubular glands are lined by mucin-containing columnar cells with basally placed, uniform vesicular nuclei.

dominate in some poorly differentiated squamous cell carcinomas, which may be confused with sarcomas {3137}. Immunolabelling for keratin and p63 may clarify the diagnosis in these spindle-cell cases. The carcinoma may arise from areas of squamous metaplasia or high-grade intraepithelial neoplasia {70}. Most gallbladder carcinomas with squamous differentiation represent adenosquamous carcinomas, and the glandular component may be very focal; thorough examination is required before a diagnosis of pure squamous cell carcinoma can be established.

Undifferentiated carcinoma

This neoplasm is more common in the gallbladder than in the extrahepatic bile ducts. Characteristically, glandular structures are few or absent. There are several histological variants: spindle cell, giant cell (including those with osteoclast-like giant cells), small cell (non-neuroendocrine), and a nodular/lobular type that superficially resembles breast carcinoma {70, 73, 721, 1085, 1124, 2231, 2298}. The recently described benign giant cell tumour of the biliary tree, a true histi-

ocytic neoplasm, can be distinguished from carcinoma with osteoclast-like giant cells by immunohistochemical assessment of CD163, CD68, HAM56, and keratins {69}.

Precursor lesions
Adenoma

Adenomas are benign neoplasms of glandular epithelium that are typically polypoid, single and well-demarcated. They are more common in women than in men, and most occur in adults {85, 3531}. They are found in 0.3–0.5% of gallbladders removed for cholelithiasis or chronic

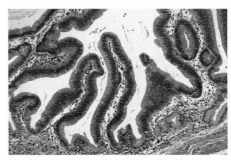

Fig. 11.13 Papillary adenoma of the gallbladder, intestinal type. Note the pseudostratified columnar cells with scattered goblet and Paneth cells.

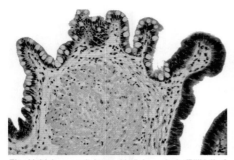

Fig. 11.14 Low-grade intraepithelial neoplasia (BilIN-1) of the gallbladder adjacent to intestinal metaplasia with numerous mature goblet cells.

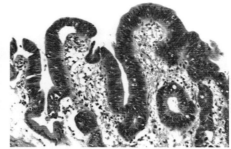

Fig. 11.15 High-grade intraepithelial neoplasia (BilIN-3) of intestinal type in the gallbladder.

cholecystitis. Adenomas are often small, asymptomatic, and usually discovered incidentally during cholecystectomy, but they can be multiple, fill the lumen of the gallbladder and be symptomatic. Occasionally, adenomas of the gallbladder occur in association with Peutz-Jeghers syndrome {884} or Gardner syndrome {3201, 3435}. While a significant number of adenomas in the gallbladder are associated with lithiasis, those of the extrahepatic bile ducts are not.

Adenomas can be divided into three types on the basis of growth pattern: tubular, papillary, and tubulopapillary {70}. Cytologically, they are classified as: pyloric-gland type, intestinal type, foveolar type and biliary type. Pyloric and intestinal-type adenomas are more common in the gallbladder than in the extrahepatic bile ducts {85}. A small proportion of adenomas progress to invasive carcinoma {85, 1540}.

Tubular adenoma, pyloric-gland type (pyloric-gland adenoma) is the most common variant of gallbladder adenoma. It is composed of lobules of closely packed pyloric-type glands, some of which may be cystically dilated, often covered by normal biliary epithelium. Squamoid morules characterized by nodular aggregates of cytologically bland spindle cells with eosinophilic cytoplasm but no keratinization are also seen {1693, 2300}. Paneth cells and neuroendocrine cells are often present. By definition, pyloric-gland adenomas have at least low-grade intraepithelial neoplasia. Larger adenomas may have high-grade intraepithelial neoplasia or may be associated with foci of invasive carcinoma. As they enlarge, some develop a pedicle and project into the lumen. Rarely, they extend into or arise from Rokitansky-Aschoff sinuses, a finding that should not be mistaken for invasive carcinoma {85}.

Intestinal-type adenoma is a rare benign neoplasm composed of dysplastic tubular glands lined by cells with an intestinal phenotype, which closely resembles colonic adenomas.

Foveolar-type adenoma has a tubulopapillary architecture and consists of tall columnar cells with small basal hyperchromatic nuclei and abundant mucin-containing cytoplasm {70}. Rarely, these adenomas arise from the epithelial invaginations of adenomyomatous hyperplasia. Foveolar-type adenomas label with antibodies to MUC5AC and occasionally MUC6.

There is also an exceedingly rare *biliary-type adenoma* lined by cytologically normal-appearing biliary epithelium.

Biliary intraepithelial neoplasia

BilINs are characterized by atypical epithelial cells with multilayering of nuclei and micropapillary projections into the gallbladder lumen {3688, 3689}. The atypical cells have an increased nucleus-to-cytoplasm ratio, partial loss of nuclear polarity, and nuclear hyperchromasia. BilIN-1 and BilIN-2 correspond to low-grade and intermediate-grade lesions and BilIN-3 corresponds to high grade lesions {3688}. The incidence of BilIN-3 parallels that of invasive carcinoma and its prevalence is higher in countries in which gallbladder carcinoma is endemic than in countries in which it is sporadic. The incidence of BilIN-3 in gallbladders with lithiasis varies from 0.5% to 3% {70}. This variation in the incidence of BilIn-3 is partially attributable to a lack of uniformity in morphological criteria and sampling methods. In addition to cholelithiasis, BilIN-3 occurs in the mucosa adjacent to most invasive carcinomas and can be found in patients with FAP, sclerosing cholangitis and pancreatobiliary reflux

{70, 239, 240, 290, 743, 991, 1139, 1492, 1729, 1910, 2234, 2253, 3137}.

BilIN is usually not recognized on macroscopic examination because it often occurs in association with chronic cholecystitis. The mucosa may be granular, nodular, plaque-like, or trabeculated. BilIN-1 and 2 of the gallbladder is characterized by mild cytoarchitectural atypia including enlargement of cells, pseudostratification of nuclei and hyperchromatism. It is typically detected incidentally and is of no established clinical significance.

BilIN-3 usually arises in a background of pyloric and intestinal metaplasia {70, 743, 1216, 1725}. Occasional goblet cells are found in one third of cases. An abrupt transition between columnar cells of normal appearance and dysplastic cells is seen in nearly all cases. Five cell phenotypes are recognized: biliary, intestinal, oncocytic, squamous and signet ring cell {70, 75, 812}. When associated with an invasive cancer, the morphological type of BilIN-3 does not always correspond with that of the carcinoma. BilIN-3 may arise from or extend into Rokitansky-Aschoff sinuses, a feature that should not be confused with stromal invasion {80}. If BilIN-3 is found, multiple sections should be taken to exclude invasive cancer. The dysplastic cells immunolabel for CEA {77}, S100 A4 {3703}, CA19-9 {70} and p53 {3530}. Cholecystectomy with negative margins is a curative surgical procedure for patients with BilIN-3 or with invasive carcinoma limited to the lamina propria {70}.

BilIN is often encountered in the setting of chronic cholecystitis and may coexist with reactive epithelial changes. In contrast to BilIN, these changes ("atypia of repair") involve a heterogeneous cell population containing columnar mucus-secreting cells, low cuboidal cells, atrophic-appearing epithelium, and pencil-like cells. In addition, reactive changes show a gradual transition between cellular abnormalities, in contrast to the abrupt transition seen in BilIN. The expression of *TP53* is more extensive and more common in BilIN than in reactive epithelia {70}.

Intracystic papillary neoplasms

Intraluminal papillary neoplasms of the extrahepatic biliary tree are referred to as "intracystic" in the gallbladder and "intraductal" in the extrahepatic bile ducts. Similar to intraductal papillary neoplasms

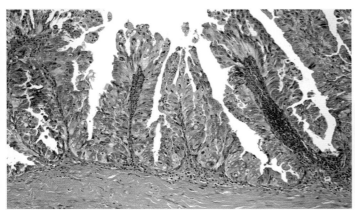
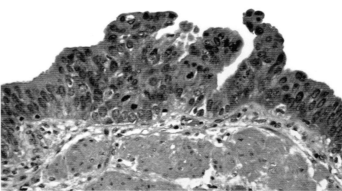

Fig. 11.16 High-grade intraepithelial neoplasia (BilIN-3) of the gallbladder, with biliary phenotype. **A** At low magnification, the dysplastic epithelium lines the mucosal villi. **B** At high magnification, there is complete loss of nuclear polarization and the round nuclei are markedly pleomorphic.

described in the extrahepatic and intra-hepatic biliary tree, intracystic papillary neoplasms of the gallbladder may occur as pancreatobiliary or intestinal pheno-types, the latter with goblet, Paneth, and/or serotonin-containing cells. Previ-ously, the low-grade lesions were some-times designated "papillary adenoma" and the high-grade lesions as "noninva-sive papillary carcinoma." These neo-plasms often arise in a background of pyloric-gland metaplasia. Intracystic pap-illary neoplasms of the gallbladder may be associated with invasive adenocarci-noma, which should be separately re-ported and staged. When an invasive carcinoma arises in association with an in-tracystic papillary neoplasm, the lesion usually has high-grade intraepithelial neo-plasia, which is characterized by complex papillary structures lined by cuboidal or low columnar biliary-type cells or colum-nar intestinal-type cells, often containing variable amounts of mucin. The invasive component is usually a tubular adenocar-cinoma, although mucinous carcinoma, undifferentiated carcinoma, small cell car-cinoma, and large cell neuroendocrine carcinoma have also been described {1215}.

Distinguishing intracystic papillary neo-plasms from papillary adenomas may be difficult. The vast majority of intracystic papillary neoplasms have a biliary phe-notype whereas papillary adenomas ex-hibit an intestinal phenotype. High-grade intracystic papillary neoplasms show greater architectural compliexity and cy-tological atypia than papillary adenomas. {74, 84, 1215}. Mitotic figures are more common in intracystic papillary neo-plasms than in adenomas.

Mucinous cystic neoplasms (MCNs)

These neoplasms resemble their intra-hepatic counterparts. MCNs are seen predominantly in adult females and are usually symptomatic. Some MCNs meas-ure up to 20 cm in diameter and cause obstructive jaundice or cholecystitis-like symptoms. More common in the extra-hepatic bile ducts than in the gallbladder, MCNs are multiloculated neoplasms that contain mucinous or serous fluid and are lined by columnar epithelium reminiscent of bile duct or foveolar gastric epithelium {706}. Neuroendocrine cells are occa-sionally present. By definition, the cellular subepithelial stroma resembles ovarian stroma and is immunoreactive for estro-gen and progesterone receptors. The stroma is also variably fibrotic. Invasive carcinomas that arise in association with MCNs of the gallbladder should be des-ignated MCN with an associated invasive carcinoma {706} and clearly described in terms of grade and extent; staging is only required for the invasive component.

Genetic susceptibility

Carcinoma of the gallbladder is concen-trated in certain racial and ethnic groups. Familial aggregation has been recorded in the USA and elsewhere {1163, 3285}. In addition, a high prevalence of gallstone disease has been associated with spe-cific human leukocyte antigen (HLA) alle-les that are more common in Native Americans {2043}. Although a person's genetic background may increase the propensity to develop gallstones and thus indirectly increase susceptibility to gall-bladder cancer, no genetic traits specific to gallbladder oncogenesis have been identified.

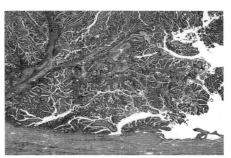

Fig. 11.17 Intracystic papillary neoplasm projecting into the lumen, but without invasion of the wall of the gallbladder.

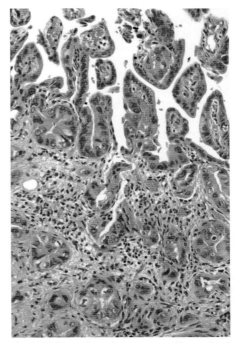

Fig. 11.18 Intracystic papillary neoplasm with associated invasive carcinoma. The noninvasive component is papillary whereas the invasive component is tubular.

Molecular pathology

Mutations of the *KRAS*, *TP53* and *CDKN2A* genes have been reported in invasive carcinomas of the gallbladder {414, 1114, 1187, 1318, 1668, 1966, 2494, 3529, 3532}. The incidence of *KRAS* mutations and loss of *SMAD4* expression is low in carcinomas arising in the gallbladder {143, 2679, 3465}, although *KRAS* mutations are more frequent in gallbladder carcinomas associated with an anomalous junction of the pancreaticobiliary duct {2634}. Amplification of the *ERBB2* gene was detected in 30 out of 43 invasive carcinomas of the gallbladder {1780}; however, there was no correlation between *ERBB2* amplification and prognosis.

The molecular pathology of adenomas of the gallbladder differs from that of invasive carcinomas. None of 16 adenomas showed *TP53* or *CDKN2A* gene mutations, which are common in carcinomas {3531}. Several studies have investigated mutations and immunohistochemical expression of β-catenin in adenomas and carcinomas of the gallbladder {482, 2634, 3612}. Mutations in β-catenin were found in 57–63% of tubular adenomas (pyloric-gland type), and in 0–9% of carcinomas {2711}. These studies provide additional support for the hypothesis that pyloric-gland adenomas play a minor role in gallbladder carcinogenesis {70}.

A high incidence of loss of heterozygosity (LOH) at the *TP53* gene locus has been reported in BilIN; other molecular abnormalities include LOH at 9p and 8p loci and the 18q gene. These abnormalities are early events and probably contribute to the pathogenesis of gallbladder carcinoma. However, no *KRAS* mutations were detected in BilIN-3 {3529, 3530}.

Prognosis and predictive factors

The prognosis for patients with carcinoma of the gallbladder depends primarily on the extent of disease and histological type {74, 85}. For example, the vast majority of adenocarcinomas of the gallbladder confined to the lamina propria do not metastasize and simple cholecystectomy appears to be curative. In contrast, the 10-year relative survival rate for invasive adenocarcinomas that extend through the entire thickness of the gallbladder wall is 30% {74, 85}. Noninvasive intracystic papillary neoplasms and minimally invasive carcinomas arising in association with such lesions, re-gardless of size, cell phenotype and degree of differentiation, rarely metastasize and therefore have the best prognosis. In contrast, carcinomas metastasize and are associated with a poor prognosis if they infiltrate the entire thickness of the gallbladder wall (10-year relative survival rate, 52% {77, 85}. The 10-year relative survival rate for patients with undifferentiated carcinoma spindle cell and giant cell types is 0% {66}.

Carcinoma of the extrahepatic bile ducts

Definition

A malignant epithelial neoplasm usually with biliary, intestinal, foveolar or squamous differentiation, arising in the extrahepatic bile ducts.

Epidemiology

Most patients with extrahepatic biliary carcinoma are in the sixth or seventh decades of life. Except for the Republic of Korea, where incidence is somewhat higher, there is no geographical variation in the incidence of extrahepatic bile-duct carcinoma. In the USA, for example, extrahepatic bile-duct carcinoma accounts for 0.16% of all invasive cancers in males and 0.15% in females in the general population {70}. From 1985 to 2005, the incidence of extrahepatic bile-duct carcinoma in the USA was 1.1 per 100 000 males and 0.7 per 100 000 females {1240}.

Etiology

Risk factors for carcinoma of the extrahepatic bile ducts include primary sclerosing cholangitis, ulcerative colitis, abnormal choledochopancreatic junction and, in south-east Asia, infestation with *Clonorchis sinensis* or *Opisthorcis viverrini* {534, 634, 1855, 3285, 3468}. Unlike in the gallbladder, choledocholithiasis does not play a role in the pathogenesis of carcinomas of the extrahepatic bile ducts. Choledochal cysts are of particular note as 2.5–15% of adult patients with choledochal cysts develop carcinomas {70}, most commonly adenocarcinoma of intestinal type.

Clinical features

Unlike those of the gallbladder, carcinomas of the extrahepatic bile ducts usually present relatively early with obstructive jaundice, which can rapidly progress or fluctuate. Jaundice usually appears while the neoplasm is relatively small and precedes widespread dissemination. Other symptoms include right upper-quadrant pain, malaise, weight loss, pruritus, anorexia, nausea, and vomiting. If cholangitis develops, chills and fever appear. In patients with carcinoma of the proximal bile ducts (right and left hepatic ducts, common hepatic duct), the intrahepatic bile ducts are dilated, the gallbladder is not palpable and the common duct often collapses. Patients with carcinoma in the common or cystic ducts have a distended and palpable gallbladder as well as a markedly dilated proximal duct system, as may be shown by ultrasonography and computed tomography. Transhepatic cholangiograms and endoscopic retrograde cholangiopancreatography (ERCP) are essential to localize carcinomas of the extrahepatic bile ducts. Like carcinoma of the gallbladder, carcinomas of the extrahepatic bile ducts may rarely present with paraneoplastic syndromes.

Macroscopy

Carcinomas of the extrahepatic bile ducts have been divided into polypoid, nodular, scirrhous constricting, and diffusely infiltrating types. While this categorization can provide a guide to the most appropriate operative procedure, extent of resection, and prognosis, it is rarely possible in practice (except for the polypoid tumours) because of overlap in the gross features of each type. The nodular and scirrhous types tend to infiltrate surrounding tissues and are difficult to resect. The diffusely infiltrating types tend to spread linearly along the ducts.

Tumour staging

The seventh edition of the TNM classification divides extrahepatic bile-duct car-

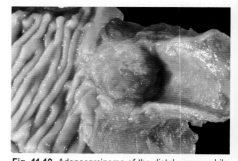

Fig. 11.19 Adenocarcinoma of the distal common bile duct infiltrating the duodenal wall.

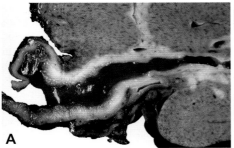 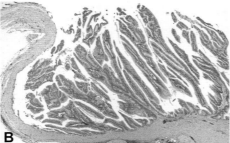 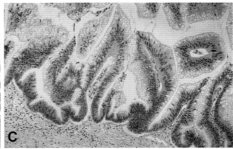

Fig. 11.20 Diffuse intraductal papillary neoplasm ("biliary papillomatosis") in the bile ducts. **A** Papillary (villous) pattern. **B** Villous pattern. **C** There is no invasive carcinoma associated with the intraductal neoplasm.

cinoma into perihilar and distal bile duct {2996}. The distal classification applies to carcinomas that are distal to the insertion of the cystic duct.

Histopathology

The WHO histological classification of carcinomas derives from prior classifications and includes the concepts of the precursor lesions intraductal papillary neoplasms and BilIN, and new entities.

Adenocarcinoma, biliary type

Extrahepatic bile-duct adenocarcinomas tend to be better differentiated and show more desmoplasia than their counterparts in the gallbladder, but are similar in all other ways, including immunoreactivity.

Adenocarcinoma, gastric foveolar type.

This unusual, distinctive, well differentiated variant is composed of tall columnar cells with basally oriented nuclei and abundant mucin-containing cytoplasm, which usually label with MUC5AC. Unlike in the gallbladder, where mixed forms are seen, the pure form of foveolar adenocarcinoma has been described in the extrahepatic bile ducts {70}.

Intestinal-type adenocarcinoma, squamous cell carcinoma, adenosquamous carcinoma, carcinosarcoma, clear cell adenocarcinoma, squamous cell carcinoma

These neoplasms share the histological and immunophenotypical characteristics of those arising in the gallbladder.

Mucinous adenocarcinoma and undifferentiated carcinoma

These carcinomas share the histological and immunophenotypical characteristics of those arising in the gallbladder, but are less common.

Precursor lesions

Two types of precursor lesions are thought to precede the development and progression of extrahepatic bile duct adenocarcinoma: BilIN and intraductal papillary neoplasms {12, 2235, 3689, 3691, 3694} (see Chapter 10).

Biliary intraepithelial neoplasia

BilINs of the extrahepatic and intrahepatic biliary tree share clinical, morphological, and immunophenotypical features.

Intraductal papillary neoplasms

Intraductal papillary neoplasms may dilate the bile ducts, and luminal accumulation of mucin may occur {2933, 3691}; the latter is much less common in biliary lesions than in pancreatic intraductal papillary mucinous neoplasms (IPMNs). As with pancreatic IPMNs, four phenotypes of epithelium are recognized: pancreatobiliary (the most common in the biliary tree), intestinal, oncocytic, and gastric types (the two latter types are rare) {1611, 2738, 2933, 3691}. The clinicopathological condition previously referred to as "biliary papillomatosis" is characterized by multiple, recurring intraductal papillary neoplasms that may involve extensive areas of the extrahepatic bile ducts and even extend into the gallbladder and intrahepatic ducts {11, 1790}. The disease affects males and females equally, most being between the ages of 50 and 70 years. In the Republic of Korea, Taiwan (China) and Japan, about 30% of cases are associated with stones and 25% with flukes {1790}. Invasive carcinoma may occur in association with intraductal papillary neoplasms {3690, 3691}. Once invasive carcinoma develops, prognosis is related to the stage of the invasive component and other conventional prognos-

tic factors. Therefore, when an invasive carcinoma is present, it should be designated (e.g. "intraductal papillary neoplasm with an associated invasive adenocarcinoma") and staged separately. The prognosis is excellent if an intraductal papillary neoplasm without an associated carcinoma is localized and can be completely resected, but more widely distributed disease may be difficult to eradicate surgically and behave more aggressively {3639}.

Molecular pathology

The incidence of *KRAS* gene mutations, immunolabelling for p53 protein, and loss of *SMAD4* expression in carcinomas of the extrahepatic bile ducts increases from proximal to distal bile duct {143, 2679, 3465}. As for IPN of the extrahepatic biliary tree, but unlike conventional adenocarcinoma of the extrahepatic bile ducts, a low frequency of *KRAS* mutations has been detected in IPNs of the extrahepatic biliary tree {12}. Microsatellite instability occurs in only 10% of IPNs of the extrahepatic bile ducts {11}.

Prognosis and predictive factors

The prognosis for patients with neoplasms of the extrahepatic biliary tract depends primarily on the extent of disease and histological type {1170, 1171, 2378, 3251}. Carcinomas arising in association with an intraductal papillary neoplasms have the potential to metastasize and are associated with a poor prognosis; when the carcinoma is localized to the ductal wall, the relative 10-year survival rate is 21% {77, 85}. Perineural invasion and lymphatic permeation are common and are significant prognostic factors {706, 2205, 3531}.

Neuroendocrine neoplasms of the gallbladder and extrahepatic bile ducts

P. Komminoth
R. Arnold
C. Capella
D.S. Klimstra
G. Klöppel

G. Rindi
J. Albores-Saavedra
E. Solcia

Definition

Neoplasms with neuroendocrine differentiation, including neuroendocrine tumours (NET) and neuroendocrine carcinomas (NEC) arising in the extrahepatic bile ducts or gallbladder. Mixed adenoneuroendocrine carcinomas (MANECs) have both exocrine and endocrine components, with each component exceeding 30%.

Synonyms

Synonyms for NETs of extrahepatic bile ducts or gallbladder include: carcinoid, well-differentiated endocrine tumour/carcinoma {3013}. Synonyms for NEC include: poorly differentiated endocrine carcinomas, high-grade neuroendocrine carcinoma, small cell and large cell endocrine carcinomas.

ICD-O codes

Neuroendocrine tumour (NET)
NET G1 (carcinoid)   8240/3
NET G2   8249/3
Neuroendocrine carcinoma (NEC)   8246/3
Large cell NEC   8013/3
Small cell NEC   8041/3
Mixed adenoneuroendocrine
carcinoma (MANEC)   8244/3
Goblet cell carcinoid   8243/3
Tubular carcinoid   8245/1

Epidemiology

NETs (carcinoids) of the bile duct and the gallbladder are very rare. There were 19 gallbladder NETs and one bile-duct NET recorded in a series of 8305 cases of all sites, representing 0.2% and 0.01% of cases {2115}. NETs are equally distributed between males and females and present at an average age of 60 years.
NECs represent 4% of all malignant neoplasms of the gallbladder {83, 2296}. NECs are slightly more common in females (male-to-female ratio, 1 : 1.8) and present at an average age of 65 years (range, 43–83 years) {2296}.

Etiology

The cause of NETs of the extrahepatic biliary tract and the gallbladder is not known. NECs (poorly differentiated endocrine carcinomas) seem to be associated with gallstones {2559}.

Localization

All types of neuroendocrine neoplasms are more commonly located in the gallbladder than in the extrahepatic bile ducts {70, 2115, 3595}. Both NETs and NECs can involve any portion of the gallbladder (fundus, body, or neck). NETs in the extrahepatic bile ducts may arise anywhere within the biliary tree, including the common hepatic duct (33%), the cystic duct (11%), and the upper or lower common bile duct (58%) {468, 774, 2590}. Involvement of the site of confluence of bile ducts (cystic duct and common hepatic duct, or right and left hepatic ducts) or origin within the intrapancreatic distal common bile duct, appear to be most common {1544}. NECs of the bile ducts tend to be located distally, only one case

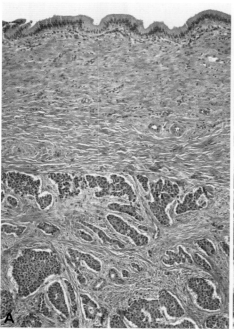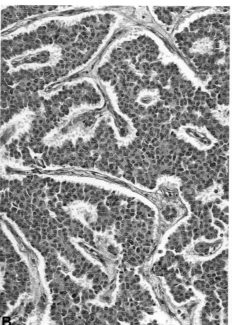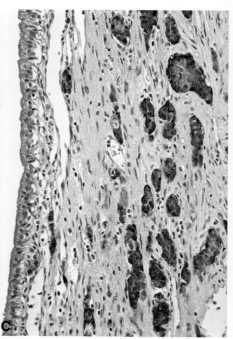

Fig. 11.21 Neuroendocrine tumour (NET) G1 (carcinoid) of the common bile duct. **A** A band of fibrous tissue separates the tumour from normal bile-duct epithelium. **B** Carcinoid cells with round nuclei and eosinophilic cytoplasm. **C** The NET cells are immunoreactive for serotonin.

has been reported in the cystic duct {1248, 3021}.

Clinical features

Gallbladder NETs usually lack specific symptoms. In most instances, they are detected incidentally after cholecystectomy. Occasionally, they cause recurrent upper-quadrant pain. NETs of the extrahepatic bile ducts typically produce either sudden onset of biliary colic or painless obstructive jaundice {2754}. Rare cases of primary, functioning, gastrin-producing NET (gastrinoma) of the common hepatic duct with Zollinger-Ellison syndrome have been reported {1988, 2590}.

The chief complaint of patients with NEC is abdominal pain. Other clinical features include abdominal mass, jaundice, and ascites {2296}. In addition, rare cases of hormonal syndromes have been reported associated with NECs, one patient with Cushing syndrome due to an adrenocorticotropic hormone (ACTH)-secreting small cell carcinoma {3039} and one suffering from paraneoplastic sensory neuropathy {3345}.

Macroscopy

NETs of the gallbladder are usually small (generally < 2 cm), grey-white or yellow, submucosal nodules or polyps, sometimes infiltrating the muscular wall {70, 774, 1957, 2388, 2754}. Some are pedunculated {1456, 2388}. Multifocality has been reported, but is rare {2425}. NETs measuring 0.3–0.5 cm can easily be overlooked on gross examination of cholecystectomy specimens {2580}.

Bile-duct NETs are usually small, submucosal nodules with variable amounts of sclerosis. Although they are often grossly circumscribed, they have infiltrative growth, grossly resembling primary adenocarcinomas of the bile ducts {1957}. There is less tendency to invade adjacent structures, however, and the size of these neoplasms averages only 2.0 cm (range, 1.1–5.4 cm) {849, 1957}. Some are polypoid, resembling papillary bile-duct neoplasms {1284, 3252}. NECs and MANECs appear as a nodular mass or neoplasm diffusely infiltrating the gallbladder or bile-duct wall {2296}. A significant proportion of NECs of both the gallbladder and bile ducts have a polypoid appearance {1420, 1560, 1685, 3595}. Although they average 3.0 cm in size {1958}, these neoplasms can be quite large and may extensively invade the liver and adjacent tissues {1535}.

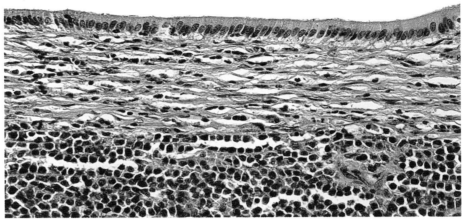
Fig. 11.22 Small cell neuroendocrine carcinoma (NEC) lying below normal gallbladder epithelium.

Histopathology

NETs

NETs are composed of cells that are uniform in size, with round or oval nuclei, inconspicuous nucleoli, and eosinophilic cytoplasm. NET cells are arranged in combined patterns with trabecular anastomosing structures, tubular structures and solid nests {529, 1028, 2754, 2999}. Tumour cells are immunoreactive for synaptophysin {1957} chromogranin A {116, 2754}, neuron-specific enolase (NSE) {116, 203, 348}, keratins (keratin 7 and AE1/AE3) {2976}, and several hormones, including serotonin {116, 203, 1957}, gastrin {201, 1957, 1972, 1988}, somatostatin {116, 1028, 1957} and pancreatic polypeptide {1183, 1647, 1957}.

Clear cell NETs of the gallbladder are characterized by cells with abundant cytoplasm containing small lipid vacuoles, imparting a foamy appearance. Periodic acid-Schiff demonstrates neither glycogen nor mucin in the clear cells. This NET variant can be either sporadic or associated with von Hippel-Lindau (VHL) disease {1647, 2976, 3252}. Neoplasms associated with VHL disease are positive for inhibin, while sporadic neoplasms are negative for inhibin {1647, 3252}.

NECs

NECs of the gallbladder and extrahepatic bile ducts encompass small cell and large cell variants. In the small cell type, the cell population and the growth pattern are similar to those of small cell carcinoma of the lung {1685, 1958, 2296}. Small cell carcinomas appear to be more common in the gallbladder than in the extrahepatic bile ducts.

Small cell NECs. These neoplasms are composed of round or fusiform cells arranged in sheets, nests, cords, and festoons. Characteristic nuclear "moulding" is demonstrable on high-power examination. Rosette-like structures and tubules are occasionally present. Extensive necrosis and subepithelial growth are constant features. In necrotic areas, intense basophilic staining of the blood vessels occurs. Tumour cells have round or ovoid hyperchromatic nuclei with inconspicuous nucleoli. Occasionally, tumour giant cells {70, 2296} and focal areas of glandular or squamous differentiation are observed {1310, 1958, 2296}. Mitotic figures are frequent and reported to range from 15 to 206 (mean, 75) per 10 high power fields (HPF) {2296}. NECs of small cell type show diffuse positivity for synaptophysin and NSE and often contain scattered chromogranin A-positive cells. In addition, tumour cells express epithelial markers such as epithelial membrane antigen (EMA), keratin AE1/AE3 and carcinoembryonic antigen (CEA). A few cells may stain for serotonin, somatostatin, and ACTH {70, 2296}. Overexpression of p53 has been detected in 83% and loss of pRb in 67% of cases {2494}. Ultrastructurally, a small number of dense-core secretory granules can be found {70, 83}.

Large cell NECs. These neoplasms display an organoid growth pattern often with rosette formation composed by large cells characterized by vesicular nuclei with prominent nucleoli and a variable amount of cytoplasm {1451, 2451}. Tumour cells are positive for keratins, chromogranin A and synaptophysin. The proliferative rate (Ki67 immunostain) is > 50%. Foci of adenocarcinoma may be present.

MANECs

A significant number of cases reported in the older literature as NETs, including the cases reviewed by Yamamoto *et al.* {3593, 3595}, are in fact MANECs. These are composite neoplasms in which areas of adenocarcinoma or squamous cell carcinoma intermingle with areas of NET or NEC, each comprising at least 30% of the neoplasm, by arbitrary definition. The neuroendocrine components display features overlapping those described in pure NETs or NECs, being formed by solid and/or trabecular structures with argyrophylic cells that are immunoreactive for NSE, chromogranin A, CD56/NCAM1, serotonin and gastrin {803, 2296, 2372, 2385, 2661, 2947, 3307, 3595}. The adenocarcinoma component is usually tubular or papillary, formed by columnar cells, goblet cells and sometimes Paneth cells. Squamous elements appear as circumscribed nests of squamous cells, sometimes with keratinization, that have an abrupt transition to the surrounding NEC elements. A case of MANEC of diffuse type with mucin-containing signet ring cells and clear neuroendocrine cells has also been reported {2454}.

Genetic susceptibility

NETs of the gallbladder and extrahepatic bile ducts are infrequently associated with VHL syndrome {2202, 2976} and multiple endocrine neoplasia type 1 (MEN1) {2590}.

Molecular pathology

Few studies have addressed genetic alterations in neuroendocrine neoplasms of the gallbladder and extrahepatic bile ducts {1848}. Mutations of *TP53*, *KRAS* and *SMAD4* appear not to play a significant role in the pathogenesis of NETs {1957}. Accumulation of p53 and inactivation of the pRb/p16 pathway has been found in most NECs of the gallbladder {2296, 2494}. Expression of SMAD4 protein is usually retained and *KRAS* mutations are rare {1958, 2494}.

Prognosis and predictive factors

In contrast to other gastrointestinal sites, there is no proposal for a TNM/staging classification of neuroendocrine neoplasms of the gallbladder and bile ducts. The relative rarity of NETs and NECs at these sites may account for this. Given the limits of differences in tumour biology, for practical purposes staging may be performed according to the TNM classification for adenocarcinomas of the gallbladder and bile duct.

Malignant behaviour of NETs of gallbladder and bile ducts is defined by the presence of regional or distant metastases {116, 2027} and/or signs of local aggressive growth, including invasion of the muscularis propria or beyond {116, 117, 2027}, and neural invasion {2027}. The risk of malignant behaviour largely depends on tumour size, since NETs measuring 0.3–0.5 cm usually do not show metastases {70}, while NETs > 2 cm often extend into the liver and/or metastasize {2294}. The percentage of gallbladder NETs showing regional and distant metastases has been estimated as approximately 44% and 11%, respectively {774, 2115}. The 5-year survival rate is 41% according to Surveillance, Epidemiology nd End Results (SEER) data for the USA. Approximately one third of patients with bile-duct NETs exhibit metastases at diagnosis {774}. Aggressive surgical therapy offers the only chance for cure and should be considered whenever possible {1092, 1373}. Five-year survival rates range from 60% to 100% {2116}.

The prognosis for patients with NEC either of small or large cell type is poor {83, 1451}. About 40–50% of patients have disseminated disease at the time of diagnosis {907}. Small cell NEC of the gallbladder appears to be highly responsive to chemotherapy as well as radiotherapy, and survival times of > 1 year have been reported using regimens similar to those used for small cell carcinoma of the lung {907}.

MANECs behave as adenocarcinomas and should be managed accordingly, being clinically more aggressive than NETs.

Mesenchymal tumours of the gallbladder and extrahepatic bile ducts

M. Miettinen
C.D.M. Fletcher
L.-G. Kindblom

ICD-O codes

Granular cell tumour	9580/0
Leiomyoma	8890/0
Kaposi sarcoma	9140/3
Leiomyosarcoma	8890/3
Rhabdomyosarcoma	8900/3

Paraganglioma

This generally benign neural tumour is composed of nests of neural cells (chief cells) often lined by Schwann cell-related sustentacular cells. The former are immunohistochemically positive for chromogranin A and synaptophysin and negative for keratins and S100 protein, whereas the latter are positive for S100 protein and often for glial fibrillary acidic protein (GFAP). The tumour is usually located in the outer wall of the gallbladder, but can also involve the extrahepatic bile ducts. It is usually an incidental microscopic finding in cholecystectomy specimens. Some cases occur in association with multiple endocrine neoplasia (MEN) syndromes {2035}. It can be difficult to distinguish between normal paraganglionic structures and a very small paraganglioma.

Granular cell tumour

Although rare, granular cell tumour is the most commonly diagnosed benign nonepithelial tumour of the gallbladder and extrahepatic biliary tract. In the gallbladder, such tumours are usually incidental microscopic findings, whereas granular cell tumours in the bile ducts can cause symptomatic biliary obstruction that clinically mimics bile duct carcinoma {3210}.

Granular cell tumours can be multicentric, involving different visceral sites as well as the skin and peripheral soft tissues. Involvement of the bile ducts often results in a concentric or eccentric mass that variably obliterates the lumen. Histologically, granular cell tumours contain clusters or sheets of polygonal cells with abundant periodic acid–Schiff (PAS)-positive granular cytoplasm and small nuclei. The cells are immunohistochemically positive for S100 protein and α-inhibin {2188}.

Ganglioneuromatosis

Diffuse ganglioneuromatosis can involve the gallbladder in patients with MEN2B. The lesions contain Schwann-cell elements admixed with scattered ganglion cells involving the entire wall of the gallbladder {437}. Diffuse or plexiform neurofibromas can also involve the biliary tract in patients with neurofibromatosis type 1 (NF1) {2095}.

Rhabdomyosarcoma

In young children, embryonal (botryoid) rhabdomyosarcoma occurs in the extrahepatic bile ducts and rarely in the gallbladder, where it can secondarily extend into the hepatic hilus and often manifests with biliary obstruction. Rhabdomyosarcoma forms a mass composed of multiple filiform, polypoid intraluminal protrusions involving the bile ducts {1714, 59A}. Rhabdomyoblastic differentiation is variable, and coexpression of desmin and myogenic regulatory proteins (MYOD1, myogenin) is diagnostic. Prognosis is reasonably good with modern combined chemotherapy and surgery regimens; in one study, the estimated 5-year survival was 66% {2278}.

Other sarcomas and benign mesenchymal tumours

Epstein-Barr virus (EBV)-associated leiomyosarcoma/smooth muscle tumour rarely involves the gallbladder wall. These tumours are described in Chapter 10. Other sarcomas involving the gallbladder and biliary ducts are undifferentiated pleomorphic sarcoma and myxofibrosarcoma (malignant fibrous histiocytoma), angiosarcoma {59A}. In addition, Kaposi sarcoma, abdominal liposarcomas and leiomyosarcomas can secondarily involve gallbladder and bile-duct system. Sarcomatoid carcinoma, (metastatic) melanoma and dedifferentiated liposarcoma have to be ruled out before diagnosing an undifferentiated sarcoma in the gallbladder. Lipomas, lymphangiomas, and haemangiomas rarely involve the gallbladder {414}. Despite occasional reports in the literature, we have doubts concerning the occurrence of true gastrointestinal stromal tumours of the gallbladder that are comparable to those found in the gastrointestinal tract.

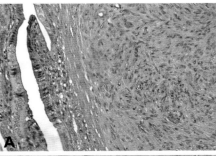
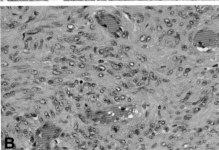

Fig. 11.23 Epstein-Barr virus-associated leiomyosarcoma. **A** The neoplasm forms a transmural mass involving the gallbladder wall. **B** It is composed of spindled to oval cells that are less differentiated than the smooth muscle in typical leiomyosarcoma.

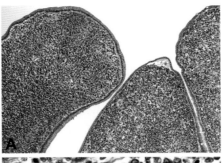
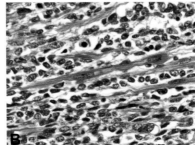

Fig. 11.24 Embryonal (botryoid) rhabdomyosarcoma. **A** The neoplasm contains multiple polypoid protrusions projecting into the bile-duct lumen. **B** At higher magnification, elongated rhabdomyoblasts can be seen as a minor component among less differentiated cells.

Lymphoma of the gallbladder and extrahepatic bile ducts

E.S. Jaffe
S. Nakamura
Y.H. Ko
H.K. Müller-Hermelink
J. Delabie

In common with lymphoma elsewhere in the digestive system, primary lymphomas of the gallbladder and extrahepatic bile ducts are defined as extranodal lymphomas arising in and localized to this region {1341}. Contiguous lymph-node involvement and distant spread may be seen, but the primary clinical presentation is in the gallbladder or, even more rarely, in the extrahepatic bile ducts. Lymphomas with this localization are extremely rare, with fewer than 40 reported cases {160, 256, 497, 1495, 2019, 2402}. A few instances of primary lymphoma of mucosa-associated lymphoid tissue (MALT) in the gallbladder have been described {256, 268, 2019}. Such tumours may arise within the context of acquired MALT lymphoma, which is frequently encountered in the gallbladder associated with chronic cholecystitis {268, 3266}.

The morphology and genetics of lymphoma of the gallbladder appear to be similar to those of gastric MALT lymphomas, including the presence of the fusion gene *BIRC3-MALT1* in at least one reported case {268}. Other types of primary gall bladder lymphoma resemble intestinal lymphomas, and have included cases of lymphomatous polypopsis, extracavitary primary effusion lymphoma and plasmablastic lymphoma {1972A}. Other lymphoma subtypes that have been reported in the gallbladder, with involvement of the extrahepatic ducts in rare instances, are follicular lymphoma and diffuse large B-cell lymphoma {843, 1282, 1412, 3118}. Rarely, other forms of lymphoma or lymphoblastic leukaemia may be seen initially at this site {1412, 2097}.

Secondary tumours and melanoma of the gallbladder and extrahepatic bile ducts

C. Iacobuzio-Donahue

Incidence and origins
Metastases to the gallbladder and extrahepatic biliary tree are uncommon. Although virtually any primary malignancy can metastasize to the gallbladder or biliary tract {725}, melanoma accounts for > 50% of all reported cases of metastasis to the gallbladder and biliary tract {442}, followed by carcinomas of the stomach and breast {725}. Secondary involvement of the gallbladder or extrahepatic biliary tract may result from transcoelomic spread in the setting of peritoneal carcinomatosis, or by direct extension from carcinomas of adjacent organs.

Primary malignant melanoma of the gallbladder or extrahepatic biliary tract is even more rare than metastatic melanoma {442, 2772, 2789, 3460}. Features that favour a primary melanoma in this location are the presence of junctional activity in the epithelium adjacent to the tumour {442, 2670}, and the absence of a primary melanoma elsewhere in the body. However, junctional activity has been reported in metastatic melanoma of the gallbladder.

Clinical features
Metastases to the gallbladder or extrahepatic biliary tract are most often asymptomatic. In patients who do have symptoms, the most common presentations are biliary colic {182}, acute cholecystitis {676, 3398}, or biliary obstruction {942, 1944}.

Macroscopy
Both intraluminal metastases and diffuse wall infiltration or stricture formation by metastases to the gallbladder have been described {1944}. Primary melanoma of the gallbladder is most often seen as an intraluminal polypoid mass {676, 2772, 2789}.

Histopathology
The features of metastases to the gallbladder and extrahepatic biliary tree are similar to those observed for metastases to other organs. Primary melanomas of the gallbladder and extrahepatic biliary tree may have evidence of melanoma *in situ* (junctional activity) adjacent to the infiltrating component {442, 2670}.

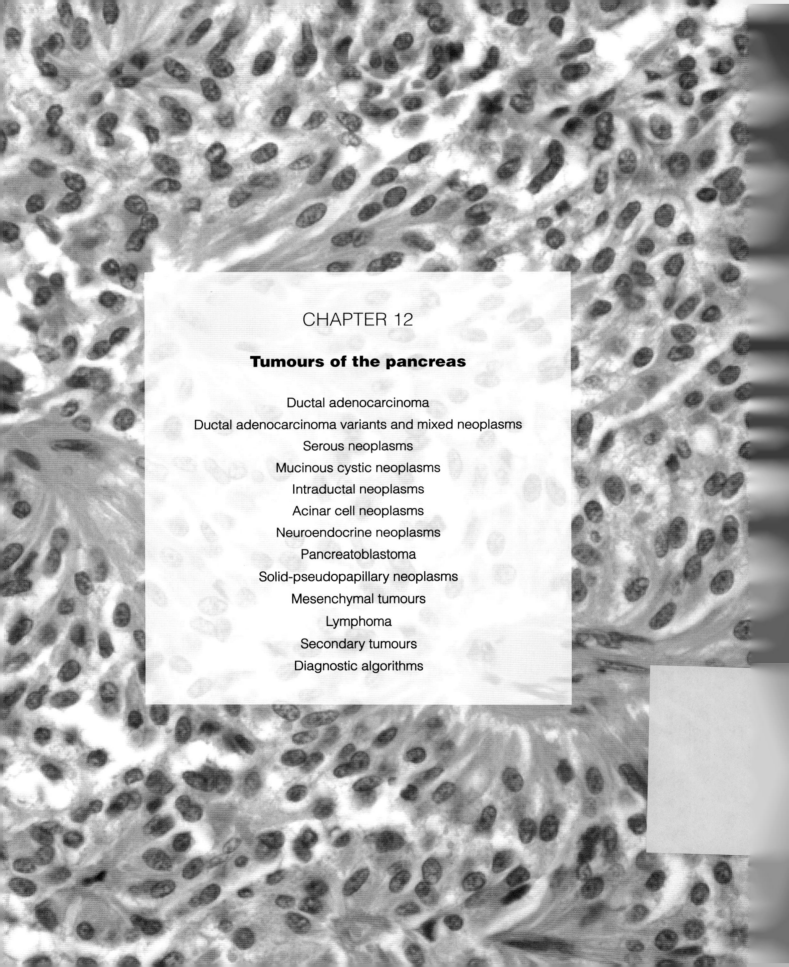

CHAPTER 12

Tumours of the pancreas

WHO classification[a] of tumours of the pancreas

Epithelial tumours

Benign

Acinar cell cystadenoma	8551/0
Serous cystadenoma	8441/0[a]

Premalignant lesions

Pancreatic intraepithelial neoplasia, grade 3 (PanIN-3)	8148/2
Intraductal papillary mucinous neoplasm with low- or intermediate-grade dysplasia	8453/0
Intraductal papillary mucinous neoplasm with high-grade dysplasia	8453/2
Intraductal tubulopapillary neoplasm	8503/2*
Mucinous cystic neoplasm with low- or intermediate-grade dysplasia	8470/0
Mucinous cystic neoplasm with high-grade dysplasia	8470/2

Malignant

Ductal adenocarcinoma	8500/3
Adenosquamous carcinoma	8560/3
Colloid carcinoma (mucinous noncystic carcinoma)	8480/3
Hepatoid carcinoma	8576/3
Medullary carcinoma	8510/3
Signet ring cell carcinoma	8490/3
Undifferentiated carcinoma	8020/3
Undifferentiated carcinoma with osteoclast-like giant cells	8035/3
Acinar cell carcinoma	8550/3
Acinar cell cystadenocarcinoma	8551/3
Intraductal papillary mucinous neoplasm with an associated invasive carcinoma	8453/3
Mixed acinar-ductal carcinoma	8552/3
Mixed acinar-neuroendocrine carcinoma	8154/3
Mixed acinar-neuroendocrine-ductal carcinoma	8154/3
Mixed ductal-neuroendocrine carcinoma	8154/3
Mucinous cystic neoplasm with an associated invasive carcinoma	8470/3
Pancreatoblastoma	8971/3
Serous cystadenocarcinoma	8441/3
Solid-pseudopapillary neoplasm	8452/3

Neuroendocrine neoplasms[b]

Pancreatic neuroendocrine microadenoma	8150/0
Neuroendocrine tumour (NET)	
Nonfunctional pancreatic NET, G1, G2	8150/3
NET G1	8240/3
NET G2	8249/3
Neuroendocrine carcinoma (NEC)	8246/3
Large cell NEC	8013/3
Small cell NEC	8041/3
EC cell, serotonin-producing NET (carcinoid)	8241/3
Gastrinoma	8153/3
Glucagonoma	8152/3
Insulinoma	8151/3
Somatostatinoma	8156/3
VIPoma	8155/3

Mature teratoma	9080/0

Mesenchymal tumours

Lymphomas

Secondary tumours

EC, enterochromaffin; VIP, vasoactive intestinal peptide. [a] The morphology codes are from the International Classification of Diseases for Oncology (ICD-O) {904A}. [b] The classification is modified from the previous WHO histological classification of tumours {691} taking into account changes in our understanding of these lesions. In the case of neuroendocrine neoplasms, the classification has been simplified to be of more practical utility in morphological classification. * These new codes were approved by the IARC/WHO Committee for ICD-O at its meeting in March 2010.

TNM classification[a] of tumours of the pancreas[b]

T – Primary tumour
TX   Primary tumour cannot be assessed
T0   No evidence of primary tumour
Tis   Carcinoma *in situ*, includes PanIN-3[c]
T1   Tumour limited to the pancreas, 2 cm or less in greatest dimension
T2   Tumour limited to the pancreas, more than 2 cm in greatest dimension
T3   Tumour extends beyond pancreas
T4   Tumour involves coeliac axis or superior mesenteric artery

N – Regional lymph nodes
NX   Regional lymph nodes cannot be assessed
N0   No regional lymph-node metastasis
N1   Regional lymph-node metastasis

M – Distant metastasis
M0   No distant metastasis
MI   Distant metastasis

Stage grouping

Stage	T	N	M
Stage 0	Tis	N0	M0
Stage IA	T1	N0	M0
Stage IB	T2	N0	M0
Stage IIA	T3	N0	M0
Stage IIB	T1, T2, T3	N1	M0
Stage III	T4	Any N	M0
Stage IV	Any T	Any N	M1

[a] {762, 2996}; [b] The classification applies to carcinomas of the exocrine pancreas and pancreatic neuroendocrine tumours; [c] PanIN, pancreatic intraepithelial neoplasia. A helpdesk for specific questions about the TNM classification is available at http://www.uicc.org.

Ductal adenocarcinoma of the pancreas

R.H. Hruban
P. Boffetta
N. Hiraoka
C. Iacobuzio-Donahue
Y. Kato
S.E. Kern
D.S. Klimstra
G. Klöppel
A. Maitra
G.J.A. Offerhaus
M.B. Pitman

Definition

An infiltrating epithelial neoplasm with glandular (ductal) differentiation, usually demonstrating luminal and/or intracellular production of mucin, and without a predominant component of any other histological type. An abundant desmoplastic stromal response is a typical feature of this neoplasm.

ICD-O codes

Ductal adenocarcinoma 8500/3
Pancreatic intraepithelial neoplasia
grade 3 (PanIN-3) 8148/2

Synonyms

Tubular adenocarcinoma, infiltrating duct carcinoma, not otherwise specified (NOS)

Epidemiology

The epidemiological study of this disease is complicated by significant geographical and temporal variations in the sensitivity and specificity of clinical diagnosis and in the proportion of cases that are histologically verified. Differences in access to health care (e.g. for different social classes or age groups) can affect reported incidence and mortality rates.

The highest rates of pancreatic ductal adenocarcinoma are recorded among African Americans (about 12 per 100 000 men and 10 per 100 000 women) and among indigenous populations in Oceania. The lowest rates (< 2 per 100 000 men and 1 per 100 000 women), which may be partly attributable to under-diagnosis, are recorded in India, northern and central Africa and south-east Asia. In the USA, rates are about 50–100% higher in African Americans than in whites living in the same areas {634}. Worldwide, there were an estimated 230 000 new cases in 2002, 60% of which occurred in high-resource countries {842}. Incidence is about 50% higher in men than in women. Most patients are between 60 and 80 years of age. Given the very poor survival, mortality rates closely parallel incidence rates.

Diagnostic improvements are partly responsible for the increase in reported incidence and mortality rates that has taken place since the 1970s, particularly in Europe; however, incidence and mortality rates in western Europe have levelled off and declined over recent years {1814}. Incidence is higher in urban populations than in rural populations, but this may reflect differences in the quality of diagnosis. Studies of migrant populations have shown that, after 15–20 years, first-generation migrants from low-risk to high-risk areas experience rates that are higher than those of the country of origin, suggesting an important role for environmental exposures occurring late in life {110}.

Etiology

The best-known risk factor for pancreatic cancer is tobacco smoking. The risk in smokers is two- to three times greater than in nonsmokers, there is a dose–response relationship, and smoking cessation has been shown to lower risk in many populations {1338}. The proportion of cases of pancreatic cancer attributable to tobacco smoking has been estimated at 20–30% in men and 10% in women {1333}. Some, but not all, of the features of the descriptive epidemiology of pancreatic cancer (i.e. the higher incidence in African Americans than in white Americans, and the higher risk in men and urban residents) can be explained by differences in smoking habits {148, 2967}. Use of smokeless tobacco products has also been linked to an increased risk of pancreatic cancer {1334}.

It has been suggested that pancreatic cancer is associated with nutritional and dietary factors, including obesity and low physical activity, high intake of fats, especially saturated fats, and low intake of vegetables and fruit {3548, 149A}.

Early reports of an association between coffee consumption and risk of pancreatic cancer were of questionable quality and have not been confirmed by larger, more recent investigations. Heavy drinking of alcohol may weakly increase risk {3286}. Of the medical conditions that have been studied {110}, a history of chronic pancreatitis is associated with an increased risk of pancreatic cancer of more than 10-fold. The risk is particularly high in individuals with hereditary pancreatitis {1901}. Diabetes mellitus has also been

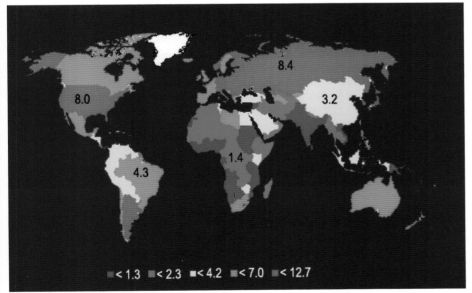

Fig. 12.01 Worldwide age-standardized annual incidence (per 100 000) of pancreatic cancer in men (2008). Note the areas of high incidence in North America, Europe, and the Russian Federation {842A}.

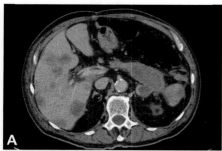

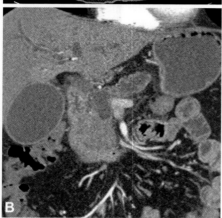

Fig. 12.02 A Computed tomography (CT) scan of a ductal adenocarcinoma of the body and tail of the pancreas with numerous liver metastases. **B** Coronal CT scan revealing a large ductal adenocarcinoma in the head of the pancreas. Note the secondary dilatation of the pancreatic and intrahepatic bile ducts, as well as the massive enlargement of the gallbladder.

associated with an increased risk of pancreatic cancer (relative risk, 1.5–2-fold). Gastrectomy patients have a three- to fivefold risk of pancreatic cancer; the association does not appear to be confounded by tobacco smoking.

Localization

Most (60–70%) pancreatic ductal adenocarcinomas arise in the head of the gland, and the remainder in the body (5–15%) or tail (10–15%). The vast majority of pancreatic cancers are solitary, but multifocal disease can occur {1270, 3012}. Very rarely, heterotopic pancreatic tissue can give rise to a carcinoma {1014, 3196}.

Clinical features

Signs and symptoms

Clinical features include back pain, unexplained weight loss, jaundice and pruritus {1229}. Diabetes mellitus is present in 70% of patients, and new-onset diabetes may be the first manifestation of pancreatic cancer {490}. Later symptoms are related to liver metastasis and/or

invasion of adjacent organs (duodenum) or involvement of the peritoneal cavity (ascites). Occasionally, patients present with acute pancreatitis {1059}, migratory thrombophlebitis {1534}, hypoglycaemia, or hypercalcaemia {2127}. Depression that is out of proportion to the severity of the disease can be a presenting symptom {434, 2497}.

Imaging and laboratory tests

Computed tomography (CT) is one of the best imaging modalities for the pancreas and pancreatic adenocarcinomas appear as hypodense masses in up to 92% of cases {286, 1461, 2775}. Diffuse tumour involvement is found in about 4% of cases. Early findings on CT include abrupt cut-off and dilatation of the pancreatic duct {940}. The "double-duct sign" – dilatation of both the biliary and pancreatic ducts – points to cancer arising in the head of the pancreas. On endoscopic ultrasonography (EUS), most ductal adenocarcinomas produce echo-poor and nonhomogeneous mass lesions. About 10% of tumours appear echo-rich. With increasing size, tumours tend to become heterogeneous, with cystic and echo-rich areas. Indirect signs of a pancreatic tumour (dilatation of pancreatic and/or common bile duct) are usually found upstream of tumours > 3 cm in size. Lymph-node metastases appear as enlarged echo-poor nodes on EUS. Biopsies performed through the endoscope can be used to establish the diagnosis.
Endoscopic retrograde cholangiopancreatography (ERCP) may demonstrate displacement, narrowing, or obstruction of the pancreatic duct.
Additional valuable techniques include magnetic resonance imaging (MRI) and serum tumour-marker determination (CA19-9, carcinoembryonic antigen [CEA]). Because of significant false-positive and false-negative rates, serum tumour markers are not useful in screening the general population.
Positron emission tomography (PET) scanning may have diagnostic value, but is of uncertain additional clinical utility beyond that of the conventional imaging modalities {2875}.
The sensitivity and specificity of any one of these tests alone range from 55% to 95%, but applying combinations can achieve accuracy rates of > 95%, although tissue diagnosis remains the gold standard {2775}.

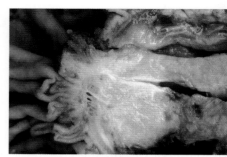

Fig. 12.03 Ductal adenocarcinoma. An ill-defined scirrhous carcinoma of the head of the pancreas infiltrating the duodenum.

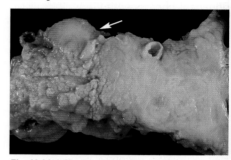

Fig. 12.04 Infiltrating ductal adenocarcinoma. Note the metastasis to a lymph node (arrow).

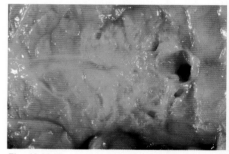

Fig. 12.05 Ductal adenocarcinoma in the tail of the pancreas. Note the normal duct (left) downstream from the carcinoma (centre), and the small retention cyst upstream from the tumour (right).

Macroscopy

Ductal adenocarcinomas are firm, sclerotic and poorly defined masses that replace the normal lobular architecture of the gland. The cut surfaces are yellow to white. Haemorrhage and necrosis are uncommon, but microcystic areas may occur, particularly in larger tumours. In surgical series, most carcinomas of the pancreatic head measure 1.5–5.0 cm, with a mean diameter of 2.5–3.5 cm, while carcinomas of the body/tail are usually larger. Cancers measuring < 2 cm are infrequent {1176} and may be difficult to recognize on gross inspection. Carcinomas of the pancreatic head usually invade the common bile duct and/or the main pancreatic duct and produce stenosis that results in proximal dilatation of both duct systems. More advanced pancreatic carcinomas in the head of the gland can involve the ampulla of Vater and/or the duodenal wall. Carcinomas in the body or tail obstruct the main pancreatic duct, but typically do not involve the common bile duct. Stenosis of the main pancreatic duct can produce secondary changes in the upstream pancreatic parenchyma, including duct dilatation, retention-cyst formation and fibrous atrophy of the parenchyma (i.e. obstructive chronic pancreatitis). Gross distinction of chronic pancreatitis from invasive ductal adenocarcinoma is often difficult, making the limits of the neoplasm hard to define.

Tumour spread and staging
At diagnosis, the vast majority of pancreatic cancers have spread beyond the pancreatic parenchyma {3007}. Carcinomas of the head commonly extend into the duodenum and the ampulla of Vater (causing ulceration), the intrapancreatic portion of the common bile duct (causing stenosis), and into peripancreatic or retroperitoneal adipose tissue. Perineural invasion is a common mechanism by which pancreatic cancers reach these structures and may precede the development of peripancreatic lymph-node metastases {1509, 2204}. Invasion into the spleen, stomach, left adrenal gland, colon, and peritoneum tends to be more common among carcinomas of the body and tail because of the proximity of these structures to the tail of the pancreas and the late stage at which such cancers are usually clinically detected {3638}. In addition to peripancreatic lymph nodes, carcinomas of the pancreatic head typically involve the chains of lymph nodes along the superior mesenteric artery, the common hepatic artery and the hepatoduodenal ligament {1577}. The carcinoma may metastasize more distantly to lymph nodes in the ligamentum hepatoduodenale, the coeliac trunk, and in para-aortic area at the level of the renal arteries. Carcinomas of the body and tail are particularly prone to metastasize to the superior and inferior body and tail lymph-node groups and to the splenic hilus lymph nodes, and may also spread via lymphatic channels to the pleura and lung {1974}. Haematogenous metastasis occurs, in decreasing order of frequency, to the liver, lungs, bones and adrenals {3573}.

Particularly problematic is the diagnosis of metastasis to the ovary, which can mimic a primary ovarian mucinous neoplasm {3374, 3375, 3632}. Pancreatic cancers metastatic to the ovary are typically cystic, large, and bilateral; they involve the surface and hilum of the ovary, and are characterized microscopically by nodularity, and a haphazard infiltrative pattern of growth {3374, 3375, 3632}. Immunolabelling with a panel of antibodies to keratins 7 and 20, SMAD4/DPC4, CDKN2A (p16) and CDX2 may help to establish the diagnosis {3374, 3375, 3632}. Pancreatic cancers are staged according to the seventh edition of the TNM system {2996}. A slightly modified classification has been proposed by the Japanese Pancreas Society {1347}.

Histopathology
Most ductal adenocarcinomas are composed of well- to moderately developed glandular and duct-like structures, which infiltrate the pancreatic parenchyma, grow in a haphazard pattern, are associated with a desmoplastic stroma and produce sialo-type and sulfated acid mucins that stain with Alcian blue and periodic acid-Schiff (PAS). Poorly differentiated ductal adenocarcinomas form small, poorly formed glands composed of cells with pleomorphic nuclei, individual infiltrating cells, and solid cellular areas. They produce much less mucin than more differentiated carcinomas.

Well-differentiated carcinomas
These carcinomas are composed of haphazardly arranged infiltrating duct-like structures and medium-sized neoplastic glands. The contours of the duct-like structures may be angular or irregular, such irregular contours are especially pronounced in the "large-duct" variant {1653}. Perineural or vascular invasion are both highly diagnostic of an invasive cancer, and "ruptured" or "incomplete" ducts (which lack a portion of epithelium and instead are partially lined by cellular stromal tissue) are highly suggestive of an invasive cancer. Non-neoplastic ducts, as well as remnants of acini and individual islets of Langerhans, are typically interspersed among the neoplastic glands, and some neoplastic glands may even infiltrate into non-neoplastic islets of Langerhans. Only in exceptional cases do neuroendocrine cells constitute a second neoplastic cell component of ductal carcinomas.

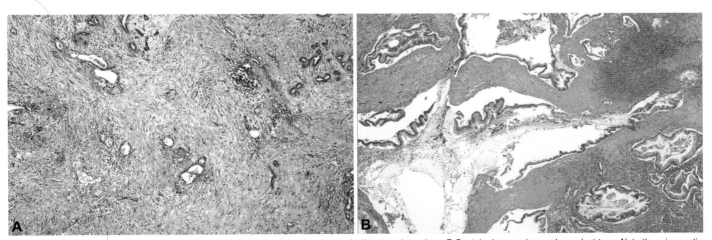

Fig. 12.06 **A** Ductal adenocarcinoma, well-differentiated, showing intensive desmoplastic stromal reaction. **B** Ductal adenocarcinoma, large-duct type. Note the microcystic well-differentiated neoplastic duct structures.

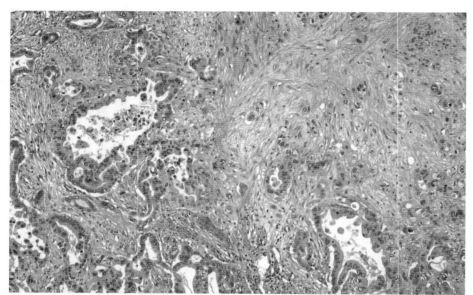

Fig. 12.07 Poorly differentiated ductal adenocarcinoma. Note the irregularly structured neoplastic glands showing distinct pleomorphism of the lining cells.

The neoplastic cells are cuboidal to columnar, and form a single cell layer, although papillary projections can be seen. The cytoplasm is usually eosinophilic, but a pale or even clear appearance may sometimes be prominent. The nuclei are round to oval and may be three to four times larger than non-neoplastic nuclei. Importantly, the size, shape, and location of the nuclei vary among cells within the individual neoplastic glands. The nuclear membranes are sharp and the distinct nucleoli are often large. Mitoses are not common.

At the time of diagnosis, virtually all carcinomas deeply infiltrate the surrounding pancreatic tissue and the adjacent peripancreatic adipose tissue. The infiltrating malignant glands are often found in abnormal locations, such as immediately adjacent to muscular blood vessels; a finding that may be diagnostically useful.

They may also invade the common bile duct, the ampulla, and the duodenal mucosa, typically following pre-existing structures such as ducts, nerves and vessels. Cancerization of the pancreatic ducts, particularly the medium-sized interlobular ducts, is not uncommon, and may extend far beyond the main neoplastic mass {1613}. In these cases, the normal epithelium is replaced by atypical columnar cells that often form papillary projections without fibrovascular stalks. This change is usually accompanied by a ductocentric desmoplasia, and can be virtually indistinguishable from high-grade pancreatic intraepithelial neoplasia (PanIN-3). Perineural invasion is seen in almost all cases within the pancreas itself, and invasive carcinoma typically extends into the retroperitoneal fatty tissue behind the head of the pancreas and around the bile duct, where nerves are abundant. In

the vast majority of cases, the neoplastic cells that invade the nerves show glandular differentiation. Benign ducts are rarely encountered in the vicinity of a nerve and a non-neoplastic glandular inclusion in a nerve is exceedingly uncommon, although non-neoplastic islet cells may involve nerves. Lymphatic invasion is another very common finding and is associated with lymph-node metastasis. Carcinoma may invade the wall of blood vessels (e.g. the portal vein), or the neoplastic cells may penetrate the lumen, causing thrombosis. In some cases, the neoplastic epithelium can entirely replace the endothelium and re-line the vessel, producing a vessel lined by well-differentiated epithelial cells; such structures can mimic PanIN.

Neoplastic glands may also infiltrate the peripancreatic adipose tissue without following pre-existing structures. Typically these glands lie individually as naked glands within the fat, either directly abutting adipocytes or surrounded by inflammatory cells. If infiltrating neoplastic glands reach the mucosa of the distal common bile duct, the ampulla and/or the duodenum, the neoplastic cells may replace the normal epithelium, mimicking a primary neoplasm of the involved site.

Moderately differentiated carcinomas

These carcinomas are largely identical to well-differentiated adenocarcinomas in growth pattern and behaviour, except that they produce a mixture of medium-sized duct-like structures and small tubular glands of variable size and shape (some are incompletely formed, others create a cribriform pattern). Moderately differentiated carcinomas are also characterized by a greater variation in nuclear size, chromatin structure and prominence of nucleoli and more mitotic figures. The cytoplasm is usually slightly eosinophilic, but clear cells are occasionally abundant. Mucin production appears to be decreased. Foci of poor and irregular glandular formation are often found at the leading edge of the neoplasm, particularly where the carcinoma invades the peripancreatic tissue.

Poorly differentiated ductal adenocarcinomas

These neoplasms are composed of a mixture of densely packed, small irregular glands, solid sheets and nests, as well as individual cells. The desmoplastic

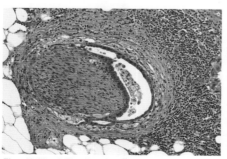

Fig. 12.08 Infiltrating ductal adenocarcinoma with perineural invasion.

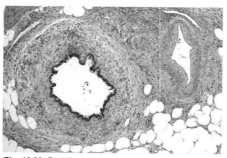

Fig. 12.09 Ductal adenocarcinoma with venous invasion, mimicking pancreatic intraepithelial neoplasia (PanIN).

response to the neoplasm can be minimal and foci of necrosis and haemorrhage may occur. The cells forming glands and solid cellular sheets show marked nuclear pleomorphism (occasionally with squamoid or spindle-cell differentiation), little or no mucin production, and brisk mitotic activity. Intraductal extension of the carcinoma is seen less often than in more differentiated carcinomas, while perineural, lymphatic, and blood-vessel invasion are equally frequent.

Many ductal adenocarcinomas obstruct the main pancreatic duct, causing upstream obstructive chronic pancreatitis. Complete obstruction usually results in the upstream duct becoming markedly dilated, the pancreatic parenchyma is atrophied, and there can be a marked clustering ("aggregation") of the residual islets, which can mimic a neuroendocrine neoplasm. The intraductal calcifications that are typically seen in alcoholic chronic pancreatitis are generally absent.

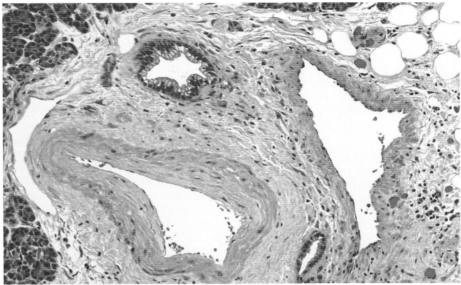

Fig. 12.10 Well-differentiated infiltrating ductal adenocarcinoma of the pancreas. Glands adjacent to muscular vessels suggest the diagnosis.

Grading

The grading of ductal adenocarcinoma is based on combined assessment of histological and cytological features and mitotic activity (see Table 12.01) {1612, 1921}. If there is intratumour heterogeneity, i.e. variation in the degree of differentiation and mitotic activity, the higher grade and activity is to be reported. This rule also applies if only a minor component (less than half the carcinoma) is of lower grade. Histological grade correlates with survival when the system illustrated is employed {1612, 1921}.

Immunohistochemistry

There is as yet no immunohistochemical marker that can be used to unequivocally distinguish pancreatic ductal adenocarcinoma from reactive glands, nor can immunostains be used to unequivocally distinguish pancreatic ductal adenocarcinoma from other extrapancreatic mucin-producing adenocarcinomas, notably bile duct carcinomas, although some markers can be useful {1270}.

Ductal adenocarcinomas express the same keratin types as normal pancreatic duct epithelium, i.e. keratins 7, 8, 18 and 19. More than 50% of ductal adenocarcinomas also express keratin 4 {2858}, while keratin 20 is often not expressed {2125}, or less widely than keratin 7. This pattern of keratin expression contrasts with that observed in non-ductal pancreatic neoplasms (i.e. acinar cell carcinomas and neuroendocrine neoplasms, which express keratins 8 and 18 and sometimes 19) and gut carcinomas (which express keratins 8, 18, 19 and 20). Most ductal adenocarcinomas express MUC1, MUC3, MUC4 and MUC5AC, but not MUC2 {2208, 3216, 3645}. They also express glycoprotein tumour antigens such as CEA, B72.3, CA125 and CA19-9 {2884, 3163}. Several of these markers also label the epithelium of normal pancreatic ducts to some extent, particularly in chronic pancreatitis.

Ductal adenocarcinomas are usually negative for vimentin {2858}. With rare exceptions (e.g. mixed ductal neuroendocrine carcinoma), they also fail to label with neuroendocrine markers such as synaptophysin and chromogranin A, although they may contain scattered non-neoplastic neuroendocrine cells in close association with neoplastic cells, particularly if the carcinoma is well-differentiated {2369}. Ductal adenocarcinomas generally do not express pancreatic exocrine enzymes such as trypsin, chymotrypsin and lipase {1235, 2161}. Immunolabelling for the SMAD4/DPC4 protein is lost in 55% of carcinomas, and the p53 protein is expressed at immunohistochemically detectable levels in most cases {1270}.

Among the growth factors and adhesion molecules that are overexpressed by pancreatic ductal adenocarcinomas are

Table 12.01 Histopathological grading of ductal adenocarcinoma of the pancreas.[a]

Tumour grade	Glandular differentiation	Mucin production	Mitoses (per 10 HPF)	Nuclear features
Grade 1	Well-differentiated	Intensive	5	Little polymorphism, polar arrangement
Grade 2	Moderately differentiated duct-like structures and tubular glands	Irregular	6–10	Moderate polymorphism
Grade 3	Poorly differentiated glands, abortive mucoepidermoid and pleomorphic structures	Abortive	> 10	Marked polymorphism and increased size

HPF, high power field. [a] Grade is assigned on the basis of the feature of highest grade {1921}.

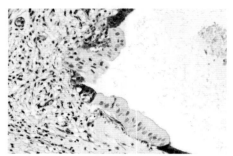

Fig. 12.11 Cancerization of preexisting duct in the pancreas. Immunolabelling for SMAD4 (DPC4) showing complete loss of expression in the neoplastic cells.

epidermal growth factor and its receptor, ERBB2 (c-erbB-2), transforming growth factors α and β {665, 2828}, platelet-derived growth factors A and B, vascular endothelial growth factor and its receptors, metallothionein {2376}, and CD44v6 {454, 3158}. A membranous pattern of labelling is usually seen with antibodies to E-cadherin; however, this expression is often lost in poorly differentiated carcinomas {3527, 2550}. Other more recently discovered markers include mesothelin, prostate stem-cell antigen, claudins 4 and 18, annexin A8, ADAM9, KOC, S100A4, S100A6 and S100P {410, 739, 1478, 2379, 2556, 2979, 3622}.

Cytopathology

Cytological diagnosis is most often obtained by fine-needle aspiration (FNA), increasingly performed endoscopically using EUS guidance {197, 3322}. Techniques of pancreatobiliary-duct brushing have improved {3326}, but brushing cytology has a lower sensitivity for malignancy than FNA, averaging 50% compared with 80% for EUS-FNA {228, 3322}.

The smear pattern of adenocarcinomas is one of scattered cellular glandular clusters admixed with single cells. This contrasts with the diffuse, uniform solid cellular smear pattern produced by the parenchymal-rich, stromal-poor neoplasms such as acinar cell carcinomas and well-differentiated neuroendocrine neoplasms {2556}.

Moderately to poorly differentiated carcinomas have overt features of malignancy. Nuclei are enlarged, hyperchromatic and display irregular nuclear membranes; the cytoplasm ranges from scant and nonmucinous to abundant and mucinous {2556, 2700, 3641}.

The recognition of well-differentiated adenocarcinoma is more challenging as the aspirated neoplastic ductal cells must be distinguished from atypical but reactive ductal cells {700, 1665}, as well as from gastrointestinal contamination from the EUS biopsy procedure {2258}. Cytological criteria for well-differentiated adenocarcinoma include irregular spacing of cells in a cohesive group, anisonucleosis of 4 : 1 in a single group, parachromatin clearing and irregular nuclear membranes {1859, 2556, 2700}. Variants such as adenosquamous carcinoma, undifferentiated carcinoma and undifferentiated carcinoma with osteoclast-like giant cells can also be recognized by their unique cytological features {1768, 2616}.

Ultrastructure

Ductal adenocarcinoma cells are characterized by mucin granules in the apical cytoplasm, irregular microvilli on the luminal surface, and a more or less polarized arrangement of the differently sized nuclei {1270}. Loss of differentiation is characterized by loss of cell polarity, disappearance of a basal lamina, appearance of irregular luminal spaces, and loss of mucin granules.

Histological variants

The variants that appear to have distinct clinical or prognostic features include adenosquamous carcinoma, colloid (mucinous noncystic) adenocarcinoma, hepatoid, medullary, signet ring cell carcinoma, undifferentiated carcinoma, and undifferentiated carcinoma with osteoclast-like giant cells. These are discussed in the next section, *Ductal adenocarcinoma variants and mixed neoplasms*. Histological types that are not considered among the variants are the ductal adenocarcinomas with a foamy gland pattern {33}, with clear cell features {1922} and with large-duct features {503, 628, 1617, 1653}; these latter types have no prognostic significance and are typically found within ductal adenocarcinomas with otherwise conventional histological features.

Differential diagnosis
Chronic pancreatitis

The most significant differential diagnosis for conventional (tubular-type) pancreatic adenocarcinoma is chronic pancreatitis {31, 1665}. From the gross perspective, chronic pancreatitis of alcoholic or obstructive etiology usually

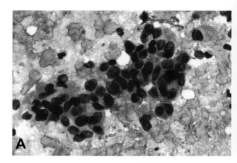

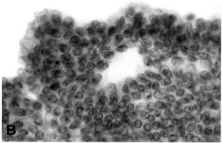

Fig. 12.12 Direct smear of ductal adenocarcinoma of the pancreas. **A** Moderately differentiated adenocarcinoma displaying enlarged, hyperchromatic, crowded and disordered nuclei with some dyshesion (Diff-Quik®). **B** Well-differentiated adenocarcinoma displaying nuclei with irregular spacing, anisonucleosis of 4 : 1, parachromatin clearing and irregular nuclear membranes (Papanicolaou).

involves the pancreas more diffusely than carcinoma. The ducts may be dilated and lithiasis can occur. The texture of the gland is more rubbery than in carcinoma, which has a more gritty consistency.

Autoimmune pancreatitis is an exception to these rules, and it can both clinically and grossly mimic pancreatic cancer, often being grossly discrete and tumourlike, and ductal dilatation is not common. The characteristic microscopic features of autoimmune pancreatitis include dense inflammation with abundant plasma cells concentrated around pancreatic ducts, a cellular fibroinflammatory stroma with a storiform appearance, and obliterative venulitis, although these features maybe less obvious in biopsies than in resection specimens. Increased numbers of plasma cells expressing IgG4 (> 10–50 cells per high power field) is typical of autoimmune pancreatitis, as are elevations in serum IgG4 {491, 703, 2163, 2617, 3700}.

The microscopic findings most helpful in distinguishing adenocarcinoma from reactive glands are the location and architecture of the glands, and the cytological features. The ductal system of the normal pancreas has a lobular architecture, and this lobular pattern is retained in chronic pancreatitis, with a central more dilated duct surrounded by a cluster of smaller ductules and atrophic acini. In contrast, carcinoma has a haphazard arrangement of glands, with loss of the normal lobularity. The abnormal presence of glands within the duodenal muscularis or submucosa, or immediately adjacent to a muscular vessel is highly suggestive of carcinoma {30, 2908}. Profound atrophy of the pancreas can juxtapose benign glands and vessels {3423}, but only in the most extreme cases of atrophic pancreatitis. Perineural and intravascular invasion are almost diagnostic of carcinoma. It is exceptional to find benign glands within the perineurium {1270}, and true vascular invasion does not occur in benign conditions. Other helpful features are "naked glands in fat" – individual glands touching adipocytes without any intervening fibrotic stroma {31, 1606} – and glands with irregular contours, luminal necrosis, and incomplete glands lacking epithelium on one edge {1606}. A nuclear size variation of 4 : 1 within a single duct is considered virtually diagnostic {1270}. Mitotic figures, especially if atypical, are also helpful, as are very prominent nucleoli. Other features that point to a malignant diagnosis are necrotic luminal debris and stromal desmoplasia (as opposed to the usually dense and hyalinized stroma of chronic pancreatitis).

Pancreatic intraepithelial neoplasia (PanIN)

The distinction between PanIN and invasive carcinoma is based on the shape and location of the glands. Distinguishing high-grade PanIN (PanIN-3) from invasive carcinoma on the basis of cytological appearance can be very difficult. Of note, it is very unusual to encounter PanIN-3 in the absence of invasive carcinoma, especially when there is a mass lesion in the pancreas.

Reactive glands and low-grade PanIN lesions do not express tumour-associated glycoproteins (CEA, B72.3, and CA125), p53, mesothelin, claudin 4, S100A4, or 14-3-3σ {41, 1133, 1242, 1270, 1956}. Positive immunolabelling for any of these markers favours a diagnosis of carcinoma, although the sensitivity of these markers varies widely. Loss of immunoexpression of SMAD4 in the face of intact expression in normal cells also strongly supports a diagnosis of carcinoma {1242, 1275}, but is only found in about half of infiltrating ductal adenocarcinomas {3202}.

Precursor lesions

The macroscopic presence of a recognized precursor (intraductal papillary mucinous neoplasm [IPMN] or mucinous cystic neoplasm [MCN]) to infiltrating carcinoma increases the chances that a solid mass may be an infiltrating carcinoma. The distinction between infiltrating carcinoma and these mass-forming cystic neoplasms (MCN and IPMN) is generally not a problem if radiographic and clinical findings are integrated with the pathology. However, some infiltrating carcinomas form massively dilated invasive glands that can simulate a cystic neoplasm. This pattern has been designated the "large-duct type" of infiltrating carcinoma {1270} and is generally not associated with gross cyst formation. The cystic glands are irregular, do not communicate with the native ducts, have an associated desmoplastic stromal response, and lack the "ovarian-like" subepithelial stroma of MCNs.

Neuroendocrine neoplasms

Paradoxically, poorly differentiated ductal adenocarcinomas can resemble well-differentiated pancreatic neuroendocrine neolasms, especially neuroendocrine neolasms with nuclear pleomorphism {3687}. The sclerotic (rather than desmoplastic) nature of the stroma, nuclear features of neuroendocrine differentiation, organoid architectural patterns, and a lack of mitotic activity all suggest that a neuroendocrine neoplasm should be considered. Immunohistochemical labelling for chromogranin and synaptophysin help to establish this diagnosis. Non-neoplastic islets in chronic pancreatitis can also simulate carcinoma, as they can assume a pseudo-infiltrative appearance within fibrotic stroma once the acinar elements have completely atrophied {205}. The nuclei remain bland, however, and immunohistochemistry is helpful in difficult cases.

Table 12.02 Morphological features of pancreatic intraepithelial neoplasia (PanIN).

Epithelial lesion	Morphological features
Normal	The normal ductal and ductular epithelium is a cuboidal to low-columnar epithelium with amphophilic cytoplasm. Mucinous cytoplasm, nuclear crowding, and atypia are not seen.
Squamous (transitional) metaplasia	A process in which the normal cuboidal ductal epithelium is replaced by mature stratified squamous or pseudostratified transitional epithelium without atypia.
PanIN-1A	These flat epithelial lesions are composed of tall columnar cells with basally located nuclei and abundant supranuclear mucin. The nuclei are small and round-to-oval in shape. When oval, the nuclei are oriented perpendicular to the basement menbrane. There may be considerable histological overlap between non-neoplastic, flat, hyperplastic lesions and flat, neoplastic lesions without atypia; the modifier term "lesion" ("PanIN/L-1A") may be used to acknowledge that the neoplastic nature of many PanIN-1A cases has not been unambiguously established.
PanIN-1B	These epithelial lesions have a papillary, micropapillary, or basally pseudostratified architecture but are otherwise identical to PanIN-1A.
PanIN-2	These mucinous epithelial lesions may be flat but are mostly papillary. By definition, PanIN-2 lesions must have some nuclear abnormalities, which may include some loss of polarity, nuclear crowding, enlarged nuclei, pseudostratification, and hyperchromatism, but to a lesser degree than in PanIN-3. Mitoses are rare, but when present are non-luminal (not apical), and are not atypical. True cribriform structures with luminal necrosis and marked cytological abnormalities are generally not seen and, when present, should suggest a diagnosis of PanIN-3.
PanIN-3	These lesions are usually papillary or micropapillary, but may rarely be flat. True cribriforming, the appearance of "budding off" of small clusters of epithelial cells into the lumen, and luminal necrosis all suggest a diagnosis of PanIN-3. PanIN-3 lesions are characterized by loss of nuclear polarity, dystrophic goblet cells (goblet cells with nuclei oriented toward the basement membrane), occasionally-abnormal mitoses, nuclear irregularities, and prominent (macro) nucleoli. Resembling carcinoma at the cytonuclear level, there is, however, no invasion of the basement membrane.

PanIN, pancreatic intraepithelial neoplasia. Adapted with permission from {1271}.

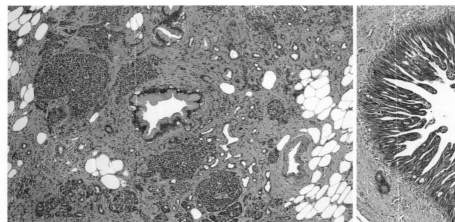 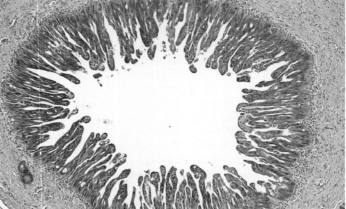

Fig. 12.13 Small low-grade pancreatic intraepithelial neoplasia (PanIN) lesion surrounded by a larger area of lobulocentric atrophy.

Fig. 12.14 High-grade pancreatic intraepithelial neoplasia (PanIN 3).

Extrapancreatic metastatic adenocarcinoma

It is not uncommon to encounter a metastatic adenocarcinoma in an extra-pancreatic location for which the pancreas appears to be a possible primary; however, there are no pancreas-specific immunohistochemical stains to prove pancreatic origin. A common immunophenotype for ductal adenocarcinomas of the pancreas is positive for keratins 7 and 19, CEA, B72.3; focally positive or negative for keratin 20, and negative for CDX2, TTF1, and hormone receptors. This labelling profile is shared by primary carcinomas of the upper gastrointestinal tract, biliary tree, gallbladder, and some pulmonary and mammary carcinomas. Immunolabelling for the SMAD4 protein can be helpful, as this is lost in 55% of invasive ductal adenocarcinomas of the pancreas, but only rarely in carcinomas arising outside of the pancreatobiliary tree.

Precursor lesions

The most common precursor lesions of pancreatic ductal adenocarcinoma are PanIN lesions. Less frequently, macroscopic (cystic) precursor lesions, including MCNs and IPMNs, may also progress to ductal adenocarcinoma.

PanINs

As defined by published consensus guidelines {1271}, PanINs are microscopic papillary or flat, noninvasive epithelial neoplasms that are usually < 5 mm in diameter and confined to the pancreatic ducts. Composed of columnar to cuboidal cells with varying amounts of mucin, PanINs are divided into three grades according to the degree of cytological and architectural atypia. Lesions with minimal, moderate or marked atypia are designated PanIN-1, PanIN-2, and PanIN-3, respectively. PanIN-1 lesions are further subdivided into flat (PanIN-1A) and papillary types (PanIN-1B).

Multiple lines of evidence support the hypothesis that PanINs are *bona fide* precursors of infiltrating ductal adenocarcinoma. PanINs (especially higher-grade lesions) are more common in pancreata with adenocarcinoma than without {108, 1662}, with at least one study identifying PanIN-3 exclusively in pancreata with an invasive carcinoma {627}. As is true for ductal adenocarcinoma, the incidence of PanINs increases with age, and PanINs are more common in the head than in the tail of the pancreas {1268, 1662}. Although rare, patients have been reported who had a residual high-grade PanIN lesion at the surgical margin of a partial pancreatectomy for benign disease and then, several months to years after surgery, developed invasive adenocarcinoma in the remnant pancreas {327, 336}. Perhaps the most compelling evidence comes from the demonstration that PanINs and invasive ductal adenocarcinomas share critical genetic abnormalities.

Lobulocentric atrophy. PanIN lesions are associated with lobulocentric atrophy in the immediately adjacent pancreatic parenchyma {353, 704, 2929}. Although the exact pathogenesis of lobulocentric atrophy remains uncertain, these foci of atrophy are larger than the PanIN lesion itself. In patients that have a familial predisposition to pancreatic cancer, PanIN lesions, and the resulting lobulocentric atrophy, tend to be multifocal in the pancreatic parenchyma {353}. It is possible to detect this distinctive change in imaging studies, such as EUS, suggesting a potential screening tool for identification of individuals with a higher risk of developing invasive carcinoma {407}.

Genetic susceptibility

Up to 10% of patients with pancreatic cancer have a family history of this disease {207, 844, 1162, 1269, 1926, 1927}. Some pancreatic cancers arise in patients with recognized genetic syndromes, but in most instances the genetic basis for the familial aggregation of pancreatic carcinomas has not yet been identified. Studies of extended families have suggested an autosomal-dominant mode of inheritance {1587}. Having one, two or three first-degree relatives with pancreatic cancer increases the risk of developing pancreatic cancer by 2.3-fold, 6-fold and 32-fold, respectively {106, 1588}. Having a member of the family with young-onset pancreatic cancer confers an added risk in kindreds in which multiple family members have been diagnosed with pancreatic cancer {354}.

FAMMM syndrome

Familial atypical multiple mole melanoma (FAMMM) is associated with germline mutations in the *CDKN2A* tumour suppressor gene on chromosome 9p. Affected individuals have an increased risk of developing both melanoma and pancreatic carcinoma {1017, 1928, 2165, 3495}.

Patients have a 20–34-fold risk of pancreatic cancer, and the risk appears to be particularly high in carriers of a specific 19-base-pair deletion in *CDKN2A* (*p16*-Leiden deletion) {678}. Carriers of this particular mutation have a 15% lifetime risk of developing pancreatic carcinoma.

BRCA2 and other Fanconi anaemia complementation (FANC) genes

The discovery of the second breast cancer gene (*BRCA2*) on chromosome 13q was made possible largely as a result of the discovery of a homozygous deletion in a pancreatic carcinoma {2859}. Pancreatic carcinomas have been reported in some kindreds with *BRCA2* gene mutations {807, 1008, 2542, 3243}, and patients with identified germline mutations in *BRCA2* have a 3- to 10-fold increased risk of pancreatic cancer {1846}. The penetrance of these germline mutations is incomplete and many patients with pancreatic ductal carcinoma who carry such mutations do not have a strong family history of breast or pancreatic carcinoma {1008}. A number of patients with *BRCA2* mutations and pancreatic cancer are of Ashkenazi Jewish descent {1008, 2426}; a founder *BRCA2* mutation, 1674 delT, is present in about 1% of the Ashkenazi Jewish population. The *BRCA2* gene interacts with the products of the *FANC* genes, and germline mutations in the *FANCC* and *FANCG* genes have been reported in young patients with pancreatic cancer {609, 3359}. Recently, *FANCN* (*PALB2*), which encodes a BRCA2-binding protein, has also been identified as a familial susceptibility gene for pancreatic cancer {1443, 3146, 3250}.

Germline *BRCA1* mutations have also been associated with an increased risk of pancreatic cancer {1846}, although some studies have not found this link to be strong {165}.

Peutz-Jeghers syndrome

Patients with Peutz-Jeghers syndrome have a highly increased risk (> 100-fold) of developing pancreatic carcinoma {977}, and bi-allelic inactivation of the *STK11* gene has been demonstrated in a pancreatic carcinoma arising in a patient with Peutz-Jeghers syndrome {980, 3105}.

Hereditary pancreatitis

This disease is caused by germline mutations in the cationic trypsinogen gene *PRSS1* or in the serine peptidase inhibitor *SPINK1* {1901, 3496}. Patients develop recurrent episodes of pancreatitis starting at a young age, and 25–40% will develop pancreatic cancer by the age of 70 years, the risk increasing if the patient is also a cigarette smoker {1902}.

Lynch syndrome

This syndrome is associated with an increased risk of developing carcinoma of the colon, endometrium, stomach, and ovary {3470}. Lynch syndrome can be caused by germline mutations in any one of a number of DNA mismatch repair genes, including *MSH2* on chromosome 2p and *MLH1* on 3p {1773, 1870, 3470}. It has been suggested that individuals with Lynch syndrome have an increased risk of pancreatic cancer, and microsatellite instability has been reported to occur in about 4% of pancreatic carcinomas {1007, 1491, 1933, 2516}. Pancreatic cancers with microsatellite instability are often microscopically distinct and have a characteristic "medullary" histological appearance.

ABO blood group

A genome-wide association study has linked variants in the ABO blood group locus to susceptibility to pancreatic cancer, with individuals with blood group O having a lower risk than those with groups A or B {105}.

Molecular pathology

The alterations reported in pancreatic cancers include losses and gains of genetic material as well as generalized chromosome instability {326, 1037, 1065, 1066, 2888}. These consist of very high rates of loss at chromosomes 18q (90% of cases), 17p (90%), 1p (60%) and 9p (85%), and moderately frequent losses at nearly a dozen additional sites (25–50% of cases). Comprehensive sequencing of the genomic exons of a series of 24 pancreatic cancers revealed that an average of five dozen intragenic mutations had accumulated in each cancer {1444}. Most of the genes mutated are infrequently involved, and thus it is assumed that most

Table 12.03 Genetic syndromes associated with an increased risk of pancreatic cancer.

Syndrome (MIM No.)[a]	Mode of inheritance	Gene (chromosome arm)	Lifetime risk of pancreatic cancer (age)	References
Lynch syndrome (120435, 609310)	Autosomal dominant	*MSH2* (2p), *MLH1* (3p) and others	1.3–4% (70 years) [b]	{1007, 1491, 1933}
Familial breast cancer and other Fanconi anaemia genes (612555, 610832, 227645)	Autosomal dominant	*BRCA2* (13q), *PALB2* (16p), *FANCC* (9q), *FANCG* (9p), and possibly *BRCA1* (17q)	3.5–10% for *BRCA2* [c]	{609, 807, 1008, 1443, 1846, 2542, 3243, 3250, 3359}
Familial pancreatic cancer (three or more relatives with pancreatic cancer)	Autosomal dominant	Unknown	9–38% (80 years) [b]	{106, 1588, 3449}
Familial atypical multiple mole melanoma, FAMMM (606719)	Autosomal dominant	*CDKN2A* (9p)	10–17% [c] (70 years)	{678, 1017, 1298, 2165, 3495}
Hereditary pancreatitis (167800, 167790)	Autosomal dominant (*PRSS1*) or autosomal recessive (*SPNK1*)	*PRSS1* (7q), *SPINK1* (5q)	25–40% (60 years)	{1264, 1901}
Peutz-Jeghers syndrome (175200)	Autosomal dominant	*STK11* (19p)	30–60% (70 years)	{977, 980, 3105}

[a] Mendelian inheritance in man (MIM): www.ncbi.nlm.nih.gov/omim; [b] Calculated empirically; [c] Extrapolated from relative rates.

Table 12.04 Genetic alterations identified in ductal adenocarcinoma of the pancreas.

Gene	Chromosome	Mechanism of alteration	Frequency
Oncogenes			
KRAS	12p	Point mutation	> 90%
MYB, AKT2, NCOA3 (AIB1)	6q, 19q, 20q	Amplification[a]	10–20%
ERBB2	17q	Overexpression	70%
Tumour-suppressor genes			
CDKN2A (p16)	9p	Homozygous deletion	40%
		LOH and intragenic mutation	40%
		Promoter hypermethylation	15%
TP53	17p	LOH and intragenic mutation	50–70%
SMAD4 (DPC4)	18q	Homozygous deletion	35%
		LOH and intragenic mutation	20%
BRCA2	13q	Inherited intragenic mutation and LOH	7%
MAP2K4 (MKK4)	17p	Homozygous deletion	4%
		LOH and intragenic mutation	
STK11 (LKB1)	19p	LOH and intragenic mutation	5%
		Homozygous deletion	
TGFBR1 (ALK5) and TGFBR2	9q, 3p	Homozygous deletion	4%
DNA mismatch-repair genes			
MSH2, MLH1, others	2p, 3p, others	Unknown	< 5%

LOH, loss of heterozygosity. [a] In cases of amplification, it is generally not possible to unambiguously identify the key oncogene due to the participation of multiple genes in an amplicon.

are "passenger mutations" accumulated before or during tumorigenesis and that they play no direct role in the disease itself.

Tumour suppressor genes

Sequencing has also identified a number of recurrent genetic abnormalities, "driver mutations" that play critical roles in the development of pancreatic neoplasia. These include CDKN2A, TP53, and SMAD4 {1444, 2888}. The CDKN2A gene is inactivated by homozygous deletion in 40% of pancreatic carcinomas, by loss of one allele coupled with an intragenic mutation in the second allele in a further 40%, and by promoter methylation in an additional 15% {398, 2860, 3509}. TP53 is inactivated by loss of one allele coupled with an intragenic mutation in the second allele in 75% of pancreatic carcinomas {2651, 2740}. The SMAD4 gene is inactivated in 55% of pancreatic carcinomas (by homozygous deletion in 35% of cases and by loss of one allele coupled with an intragenic mutation in the second allele in 20% of cases) {1100}. The consequent loss of SMAD4 protein is essentially cancer-specific and thus serves as a diag-

nostic aid in the histopathological evaluation of pancreatic biopsies {3511}. The BRCA2 gene is involved in DNA repair as an effector in the FANC anaemia signal-transduction pathway {1264}. BRCA2 is inactivated in about 7% of pancreatic carcinomas {1008, 2426, 2859}; remarkably, in almost all these cases one allele of BRCA2 has been inactivated by a germline mutation {1008}.

Other tumour-suppressor genes that have been shown to be occasionally inactivated in pancreatic carcinoma include MKK4, STK11, transforming growth factor β receptors I and II, and the FANC pathway genes FANCC, FANCG, and FANCN {1009, 1443, 3104, 3105, 3359}. It is thought that inactivation of the FANC pathway increases sensitivity to treatment by DNA-crosslinking agents or poly-(ADP-ribose) polymerase (PARP) enzyme-inhibiting drugs {878, 3358}.

Oncogenes

Oncogenes that have been shown to be activated in ductal adenocarcinomas of the pancreas include KRAS on chromosome 12p, which is activated by point mutations in > 90% of these carcinomas,

occasional mutation or amplification of various growth-stimulating genes, and overexpression of ERBB2 on chromosome 17q in 70% of pancreatic carcinomas {97, 517, 665, 971, 1279, 1444, 2100}. Mutations of KRAS2 have been detected in stool, pancreatic juice, cytology and/or blood samples from patients with proven ductal adenocarcinoma of the pancreas {399, 1643, 3102, 3153}, but the diagnostic value of these mutations in daily clinical practice is uncertain.

DNA mismatch repair

Microsatellite instability has been identified in 4% of pancreatic carcinomas {1007}; these carcinomas are also characterized by wild-type KRAS, frequent BRAF gene mutations and a distinctive "medullary" histological appearance.

Molecular pathology of precursor lesions

The histological progression of PanIN lesions to invasive cancer is usually mirrored by genetic and epigenetic progression, with the frequency of individual molecular aberrations being higher in higher-grade precursors {922, 2821}. For example, mutations of the KRAS gene are found in 36%, 44%, and 87% of PanIN-1A, PanIN-1B and PanIN-2/3 lesions, respectively {1886}. Although the precise sequence of alterations is not well-defined, and not every mutation is found in all PanIN lesions, certain genetic abnormalities, such as activating mutations of KRAS and telomere shortening, are "early" changes that are likely to contribute to disease initiation. Mutations of CDKN2A occur in intermediate-grade (PanIN-2) lesions, while inactivating mutations of TP53, BRCA2 and SMAD4 (DPC4) are typically observed in higher-grade lesions (most often, PanIN-3) or invasive cancers, suggesting an association between these "late" changes and disease progression.

PanINs differ genetically from IPMNs in that they express the apomucin MUC1, but not MUC2, while the reverse is true for intestinal-type IPMNs {1813}. Certain genetic alterations, such as activating mutations of the PIK3CA gene, which encodes a protein in the oncogenic AKT signalling pathway, appear to be restricted to IPMNs {2853}. In conjunction with the finding that a subset of IPMN-associated invasive carcinomas tends to have an overall better prognosis than adenocarcinomas arising in the setting of PanINs, an emerging consensus suggests that there are two major avenues to invasive carcinoma in the pancreas: one that is more "aggressive" (via PanIN and pancreatobiliary-type IPMN precursors) and a second that is more "indolent" (via intestinal-type IPMN precursors) {1266}, although PanINs and IPMNs can be found in the same pancreas.

Prognosis and predictive factors

Ductal adenocarcinoma is fatal in almost all cases {1413}. The mean survival time for untreated patients is 3–5 months, while the mean survival after surgical resection ranges from 10 to 20 months {589, 1168, 1347, 1360, 1674, 2267}. Only 10–20% of patients or fewer have surgically resectable carcinomas at the time of diagnosis {589, 590, 2876, 3041}. Carcinomas of the body or tail of the pancreas tend to present at a more advanced stage than those of the head {937, 2939, 3290, 3308, 3316}.

Resectability is the most important determinant of prognosis. The overall 5-year survival rate is 3–5% {1413}, while that for patients treated by curative resection is 15–25% {848, 1252, 1675, 3525}. Unfortunately, most (70–90%) carcinomas recur within 2 years after curative resection {208, 3357}, often local-regionally and in the liver. The peritoneal cavity or lymph nodes are also common sites of recurrence {208, 3357}. Adjuvant chemotherapy with gemcitabine or 5-fluorouracil prolongs survival time only slightly {2266, 2268, 2357}.

Survival is longer in patients with carcinomas that are confined to the pancreas and < 30 mm in diameter than it is in patients with tumours that extend beyond the gland and are > 30 mm {1175, 1853, 2941, 3007, 3634}.

Patients with no residual tumour after resection (R0) have the most favourable prognosis of those who are treated surgically {1175, 2267, 3514, 3525}. This implies that local spread to peripancreatic tissues, i.e. the retroperitoneal resection margin, is of critical importance in terms of prognosis {1923}. The presence of lymph-node metastases significantly worsens prognosis {1202, 1252, 1853, 2849, 3007, 3290, 3634}. The status of the lymph nodes correlates with both short-term (< 5 years) and long-term survival (≥ 5 years) after surgical resection {2849}. The lymph-node ratio, i.e. the ratio of the number of nodes harbouring a metastasis to the total number of nodes examined, is one of the most powerful predictors of postoperative survival {2505}.

Histological features are less significant prognostic factors than stage, but tumour grade, mitotic index, and severity of cellular atypia have been correlated with postoperative survival {1612, 1921}. Major vessel involvement {2239}, vascular invasion and perineural invasion {2098, 2240, 2422} are also prognostic indicators.

Molecular prognostic factors

None of the many molecular prognostic indicators reported has yet become established in routine clinical practice. Loss of SMAD4 expression and *SMAD4* mutations have been correlated with poor survival after surgery {273, 3203, 3699}, and an autopsy study reported that pancreatic cancers with loss of SMAD4 expression were more likely to have widespread metastases than those with intact expression {1300}. Down-regulation of E-cadherin and up-regulation of dysadherin have been reported to be significantly associated with poorer survival and to be independent prognostic indicators {2943, 3527}.

Ductal adenocarcinoma variants and mixed neoplasms of the pancreas

N. Fukushima
R.H. Hruban
Y. Kato
D.S. Klimstra
G. Klöppel
M. Shimizu
B. Terris

This category includes mixed neoplasms and histological variants of ductal adenocarcinoma of the pancreas that have distinct clinical or prognostic significance.

ICD-O codes

Adenosquamous carcinoma	8560/3
Colloid carcinoma (mucinous noncystic carcinoma)	8480/3
Hepatoid carcinoma	8576/3
Medullary carcinoma	8510/3
Mixed acinar-ductal carcinoma	8552/3
Mixed acinar-neuroendocrine carcinoma	8154/3
Mixed acinar-neuroendocrine-ductal carcinoma	8154/3
Mixed ductal-neuroendocrine carcinoma	8154/3
Signet ring cell carcinoma	8490/3
Undifferentiated carcinoma	8020/3
Undifferentiated carcinoma with osteoclast-like giant cells	8035/3

Adenosquamous carcinoma

Adenosquamous carcinoma is a malignant epithelial neoplasm of the pancreas that has both significant ductal and significant squamous differentiation. The squamous component should account for at least 30% of the neoplasm. Neoplasms with these features were previously designated adenoacanthoma, mixed squamous and adenocarcinoma, and mucoepidermoid carcinoma. Adenosquamous carcinomas account for only 1–4% of exocrine pancreatic malignancies {1273, 1945}. Pure squamous carcinoma of the pancreas is very rare, and a metastasis from another site (e.g. lung) should be excluded if a neoplasm has purely squamous differentiation. Even focal glandular differentiation in a carcinoma with predominant squamous differentiation warrants a diagnosis of adenosquamous carcinoma.

Macroscopy

Macroscopically, most adenosquamous carcinomas are infiltrative yellow-white to grey firm masses; however, some are multinodular and others are cystic {1482}.

Histopathology

Histologically, the adenocarcinoma component forms ductal or glandular structures with focal to abundant intra- and/or extracellular mucin. Squamous differentiation is characterized by an infiltrating sheet-like arrangement of polygonal cells with distinct cellular borders, prominent intracellular junctions, hard eosinophilic cytoplasm and varying degrees of keratinization.

Molecular pathology

Most cases harbour KRAS2 mutations at codon 12, and immunohistochemically show loss of CDKN2A (p16) protein expression, loss of SMAD4 (DPC4) protein and strong nuclear p53 immunoreactivity, similar to the molecular signature found in pancreatic ductal adenocarcinomas {337, 1482}. The squamous component often expresses p63 {337}.

Prognosis and predictive factors

Patients with resected adenosquamous carcinoma have a poorer prognosis (median survival, 7–11 months) than do those with pure adenocarcinoma {1482, 2383, 3419}. The presence of any squamous component in the neoplasm appears to portend a worse prognosis {3419}.

Carcinomas with mixed differentiation

Carcinomas with mixed differentiation are malignant epithelial neoplasms of the pancreas with significant components of more than one distinct direction of differentiation {1235, 1238, 2857, 3340}. "Collision tumours" composed of two topographically separate neoplasms are not included in the mixed differentiation. Rare acinar neoplasms have a substantial proportion (> 30%) of more than one cell type {1270, 1710, 2313, 2369, 3405}. Of these, the best characterized is mixed acinar-neuroendocrine carcinoma {1710}. This carcinoma has also been referred to as mixed carcinoid-adenocarcinoma, mucinous carcinoid tumour, or simply mixed exocrine-endocrine tumour {1106}. Patients with mixed ductal-neuroendocrine carcinoma are usually older adults and present with nonspecific symptoms. This neoplasm is characterized by an intimate admixture of neoplastic ductal and neoplastic neuroendocrine cells in the primary neoplasm as well as in its metastases. Two patterns can be distinguished, one consisting of intermingled neoplastic ductal and neuroendocrine cells forming glandular (occasionally also squamoid) and solid structures, and another consisting of moderately differentiated

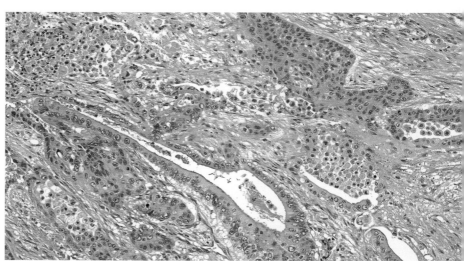

Fig. 12.15 Adenosquamous carcinoma. Both glandular and squamous differentiation are present.

neoplastic ductal structures embedded in a solid neuroendocrine cell compartment {1270, 2368}. By definition, each component should comprise at least one third of the neoplastic tissue. Ductal differentiation is defined by mucin production and the expression of ductal markers such as carcinoembryonic antigen (CEA) or MUC1. The neoplastic neuroendocrine cells are typically of high grade on the basis of mitotic rate and express neuroendocrine markers such as synaptophysin, chromogranin A, and pancreatic hormones.

As defined above, these neoplasms are exceptionally rare in the pancreas {2368, 2884, 3012}. It is much more common to find a neuroendocrine neoplasm that has entrapped non-neoplastic ductal cells {2318, 3261, 3361}. The trapped ductal cells are cytologically benign and limited by the well-demarcated edges of the underlying neuroendocrine neoplasm. The latter behave like pure neuroendocrine neoplasms, while true mixed ductal-neuroendocrine carcinomas behave like the usual ductal adenocarcinoma.

Mixed ductal-neuroendocrine carcinomas should also be distinguished from ductal adenocarcinomas with reactive non-neoplastic neuroendocrine cells {2368}. Scattered non-neoplastic neuroendocrine cells are found in 40–80% of ductal adenocarcinomas and seem to be particularly frequent in well-differentiated adenocarcinomas, where they tend to either line up along the base of the neoplastic ductal structures or lie between the neoplastic columnar cells {504, 2368}.

Mixed acinar-neuroendocrine carcinoma

In many of these neoplasms, the only evidence for divergent differentiation is provided by immunohistochemical labelling. Although different regions of the neoplasm may suggest acinar or neuroendocrine differentiation morphologically, many areas have intermediate features, and immunohistochemistry generally shows a mixture of cells expressing acinar or neuroendocrine markers (or both). Most reported acinar-neuroendocrine carcinomas have been composed predominantly of acinar elements {1710}.

Mixed acinar-ductal carcinoma

These neoplasms have one of two different patterns {1270, 3070, 3073}. Some exhibit extensive intra- or extracellular mucin accumulation in association with acinar elements. There may be nests of acinar cells floating in colloid-like pools of mucin, or the neoplastic elements may have a combination of typical acinar elements mixed with columnar or signet ring-like cells with cytoplasmic mucin. Mucin staining (mucicarmine or Alcian blue) is positive, as is immunohistochemical labelling for trypsin and chymotrypsin. Individual cells can have multiple directions of differentiation. Other mixed acinar-ductal carcinomas have an individual gland pattern of infiltration with an associated desmoplastic stromal response, reminiscent of infiltrating ductal adenocarcinoma, but nonetheless show significant acinar differentiation by immunohistochemistry.

Mixed acinar-neuroendocrine-ductal carcinoma

These are extremely rare and poorly documented, but show mixed morphology, with acinar patterns, cells with neuroendocrine differentiation and areas simulating infiltrating ductal adenocarcinoma {3073}. Immunohistochemistry is positive for acinar, neuroendocrine, and ductal markers, and mucin production is also evident. One of the reported cases arose in association with high-grade pancreatic intraepithelial neoplasia (PanIN) {1270}.

There is an insufficient number of recorded cases to define the biological behaviour of mixed acinar carcinomas, but, like pure acinar cell carcinomas, they appear to be aggressive {2369}.

Colloid carcinoma

Synonym
Mucinous noncystic adenocarcinoma

Colloid carcinoma is an infiltrating ductal epithelial neoplasm of the pancreas characterized by the presence, in at least 80% of the neoplasm, of large extracellular stromal mucin pools containing suspended neoplastic cells {37}. Colloid carcinomas tend to be large and well-demarcated and almost always arise in association with an intestinal-type intraductal papillary mucinous neoplasm (IPMN) {2868}. The large pools of mucin are partially lined by well-differentiated cuboidal to columnar neoplastic cells and contain clumps or strands of neoplastic cells. Some floating cells may be of the

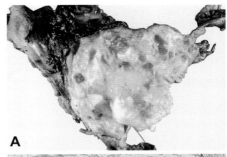

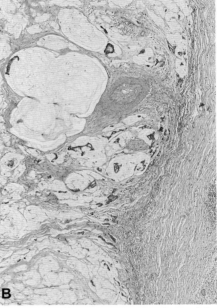

Fig 12.16 Colloid carcinoma. **A** Arising in association with an intraductal papillary mucinous neoplasm (IPMN). **B** Note the neoplastic cells "floating" in large stromal pools of mucin.

signet-ring type. The neoplastic cells of colloid carcinoma show intestinal differentiation; there is strong expression of CDX2 and MUC2, which are not significantly expressed in conventional ductal adenocarcinoma.

Two features help to distinguish benign spillage of mucin into the extraductal stroma caused by rupture of the dilated pancreatic duct occupied by an IPMN from true tissue invasion by a colloid carcinoma. Neoplastic cells "floating" in pools of stromal mucin, and neoplastic cells in an abnormal location, such as in the perineurium, help identify the lesion as a colloid carcinoma. In contrast, benign mucin spillage will consist of mucus lakes adjacent to a pancreatic branch duct without "floating" neoplastic cells.

Pseudomyxoma peritonei can be a rare complication of this carcinoma. Colloid carcinomas seem to have a more favourable prognosis than conventional ductal adenocarcinomas {2575B}.

Hepatoid carcinoma

Hepatoid carcinoma of the pancreas is an extremely rare malignant epithelial neoplasm with a significant component of hepatocellular differentiation. Hepatoid differentiation can occur in a pure form, or in association with a ductal adenocarcinoma, an acinar or a neuroendocrine neoplasm {1285, 2443, 3200, 3618}. Hepatoid carcinomas are composed of large polygonal cells with abundant eosinophilic cytoplasm. Most express α-fetoprotein (AFP); however, AFP secretion can also be observed in pancreatoblastomas and in acinar, neuroendocrine, and ductal neoplasms without hepatoid features {564, 1505}. The expression of hepatocyte-specific antigen (hepatocyte paraffin-1) is more specific for hepatocellular differentiation. A canalicular pattern of labelling with antibodies to polyclonal CEA and CD10 can help establish the diagnosis in some cases {630, 1103}. Hepatocellular carcinoma arising from ectopic liver tissue should not be included in this category. Pancreatic metastases from an occult hepatocellular carcinoma are probably much more common than are primary hepatoid carcinomas of the pancreas, and a metastasis to the pancreas needs to be excluded, usually on clinical grounds, before establishing the diagnosis of a hepatoid carcinoma primary to the pancreas. Data on the prognosis of hepatoid carcinomas are minimal.

Medullary carcinoma

Medullary carcinoma is a malignant epithelial neoplasm characterized by poor differentiation, limited gland formation, pushing borders at the interface between the neoplasm and non-neoplastic tissues and a prominent syncytial growth pattern {1007, 3510}. Increased numbers of tumour-infiltrating leukocytes (CD3+) are present in some cases {2244}. Because of the histological overlap with acinar cell carcinoma, acinar differentiation should be excluded by immunolabelling for trypsin or chymotrypsin. Medullary carcinomas express keratin, and immunohistochemistry will often demonstrate the loss of expression of one of the DNA mismatch repair genes {190, 1640, 2243, 3510}.
Medullary carcinomas may arise sporadically or in patients with Lynch syndrome {190, 3591}. It has been reported that patients with medullary carcinoma of the pancreas are more likely to have a family history of cancer than are patients with ductal adenocarcinoma of the pancreas {3510}. The age and sex distributions are similar to those for ductal adenocarcinoma {2244, 3510}.
Medullary carcinomas in patients with Lynch syndrome harbour biallelic mutations (one germline, the second somatic) in one of the DNA mismatch repair genes (i.e. *MLH1* and *MSH2* {190}). Most medullary carcinomas are microsatellite-unstable (MSI+) {3510} and, as one would expect in an MSI+ neoplasm, most are wild-type for the *KRAS2* gene, and diploid (no loss of heterozygosity) {1007, 3510}. Medullary carcinomas also can harbour *BRAF* mutations, *FHIT* homozygous deletions, and biallelic inactivating mutations of the *ACVR2* and *TGFBR2* genes {400,

1007, 1165, 1193, 3103, 3591}. A medullary carcinoma with Epstein-Barr virus (EBV) infection of the neoplastic cells has been reported {3510}.
Despite poor differentiation, the prognosis for patients with medullary carcinomas is better than for those with ductal adenocarcinomas {2243, 2244, 3510, 3591}. On the basis of extensive experience with MSI+ colorectal carcinomas, it is likely that medullary carcinomas of the pancreas will not respond to 5-fluorouracil therapy {698}.

Signet ring cell carcinoma

The extremely rare signet-ring cell carcinoma is an adenocarcinoma composed almost exclusively of poorly cohesive neoplastic epithelial cells containing intracytoplasmic mucin that displaces the nuclei towards the periphery, infiltrating in an individual cell pattern {813, 3284}. A variable amount of extracellular mucin is usually present. The prognosis is extremely poor. A gastric or breast primary should always be excluded before making this diagnosis.

Undifferentiated (anaplastic) carcinoma

Synonyms
Anaplastic carcinoma, pleomorphic carcinoma, pleomorphic large cell carcinoma, pleomorphic giant cell carcinoma, spindle cell carcinoma, sarcomatoid carcinoma and carcinosarcoma.
Undifferentiated carcinoma is a malignant epithelial neoplasm in which a significant component of the neoplasm does not

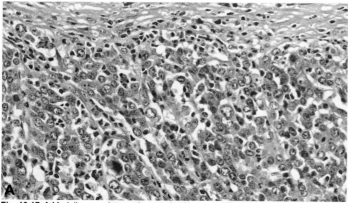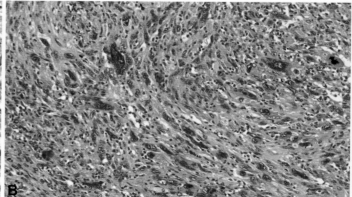

Fig. 12.17 A Medullary carcinoma characterized by poor differentiation, a syncytial growth pattern, pushing borders, and tumour-infiltrating lymphocytes. **B** Undifferentiated carcinoma with spindle cells, pleomorphic nuclei, and mitoses.

show a definitive direction of differentiation. These neoplasms usually occur in elderly people, and males and females are equally affected.

Three histological variants have been described. Anaplastic giant cell carcinomas are composed of pleomorphic mononuclear cells admixed with bizarre-appearing giant cells with eosinophilic cytoplasm. Cells with spindle-cell morphology predominate in the sarcomatoid carcinoma, and carcinosarcomas have cells recognizable as adenocarcinoma as well as a high-grade spindle-cell component. In contrast to ductal adenocarcinoma, undifferentiated carcinomas are poorly cohesive, cellular and often have only scant stroma {628, 1604, 3299}. Nuclear pleomorphism, mitoses as well as perineural, lymphatic, and vascular invasion are easily identified. Immunohistochemically, most of these carcinomas express keratin and vimentin but not E-cadherin {1236, 2428, 3527}. Electron microscopy reveals epithelial differentiation, microvilli and occasional mucin in some cases {628}. The prognosis is extremely poor, and average survival is just 5 months {1236, 2428, 3299}.

Undifferentiated carcinoma with osteoclast-like giant cells

This is a rare neoplasm composed of round to spindle-shaped, highly pleomorphic neoplastic mononuclear cells and large, non-neoplastic multinucleated, histiocytic giant cells. The latter usually contain > 20 uniform and small nuclei, and are often found in areas adjacent to haemorrhage or necrosis. In most cases there is an associated *in situ* or invasive adenocarcinoma or an associated mucinous cystic neoplasm (MCN) {2124, 3493, 3673}. The osteoclast-like giant cells can be phagocytically active and may contain haemosiderin. Some of the mononuclear cells are atypical, while others can be histiocyte-like {2778}. Immunohistochemically, most of the neoplastic mononuclear cells express vimentin, some express keratin, and some label with antibodies to p53. On the other

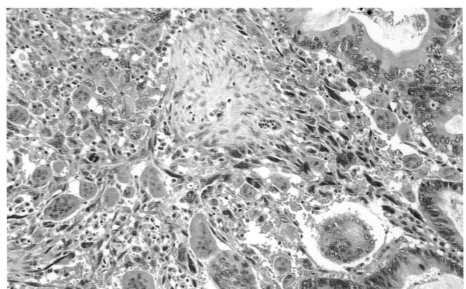

Fig. 12.18 Undifferentiated carcinoma with osteoclast-like giant cells. A component of ductal adenocarcinoma is also seen (right).

hand, osteoclast-like giant cells, and a subset of the mononuclear cells, express CD68, vimentin, and leukocyte common antigen, but are negative for keratin and do not label with antibodies to p53 {1236, 1912, 2124, 3493}. These immunolabelling studies, when combined with molecular analyses, have shown that the pleomorphic mononuclear cells are the neoplastic cells, while the osteoclast-like giant cells are reactive non-neoplastic cells {3493}.

The mean age of patients with an undifferentiated carcinoma with osteoclast-like giant cells is 62 years, but there is a wide range (32–93 years) {1270, 2314}. Recent studies have shown that the prognosis is poor and mean survival is only 12 months {628, 1270}. Interestingly, *in situ* as well as early-stage undifferentiated carcinomas with osteoclast-like giant cells have also been reported {237, 3225}.

Other entities

A number of rare entities of uncertain clinical significance have been reported. Those carcinomas of probable ductal phenotype include oncocytic carcinoma {2452, 3012}, non-mucinous, glycogen-poor cystadenocarcinoma {896}, choriocarcinoma {3012, 3668}, clear cell carcinoma {628, 1470, 1556, 1604, 1896, 1922, 3012, 3212}, ciliated cell adenocarcinoma {2154} and microadenocarcinoma {628, 1604}. Although most of these neoplasms are reported to have a distinctive histological appearance, their clinical/biological significance is not well defined, and they are therefore not considered as separate entities at this time. Some have been reclassified immunohistochemically as adenocarcinoma, acinar cell carcinomas and neuroendocrine carcinoma, and others are regarded as patterns of growth rather than distinctive entities.

Serous neoplasms of the pancreas

B. Terris
N. Fukushima
R.H. Hruban

Serous cystic neoplasms are usually cystic epithelial neoplasms composed of cuboidal, glycogen-rich, epithelial cells that produce a watery fluid similar to serum. Most are benign (serous cystadenomas), and only rare cases metastasize (serous cystadenocarcinoma). In addition to the most common microcystic type, four variants of serous cystic neoplasm have been described: macrocystic serous cystic neoplasm, solid serous neoplasm, von Hippel-Lindau (VHL)-associated serous cystic neoplasm, and mixed serous-neuroendocrine neoplasm.

Serous adenoma

Definition

A benign neoplasm composed of uniform glycogen-rich cuboidal epithelial cells that usually form cysts containing serous fluid. The term "serous cystadenoma" refers to the microcystic form of the neoplasm unless otherwise specified.

ICD-O code

Serous cystadenoma   8441/0
Serous cystadenocarcinoma   8441/3

Epidemiology

This is a relatively uncommon neoplasm, accounting for 1–2% of all pancreatic neoplasms {1270, 1655}. The mean age at presentation is 60 years (range, 26–91 years), with a slight predominance in

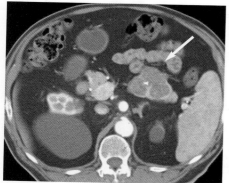

Fig. 12.20 Axial CT scan of a serous cystadenoma in the tail of the pancreas (arrow). Note the central calcified scar.

women (67–80%) {584, 585, 934, 1655, 3647}. As many as 90% of patients with the von Hippel-Lindau (VHL) syndrome develop serous cystic neoplasms {585, 1109, 2123, 3421}.

Localization

These neoplasms occur most frequently (50–75%) in the body or tail of the pancreas; the remaining tumours involve the pancreatic head {584, 585, 934, 1655, 3647}. They are only rarely multifocal, large, or involve almost the full length of the pancreas.

Clinical features

Approximately 40% of resected serous neoplasms present as an incidental finding at routine physical examination {584, 934, 3647}. Other patients exhibit symptoms related to local mass effects, including abdominal pain, palpable mass, nausea and vomiting, and weight loss {584, 934, 3647}. Jaundice caused by obstruction of the common bile duct is unusual, even in neoplasms originating in the head of the pancreas.

Imaging

Serum tumour markers are generally normal. Endoscopic ultrasonography (EUS) and computed tomography (CT) reveal a well-circumscribed, multilocular mass, occasionally with evident prominent central stellate scar with a sunburst-type pattern of calcification {944, 1551}. On magnetic resonance imaging (MRI), serous cystic neoplasms are predominantly hypointense in T1-weighted images and hyperintense in T2-weighted images, a manifestation of of the fluid content of the small cysts {3708}. Any areas of haemorrhage are hyperintense on T1-weighted sequences {3708}. Angiographically, these neoplasms are usually hypervascular. The cysts do not communicate with the pancreatic duct system.

Macroscopy

Serous cystadenomas are usually single, well-circumscribed, slightly bosselated, round lesions 1–25 cm in diameter (mean,

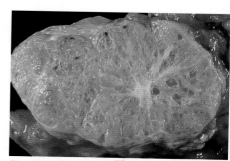

Fig. 12.19 Gross appearance of microcystic serous cystadenoma. Note the central stellate scar and sponge-like appearance.

6 cm) {585, 934, 1655}. On cross-section, serous cystadenomas are sponge-like and composed of numerous tiny cysts (usually < 2 mm to 10 mm) filled with serous (clear watery) fluid. The cysts do not communicate with the larger pancreatic ducts, and often are arranged around a central, dense fibronodular scar from which thin fibrous septa radiate to the periphery. The cysts at the periphery are often larger than those near the centre of the tumour. The central scar may be calcified.

Histopathology

The cysts are lined by a single layer of cuboidal or flattened epithelial cells. Their cytoplasm is almost always clear, but can rarely be eosinophilic (oncocytic) and granular. The nuclei are centrally located, round to oval, uniform, and have an inconspicuous nucleolus. Owing to the presence of abundant intracytoplasmic glycogen, the periodic acid-Schiff (PAS) stain without diastase digestion is positive, whereas PAS-diastase and Alcian blue stains are negative. Nuclear atypia and mitoses are practically absent. Occasionally, the neoplastic cells form intracystic papillary projections, usually without a fibrovascular stalk. The central fibrous stellate core is composed of relatively acellular hyalinized tissue admixed with a few clusters of tiny cysts.

Immunohistochemistry

Serous cystadenoma and its variants have a similar immunoprofile. The epithelial nature of these neoplasms is reflected in their immunoreactivity with antibodies to epithelial membrane antigen and keratins 7, 8, 18, and 19. In addition, the neoplastic cells express neuron-specific enolase, but immunolabelling for antigens that are more specific for neuroendocrine differentiation (e.g. chromogranin or synaptophysin) is uniformly negative {1657}. α-Inhibin, MUC6 and MUC1 are expressed in 82%, 70% and 34% of serous cystadenomas, respectively. This mucin expression profile supports a centroacinar differentiation. Serous cystic neoplasms occurring sporadically or in association with VHL disease show a dysregulation of VHL/hypoxia-inducible factor (HIF) pathway with the expression of HIF-1α and carbonic anhydrase 9 (CA9) {2524}.

Cytopathology

Fine-needle aspiration (FNA) biopsy is usually paucicellular. The neoplastic epithelial cells are rarely identified on CT or EUS-guided FNA biopsy. Any cells observed form sheets or small clusters. They have moderate to scant cytoplasm and round uniform nuclei {229, 1728}. Nuclei without associated cytoplasm (naked nuclei) are occasionally present. The stroma is relatively acellular, and calcifications can be seen in some cases {229}.

Ultrastructure

Electron microscopy shows a single row of uniform epithelial cells lining the cysts and resting on a basal lamina {99, 2799}. Many small blood vessels are intimately associated with the neoplastic epithelial cells {3607}. The apical surfaces have poorly developed or no microvilli. The cytoplasm contains numerous glycogen granules. Zymogen granules and neurosecretory granules are absent.

Histological variants

Four variants of serous adenoma have been characterized. The serous epithelial component of these variants is cytologically identical to the epithelial component of serous cystadenomas.

Macrocystic serous cystadenoma

This category includes entities previously classified as serous oligocystic and ill-demarcated serous adenoma {766, 1655, 1657}. These benign neoplasms are composed of a few large cysts and may even be unilocular. Macrocystic serous cystadenomas are much less common than serous cystadenomas and occur more frequently in males {1655}. Most patients are > 60 years of age (age range, 28–85 years; mean, 65 years); however, these neoplasms have also been described in infants as young as 2–16 months of age {2131}. Most macrocystic serous cystadenomas are located in the head of the pancreas {1655} where they may obstruct the periampullary portion of the common bile duct. Grossly, these lesions appear as a cystic mass with a diameter of 2–14 cm (mean, 7.2 cm) {1655}. They are composed of few or only one macroscopically visible cyst(s) filled with watery clear or light-brown fluid. The cysts usually vary between 1 and 3 cm in diameter, but cysts as large as 8 cm have been reported {1820}. They are irregularly arranged, sometimes separated by broad septa, and lie within a fibrous stroma that lacks a central stellate scar. The cysts and the supporting fibrous tissue may extend into the adjoining pancreatic tissue so that the neoplasms are poorly demarcated. Microscopically, macrocystic variants are composed of the same glycogen-rich cells as are serous cystadenomas. Occasionally, however, the lining epithelium may be more cuboidal and less flattened, and the nuclei are generally larger. The cytoplasm is usually clear, owing to the presence of glycogen, but may be eosinophilic. Smaller microscopic cysts may be present in the wall of unilocular lesions. The stromal framework is well developed and often hyalinized. The tumour border is not well defined and small cysts often extend into the adjoining pancreatic tissue. The immunohistochemical and ultrastructural features are the same as for serous cystadenoma {1657}. These lesions are entirely benign.

Solid serous adenoma

These well-circumscribed neoplasms have a solid gross appearance, similar to well-differentiated pancreatic neuroendocrine neoplasms, and are usually smaller than serous cystadenomas, measuring 2–4 cm {449}. The cells are arranged in small acini with no or minute central lumina, resembling a solid tumour. These neoplasms otherwise share the cytological and immunohistological features of serous cystadenoma.

VHL-associated serous cystic neoplasm

Multiple serous cystadenomas and macrocystic variants are the most common

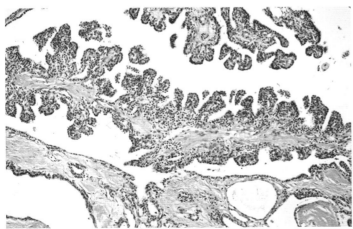

Fig. 12.21 Microcystic serous cystadenoma. Characteristic cuboidal epithelium focally forming intracystic papillary structures.

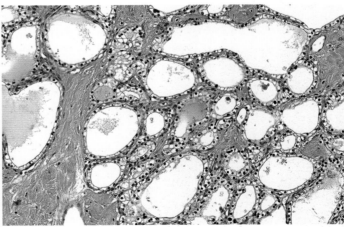

Fig. 12.22 Microcystic serous cystadenoma: the cysts are lined by a single layer of clear cuboidal epithelial cells with round, hyperchromatic, uniform nuclei.

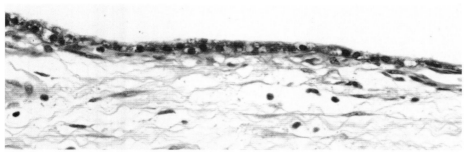

Fig. 12.23 Microcystic serous cystadenoma. The cytoplasm shows granular periodic acid-Schiff (PAS) positivity.

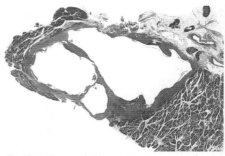

Fig. 12.24 Macrocystic (oligocystic) serous cystadenoma.

pancreatic lesions in VHL patients, occurring in 35–90% of patients {1109, 1249}. Microscopically, these cysts are virtually indistinguishable from those occurring sporadically. In VHL patients, however, serous cystic neoplasms typically involve the pancreas diffusely or in a patchy fashion rather than forming a distinct, well-demarcated tumour. The lesions vary from single and minute cystic dilatations of the centroacinar lumen to involvement of the entire pancreatic gland.

Mixed serous neuroendocrine neoplasm

In rare cases, serous cystadenomas are associated with pancreatic neuroendocrine neoplasms. The neuroendocrine proliferation can be independent or intermingled with the cysts. Such an association is highly suggestive of VHL syndrome; 10–17% of patients with VHL have been reported to have neuroen-

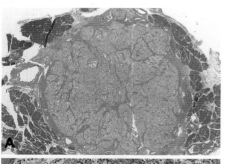

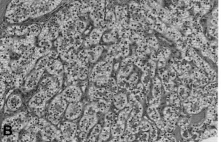

Fig. 12.25 Solid serous adenoma. **A** Whole mount. **B** Microscopic pattern.

docrine neoplasms and 70% have neuroendocrine microadenomatosis {1109, 1909, 2524}. In a few cases, however, no genetic syndrome is found {279}.

Differential diagnosis

Serous cystadenomas are usually so characteristic that they do not present a significant diagnostic challenge. When the lesion is not a classic example, the main entities to consider in the differential diagnosis are lymphangioma, haemangioma and metastatic renal cell carcinoma. Immunostains for epithelial and vascular markers can help to distinguish serous cystic neoplasms from vascular tumours, and immunolabelling for PAX8 and a good clinical history can identify renal metastases. In contrast, variant forms can be more challenging and have a broader differential diagnosis.

Macrocystic variants closely mimic mucinous cystic neoplasms (MCN) and pseudocysts both radiologically and macroscopically. This may also be the case on microscopic examination, as epithelial denudation occurs frequently both in serous and in mucinous cysts. Identification of small conserved microscopic cysts within the wall of the macrocystic variant can be used to establish the diagnosis {495}.

Solid serous adenoma can be difficult to distinguish from pancreatic neuroendocrine neoplasms, metastatic renal cell carcinoma and clear cell sugar tumour. The use of immunohistochemistry helps to differentiate these different entities. It can be particularly difficult to distinguish between a VHL-associated serous cystic neoplasm and a well-differentiated neuroendocrine neoplasm in patients with VHL, as the syndrome predisposes to both entities and well-differentiated neuroendocrine neoplasms in patients with VHL are often composed of cells with clear cytoplasm {1909}.

Genetic susceptibility

Pancreatic serous cystadenomas and macrocystic variants are observed in 35–90% of patients with VHL syndrome {1109, 1249}. Pancreatic involvement is the first manifestation of this syndrome in 8% of patients with VHL.

Molecular pathology

Loss of heterozygosity at the *VHL* gene locus, mapped to chromosome 3p25, has been reported in two of two serous cystadenomas associated with VHL disease and in 40–70% of sporadic cases {2123, 2142}. Somatic inactivating mutations in the *VHL* gene have been reported in a minority (22%) of sporadic cases. In contrast to ductal adenocarcinomas, no mutations in *KRAS* or *TP53* have been reported in serous cystadenomas {2142}.

Prognosis and predictive factors

The prognosis for patients with serous cystadenoma is excellent. These neoplasms grow slowly, and there is minimal risk of malignant transformation. In a study in which 24 patients were followed with serial radiographic imaging, the annual median growth rate was only 0.6 cm, and none of the neoplasms metastasized {3300}. Because serous cystic neoplasms grow and because complete surgical resection is curative, most institutions recommend the removal of these neoplasms {3300}. However, conservative management has been proposed when serous cystadenomas are small, not clinically complicated and show typical morphological characteristics on radiological examination. This course of action is supported by the benign nature of the vast majority of serous cystadenomas and by the potentially significant postoperative morbidity and mortality, particularly in elderly patients.

Although not technically classified as malignant, serous cystic neoplasms with locally aggressive features, such as direct extension into adjacent structures, can rarely recur or even metastasize {934}; clinical postoperative follow-up of patients with such neoplasms is therefore warranted {934}.

Serous cystadenocarcinoma

Definition
A malignant neoplasm composed of uniform glycogen-rich cuboidal epithelial cells that usually form cysts containing serous fluid. Malignancy is defined by the presence of distant metastases.

Epidemiology
Some 1–3% of serous cystic neoplasms are malignant, and only about 25 cases have been reported {934, 1571}. These patients were between 52 and 81 years of age; two thirds were women and one third were men {1571}.

Localization
Serous cystadenocarcinomas usually arise in the tail of the gland.

Clinical features
Presenting signs and symptoms include abdominal pain, upper gastrointestinal bleeding, jaundice, weight loss and a palpable upper abdominal mass. Imaging typically reveals a large cystic mass.

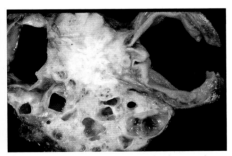

Fig. 12.27 Mixed serous neuroendocrine neoplasm. The serous cystadenoma is juxtaposed with a pancreatic neuroendocrine neoplasm in this patient with von Hippel-Lindau (VHL) syndrome.

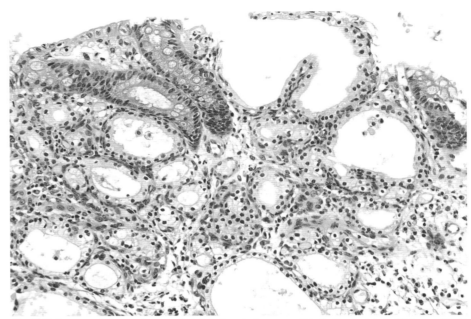

Fig. 12.26 Serous cystadenocarcinoma metastatic to the colonic mucosa. Note the bland cytological features, virtually indistinguishable from an ordinary serous cystadenoma.

Serum CEA and CA19-9 levels are usually normal or only slightly increased.

Macroscopy
These neoplasms are grossly similar to benign serous cystic neoplasms, except that they tend to be larger (mean diameter, 10 cm), and some, but not all, are locally aggressive {1571}. Direct invasion into lymph nodes, the spleen, stomach, small intestines and adrenal gland has been observed {934, 1571, 3557}.

Histopathology
The histological features of the primary as well as the metastases are remarkably similar to those of benign serous neoplasms. The neoplastic cells are uniform and most serous cystadenocarcinomas do not have an increased mitotic rate. Vascular and perivascular invasion have been reported. As is true for their benign counterparts, serous cystadenocarcinomas express keratins (keratins 7,8,18 and 19), α-inhibin, MUC6, and neuron-specific enolase {1657}.

Differential diagnosis
Benign serous cystadenoma is the primary differential diagnosis. Clinical behaviour is the only established way to distinguish the two entities. By definition, distant metastases need to be present to establish the diagnosis of serous cystadenocarcinoma.

Prognosis and predictive factors
Serous cystadenocarcinomas are slowly growing neoplasms and palliative resection may be helpful even at an advanced stage. With a mean follow-up of 36 months, most patients were still alive at the time their cases were reported {1571}.

Mucinous cystic neoplasms of the pancreas

G. Zamboni
N. Fukushima
R.H. Hruban
G. Klöppel

Definition

A cyst-forming epithelial neoplasm that usually does not communicate with the pancreatic ductal system, and is composed of columnar, mucin-producing epithelium associated with ovarian-type subepithelial stroma {1106, 1270}. This neoplasm occurs almost exclusively in women.

Noninvasive mucinous cystic neoplasms (MCN) are categorized as MCN with low-grade, intermediate-grade or high-grade dysplasia. If there is a component of invasive carcinoma, the lesions are designated as MCN with an associated invasive carcinoma.

ICD-O codes

MCN with low- or intermediate-grade
  dysplasia   8470/0
MCN with high-grade dysplasia   8470/2
MCN with an associated invasive
  carcinoma   8470/3

Synonyms

Terms that are no longer to be used: mucinous cystadenoma, not otherwise specified (NOS); mucinous cystadenocarcinoma, noninvasive; mucinous cystadenocarcinoma, NOS.

Epidemiology

MCNs are relatively rare, accounting for about 8% of surgically resected cystic lesions of the pancreas {1655}. Poorly defined diagnostic criteria may have led to over-representation of MCNs in older histopathology series, while the recent rise in the incidence of these lesions is most likely attributable to advances in imaging and other diagnostic techniques.

The vast majority of MCNs occur in women, with a female-to-male ratio of 20 : 1 {618, 2809}. The mean age at diagnosis is between 40 and 50 years in most series, with a range of 14–95 years {618, 1010, 1270}. Patients with MCNs with an associated invasive carcinoma are 5–10 years older, on average, than are patients with noninvasive MCNs, suggesting that progression from a noninvasive curable neoplasm to an invasive cancer occurs over a period of years {1655}.

The incidence of MCNs does not vary according to ethnic group.

Localization

Most cases (> 95%) occur in the body and tail of the pancreas {3239, 3578, 3673}. The head is only rarely involved {618, 1010, 3239, 3673}.

Clinical features

Clinical presentation depends on the size of the tumour. Small tumours (< 3 cm) are usually found incidentally. Larger tumours may produce symptoms that are usually secondary to compression of adjacent structures, and are often accompanied by a palpable abdominal mass. In rare cases, patients present with symptoms related to cancerous invasion of the bile duct, stomach, colon, peritoneal cavity or liver metastasis. Some patients present with new-onset diabetes mellitus {3012}. Serum tumour and cyst-fluid markers, in-

cluding carcinoembryonic antigen (CEA), and CA19-9, are useful but imperfect markers for distinguishing mucinous from non-mucinous cystic lesions and for predicting the presence of a malignant component (since they are not sufficiently reliable in individual cases). The highest levels of tumour markers are seen in MCNs with an associated invasive carcinoma {1821, 3042}. Cyst-fluid amylase activity is usually low as the cysts of MCNs do not communicate with the larger pancreatic ducts. Recent studies have shown that exopeptidases may hamper the proteomic analysis of pancreatic cystic fluids {1510}.

An MCN should be suspected whenever a cystic lesion is seen by endoscopic ultrasonography (EUS), computed tomography (CT) or magnetic resonance imaging (MRI) in the pancreatic body–tail of a young or middle-aged woman, especially in the absence of a history of pancreatitis. The morphological features revealed by radiography and EUS include a sharply demarcated lesion with one or more thick-walled large loculations {2366}. The cysts do not communicate with the main pancreatic duct {2366}. Features suggestive of an associated invasive carcinoma include large size, an irregular thickening of the cyst wall, mural nodules and/or papillary excrescences projecting into the cyst {362, 3458}.

Macroscopy

MCNs typically present as a single spherical mass with a smooth surface and a fibrous pseudocapsule of variable thickness and occasional calcifications. The size of the tumour ranges from 2 to 35 cm in diameter (average, 6–10 cm). On the cut surface, the tumours are either unilocular or multilocular, with cysts ranging from a few millimetres to several centimetres in diameter. The cysts contain either thick mucin or a mixture of mucin and haemorrhagic-necrotic material. The internal surface of unilocular tumours is usually smooth and glistening, whereas higher-grade neoplasms often have papillary projections.

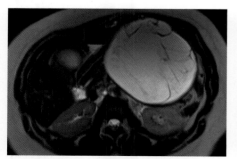

Fig. 12.28 MRI of a mucinous cystic neoplasm. Note the large septated and fluid-filled mass.

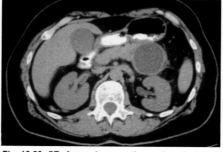

Fig. 12.29 CT of a mucinous cystic neoplasm in the tail of the pancreas.

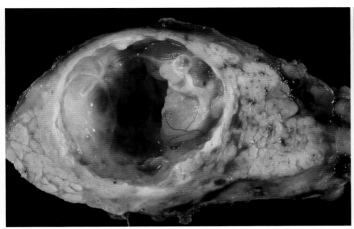

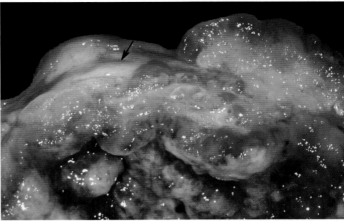

Fig. 12.30 Mucinous cystic neoplasm. Gross appearance, with glistening mucin.

Fig. 12.31 Mucinous cystic neoplasm with an associated invasive carcinoma (upper right). Note that the neoplasm does not involve the pancreatic duct (arrow).

MCNs with an associated invasive carcinoma are usually large and multilocular, and the locules often contain papillary projections and/or mural nodules {3673}. Associated infiltrating carcinomas may also infiltrate the adjacent organs. Unless there is fistula formation, there is no communication between the locules of MCNs and the pancreatic duct system {211}.

Tumour spread and staging

MCNs with an associated invasive adenocarcinoma follow the same pathways of local spread as invasive ductal adenocarcinoma. The first metastases are typically found in the regional peripancreatic lymph nodes and the liver. Staging follows the protocol for ductal adenocarcinoma.

Histopathology

MCNs have two distinct components – an epithelial lining and an underlying ovarian-type stromal component. The cysts are lined by tall, columnar, mucin-producing cells that stain with diastase-resistant periodic acid-Schiff (PAS) and Alcian blue. Pseudopyloric, gastric foveolar, small- and large-intestinal, and rarely even squamous differentiation can also be found. Atypia exhibited by the columnar cells in a single neoplasm may vary widely from uniform benign-appearing to severely atypical. On the basis of the highest degree of architectural and cytological atypia (dysplasia), noninvasive MCNs are categorized as MCN with low-grade dysplasia, intermediate-grade dysplasia, or high-grade dysplasia {1270}.

In MCN with low-grade dysplasia, the columnar epithelium has only minimal to mild architectural and cytological atypia

with a slight increase in the size of the basally located nuclei; mitoses are absent. MCNs with intermediate-grade dysplasia have mild-to-moderate architectural and cytological atypia with papillary projections or crypt-like invaginations, cellular pseudostratification caused by crowding of slightly enlarged nuclei, and occasional mitoses. MCNs with high-grade dysplasia are characterized by significant architectural and cytological atypia, with the formation of papillae with irregular branching and budding, nuclear stratification with loss of polarity, pleomorphism and prominent nucleoli. Mitoses are frequent and can be atypical.

Up to one third of MCNs have an associated invasive carcinoma. The invasive component can be focal, and MCNs therefore require careful and extensive histological examination. The presence of a stromal desmoplastic reaction can be useful in the differential diagnosis between invasive carcinoma and trapped non-neoplastic glands {1270}. The invasive component usually resembles the common infiltrating ductal adenocarcinoma, forming tubular and duct-like structures. However, other rare variants of invasive carcinoma have been described, including adenosquamous carcinoma, undifferentiated carcinoma and undifferentiated carcinoma with osteoclast-like giant cells {283, 945, 2581, 3668}.

The distinctive ovarian-type stroma underlying the epithelium consists of densely packed spindle-shaped cells with round or elongated nuclei and sparse cytoplasm. This type of stroma is an entity-defining feature of MCNs, and its presence has become a requirement for

diagnosis {3185}. It can be particularly useful in cases in which the epithelial lining is extensively denuded. In such cases, histological examination of the entire lesion and scrutiny of the epithelial lining in the smaller cysts will usually lead to the correct diagnosis. The stroma frequently displays a variable degree of luteinization, characterized by the presence of single or clusters of epithelioid cells with round to oval nuclei and abun-

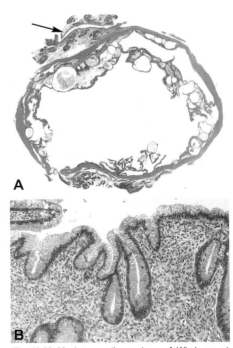

Fig. 12.32 Mucinous cystic neoplasm. **A** Whole-mount section. Note that the cysts do not communicate with the pancreatic duct (arrow). **B** The columnar, mucin-containing epithelium displays low-grade dysplasia and ovarian-type subepithelial stroma.

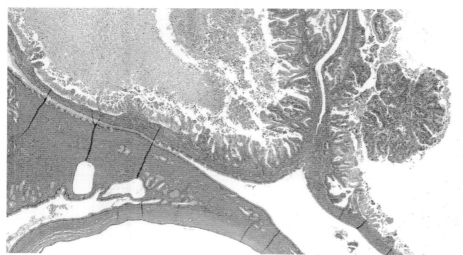

Fig. 12.33 Mucinous cystic neoplasm. Note the abrupt transition from low-grade (lower left) to high-grade (upper right) dysplasia.

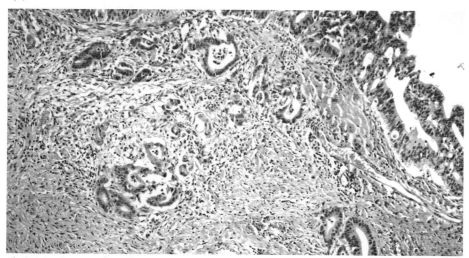

Fig. 12.34 Mucinous cystic neoplasm with an associated invasive, tubular-type adenocarcinoma (centre).

dant clear or eosinophilic cytoplasm. Occasionally, these cells, resembling ovarian hilar cells, can be found associated with (or present in) nerve trunks. The frequency of stromal luteinization decreases as the degree of dysplasia increases {3668}. In large MCNs, the stroma may become fibrotic and hypocellular, and some foci have the appearance of corpora albicantia. Uncommonly, the ovarian-type stroma predominates over the epithelial component, creating a solid mass {1117, 1792}. The adjoining pancreatic tissue may show fibrous atrophy owing to obstruction of the main pancreatic duct by the tumour.

Immunohistochemistry

The neoplastic epithelial cells are immunoreactive with keratins 7, 8, 18 and 19 {3239, 3673}, epithelial membrane antigen (EMA), CEA, and express the gastric-type mucin marker MUC5AC {919, 2884} and the pancreatic-type mucin markers DUPAN-2 and CA19-9. Scattered goblet-like cells express the intestinal mucin marker MUC2 {919, 1270, 2884}, and scattered intraepithelial chromogranin A-positive neuroendocrine cells express serotonin followed by somatostatin, pancreatic polypeptide and gastrin {1918, 3239, 3673}. With increasing epithelial atypia, the mucin that is produced changes from sulfated to sialated or neutral {3239} and nuclear p53 protein immunoreactivity occurs {1918, 3673}. While most noninvasive MCNs express SMAD4 (DPC4) protein, but not MUC1, MCNs with an invasive ductal adenocarcinoma component may lose the expression of SMAD4 and express MUC1 {1302, 1918, 1918}.

The subepithelial ovarian-type stroma expresses smooth muscle actin (SMA), progesterone receptors (60–90%) and estrogen receptors (30%) {919, 3673}. Luteinized cells label with antibodies to tyrosine hydroxylase, calretinin and α-inhibin {3673, 3707}. In addition, steroidogenic acute regulatory (STAR) protein, 3-β-hydroxysteroid dehydrogenase (3βHSD) and 17-α-hydroxylase (17αH) are occasionally expressed in luteinized cells of the MCN, suggesting that such cells are capable of steroidogenesis {921, 1355}.

Cytopathology

Aspirates contain varying amounts of mucin and often only few epithelial cells. The epithelium is mucin-producing and can have varying degrees of architectural and cytological atypia {1270, 1756, 2648, 2948}. The neoplastic cells form sheets and small clusters, the nuclei are usually basally located and the cytoplasm contains mucin. The degree of dysplasia in cytological samples often underestimates that observed histologically when the lesion is resected {1270}. The ovarian-type stroma is often not present in aspirates and, in such cases, only the nonspecific diagnosis of mucin-producing cystic neoplasm can be made {1270, 2648}.

Ultrastructure

Electron microscopy reveals columnar epithelial cells resting on a thin basement membrane. The cells may have well-developed microvilli and mucin granules {65}. The ovarian-type stroma has a myofibroblastic differentiation {2952}.

Differential diagnosis

The differential diagnosis of MCN includes other cystic neoplasms of the pancreas and pseudocysts. The best approach to obtaining an accurate diagnosis is the combined evaluation of all available clinical, serological, radiological and morphological findings.

It is usually easy to distinguish MCNs from entities that do not have a mucin-producing epithelium, i.e. serous cystic neoplasms, acinar cell cystadenocarcinoma, solid-pseudopapillary neoplasm and cystic neuroendocrine neoplasms.

The differential diagnosis also includes mucinous non-neoplastic cysts, characterized by the presence of mucin-producing cells without atypia. The correct diagnosis is established considering the equal prevalence in males and females, the more common involvement of the head of the pancreas, and microscopically by the lack of the ovarian-type stroma {1652, 1655}.

Differentiating a pseudocyst from an MCN may not only be a clinical problem but also a morphological one, since some MCNs can have significant degenerative changes, including denuded epithelium and haemorrhagic cyst contents. Extensive sampling to identify one of the two morphological diagnostic features of an MCN (the mucin-producing epithelial lining or the ovarian-type stroma) is often needed {1270}.

The differential diagnosis with intraductal papillary mucinous neoplasms (IPMNs) can be relatively straightforward for main duct-type IPMNs, but may be difficult for "branch duct-type" IPMNs. Two features distinguish these entities: MCNs do not grow significantly within the pancreatic duct system and contain, by definition, an ovarian-type stroma {1106, 3185}.

Pathogenesis

Pancreatic MCNs share many clinicopathological features with their counterparts in the ovary, hepatobiliary tree, mesentery, retroperitoneum and with the mixed epithelial stromal (MEST) tumour of the kidney {367, 2002, 2053, 2952, 3227, 3320, 3673, 3711}. The possibility that the stromal component of MCNs is derived from ovarian primordium is supported by morphology, tendency to undergo luteinization, presence of hilar-like cells, and immunophenotypic sex cord–stromal differentiation. It is conceivable that ectopic ovarian stroma incorporated during embryogenesis in the pancreas, hepatobiliary tree, retroperitoneum or kidney, may

become activated in the setting of a hormonal imbalance, releasing hormones and growth factors causing nearby epithelium to proliferate and form cystic neoplasms {800, 1374, 3673}. This hypothesis could explain the predilection of pancreatic MCNs for the body–tail region (which is in close proximity to the left primordial gonads) {800, 3317, 3673}. Of course, this hypothesis cannot account for MCNs in males. Another possibility is that the ovarian-type stroma represents a fetal primitive mesenchyme, which responds and proliferates in response to hormonal stimulation {1270}.

Molecular pathology

Activating point mutations in codon 12 of the *KRAS* gene have been observed in both noninvasive and invasive MCNs, with the prevalence of mutations increasing with increasing degree of dysplasia {206, 1430, 1558}. Alterations of *TP53*, *CDKN2A* (*p16*) and *SMAD4* (*DPC4*) tumour-suppressor genes are more frequent in cases with an associated invasive component {206, 968}. Aberrant hypermethylation of the *CDKN2A* gene has been reported in about 15% of MCNs with low- to intermediate-grade dysplasia {1558}.

Rare examples of MCNs with a sarcomatous stroma have been reported and molecular genetic analyses of these cases have revealed that the epithelial and "sarcomatous" components have a clonal origin {3355}. These lesions are therefore best categorized as undifferentiated carcinomas arising in association with MCNs {3355}.

Prognosis and predictive factors

Surgical resection is curative for almost all patients with a noninvasive MCN {618, 2809, 3508, 3673}. The prognosis for pa-

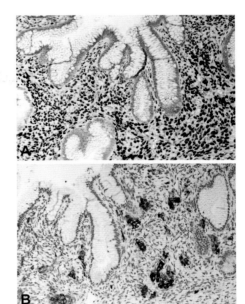

Fig. 12.35 Mucinous cystic neoplasm, with immunolabelling for progesterone receptors (**A**) and α-inhibin (**B**).

tients with an MCN with an associated invasive carcinoma depends on the extent (depth) of the invasive component, tumour stage (lymph-node and distant metastasis), and resectability {3673}. The 2-year survival rate for patients with a surgically resected MCN with an associated invasive carcinoma is about 67%, and the 5-year survival rate is about 50% {618, 1270, 1771, 3508}. Recurrence of the carcinoma and poor outcome correlate with invasion of the carcinoma beyond the tumour wall and into peritumoral tissue. Patients aged > 50 years appear to have a lower survival rate {3673}.

Intraductal neoplasms of the pancreas

N.V. Adsay
N. Fukushima
T. Furukawa
R.H. Hruban
D.S. Klimstra

G. Klöppel
G.J.A. Offerhaus
M.B. Pitman
M. Shimizu
G. Zamboni

Introduction

The intraductal neoplasms discussed in the following section, intraductal papillary mucinous neoplasms (IPMNs) and intraductal tubulopapillary neoplasms (ITPNs; previously designated as intraductal tubular neoplasms), are defined as macroscopic (cystic or mass-forming) epithelial neoplasms with ductal differentiation that characteristically grow primarily within the ductal system of the pancreas {211, 1270, 3156, 3185, 3580}. These lesions are distinct from pancreatic intraepithelial neoplasia (PanIN), which is a microscopic lesion that is not usually macroscopically detectable. Intraductal growth of neoplasms with non-ductal directions of differentiation, such as acinar cell carcinomas, are not included in this category {1271}.

Both IPMNs and ITPNs form intraductal masses that are radiographically and grossly detectable. These neoplasms, due to their relatively slow-growing nature, often achieve fairly large sizes before they come to clinical attention, and both IPMNs and ITPNs may be associated with (or progress to) invasive carcinoma. While some invasive carcinomas arising within these neoplasms are morphologically indistinguishable from conventional ductal adenocarcinomas, many are distinctive enough to be classified as separate variants of adenocarcinoma, including colloid carcinoma {37}.

Both IPMNs and ITPNs can form tubules and papillary growths. The major features that distinguish these two groups of intraductal neoplasms are: (1) IPMNs are commonly assoicated with significant luminal accumulation of mucin, whereas ITPNs have minimal luminal mucin and also commonly lack obvious intracellular mucin; (2) most IPMNs have a predominantly papillary histological growth patterns, whereas ITPNs are predominantly tubular in architecture; (3) grossly or histologically evident necrosis, often with a comedo-like pattern, may be found in ITPNs and is not typical of IPMNs; and (4) immunolabelling of MUC5AC is common in IPMNs, but negative in the vast majority of ITPNs {3156, 3580}.

An arbitrary minimal size criterion of 1 cm has been suggested to define this family, underlining the mass-forming nature (gross and radiographic detectability) of the intraductal neoplasms and distinguishing them from the smaller PanINs {1271}.

ICD-O codes

IPMN with low- or intermediate-
grade dysplasia   8453/0
IPMN with high-grade dysplasia   8453/2
IPMN with an associated invasive
carcinoma   8453/3
Intraductal tubulopapillary neoplasm
                                                  8503/2

Intraductal papillary mucinous neoplasm (IPMN)

Definition

An intraductal grossly-visible (typically ≥ 1.0 cm) epithelial neoplasm of mucin-producing cells, arising in the main pancreatic duct or its branches {1271, 3185}.

The neoplastic epithelium is usually papillary, and the degrees of mucin secretion, duct dilatation (cyst formation), and dysplasia are variable. Noninvasive IPMNs are classified into three categories on the basis of the highest degree of cytoarchitectural atypia: low-grade dysplasia, intermediate-grade dysplasia and high-grade dysplasia {1270}. The presence of a component of invasive carcinoma leads to the designation "IPMN with an associated invasive carcinoma."

Synonyms

Before they were unified under the heading of "intraductal papillary mucinous neoplasms," these neoplasms were variably designated as "mucin-producing tumour" {3578, 3588}, "mucinous duct ectasia", "ductectatic mucinous cystadenoma/cystadenocarcinoma" {3611}, "villous adenoma" {2506} or "papillary adenoma/carcinoma" {2160} of pancreatic ducts, each term reflecting a different but important facet of this entity. These designations are no longer employed.

The names given to three of the four categories of IPMN have been updated such that the nomenclature presented here parallels that used in other organs and in the fourth series of the Armed Forces Institutes of Pathology Atlas of Tumor Pathology {1270}. The entity previously classified as "intraductal papillary mucinous adenoma" is now designated "intraductal papillary mucinous neoplasm with low-grade dysplasia." "Intraductal papillary mucinous neoplasm with moderate dysplasia" has been changed to "intraductal papillary mucinous neoplasm with intermediate-grade dysplasia;" the old term "borderline" used synonymously for this group has been eliminated. "Intraductal papillary mucinous carcinoma, noninvasive" is now designated "intraductal papillary mucinous neoplasm with high-grade dysplasia," and "intraductal papillary mucinous carcinoma, invasive" is now designated "intraductal papillary mucinous neoplasm with an associated invasive carcinoma."

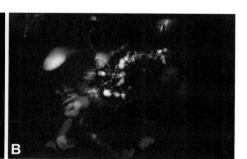

Fig. 12.36 Imaging of IPMNs. **A** Axial CT: note the dilatation of the pancreatic duct. **B** Magnetic resonance cholangiopancreatography (MRCP): numerous branch-duct type IPMNs are highlighted.

Epidemiology

The incidence of IPMNs in the general population is poorly defined because most are asymptomatic. The apparent rise in the reported incidence of IPMNs is mostly attributable to increased recognition secondary to better characterization of this entity {3255}. Another established factor is the advancement and widespread use of imaging modalities with which small IPMNs are detected incidentally during the evaluation of patients for other conditions {3526}.

IPMNs are fairly common, particularly in the elderly. Asymptomatic cysts, most of which were presumably small IPMNS, were identified in 2.8% of 2832 consecutive CT scans performed in 1 year at a single institution {1717}. This rose to 8.7% in individuals of > 80 years {1717}. IPMNs are currently estimated to account for 1–3% of exocrine pancreatic neoplasms, and for 20% of all cystic neoplasms of the pancreas {211}, but these figures represent older surgical data, and both numbers are increasing {1894, 2159, 3185}. Two studies provide some evidence that the incidence may be higher among Asians than among whites, but issues of consistency of classification require that these associations be further evaluated {1604, 1894}.

Etiology

There are no well established environmental etiological factors. In one series, most patients with IPMNs were cigarette smokers {920}. IPMNs have been reported in patients with Peutz-Jeghers syndrome and in patients with familial adenomatous polyposis (FAP) {1955, 3105}. Some studies have suggested that IPMNs may be particularly common among the neoplasms arising in patients with a family history of pancreatic carcinoma {407, 2571, 2930}.

Localization

Although IPMNs can occur throughout the pancreas, most are located in the head of the gland {169, 211, 588, 3012}. Branch-duct type IPMNs usually form a cystic mass in the uncinate process {3611}. Main-duct type IPMNs can be diffuse, involving the entire length of the main pancreatic duct {1893, 2957, 3287}. Multicentricity, depending upon the definition thereof, is observed in up to 40% of cases {1883, 2512, 3006}. Some main-duct IPMNs limited to the head of the gland are associated with obstructive dilatation of the entire length of the pancreatic duct, although not all of the dilated ducts are involved by the neoplasm. IPMNs may extend to the ampulla of Vater, and some IPMNs extend into the common bile duct {3012}.

Clinical features

IPMNs are found at a broad age range (30–94 years); however, they are significantly more common in the elderly, with a median age at diagnosis of about 66 years {32, 931, 2429, 2848, 3578}. The mean age of patients with IPMNs without an associated invasive carcinoma is 3–5 years younger than the mean age of patients with IPMNs with an associated invasive carcinoma, suggesting that progression from a noninvasive curable neoplasm to an invasive cancer occurs over a period of years {2787, 3005}. IPMNs occur slightly more frequently in males than in females {1946, 2787, 3005, 3578}. Clinical symptoms include epigastric pain, chronic pancreatitis, weight loss, diabetes mellitus, and jaundice {1605, 2787, 3005, 3287, 3626}. Many cases are detected incidentally during clinical evaluation for other conditions {1717}. The incidence of synchronous and metachronous neoplasms of other organs appear to be high {216, 768, 1468, 2655, 3122}. Some patients have a history of many years of chronic pancreatitis, suggesting that IPMNs can be present for years before they are diagnosed. Serum amylase and lipase levels are commonly elevated. Serum tumour markers such as CEA and CA19-9 are generally not of value, but are often elevated in patients with an associated invasive carcinoma {3287, 3578}.

CT, MRI and EUS are commonly used to visualize IPMNs. IPMNs typically appear as cystic lesions communicating with the pancreatic duct system. By imaging, two distinct types of IPMN can be discerned {1506, 1630}. Most of those detected incidentally are branch-duct type IPMNs, which are cystic lesions that do not affect the main pancreatic duct, but instead involve the smaller, secondary pancreatic ducts {2512, 2787, 2848, 3005}. Branch-duct type IPMNs typically arise in the head of the pancreas, in particular, in the uncinate region. In contrast, symptomatic patients often have a main-duct type IPMN {2787, 3123, 3185}, which are characterized by primary involvement of the main pancreatic duct with distension of the main pancreatic duct, sometimes also with dilated secondary branches.

More advanced IPMNs are more complex and can have mural nodules and irregularities in the duct contours, mostly reflecting the papillary component of the neoplasm, and in some cases, corresponding to an invasive component {930, 1631}. Endoscopically, mucin extrusion from the ampulla of Vater (or even the minor papilla, in rare cases) is characteristic, but not always present {3588}.

Macroscopy

Proper macroscopic examination and sampling is important; bisecting resected pancreata along a plane created by

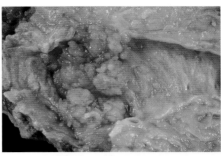

Fig. 12.37 IPMN involving the main pancreatic duct.

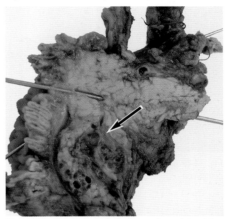

Fig. 12.38 IPMN, branch-duct type (arrow) involving uncinate process. The probe is in the main pancreatic duct.

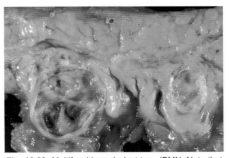

Fig. 12.39 Multifocal branch-duct type IPMN. Note that the main pancreatic duct is not involved.

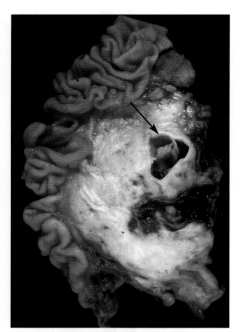

Fig. 12.40 IPMN (arrow) with an associated invasive carcinoma.

placing a probe in the main pancreatic duct is the best way to define the pattern of ductal involvement.

The subtypes of IPMNs recognized by imaging studies, namely the branch-duct; and main-duct types, are also identifiable by macroscopic examination; however, many IPMNs involve both the main and branch ducts {2512, 2787, 2848, 3005, 3123, 3185}. When both are significantly involved, the neoplasms are designated "combined" type. Since the clinical behaviour of combined-type IPMNs mirrors that of main-duct type IPMNs, it would be reasonable to consider them in the predominantly main-duct type category.

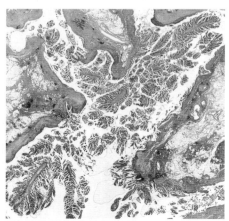

Fig. 12.41 IPMN within the dilated main pancreatic duct and branch ducts.

Main-duct type IPMNs

In this type, the main pancreatic duct is typically diffusely dilated. The duct is often filled with mucin, and is tortuous and irregular. Main duct IPMNs usually arise in the head of the gland and progress along the main duct. In some cases, the entire pancreas is involved. The neoplasm may even extend to involve the major and/or minor papillae, leading in some cases to mucin extrusion from a patulous ampullary orifice into the duodenum {3588}. The documentation of involvement of the main pancreatic duct has clinical significance because this type is associated with a higher risk of high-grade dysplasia and invasive carcinoma. In main duct-type IPMNs, the uninvolved pancreas is often pale and firm, reflecting changes of extensive chronic obstructive pancreatitis {1883}.

Branch-duct type IPMNs

IPMNs of this type arise most often in the uncinate process {3611}. Branch-duct IPMNs form multicystic, grape-like structures. The cystically dilated ducts, range from 1 to 8–10 cm, and are filled with tenacious mucin. The cyst walls are usually thin, and they can have either a flat or papillary lining. The individual cysts may be separated by intervening normal pancreatic parenchyma, giving the impression of separate individual cysts on cut sections. The number and size of papillae vary from case to case and region to region, but grossly visible papillae are present in most resected branch-duct type IPMNs if inspected carefully. The adjacent pancreas is generally normal in branch-duct type IPMNs.

Oncocytic-type IPMNs

IPMNs with predominantly oncocytic morphology, also known as intraductal oncocytic papillary neoplasms (IOPNs), can have a distinctive gross appearance. They typically form large (5–6 cm), tan-brown friable nodular papillary growths in the larger pancreatic ducts {27, 28}.

Invasive carcinoma

If present, invasive carcinoma produces irregular, heterogeneous thickening of the cyst walls, fibrotic foci in endoluminal papillary-nodular vegetations, or gelatinous stromal masses. The latter appearance is characteristic of colloid carcinoma (see *Ductal adenocarcinoma variants and mixed neoplasms*) {37}.

Small invasive carcinomas may be macroscopically undetectable, and thorough histological sampling is needed to rule out invasion.

Large advanced IPMNs can fistulize into adjacent organs (duodenum, bile duct, and stomach), and neoplastic papillae may develop in these secondary sites. Whether fistuli are sufficient evidence to diagnose invasive carcinoma is controversial {2252, 3072}.

Tumour spread and staging

Intraductal components of IPMNs can extend along the ductal system into the adjacent pancreas, as well as into the ampulla. Occasionally, an IPMN may be associated with fistulas, and the neoplastic cells may spread along these fistula tracks {2252, 3072}.

IPMN with high-grade dysplasia is staged as Tis. Since invasive carcinoma can be small and occult, careful evaluation is necessary before classifying a case as Tis. The adverse outcome reported in some cases classified as Tis have been at least partially attributed to sampling or evaluation errors.

The pattern of spread of invasive carcinomas arising in association with IPMNs is similar to that of ductal adenocarcinoma. Regardless of type, whether colloid or ductal, invasive carcinomas arising in association with IPMNs often show perineural invasion. The lymph nodes are the

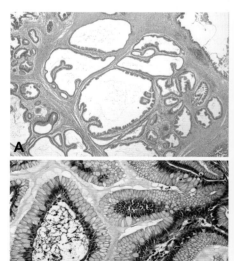

Fig. 12.42 Gastric-type IPMN. **A** With low-grade dysplasia. **B** The epithelium is reminiscent of gastric foveolar epithelium.

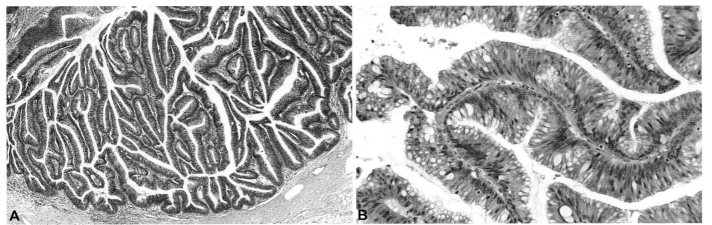

Fig. 12.43 Intestinal-type IPMN. **A** Pseudostratified tall columnar cells line papillae. **B** Note the goblet cells.

most common site of metastases and are seen in 30% of resected IPMNs with invasive carcinoma, in contrast to 75% in resected conventional ductal adenocarcinomas of the pancreas without an accompanying IPMN {492}. The liver is the main site of distant metastasis. IPMNs associated with an invasive carcinoma are staged on the basis of the characteristics of the invasive component only, and the conventional staging system for ductal adenocarcoma is employed.

Histopathology

IPMNs are characterized by the intraductal proliferation of columnar mucin-producing cells. The intraductal nature of these neoplasms can be appreciated by their involvement of the branching duct system. IPMNs lack the "ovarian-type" hypercellular periductal stroma that characterizes mucinous cystic neoplasms (MCNs) {3185}.

Architecturally, the epithelium of IPMNs can be flat or form papillae with fibrovascular cores. The papillae range from microscopic folds of neoplastic epithelium to grossly visible finger-like projections that measure up to several centimetres. The papillae may be simple and villous-like, or complex and branching. The lesion can be focal (localized), multifocal (in up to 40% of cases {2512}), or diffuse. In general, the leading edges of IPMNs tend to be relatively ill-defined, and IPMNs often extend microscopically beyond the grossly visible mass lesion. The neoplastic epithelium can extend into the smaller pancreatic ducts, mimicking pancreatic intraepithelial neoplasia.

The neoplastic epithelium can show a variety of directions of differentiation {36,

184, 929}. On the basis of the predominant architectural and cell differentiation pattern, IPMNs can be subclassified into four types: gastric, intestinal, pancreatobiliary and oncocytic {28, 36, 184, 562, 929, 1270}.

Gastric-type IPMN

The gastric type is characteristically found in the branch-duct IPMNs. The epithelium lining gastric IPMNs is composed of innocuous, tall columnar cells with basally oriented nuclei and abundant pale mucinous cytoplasm, reminiscent of gastric foveolar epithelium. The peripheral portions of the lesion often form pyloric-like glands {184}. This latter finding may be prominent in some cases and has been designated as "pyloric gland adenoma" by some authors {79, 522, 2246}. Generally, the gastric-type IPMN proves to have only low- or intermediate-grade dysplasia. Scattered goblet cells can be seen.

Intestinal-type IPMN

This type is characterized by main-duct involvement, the formation of tall papillae lined by columnar cells with pseudostratified, cigar-shaped nuclei, and basophilic cytoplasm with variable amount of apical mucin. The overall picture is highly reminiscent of colonic villous adenomas {36}. Some examples are composed predominantly of goblet-like cells with micropapillary features {929}. The epithelial cells in intestinal-type IPMNs usually have intermediate- or high-grade dysplasia.

Pancreatobiliary-type IPMN

The pancreatobiliary type of IPMN {36} occurs less frequently than the others,

and is less well-characterized. Pancreatobiliary-type IPMNs typically involve the main pancreatic duct, and form thin, branching papillae with high-grade dysplasia. The neoplastic cells are cuboidal, with round, hyperchromatic nuclei, prominent nucleoli, moderately amphophilic cytoplasm, and have a less mucinous appearance. Some cases have overlapping features with intraductal oncocytic papillary neoplasms, and some with intraductal tubulopapillary neoplasms.

Oncocytic-type IPMN

The oncocytic type of IPMN usually has complex and arborizing papillae with delicate stroma. The papillae are lined by two to five layers of cuboidal to columnar cells with abundant eosinophilic granular cytoplasm. The nuclei are round, large, and fairly uniform and typically contain single, prominent, eccentrically located nucleoli. Goblet cells may be interspersed among the oncocytic cells. The neoplastic cells often form intraepithelial lumina, which are spaces about one quarter the size of the cells, but which merge to form multicell-sized punched-out spaces within the epithelium. In some cases, these intraepithelial lumina produce a cribriform pattern, and in others the epithelium of adjacent papillae may fuse, producing a solid growth pattern punctuated by small vessels. The intraductal nature of oncocytic-type IPMNs with extensive solid areas may be difficult to recognize. Most oncocytic-type IPMNs have sufficient cytoarchitectural atypia to be calssified as having high-grade dysplasia.

Several directions of differentiation can be seen in an individual IPMN. In particular,

Table 12.05 Differential immunolabelling of intraductal neoplasms of the exocrine pancreas.

Histopathological type		MUC1	MUC2	MUC5AC	MUC6	CDX2
IPMN	Intestinal	–	++	++	–	++
	Pancreatobiliary	++	–	++	+	–
	Gastric	–	–	++	–	–
	Oncocytic	+	–	+	++	–
ITPN		+	–	–	++	–

IPMN, intraductal papillary mucinous neoplasm; ITPN, intraductal tubulopapillary neoplasm.
– no labelling; +, may be positive; ++, usually positive

the gastric type of epithelium can be seen in the less papillary regions of all IPMNs {36}. In fact, some authors believe that the pancreatobiliary type of IPMNs is a high-grade transformation of the gastric type {184}. However, it is uncommon to find both intestinal and pancreatobiliary epithelium within the same IPMN {929, 1270}.

Degree of dysplasia
Noninvasive IPMNs are classified as having low-grade, intermediate-grade, or high-grade dysplasia on the basis of the highest degree of architectural and cytological atypia (dysplasia) identified {1270}. IPMNs with low-grade dysplasia are characterized by a single layer of well-polarized cells, small and uniform nuclei with only mild pleomorphism, and rare mitoses. IPMNs with intermediate-grade dysplasia have nuclear stratification, crowding, and loss of polarity. The nuclei are enlarged and moderately hyperchromatic. The papillae maintain identifiable stromal cores. IPMNs with high-grade dysplasia are characterized by severe architectural and cytological atypia, with the formation of irregular branching papillae and sometimes cribriform growth. The epithelial cells lack polarity, and the nuclei are stratified, hyperchromatic, and pleomorphic. Mitoses are frequently found, and can even be found near the luminal surface.

Associated invasive carcinoma
Approximately 30% of resected IPMNs have an associated invasive carcinoma, which can be unifocal or multifocal. This figure is decreasing with the increased diagnosis of earlier, incidental lesions. Most invasive carcinomas arise in association with main-duct type IPMNs with high-grade dysplasia {2786, 2787, 3123, 3199, 3222}. Two distinct types of invasive carcinoma can be seen. Invasive colloid carcinoma usually arises in association with intestinal-type IPMNs {37, 2868}. Tubular (conventional ductal) adenocarcinoma, which is morphologically similar to usual ductal adenocarcinoma not arising in association with an IPMN, arises in association with either pancreatobiliary-type or intestinal-type IPMNs. Invasive carcinomas occurring in IOPNs are typically of the tubular type, closely resembling conventional ductal adenocarcinomas, but displaying more oncocytic features.
The pathology report of IPMNs with an associated invasive carcinoma should specify the type, grade, size and stage of the invasive component {211, 1493}. All other parameters typically documented for invasive carcinomas, such as vascular and perineural invasion, should also be documented.

Immunohistochemistry
Ductal markers including keratins 7 and 19, CA19-9, B72.3, and CEA are strongly expressed in most IPMNs {3214, 3215}. The expression of mucin glycoproteins (MUCs) is useful for distinguishing the morphological subtypes {28, 35, 36, 929, 3645, 3646}. Gastric-type IPMNs label for MUC5AC, but not MUC1 or MUC2 (with the exception of scattered goblet cells highlighted by MUC2). The intestinal-type IPMNs consistently label diffusely and strongly for intestinal-differentiation markers, MUC2 and CDX2 {36}, in addition to MUC5AC, but not MUC1. In contrast, the pancreatobiliary-type IPMNs express MUC5AC and MUC1 but not MUC2 or CDX2 {36, 184, 929, 1352, 2212}. IPMNs with oncocytic differentiation diffusely label with antibodies to mitochondrial elements, such as 111.3, and express MUC6 and MUC5AC (focal) {28}. Most IPMNs with onocytic differentiation are negative for MUC2 and CDX2. MUC6, the pyloric-type mucin, is consistently expressed in the pyloric-type glands that can occur in low-grade dysplasia and

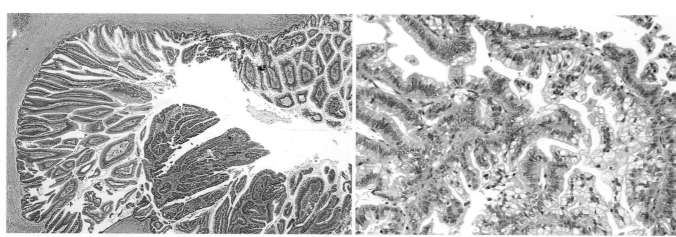

Fig. 12.44 Intestinal-type IPMN, with progression of intermediate-grade dysplasia (left) to high-grade dysplasia (centre right).

Fig. 12.45 Pancreatobiliary-type IPMN, with high-grade dysplasia.

cystic components of any subtype of IPMNs; however, it is mostly confined to pancreatobiliary-type IPMNs, and is not detected in intestinal or gastric types {212}.

Epidermal growth factor receptor (EGFR) is expressed relatively frequently in IPMNs, especially in those with high-grade dysplasia {3631}. *ERBB2* is commonly overexpressed in IPMNs {665, 2827, 2886}. The Ki67 labelling index is associated with grade of dysplasia in IPMNs, being higher in IPMNs with a more significant degree of dysplasia {1363, 1432, 3214}. Loss of expression of *CDKN2A* increases in frequency from IPMNs with low-grade dysplasia to those with high-grade dysplasia {254, 928}. Abnormal labelling with antibodies to p53 has been observed in a small fraction (5–19%) of IPMNs with high-grade dysplasia, but not in those with low-grade dysplasia {928, 1503}. Expression of *SMAD4* (*DPC4*) is preserved in most IPMNs with any grade of dysplasia; this contrasts with the high frequency of loss of expression in high-grade pancreatic intraepithelial neoplasia and in infiltrating ductal adenocarcinoma {254, 928, 1301}.

Cytopathology

On cytological preparations, the findings for IPMNs and MCNs are nearly identical, and the generic cytological diagnosis of "mucinous cyst" is often used to refer to cytological findings consistent with either of these neoplasms. Cyst fluid aspirated from an IPMN can contain highly variable amounts of extracellular mucin and neoplastic epithelium {197, 788, 906, 1769, 2060, 2558, 2648, 3015, 3074}. In many cases, the aspirate is composed only of mucinous material, without a cellular component. Thus, if gastrointestinal contamination can be ruled out, the presence of mucin may be the only manifestation that the lesion is in fact a "mucinous cyst." In such cases, the imaging findings, stains for mucin, and elevated levels of CEA in the cyst fluid {1204}, with or without elevated levels of exocrine enzymes, may be needed to verify the diagnosis of IPMN. As IPMNs connect with the duct system, it has been suggested that cytology of the pancreatic juice may also be useful {1186}.

Owing to sampling phenomena, cytology tends to underestimate the highest histological grade of dysplasia {211, 2060, 2558}. The oncocytic nature of IPMNs

with oncocytic differentiation is reflected in the cytoplasm of the aspirated cells. The presence of small clusters of atypical epithelial cells with irregular nuclei and a high nucleus-to-cytoplasm ratio, with or without visible cytoplasmic mucin, correlates with an increased risk of malignancy, even when these clusters are very few in number {2060, 2558, 2917}. A diagnosis of malignancy is rendered with sufficient quality and quantity of an atypical epithelial component, generally composed of crowded groups of cells with parachromatin clearing, irregular nuclear membranes and nucleoli {1859, 2060, 2700}. Whether the malignant cells represent high-grade dysplasia or invasive carcinoma is often difficult to determine. The association of such cells with abundant acute inflammation or necrosis suggests an associated invasive carcinoma {2060}.

Ultrastructure

IPMN has no specific ultrastructural features {2160}. The neoplastic cells lie on a basement membrane and have numerous microvilli on the apical surface, a number of mitochondria, a well-developed rough endoplasmic reticulum and Golgi apparatus. Mucin droplets of variable size and electron density are present {2160}. Oncocytic-type IPMNs contain numerous mitochondria that exclude other organelles.

Differential diagnosis

The differential diagnosis for larger IPMNs includes other macrocystic (oligocystic) lesions, in particular, MCNs and macrocystic serous cystadenomas {211}. The differential for small IPMNs primarily includes PanIN and retention cysts {35, 1271}.

MCN. MCNs can closely mimic branch-duct type IPMNs {211, 3185}. MCNs typically occur in women with a median age in the fifth decade of life, and almost all

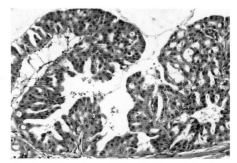

Fig. 12.46 Oncocytic-type IPMN, with high-grade dysplasia.

MCNs are located in the tail or body of the pancreas. The vast majority of MCNs do not communicate with the pancreatic duct system. MCNs contain a cellular "ovarian-type" stroma that expresses hormone receptors by immunohistochemistry. In contrast, IPMNs occur in men slightly more often than women, in a slightly older age group, involving the head of the gland more frequently than the tail, always communicating with the duct system, and do not have ovarian-type stroma.

Macrocystic serous cystadenomas. Macro (oligocystic) serous cystic neoplasms {211} form larger and less defined cysts than the more common microcystic serous cystic neoplasms; they may thus resemble branch-duct IPMNs. However, the epithelial cells of macrocystic serous cystic neoplasms are cuboidal and have glycogen-rich clear cytoplasm, with no mucin and no significant nuclear atypia.

PanIN. PanINs should be distinguished from small IPMNs. Most PanINs are < 0.5 cm in greatest ductal diameter, whereas IPMNs are defined to be grossly detectable cystic lesions that typically measure ≥ 1.0 cm {1271}. Lesions measuring 0.5–1.0 cm with mucinous epithelium are intermediate-grade lesions. PanINs tend to have short stubby papillae, while IPMNs often have long finger-

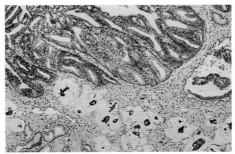 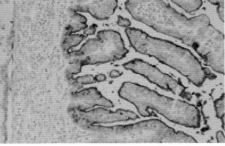

Fig. 12.47 A Intestinal-type IPMN, with an invasive colloid carcinoma. Immunolabelling for MUC2 labels both components. **B** Pancreatobiliary-type IPMN, with high-grade dysplasia. Immunolabelling for MUC1 reveals a cell-surface pattern of expression.

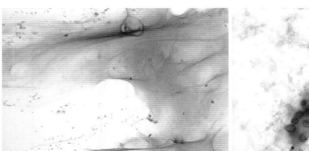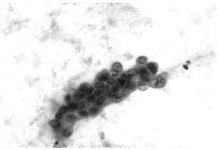

Fig. 12.48 Fine-needle aspiration cytology of IPMN (Papanicolaou stain). **A** Thick extracellular mucin is typical. **B** The presence of parachromatin clearing, irregular nuclear membranes and nucelar-size variation correlates with high-grade dysplasia.

like papillae. The presence of abundant luminal mucin and the expression of MUC2 suggests a diagnosis of IPMN {35, 1271}. However, there is histological overlap, and the distinction between these two lesions can be nearly impossible in cases measuring between 0.5 and 1.0 cm.

Retention cysts. These are usually unilocular and are lined by a flat single layer of ductal epithelium without nuclear atypia. Mucinous cytoplasm is typically lacking, although retention cysts can be focally involved by PanIN {1652}.

ITPN. ITPNs may resemble IPMNs of the pancreatobiliary type {1646, 3157, 3580}. IPMNs are distinguished by more complex papillary architecture, fewer tubular structures, and evident intracellular mucin. The similarities between pancreatobiliary variant of IPMN and intraductal tubulopapillary neoplasms include expression of MUC6 {212}.

Acinar cell carcinoma. Some acinar cell carcinomas have a prominent intraductal pattern of growth and contain papilla, and can resemble IPMNs {213}. The cells of these carcinomas contain abundant apical, acidophilic zymogen granules, and immunolabelling reveals the expression of pancreatic exocrine enzymes {213, 3254}.

Oncocytic variants. The differential diagnosis of rare solid examples of oncocytic-type IPMN include occasional oncocytic variants of pancreatic neoplasms, such as oncocytic neuroendocrine neoplasms, and rare oncocytic solid-pseudopapillary neoplasms; however, careful sampling allows for the recognition of the characteristic features of the respective entities in each case.

Pseudoinvasion. The distinction between an invasive carcinoma arising in association with an IPMN and pseudoinvasion is critically important. In particular, benign mucin spillage into the stroma that presumably occurs owing to rupture of involved distended duct can mimic an invasive colloid carcinoma. Mucin spillage is characterized by stromal dissection by acellular mucin and is usually associated with a brisk inflammatory reaction. In contrast, the stromal mucin of invasive carcinoma contains neoplastic cells and is usually not associated with intense inflammation; however, any mucin in the stroma should be evaluated carefully as being suspicious for invasion. Similarly, IPMN extending along branch ducts or tributary ductules may create the impression of early invasion. The lobular architecture, smooth contours of the units, and morphological similarity to the larger lesion are the main features that help distinguish this pattern of growth from invasive carcinoma.

Genetic susceptibility

Some patients with a strong family history of pancreatic cancer develop an IPMN, suggesting that IPMNs may be part of a genetic susceptibility syndrome {4, 407}. Although the gene in most cases is not known, IPMNs have been reported in individuals with the Peutz-Jeghers syndrome, and genetic analyses have revealed biallelic inactivation of the *STK11* gene in these neoplasms, suggesting a causal link between Peutz-Jeghers and IPMNs {2822}. Also, excessive rates of synchronous and metachronous gastric and colonic epithelial neoplasms have been reported in patients with IPMNs {216, 768, 1468, 2655, 3122}. This finding suggests the possibility of genetic predisposition, but no specific hereditary syndrome linking IPMNs with other cancers has been established.

Molecular pathology

Activating point mutations in codon 12 of the *KRAS* oncogene have been reported in 30–80% of IPMNs, and the prevalence of these mutations increases with increasing degree of dysplasia {2852, 3333}. Heterogeneous mutations in *KRAS* have been identified in multicentric IPMNs, helping to establish these lesions as polyclonal {353, 1580}. *KRAS* mutations have not been reported in IPMNs with oncocytic differentiation {562}. *PIK3CA* gene mutations occur in about 10% of IPMNs, which is in contrast to pancreatic ductal adenocarcinoma, in which no mutations in *PIK3CA* have so far been found {1818, 2853}. Mutations in the *BRAF* gene are found in a small fraction of IPMNs {2852}. Allelic losses involving loci of tumour-suppressor genes, including *CDKN2A*, *TP53*, and *SMAD4*, are found in up to 40% of IPMNs, and these losses increase with increasing degree of dysplasia {4, 908, 3424}. Although mutations in *CDKN2A* are not common, methylation of the *CDKN2A* promoter, resulting in loss of expression, is more frequently found in IPMNs {2176, 2823}. *TP53* gene mutations have been reported in IPMNs with high-grade dysplasia {465, 2176}. Despite the high frequency of allelic loss involving the *SMAD4* locus, mutations in the *SMAD4* gene are rare, and expression of the SMAD4/DPC4 protein is preserved in most noninvasive IPMNs {1301, 1330}.

Prognosis and predictive factors

It is generally agreed that all main-duct IPMNs should be surgically resected because of the significant risk of high-grade dysplasia or an invasive carcinoma {2786, 2787, 3123, 3185, 3199, 3222}. Branch-duct IPMNs are less likely to harbour high-grade dysplasia or an associated invasive carcinoma {2512, 2786, 2787, 2848, 3005, 3123, 3199, 3222}. International consensus guidelines defining the indications for the surgical resection of branch-duct IPMNs were published by the International Association of Pancreatology {3185}. These guidelines recommend that patients with symptoms related to their IPMN, those with main-duct dilatation, and those with a branch-duct IPMNs of > 30 mm or with a mural nodule should undergo resection. Smaller branch-duct IPMNs without these features can be followed using imaging such as CT and MRI {3185}. These criteria have

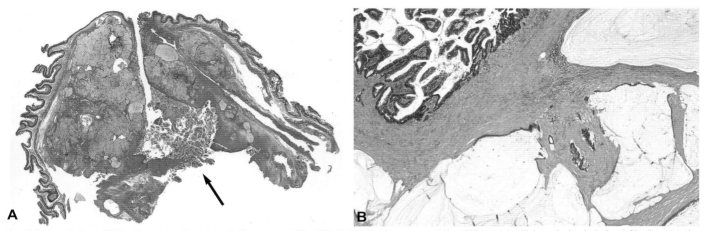

Fig. 12.49 Intestinal-type IPMN with associated invasive colloid carcinoma. **A** The IPMN is indicated by an arrow. **B** The IPMN contains high-grade dysplasia (top left) adjacent to the invasive colloid carcinoma (bottom right).

recently been validated in several retrospective and prospective studies {1779, 2512, 2704, 2771, 2848, 3124, 3185, 3199}. That most IPMNs occur in older age groups with several comorbities is a major confounding factor in the management of these patients.

Another subclassification of IPMNs with some predictive value for clinical outcome is based on the phenotype of the neoplastic cells {36, 1352}. Gastric-type IPMNs are often noninvasive lesions, and most reveal low-grade dysplasia. Most branch-duct IPMNs are of this type. In contrast, intestinal-type IPMNs tend to be large, often of the main-duct type, and commonly harbour high-grade dysplastic changes. Invasive carcinomas arising from this type are more commonly colloid carcinomas. Pancreatobiliary-type IPMN, the least common type, tends to have high-grade dysplasia, and invasive carcinomas associated with this phenotype are usually of tubular type.

The main determinant of outcome for surgically resected IPMNs is the presence or absence of an associated invasive carcinoma. IPMNs without an associated invasive component are often curable; the 5-year survival rate for patients with resected noninvasive IPMNs is 90–95% {492, 3005}. While some of the mortality in this group represents deaths from other causes and the presence of residual neoplasm at a margin {3287, 3497}, the observation that patients with noninvasive IPMNs who undergo a total pancreatectomy have a nearly 100% survival rate suggests that metachronous multifocal disease remains a significant risk for these patients. Certainly, these data sug-

gest that careful clinical follow-up is warranted following the surgical resection of a noninvasive IPMN, even if the margins are not involved {3497}. It should be kept in mind that invasive carcinoma may develop in parts of the pancreas grossly separate from the main IPMN {3587}.

The prognosis for IPMNs with an associated invasive carcinoma is significantly worse than for noninvasive IPMNs; the 5-year survival rates for IPMNs with an associated invasive carcinoma are reported to be between 27% and 60%, depending upon the extent and histological type of the invasive component {492, 816, 1579, 1723, 2787, 2848, 2940, 3005, 3497}. Patients with a colloid (mucinous noncystic) type of invasive carcinoma have a better prognosis than do those with a ductal (tubular) type of invasive cancer {36, 2575B}. Those with invasion of < 5 mm have an excellent prognosis {2252}, whereas the prognosis for advanced-stage invasive carcinomas arising in association with IPMNs (i.e. with metastasis to the lymph nodes or other sites) is as poor as for invasive ductal adenocarcinoma {2252, 2848, 2757B}.

Intraductal tubulopapillary neoplasm (ITPN)

Definition

An intraductal, grossly visible, tubule-forming epithelial neoplasm with high-grade dysplasia and ductal differentiation without overt production of mucin {1597, 3112, 3156, 3580}. Focal tubulopapillary growth may be seen. If there is a component of invasive carcinoma, the lesions

are designated "intraductal tubulopapillary neoplasm with an associated invasive carcinoma".

Epidemiology

Intraductal tubulopapillary neoplasms (ITPNs) are rare neoplasms accounting for < 1% of all pancreatic exocrine neoplasms and only 3% of intraductal neoplasms of the pancreas {3580}. Although data on this entity are still limited, ITPNs occur equally frequently in males and females. The age range of reported cases has been between 35 and 84 years, with a mean age of 56 years.

Clinical features

Patients present with nonspecific symptoms including abdominal pain, vomiting, weight loss, steatorrhea, and diabetes mellitus. Obstructive jaundice is uncommon. Some patients are asymptomatic, and their neoplasms are detected incidentally during the clinical evaluation for other conditions. Laboratory tests, including those for cancer antigens in the blood, are nonspecific. Imaging studies,

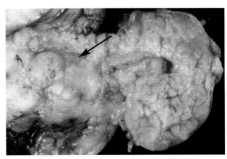

Fig. 12.50 ITPN, gross appearance. Note the polypoid component within the main pancreatic duct (arrow).

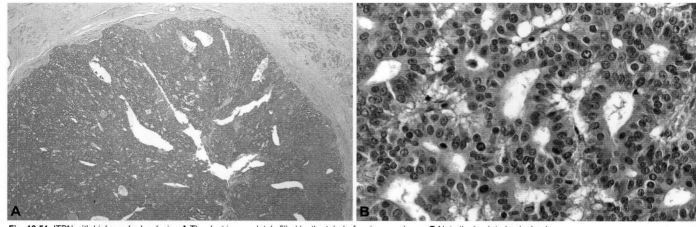

Fig. 12.51 ITPN with high-grade dysplasia. **A** The duct is completely filled by the tubule-forming neoplasm. **B** Note the back-to-back glands.

particularly CT, endoscopic ultrasonography and endoscopic retrograde cholangiopancreatography (ERCP), may be helpful in demonstrating the intraductal location of the lesion. Preoperatively, most ITPNs are indistinguishable from IPMNs. About half of ITPNs occur in the head of the pancreas; a third diffusely involve the gland, and 15% are localized to the tail.

Macroscopy

Grossly, ITPNs form solid, nodular masses within dilated pancreatic ducts {1209, 1597, 3112, 3580}. The nodules are large (up to 9 cm), dense and fleshy to rubbery. Cyst formation is often less evident than in IPMNs. Mucinous secretions are not present in the dilated ducts of ITPNs. The intraductal location of the tumour can usually be confirmed by a careful dissection of the ductal system. The average ITPN is 6 cm in diameter (range, 0.8–15.0 cm). The surrounding pancreatic tissue is usually densely sclerotic.

Histopathology

ITPNs form nodules of back-to-back tubular glands with occasional papillary elements, resulting in large cribriformed structures within dilated pancreatic ducts {1597, 3156, 3580}. Mucin is typically not detectable, or, is minimal at most. While most ITPNs are predominantly or exclusively tubular, papillae may be present in some {3580}. Solid areas with abortive glandular arrangements may also be seen. Some of the neoplastic nodules obliterate the ductal lumen, appearing as sharply circumscribed nests of cells surrounded by fibrotic stroma. ITPNs are architecturally complex and typically have

high-grade dysplasia. Each neoplastic nodule consists of tightly packed small acinar glands lined by predominantly cuboidal cells with modest amounts of eosinophilic to amphophilic cytoplasm. In some cases, apocrine snout-like formations are noted in the apical surface of the cells. Intraluminal secretions may be seen. Cases with more papillary growth also tend to be complex {1646, 3580}. The nuclei are round to oval and moderately to markedly atypical. Mitotic figures are often readily identifiable (range, 0–9 per 10 high power fields) {3580}. Some cases contain foci of necrosis or desmoplastic stroma within the intraductal, polypoid neoplastic nodules. Occasionally, a comedocarcinoma-like pattern is noted. In general, cyst formation is less prominent than in IPMNs.

ITPNs typically have a relatively homogeneous appearance, and there are no transitions to areas with less marked cytoarchitectural atypia, or to IPMNs {3156, 3157, 3580}.

Invasive carcinoma is found in association with about 40% of cases and the invasive component is usually limited in extent {1597, 3112, 3580}. Because many of the individual neoplastic nodules lack a peripheral rim of non-neoplastic ductal epithelium, it can be difficult to recognize invasive carcinoma. Thin strands of cells extending into the stroma surrounding the circumscribed neoplastic nodules represent invasive carcinoma. The cytological appearance of the invasive elements is similar to that of the intraductal portion, and typically exhibits a tubular pattern.

Immunohistochemistry

The immunohistochemical labelling profile of ITPNs confirms their ductal nature. The neoplastic cells commonly label for keratins 7 and 19, in addition to displaying consistent positivity for pankeratins. Labelling for the acinar marker, trypsin, and endocrine markers chromogranin and synaptophysin, is negative. Mucin-related glycoproteins are typically expressed at lower levels than in mucinous ductal neoplasms: CA19-9 is commonly detected but only as a focal finding. B72.3, CEA and CA125/MUC16 are detected in less than half of cases and typically as a very focal finding. Neither MUC5AC, which is a consistent marker of IPMNs regardless of type, nor MUC2, which is expressed in intestinal-type IPMNs, are expressed in ITPNs. MUC1 is expressed in 90% and MUC6 in 60% of ITPNs. The expression of SMAD4/DPC4 is retained in most cases. Immunohistochemical expression of p53 and CDKN2A/p16 are detected in 20% and 54% of cases, respectively. The Ki67 labelling index varies from case to case (range, 6–43%). β-Catenin nuclear expression and loss of E-cadherin expression are reported in < 10% of ITPNs.

Cytopathology

There have been no systematic analyses of cyst fluid in patients with ITPN. In a case report {155}, prominent tubular growth was documented in cytological smears from an endoscopic ultrasound-guided biopsy of an ITPN.

Differential diagnosis

On clinical grounds, the main differential diagnosis of ITPNs is with IPMNs. Both may present with intraductal lesions showing solid and cystic areas. ITPNs appear to occur in younger patients (average age is a decade younger than that of patients with IPMNs). The presence of copious mucin is characteristic of IPMN, and prominent cystic change is also more common in IPMNs. On microscopic examination, IPMNs of gastric and intestinal types are easy to distinguish from ITPNs by their mucinous nature in parallel with their MUC-immunolabelling profile showing MUC5AC and MUC2 expression, respectively, as well as the presence of a spectrum of neoplastic changes that contrast with the more uniform appearance of ITPNs. Some pancreatobiliary-type IPMNs may be difficult to distinguish from ITPNs. Significant amounts of mucin, the presence of a component with low-grade dysplasia, and the expression of MUC5AC would all favour a diagnosis of pancreatobiliary-type IPMN.

It has been suggested that some ITPNs have a predominantly papillary growth pattern, an area that deserves further study {3580}.

On histological sections, more tubular examples of ITPN can be difficult to distinguish from acinar cell carcinomas, which may also grow intraductally {213}. In contrast with ITPNs, acinar cell carcinomas often have apical acidophilic granules, which can be highlighted by PAS stain, and occasionally display intraluminal crystals (enzymatic concretions). Immunohistochemical labelling for markers of pancreatic exocrine enzymes, such as chymotrypsin, may be crucial in this differential diagnosis.

Prognosis and predictive factors

The limited data in the literature regarding the prognosis for patients with ITPNs suggest that these neoplasms are relatively indolent neoplasms, with a prognosis that is significantly better than that of infiltrating ductal adenocarcinoma of the pancreas {1597, 3112, 3156, 3580}. Survival beyond 5 years is noted in more than a third of the patients reported {1597}. Recurrence and metastasis to lymph nodes or to the liver are reported in about a third of cases, and even these patients sometimes experience a protracted clinical course over > 2 years, which would be unusual for conventional ductal adenocarcinoma. In one study {1597}, no significant correlation between invasion and survival was identified, which was attributed to the microscopic nature of the invasion detected in most cases, and also partly to the fact that inadequate sampling may have missed small foci of invasion in the neoplasms classified as noninvasive. We recommend that the invasive carcinomas associated with these neoplasms be reported and staged separately, as is done for IPMNs.

Acinar cell neoplasms of the pancreas

D.S. Klimstra
R.H. Hruban
G. Klöppel
T. Morohoshi
N. Ohike

Introduction

Acinar cell neoplasms are epithelial neoplasms defined by their morphological resemblance to acinar cells and the production of pancreatic exocrine enzymes. Most are solid malignant neoplasms (acinar cell carcinoma). A rare benign cystic lesion (acinar cell cystadenoma) and rare malignant cystic (acinar cell cystadenocarcinoma) and mixed carcinomas (mixed acinar-neuroendocrine carcinoma, mixed acinar-ductal carcinoma, and mixed acinar-neuroendocrine-ductal carcinoma) also exist.

ICD-O codes

Acinar cell cystadenoma	8551/0
Acinar cell carcinoma	8550/3
Acinar cell cystadenocarcinoma	8551/3
Mixed acinar-neuroendocrine carcinoma	8154/3
Mixed acinar-neuroendocrine-ductal carcinoma	8154/3
Mixed acinar-ductal carcinoma	8552/3

Acinar cell cystadenoma

Definition

Acinar cell cystadenoma is a benign cystic epithelial lesion lined by cells with morphological resemblance to acinar cells and with evidence of pancreatic exocrine enzyme production.

Epidemiology

The lesion is too rare to establish epidemiological associations.

Localization

Acinar cell cystadenomas may involve any portion of the pancreas, but are more common in the head, and some involve the entire gland {3674}.

Clinical features

Cases are divided into two categories: clinically recognized macroscopic lesions and incidental microscopic findings. Clinically recognized cases may present with abdominal pain or, in one case, polyarthralgia, or they may be detected by radiographic imaging in asymptomatic patients {3674}. Incidental cases are identified only microscopically in pancreata removed for other reasons.

Macroscopy

Clinically recognized acinar cell cystadenomas range from 1.5 to 10.0 cm in diameter (mean, 6 cm) and form unilocular or multilocular cystic masses that are usually grossly circumscribed {64, 496, 3674}. Individual cysts range from 1 mm to several cm. The cysts contain watery fluid and have a smooth lining. Communication with the ductal system of the pancreas is rare. Some cases are multicentric and others diffusely involve the entire gland, with islands of parenchyma between the cysts. Incidentally detected acinar cell cystadenomas are usually < 1.0 cm and unilocular, and some are not apparent grossly.

Histopathology

Acinar cell cystadenomas produce variably sized cysts; some are little more than slightly dilated acinar-like spaces, whereas others are more substantial. Most of the cysts are lined by well-differentiated cells with acinar differentiation, either in a single layer or forming small clusters of cells surrounding the lumen {64, 496, 3674}. Residual pancreatic elements are present between the larger cysts, and some of the adjacent acini may be dilated. The lesional cells have basally situated, uniform nuclei, apical granular eosinophilic cytoplasm, and basal cytoplasmic basophilia, resembling non-neoplastic acinar cells. In some cases, the cysts are partially lined by cuboidal cells that lack cytoplasmic granules and that instead resemble normal ductal epithelium. Incidental microscopic cases may consist of a single cyst lined by cells with acinar differentiation. Transitions to ductal epithelium including cells with columnar, mucinous cytoplasm (low-grade pancreatic intraepithelial neoplasia, PanIN) may be found. The cyst lumina may contain inspissated eosinophilic enzymatic secretions. The surrounding pancreatic parenchyma is typically fibrotic and atrophic. The lining cells stain with periodic acid–Schiff and are resistant to diastase. Staining for mucins is negative.

Immunohistochemistry

Acinar cell cystadenomas express pancreatic exocrine enzymes, including trypsin, chymotrypsin, and lipase {64, 496, 3674}. Most cases show diffuse labelling of the lesional cells and the luminal secretions, although some with a greater

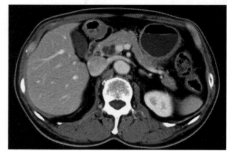

Fig. 12.52 CT scan of an acinar cell cystadenoma.

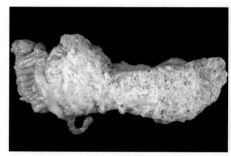

Fig. 12.53 Acinar cell cystadenoma involving the entire length of the pancreas.

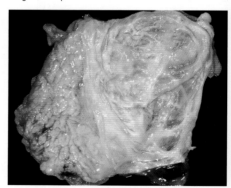

Fig. 12.54 Acinar cell cystadenoma. In contrast to Fig. 12.50, this lesion is localized.

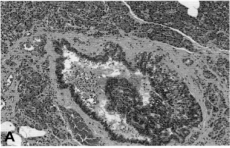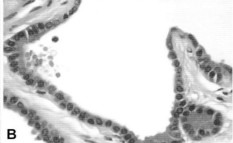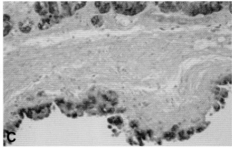

Fig. 12.55 Acinar cell cystadenoma. **A** Small acinar cell cystadenoma. **B** Cystic structures are lined by acinar cells. **C** The lesion displays granular labelling for trypsin.

proportion of duct-like cells only label focally. Keratins (e.g. keratin 8 and 18) are also expressed {3674}.

Differential diagnosis

Small, incidental acinar cell cystadenomas can resemble PanINs. Recognition of the granular eosinophilic cytoplasm and the absence of mucin help confirm the diagnosis of acinar cell cystadenoma. Larger acinar cell cystadenomas can be confused with serous cystic neoplasms, squamoid cyst of pancreatic ducts, or mucinous cystic neoplasms (MCNs). Again, recognition of acinar differentiation is very helpful. Acinar cell cystadenomas lack the clear cells of serous cystic neoplasms, the squamous differentiation of squamoid cysts, and the mucinous cells and ovarian-type stroma of MCNs {2414}.

Prognosis and predictive factors

All acinar cell cystadenomas reported to date have been clinically benign, and there is no evidence of malignant transformation or association with acinar cell carcinoma {64, 496, 3674}. In fact, some authorities have questioned the neoplastic nature of acinar cell cystadenoma, especially of the incidental microscopic examples. Cases involving the entire pancreas present a management dilemma, given the radical nature of the operation necessary to completely remove the lesion.

Acinar cell carcinoma

Definition

Acinar cell carcinoma is a malignant epithelial neoplasm composed of cells with morphological resemblance to acinar cells and with evidence of pancreatic exocrine enzyme production. Cases with significant endocrine or ductal components (i.e. > 25% of the neoplasm) are regarded as mixed carcinomas (mixed

acinar-neuroendocrine carcinoma, mixed acinar-ductal carcinoma, or mixed acinar-neuroendocrine-ductal carcinoma) {1270, 3070, 3073}. Rare cases with macroscopic, nondegenerative cyst formation have been reported as acinar cell cystadenocarcinoma {408, 583, 1235, 1376, 3054}.

Epidemiology

Acinar cell carcinomas represent 1–2% of all exocrine pancreatic neoplasms in adults {1235, 1598} and 15% of those in children {1227, 1235, 1598}. Most occur in late adulthood, with a mean age of 58 years (range, 10–87 years) {1376, 1682, 3474}. Paediatric cases account for only 6% of acinar cell carcinomas, usually in patients of 8–15 years of age {1682, 2161}. Males are affected more frequently than females, with a male-to-female ratio of 3.6 : 1 {1235, 1598}. There are no known racial associations.

Localization

Acinar cell carcinomas may arise in any portion of the pancreas, but are somewhat more common in the head.

Clinical features

Most acinar cell carcinomas present with nonspecific symptoms including abdominal or back pain, weight loss, nausea, or diarrhoea {1235, 1598, 1682, 2001, 3474}. Since they generally compress rather than infiltrate into adjacent structures, biliary obstruction and jaundice are infrequent presenting complaints.

Hypersecretion syndrome

The lipase hypersecretion syndrome occurs in 10–15% of patients {377, 1598, 1673, 3012}. It is more commonly encountered in patients with hepatic metastases and is caused by the release into the serum of excessive amounts of lipase by the neoplasm, with clinical symptoms

including subcutaneous fat necrosis and polyarthralgia. Peripheral blood eosinophilia may also be noted. In some patients, lipase hypersecretion syndrome is the first presenting sign of the carcinoma, while in others it develops after tumour recurrence. Successful surgical removal of the neoplasm may result in the normalization of the serum lipase levels and resolution of the symptoms. Other than an elevation of serum lipase levels associated with the lipase hypersecretion syndrome, there are no specific laboratory abnormalities in patients with acinar cell carcinoma. Serum α-fetoprotein levels are elevated in some patients {1365, 2313, 2403, 2949}.

Imaging

Radiographically, acinar cell carcinomas are generally bulky, with a mean size of 11 cm, and cases of < 2 cm are rare {1682}. On abdominal computed tomography (CT) scans, they are circumscribed and enhance homogeneously, although less than the surrounding pancreas {3205}. Cystic change attributable to necrosis can occur. Owing to their larger size and relatively sharp circumscription, acinar cell carcinomas can generally be distinguished from ductal adenocarcinomas radiographically.

Macroscopy

Acinar cell carcinomas are generally softer and more circumscribed than ductal adenocarcinomas. They may be multinodular {1235, 1598}. Individual nodules are soft and vary from yellow to brown. Areas of necrosis and cystic degeneration may be present. Extension into adjacent structures, such as duodenum, spleen, or major vessels may occur. Some acinar cell carcinomas grossly involve the ductal system, with polypoid nodules projecting into dilated pancreatic ducts {213, 810, 3254}.

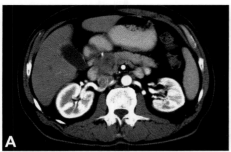 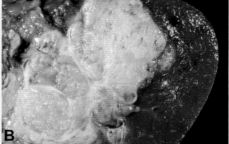

Fig. 12.56 Acinar cell carcinoma. **A** CT of an acinar cell carcinoma in the head of the pancreas. **B** Acinar cell carcinoma in the tail of the pancreas.

Tumour spread and staging

Metastases are found in half of patients at presentation and another 25% develop them following surgical resection of the primary carcinoma {1598}. Most commonly metastases involve regional lymph nodes and the liver, although metastatic spread to other organs occurs occasionally, and some patients present with distant metastases as the first manifestation of the disease {3348}. Acinar cell carcinomas are staged using the same protocol as ductal adenocarcinomas.

Histopathology

Acinar cell carcinomas are highly cellular, with a high neoplastic-cell-to-stroma ratio. These neoplasms are composed of large circumscribed nodules of neoplastic cells separated by hypocellular fibrous bands {1235, 1598}. The desmoplastic stroma characteristic of ductal adenocarcinomas is generally absent. Tumour necrosis may occur and is generally infarct-like in appearance. Numerous small vessels surround the nests of neoplastic cells.

Architectural patterns

Of the several architectural patterns described {1598}, the most characteristic is the acinar pattern, with neoplastic cells arranged in small acinar units; there are numerous small lumina within each island of cells, producing a cribriform appearance. In some instances, the lumina are more dilated, resulting in the glandular pattern, although individual glandular units, each surrounded by stroma, are not commonly encountered. A number of the microglandular carcinomas previously reported as "microadenocarcinoma" were more recently shown to have been acinar cell carcinomas {1890}. The second most common pattern is the solid pattern: solid nests of neoplastic cells lacking luminal formations separated by small vessels.

Within these nests, cellular polarization is generally not evident, but there may be an accentuation of polarization at the interface with the vessels, resulting in basal nuclear localization in these regions and a palisading of nuclei along the microvasculature. In rare instances, a trabecular arrangement of neoplastic cells may be present, with exceptional cases also showing a gyriform appearance {1598}.

Recently, intraductal and papillary variants of acinar cell carcinoma have been reported {213, 810, 3254}. These neoplasms are composed of polypoid growths of neoplastic cells histologically similar to conventional acinar cell carcinoma projecting into dilated ducts, some of which retain a layer of normal ductal epithelium surrounding the carcinomatous polyp. In rare cases, true papillae may be found, with fibrovascular cores lined by neoplastic cells with acinar differentiation. Most such cases have areas with conventional histological features elsewhere in the neoplasm.

High magnification

At high magnification, the neoplastic cells of acinar cell carcinoma contain minimal to moderate amounts of cytoplasm that may be more abundant in cells lining lumina. The cytoplasm varies from amphophilic to eosinophilic and is characteristically finely granular, reflecting the presence of zymogen granules (although only minimal cytoplasmic granularity may be detectable in many cases). The nuclei are generally round to oval and relatively uniform, with marked nuclear pleomorphism being exceptional {1595, 2518}. A single, prominent, central nucleolus is characteristic but not invariably present. The mitotic rate ranges from 0 to more than 50 per 10 high power fields (mean, 14 per 10 high power fields).

Zymogen granules are weakly positive with PAS staining, and resistant to diastase. Mucin production is generally not detectable with mucicarmine or Alcian blue stains and, if present, is limited to the luminal membrane in acinar or glandular formations. Owing to the scarcity of zymogen granules in many examples of acinar cell carcinoma, histochemical stains are relatively insensitive for documenting acinar differentiation, and very focal staining may be difficult to interpret.

Immunohistochemistry

Immunohistochemical detection of the production of pancreatic exocrine enzymes (e.g. trypsin, chymotrypsin, lipase, and elastase) is helpful in confirming the diagnosis of acinar cell carcinoma {1235, 1356, 1598, 2161}. Both trypsin and chymotrypsin are detectable in > 95% of cases; lipase is less commonly identified (approximately 70% of cases) {1598}. In solid areas, immunohistochemical labelling for these enzymes may show diffuse cytoplasmic positivity, whereas the reaction product is restricted to the apical cytoplasm in acinar areas. Pancreatic stone protein, pancreatic secretory trypsin inhibitor, phospholipase A2, and BCL10 are also commonly expressed

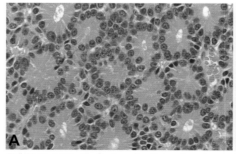 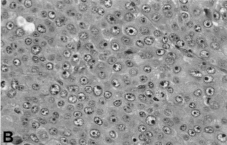

Fig. 12.57 Architectural patterns in acinar cell carcinoma. **A** Acinar pattern. Note the granular, eosinophilic cytoplasm and single, prominent nucleoli. **B** Solid pattern. Note the single prominent nucleoli, obvious mitotic figures, and cytoplasmic basophilia.

{1235, 1682, 1704, 3012}. Acinar cell carcinomas express keratins 8 and 18, but usually do not label with antibodies to keratins 7, 19, or 20 {2406}.

Scattered individual cells labelling for chromogranin A or synaptophysin are found in more than one third of acinar cell carcinomas. More than half focally express carcinoembryonic antigen (CEA) and B72.3 {1235, 1598}. Uncommonly, there is immunohistochemical positivity for α-fetoprotein, mostly in younger patients and in cases associated with elevations in serum α-fetoprotein {564, 1365}.

Reflecting abnormalities in the APC/β-catenin pathway, some acinar cell carcinomas show nuclear immunolabelling for β-catenin that can be patchy or diffuse {586}. There is also strong membranous expression of claudin 7 and absence of claudin 5 {586}.

Cytopathology

Fine-needle aspirates are usually highly cellular {1356, 1710, 2791, 3070, 3405}. The neoplastic cells are arranged in irregular solid sheets, small glandular clusters, and individually. The cytological appearance of acinar cell carcinoma closely mimics that of pancreatic neuroendocrine neoplasm, although smears from the latter are more likely to contain uniform plasmacytoid cells and speckled chromatin. Coarsely clumped chromatin and prominent nucleoli are typical of acinar cell carcinoma. Immunohistochemistry may be used on cytological specimens to confirm acinar differentiation {1710}.

Ultrastructure

Exocrine secretory features are consistently found, with abundant rough endoplasmic reticulum arranged in parallel arrays and relatively abundant mitochondria {716, 1132, 1598, 3318}. Most acinar cell carcinomas contain electron-dense zymogen granules ranging in size from 125 to 1000 nm. A second granule type, the irregular fibrillary granule, is detected ultrastructurally in many cases {538, 1598, 1601, 2496}.

Histological variants

Acinar cell cystadenocarcinoma

Acinar cell cystadenocarcinomas are rare, grossly cystic neoplasms with acinar differentiation {408, 583, 1235, 1376, 3054}. Most cases are large tumours (mean, 24 cm) with variably sized cysts

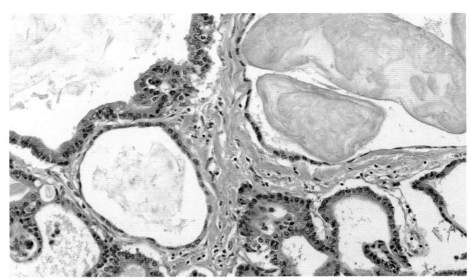

Fig. 12.58 Acinar cell cystadenocarcinoma.

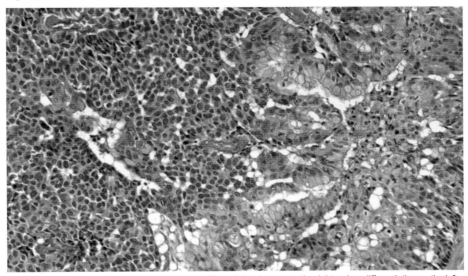

Fig. 12.59 Mixed acinar-ductal carcinoma. Ductal differentiation is seen on the right, acinar differentiation on the left.

that are often < 1 cm in diameter. The cysts are lined by layers of neoplastic cells with acinar morphology that immunolabel for pancreatic exocrine enzymes. The clinical behaviour of these neoplasms is not different from that of conventional acinar cell carcinoma.

Mixed acinar carcinomas

Rare neoplasms have shown a substantial (> 30%) proportion of more than one cell type. These "mixed acinar carcinomas" have been designated, depending upon the cell types identified, as "mixed acinar-neuroendocrine carcinoma", "mixed acinar-ductal carcinoma", or "mixed acinar-neuroendocrine-ductal carcinoma" {1270, 1710, 2313, 2369, 3405}. These mixed

acinar carcinomas are described in greater detail in *Ductal adenocarcinoma variants and mixed neoplasms*.

Differential diagnosis

Other pancreatic neoplasms with a solid, cellular appearance should be considered in the differential diagnosis with acinar cell carcinoma. These include pancreatic neuroendocrine tumours (NETs), pancreatoblastoma, and solid-pseudopapillary neoplasm {1594, 1600}. *Pancreatic neuroendocrine tumours (NETs).* These neoplasms are commonly confused with acinar cell carcinomas because they share certain architectural patterns (nesting, trabecular) and cytological features (uniform nuclei,

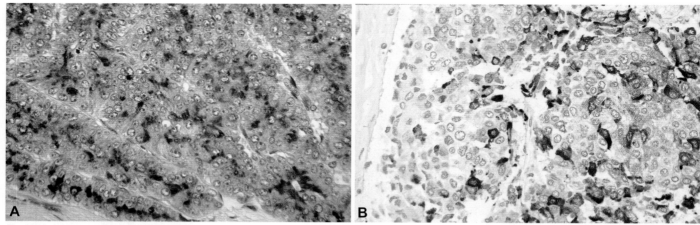

Fig. 12.60 **A** Acinar cell carcinoma with immunohistochemical labelling for trypsin. **B** Mixed acinar-neuroendocrine carcinoma showing immunoreactivity for chromogranin.

eosinophilic to amphophilic cytoplasm) and because acinar cell carcinomas may have focal or (in the case of mixed acinar-neuroendocrine carcinomas) widespread labelling for chromogranin and synaptophysin. Features that favour a diagnosis of acinar cell carcinoma include single prominent nucleoli, granular eosinophilic cytoplasm, basal nuclear polarization, abundant acinar formations, absolutely no fibrotic stroma within neoplastic nodules, an elevated mitotic rate, and limited labelling for neuroendocrine markers {1270}. If the diagnosis of acinar cell carcinoma is considered, immunohistochemical labelling for trypsin and chymotrypsin are usually sufficient to establish the diagnosis, although it should be noted that scattered trypsin-expressing cells can be found in pancreatic NETs {3622}.

Pancreatoblastomas. Pancreatoblastomas share with acinar cell carcinomas the consistent presence of acinar differentiation, both at the histological and immunohistochemical levels {2980}. Pancreatoblastomas most commonly affect children < 10 years of age, although cases in adulthood have been reported {1602}. The characteristic feature of pancreatoblastoma is the squamoid nests. Squamoid nests are circumscribed islands of larger, spindled cells that may show keratinization. There is also more pronounced lobulation in pancreatoblastomas, and the stromal bands separating the lobules are hypercellular.

Solid-pseudopapillary neoplasms. These neoplasms typically affect young females and are composed of uniform, poorly cohesive polygonal cells arranged in solid sheets and degenerative pseudopapillae supplied by an abundant network of small delicate vessels {1603}. True glands or acini are not present. Solid-pseudopapillary neoplasms usually contain aggregates of large eosinophilic hyaline globules, foamy histiocytes and cholesterol clefts. The mitotic rate is usually very low. Immunohistochemically, solid-pseudopapillary neoplasms do not express trypsin, chymotrypsin, lipase, or chromogranin, although synaptophysin and CD56 (NCAM1) may be positive. Solid-pseudopapillary neoplasms will also express vimentin, CD10, α-1-antitrypsin, and β-catenin (nuclear){8}.

Molecular pathology

In contrast to ductal adenocarcinomas, acinar cell carcinomas very rarely have *KRAS* gene mutations, p53 immunoreactivity, loss of *SMAD4* (*DPC4*) expression, or *CDKN2A* (*p16*) abnormalities {18, 1235, 2141, 2513, 3218, 3219}. Half of acinar cell carcinomas have losses of heterozygosity (LOH) on chromosome arm 11p and 25% have abnormalities in the APC/β-catenin pathway, either activating mutations in the β-catenin gene, *CTNNB1*, or truncating mutations in the *APC* gene {18}. Immunolabelling for the β-catenin protein can show a normal membranous pattern of labelling, diffuse abnormal nuclear labelling, or a peculiar mosiac pattern with some cells showing nuclear labelling and others showing membranous labelling.

Prognosis and predictive factors

Acinar cell carcinomas are aggressive; however, outcome is better than that for stage-matched infiltrating ductal adenocarcinomas, with 5-year survival figures of 25–50% depending on stage at diagnosis {1576, 2001, 2844, 3528}. There are reports of survival for several years in the presence of metastatic disease, and responses to chemotherapy have been noted {1598}. Thus, the prognosis for acinar cell carcinoma is somewhat less poor than that of ductal adenocarcinoma.

The most important prognostic factor is stage, with patients lacking lymph-node or distant metastases surviving longer than patients with metastases {1598}. Being < 65 years of age and negative surgical resection margins also predict a better outcome {2844}. Patients with the lipase hypersecretion syndrome have a particularly short survival because most of these patients have hepatic metastases. No specific grading system for acinar cell carcinomas has been proposed. In particular, no association between the extent of acinus formation and prognosis has been observed.

There is an insufficient number of paediatric acinar cell carcinomas to allow an accurate assessment of the biological behaviour of this neoplasm in children, but available data suggest that acinar cell carcinomas occurring in patients < 20 years of age may be less aggressive than their adult counterparts {1598, 2436, 2958}.

Pancreatoblastoma

T. Morohoshi
R.H. Hruban
D.S. Klimstra
N. Ohike
B. Terris

Definition

An uncommon malignant epithelial neoplasm characterized by neoplastic cells with acinar differentiation and distinctive squamoid nests. Endocrine and ductal differentiation also occur but are typically less extensive. These neoplasms rarely contain a discrete mesenchymal component. Pancreatoblastoma usually occurs in childhood.

ICD-O code   8971/3

Epidemiology

Although pancreatoblastoma is a rare neoplasm, with < 200 cases reported, it is one of the most frequent pancreatic neoplasms in childhood, accounting for approximately 25% of pancreatic neoplasms occurring in the first decade of life {2958}. The great majority of pancreatoblastomas occur in children, mostly < 10 years of age. The median age of paediatric patients is approximately 4 years. Rare cases have been reported in association with Beckwith-Wiedemann syndrome {2177}.

Exceptionally, pancreatoblastomas can be encountered in adults. More than twenty cases have been reported in patients of between 18 and 78 years of age {458}. There is a slight male predominance, with a male-to-female ratio of 1.3 : 1. Approximately half of the cases reported to date have been in Asians {1270}.

Localization

Pancreatoblastomas do not preferentially localize to any particular part of the pancreas {1238}. The cases reported to date are almost evenly distributed between the head and the body–tail of the gland.

Clinical features

The presenting features of pancreatoblastoma are nonspecific and many cases are discovered incidentally. Common symptoms typically include abdominal pain, weight loss, nausea and diarrhoea. Less common presentations include jaundice, gastrointestinal bleeding and bowel obstruction. An abdominal mass is often palpable on physical examination, especially in children. Isolated case reports have described patients with Cushing syndrome secondary to the inappropriate secretion of adrenocorticotropic hormone by the tumour {1590}. Radiologically, pancreatoblastomas are large, well-defined, heterogeneous masses that may contain calcifications {2130, 2709}.

A quarter of all patients have elevated serum α-fetoprotein levels, a marker that, when present, can be used to monitor the effectiveness of therapy.

Macroscopy

Pancreatoblastomas are usually large at presentation; reported cases have measured 1.5–20 cm and the mean size is 11 cm. Most are solitary, circumscribed, solid neoplasms composed of well-defined lobules of soft, fleshy tissue separated by fibrous bands. Areas of necrosis may be prominent. Uncommonly the tumours are grossly cystic, a phenomenon reported in all cases arising in patients with the Beckwith-Wiedeman syndrome {741}.

Tumour spread and staging

These are fully malignant neoplasms and should be staged as one would stage a ductal adenocarcinoma. Pancreatoblastomas can invade adjacent structures. Metastases are present in 17–35% of patients at the time of diagnosis, and additional patients will develop metastases later in the course of their disease {711}. The liver is the most common site of metastases, followed by the lymph nodes and lung. Bone metastases are rare.

Histopathology

The epithelial elements of pancreatoblastomas are highly cellular and are arranged in well-defined islands separated by stromal bands, producing a geographic low power appearance. By definition, these neoplasms have both acinar differentiation and squamoid nests (corpusels). Solid, hypercellular nests of polygonal-shaped cells alternate with regions showing more obvious acinar differentiation. The cells with acinar differentiation are polarized around small lumina and have nuclei with single prominent nucleoli. Nuclear atypia is generally modest.

A characteristic feature of pancreatoblastoma is the squamoid nest. These enigmatic structures vary from large islands of plump, epithelioid cells to whorled nests of spindled cells to frankly keratinizing squamous islands. The nuclei of the squamoid nests are larger and more oval than those of the surrounding cells. The nuclei in the squamoid nests may be clear owing to the intranuclear accumulation of biotin {1130, 3188}. The prominent nucleoli of the solid and acinar regions are not seen in the cells of the squamoid nests. The density and composition of the squamoid nests varies in different regions of the neoplasm and among different cases, but these structures are regarded as

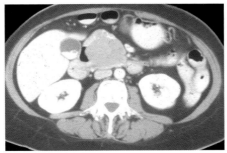

Fig. 12.61 Pancreatoblastoma seen on a CT scan.

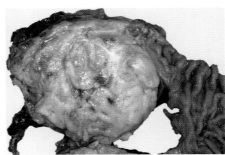

Fig. 12.62 Pancreatoblastoma. The cut section of the neoplasm reveals the lobulated surface.

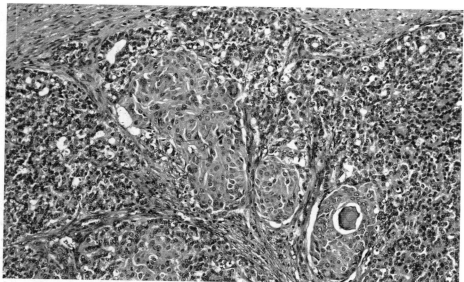

Fig. 12.63 Pancreatoblastoma. Note the prominent squamoid nests.

a defining component of pancreatoblastoma and serve to distinguish it from acinar cell carcinoma and other related entities.

In addition to cells with acinar differentiation and the squamoid nests, cells in the solid areas may have nuclear features suggestive of endocrine differentiation, although the morphological features do not strongly correlate with immunohistochemical labelling. A more primitive-appearing small-cell component may also occur, and in rare neoplasms, glandular spaces lined by mucin-containing cells may be seen.

The stroma of pancreatoblastomas is often hypercellular, in some instances achieving a neoplastic appearance. Rarely, heterologous stromal elements, including neoplastic bone and cartilage, have been reported {233}.

Pancreatoblastomas in adults have similar histological features to those in children, including the presence of squamoid nests {458}; however, the stromal bands may be less abundant and the stroma can be less cellular than in paediatric cases.

Immunohistochemistry

Pancreatoblastomas express keratins by immunohistochemistry, including keratins 7, 8, 18, and 19. They also exhibit evidence of acinar differentiation in the form of periodic acid–Schiff (PAS)-positive, diastase-resistant cytoplasmic granules and immunohistochemical labelling for pancreatic enzymes, including trypsin, chymotrypsin, and lipase. The labelling may be focal, sometimes limited to areas of the neoplasm with acinar formations. At least focal immunoreactivity for markers of endocrine differentiation (chromogranin or synaptophysin) is found in more than two thirds of cases, usually in scattered clusters of cells. Specific peptide hormones are not usually expressed. Expression of markers of ductal differentiation such as CEA, DUPAN-2, or

B72.3 can also be seen in more than half of cases. In most cases, the proportion of cells expressing acinar markers outnumbers the proportion expressing endocrine or ductal markers. Immunohistochemical positivity for α-fetoprotein is found in 20% of pancreatoblastomas, especially cases associated with elevations in the serum levels of α-fetoprotein {1348}. Immunohistochemical evaluation of the squamoid nests has failed to define a reproducible direction of differentiation for this component, {1602, 2303}. The nuclei of the cells in the squamoid nests contain abundant biotin, and can nonspecifically label with a number of antibodies, a feature that can help highlight these nests in some cases. Loss of expression of SMAD4 (DPC4) is found in up to 22% of pancreatoblastomas and p53 is usually not expressed at immunohistochemically detectable levels {19}. Consistent with the involvement of the WNT pathway in tumorigenesis, pancreatoblastomas may show nuclear immunolabelling for β-catenin, although in some cases the nuclear labelling is patchy or limited to the squamoid nests {19, 586, 3070, 3190}. The downstream target of β-catenin, cyclin D1, is also overexpressed in the squamoid nests {3190}. Pancreatoblastomas have diffuse membranous immunoexpression of claudin 7 but lack claudin 5, in contrast to solid-pseudopapillary neoplasms, which have the opposite profile for these markers {586}.

Cytopathology

Fine-needle aspiration biopsy has been performed for only a few cases. Aspiration smears show both a noncohesive and a clustered cellular pattern. Most of the neoplastic cells are polygonal with round to oval nuclei, one or more small nucleoli, and granular, amphophilic or eosinophilic cytoplasm {1130, 2776, 2968, 3716}. These nuclear features are similar to those of acinar cell carcinoma. The squamoid nests are usually more difficult to appreciate, and are best seen in cell-block preparations {1167, 2557}. Optically clear nuclei may be recognized in some of the neoplastic cells forming the squamoid nests {1130}.

Ultrastructure

Pancreatoblastomas have only rarely been examined ultrastructurally {357, 752, 1504, 2303, 2920}. The predominant cells have acinar differentiation, with well-

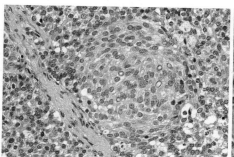 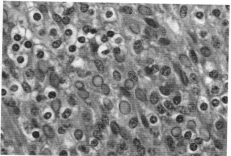

Fig. 12.64 Pancreatoblastoma. A Squamoid nest with biotin-rich, optically clear nuclei. This biotin may cause nonspecific nuclear immunolabelling. B Close-up of a squamoid nest. Note the clearing of some of the nuclei secondary to the accumulation of biotin.

developed organelles, including prominent rough endoplasmic reticulum, and numerous zymogen granules (400–800 nm in size). Additionally, the large irregular fibrillary granules characteristic of acinar cell carcinoma may be recognized. Cells with small dense-core endocrine granules (125–250 nm in size) are often present, as are glandular cells with relatively large mucinous granules (500–900 nm in size). The cells of the squamoid nests contain numerous desmosomes but only focally well-developed desmosome-tonofilament complexes {2303}. These cells have no other features to suggest a direction of differentiation.

Differential diagnosis

The differential diagnosis should include acinar cell carcinoma (including mixed acinar-neuroendocrine carcinoma), pancreatic NET, ductal adenocarcinoma in childhood, and solid-pseudopapillary neoplasm. Although extremely rare, metastases to the pancreas, such as neuroblastoma, Wilms tumour, hepatoblastoma, should also be considered if clinically indicated. The clinical and morphological features of pancreatoblastoma extensively overlap with those of acinar cell carcinoma {1598, 2162}. Both neoplasms are often associated with elevation of serum α-fetoprotein levels {564}, and they both are composed of cells with predominantly acinar differentiation. Squamoid nests are the most useful feature for distinguishing these two entities.

Genetic susceptibility

Pancreatoblastoma has been reported in infants with Beckwith-Wiedemann syndrome {1523}, which is characterized by hemihypertrophy, macroglossia, macrosomia, midline abdominal-wall defects, neonatal hypoglycaemia, abnormalities of chromosome 11p15.5, and an increased risk of developing embryonal neoplasms. A pancreatoblastoma has also been reported in an adult patient with familial adenomatosis polyposis (FAP) {19}.

Molecular pathology

The most common genetic alteration identified to date is loss of heterozygosity (LOH) of the short arm of chromosome 11p {19, 1523}. The allele lost is typically

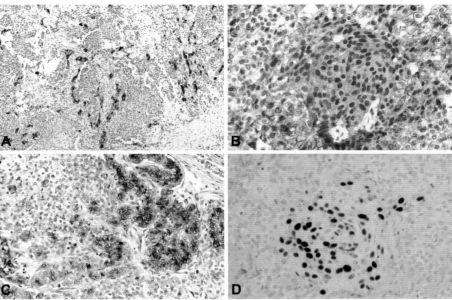

Fig. 12.65 Pancreatoblastoma. **A** Immunolabelling for chromogranin. **B** Immunolabelling for β-catenin. Note the mosaic pattern of membranous and nuclear labelling. **C** Immunolabelling for trypsin. **D** Nonspecific nuclear labelling of the biotin-rich nuclei in a squamoid nest.

the maternal allele {1523}. These findings are identified in other embryonal neoplasms that arise in association with the Beckwith-Wiedemann syndrome, including Wilms tumour and hepatoblastoma. Alterations in the β-catenin/APC pathway have been reported in 50–80% of pancreatoblastomas {19, 3190}. Most often these involve mutation of the β-catenin gene (*CTNNB1*), which results in abnormal nuclear accumulation of the β-catenin protein. Biallelic inactivation of the *APC* gene was identified in the pancreatoblastoma reported in an FAP patient {19}. Mutations in *KRAS2* and accumulation of p53 protein, typically found in ductal adenocarcinoma of the pancreas, are not detected {19, 1234}.

Prognosis and predictive factors

Overall survival is approximately 50% in patients with pancreatoblastoma. Postoperative prognosis in patients with localized surgically resectable disease is favourable, with a 5-year survival of 65%, while patients with non-resectable disease usually do not survive beyond 5 years {711}. After complete resection, 18% of patients with pancreatoblastoma develop local recurrence at a median of 20 months, and 26% develop metachro-

nous metastases. Factors associated with a worse prognosis are metastases and non-resectable disease {711}. The outcome in children may be more favourable than in adults {711}. One of the reasons appears to be that children often present with non-metastatic and well-encapsulated neoplasms with an indolent course. Even adults can achieve long-term disease-free survival when these features are present {458, 1234, 2370}. Chemotherapy and radiotherapy may have a role in the treatment of recurrent, residual, unresectable and metastatic disease.

Neuroendocrine neoplasms of the pancreas

D.S. Klimstra   P. Komminoth
R. Arnold   E. Solcia
C. Capella   G. Rindi
R.H. Hruban
G. Klöppel

Definition

A neoplasm arising in the pancreas that has predominantly neuroendocrine differentiation. This includes well-differentiated (low- to intermediate-grade) neuroendocrine tumours (NETs) and poorly differentiated (high-grade) neuroendocrine carcinomas (NECs); NECs, defined by the presence of > 20 mitoses per 10 high power fields, are divided into large cell NEC and small cell NEC. Mixed adenoneuroendocrine carcinoma (MANEC) has both an exocrine and a neuroendocrine component, with each component exceeding 30%, and include mixed acinar-neuroendocrine carcinoma, mixed ductal-neuroendocrine carcinoma, and mixed acinar-neuroendocrine-ductal carcinoma. Nonfunctional (nonsyndromic) pancreatic NETs measuring < 0.5 cm are termed pancreatic neuroendocrine microadenomas.

ICD-O codes

Pancreatic neuroendocrine microadenoma	8150/0
Neuroendocrine tumour (NET)	
NET G1	8240/3
NET G2	8249/3
Nonfunctional pancreatic NET, G1, G2	8150/3
Neuroendocrine carcinoma (NEC)	8246/3
Large cell NEC	8013/3
Small cell NEC	8041/3
EC cell, serotonin-producing NET (carcinoid)	8241/3
Gastrinoma	8153/3
Glucagonoma	8152/3
Insulinoma	8151/3
Somatostatinoma	8156/3
VIPoma	8155/3

Synonyms

Synonyms for pancreatic NETs include "islet cell tumour," "APUDoma" (obsolete), well-differentiated pancreatic endocrine neoplasm, neuroendocrine neoplasm and well-differentiated pancreatic endocrine carcinoma. Synonyms for NEC include high-grade neuroendocrine carcinoma and poorly differentiated endocrine carcinoma.

Classification

Pancreatic NETs and NECs are classified on the basis of criteria similar to those for other neuroendocrine neoplasms of the gastrointestinal tract (Chapter 1). Pancreatic NETs can be associated with characteristic clinical syndromes owing to hormone hypersecretion ("functioning NETs" or "syndromic NETs") or they can be nonfunctioning ("nonsyndromic NETs". Although routine immunohistochemical staining for peptide hormones is not suggested for clinically nonfunctional pancreatic NETs, for cases in which the production of a specific hormone has been demonstrated in the majority of the neoplastic cells, it is acceptable to supplement the diagnosis of pancreatic NET to reflect the corresponding cell type (e.g. "α cell/glucagon-producing NET," "β cell/insulin-producing NET," "G cell/gastrin-producing NET"), but specific functional terms (e.g. "glucagonoma," "insulinoma," "gastrinoma") should not be used in the absence of a hormonal syndrome. Changes to the classification of pancreatic neuroendocrine neoplasms since the third edition of the *WHO Classification of Tumours* include the use of "neuroendocrine" rather than "endocrine" (to parallel the terminology of the remainder of the gastrointestinal tract) and the replacement of the hybrid grade- and stage-based classification system with a purely grade-based system determined by proliferative rate. Pancreatic NETs should also now be staged, since stage is an independent prognostic indicator.

Epidemiology

Incidence

Pancreatic NETs are uncommon and represent 1–2% of all pancreatic neoplasms. Their prevalence has been estimated to be 0.2–2 per million persons per year {3012}. Based on surgical series, 30–40% of all pancreatic NETs are nonfunctioning {346, 1522, 1609, 3012}, although the increasing detection of incidental nonfunctioning NETs during imaging procedures is expected to increase their numbers relative to functioning pancreatic NETs. Pan-

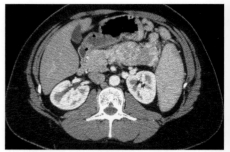

Fig. 12.66 CT scan of a pancreatic NET.

creatic neuroendocrine microadenomas are usually clinically unrecognized and asymptomatic and have been found in 0.4–1.5% of unselected autopsies {1068, 1567, 1660, 1907, 2735, 3013}. High-grade pancreatic NECs are rare tumours accounting for < 1% of pancreatic carcinomas {2159, 2338} and no more than 2–3% of all pancreatic NETs {3012}. An association with cigarette smoking has been reported for high-grade pancreatic NECs {521}.

Age and sex distribution

Pancreatic NETs may occur at any age, but are rare in childhood {2958}. The peak incidence is between 30 and 60 years and the mean age at presentation is 50 years {719, 759, 1522, 1874, 3390}. Pancreatic NETs in patients with specific genetic backgrounds (multiple endocrine neoplasia type 1 [MEN1], and von Hippel Lindau [VHL]) occur at a younger age. Both sexes are equally affected (the male-to-female ratio is 1 : 1.15).

High-grade pancreatic NECs usually arise in older patients, mostly males of > 40 years of age {2665}.

Localization

Pancreatic NETs can occur anywhere in the pancreas, and some functional types are slightly more common in the head (e.g. gastrinoma) or tail (e.g. VIPoma) {691}. Approximately two thirds of surgically resected nonfunctioning pancreatic NETs arise in the head of the pancreas {719, 759, 1522, 1874, 3390}; because these neoplasms are hormonally silent, those lesions that cause local symptoms (i.e. those in the head of the gland) are most commonly detected. Pancreatic high-grade NECs are also more common in the head of the gland {2665}.

Clinical features
NETs
Functioning pancreatic NETs are associated with clinical syndromes caused by hypersecretion of hormones either appropriate to the endocrine pancreas (insulin, glucagon, and somatostatin) or inappropriate (e.g. gastrin, vasoactive intestinal peptide [VIP], growth hormone-releasing factor, adrenocorticotropic hormone [ACTH]). Within this group are insulinomas, glucagonomas, somatostatinomas, gastrinomas, VIPomas, and other less common pancreatic NETs. These designations should only be used when the hormone production produces a clinical syndrome ("syndromic" or "functional"). The clinical and pathological features of the specific functioning pancreatic NETs are described elsewhere {691}. Pancreatic neuroendocrine microadenomas are, by definition, nonfunctioning.

By definition, nonfunctioning (or inactive, clinically silent, nonsyndromic) tumours are not associated with a distinct clinical hormonal syndrome, but may still be associated with elevated hormone levels in the blood and hormone immunoreactivity in tissue sections. Neoplasms in which the majority of cells express (and often secrete) pancreatic polypeptide (PP) or neurotensin are included in the group of nonfunctioning neoplasms (as are many delta [D] cell or somatostatin-producing cell tumours and the rare ghrelin cell tumours), because they do not cause a distinct hormonal syndrome. Nonfunctioning tumours only become clinically apparent when they become large and invade adjacent organs, or when they metastasize. They rarely present with acute pancreatitis. Increasingly, they are detected on imaging tests as incidental findings.

NECs
High-grade pancreatic NECs may present with symptoms similar to those of the exocrine pancreatic neoplasms {682, 1419, 1522}. Presentation with widespread metastases may occur. Lesions in the pancreatic head may induce back pain and jaundice owing to obstruction of the common bile duct. Individual cases have been associated with Cushing syn-

drome {605}, carcinoid syndrome {1033} and hypercalcaemia {1218}.

Macroscopy
NETs
Most pancreatic NETs are well-demarcated, solitary, and white-yellow or pink-brown. They can be soft and fleshy or densely fibrotic. Areas of haemorrhage or necrosis can occur, usually in larger neoplasms. Rarely, pancreatic NETs are cystic {1850}. Among the functioning neoplasms, insulinomas are usually smaller (< 2 cm in diameter) than glucagonomas, somatostatinomas, gastrinomas or VIPomas, but the size of the tumours is not related to the severity of the hormonally induced symptoms. Nonfunctioning NETs are generally > 2 cm in diameter (often 5 cm or more); in part, their larger size can be attributed to later detection.
NECs
Pancreatic NECs have an average diameter of approximately 4 cm {2665}. They are firm, white-grey masses with ill-defined borders, often showing areas of necrosis and haemorrhage.

Histopathology
NETs
Pancreatic NETs are well-differentiated by definition and show various "organoid" histological patterns, characterized by a nesting, trabecular, glandular, gyriform, tubuloacinar or pseudorosette arrangements of their cells. The cells are relatively uniform, show finely granular amphophilic to eosinophilic cytoplasm and a centrally located round to oval nucleus that may display a distinct nucleolus. The chromatin pattern is characteristically coarsely clumped ("salt and pepper"). Occasionally, clear cells, vacuolated lipid-rich cells, oncocytes, or "rhabdoid" features {443, 1040, 1214, 2523, 2614} may be observed. Pancreatic NETs with marked nuclear enlargement and irregularities have been termed "pleomorphic" pancreatic NETs {3686}.

Non-neoplastic ductules may be trapped in the tumour, and the neoplastic cells may even form glands, but these features do not indicate a diagnosis of mixed ductal-neuroendocrine carcinoma unless a separate component of histologically typical infiltrating ductal adenocarcinoma is present.

By definition, pancreatic NETs have < 20 mitoses per 10 HPF; most cases have < 10 per 10 HPF, and in many cases mi-

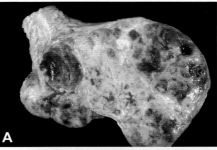
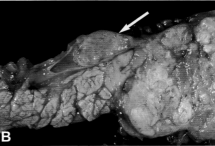

Fig. 12.67 Macroscopy of well-differentiated pancreatic neuroendocrine tumours (NETs). **A** This large soft fleshy tumour has areas of degeneration and haemorrhage. The normal pancreas is in the upper left. **B** Invasion of a large vessel (arrow) in a well-differentiated NET.

toses are nearly undetectable. The mitotic rate is a critical component of grading.

The amount of stroma and degree of fibrosis vary. Necrosis is usually limited and may be comedo-like. In general, the histological pattern of a neoplasm does not indicate its functional state or type of hormone produced. There are two exceptions to this rule: amyloid deposits are more typical of insulinomas, and glandular structures containing psammoma bodies are commonly observed in somatostatin cell tumours, usually not primary in the pancreas but rather in the periampullary duodenum.

NECs
Pancreatic high-grade NECs commonly consist of tightly packed nests or diffuse, irregular sheets of cells, often, with extensive necrosis. NECs are classified as small cell NEC or large cell NEC depending upon the size of the neoplastic cells, the prominence of nucleoli and the amount of cytoplasm, using similar criteria to those used for NECs of the lung {2665, 3012, 3288}. In the pancreas, large cell NECs are more common than small cell NECs. By definition, mitoses are abundant (> 20 per 10 HPF). Most cases have > 40–50 per 10 HPF and necrosis is frequent and often geographic. Neoplasms with an organized pattern of

growth, uniform nuclei with salt-and-pepper chromatin, and with > 20 mitoses per HPF are currently classified as NEC based solely on the mitotic count. Further studies are necessary, however, to establish the clinical behaviour of such neoplasms.

Immunohistochemistry
NETs
Pancreatic NETs can be identified by using antibodies against chromogranin A and synaptophysin, which are strongly expressed in the vast majority of cases {2735, 3013}. Synaptophysin expression is often more diffuse than chromogranin A, which can be focal or patchy. Also expressed are protein gene product (PGP) 9.5 and neural cell adhesion molecule (NCAM1/CD56), but these are considered less specific {1156, 1876, 2178}. Pancreatic NETs also contain keratins 8 and 18, and keratin 19 may also be expressed, especially in more aggressive cases. Lineage markers including PDX1 and Isl1 may be expressed and can indicate a pancreatic origin for NETs of unknown primary {832, 2846, 3052}. CDX2 expression can also occur, but is not specific for pancreatic origin {2801, 3052}.

Peptide hormones (e.g. insulin, glucagon) are generally detectable in the corresponding functioning pancreatic NETs. It is important to recognize that functioning NETs are defined on the basis of clinical symptoms rather than immunohistochemical findings, and the immunohistochemical detection of peptide hormones in nonfunctioning pancreatic NETs has no clinical significance. The expression of different hormones by distinct cells within a NET can occur, and metastases may produce hormones other than those found in the primary {1219, 1747, 3012, 3013}. Clinically nonfunctioning NETs with immunolabelling for pancreatic polypeptide (PP) in the majority of cells have been designated as "PPomas" {1748, 3262, 3263}. Microadenomas are more likely to show diffuse expression of a single peptide, most often glucagon or PP {3012}.

Many pancreatic NETs also express glycoproteins including carcinoembryonic antigen(CEA) and CA19-9 {1219, 1467}. Neoplasms with gland formation are particularly likely to stain for glycoproteins. Focal acinar differentiation may also be detected, generally in single widely scattered cells (less than one third) that stain for trypsin or chymotrypsin {1467}. Expression of progesterone receptors and CD99 is found in a subset of normal islet cells and also in some pancreatic NETs. Immunohistochemical labelling for Ki67 with MIB1 antibody may be used to determine the proliferative rate of pancreatic NETs. Most have a low proliferative rate, with a labelling index of 1–5%, but values of up to 20% are acceptable, although rarely observed {3012}. A greater percentage of immunoreactivity for MIB1 indicates a diagnosis of high-grade NEC.

NECs
It is necessary to demonstrate immunolabelling for general neuroendocrine markers (chromogranin A and synaptophysin) to establish a diagnosis of large cell NEC of the pancreas, and therefore a variable proportion of the neoplastic cells label in all cases, usually with less intensity than in well-differentiated NETs {1110}.

Cytologically, classic small cell NECs may not express neuroendocrine markers and, following the definition used in the lung, this does not preclude the diagnosis so long as alternative diagnostic considerations are excluded. As a rule, no reactivity for peptide hormones is found in pancreatic NECs. Abnormal nuclear accumulation of p53, a feature virtually absent in NETs, is commonly although not invariably found in NECs. The Ki67-MIB1 labelling index is consistently > 20% and often exceeds 50%.

Cytopathology
Fine-needle aspiration (FNA) is a useful method for diagnosing pancreatic NETs and their metastases. Smears are usually uniformly cellular and composed of a relatively monotonous population of cells predominantly arranged singly, but also in loose clusters or pseudorosettes {59, 226, 581, 2992}. The round to ovoid, smoothly contoured nuclei demonstrate a salt-and-pepper chromatin pattern. The cytoplasm is amphophilic and varies in quantity and density. Some cells may be stripped of their cytoplasm whereas others may have abundant cytoplasm, and a plasmacytoid appearance is highly characteristic. Immunocytochemical techniques may effectively be applied to cytology samples.

Differential diagnosis
NETs
Most pancreatic NETs are recognizable without much difficulty. The use of immunohistochemical markers of the neuroendocrine phenotype can often establish the diagnosis. Primary pancreatic neoplasms that must be distinguished from NETs include solid-

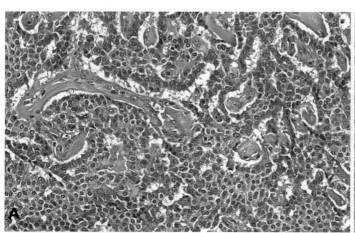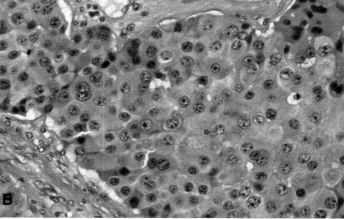

Fig. 12.68 Well-differentiated pancreatic neuroendocrine tumour (NET). **A** Trabecular and nesting growth. **B** Note the "salt and pepper" nuclei.

pseudopapillary neoplasm, acinar cell carcinoma and pancreatoblastoma, primitive neuroectodermal tumour, and ductal adenocarcinoma.

Solid-pseudopapillary neoplasms can morphologically resemble NETs, and both neoplasms can immunolabel for CD56 (NCAM1), neuron-specific enolase (NSE) and synaptophysin. Findings that favour a diagnosis of solid-pseudopapillary neoplasm include poorly cohesive cells with degenerative pseudopapilla formation, longitudinal nuclear grooves, and aggregates of PAS-positive, diastase-resistant hyaline globules. Immunoreactivity for vimentin, CD10, α-1-antitrypsin, and β-catenin (nuclear) are also features of solid-pseudopapillary neoplasm.

Immunolabelling for trypsin and chymotrypsin can be used to distinguish acinar cell carcinomas from pancreatic NETs. The same is true for pancreatoblastomas, which have the additional distinguishing histological feature of squamoid nests. Both neoplasms may contain scattered neuroendocrine cells. True mixed acinar-neuroendocrine carcinomas are very rare. In these carcinomas, the neuroendocrine-cell component should account for at least one third of the entire cell population.

Poorly differentiated ductal adenocarcinomas may have a solid growth pattern, resembling a NET, but they have more pleomorphism and mitotic activity and usually demonstrate focal production of mucin; immunolabelling for neuroendocrine markers is not found. The occasional nuclear pleomorphism that can occur in pancreatic NETs may lead to confusion with poorly differentiated adenocarcinoma.

Primary primitive neuroectodermal tumours are rare in the pancreas {1920, 2170}. Since reported cases in this location may strongly express keratin and because pancreatic NETs often express CD99, these entities can be confused. Molecular or cytogenetic evidence of the characteristic 11;22 chromosomal translocation is helpful in the diagnosis of primitive neuroectodermal tumour.

NECs

Prominent cytological atypia, extensive necrosis, a Ki67 index of > 20% and diffuse nuclear expression of p53 (when present) are useful in differentiating high-grade NECs with intermediate-sized cells from well-differentiated pancreatic NETs.

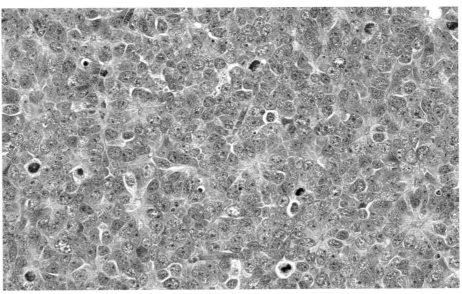

Fig. 12.69 Pancreatic neuroendocrine carcinoma (NEC). Note the very high mitotic rate.

Expression of neuroendocrine markers is needed to distinguish NECs from poorly differentiated ductal adenocarcinomas. Acinar cell carcinomas share with NECs a relatively high mitotic rate, and since they are much more frequent pancreatic primaries, they should be ruled out using immunolabelling for trypsin and chymotrypsin in all cases. The possibility of a metastasis from an extrapancreatic NEC should always be excluded, especially in the case of small cell carcinoma. Immunolabelling for TTF1 may not be helpful, since the expression of this marker is well described in extrapulmonary small cell carcinomas as well as in lung primaries.

Genetic susceptibility

Pancreatic NETs are a major component of the multiple endocrine neoplasia type 1 (MEN1) syndrome and NETs are also found in patients with von Hippel Lindau (VHL) syndrome. The underlying germline genetic abnormalities of these syndromes (in the *MEN1* and *VHL* genes, respectively) are known to play a role in the development of pancreatic NETs in these patients. A few cases have been associated with tuberous sclerosis, especially in children {885, 3395}. The somatostatinomas associated with neurofibromatosis (NF) are almost exclusively duodenal. Rare examples of insulinomas have also been described in patients suffering from NF1 {923}.

Pancreatic NETs are found in 60–70% of patients with MEN1, and most affected patients have at least one functioning pancreatic NET. Gastrinomas, almost exclusively of the duodenum, are the most frequent functioning gastroenteropancreatic tumour in MEN1 patients; pancreatic insulinomas are the next most frequent {1049, 1660, 1770, 2807, 2883}. Pancreatic NETs in MEN1 patients usually arise in a background of multiple neuroendocrine microadenomas and other abnormalities of the islets (hypertrophy or hyperplasia). Between 12% and 17% of patients with VHL develop pancreatic NETs, most of which are nonfunctioning {1909}. Background abnormalities in the islets have only recently been reported in VHL patients {2524}.

In contrast to well-differentiated pancreatic NETs, high-grade NECs are very infrequently associated with MEN1 {2334}.

Molecular pathology

Whereas the molecular basis of familial pancreatic NETs associated with MEN1 and VHL syndromes has been established {477, 1753}, little is known about the molecular basis for sporadic tumours. It appears that activation of oncogenes is not a common event in pancreatic NETs {1224, 1369, 1885}. In particular, the common genetic mutations identified in pancreatic ductal adenocarcinomas (e.g. *TP53*, *KRAS*, *CDKN2A/p16*, *SMAD4/DPC4*) are not found with any significant frequency in pancreatic NETs {560, 1036, 1267, 2141, 2530, 2881}. Somatic *MEN1* mutations are present in about 20% of sporadic pancreatic NETs, and 68% harbour losses of 11q13 or more distal parts of the long arm of chromosome 11, indicating that another yet unknown tumour suppressor gene might be involved {633, 641, 1036, 1181, 1182, 2140, 2529, 2676, 2900, 3442, 3718}. Point mutations in the *VHL* gene appear to be extremely rare in sporadic pancreatic NETs (1–3%) {560, 1036, 2141, 2530, 2881}.

Staging, prognosis and predictive factors

NETs and NECs should be staged using the TNM (tumour, node, metastasis) system for ductal adenocarcinoma of the pancreas. The issue of TNM/staging classification for NETs is controversial. The classification presented in this book follows that of the American Joint Committee on Cancer/ Internation Union Against Cancer (AJCC/UICC) and is the same for adenocarcinoma and NETs, including "carcinoids," i.e. well-differentiated lesions only {762, 2996}. Conversely, the classification proposed by the European Neuroendocrine Tumor Society (ENETS) is also meant for high-grade neuroendocrine neoplasms, has different T (tumour) definitions and stage groupings {2684, 2685, 2832A}.

NETs

Other than neuroendocrine microadenomas, which are benign neoplasms {3012} (there being no evidence for progression to clinically relevant malignant NETs outside the setting of MEN1), all pancreatic NETs are regarded to have malignant potential. Most clinically functioning insuli-nomas are very small (often < 1.0 cm) at diagnosis, and probably for this reason they pursue a benign clinical course, even when treated by enucleation. The percentage of insulinomas with malignant behaviour ranges from 2.4% to 17.9% with an average of 8.4% {935, 986, 998, 1772, 2882, 3002, 3065, 3366}. Most other functioning and nonfunctioning pancreatic NETs are relatively aggressive neoplasms.

Approximately 65–80% of cases are associated with clear-cut evidence of malignant behaviour (gross invasive growth or metastasis), and tumour recurrence following resection is common {719, 759, 1190, 1522, 2591, 2762, 3012, 3390}. Once distant metastases occur, cure is highly unlikely, although the rate of tumour progression may be slow. Following surgical resection, the 5-year survival for patients with pancreatic NETs other than insulinomas is reportedly 65%, and 10-year survival is only 45% {1219}. A sizeable proportion of patients with nonfunctioning pancreatic NETs initially present with distant metastases, perhaps because there is no hormonal syndrome to draw clinical attention to the neoplasm early in its course.

A variety of prognostic factors can be used to stratify pancreatic NETs into different risk groups, but stage (extent of disease) and grade (based on proliferative rate) have emerged as the most potent predictive features in most studies {772, 850, 868, 1219, 1705, 2449, 2845}. Staging and grading information should therefore be provided separately.

The proliferative rate based on mitotic count or Ki67 index has been shown to be prognostically relevant in many studies {570, 2514, 3412}. The most widely used proliferative rate-based grading system is that of ENETS, which separates pancreatic NETs into low-grade (G1) and intermediate-grade (G2) categories based on mitoses (0–1 vs 2–20 per 10 HPF) and Ki67 labelling rate (0–2% versus 3–20%). This system strongly correlates with outcome {772, 868, 1705, 2449}.

In nonfunctioning pancreatic NETs, production of specific peptides has no impact on survival {1219}. Some studies have demonstrated a correlation between overall nuclear grade and prognosis {1219}. Other factors reportedly predictive of more aggressive behaviour include necrosis, loss of progesterone-receptor expression {2514, 3401}, aneuploidy {1521}, increased fractional allelic loss {2676}, upregulated expression of CD44 isoforms {1322}, and immunohistochemical expression of keratin 19 {701}.

NECs

The highly aggressive behaviour of high-grade pancreatic NECs and the usually advanced and unresectable stage at the time of diagnosis make mortality from these tumours virtually 100%. Invasion of the adjacent duodenum or of other peripancreatic tissues is frequent. Extensive, widespread metastases are the rule, involving regional and distant lymph nodes, as well as intra- and extra-abdominal organs such as liver and lung {2665, 3012}. Survival ranges from 1 month to 1 year, despite some initial favourable responses to chemotherapy {2146, 2338}.

Solid-pseudopapillary neoplasm of the pancreas

G. Klöppel
R.H. Hruban
D.S. Klimstra
A. Maitra
T. Morohoshi

K. Notohara
M. Shimizu
B. Terris

Definition

A low-grade malignant neoplasm composed of poorly cohesive monomorphic epithelial cells forming solid and pseudopapillary structures. These neoplasms frequently undergo haemorrhagic-cystic degeneration, and occur predominantly in young women.

Synonyms

Synonyms that should no longer be used include solid-pseudopapillary tumour, solid-cystic tumour {1615}, papillary-cystic tumour {301}, solid and papillary epithelial neoplasm {1845}, and Frantz tumour {313}.

ICD-O code   8452/3

Epidemiology

Solid-pseudopapillary neoplasms are rare, accounting for 0.9–2.7% of all exocrine pancreatic neoplasms and only 5% of cystic neoplasms {1270, 1654}. They occur predominantly in adolescent girls and young women (female, 90%; mean, 28 years; range, 7–79 years) {3012} and are rare in men (mean, 35 years; range, 25–72 years) {1270, 1614, 1656, 2009, 3315}. It should therefore not be surprising that solid-pseudopapillary neoplasms account for 30% of all pancreatic neoplasms in patients < 40 years

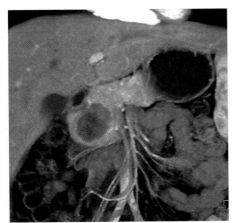

of age {3012}. There is no apparent ethnic predilection {1680, 2356} or any established association with recognized clinical or genetic syndromes, although very rare cases have been reported in the setting of familial adenomatous polyposis (FAP) {2758}.

Localization

There is no preferential localization within the pancreas {1270, 1656, 2297}. Origin outside of the pancreas is uncommon, but solid-pseudopapillary neoplasms have been reported in the retropancreatic tissue and in the mesocolon {1270, 1359, 1564, 1614}. Invasion of adjacent organs or the portal vein is rare {2864}.

Clinical features

Solid-pseudopapillary neoplasms are usually found incidentally on routine physical examination or imaging for another indication. If symptomatic, they cause abdominal discomfort, early satiety, nausea, vomiting and pain {2297}. Intratumoral haemorrhage following abdominal trauma can produce an acute abdomen {1614}. Jaundice is rare even in cases that originate in the head of the pancreas. Blood tumour markers are normal and the neoplasms have not been associated with a functional endocrine syndrome.

Endoscopic ultrasonography (EUS) and computed tomography (CT) reveal a sharply demarcated, heterogeneous (i.e. variably solid and cystic) mass without internal septations {533}. The tumour margin may contain calcifications. Administration of contrast medium results in enhancement of the solid components. On angiography, solid-pseudopapillary neoplasms are usually hypovascular or mildly hypervascular lesions that displace surrounding vessels {3585}.

Macroscopy

Solid-pseudopapillary neoplasms usually form large, round, solitary masses (average size, 8–10 cm; range, 0.5–25.0 cm) {1270}, and are often fluctuant. They are well-demarcated from the surrounding pancreas and may appear to be encap-

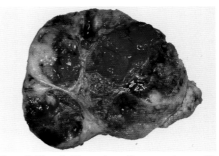

Fig. 12.70 Solid-pseudopapillary neoplasm with lobulated, fleshy surface showing marked haemorrhage and degenerative changes.

sulated. Multiple tumours are exceptional {2407}. The cut section reveals lobulated, light brown to yellow solid areas and zones of haemorrhage, necrosis, and cystic degeneration filled with necrotic debris. The contribution of each component varies greatly. Small tumours tend to be more solid than larger examples. Solid-pseudopapillary neoplasms are usually very soft, although some cases are firm and sclerotic. Occasionally, the haemorrhagic-cystic changes may be so extensive as to mimic a pseudocyst. The wall of the neoplasm may contain calcifications {2297}.

Tumour spread and staging

Rarely, these neoplasms may directly extend into the stomach, duodenum and spleen. Metastases occur in 5–15% of cases, usually to the peritoneum and liver. Lymph nodes and skin are exceptionally rare sites of metastatic disease {533, 1185, 2297, 3721}. Staging follows that for other carcinomas of the exocrine pancreas.

Histopathology

Solid-pseudopapillary neoplasms have a distinctive microscopic appearance. The growth pattern is heterogeneous, with a combination of solid, pseudopapillary and haemorrhagic-necrotic, pseudocystic structures in various proportions. The solid areas, which in large haemorrhagic-cystic neoplasms are only found at the periphery of the tumour, are composed of

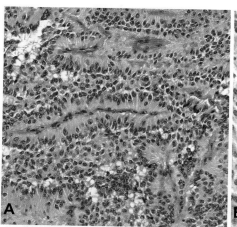
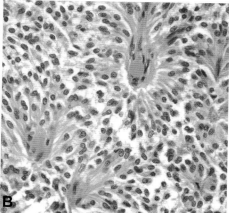

Fig. 12.72 Solid-pseudopapillary neoplasm. **A** Note the delicate vessels surrounded by loosely cohesive cells. **B** Delicate pseudopapillae and uniform loosely cohesive cells.

poorly cohesive monomorphic cells that are admixed with hyalinized to myxoid stromal bands containing thin-walled blood vessels. Pseudopapillae are formed when the poorly cohesive neoplastic cells drop away, leaving variable aggregates of loosely cohesive cells between the fibrovascular stalks. Touch preparations at the time of intraoperative frozen section can highlight the pattern of delicate branching vessels and loosely cohesive cells. Sometimes the neoplastic cells are arranged radially around the minute fibrovascular stalks thereby resembling "ependymal" rosettes. True gland formation is not seen. The solid parts may contain aggregates of neoplastic cells with foamy cytoplasm and often include cholesterol crystals surrounded by foreign-body giant cells. The pseudopapillary areas are usually associated with blood lakes. Foci of calcification and even ossification may be seen in the hyalinized connective tissue {2009}. Although the tumour is in most cases grossly well-demarcated from the normal pancreas, often by a fibrous capsule, microscopically the neoplastic cells delicately infiltrate into the surrounding pancreatic tissue, entrapping acinar cells and islets {2009, 2297}. Vascular and perineural invasion are rare {3552}.

The neoplastic cells have either eosinophilic or clear vacuolated cytoplasm. A few neoplasms are almost entirely composed of either eosinophilic cells or multivacuolated clear cells {82, 1018}. Some of the neoplastic cells contain eosinophilic, diastase-resistant PAS-positive globules of varying size, which may also occur extracellularly, sometimes in large amounts. Glycogen is not prominent and mucin is absent. The round to oval nuclei of the neoplastic cells have finely dispersed chromatin and the nuclei are often grooved or indented. Bizarre, presumably degenerative, nuclei may occasionally occur. Mitoses are usually rare, but in a few instances prominent mitotic activity has been observed {2297}. If there are metastases, they have largely the same morphological appearance as the primary neoplasm, but the cells may be more pleomorphic and show more mitoses.

Perineural invasion, angioinvasion, or deep infiltration of the surrounding acinar tissue do not indicate an accelerated malignant behaviour, because solid-pseudopapillary neoplasms in which the above-mentioned histological criteria of agressive behaviour are not detected may also metastasize. Consequently, all solid-pseudopapillary neoplasms are currently classified as low-grade malignant neoplasms.

Immunohistochemistry

Almost all solid-pseudopapillary neoplasms express α-1-antitrypsin, α-1-antichymotrypsin, NSE, vimentin, progesterone receptors, CD10, CD56, claudins 5 and 7, galectin 3, cyclin D1, and nuclear/cytoplasmic β-catenin {541, 586, 775, 956, 1614, 1656, 2071, 2161, 2324, 3247}. Immunoreactivity for α-1-antitrypsin and α-1-antichymotrypsin is always intense, but only involves small cell clusters or single cells, a finding that is characteristic of this neoplasm, and the distribution parallels that of the hyaline globules. Staining for NSE and vimentin, in contrast, is usually diffuse. Labelling using antibodies to the extracellular domain of E-cadherin shows complete loss of expression, while labelling with antibodies to the intracellular domain of the protein produces an abnormal cytoplasmic/nuclear pattern of labelling {2880}. Inconsistent results have been reported for epithelial markers, synaptophysin, and other antigens such as CEA or CA19-9. Antibodies to chromogranin A, exocrine enzymes (trypsin, chymotrypsin, and lipase), pancreatic hormones, estrogen receptors α, and α-fetoprotein do not label the neoplastic cells. Keratin is detected in 30–70% of cases {1615, 1656, 3669}, depending on the method of antigen retrieval applied. Usually, labelling for keratins (7, 8, 18 and 19) is focal and faint.

As solid-pseudopapillary neoplasms express so many diverse antigens, a core panel of markers that includes β-catenin, CD10, chromogranin and vimentin is recommended for establishing the diagnosis.

Ultrastructure

The neoplastic cells contain abundant cytoplasm, which is rich in mitochondria. Zymogen-like granules of variable sizes (500–3000 nm) are conspicuous, probably representing deposits of α-1-antitrypsin. The contents of these granules commonly disintegrate, forming multilamellated vesicles and lipid droplets {1615, 1775, 2071, 3586}. Neurosecretory-like granules have been described in a few neoplasms {1448, 1466, 2843, 3522, 3575}. Intermediate cell junctions are rarely observed and microvilli are lacking, but small intercellular spaces are frequent.

Cytopathology

Fine-needle aspiration cytology usually shows small monomorphic cells loosely adherent to thin branching vessels {417, 1270, 3522, 3552}. Poorly cohesive neoplastic cells fill the spaces between the vessels, and naked nuclei stripped of cytoplasm are usually abundant. The background often contains haemorrhagic debris, foamy histiocytes and multinucleated giant cells. The neoplastic cells have round nuclei with indented or grooved nuclear membranes and eosinophilic or foamy cytoplasm. The presence of intracytoplasmic hyaline globules can aid the diagnosis.

Histological variants

Solid-pseudopapillary neoplasms with apparent high-grade malignant transformation have been reported. In addition to areas with the appearance of a conventional solid-pseudopapillary neoplasm, these neoplasms contained foci with a diffuse solid growth pattern, increased nuclear atypia, and relatively abundant mitoses. One case contained a focus of sarcomatoid (spindle cell) carcinoma {3191}. These neoplasms were clinically extremely aggressive.

Differential diagnosis

Macroscopically, solid-pseudopapillary neoplasms may be mistaken for pseudocysts. They can be clearly separated from other cystic neoplasms of the pancreas by the yellow to haemorrhagic appearance of their cut surface. Microscopically the main differential diagnosis is with well-differentiated pancreatic neuroendocrine neoplasms and acinar cell carcinomas. Pseudocysts occur in males and females, usually with a history of pancreatitis and pain. In contrast, solid-pseudopapillary neoplasms are often found incidentally and occur predominantly in young women.

Histologically, pseudocysts are easily distinguished from solid-pseudopapillary neoplasms by the absence of epithelial lining of the inner cyst surface, but it should be noted that some solid-pseudopapillary neoplasms are extensively necrotic and viable epithelium can

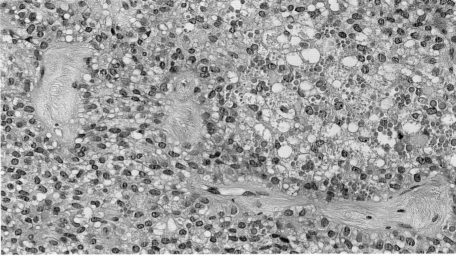

Fig. 12.73 Solid-pseudopapillary neoplasm showing numerous hyaline globules (haematoxylin phloxine saffron stain).

be hard to identify on cursory examination. Occasionally, "ghosts" of necrotic pseudopapillary structures may be visible in the periphery of such lesions.

Solid-pseudopapillary neoplasms may be confused with well-differentiated pancreatic neuroendocrine neoplasms or with acinar cell carcinomas, particularly if the solid-pseudopapillary neoplasm displays a predominantly solid growth pattern and lacks pseudopapillary structures, eosinophilic globules, foam cells and hyalinized fibrovascular stalks. In these cases, immunohistochemical expression of CD10 and vimentin, abnormal nuclear labelling with antibodies to β-catenin, and negativity for chromogranin A and exocrine enzymes (trypsin and chymotrypsin in particular) may be helpful in establishing the diagnosis of a solid-pseudopapillary neoplasm.

Molecular pathology

Almost all solid-pseudopapillary neoplasms harbour somatic point mutations in exon 3 of *CTNNB1*, the gene encoding β-catenin {8, 3189}. This mutation leads to a β-catenin protein that escapes intracytoplasmic phosphorylation and subsequent degradation and that therefore binds to the T-cell transcription factor (Tcf)/lymphoid enhancer-binding factor (Lef). The β-catenin-Tcf/Lef complex is then abnormally translocated to the nucleus, as indicated by nuclear expression of β-catenin on immunohistochemistry {8, 3189}. In the nucleus, the β-catenin-Tcf/Lef complex activates the transcription of several oncogenic genes, among them *MYC* and cyclin D1 {2181}. This leads to activation of the Wnt/β-catenin signalling pathway. Although this activation increases proliferation in other neoplasms, in solid-pseudopapillary neoplasms the signalling cascade may be interrupted by an as yet unexplained overexpression of p21 and p27 {3247}, resulting in a very low proliferation rate.

Alterations in the *KRAS*, *CDKN2A/p16*, *TP53* and *SMAD4/DPC4* genes, frequently found in ductal adenocarcinomas, have not been reported in solid-pseudopapillary neoplasms. A study using fluorescent *in situ* hybridization (FISH) and comparative genomic

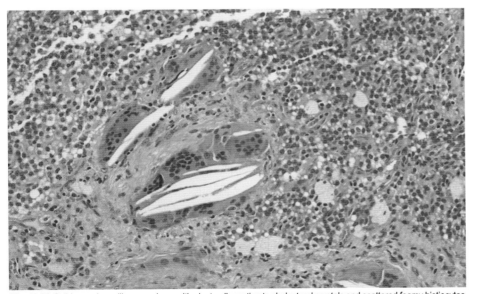

Fig. 12.74 Solid-pseudopapillary neoplasm with giant-cell reaction to cholesterol crystals and scattered foamy histiocytes in the background.

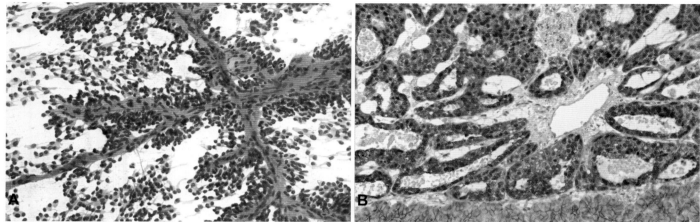

Fig. 12.75 Solid-pseudopapillary neoplasm. **A** Cytological preparation: note the delicate branching vessels and poorly cohesive uniform cells. **B** The neoplastic cells show nuclear immunolabelling for β-catenin: note the normal membranous labelling of the non-neoplastic acinar cells (bottom).

hybridization detected neither *EWS/FLI1* translocations nor any gross chromosomal gains or losses {3248}. Although up to 50% of solid-pseudopapillary neoplasms diffusely express the KIT (CD117) antigen on immunohistochemistry, this finding is not associated with underlying mutations of the *KIT* gene {409}. A study of global gene expression revealed a gene expression profile that is distinct from that of ductal adenocarcinomas and from neuroendocrine neoplasms, and demonstrated the involvement of the Wnt/β-catenin and the Notch signalling pathways {459}.

The striking sex and age distribution suggest genetic and hormonal factors, but there are no reports indicating an association with endocrine disturbances, including overproduction of estrogen or progesterone. Moreover, only very few women develop a solid-pseudopapillary neoplasm after long-term use of hormonal contraceptives {744}.

Prognosis and predictive factors

After complete surgical resection, 85–95% of patients are cured. Local spread or dissemination to the peritoneal cavity has been reported in the context of abdominal trauma and rupture of the tumour {1819}. Even in patients who had local spread, recurrences, or metastases, long disease-free periods have been recorded after initial diagnosis and resection {1713, 2007, 2649, 2760}. Only a few patients have died of a metastastic solid-pseudopapillary neoplasm, mostly those patients whose tumours harboured an undifferentiated component {2007, 2356, 2649, 3191}. There are no proven biological or morphological predictors of outcome, although it has been suggested that older patients do worse than younger patients, that patients with neoplasms with an aneuploid DNA content do worse than those with diploid tumours, and that an elevated mitotic rate and certain nuclear features of the neoplastic cells, such as mean nuclear diameter and size, are associated with the presence of metastases {2297, 3191}.

Mesenchymal tumours of the pancreas

M. Miettinen
C.D.M. Fletcher
L.-G. Kindblom
W.M.S. Tsui

Introduction

Although some mesenchymal tumours occur primarily in the pancreas, most are extrapancreatic lesions that have invaded the pancreas.

Extrapancreatic mesenchymal tumours

Such tumours can involve the pancreas. For example, gastrointestinal stromal tumours (GISTs) of the second part of the duodenum can infiltrate the pancreatic head, and gastric GISTs can extend into the pancreatic body and tail. The same is true for retroperitoneal and gastrointestinal leiomyosarcomas, liposarcomas, and intra-abdominal desmoids. Whenever an intrapancreatic sarcoma (GIST, leiomyosarcoma) is encountered, a search for an extrapancreatic primary is necessary.

Primary mesenchymal neoplasms

The mesenchymal neoplasms that occur primarily in the pancreas include most of the entities occurring primarily in soft tissues, but several deserve special note {2184}.

Lymphangiomas. A small number of lymphangiomas of the pancreas have been reported, most commonly centred in the peripancreatic tissues. These neoplasms often occur in young adults and tend to be cystic {1307, 3129}. Lymphangiomas should be distinguished from serous cystadenomas of the pancreas. Serous cystic neoplasms will express keratins 7, 8, 18 and 19, while lymphangiomas express CD31.

Lipomas. Lipomas of the pancreas have been reported, and should be distinguished from non-neoplastic fat accumulation. These lesions are particularly problematic because their low attenuation on computed tomography (CT) imaging can mimic a pancreatic cancer {1507}. In most cases, magnetic resonance imaging (MRI) can detect the lipomatous nature of these lesions.

Solitary fibrous tumour. This neoplasm, more commonly seen on the serosal surfaces of the peritoneum, has been described as an intrapancreatic mass {1919}. It is composed of bland spindle cells in a variably collagenous to focally myxoid background, and a haemangiopericytoma-like vascular pattern is a usual finding. The neoplastic cells are positive for CD34 and negative for KIT and desmin.

Perivascular epithelioid cell neoplasms (PEComas). PEComas have been reported in the pancreas {1197, 2629, 3672}. These well-vascularized neoplasms are composed of large, clear, epithelioid smooth-muscle cells. They variably express HMB45 and smooth muscle actin, but not keratins.

Ewing sarcoma. Tumours of this family (peripheral primitive neuroectodermal tumours [PNETs]) have been reported in the pancreas {2170}. These small round blue cell tumours have rearrangement of the *EWSR1* gene, usually a *EWSR1-FLI1* fusion with t(11;22) translocation, and are strongly immunoreactive for CD99. They often express synaptophysin, and occasionally keratins. Before making a diagnosis of Ewing sarcoma, other small round blue cell tumours and pancreatic neuroendocrine neoplasms must be excluded {1270}.

Desmoplastic small round cell tumours. These are small round blue cell tumours characterized by a distinctive desmoplastic stroma {1270, 2764} and can occur adjacent to the pancreas. They have divergent differentiation, and express keratins, desmin, and neuron-specific enolase (NSE) {1270}. Unlike PNETs, desmoplastic small round cell tumours do not strongly express CD99. These tumours typically harbour the *EWSR1-WT1* gene fusion.

Others. Cystic schwannomas can clinically mimic cystic epithelial neoplasms of the pancreas {1087}. Both cystic and solid hamartomas have been reported in the pancreas {1270, 2209, 2503}. These well-circumscribed lesions, composed of cystically dilated ducts, acini and fibroblastic stroma, are important to recognize because they can mimic mesenchymal and epithelial neoplasms of the pancreas {1270, 2209, 2503}.

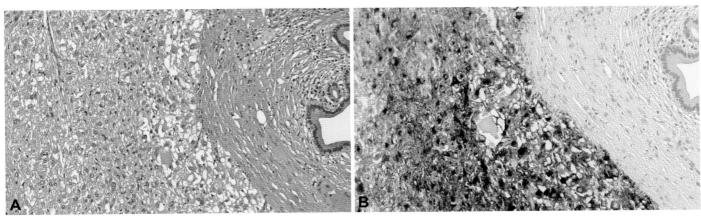

Fig. 12.76 Perivascular epithelioid cell neoplasm (PEComa). **A** PEComa involving the pancreas. **B**. Immunolabelling for HMB45.

Lymphoma of the pancreas

E.S. Jaffe
H.K. Müller-Hermelink
J. Delabie
Y.H. Ko
S. Nakamura

Definition
Primary lymphoma of the pancreas is an extranodal lymphoma arising in the pancreas, with the bulk of the disease localized to this site. Contiguous lymph-node involvement and distant spread may be seen, but the primary clinical presentation is in the pancreas.

Epidemiology
Primary lymphoma of the pancreas is very rare, accounting for < 0.5% of pancreatic tumours. As with primary lymphomas occurring elsewhere in the digestive tract, patients are more frequently elderly {1341}.

Etiology
Pancreatic lymphomas may be associated with immunodeficiency; they may be iatrogenic following solid-organ transplantation {423}, and they can arise in the setting of infection with human immunodeficiency virus (HIV) {1445}. Pancreatic lymphoma has also been described in a patient with short-bowel syndrome {1527}.

Clinical features
The presentation of primary pancreatic lymphoma may mimic that of an epithelial neoplasm or pancreatitis {423}. Pain-free jaundice can occur {2260}. Ultrasonography may show an echo-poor lesion {2260}.

Histopathology
Primary pancreatic lymphomas are usually of B phenotype. Lymphomas of various types have been described, including follicular lymphoma {2091, 2260, 2816}, lymphoma of mucosa-associated lymphoid tissue (MALT lymphoma)

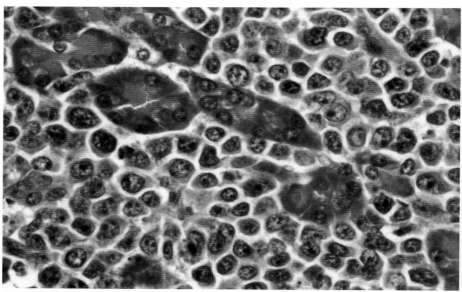

Fig. 12.77 Diffuse large B-cell lymphoma involving the parenchyma of the pancreas.

{3234}, and diffuse large B-cell lymphoma (DLBCL) {1382, 2579}. Only extremely rare cases of T-cell lymphomas presenting with pancreatic involvement have been reported {1996, 2374}. The histology of these cases varies little from that seen elsewhere in the body.

Differential diagnosis
Autoimmune pancreatitis should be considered in the differential diagnosis of MALT lymphoma {2617}. Autoimmune pancreatitis is associated with increased levels of IgG4 in the serum. Histologically, autoimmune pancreatitis is characterized by a duct-centric mixed inflammatory cell infiltrate and venulitis. Large numbers of the infiltrating plasma cells in autoimmune pancreatitis often express IgG4.

Prognosis
The distinction between lymphoma and carcinoma is important, as pancreatic lymphomas are associated with better prognosis and may be curable even at an advanced stage. Surgical resection does not play a role in clinical management of lymphoma of the pancreas. Therefore, diagnosis before pancreatic resection is important. Fine-needle aspiration or biopsy with ancillary studies of immunophenotype and molecular genetics can often lead to accurate diagnosis.

Secondary tumours of the pancreas

C. Iacobuzio-Donahue
N. Fukushima

Definition
Neoplasms that have spread to the pancreas from an extra-pancreatic primary.

Origin
Both epithelial and nonepithelial neoplasms can metastasize to the pancreas. The pancreas may be involved by direct extension, or by lymphatic or haematogenous spread from distant sites. Cancers of the ampulla of Vater, duodenum and distal common bile duct often involve the pancreas by direct extension. The most common more distant malignancies that metastasize to the pancreas are renal cell carcinomas, melanomas, colorectal carcinomas, breast carcinomas and sarcomas {2650}. Occasionally, neoplasms may metastasize to the pancreas many years after diagnosis of the primary neoplasm {53, 1120}.

Epidemiology
Secondary neoplasms of the pancreas account for 4-15% of all malignancies in the pancreas found at autopsy {29, 617, 2213}. Secondary neoplasms affect males and females equally. As is true for metastases in general, the highest incidence is in the sixth and seventh decades of life.

Localization
Any anatomical region of the pancreas may be involved and there is no site predilection {1589}. Although usually multiple, metastases to the pancreas can also be solitary, or they may diffusely involve the gland {1589}.

Clinical features
Similar to primary pancreatic neoplasms, the early signs and symptoms of isolated pancreatic metastases are often nonspecific and subtle. The most common symptoms are abdominal pain, jaundice and gastrointestinal bleeding {2650}. Many lesions are asymptomatic and detected on imaging studies performed to follow-up the patient's original primary neoplasm.

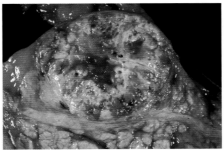

Fig. 12.78 Renal cell carcinoma metastatic to the pancreas.

Macroscopy
Metastases to the pancreas are most often seen as circumscribed masses that may have extensive haemorrhage and/or a cystic component {29}. Pigmented melanomas can form discrete black or brown masses surrounded by normal pancreatic parenchyma; renal cell carcinomas often have a yellow-orange cut surface.

Histopathology
The diagnosis of a secondary neoplasm of the pancreas is often straightforward as most patients will have a known history of an extra-pancreatic primary malignancy. Metastases to the pancreas are histologically similar to their primary tumour of origin. Multiple tumour foci with an abrupt transition from normal pancreas to the neoplastic tissue without signs of chronic pancreatitis in the surrounding parenchyma support metastatic origin {29}. As expected, renal cell carcinomas metastatic to the pancreas often have clear cytoplasm, while the cells of metastatic melanoma may produce melanin and have prominent nucleoli.

Immunohistochemistry
A panel of immunohistochemical markers can be employed to narrow possible organs of origin in problematic cases or to validate a clinical impression.

Cytopathology
Endoscopic ultrasound (EUS)-guided fine-needle aspirations have a high sensitivity in diagnosing a pancreatic metas-

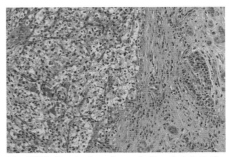

Fig. 12.79 Renal cell carcinoma (left) metastatic to the pancreas. A residual islet of Langerhans can be seen (right)

tasis, even after a previously negative or inconclusive imaging study {709, 3409}. Lesions with the impression of having well-defined borders by EUS are more likely to be a secondary tumour {709}.

Differential diagnosis
The most problematic secondary neoplasms to differentiate from a primary pancreatic neoplasm are metastases from the gastrointestinal tract, renal cell carcinomas and melanomas. Renal cell carcinomas can be difficult to distinguish from well-differentiated pancreatic neuroendocrine neoplasms, especially in patients with von Hippel-Lindau syndrome {584, 1214}. Melanomas may mimic solid pancreatic neoplasms with brisk mitotic activity and nuclei with single prominent nucleoli, such as acinar cell carcinomas or medullary carcinomas of the pancreas {29}. Breast cancer metastatic to the pancreas is important to recognize because of the specific therapies available to treat some metastatic breast cancers. The patient's history and immunolabelling studies can help establish the correct diagnosis.

Prognosis and predictive factors
Since in most cases pancreatic metastases indicate an advanced stage of disease, the prognosis is generally poor. Surgical resection may be beneficial in selected patients {2650}.

Diagnostic algorithms for tumours of the pancreas

D.S. Klimstra
N. Fukushima
R.H. Hruban
G. Klöppel

Introduction

A simple diagnostic algorithm that integrates gross and radiographic features with histological and immunohistochemical findings can help classify neoplasms of the pancreas {1600}. Most pancreatic neoplasms can be accurately diagnosed using the process detailed below, although some exceptions occur because rare, and occasionally also some common neoplasms, may demonstrate unusual features.

The basis for classifying pancreatic neoplasms

The classification of pancreatic epithelial neoplasms appears to be long and complex. However, it can be distilled into a much shorter list if only the commonly encountered entities that encompass > 98% of all pancreatic neoplasms are considered (Table 12.07). Most pancreatic neoplasms are infiltrating ductal adenocarcinomas {1270}. Each of the other more commonly encountered entities makes up only 1–5% of pancreatic neoplasms, but these entities include some of the most treatable pancreatic neoplasms, so their proper recognition is very important.

The classification of pancreatic neoplasms is based on: (1) the gross appearance of the tumour (solid, cystic, or intraductal) (Table 12.06); and (2) the line(s) of cellular differentiation of the neoplastic cells (ductal, acinar, or endocrine)

{1596}. The differentiation present in a pancreatic neoplasm may be obvious histologically, but additional studies such as immunohistochemistry are needed in some cases (Table 12.09).

Gross appearance

Most pancreatic neoplasms (ductal adenocarcinoma, pancreatic neuroendocrine neoplasm, acinar cell carcinoma, pancreatoblastoma) typically form a solid mass. Cystic neoplasms are less common, but are increasingly recognized owing to the use of sensitive imaging techniques {34, 1655, 1717}.

Cystic change can occur via several mechanisms {1270}. The cysts of "true" cystic neoplasms are lined by a continuous layer of neoplastic epithelium. Other neoplasms develop secondary cystic changes because of degeneration or necrosis; this type of cystic change is characteristic in certain entities (solid-pseudopapillary neoplasm) but uncommonly may also affect most typically solid neoplasms. Intraductal neoplasms can appear cystic due to dilatation of the native pancreatic ducts {34, 929}.

When present, the intraductal nature of a cystic neoplasm is important to recognize. Careful gross evaluation and radiographic images can help define the relationship between the duct system and the neoplastic cysts. By probing the larger pancreatic ducts, one can determine the presence or absence of connectivity between the native duct system and a cystic lesion.

Line of differentiation

The most common cellular differentiation in pancreatic neoplasms is ductal {1592}. Mucin can be demonstrated histochemically (periodic-acid-Schiff, or mucicarmine), and with immunohistochemical markers, which detect mucin-related antigens including CA19-9, carcinoembryonic antigen (CEA), and MUC1 {1600, 2126}. Finally, expression of keratins 7 and 19 are most typical of ductal differentiation {1785}, although these keratins, particularly 19, are also found in a subset of pancreatic neuroendocrine neoplasms {90}.

Neuroendocrine differentiation is usually suggested by an organoid growth pattern (nests and trabeculae) and typical nuclear features ("salt and pepper" chromatin). Endocrine differentiation can be demonstrated by immunohistochemical labelling with antibodies against the general neuroendocrine markers chromogranin A and synaptophysin {1876}. Acinar differentiation may be suspected from the growth pattern (formation of acini) and nuclear features (single prominent nucleoli), but immunohistochemical labelling using antibodies against the enzymes trypsin and chymotrypsin is the most sensitive and specific tool {1598, 1601}.

Table 12.07 Frequency of selected pancreatic epithelial neoplasms.

Entity	Frequency
Ductal adenocarcinoma	85%
Intraductal papillary mucinous neoplasm	3–5%
Pancreatic neuroendocrine neoplasm	3–4%
Serous cystadenoma	1–2%
Mucinous cystic neoplasm	1–2%
Acinar cell carcinoma	1–2%
Solid-pseudopapillary neoplasm	1–2%
Pancreatoblastoma	< 1%

Table 12.06 Gross configuration of common pancreatic neoplasms.

Gross configuration	Type	Neoplasm
Solid	—	Ductal adenocarcinoma, acinar cell carcinoma, pancreatoblastoma, pancreatic neuroendocrine neoplasm (solid-pseudopapillary neoplasm)[a]
Cystic	True cysts	Serous cystadenoma, mucinous cystic neoplasm
	Intraductal	Intraductal papillary mucinous neoplasm
	Degenerative	Solid-pseudopapillary neoplasm (ductal adenocarcinoma, acinar cell carcinoma, pancreatic neuroendocrine neoplasm)[a]

[a] Entities in parentheses also uncommonly exhibit this gross configuration.

Diagnostic clues from the clinical presentation

Clinical findings that can aid in the diagnosis of pancreatic neoplasms are age and sex of the patient, location of the neoplasm within the pancreas (head or tail), and presenting symptoms. For example, a young woman with a cystic neoplasm in the tail of the pancreas is likely to have either a mucinous cystic neoplasm or a solid-pseudopapillary neoplasm. An older individual with a cystic lesion in the head of the gland is more likely to have a serous cystic neoplasm or an intraductal papillary mucinous neoplasm. Older adults with solid neoplasms in the head of the pancreas associated with jaundice, back pain, and weight loss have infiltrating ductal adenocarcinomas until proven otherwise. Pancreatic neoplasms presenting in the first decade of life are most commonly pancreatoblastomas, whereas teenagers usually develop solid-pseudopapillary neoplasms or pancreatic neuroendocrine neoplasms {2958}. When there is a pancreatic mass associated with endocrine paraneoplastic syndromes, such as hyperinsulinaemic hypoglycaemia or Zollinger-Ellison syndrome, a well-differentiated pancreatic neuroendocrine neoplasm is usually the diagnosis, whereas subcutaneous fat necrosis and polyarthralgia occur in association with acinar cell carcinoma {1598}. Trousseau syndrome is a classic presentation of ductal adenocarcinoma {1253}.

The diagnostic algorithm

A simple diagnostic algorithm is illustrated here {1270}. The first step in the evaluation of a pancreatic neoplasm is to determine whether the lesion is solid or cystic. The entities included in the cystic category should have a predominantly cystic appearance that is obvious on gross examination or radiographic images, since some solid neoplasms can contain small cysts caused by necrosis or dilated, obstructed ducts.

Solid neoplasms

For solid neoplasms, the next step is to determine the density of the neoplastic cells relative to the stroma, and the character of the stromal component. Is the neoplasm composed of relatively few neoplastic elements associated with abundant stroma, or is it predominantly neoplastic cells with little stroma? If the neoplasm is composed of individually arranged mucin-producing glands with a prominent desmoplastic stroma, it is likely to be an infiltrating ductal adenocarcinoma. The most important differential diagnosis in this case is chronic pancreatitis {1606}. The presence of haphazardly arranged glands in abnormal locations (within the perineurium or vascular spaces, or adjacent to muscular vessels or adipocytes,) and cytological atypia (nuclear enlargement, loss of polarity, and variation in size and shape of nuclei among cells within a gland) all point to a diagnosis of carcinoma.

If the solid neoplasm is composed predominantly of neoplastic elements with little stroma, it will have a more cellular low power appearance, and the differential diagnosis of these "solid, cellular pancreatic neoplasms" includes pancreatic neuroendocrine neoplasm, acinar cell carcinoma, pancreatoblastoma, and solid-pseudopapillary neoplasm {1592}. These four neoplasms are distinguished by their direction of differentiation. The next step in the algorithm is therefore to determine the line(s) of differentiation for the solid cellular neoplasm. Neoplasms with neuroendocrine differentiation, expressing chromogranin A and synaptophysin,

Table 12.08 Sex ratio and location of common pancreatic neoplasms.

Entity	Males : Females	Location
Ductal adenocarcinoma	1.3 : 1.0	Head > tail
Intraductal papillary mucinous neoplasm	1.5 : 1.0	Head > tail
Pancreatic neuroendocrine neoplasm	1.0 : 1.0	Head = tail
Serous cystadenoma	1.0 : 2.3	Head = tail
Mucinous cystic neoplasm	1.0 : 20.0	Tail >>> head
Acinar cell carcinoma	3.6 : 1.0	Head = tail
Solid-pseudopapillary neoplasm	1.0 : 9.0	Head = tail
Pancreatoblastoma	1.7 : 1.0	Head = tail

Table 12.09 Immunohistochemical labelling of common pancreatic neoplasms.

Label	Pancreatic neuroendocrine neoplasms	Acinar cell carcinoma	Pancreatoblastoma	Solid-pseudopapillary neoplasms	Ductal neoplasms[b]
Keratins 8/18	++	++	++	F	++
Keratin 19	+	–	+	–	++
Vimentin	–	–	–	+	–
Trypsin/chymotrypsin	–	++	++	–	–
Chromogranin	++	F	+	–	F
Synaptophysin	++	F	+	+	F
CD10	–	–	–	++	+
β-Catenin[a]	–	+	+	++	–

++, usually positive; +, may be positive; F, may be focally positive; –, usually negative.
[a] Nuclear labelling.
[b] Ductal neoplasms include infiltrating ductal adenocarcinoma, mucinous cystic neoplasm, intraductal papillary mucinous neoplasm and serous cystic neoplasms.

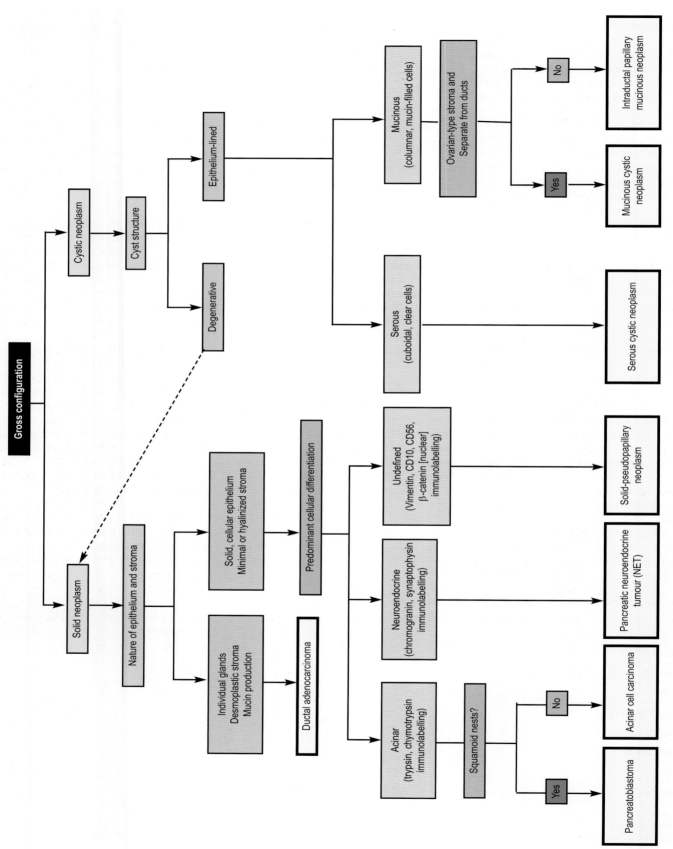

Fig 12.80 Simple algorithm for the diagnostic evaluation of pancreatic neoplasms {1270}.

are usually well-differentiated pancreatic neuroendocrine neoplasms. Neoplasms with acinar differentiation are usually acinar cell carcinomas or pancreatoblastomas {1598, 1602} and consistently express trypsin and chymotrypsin {1235, 1598}. Although most pancreatoblastomas arise in young children and acinar cell carcinoma affect adults, exceptions occur, and the histological and immunohistochemical features of acinar cell carcinoma and pancreatoblastoma overlap extensively.

The single histological feature that most distinguishes pancreatoblastoma is the squamoid nest (corpuscle), which can be composed of vaguely whorled nests of cells with elongate nuclei and more cytoplasm than the surrounding acinar elements, or of spindled cells with keratinization {1602}.

Cellular neoplasms composed of poorly cohesive cells lacking a clearly definable line of differentiation and expressing CD10, CD56 (NCAM1), α-1-antitrypsin, and β-catenin (nuclear) are likely to be solid-pseudopapillary neoplasms {8, 1603, 2324}. Other histological features of solid-pseudopapillary neoplasms include degenerative pseudopapillae, loosely cohesive cells with grooved nuclei, aggregates of large hyaline globules, and a giant-cell reaction to cholesterol crystals.

Cystic neoplasms

If a pancreatic neoplasm is cystic, the first step is to determine whether the cystic change is degenerative in nature or whether the cysts are lined by continuous epithelium (truly cystic or intraductal). If the cystic change is degenerative, the noncystic regions of the neoplasm should be evaluated as though the tumour were solid. Degenerative cystic change is usually extensive in solid-pseudopapillary neoplasm, and this is the solid neoplasm that would most often be placed (initially) on the cystic arm of the algorithm.

If the cysts are lined by neoplastic epithelium, then the nature of the neoplastic cells should be determined. Serous, cuboidal, clear cells with uniform, round hyperchromatic nuclei indicate either a microcystic or macrocystic serous cystadenoma {1610}. Mucin stains are negative in serous cystadenomas, and periodic acid-Schiff (PAS) stain will reveal intracellular glycogen, which is sensitive to digestion with diastase. If mucinous cells are present, then the next step is to determine whether the lesion is a true cystic neoplasm or an intraductal neoplasm {1270}. True cystic neoplasms that are separate from the ductal system and also have cellular, ovarian-type subepithelial stroma are mucinous cystic neoplasms {3673}. Immunohistochemical labelling for estrogen and progesterone receptors can be used to demonstrate this stroma, which is considered a requisite feature for the diagnosis of mucinous cystic neoplasm {3239, 3673}. These neoplasms occur almost exclusively in females (female to male ratio, at least 20 : 1) and nearly always arise in the tail of the pancreas.

Neoplastic mucinous epithelium involving the duct system without associated ovarian-type stroma is characteristic of an intraductal papillary mucinous neoplasm (IPMN) {1106, 1271}. When an IPMN involves one of the major pancreatic ducts, it is relatively easy to confirm that the neoplasm is intraductal. For branch-duct IPMNs {3222}, it can be more difficult to recognize grossly that the cystic structures represent dilated ducts, but microscopically there are periductal glands surrounding the cysts, and the cysts are separated by other pancreatic elements (islets, non-neoplastic ducts, or acinar cells). IPMNs appear as multiple separate cysts on cross section, whereas mucinous cystic neoplasms are single, multilocular cysts usually surrounded by a fibrous pseudocapsule. Most importantly, the hypercellular ovarian-type subepithelial stroma of mucinous cystic neoplasms is not found in IPMNs.

Exceptions to the rules

Rare neoplasms are not included in the algorithm to prevent it from becoming unwieldy. Also, some of the neoplasms in the algorithm have uncommon variants with fundamentally different features that would place them elsewhere in the algorithm. For example, acinar cell cystadenocarcinoma {408} is an inherently cystic neoplasm with acinar differentiation. Similarly, an intraductal growth pattern can also occur rarely in acinar cell carcinomas {213} as well as in pancreatic neuroendocrine neoplasms. Pathologists need to keep these rarer lesions in mind, especially when dealing with a neoplasm that does not fit cleanly into one of the more common categories covered in the algorithm.

As previously mentioned, rare pancreatic neoplasms have significant components of more than one cell type. For example, although they are predominantly acinar, pancreatoblastomas often have endocrine and ductal differentiation. Rare carcinomas have been described with all different combinations of differentiation (acinar-neuroendocrine, ductal-neuroendocrine, acinar-ductal, and acinar-neuroendocrine-ductal) {182, 691, 1270, 2369}. These are not included in the algorithm. A final note is that metastases to the pancreas from other organs (lung, ovary, breast, melanoma and kidney in particular) do occur, although usually in the context of widespread disease {29}. Some metastatic carcinomas have overlapping features with primary pancreatic neoplasms, and in the case of infiltrating ductal adenocarcinoma, there is no pancreas-specific immunohistochemical marker to allow easy distinction from a metastatic adenocarcinoma.

Contributors

Dr N. Volkan ADSAY*
Department of Pathology
Emory University Hospital
1364 Clifton Road, NE, Room H180-B
Atlanta, GA 30322
USA
Tel. +1 404 712 4179
Fax. +1 404 727 2519
volkan.adsay@emory.edu

Dr Dennis J. AHNEN
Department of Medicine
Denver Dept of Veterans Affairs Medical Center
and University of Colorado School of Medicine
Denver, CO 80220
USA
Tel. +1 303 399 8020
Fax. +1 303 393 4168
dennis.ahnen@ucdenver.edu

Dr Jorge ALBORES-SAAVEDRA*
Department of Pathology
Instituto Nacional de Ciencias Medicas
y Nutricion Salvador Zubiran
Vasco de Quiroga 15, Col. Seccion XVI
Talpan 14000, CP 14400 Mexico D.F.
MEXICO
Tel. +52 55 548 70900
Fax. +52 55 548 53489
alboresjorge@yahoo.com

Dr Stefan ARETZ
Institute of Human Genetics
Biomedical Center, University Hospital Bonn
Sigmund-Freud Strasse 25
53127 Bonn
GERMANY
Tel. +49 228 287 51009
Fax. +49 228 287 51011
Stefan.Aretz@uni-bonn.de

Dr Rudolf ARNOLD
Wittelsbacherstrasse 6
80469 Munich
GERMANY
Tel. + 49 892 016 359
Fax. + 49 892 020 5564
arnoldr@mailer.uni-marburg.de

Dr Charles BALABAUD
Department of Hepatology
Hôpital Saint André
INSERM U889, Université Bordeaux 2
Place Amélie-Raba-Léon
33076 Bordeaux Cedex
FRANCE
Tel. +33 5 57 57 17 71 (ext 76769)
Fax. +33 5 56 51 40 77
charles.balabaud@chu-bordeaux.fr

Dr Marc BILLAUD
Laboratoire Génétique Moléculaire
Signalisation et Cancer, CNRS UMR5201
Centre Léon Bérard, Bâtiment Cheney D
28, rue Laënnec, 69008 Lyon
FRANCE
Tel: +33 4 69 16 66 56
Fax: +33 4 69 16 66 60
billaud@lyon.fnclcc.fr

Dr Paulette BIOULAC-SAGE*
Department of Pathology, Hopital Pellegrin
Centre Hospitalier Universitaire Bordeaux
INSERM U889, Université Bordeaux 2
Place Amélie-Raba-Léon
33076 Bordeaux Cedex
FRANCE
Tel. +33 5 56 79 56 02
Fax. +33 5 56 79 60 88
paulette.bioulac-sage@chu-bordeaux.fr

Dr Paolo BOFFETTA
Section of Environment
International Agency for Research
on Cancer (IARC)
150 cours Albert Thomas
69372 Lyon cedex 08
FRANCE
paolo.boffetta@mssm.edu

Dr Fredrik T. BOSMAN*
University Institute of Pathology
Rue du Bugnon 25
1011 Lausanne
SWITZERLAND
Tel. +41 21 314 7202
Fax. +41 21 314 7205
fred.bosman@chuv.ch

Dr Randall W. BURT
Huntsman Cancer Institute
University of Utah
Salt Lake City, UT 84112
USA
Tel. +1 801 585 3281
Fax. +1 801 581 3389
randall.burt@hci.utah.edu

Dr Carlo CAPELLA
Department of Pathology
Ospedale di Circolo
Viale Borri 57
21100 Varese
ITALY
Tel. +39 0332 270 601
Fax. +39 0332 270 600
carlo.capella@ospedale.varese.it

Dr Fátima CARNEIRO*
Institute of Molecular Pathology and Immunology
of the University of Porto (IPATIMUP)
and University Hospital S.João/Faculty
of Medicine of the University of Porto,
Rua Dr Roberto Frias s/n, 4200-465 Porto
PORTUGAL
Tel. +351 225 570 700
Fax. +351 225 570 799
fcarneiro@ipatimup.pt

Dr Norman J. CARR
School of Medicine
University of Southampton
Mailpoint 801, Southampton General Hospital
Tremona Road,
Southampton S016 6YD
UK
Tel. +44 23 8079 5107
Fax. +44 23 8079 4760
carrnj@doctors.org.uk

Dr Parakrama CHANDRASOMA
Keck School of Medicine
University of Southern California
LAC-USC Medical Center CT-7A-121
1100 N State Street, Los Angeles, CA 90033
USA
Tel. +1 323 409 4600
Fax. +1 323 441 8183
ptchandr@usc.edu

*The asterisk indicates participation in the
Working Group Meeting on the Classification
of Tumours of the Digestive System that was
held in Lyon, France, December 10–12, 2009

Dr Amanda CHARLTON
Dept of Molecular Medicine and Pathology
Faculty of Medical and Health Sciences
University of Auckland
Private Bag 92019
Auckland
NEW ZEALAND
Tel. +64 9 373 7599
a.charlton@auckland.ac.nz

Dr James M. CRAWFORD
Dept of Pathology and Laboratory Medicine
North Shore-LIJ Health System
North Shore-LIJ Core Laboratory
10 Nevada Drive,
Lake Success, NY 11042-1114
USA
Tel. +1 516 719 1060
Fax. +1 516 719 1061
jcrawford1@nshs.edu

Dr Maria-Paula CURADO
Section of Cancer Information
International Agency for Research
on Cancer (IARC)
150 cours Albert Thomas
69372 Lyon cedex 08
FRANCE

Dr Yataro DAIGO
Laboratory of Molecular Medicine
Human Genome Center
Institute of Medical Science, University of Tokyo
4-6-1 Shirokanedai Minato-ku
108-8639 Tokyo
JAPAN
Tel. +81 3 5449 5457
Fax. +81 3 5449 5406
ydaigo@ims.u-tokyo.ac.jp

Dr Jan DELABIE
Department of Pathology
The Norwegian Radium Hospital
University of Oslo
0310 Oslo
NORWAY
Tel. +47 22934879
Fax. +47 22730164
jan.delabie@labmed.uio.no

Dr Cathy ENG
Dept of Gastrointestinal Medical Oncology
University of Texas MD Anderson Cancer Center
1515 Holcombe Blvd, Unit 426
Houston, TX 77030
USA
Tel. +1 713 792 2828
Fax. +1 713 794 1873
ceng@mdanderson.org

Dr Charis ENG
Genomic Medicine Institute
Cleveland Clinic
9500 Euclid Avenue, NE-50
Cleveland, OH 44195
USA
Tel. +1 216 444 3440
Fax. +1 216 636 0655
engc@ccf.org

Dr Linda FERRELL
Department of Anatomic Pathology
University of California, San Francisco
505 Parnassus Avenue, M-590, Box 0102
San Francisco, CA 94143
USA
Tel. +1 415 353 1090
Fax. +1 415 353 1200
linda.ferrell@ucsf.edu

Dr John K. FIELD
Roy Castle Lung Cancer Research Programme
University of Liverpool, Cancer Research Centre
Roy Castle Building
200 London Road
Liverpool, L3 9TA
UK
Tel. + 44 151 794 8901/8900
Fax. + 44 151 794 8989
j.k.field@liv.ac.uk

Dr Jean-François FLÉJOU*
Service d'Anatomie Pathologique
Hôpital Saint-Antoine
Faculté de Médecine Pierre et Marie Curie
184, rue du Faubourg Saint-Antoine
75571 Paris Cedex 12
FRANCE
Tel. + 33 1 49 28 30 12
Fax. + 33 1 49 28 28 78
jean-francois.flejou@sat.aphp.fr

Dr Christopher D.M. FLETCHER
Department of Pathology
Brigham and Women's Hospital
and Harvard Medical School
75 Francis Street
Boston, MA 02115
USA
Tel. +1 617 732 8558
Fax. +1 617 566 3897
cfletcher@partners.org

Dr Silvia FRANCESCHI
Section of Infections
International Agency for Research on Cancer
(IARC)
150 cours Albert Thomas
69372 Lyon cedex 08
FRANCE
Tel. +33 4 72 73 84 02
Fax.+33 4 72 73 83 45
franceschi@iarc.fr

Dr Noriyoshi FUKUSHIMA*
Department of Pathology
Jichi Medical University
3311-1 Yakushiji, Shimotsuke-shi
329-0498 Tochigi
JAPAN
Tel. +81 285 58 7330
Fax. +81 285 44 8467
nfukushima@jichi.ac.jp

Dr Toru FURUKAWA
Institute for Integrated Medical Sciences
Tokyo Women's Medical University
8-1 Kawada-cho, Shinjuku-ku
162-8666 Tokyo
JAPAN
Tel. +81 3 3353 8111 Ext 29675
Fax. +81 3 3352 3088
toru.furukawa@twmu.ac.jp

Dr Karel GEBOES
Department of Pathology
University Hospital, K.U. Leuven
Minderbroedersstraat 12
3000 Leuven
BELGIUM
Tel. + 32 16 33 65 84
Fax. + 32 16 33 65 48
karel.geboes@uz.kuleuven.ac.be

Dr Robert M. GENTA
Department of Pathology
Dallas Veterans Affairs Medical Center
University of Texas Southwestern Medical School
5323 Harry Hines Blvd
Dallas, TX 75390-9072
USA
Tel. +1 214 596 7440
Fax. +1 214 596 2297
robert.genta@utsouthwestern.edu

Dr Francis M. GIARDIELLO
The Johns Hopkins Hospital
1830 E Monument Street
Baltimore, MD 21205
USA
Tel. +1 410 955 2635
Fax. +1 410 614 8337

Dr Gregory GORES
Division of Gastroenterology and Hepatology
Mayo Clinic College of Medicine
200 1st Street SW
Rochester, MN 55905
USA
Tel. +1 507 284 0686
Fax. + 1 507 284 0762
gores.gregory@mayo.edu

Dr David Y. GRAHAM
Dept of Medicine/Gastroenterology
Michael E DeBakey VA Medical Center
and Baylor College of Medicine
Rm 3A-320 (111D) 2002 Holcombe Blvd
Houston, TX 77030
USA
Tel. +1 713 794 7280
Fax. +1 713 795 4471
dgraham@bcm.tmc.edu

Dr Gabriel M. GROISMAN
Department of Pathology
Hillel Yaffe Medical Center
Hadera 38100
ISRAEL
Tel. +972 4 630 4627
Fax. +972 4 630 4630
groisman@hy.health.gov.il

Dr Stephen B. GRUBER
Division of Molecular Medicine and Genetics
University of Michigan
4301 MSRB III
Ann Arbor, MI 48109-0652
USA
Tel. +1 734 615 9712
Fax. +1 734 647 7950
sgruber@umich.edu

Dr Stanley R. HAMILTON*
Division of Pathology and Laboratory Medicine
University of Texas MD Anderson Cancer Center
1515 Holcombe Blvd, Unit 85
Houston,TX 77030
USA
Tel. + 1 713 792 2040
Fax. +1 713 792 4094
shamilto@mdanderson.org

Dr Takanori HATTORI
Shiga University of Medical Science
Seta Tsukinowa-Cho, Ohtsu
520-2192 Shiga
JAPAN
Tel. +81 77 548 2002
Fax. +81 77 543 9880
hattori@belle.shiga-med.ac.jp

Dr Nobuyoshi HIRAOKA
Pathology Division
National Cancer Center Research Institute
5-1-1 Tsukiji, Chuo-ku
104-0045 Tokyo
JAPAN
Tel. +81 3 3542 2511
Fax. +81 3 3248 2463
nhiraoka@gan2.res.ncc.go.jp

Dr Heinz HÖFLER
Department of Pathology
Technical University of Munich
Ismaningerstrasse 22
81675 Munich
GERMANY
Tel. +49 89 4140 4160
Fax. +49 89 4140 4865
hoefler@lrz.tum.de

Dr James R. HOWE
Department of Surgery
University of Iowa College of Medicine
Iowa City, IA 52242-1086
USA
Tel. +1 319 356 1727
Fax. +1 319 353 8940
james-howe@uiowa.edu

Dr Ralph H. HRUBAN*
Department of Pathology
The Sol Goldman Pancreatic Cancer Research
Center, Johns Hopkins Medical Institutions
401 N. Broadway, Weinberg 2242
Baltimore, MD 21231-2410
USA
Tel. +1 410 955 9132
Fax. +1 410 955 0115
rhruban@jhmi.edu

Dr David G. HUNTSMAN
Department of Pathology
British Columbia Cancer Agency - CTAG Lab
3427-600 West 10th Avenue
Vancouver, BC V5Z 4E6
CANADA
Tel. +1 604 877 6000 Ext 2148
Fax. +1 604 877 6089
dhuntsma@bccancer.bc.ca

Dr Prodromos HYTIROGLOU*
Department of Pathology
Aristotle University Medical School
54006 Thessaloniki
GREECE
Tel. +302 310 999 218
Fax. +302 310 999 229
phitir@med.auth.gr

Dr Christine IACOBUZIO-DONAHUE
Department of Pathology
The Sol Goldman Pancreatic Cancer Research
Center, Johns Hopkins Medical Institutions
1550 Orleans Street, CRB II Room 343
Baltimore, MD 21231
USA
Tel. +1 410 955 3511
Fax. +1 410 614 0671
ciacobu@jhmi.edu

Dr Mohammad ILYAS
School of Molecular Medical Sciences
Faculty of Medicine & Health Sciences
University of Nottingham
Level A, West Block, Queens Medical Centre
Nottingham NG7 2UH
UK
Tel. +44 115 8230735
Fax. +44 115 823 0759
mohammad.ilyas@nottingham.ac.uk

Dr Elaine S. JAFFE
Hematopathology Section, Laboratory
of Pathology, Center for Cancer Research
National Cancer Institute
10 Center Drive MSC 1500
Bethesda, MD 20892
USA
Tel. +1 301 496 0183
Fax. +1 301 402 2415
elainejaffe@nih.gov

Dr Heikki J. JÄRVINEN
Department of Surgery
Helsinki University Central Hospital
Haartmaninkatu 4, PO Box 340
00029 HUS Helsinki
FINLAND
Tel. +358 947173852
Fax. +358 947174675
heikki.jarvinen@hus.fi

Dr Yo KATO
Department of Pathology
Cancer Institute, JFCR
3-10-6 Ariake, Koto-ku
135-8550 Tokyo
JAPAN
Tel. +81 3 3520 0111
Fax. +81 3 3570 0558 / +81 3 5879 8846
kato@jfcr.or.jp

Dr Scott E. KERN
Department of Oncology
Johns Hopkins University
1650 N. Orleans Street, CRB 451
Baltimore, MD 21231
USA
Tel. +1 410 614 3314
Fax. +1 443 287 4653
skern1@jhmi.edu

Dr Lars-Gunnar KINDBLOM
Department of Musculoskeletal Pathology
Royal Orthopaedic Hospital NHS Trust
University of Birmingham Medical School
Bristol Road South, Northfield
Birmingham B31 2AP
UK
Tel. + 44 12 1414 7643
Fax. + 44 12 1414 7640
lars.kindblom@roh.nhs.uk

Dr David S. KLIMSTRA*
Department of Pathology
Memorial Sloan-Kettering Cancer Center
1275 York Avenue
New York, NY 10065
USA
Tel. +1 212 639 2410
Fax. +1 646 422 2016
klimstrd@mskcc.org

Dr Günter KLÖPPEL*
Department of Pathology
TU-Munich
Ismaningerstrasse 22
81675 Munich
GERMANY
Tel. +49 89 4140 6158
Fax. +49 89 4140 4865
Guenter.Kloeppel@lrz.tu-muenchen.de

Dr Young Hyeh KO
Department of Pathology
Samsung Medical Center
Sungkyunkwan University
Gangnam-gu, Irwondong 50
135-710 Seoul
REPUBLIC OF KOREA
Tel. +82 02 3410 2762
Fax. +82 02 3410 0025
yhko310@skku.edu

Dr Paul KOMMINOTH
Institute of Pathology, Stadtspital Triemli
Birmendorferstrasse 497
CH-8063 Zurich
SWITZERLAND
Tel. +41 444 662122
Fax. +41 444 662138
paul.komminoth@triemli.stzh.ch

Dr Masatoshi KUDO
Department of Gastroenterology and Hepatology
Kinki University School of Medicine
377-2, Ohno-Higashi
Osaka-Sayama
589-8511 Osaka
JAPAN
Tel. +81 72 366 0221
Fax. +81 72 367 2880
m-kudo@med.kindai.ac.jp

Dr Sunil R. LAKHANI*
Molecular and Cellular Pathology
The University of Queensland Centre for
Clinical Research and School of Medicine
The Royal Brisbane & Women's Hospital
Herston, 4029, Brisbane QLD
AUSTRALIA
Tel. +61 7 3346 6052
Fax. +61 7 3346 5596
s.lakhani@uq.edu.au

Dr René LAMBERT
Section of Early Detection and Prevention
International Agency for Research on Cancer
(IARC)
150 cours Albert Thomas
69372 Lyon cedex 08
FRANCE
Tel. +33 4 72 73 84 99
Fax: + 33 4 72 73 85 18
lambert@iarc.fr

Dr Gregory Y. LAUWERS*
Department of Pathology
Massachusetts General Hospital
and Harvard Medical School
55 Fruit Street
Boston, MA 02114-2696
USA
Tel. +1 617-726-0931
Fax. +1 617-726-0982
glauwers@partners.org

Dr Anirban MAITRA
Department of Pathology
The Sol Goldman Pancreatic Cancer Research
Center, Johns Hopkins Medical Institutions
1550 Orleans Street, CRB II, Room 345
Baltimore, MD 21231
USA
Tel. +1 410 955 3511
Fax. +1 410 614 0671
amaitra1@jhmi.edu

Dr Markku MIETTINEN
Department of Soft Tissue
and Orthopedic Pathology
Armed Forces Institute of Pathology
6825 16th Street NW Bldg 54
Washington, DC 20306-6000
USA
Tel. +1 202 782 1575
Fax. +1 202 782 9182
Markku.Miettinen@us.army.mil

Dr Elizabeth MONTGOMERY*
Department of Pathology
Johns Hopkins Medical Institutions
401 N Broadway, Weinberg 2242
Baltimore, MD 21231-2410
USA
Tel. +1 410 614 2308
Fax. +1 443 287 3818
emontgom@jhmi.edu

Dr Toshio MOROHOSHI
First Department of Pathology
Showa University School of Medicine
1-5-8 Hatanodai, Shinagawa-ku
142-8555 Tokyo
JAPAN
Tel. +81 3 3784 8118
Fax. +81 3 3784 8249
moro@med.showa-u.ac.jp

Dr Hans MORREAU*
Department of Pathology
Leiden University Medical Center
Albinusdreef 2,
PO Box 9600
2333 ZA Leiden
THE NETHERLANDS
Tel. +31 71 526 6630
Fax. +31 71 526 6952
j.morreau@lumc.nl

Dr Hans Konrad MÜLLER-HERMELINK
Institute of Pathology
University of Würzburg
Josef Schneider Srt. 2
97080 Würzburg
GERMANY
Tel. +49 931 2014 7776/+49 931 2014 7427
Fax. +49 931 2014 7440
Konrad.mh@mail.uni-wuerzburg.de

Dr Shin-ichi NAKAMURA*
Diagnostic Pathology Research Co., Ltd
10-53 Mitake 4
020-0122 Morioka
JAPAN
Tel. +81 19 648 1432
Fax. +81 19 648 1386
nakamurashin@grace.ocn.ne.jp

Dr Shigeo NAKAMURA
Department of Pathology
and Laboratory Medicine
Nagoya University Hospital
65 Tsurumai-cho, Showa-ku
466-8550 Nagoya
JAPAN
Tel. +81 52 744 2896
Fax. +81 52 744 2897
snakamur@med.nagoya-u.ac.jp

Dr Yasuni NAKANUMA
Department of Human Pathology
Kanazawa University
Graduate School of Medicine
Takaramachi 13-1
920-8640 Kanazawa
JAPAN
Tel. +81 076 265 2195
Fax. +81 076 234 4229
pbcpsc@kenroku.kanazawa-u.ac.jp

Dr Osamu NAKASHIMA
Department of Pathology
Kurume University School of Medicine
67 Asahi-machi
830-0011 Kurume-shi
JAPAN
Tel. +81 942 31 7546
Fax. +81 942 32 0905
osamu31@med.kurume-u.ac.jp

Dr Amy E. NOFFSINGER
Department of Pathology
and Laboratory Medicine
University of Cincinnati
234 Goodman Ave ML 0533
Cincinnati, OH 45219
USA
Tel.   +1 513 584 3837
Fax. +1 513 584 3892
amy.noffsinger@uc.edu

Dr Kenji NOTOHARA
Department of Pathology
Kurashiki Central Hospital
1-1-1 Miwa, Kurashiki
710-8602 Okayama
JAPAN
Tel. +81 86 422 0210
Fax. +81 86 421 3424
notohara@kchnet.or.jp

Dr Robert D. ODZE*
Pathology Department
Brigham and Women's Hospital
Harvard Medical School
75 Francis Street
Boston, MA 02115
USA
Tel. +1 617 732 7549
Fax. +1 617 278 6950
rodze@partners.org

Dr G. Johan A. OFFERHAUS*
Department of Pathology
University Medical Center Utrecht
PB 85500
3508 GA Utrecht
THE NETHERLANDS
Tel. +31 88 7556561
Fax. +31 30 2544990
g.j.a.offerhaus@umcutrecht.nl

Dr Hiroko OHGAKI*
Section of Molecular Pathology
International Agency for Research on Cancer
(IARC)
150 cours Albert Thomas
69372 Lyon cedex 08
FRANCE
Tel. +33 4 72 73 85 34
Fax. +33 4 72 73 86 98
ohgaki@iarc.fr

Dr Nobuyuki OHIKE
First Department of Pathology
Showa University School of Medicine
1-5-8 Hatanodai, Shinagawa-ku
142-8555 Tokyo
JAPAN
Tel. + 81 3 3784 8118
Fax. +81 3 3784 8249
ohike@med.showa-u.ac.jp

Dr Valérie PARADIS
Service d'Anatomie Pathologique
Hôpital Beaujon
100 Boulevard Général Leclerc
92118 Clichy
FRANCE
Tel. +33 1 40 87 54 63
Fax. +33 1 40 87 00 77
vparadis@teaser.fr

Dr Young Nyun PARK
Department of Pathology and Severance
Medical Research Institute
Yonsei University College of Medicine
CPO Box 8044 Seoul
REPUBLIC OF KOREA
Tel. +82 2 2228 1768
Fax. +82 2 362 0860
young0608@yuhs.ac

Dr Paivi PELTOMAKI
Department of Medical Genetics
Haartman Institute
P.O. Box 63, Haartmaninkatu 8
FI-00014 University of Helsinki
FINLAND
Tel. +358 9 1912 5092
Fax. +358 9 1912 5105
paivi.peltomaki@helsinki.fi

Dr Martha Bishop PITMAN
Department of Pathology
Harvard Medical School
Massachusetts General Hospital
55 Fruit Street, WRN 2
Boston MA 02114
USA
Tel. +1 617 726 3185
Fax. +1 617 724 6564/+1 617 726 7474
mpitman@partners.org

Dr Phil QUIRKE
Wellcome Trust Brenner Building
Leeds Institute of Molecular Medicine
University of Leeds St James's University Hospital
Beckett Street
Leeds, LS9
UK
Tel. +44 113 343 8407
Fax. +44 113 34 38 431
P.Quirke@leeds.ac.uk

Dr Elio RIBOLI
Dept of Epidemiology and Public Health
Imperial College, St Mary's Campus
Norfolk Place
Paddington
London W2 1PG
UK
Tel. +44 20 7594 1913
Fax. +44 20 7262 1034
e.riboli@imperial.ac.uk

Dr Robert H. RIDDELL*
Department of Pathology
and Laboratory Medicine, Mount Sinai Hospital
Joseph & Wolf Lebovic Health Complex
600 University Ave
Ontario, M5G 1X5 Toronto
CANADA
Tel. +1 416 586 4768
Fax. +1 416 586 8481
RRiddell@mtsinai.on.ca

Dr Guido RINDI*
Institute of Anatomic Pathology
Catholic University Sacro Cuore
Policlinico A. Gemelli
Largo A. Gemelli, 8
00168 Rome
ITALY
Tel. +39 06 3015 5883
Fax. +39 06 3015 7008
guido.rindi@rm.unicatt.it

Dr Massimo RUGGE
Department of Pathology
University of Padova
Via Aristide Gabelli, 61
35100 Padova
ITALY
Tel. + 39 049 827 2248
Fax. + 39 049 827 2277
massimo.rugge@unipd.it

Dr Michiie SAKAMOTO*
Department of Pathology
Keio University School of Medicine
35 Shinanomachi, Shinjuku-ku
160-8582 Tokyo
JAPAN
Tel. +81 3 5363 3762
Fax. +81 3 3353 3290
msakamot@sc.itc.keio.ac.jp

Dr Romil SAXENA*
Clarian Pathology Laboratory
Indiana University
350 West 11th Street, Room 4056
Indianapolis, IN 46202-4108
USA
Tel. +1 317 491 6487
Fax. +1 317 491 6419
rsaxena@iupui.edu

Dr Neil A. SHEPHERD
Gloucestershire Cellular Pathology Laboratory
Cheltenham General Hospital
Sandford Road
Cheltenham
Gloucestershire GL53 7AN
UK
Tel. +44 8454 223304
Fax. +44 8454 223318
neil.shepherd@glos.nhs.uk

Dr Michio SHIMIZU
Department of Pathology
Saitama International Medical Center
1397-1 Yamane Hidaka-shi
Saitama
JAPAN
Tel. +81 42 984 4625
Fax. +81 42 984 0609
shimizu@saitama-med.ac.jp

Dr Tadakazu SHIMODA*
Cancer Control and Information Services
National Cancer Center
5-1-1 Tsukiji Chuo Ku
104-0045 Tokyo
JAPAN
Tel. +813 3542 2511
Fax. +813 3457 5013
tshimoda@ncc.go.jp

Dr Dale C. SNOVER*
Department of Pathology
Fairview Southdale Hospital
6401 France Ave S
Minneapolis, MN 55435
USA
Tel. +1 952 924 5152
Fax. +1 952 924 5256
snoverd@umn.edu

Dr Leslie H. SOBIN*
Division of Gastrointestinal Pathology
Armed Forces Institute of Pathology
Washington, DC 20306
USA
Tel. +1 202 364 8358
sobin@uicc.org

Dr Enrico SOLCIA
Department of Human Pathology and Genetics
University of Pavia and IRCCS
Policlinico San Matteo
Via Forlanini 16
27100 Pavia
ITALY
Tel. +39 0382 528 474-5-6-7
Fax. +39 0382 525 866
solciae@smatteo.pv.it

Dr Stuart Jon SPECHLER
Division of Gastroenterology
UT Southwestern Medical Center at Dallas
4500 South Lancaster Road
Dallas, TX 75216
USA
Tel. +1 214 374 7799
Fax. +1 214 857 1571
sjspechler@aol.com

Dr Banchob SRIPA
Department of Pathology
Faculty of Medicine
Khon Kaen University
123 Mitraparp Road
40002 Khon Kaen
THAILAND
Tel. +66 43 363113
Fax. +66 43 202024
banchob@kku.ac.th

Dr Masae TATEMATSU
Division of Oncological Pathology
Aichi Cancer Center Research Institute
1-1 Kanokoden, Chikusa-ku
464-8681 Nagoya
JAPAN
Tel. +81 052 802 8600
Fax. +81 052 802 8700
mtate821@dream.ocn.ne.j

Dr Benoit TERRIS*
Service d'Anatomie Pathologique
Hôpital Cochin
27 rue du Faubourg Saint-Jacques
75679 Paris cedex 14
FRANCE
Tel. +33 1 58 41 14 79
Fax. +33 1 58 41 14 80
benoit.terris@cch.ap-hop-paris.fr

Dr Neil D. THEISE*
Division of Digestive Diseases
Beth Israel Medical Center
First Avenue at 16th Street
New York, NY 10003
USA
Tel. +1 212 420 2211/+1 212 420 4246
Fax. +1 212 420 4373
ntheise@chpnet.org

Dr Michael TORBENSON
Department of Pathology
The Johns Hopkins University School
of Medicine
1503E Jefferson (Bond Street Building)
Baltimore, MD 21231
USA
Tel. +1 443 287 4730
Fax. +1 410 502 5158
mtorben@jhmi.edu

Dr Wilson M.S. TSUI
Departement of Pathology
Caritas Medical Centre
Wing Hong Street, Shamshuipo
Kowloon
Hong Kong SAR
CHINA
Tel. +852 3408 7961
Fax. +852 2745 1804
mstsui@ha.org.hk

Dr J. Han VAN KRIEKEN
Department of Pathology, 824 PA
Radboud University Nijmegen Medical Centre
PO Box 9101
NL-6500HB Nijmegen
THE NETHERLANDS
Tel. +31 24 361 4352
Fax. +31 24 366 8750
J.vanKrieken@pathol.umcn.nl

Dr Hans F.A. VASEN
The Netherlands Foundation for the Detection
of Hereditary Tumours & Department
of Gastroenterology and Hepatology
Leiden University Medical Center
2300 RC Leiden
THE NETHERLANDS
Tel. +31 71 52 62 687
Fax.+ 31 71 52 12 137
hfavasen@stoet.nl

Dr Michael VIETH
Institute of Pathology, Klinikum Bayreuth
Preuschwitzer Strasse 101
95445 Bayreuth
GERMANY
Tel. +49 921 400 502
Fax. +49 921 400 5609
vieth.lkpathol@uni-bayreuth.de

Dr Ian WANLESS
MacKenzie Building, 7th floor
QEII HSC, Anatomic Pathology
740-5788 University Avenue
Halifax, Nova Scotia, B3H 1V8
CANADA
Tel. +1 902 473 7713/+1 902 473 5236
Fax. +1 902 473 1049
ian.wanless@cdha.nshealth.ca

Dr Bryan F. WARREN
Cellular Pathology
John Radcliffe Hospital
Oxford OX3 9DU
UK
Tel. +44 1865 220499
Fax.+44 1865 220519
wbf7warren@aol.com

Dr Aileen WEE
Department of Pathology
Yong Loo Lin School of Medicine
National University of Singapore
National University Hospital
Main Building, Level 3, Singapore 119074
SINGAPORE
Tel. +65 6772 4305
Fax. +65 6778 0671
aileen_wee@nuhs.edu.sg

Dr Mark Lane WELTON
Department of Surgery
Stanford University School of Medicine
875 Blake Wilbur Drive, Rm CC2213
Stanford, CA 94305-5820
USA
Tel. +1 650 721 1792
Fax. +1 650 736 8136
MWelton@Stanfordmed.org

Dr Giuseppe ZAMBONI*
Department of Pathology
University of Verona
Ospedale Sacro Cuore-Don Calabria
Via don Sempreboni 5
37024 Negrar-Verona
ITALY
Tel. +39 045 6013 415
Fax. +39 045 7500 480
giuseppe.zamboni@sacrocuore.it

Dr Arthur ZIMMERMANN
Institute of Pathology of the University
Murtenstrasse 31
P.O. Box 62
CH – 3010 Bern
SWITZERLAND
Tel. +41 31 632 32 22 / 632 99 50
Fax. +41 31 632 49 95
zimmerma@patho.unibe.ch

IARC/WHO Committee for the International Classification of Diseases for Oncology (ICD-O)

Dr Jean FAIVRE
Registre Bourguignon des Cancers Digestifs
Faculté de Médecine
7 boulevard Jeanne d'Arc
21079 Dijon cedex
FRANCE
Tel. +33 3 80 39 33 40
Fax +33 3 80 66 82 51
jean.faivre@u-bourgogne.fr

Dr David FORMAN
Section of Cancer Information
International Agency for Research on Cancer
(IARC)
150 cours Albert Thomas
69372 Lyon cedex 08
FRANCE
Tel. +33 4 72 73 80 56
Fax +33 4 72 73 86 96
formand@iarc.fr

Mrs April FRITZ
April Fritz and Associates, LLC
21361 Crestview Road
Reno, NV 89521
USA
Tel. +1 775 636 7243
Fax +1 888 891 3012
april@afritz.org

Dr Elaine S. JAFFE
Hematopathology Section
Laboratory of Pathology
Center for Cancer Research
National Cancer Institute
10 Center Drive MSC 1500
Bethesda, Maryland 20892
USA
Tel. +1 301 496 01 83
Fax +1 301 402 24 15
elainejaffe@nih.gov

Dr Robert JAKOB
Classifications and Terminologies
Evidence and Information for Policy
World Health Organization (WHO)
20 Avenue Appia
1211 Geneva 27
SWITZERLAND
Tel. +41 22 791 58 77
Fax +41 22 791 48 94
jakobr@who.int

Dr Paul KLEIHUES
Department of Pathology
University Hospital Zurich
Schmelzbergstrasse 12
8091 Zurich
SWITZERLAND
Tel. +41 44 255 2502
Fax +41 44 255 2525
paul.kleihues@usz.ch

Dr Hiroko OHGAKI
Section of Molecular Pathology
International Agency for Research on Cancer
(IARC)
150 Cours Albert Thomas
69372 Lyon cedex 08
FRANCE
Tel. +33 4 72 73 85 34
Fax +33 4 72 73 86 98
ohgaki@iarc.fr

Dr D. Maxwell PARKIN
Clinical Trials Service and Epidemiology
    Studies Unit
University of Oxford
Richard Doll Building, Old Road Campus
Roosevelt Drive, Headington
Oxford OX3 7LF
UK
Tel. +44 1865 743663
Fax +44 1865 743985
ctsu0138@herald.ox.ac.uk

Dr Kanagaratnam SHANMUGARATNAM
Department of Pathology
National University Hospital
5 Lower Kent Ridge Road
Singapore 119074
SINGAPORE
Tel. +65 67724312
Fax +65 6773 6021
k_shanmugaratnam@nuhs.edu.sg

Dr Leslie H. SOBIN
Division of Gastrointestinal Pathology
Armed Forces Institute of Pathology
Washington, DC 20306
USA
Tel. +1 202 364 8358
sobin@uicc.org

Source of charts and photographs

2.01 A	IARC {842A}
2.01 B	IARC {842}
2.02	Japanese Esophageal Cancer Society {1388}
2.03 A,B	Shimoda T.
2.04 A-C	Shimoda T.
2.05 A	Shimizu M.
2.05 B	Gabbert H.E. Institute of Pathology, Heinrich Heine University, Dusseldorf, Germany
2.06	Montgomery E.
2.07 A,B	Shimoda T.
2.08 A-C	Shimizu M.
2.09 A,B	Shimoda T.
2.10 A-C	Dunbar K.B. Johns Hopkins School of Medicine, Baltimore, MD, USA
2.11 A,B	Fléjou J.-F.
2.12 A	Odze R.
2.12 B	Montgomery E.
2.13 A,B	Fléjou J.-F.
2.14	Fenoglio-Preiser C.M. Gastrointestinal Pathology University of Cincinnati, OH, USA
2.15 A,B	Montgomery E.
2.16	Anthony P.P. Histopathology Dept, Royal Devon and Exeter Hospital, UK
2.17	Klöppel G.
2.18	Klöppel G.
2.19	Miettinen M.
2.20 A,B	Miettinen M.
2.21 A,B	Miettinen M.
2.22 A,B	Miettinen M.
2.23	Fenger C. University Hospital Odense, Denmark
2.24	Carr N.J.
3.01	Spechler S.J. {3033}
3.02	Lambert R.
3.03	Odze R.
3.04	Rubio C.A., Dept of Pathology, Karolinska Institute, Stockholm, Sweden
3.05 A,B	Odze R.
4.01	Graham D.Y.
4.02 A,B	IARC {842A}
4.03 A,B	Kato M. Division of Endoscopy, Hokkaido University Hospital, Sapporo, Japan
4.04 A,B	Shimoda T.
4.05	Lauwers G.Y.
4.06 A-C	Shimoda T.
4.07 A	Lauwers G.Y.
4.07 B	Carneiro F.

4.08 A,B	Lauwers G.Y.
4.09	Fenoglio-Preiser C.
4.10	Lauwers G.Y.
4.11 A,B	Lauwers G.Y.
4.12	Lauwers G.Y
4.13 A-D	Hattori T.
4.14 A,B	Lauwers G.Y.
4.15	Lauwers G.Y.
4.16	Lauwers G.Y.
4.17 A,B	Shimoda T.
4.18 A	Charlton A. {493}
4.18 B	Charlton A.
4.19 A	Shaw D. {2910}
4.19 B	Charlton A.
4.20	Charlton A.
4.21	Carneiro F.
4.22	Carneiro F.
4.23	Carneiro F.
4.24	Carneiro F.
4.25	Charlton A.
4.26 A,B	Carneiro F.
4.27	Olivera C. & Seruca R. IPATIMUT, Porto, Portugal
4.28	Capella C.
4.29 A	Hamilton S.R.
4.29 B	Capella C.
4.30 A	Jass J.R.
4.30 B	Capella C.
4.31	Capella C.
4.32 A,B	Nakamura S.
4.33 A,B	Nakamura S.
4.34	Nakamura S.
4.35	Nakamura S.
4.36 A,B	Nakamura S.
4.37 A-D	Nakamura S.
4.38	Nakamura S.
4.39 A,B	Nakamura S.
4.40	Nakamura S.
4.41 A,B	Miettinen M.
4.42 A-D	Miettinen M.
4.43 A-D	Miettinen M.
4.44 A-F	Miettinen M.
4.45	Lasota J. AFIP, Washington, DC, USA
4.46	Miettinen M.
4.47 A,B	Miettinen M.
4.48 A,B	Miettinen M.
4.49 A,B	Miettinen M.
4.50	Miettinen M.
4.51	Sobin L.H.
4.52	Ishak K. AFIP, Washington, DC, USA
4.53 A,B	Iacobuzio-Donahue C.
5.01	Klimstra D.S.
5.02	Klimstra D.S.
5.03 A,B	Klimstra D.S.
5.04 A,B	Albores-Saavedra J.
5.05 A,B	Klimstra D.S.
5.06	Klimstra D.S.
5.07	Albores-Saavedra J.
5.08 A,B	Albores-Saavedra J.
5.09	Albores-Saavedra J.

5.10 A,B	Albores-Saavedra J.
5.11 A,B	Albores-Saavedra J.
5.12	Albores-Saavedra J.
5.13 A,B	Albores-Saavedra J.
5.14	Klöppel G.
5.15 A,B	Klöppel G.
5.16	Klöppel G.
5.17 A,B	Klöppel G.
5.18	Albores-Saavedra J.
5.19	Albores-Saavedra J.
6.01	Fenoglio-Preiser C.
6.02	Shepherd N.A.
6.03	Shepherd N.A.
6.04 A	Sobin L.H.
6.04 B	Carr N.J.
6.05 A,B	Carr N.J.
6.06 A	Sobin L.H.
6.06 B	Carr N.J.
6.07	Klöppel G.
6.08 A,B	Capella C. & La Rosa S.
6.09	Capella C. & La Rosa S.
6.10	Vogt P. Dept of Pathology, University Hospital Zurich, Switzerland
6.11 A,B	Capella C. & La Rosa S.
6.12	Capella C. & La Rosa S.
6.13	Capella C. & La Rosa S.
6.14	Oda Y. Kyushu University, Japan
6.15	Sobin L.H.
6.16	Nakamura S.
6.17 A,B	Nakamura Sh. Dept of Gastroenterology, Kyushu University Hospital, Japan
6.18	Sobin L.H.
6.19	Futamura S. Fukuoka University, Japan
6.20	Nakamura S.
6.21	Jass J.R.
6.22	Muller-Hermelink H.K.
6.23 A-D	Isaacson P.G. Dept of Histopathology, University College Medical School, London, UK
6.23 B	Brunning R.D.
6.24 A-D	Muller-Hermelink H.K.
6.25	Muller-Hermelink H.K.
6.26 A-D	Muller-Hermelink H.K.
6.27 A-C	Miettinen M.
6.28 A,B	Miettinen M.
6.29 A,B	Miettinen M.
6.30	Miettinen M.
6.31	Miettinen M.
6.32	Hruban R.H.
6.33	Iacobuzio-Donahue C.
6.34	Iacobuzio-Donahue C. {735}
6.35 A	Talbot I.C.
6.35 B	Sobin L.H.
6.36 A,B	Fenoglio-Preiser C.
6.37	Sobin L.H.

6.38	Niederau C., Dept of Medicine, St Joseph Hospital, Oberhausen, Germany.	8.28 A	Talbot I.C.	9.01	Fenger C. Reproduced with permission from {835}.
		8.28 B	Fenger C.	9.02	Fenger C.
		8.29	Talbot I.C.	9.03	Fenger C.
7.01	Carr N.J.	8.30	Offerhaus J.G.A.	9.04	Fenger C.
7.02 A,B	Carr N.J.	8.31	Talbot I.C.	9.05 A,B	Fenger C.
7.03	Carr N.J.	8.32	Jarvinen H., Dept of Surgery, Helsinki University Central Hospital, Finland	9.06	Sobin L.H.
7.04	Carr N.J.			9.07	Talbot I.C.
7.05 A	Sobin L.H.			9.08	Fenger C.
7.05 B	Jass J.R.	8.33	Giardiello F.M.	9.09	Jass J.R.
7.05 C	Sobin L.H.	8.34	Jass J.R.	9.10	Sobin L.H.
7.06	Carr N.J.	8.35 A,B	Jass J.R.	9.11	Talbot I.C.
7.07	Sobin L.H.	8.36 A,B	Jass J.R.	9.12 A,B	Talbot I.C.
7.08	Jass J.R.	8.37	Sampson J.R & Jones N. {2790}	9.13	Sobin L.H.
7.09	Fenger C.	8.38	Ponti et al. {2575A}		
7.10	Komminoth P.	8.39 A	Nielsen et al. {2283}	10.01A-C	Bioulac-Sage P.
7.11A	Komminoth P.	8.39 B	Morreau H. & Nielsen M.	10.02	Bioulac-Sage P.
7.11 B	Tang L. Memorial Sloan Kettering, New York, NY, USA	8.40	Cheadle J.P. & Sampson N. {499A}	10.03	Bioulac-Sage P.
		8.41	Burt R.W.	10.04	Bioulac-Sage P.
		8.42 A,B	Snover D.C.	10.05	Bioulac-Sage P.
7.12 A	Rindi G.	8.43 A-C	Snover D.C.	10.06 A,B	Bioulac-Sage P.
7.12 B	Carr N.J.	8.44 A,B	Snover D.C.	10.07 A,B	Bioulac-Sage P.
7.13 A,B	Nakamura S.-I.	8.45 A,B	Snover D.C.	10.08 A-C	Bioulac-Sage P.
7.14	Carr N.J.	8.46 A-C	Snover D.C.	10.09	Bioulac-Sage P.
7.15	Snover D.C.	8.47 A-D	Snover D.C.	10.10	Bioulac-Sage P.
		8.48	Jass J.R.	10.11	Bioulac-Sage P.
8.01 A	IARC {842A}	8.49	Snover D.C.	10.12	Bioulac-Sage P.
8.01 B	IARC {842}	8.50	Jass J.R.	10.13	Bioulac-Sage P.
8.02 A,B	Kudo S., Showa University & Northern Yokohama Hospital, Japan.	8.51 A	Sobin L.H.	10.14	Bioulac-Sage P.
		8.51 B	Talbot I.C.	10.15	Bioulac-Sage P.
		8.52	Talbot I.C.	10.16	Bioulac-Sage P.
8.02 C	Gabbert H.E.	8.53	Talbot I.C.	10.17	Bioulac-Sage P.
8.03 A,B	Hamilton S.R.	8.54 A	Offerhaus G.J.A.	10.18	IARC {842A}
8.04 A	Fogt F., Dept of Pathology, Medical Center, University of Pennsylvania, Philadelphia, PA, USA	8.54 B	Sobin L.H.	10.19	IARC {842A}
		8.55 A,B	Sobin L.H.	10.2 A	Kadar A.
		8.56	Sobin L.H.	10.2 B, C	Hirohashi S.
		8.57 A,B	Snover D.C.	10.20 D	Sakamoto M.
		8.58 A,B	Snover D.C.	10.21	Sakamoto M.
8.04 B,C	Jass J.R.	8.59 A	Jass J.R.	10.22	Wee A.
8.05	Talbot I.C.	8.59 B	Talbot I.C.	10.23	Wee A.
8.06	Fenoglio-Preiser C.	8.60	Reprinted by permission from Macmillan Publishers Ltd: European Journal of Human Genetics, Blumenthal GM et al. {287A}, Copyright 2008.	10.24	Wee A.
8.07	Hamilton S.R.			10.25	Wee A.
8.08 A-C	Hamilton S.R.			10.26 A,B	Hirohashi S.
8.09	Nakamura S.-I.			10.27 A,B	Hirohashi S.
8.10 A,B	Kudo S.			10.28 A	Hirohashi S.
8.11 A,B	Rubio C.A.	8.61	Rindi G.	10.28 B	Fischer H.P.
8.12 A,B	Kudo S.	8.62	Tang L.	10.29 A,B	Hirohashi S.
8.13	Hamilton S.R.	8.63	Sobin L.H.	10.30	Wee A.
8.14 A	Talbot I.C.	8.64	Snover D.C.	10.31	Ishak K.
8.14 B	Sobin L.H.	8.65 A	Sobin L.H.	10.32 A,B	Torbenson M.
8.15	Rubio C.A.	8.65 B	Fenoglio-Preiser C.	10.33	Torbenson M.
8.16 A	Jass J.R.	8.66	Rindi G.	10.34	Park Y.N.
8.16 B	Rubio C.A.	8.67	Talbot I.C.	10.35	Park Y.N.
8.17	Kudo S.	8.68	Sobin L.H.	10.36	Park Y.N.
8.18 A	Jass J.R.	8.69	Talbot I.C.	10.37	Park Y.N.
8.18 B	Rubio C.A.	8.70	Wotherspoon A. Histopathology Dept, Royal Marsden Hospital, London, UK	10.38 A	Park Y.N.
8.18 C	Sobin L.H.			10.38 B	Hirohashi S.
8.19 A	Talbot I.C.			10.38	Hytiroglou P.
8.19 B	Jass J.R.			10.39	Kudo M.
8.20 A,B	Nakamura S.-I.	8.71	Jass J.R.	10.40 A,B	Sakamoto M.
8.21	Talbot I.C.	8.72 A,B	Miettinen M.	10.41	Hytiroglou P.
8.22	Talbot I.C.	8.73	Miettinen M.	10.42	Hytiroglou P.
8.23	Talbot I.C.	8.74	Miettinen M.	10.43 A,B	Sakamoto M.
8.24	Fenoglio-Preiser C.	8.75	Fletcher C.D.M.	10.43 C	Hirohashi S.
8.25	Sobin L.H.	8.76 A,B	Miettinen M.	10.44 A-C	Nakanuma Y.
8.26	Rubio C.A.	8.77	Fenger C.	10.45 A-D	Nakanuma Y.
8.27 A,B	Nakamura S.-I.	8.78	Sobin L.H.	10.46	Nakanuma Y.
				10.47 A-D	Nakanuma Y.

10.48 A-D	Nakanuma Y.
10.49 A-D	Nakanuma Y.
10.50 A,B	Nakanuma Y.
10.51 A,B	Nakanuma Y.
10.52 A-H	Nakanuma Y.
10.53	Nakanuma Y.
10.54 A-D	Nakanuma Y.
10.55 A,B	Nakanuma Y.
10.56 A,B	Ishak K.
10.57	Theise N.
10.58 A-D	Nakanuma Y.
10.59 A-D	Park Y.N.
10.60 A-I	Nakashima O.
10.61	Stocker J.T.
10.62 A,B	Stocker J.T.
10.63	Stocker J.T.
10.64	Zimmermann A.
10.65	Ishak K.
10.66	Stocker J.T.
10.67 A,B	Zimmermann A.
10.68 A	Stocker J.T.
10.68 B	Zimmermann A.
10.69 A-C	Zimmermann A.
10.70 A,B	Zimmermann A.
10.71	Zimmermann A.
10.72	Zimmermann A.
10.73 A-C	Zimmermann A.
10.74 A-C	Zimmermann A.
10.75	Tsui W.M.S.
10.76	Tsui W.M.S.
10.77 A-D	Tsui W.M.S.
10.78 A,B	Tsui W.M.S.
10.79 A-C	Tsui W.M.S.
10.80 A,B	Tsui W.M.S.
10.81 A,B	Nakanuma Y.
10.82	Tsui W.M.S.
10.83 A,B	Jaffe E.S.
10.84	Jaffe E.S.
10.85 A,B	Jaffe E.S.
10.86 A	Stocker J.T.
10.86 B-D	Ishak K.
10.87 A,B	Ishak K.
10.88 A,B	Ishak K.
10.89 A	Tsui W.M.S.
10.89 B,C	Ishak K.
10.90	Anthony P.
10.91	Ishak K.
10.92 A-H	Tsui W.M.S.
10.93 A,B	Tsui W.M.S.
10.94 A-D	Tsui W.M.S.
10.95 A-D	Miettinen M.
10.96 A,B	Ishak K.
10.97	Miettinen M.
10.98	Miettinen M.
10.99 A,B	Zimmermann A.
10.100 A-D	Zimmermann A.
10.101	DiSibio G et al. {725}
10.102 A,B,D	Anthony P.P.
10.103 C	Fenoglio-Preiser C.
10.103	Anthony P.
10.104	Saxena R.
10.105	Saxena R.
11.01	Albores-Saavedra J.
11.02	Albores-Saavedra J.
11.03 A,B	Albores-Saavedra J.
11.04	Albores-Saavedra J.
11.05	Albores-Saavedra J.

11.06	Albores-Saavedra J.
11.07	Albores-Saavedra J.
11.08	Albores-Saavedra J.
11.09	Albores-Saavedra J.
11.10	Albores-Saavedra J.
11.11	Albores-Saavedra J.
11.12 A,B	Albores-Saavedra J.
11.13	Albores-Saavedra J.
11.14	Albores-Saavedra J.
11.15	Albores-Saavedra J.
11.16 A,B	Albores-Saavedra J.
11.17	Albores-Saavedra J.
11.18	Albores-Saavedra J.
11.19	Albores-Saavedra J.
11.20 A-C	Fischer H.P.
11.21 A-C	Albores-Saavedra J.
11.22	Albores-Saavedra J.
11.23 A,B	Miettinen M.
11.24 A,B	Miettinen M.
12.01	IARC {842A}
12.02 A	Zamboni G.
12.02 B	Kawamoto S.
12.03	Klöppel G.
12.04	Terris B.
12.05	Hruban R.H.
12.06 A,B	Klöppel G.
12.07	Klöppel G.
12.08	Hruban R.H.
12.09	Hruban R.H.
12.10	Hruban R.H.
12.11	Pathology AMC
12.12 A,B	Bishop Pitman M.
12.13	Maitra A.
12.14	Klimstra D.S.
12.15	Fukushima N.
12.16 A	Klimstra D.S.
12.16 B	Zamboni G.
12.17 A	Hruban R.H.
12.17 B	Shimizu M.
12.18	Shimizu M.
12.19	Terris B.
12.20	Kawamoto S., Johns Hopkins, USA
12.21	Klöppel G.
12.22	Terris B.
12.23	Fukushima N.
12.24	Zamboni G.
12.25 A	Zamboni G.
12.25 B	Terris B.
12.26	Adsay N.V.
12.27	Adsay N.V.
12.28	Klimstra D.S.
12.29	Klöppel G.
12.30	Zamboni G.
12.31 A,B	Zamboni G.
12.32	Zamboni G.
12.33	Zamboni G.
12.34 A,B	Zamboni G.
12.35 A	Kawamoto S., Johns Hopkins, USA
12.35 B	Zamboni G.
12.36	Terris B.
12.37	Klöppel G.
12.38	Hruban R.H.
12.39	Klöppel G.
12.40	Zamboni G.
12.41 A	Klöppel G.

12.41 B	Klimstra D.S.
12.42 A,B	Klimstra D.S.
12.43 A	Adsay N.V.
12.43 B	Zamboni G.
12.44	Adsay N.V.
12.45	Zamboni G.
12.46	Adsay N.V.
12.47 A	Adsay N.V.
12.47 B	Zamboni G.
12.48 A,B	Bishop Pitman M.
12.49 A	Klimstra D.S.
12.49 B	Klöppel G.
12.50	Klöppel G.
12.51 A,B	Adsay N.V.
12.52	Ohike N.
12.53	Klimstra D.S.
12.54	Hruban R.H.
12.55 A	Klöppel G.
12.55 B	Terris B.
12.55 C	Zamboni G.
12.56 A	Tang L.
12.56 B	Hruban R.H.
12.57 A	Adsay N.V.
12.57 B	Klimstra D.S.
12.58	Klimstra D.S.
12.59	Klimstra D.S.
12.60 A	Klimstra D.S.
12.60 B	Zamboni G.
12.61	Klimstra D.S.
12.62	Zamboni G.
12.63	Klimstra D.S.
12.64 A	Ohike N.
12.64 B	Hruban R.H.
12.65 A,C	Klimstra D.S.
12.65 B	Ohike N.
12.65 D	Hruban R.H.
12.66	Tang L.
12.67 A	Klimstra D.S.
12.67 B	Hruban R.H.
12.68 A,B	Klimstra D.S.
12.69	Klimstra D.S.
12.70	Klöppel G.
12.71	Kawamoto S., Johns Hopkins, USA
12.72 A	Klimstra D.S.
12.72 B	Klöppel G.
12.73	Terris B.
12.74	Hruban R.H.
12.75 A	Hruban R.H.
12.75 B	Klöppel G.
12.76 A	Zamboni G.
12.76 B	Zamboni G.
12.77	Hruban R.H.
12.78	Iacobuzio-Donahue C.
12.79	Hruban R.H.
12.80	Hruban R.H. {1270}

References

1.   Aaltonen L, Johns L, Jarvinen H, Mecklin JP, Houlston R (2007). Explaining the familial colorectal cancer risk associated with mismatch repair (MMR)-deficient and MMR-stable tumors. Clin Cancer Res 13: 356-361.

2.   Aaltonen LA, Salovaara R, Kristo P, Canzian F, Hemminki A, Peltomaki P et al. (1998). Incidence of hereditary nonpolyposis colorectal cancer and the feasibility of molecular screening for the disease. N Engl J Med 338: 1481-1487.

3.   Abdul-Al HM, Makhlouf HR, Goodman ZD (2007). Expression of estrogen and progesterone receptors and inhibin-alpha in hepatobiliary cystadenoma: an immunohistochemical study. Virchows Arch 450: 691-697.

4.   Abe T, Fukushima N, Brune K, Boehm C, Sato N, Matsubayashi H et al. (2007). Genome-wide allelotypes of familial pancreatic adenocarcinomas and familial and sporadic intraductal papillary mucinous neoplasms. Clin Cancer Res 13: 6019-6025.

5.   Abel ME, Chiu YS, Russell TR, Volpe PA (1993). Adenocarcinoma of the anal glands. Results of a survey. Dis Colon Rectum 36: 383-387.

6.   Abenoza P, Manivel JC, Wick MR, Hagen K, Dehner LP (1987). Hepatoblastoma: an immunohistochemical and ultrastructural study. Hum Pathol 18: 1025-1035.

7.   Aberle H, Bauer A, Stappert J, Kispert A, Kemler R (1997). Beta-catenin is a target for the ubiquitin-proteasome pathway. EMBO J 16: 3797-3804.

8.   Abraham SC, Klimstra DS, Wilentz RE, Yeo CJ, Conlon K, Brennan M et al. (2002). Solid-pseudopapillary tumors of the pancreas are genetically distinct from pancreatic ductal adenocarcinomas and almost always harbor beta-catenin mutations. Am J Pathol 160: 1361-1369.

9.   Abraham SC, Krasinskas AM, Correa AM, Hofstetter WL, Ajani JA, Swisher SG et al. (2007). Duplication of the muscularis mucosae in Barrett esophagus: an underrecognized feature and its implication for staging of adenocarcinoma. Am J Surg Pathol 31: 1719-1725.

10.   Abraham SC, Krasinskas AM, Hofstetter WL, Swisher SG, Wu TT (2007). "Seedling" mesenchymal tumors (gastrointestinal stromal tumors and leiomyomas) are common incidental tumors of the esophagogastric junction. Am J Surg Pathol 31: 1629-1635.

11.   Abraham SC, Lee JH, Boitnott JK, Argani P, Furth EE, Wu TT (2002). Microsatellite instability in intraductal papillary neoplasms of the biliary tract. Mod Pathol 15: 1309-1317.

12.   Abraham SC, Lee JH, Hruban RH, Argani P, Furth EE, Wu TT (2003). Molecular and immunohistochemical analysis of intraductal papillary neoplasms of the biliary tract. Hum Pathol 34: 902-910.

13.   Abraham SC, Montgomery EA, Singh VK, Yardley JH, Wu TT (2002). Gastric adenomas: intestinal-type and gastric-type adenomas differ in the risk of adenocarcinoma and presence of background mucosal pathology. Am J Surg Pathol 26: 1276-1285.

14.   Abraham SC, Nobukawa B, Giardiello FM, Hamilton SR, Wu TT (2000). Fundic gland polyps in familial adenomatous polyposis: neoplasms with frequent somatic adenomatous polyposis coli gene alterations. Am J Pathol 157: 747-754.

15.   Abraham SC, Nobukawa B, Giardiello FM, Hamilton SR, Wu TT (2001). Sporadic fundic gland polyps: common gastric polyps arising through activating mutations in the beta-catenin gene. Am J Pathol 158: 1005-1010.

16.   Abraham SC, Park SJ, Mugartegui L, Hamilton SR, Wu TT (2002). Sporadic fundic gland polyps with epithelial dysplasia: evidence for preferential targeting for mutations in the adenomatous polyposis coli gene. Am J Pathol 161: 1735-1742.

17.   Abraham SC, Singh VK, Yardley JH, Wu TT (2001). Hyperplastic polyps of the stomach: associations with histologic patterns of gastritis and gastric atrophy. Am J Surg Pathol 25: 500-507.

18.   Abraham SC, Wu TT, Hruban RH, Lee JH, Yeo CJ, Conlon K et al. (2002). Genetic and immunohistochemical analysis of pancreatic acinar cell carcinoma: frequent allelic loss on chromosome 11p and alterations in the APC/beta-catenin pathway. Am J Pathol 160: 953-962.

19.   Abraham SC, Wu TT, Klimstra DS, Finn LS, Lee JH, Yeo CJ et al. (2001). Distinctive molecular genetic alterations in sporadic and familial adenomatous polyposis-associated pancreatoblastomas : frequent alterations in the APC/beta-catenin pathway and chromosome 11p. Am J Pathol 159: 1619-1627.

20.   Abu-Farsakh H, Fraire AE (1991). Adenocarcinoma and (extragonadal) choriocarcinoma of the gallbladder in a young woman. Hum Pathol 22: 614-615.

21.   Acharya S, Wilson T, Gradia S, Kane MF, Guerrette S, Marsischky GT et al. (1996). hMSH2 forms specific mispair-binding complexes with hMSH3 and hMSH6. Proc Natl Acad Sci U S A 93: 13629-13634.

22.   Achille A, Baron A, Zamboni G, Orlandini S, Bogina G, Bassi C et al. (1998). Molecular pathogenesis of sporadic duodenal cancer. Br J Cancer 77: 760-765.

23.   Achille A, Scupoli MT, Magalini AR, Zamboni G, Romanelli MG, Orlandini S et al. (1996). APC gene mutations and allelic losses in sporadic ampullary tumours: evidence of genetic difference from tumours associated with familial adenomatous polyposis. Int J Cancer 68: 305-312.

24.   Adachi E, Hashimoto H, Tsuneyoshi M (1993). Proliferating cell nuclear antigen in hepatocellular carcinoma and small cell liver dysplasia. Cancer 72: 2902-2909.

25.   Adesina AM, Lopez-Terrada D, Wong KK, Gunaratne P, Nguyen Y, Pulliam J et al. (2009). Gene expression profiling reveals signatures characterizing histologic subtypes of hepatoblastoma and global deregulation in cell growth and survival pathways. Hum Pathol 40: 843-853.

26.   Adesina AM, Nguyen Y, Guanaratne P, Pulliam J, Lopez-Terrada D, Margolin J et al. (2007). FOXG1 is overexpressed in hepatoblastoma. Hum Pathol 38: 400-409.

27.   Adsay NV (2007). Cystic lesions of the pancreas. Mod Pathol 20 Suppl 1: S71-S93.

28.   Adsay NV, Adair CF, Heffess CS, Klimstra DS (1996). Intraductal oncocytic papillary neoplasms of the pancreas. Am J Surg Pathol 20: 980-994.

29.   Adsay NV, Andea A, Basturk O, Kilinc N, Nassar H, Cheng JD (2004). Secondary tumors of the pancreas: an analysis of a surgical and autopsy database and review of the literature. Virchows Arch 444: 527-535.

30.   Adsay NV, Bandyopadhyay S, Basturk O (2006). Duct adjacent to a thick-walled medium-sized muscular vessel in the pancreas is often indicative of invasive adenocarcinoma. Am J Surg Pathol 30: 1203-1205.

31.   Adsay NV, Bandyopadhyay S, Basturk O, Othman M, Cheng JD, Klöppel G et al. (2004). Chronic pancreatitis or pancreatic ductal adenocarcinoma? Semin Diagn Pathol 21: 268-276.

32.   Adsay NV, Conlon KC, Zee SY, Brennan MF, Klimstra DS (2002). Intraductal papillary-mucinous neoplasms of the pancreas: an analysis of in situ and invasive carcinomas in 28 patients. Cancer 94: 62-77.

33.   Adsay NV, Logani S, Sarkar F, Crissman J, Vaitkevicius V (2000). Foamy gland pattern of pancreatic ductal adenocarcinoma: a deceptively benign-appearing variant. Am J Surg Pathol 24: 493-504.

34.   Adsay NV, Longnecker DS, Klimstra DS (2000). Pancreatic tumors with cystic dilatation of the ducts: intraductal papillary mucinous neoplasms and intraductal oncocytic papillary neoplasms. Semin Diagn Pathol 17: 16-30.

35.   Adsay NV, Merati K, Andea A, Sarkar F, Hruban RH, Wilentz RE et al. (2002). The dichotomy in the preinvasive neoplasia to invasive carcinoma sequence in the pancreas: differential expression of MUC1 and MUC2 supports the existence of two separate pathways of carcinogenesis. Mod Pathol 15: 1087-1095.

36.   Adsay NV, Merati K, Basturk O, Iacobuzio-Donahue C, Levi E, Cheng JD et al. (2004). Pathologically and biologically distinct types of epithelium in intraductal papillary mucinous neoplasms: delineation of an "intestinal" pathway of carcinogenesis in the pancreas. Am J Surg Pathol 28: 839-848.

37.   Adsay NV, Pierson C, Sarkar F, Abrams J, Weaver D, Conlon KC et al. (2001). Colloid (mucinous noncystic) carcinoma of the pancreas. Am J Surg Pathol 25: 26-42.

38.   Agaimy A, Pelz AF, Wieacker P, Roessner A, Wunsch PH, Schneider-Stock R (2008). Gastrointestinal stromal tumors of the vermiform appendix: clinicopathologic, immunohistochemical, and molecular study of 2 cases with literature review. Hum Pathol 39: 1252-1257.

39.   Agaimy A, Wunsch PH, Dirnhofer S, Bihl MP, Terracciano LM, Tornillo L (2008). Microscopic gastrointestinal stromal tumors in esophageal and intestinal surgical resection specimens: a clinicopathologic, immunohistochemical, and molecular study of 19 lesions. Am J Surg Pathol 32: 867-873.

40.   Agaram NP, Baren A, Antonescu CR (2006). Pediatric and adult hepatic embryonal sarcoma: a comparative ultrastructural study with morphologic correlations. Ultrastruct Pathol 30: 403-408.

41.   Agarwal B, Ludwig OJ, Collins BT, Cortese C (2008). Immunostaining as an adjunct to cytology for diagnosis of pancreatic adenocarcinoma. Clin Gastroenterol Hepatol 6: 1425-1431.

42.   Agarwal SK, Guru SC, Heppner C, Erdos MR, Collins RM, Park SY et al. (1999). Menin interacts with the AP1 transcription factor JunD and represses JunD-activated transcription. Cell 96: 143-152.

43.   Agoff SN, Crispin DA, Bronner MP, Dail DH, Hawes SE, Haggitt RC (2001). Neoplasms of the ampulla of vater with concurrent pancreatic intraductal neoplasia: a histological and molecular study. Mod Pathol 14: 139-146.

44.   Ahlman H, Wangberg B, Nilsson O (1993). Growth regulation in carcinoid tumors. Endocrinol Metab Clin North Am 22: 889-915.

45.   Ahmadi A, Polyak S, Draganov PV (2009). Colorectal cancer surveillance in inflammatory bowel disease: the search continues. World J Gastroenterol 15: 61-66.

46.   Ahn MJ, Park YW, Han D, Choi JH, Shin SJ, Yoon BC et al. (2000). A case of primary intestinal T-cell lymphoma involving entire gastrointestinal tract: esophagus to rectum. Korean J Intern Med 15: 245-249.

47.   Aikou T, Shimazu H (1989). Difference in main lymphatic pathways from the lower esophagus and gastric cardia. Jpn J Surg 19: 290-295.

48.   Aishima S, Nishihara Y, Tsujita E, Taguchi K, Soejima Y, Taketomi A et al. (2008). Biliary neoplasia with extensive intraductal spread associated with liver cirrhosis: a hitherto unreported variant of biliary intraepithelial neoplasia. Hum Pathol 39: 939-947.

49.   Akagi T, Motegi M, Tamura A, Suzuki R, Hosokawa Y, Suzuki H et al. (1999). A novel gene, MALT1 at 18q21, is involved in t(11;18) (q21;q21) found in low-grade B-cell lymphoma of mucosa-associated lymphoid tissue. Oncogene 18: 5785-5794.

50.   Akama Y, Yasui W, Yokozaki H, Kuniyasu H, Kitahara K, Ishikawa T et al. (1995). Frequent amplification of the cyclin E gene in human gastric carcinomas. Jpn J Cancer Res 86: 617-621.

51.   Akatsu T, Aiura K, Takahashi S, Kameyama K, Kitajima M, Kitagawa Y (2007). Signet-ring cell carcinoma of the ampulla of Vater: report of a case. Surg Today 37: 1110-1114.

52.   Akatsu T, Kameyama K, Kawachi S, Tanabe M, Aiura K, Wakabayashi G et al. (2006). Gallbladder carcinoma with osteoclast-like giant cells. J Gastroenterol 41: 83-87.

53.   Akatsu T, Shimazu M, Aiura K, Ito Y, Shinoda M, Kawachi S et al. (2007). Clinicopathological features and surgical outcome of isolated metastasis of renal cell carcinoma. Hepatogastroenterology 54: 1836-1840.

54.   Akcali Z, Ozyilkan O, Sakalli H, Bal N, Noyan T (2005). Gallbladder adenosquamous cell carcinoma: report of two cases. Acta Gastroenterol Belg 68: 440-442.

55.   Akishima-Fukasawa Y, Nakanishi Y, Ino Y, Moriya Y, Kanai Y, Hirohashi S (2009). Prognostic significance of CXCL12 expression in patients with colorectal carcinoma. Am J Clin Pathol 132: 202-210.

56.   Akiyama H, Tsurumaru M, Udagawa H, Kajiyama Y (1994). Radical lymph node dissection for cancer of the thoracic esophagus. Ann Surg 220: 364-372.

57.   Akiyama T, Okino T, Konishi H, Wani Y, Notohara K, Tsukayama C et al. (2008). CD8+,

CD56+ (natural killer-like) T-cell lymphoma involving the small intestine with no evidence of enteropathy: clinicopathology and molecular study of five Japanese patients. Pathol Int 58: 626-634.
58. Aktas D, Ayhan A, Tuncbilek E, Ozdemir A, Uzunalimoglu B (1998). No evidence for over-expression of the p53 protein and mutations in exons 4-9 of the *p53* gene in a large family with adenomatous polyposis. Am J Gastroenterol 93: 1524-1526.
59. Al Kaisi N, Weaver MG, Abdul-Karim FW, Siegler E (1992). Fine needle aspiration cytology of neuroendocrine tumors of the pancreas. A cytologic, immunocytochemical and electron microscopic study. Acta Cytol 36: 655-660.
59A Al-DarajiWI, Makhlouf HR, Miettinen M, Montgomery EA, Goodman ZD, Marwaha JS and Fanburg-Smith JC (2009). Primary gallbladder sarcoma: a clinicopathologic study of 15 cases, heterogeneous sarcomas with poor outcome, except pediatric botryoid rhabdomyosarcoma. Am J Surg Pathol. 33: 826-834.
60. Al-Tassan N, Chmiel NH, Maynard J, Fleming N, Livingston AL, Williams GT et al. (2002). Inherited variants of MYH associated with somatic G:C—>T:A mutations in colorectal tumors. Nat Genet 30: 227-232.
61. Alarcon FJ, Burke CA, Church JM, van Stolk RU (1999). Familial adenomatous polyposis: efficacy of endoscopic and surgical treatment for advanced duodenal adenomas. Dis Colon Rectum 42: 1533-1536.
62. Albert JG, Gimm O, Stock K, Bilkenroth U, Marsch WC, Helmbold P (2007). Small-bowel endoscopy is crucial for diagnosis of melanoma metastases to the small bowel: a case of metachronous small-bowel metastases and review of the literature. Melanoma Res 17: 335-338.
63. Alberts DS, Martinez ME, Roe DJ, Guillen-Rodriguez JM, Marshall JR, van Leeuwen JB et al. (2000). Lack of effect of a high-fiber cereal supplement on the recurrence of colorectal adenomas. Phoenix Colon Cancer Prevention Physicians' Network. N Engl J Med 342: 1156-1162.
64. Albores-Saavedra J (2002). Acinar cystadenoma of the pancreas: a previously undescribed tumor. Ann Diagn Pathol 6: 113-115.
65. Albores-Saavedra J, Angeles-Angeles A, Nadji M, Henson DE, Alvarez L (1987). Mucinous cystadenocarcinoma of the pancreas. Morphologic and immunocytochemical observations. Am J Surg Pathol 11: 11-20.
66. Albores-Saavedra J, Batich K, Hossain S, Henson DE, Schwartz AM (2009). Carcinoid tumors and small cell carcinomas of the gallbladder and extrahepatic bile ducts: a comparative study based on 221 cases from the SEER program. Ann Diagn Pathol 13:378-383.
67. Albores-Saavedra J, Delgado R, Henson DE (1999). Well-differentiated adenocarcinoma, gastric foveolar type, of the extrahepatic bile ducts: A previously unrecognized and distinctive morphologic variant of bile duct carcinoma. Ann Diagn Pathol 3: 75-80.
68. Albores-Saavedra J, Galliani C, Chable-Montero F, Batich K, Henson DE (2009). Mucin-containing Rokitansky-Aschoff sinuses with extracellular mucin deposits simulating mucinous carcinoma of the gallbladder. Am J Surg Pathol 33:1633-1638.
69. Albores-Saavedra J, Grider DJ, Wu J, Henson DE, Goodman ZD (2006). Giant cell tumor of the extrahepatic biliary tree: a clinicopathologic study of 4 cases and comparison with anaplastic spindle and giant cell carcinoma with osteoclast-like giant cells. Am J Surg Pathol 30: 495-500.
70. Albores-Saavedra J, Henson DE, and Klimstra DS (eds) (2000). Tumors of the Gallbladder, Extrahepatic Bile Ducts, and Ampulla of Vater. Armed Forces Institute of Pathology: Washington, DC.
71. Albores-Saavedra J, Henson DE, Moran-Portela D, Lino-Silva S (2008). Cribriform carcinoma of the gallbladder: a clinicopathologic study of 7 cases. Am J Surg Pathol 32: 1694-1698.
72. Albores-Saavedra J, Henson DE, and Sobin LH (eds) (1991). Histological Typing of Tumours of the Gallbladder and Extrahepatic Bile Ducts. Springer-Verlag: Berlin.
73. Albores-Saavedra J, Molberg K, Henson DE (1996). Unusual malignant epithelial tumors of the gallbladder. Semin Diagn Pathol 13: 326-338.
74. Albores-Saavedra J, Murakata L, Krueger JE, Henson DE (2000). Noninvasive and minimally invasive papillary carcinomas of the extrahepatic bile ducts. Cancer 89: 508-515.
75. Albores-Saavedra J, Nadji M, Henson DE (1986). Intestinal-type adenocarcinoma of the gallbladder. A clinicopathologic study of seven cases. Am J Surg Pathol 10: 19-25.
76. Albores-Saavedra J, Nadji M, Henson DE, Angeles-Angeles A (1988). Enteroendocrine cell differentiation in carcinomas of the gallbladder and mucinous cystadenocarcinomas of the pancreas. Pathol Res Pract 183: 169-175.
77. Albores-Saavedra J, Nadji M, Morales AR, Henson DE (1983). Carcinoembryonic antigen in normal, preneoplastic and neoplastic gallbladder epithelium. Cancer 52: 1069-1072.
78. Albores-Saavedra J, Schwartz AM, Batich K, Henson DE (2009). Cancers of the ampulla of vater: Demographics, morphology, and survival based on 5625 cases from the SEER program. J Surg Oncol 100: 598-605.
79. Albores-Saavedra J, Sheahan K, O'Riain C, Shukla D (2004). Intraductal tubular adenoma, pyloric type, of the pancreas: additional observations on a new type of pancreatic neoplasm. Am J Surg Pathol 28: 233-238.
80. Albores-Saavedra J, Shukla D, Carrick K, Henson DE (2004). *In situ* and invasive adenocarcinomas of the gallbladder extending into or arising from Rokitansky-Aschoff sinuses: a clinicopathologic study of 49 cases. Am J Surg Pathol 28: 621-628.
81. Albores-Saavedra J, Simpson K, Dancer YJ, Hruban R (2007). Intestinal type adenocarcinoma: a previously unrecognized histologic variant of ductal carcinoma of the pancreas. Ann Diagn Pathol 11: 3-9.
82. Albores-Saavedra J, Simpson KW, Bilello SJ (2006). The clear cell variant of solid pseudopapillary tumor of the pancreas: a previously unrecognized pancreatic neoplasm. Am J Surg Pathol 30: 1237-1242.
83. Albores-Saavedra J, Soriano J, Larraza-Hernandez O, Aguirre J, Henson DE (1984). Oat cell carcinoma of the gallbladder. Hum Pathol 15: 639-646.
84. Albores-Saavedra J, Tuck M, McLaren BK, Carrick KS, Henson DE (2005). Papillary carcinomas of the gallbladder: analysis of noninvasive and invasive types. Arch Pathol Lab Med 129: 905-909.
85. Albores-Saavedra J, Vardaman CJ, Vuitch F (1993). Non-neoplastic polypoid lesions and adenomas of the gallbladder. Pathol Annu 28 Pt 1: 145-177.
86. Alessi DR, Sakamoto K, Bayascas JR (2006). LKB1-dependent signaling pathways. Annu Rev Biochem 75: 137-163.
87. Alexander HR, Grem JL, Hamilton JM, Pass HI, Hong M, Fraker DL et al. (1995). Thymidylate synthase protein expression: Association with response to neoadjuvant chemotherapy and resection for locally advanced gastric and gastroesophageal adenocarcinoma. Cancer J Sci Am 1: 49-54.
88. Alexander JR, Andrews JM, Buchi KN, Lee RG, Becker JM, Burt RW (1989). High prevalence of adenomatous polyps of the duodenal papilla in familial adenomatous polyposis. Dig Dis Sci 34: 167-170.
89. Alhopuro P, Phichith D, Tuupanen S, Sammalkorpi H, Nybondas M, Saharinen J et al. (2008). Unregulated smooth-muscle myosin in human intestinal neoplasia. Proc Natl Acad Sci U S A 105: 5513-5518.
90. Ali A, Serra S, Asa SL, Chetty R (2006). The predictive value of CK19 and CD99 in pancreatic endocrine tumors. Am J Surg Pathol 30: 1588-1594.
91. Alinari L, Castellucci P, Elstrom R, Ambrosini V, Stefoni V, Nanni C et al. (2006). 18F-FDG PET in mucosa-associated lymphoid tissue (MALT) lymphoma. Leuk Lymphoma 47: 2096-2101.
92. Alison MR, Islam S (2009). Attributes of adult stem cells. J Pathol 217: 144-160.
93. Allen NE, Beral V, Casabonne D, Kan SW, Reeves GK, Brown A et al. (2009). Moderate alcohol intake and cancer incidence in women. J Natl Cancer Inst 101: 296-305.
94. Allgaier HP, Deibert P, Olschewski M, Spamer C, Blum U, Gerok W et al. (1998). Survival benefit of patients with inoperable hepatocellular carcinoma treated by a combination of transarterial chemoembolization and percutaneous ethanol injection—a single-center analysis including 132 patients. Int J Cancer 79: 601-605.
95. Allison KH, Yoder BJ, Bronner MP, Goldblum JR, Rubin BP (2004). Angiosarcoma involving the gastrointestinal tract: a series of primary and metastatic cases. Am J Surg Pathol 28: 298-307.
96. Ally MR, Veerappan GR, Maydonovitch CL, Duncan TJ, Perry JL, Osgard EM et al. (2009). Chronic proton pump inhibitor therapy associated with increased development of fundic gland polyps. Dig Dis Sci 2617-2622.
97. Almoguera C, Shibata D, Forrester K, Martin J, Arnheim N, Perucho M (1988). Most human carcinomas of the exocrine pancreas contain mutant *c-K-ras* genes. Cell 53: 549-554.
98. Alonsozana EL, Stamberg J, Kumar D, Jaffe ES, Medeiros LJ, Frantz C et al. (1997). Isochromosome 7q: the primary cytogenetic abnormality in hepatosplenic gammadelta T cell lymphoma. Leukemia 11: 1367-1372.
99. Alpert LC, Truong LD, Bossart MI, Spjut HJ (1988). Microcystic adenoma (serous cystadenoma) of the pancreas. A study of 14 cases with immunohistochemical and electron-microscopic correlation. Am J Surg Pathol 12: 251-263.
100. Alsaad KO, Serra S, Schmitt A, Perren A, Chetty R (2007). Cytokeratins 7 and 20 immunoexpression profile in goblet cell and classical carcinoids of appendix. Endocr Pathol 18: 16-22.
101. Alvarez-Canas MC, Fernandez FA, Rodilla IG, Val-Bernal JF (1996). Perianal basal cell carcinoma: a comparative histologic, immunohistochemical, and flow cytometric study with basaloid carcinoma of the anus. Am J Dermatopathol 18: 371-379.
102. Alves A, Adam R, Majno P, Delvart V, Azoulay D, Castaing D et al. (2003). Hepatic resection for metastatic renal tumors: is it worthwhile? Ann Surg Oncol 10: 705-710.
103. Aly EH (2009). Laparoscopic colorectal surgery: summary of the current evidence. Ann R Coll Surg Engl 91: 541-544.
104. Amieva MR, El-Omar EM (2008). Host-bacterial interactions in *Helicobacter pylori* infection. Gastroenterology 134: 306-323.
105. Amundadottir L, Kraft P, Stolzenberg-Solomon RZ, Fuchs CS, Petersen GM, Arslan AA et al. (2009). Genome-wide association study identifies variants in the ABO locus associated with susceptibility to pancreatic cancer. Nat Genet 41: 986-990.
106. Amundadottir LT, Thorvaldsson S, Gudbjartsson DF, Sulem P, Kristjansson K, Arnason S et al. (2004). Cancer as a complex phenotype: pattern of cancer distribution within and beyond the nuclear family. PLoS Med 1: e65
107. Anagnostopoulos GK, Arvanitidis D, Sakorafas G, Pavlakis G, Kolilekas L, Arkoumani E et al. (2004). Combined carcinoid-adenocarcinoma tumour of the anal canal. Scand J Gastroenterol 39: 198-200.
108. Andea A, Sarkar F, Adsay VN (2003). Clinicopathological correlates of pancreatic intraepithelial neoplasia: a comparative analysis of 82 cases with and 152 cases without pancreatic ductal adenocarcinoma. Mod Pathol 16: 996-1006.
109. Anderson JR, Wilson BG (1985). Carcinoid tumours of the appendix. Br J Surg 72: 545-546.
110. Anderson KE, Mack TM, Silverman DT (2006). Cancer of the pancreas. In: Cancer Epidemiology and Prevention. Schottenfeld D, Fraumeni JF, eds. Oxford University Press: Oxford, pp. 721-762.
111. Andersson JL, Sundin A, Valind S (1995). A method for coregistration of PET and MR brain images. J Nucl Med 36: 1307-1315.
112. Ando N, Ozawa S, Kitagawa Y, Shinozawa Y, Kitajima M (2000). Improvement in the results of surgical treatment of advanced squamous esophageal carcinoma during 15 consecutive years. Ann Surg 232: 225-232.
113. Andoh A, Takaya H, Bamba M, Sakumoto H, Inoue T, Tujikawa T et al. (1998). Primary gastric Burkitt's lymphoma presenting with *c-myc* gene rearrangement. J Gastroenterol 33: 710-715.
114. Andres E, Herbrecht R, Campos F, Marcellin L, Oberling F (1997). Primary hepatic lymphoma associated with chronic hepatitis C. Ann Med Interne (Paris) 148: 280-283.
115. Andreyev HJ, Norman AR, Cunningham D, Oates JR, Clarke PA (1998). Kirsten ras mutations in patients with colorectal cancer: the multicenter "RASCAL" study. J Natl Cancer Inst 90: 675-684.
116. Angeles-Angeles A, Quintanilla-Martinez L, Larriva-Sahd J (1991). Primary carcinoid of the common bile duct. Immunohistochemical characterization of a case and review of the literature. Am J Clin Pathol 96: 341-344.
117. Anjaneyulu V, Shankar-Swarnalatha G, Rao SC (2007). Carcinoid tumor of the gall bladder. Ann Diagn Pathol 11: 113-116.
118. Anlauf M, Enosawa T, Henopp T, Schmitt A, Gimm O, Brauckhoff M et al. (2008). Primary lymph node gastrinoma or occult duodenal microgastrinoma with lymph node metastases in a MEN1 patient: the need for a systematic search for the primary tumor. Am J Surg Pathol 32: 1101-1105.
119. Anlauf M, Garbrecht N, Henopp T, Schmitt A, Schlenger R, Raffel A et al. (2006). Sporadic versus hereditary gastrinomas of the duodenum and pancreas: distinct clinico-pathological and epidemiological features. World J Gastroenterol 12: 5440-5446.
120. Anlauf M, Perren A, Henopp T, Rudolf T, Garbrecht N, Schmitt A et al. (2007). Allelic deletion of the *MEN1* gene in duodenal gastrin and somatostatin cell neoplasms and their precursor lesions. Gut 56: 637-644.
121. Annibale B, Azzoni C, Corleto VD, di GE, Caruana P, D'Ambra G et al. (2001). Atrophic body gastritis patients with enterochromaffin-like cell dysplasia are at increased risk for the development of type I gastric carcinoid. Eur J Gastroenterol Hepatol 13: 1449-1456.
122. Anon. (1998). Age-adjusted death rates by prefecture, Special Report on Vital Statistics.

Statistics and Information Department, Minister's Secretariat, Ministry of Health and Welfare, Health and Welfare Statistics Association. -

123. Anon. (2001). Prognostic significance of cyclin D1 and E-cadherin in patients with esophageal squamous cell carcinoma: multiinstitutional retrospective analysis. Research Committee on Malignancy of Esophageal Cancer, Japanese Society for Esophageal Diseases. J Am Coll Surg 192: 708-718.

124. Anon. (2003). The Paris endoscopic classification of superficial neoplastic lesions: esophagus, stomach, and colon: November 30 to December 1, 2002. Gastrointest Endosc 58: S3-43.

125. Anon. (The International Consensus Group for Hepatocellular Neoplasia) (2009). Pathologic diagnosis of early hepatocellular carcinoma: a report of the international consensus group for hepatocellular neoplasia. Hepatology 49: 658-664.

126. Ansorge WJ (2009). Next-generation DNA sequencing techniques. N Biotechnol 25: 195-203.

127. Anthony PP, Drury RA (1970). Elastic vascular sclerosis of mesenteric blood vessels in argentaffin carcinoma. J Clin Pathol 23: 110-118.

128. Anthony PP, Vogel CL, Barker LF (1973). Liver cell dysplasia: a premalignant condition. J Clin Pathol 26: 217-223.

129. Anthony T, Simmang C, Lee EL, Turnage RH (1997). Perianal mucinous adenocarcinoma. J Surg Oncol 64: 218-221.

130. Antonescu CR, Nafa K, Segal NH, Dal CP, Ladanyi M (2006). *EWS-CREB1*: a recurrent variant fusion in clear cell sarcoma—association with gastrointestinal location and absence of melanocytic differentiation. Clin Cancer Res 12: 5356-5362.

131. Aoki K, Taketo MM (2007). Adenomatous polyposis coli (APC): a multi-functional tumor suppressor gene. J Cell Sci 120: 3327-3335.

132. Aoki S, Okayama Y, Kitajima Y, Hayashi K, Imai H, Okamoto T et al. (2005). Intrahepatic biliary papilloma morphologically similar to biliary cystadenoma. J Gastroenterol Hepatol 20: 321-324.

133. Appelman HD, Helwig EB (1969). Glomus tumors of the stomach. Cancer 23: 203-213.

134. Arai M, Shimizu S, Imai Y, Nakatsuru Y, Oda H, Oohara T et al. (1997). Mutations of the *Ki-ras*, *p53* and *APC* genes in adenocarcinomas of the human small intestine. Int J Cancer 70: 390-395.

135. Aramendi T, Fernandez-Acenero MJ, Villanueva MC (2003). Carcinosarcoma of the colon: report of a rare tumor. Pathol Res Pract 199: 345-348.

136. Aranha GV, Reyes CV, Greenlee HB, Field T, Brosnan J (1980). Squamous cell carcinoma of the proximal bile duct—a case report. J Surg Oncol 15: 29-35.

137. Aravalli RN, Steer CJ, Cressman EN (2008). Molecular mechanisms of hepatocellular carcinoma. Hepatology 48: 2047-2063.

138. Arber N, Lightdale C, Rotterdam H, Han KH, Sgambato A, Yap E et al. (1996). Increased expression of the cyclin D1 gene in Barrett's esophagus. Cancer Epidemiol Biomarkers Prev 5: 457-459.

139. Archer HA, Owen WJ (2000). Primary malignant melanoma of the esophagus. Dis Esophagus 13: 320-323.

140. Aretz S, Stienen D, Friedrichs N, Stemmler S, Uhlhaas S, Rahner N et al. (2007). Somatic APC mosaicism: a frequent cause of familial adenomatous polyposis (FAP). Hum Mutat 28: 985-992.

141. Aretz S, Stienen D, Uhlhaas S, Stolte M, Entius MM, Loff S et al. (2007). High proportion of large genomic deletions and a genotype phenotype update in 80 unrelated families with juvenile polyposis syndrome. J Med Genet 44: 702-709.

142. Aretz S, Uhlhaas S, Goergens H, Siberg K, Vogel M, Pagenstecher C et al. (2006). MUTYH-associated polyposis: 70 of 71 patients with biallelic mutations present with an attenuated or atypical phenotype. Int J Cancer 119: 807-814.

143. Argani P, Shaukat A, Kaushal M, Wilentz RE, Su GH, Sohn TA et al. (2001). Differing rates of loss of DPC4 expression and of p53 overexpression among carcinomas of the proximal and distal bile ducts. Cancer 91: 1332-1341.

144. Argatoff LH, Connors JM, Klasa RJ, Horsman DE, Gascoyne RD (1997). Mantle cell lymphoma: a clinicopathologic study of 80 cases. Blood 89: 2067-2078.

145. Armitage NC, Jass JR, Richman PI, Thomson JP, Phillips RK (1989). Paget's disease of the anus: a clinicopathological study. Br J Surg 76: 60-63.

146. Arnold CN, Sosnowski A, Schmitt-Graff A, Arnold R, Blum HE (2007). Analysis of molecular pathways in sporadic neuroendocrine tumors of the gastro-entero-pancreatic system. Int J Cancer 120: 2157-2164.

147. Arnold GL, Mardini HE (2002). Barrett's esophagus-associated polypoid dysplasia: a case report and review of the literature. Dig Dis Sci 47: 1897-1900.

148. Arnold LD, Patel AV, Yan Y, Jacobs EJ, Thun MJ, Calle EE et al. (2009). Are racial disparities in pancreatic cancer explained by smoking and overweight/obesity? Cancer Epidemiol Biomarkers Prev 18: 2397-2405.

149. Arnold R, Rinke A, Klose KJ, Muller HH, Wied M, Zamzow K et al. (2005). Octreotide versus octreotide plus interferon-alpha in endocrine gastroenteropancreatic tumors: a randomized trial. Clin Gastroenterol Hepatol 3: 761-771.

149A. Arslan AA, Helzlsouer KJ, Kooperberg C, Shu XO, Steplowski E, Bueno-de-Mesquita HB et al. (2010). Anthropometric measures, body mass index, and pancreatic cancer: a pooled analysis from the Pancreatic Cancer Cohort Consortium (PanScan). Arch Intern Med 170: 791–802.

150. Asano N, Yamamoto K, Tamaru J, Oyama T, Ishida F, Ohshima K et al. (2009). Age-related Epstein-Barr virus (EBV)-associated B-cell lymphoproliferative disorders: comparison with EBV-positive classic Hodgkin lymphoma in elderly patients. Blood 113: 2629-2636.

151. Ascano JJ, Frierson H, Jr., Moskaluk CA, Harper JC, Roviello F, Jackson CE et al. (2001). Inactivation of the E-cadherin gene in sporadic diffuse-type gastric cancer. Mod Pathol 14: 942-949.

152. Ascoli V, Lo CF, Artini M, Levrero M, Martelli M, Negro F (1998). Extranodal lymphomas associated with hepatitis C virus infection. Am J Clin Pathol 109: 600-609.

153. Ashida K, Terada T, Kitamura Y, Kaibara N (1998). Expression of E-cadherin, alpha-catenin, beta-catenin, and CD44 (standard and variant isoforms) in human cholangiocarcinoma: an immunohistochemical study. Hepatology 27: 974-982.

154. Ashton-Key M, Diss TC, Pan L, Du MQ, Isaacson PG (1997). Molecular analysis of T-cell clonality in ulcerative jejunitis and enteropathy-associated T-cell lymphoma. Am J Pathol 151: 493-498.

155. Aslan DL, Jessurun J, Gulbahce HE, Pambuccian SE, Adsay V, Mallery JS (2008). Endoscopic ultrasound-guided fine needle aspiration features of a pancreatic neoplasm with predominantly intraductal growth and prominent tubular cytomorphology: intraductal tubular carcinoma of the pancreas? Diagn Cytopathol 36: 833-839.

156. Atherton JC, Cao P, Peek RM, Jr., Tummuru MK, Blaser MJ, Cover TL (1995). Mosaicism in vacuolating cytotoxin alleles of *Helicobacter pylori*. Association of specific vacA types with cytotoxin production and peptic ulceration. J Biol Chem 270: 17771-17777.

157. Attanoos R, Williams GT (1991). Epithelial and neuroendocrine tumors of the duodenum. Semin Diagn Pathol 8: 149-162.

158. Attar BM, Levendoglu H, Rhee H (1990). Small cell carcinoma of the esophagus. Report of three cases and review of the literature. Dig Dis Sci 35: 145-152.

159. Attard TM, Giardiello FM, Argani P, Cuffari C (2001). Fundic gland polyposis with high-grade dysplasia in a child with attenuated familial adenomatous polyposis and familial gastric cancer. J Pediatr Gastroenterol Nutr 32: 215-218.

160. Au E, Ang PT, Tan P, Sng I, Fong CM, Chua EJ et al. (1997). Gastrointestinal lymphoma—a review of 54 patients in Singapore. Ann Acad Med Singapore 26: 758-761.

161. Auer IA, Gascoyne RD, Connors JM, Cotter FE, Greiner TC, Sanger WG et al. (1997). t(11;18)(q21;q21) is the most common translocation in MALT lymphomas. Ann Oncol 8: 979-985.

162. Avery AK, Beckstead J, Renshaw AA, Corless CL (2000). Use of antibodies to RCC and CD10 in the differential diagnosis of renal neoplasms. Am J Surg Pathol 24: 203-210.

163. Avezzu A, Agostini M, Pucciarelli S, Lise M, Urso ED, Mammi I et al. (2008). The role of MYH gene in genetic predisposition to colorectal cancer: another piece of the puzzle. Cancer Lett 268: 308-313.

164. Avidan B, Sonnenberg A, Schnell TG, Chejfec G, Metz A, Sontag SJ (2002). Hiatal hernia size, Barrett's length, and severity of acid reflux are all risk factors for esophageal adenocarcinoma. Am J Gastroenterol 97: 1930-1936.

165. Axilbund JE, Argani P, Kamiyama M, Palmisano E, Raben M, Borges M et al. (2009). Absence of germline *BRCA1* mutations in familial pancreatic cancer patients. Cancer Biol Ther 8: 131-135.

166. Ayala AG, Ro JY (2007). Prostatic intraepithelial neoplasia: recent advances. Arch Pathol Lab Med 131: 1257-1266.

167. Ayantunde AA, Agrawal A, Parsons SL, Welch NT (2007). Esophagogastric cancers secondary to a breast primary tumor do not require resection. World J Surg 31: 1597-1601.

168. Ayhan A, Yasui W, Yokozaki H, Seto M, Ueda R, Tahara E (1994). Loss of heterozygosity at the *bcl-2* gene locus and expression of bcl-2 in human gastric and colorectal carcinomas. Jpn J Cancer Res 85: 584-591.

169. Azar C, Van de Stadt J, Rickaert F, Deviere M, Baize M, Klöppel G et al. (1996). Intraductal papillary mucinous tumours of the pancreas. Clinical and therapeutic issues in 32 patients. Gut 39: 457-464.

170. Azuma M, Sunagawa M, Shida S (1994). [Metastatic carcinoma of the appendix]. Nippon Rinsho Suppl 6: 725-727.

171. Azzoni C, Bottarelli L, Pizzi S, D'Adda T, Rindi G, Bordi C (2006). Xq25 and Xq26 identify the common minimal deletion region in malignant gastroenteropancreatic endocrine carcinomas. Virchows Arch 448: 119-126.

172. Baba Y, Nosho K, Shima K, Freed E, Irahara N, Philips J et al. (2009). Relationship of CDX2 loss with molecular features and prognosis in colorectal cancer. Clin Cancer Res 15: 4665-4673.

173. Bacq Y, Jacquemin E, Balabaud C, Jeannot E, Scotto B, Branchereau S et al. (2003). Familial liver adenomatosis associated with hepatocyte nuclear factor 1alpha inactivation. Gastroenterology 125: 1470-1475.

174. Baert AL, Casteels-Van DM, Broeckx J, Wijndaele L, Wilms G, Eggermont E (1983). Generalized juvenile polyposis with pulmonary arteriovenous malformations and hypertrophic osteoarthropathy. AJR Am J Roentgenol 141: 661-662.

175. Bagdi E, Diss TC, Munson P, Isaacson PG (1999). Mucosal intra-epithelial lymphocytes in enteropathy-associated T-cell lymphoma, ulcerative jejunitis, and refractory celiac disease constitute a neoplastic population. Blood 94: 260-264.

176. Baggens (1938). Major duodenal papilla. Variations of pathologic interest and lesions of the mucosa. Arch Pathol 26: 853-868.

177. Baglietto L, Jenkins MA, Severi G, Giles GG, Bishop DT, Boyle P et al. (2006). Measures of familial aggregation depend on definition of family history: meta-analysis for colorectal cancer. J Clin Epidemiol 59: 114-124.

178. Baglietto L, Lindor NM, Dowty JG, White DM, Wagner A, Gomez Garcia EB et al. (2010). Risks of Lynch syndrome cancers for *MSH6* mutation carriers. J Natl Cancer Inst 102: 193-201.

178A. Balachandra B, Marcus V, Jass JR (2007). Poorly differentiated tumours of the anal canal: a diagnostic strategy for the surgical pathologist. Histopathology 50: 163-174.

179. Balachandran P, Sikora SS, Kapoor S, Krishnani N, Kumar A, Saxena R et al. (2006). Long-term survival and recurrence patterns in ampullary cancer. Pancreas 32: 390-395.

180. Balaguer F, Castellvi-Bel S, Castells A, Andreu M, Munoz J, Gisbert JP et al. (2007). Identification of *MYH* mutation carriers in colorectal cancer: a multicenter, case-control, population-based study. Clin Gastroenterol Hepatol 5: 379-387.

181. Bale SJ, Bale AE, Stewart K, Dachowski L, McBride OW, Glaser T et al. (1989). Linkage analysis of multiple endocrine neoplasia type 1 with *INT2* and other markers on chromosome 11. Genomics 4: 320-322.

182. Ballas KD, Rafailidis SF, Demertzidis C, Alatsakis MB, Pantzaki A, Sakadamis AK (2005). Mixed exocrine-endocrine tumor of the pancreas. JOP 6: 449-454.

183. Bamboat ZM, Berger DL (2006). Is right hemicolectomy for 2.0-cm appendiceal carcinoids justified? Arch Surg 141: 349-352.

184. Ban S, Naitoh Y, Mino-Kenudson M, Sakurai T, Kuroda M, Koyama I et al. (2006). Intraductal papillary mucinous neoplasm (IPMN) of the pancreas: its histopathologic difference between 2 major types. Am J Surg Pathol 30: 1561-1569.

185. Banerjee SS, Eyden BP, Wells S, McWilliam LJ, Harris M (1992). Pseudoangiosarcomatous carcinoma: a clinicopathological study of seven cases. Histopathology 21: 13-23.

186. Bani-Hani K, Martin IG, Hardie LJ, Mapstone N, Briggs JA, Forman D et al. (2000). Prospective study of cyclin D1 overexpression in Barrett's esophagus: association with increased risk of adenocarcinoma. J Natl Cancer Inst 92: 1316-1321.

187. Banks ER, Frierson HF, Jr., Mills SE, George E, Zarbo RJ, Swanson PE (1992). Basaloid squamous cell carcinoma of the head and neck. A clinicopathologic and immunohistochemical study of 40 cases. Am J Surg Pathol 16: 939-946.

188. Banks PM, Chan J, Cleary ML, Delsol G, De Wolf-Peeters C, Gatter K et al. (1992). Mantle cell lymphoma. A proposal for unification of morphologic, immunologic, and molecular data. Am J Surg Pathol 16: 637-640.

189. Bansal M, Fenoglio CM, Robboy SJ, King DW (1984). Are metaplasias in colorectal adenomas truly metaplasias? Am J Pathol 115: 253-265.

190. Banville N, Geraghty R, Fox E, Leahy DT, Green A, Keegan D et al. (2006). Medullary carcinoma of the pancreas in a man with hereditary nonpolyposis colorectal cancer due to a mutation of the *MSH2* mismatch repair gene. Hum Pathol 37: 1498-1502.
191. Barakat J, Dunkelberg JC, Ma TY (2006). Changing patterns of gallbladder carcinoma in New Mexico. Cancer 106: 434-440.
192. Baratti D, Kusamura S, Nonaka D, Cabras AD, Laterza B, Deraco M (2009). Pseudomyxoma peritonei: biological features are the dominant prognostic determinants after complete cytoreduction and hyperthermic intraperitoneal chemotherapy. Ann Surg 249: 243-249.
193. Barbareschi M, Roldo C, Zamboni G, Capelli P, Cavazza A, Macri E et al. (2004). *CDX-2* homeobox gene product expression in neuroendocrine tumors: its role as a marker of intestinal neuroendocrine tumors. Am J Surg Pathol 28: 1169-1176.
194. Barber M, Murrell A, Ito Y, Maia AT, Hyland S, Oliveira C et al. (2008). Mechanisms and sequelae of E-cadherin silencing in hereditary diffuse gastric cancer. J Pathol 216: 295-306.
195. Barber ME, Save V, Carneiro F, Dwerryhouse S, Lao-Sirieix P, Hardwick RH et al. (2008). Histopathological and molecular analysis of gastrectomy specimens from hereditary diffuse gastric cancer patients has implications for endoscopic surveillance of individuals at risk. J Pathol 216: 286-294.
196. Bardales RH, Stanley MW, Simpson DD, Baker SJ, Steele CT, Schaefer RF et al. (1998). Diagnostic value of brush cytology in the diagnosis of duodenal, biliary, and ampullary neoplasms. Am J Clin Pathol 109: 540-548.
197. Bardales RH, Stelow EB, Mallery S, Lai R, Stanley MW (2006). Review of endoscopic ultrasound-guided fine-needle aspiration cytology. Diagn Cytopathol 34: 140-175.
198. Bariol C, Hawkins NJ, Turner JJ, Meagher AP, Williams DB, Ward RL (2003). Histopathological and clinical evaluation of serrated adenomas of the colon and rectum. Mod Pathol 16: 417-423.
199. Barnhill M, Hess E, Guccion JG, Nam LH, Bass BL, Patterson RH (1994). Tripartite differentiation in a carcinoma of the duodenum. Cancer 73: 266-272.
200. Baron TH, Harewood GC, Rumalla A, Pochron NL, Stadheim LM, Gores GJ et al. (2004). A prospective comparison of digital image analysis and routine cytology for the identification of malignancy in biliary tract strictures. Clin Gastroenterol Hepatol 2: 214-219.
201. Barone GW, Schaefer RF, Counce JS, Eidt JF (1992). Gallbladder and gastric argyrophil carcinoid associated with a case of Zollinger-Ellison syndrome. Am J Gastroenterol 87: 392-394.
202. Barrett WL, Callahan TD, Orkin BA (1998). Perianal manifestations of human immunodeficiency virus infection: experience with 260 patients. Dis Colon Rectum 41: 606-611.
203. Barron-Rodriguez LP, Manivel JC, Mendez-Sanchez N, Jessurun J (1991). Carcinoid tumor of the common bile duct: evidence for its origin in metaplastic endocrine cells. Am J Gastroenterol 86: 1073-1076.
204. Barros-Silva JD, Leitao D, Afonso L, Vieira J, Dinis-Ribeiro M, Fragoso M et al. (2009). Association of ERBB2 gene status with histopathological parameters and disease-specific survival in gastric carcinoma patients. Br J Cancer 100: 487-493.
205. Bartow SA, Mukai K, Rosai J (1981). Pseudoneoplastic proliferation of endocrine cells in pancreatic fibrosis. Cancer 47: 2627-2633.
206. Bartsch D, Bastian D, Barth P, Schudy A, Nies C, Kisker O et al. (1998). K-ras oncogene mutations indicate malignancy in cystic tumors of the pancreas. Ann Surg 228: 79-86.
207. Bartsch DK, Kress R, Sina-Frey M, Grutzmann R, Gerdes B, Pilarsky C et al. (2004). Prevalence of familial pancreatic cancer in Germany. Int J Cancer 110: 902-906.
208. Barugola G, Falconi M, Bettini R, Boninsegna L, Casarotto A, Salvia R et al. (2007). The determinant factors of recurrence following resection for ductal pancreatic cancer. JOP 8: 132-140.
209. Basik M, Rodriguez-Bigas MA, Penetrante R, Petrelli NJ (1995). Prognosis and recurrence patterns of anal adenocarcinoma. Am J Surg 169: 233-237.
210. Basso D, Zambon CF, Letley DP, Stranges A, Marchet A, Rhead JL et al. (2008). Clinical relevance of *Helicobacter pylori cagA* and *vacA* gene polymorphisms. Gastroenterology 135: 91-99.
211. Basturk O, Coban I, Adsay NV (2009). Pancreatic cysts: pathologic classification, differential diagnosis, and clinical implications. Arch Pathol Lab Med 133: 423-438.
212. Basturk O, Khayyata S, Klimstra DS, Hruban RH, Zamboni G, Coban I et al. (2010). Preferential expression of MUC6 in oncocytic and pancreatobiliary types of intraductal papillary neoplasms highlights a pyloropancreatic pathway, distinct from the intestinal pathway, in pancreatic carcinogenesis. Am J Surg Pathol 34: 364-370.
213. Basturk O, Zamboni G, Klimstra DS, Capelli P, Andea A, Kamel NS et al. (2007). Intraductal and papillary variants of acinar cell carcinomas: a new addition to the challenging differential diagnosis of intraductal neoplasms. Am J Surg Pathol 31: 363-370.
214. Batheja N, Suriawinata A, Saxena R, Ionescu G, Schwartz M, Thung SN (2000). Expression of p53 and PCNA in cholangiocarcinoma and primary sclerosing cholangitis. Mod Pathol 13: 1265-1268.
215. Battles OE, Page DL, Johnson JE (1997). Cytokeratins, CEA, and mucin histochemistry in the diagnosis and characterization of extramammary Paget's disease. Am J Clin Pathol 108: 6-12.
216. Baumgaertner I, Corcos O, Couvelard A, Sauvanet A, Rebours V, Vullierme MP et al. (2008). Prevalence of extrapancreatic cancers in patients with histologically proven intraductal papillary mucinous neoplasms of the pancreas: a case-control study. Am J Gastroenterol 103: 2878-2882.
217. Bayon LG, Izquierdo MA, Sirovich I, van Rooijen N, Beelen RH, Meijer S (1996). Role of Kupffer cells in arresting circulating tumor cells and controlling metastatic growth in the liver. Hepatology 23: 1224-1231.
218. Beck PL, Gill MJ, Sutherland LR (1996). HIV-associated non-Hodgkin's lymphoma of the gastrointestinal tract. Am J Gastroenterol 91: 2377-2381.
219. Becker K, Mueller JD, Schulmacher C, Ott K, Fink U, Busch R et al. (2003). Histomorphology and grading of regression in gastric carcinoma treated with neoadjuvant chemotherapy. Cancer 98: 1521-1530.
220. Becker KF, Atkinson MJ, Reich U, Becker I, Nekarda H, Siewert JR et al. (1994). E-cadherin gene mutations provide clues to diffuse type gastric carcinomas. Cancer Res 54: 3845-3852.
221. Becker KF, Keller G, Hoefler H (2000). The use of molecular biology in diagnosis and prognosis of gastric cancer. Surg Oncol 9: 5-11.
222. Beckers A, Abs R, Reyniers E, De BK, Stevenaert A, Heller FR et al. (1994). Variable regions of chromosome 11 loss in different pathological tissues of a patient with the multiple endocrine neoplasia type I syndrome. J Clin Endocrinol Metab 79: 1498-1502.
223. Beghelli S, de MG, Barbi S, Tomezzoli A, Roviello F, Di GC et al. (2006). Microsatellite instability in gastric cancer is associated with better prognosis in only stage II cancers. Surgery 139: 347-356.
224. Behrens J, Jerchow BA, Wurtele M, Grimm J, Asbrand C, Wirtz R et al. (1998). Functional interaction of an axin homolog, conductin, with beta-catenin, APC, and GSK3beta. Science 280: 596-599.
225. Belhadj K, Reyes F, Farcet JP, Tilly H, Bastard C, Angonin R et al. (2003). Hepatosplenic gammadelta T-cell lymphoma is a rare clinicopathologic entity with poor outcome: report on a series of 21 patients. Blood 102: 4261-4269.
226. Bell DA (1987). Cytologic features of islet-cell tumors. Acta Cytol 31: 485-492.
227. Bellizzi AM, Frankel WL (2009). Colorectal cancer due to deficiency in DNA mismatch repair function: a review. Adv Anat Pathol 16: 405-417.
228. Bellizzi AM, Stelow EB (2009). Pancreatic cytopathology: a practical approach and review. Arch Pathol Lab Med 133: 388-404.
229. Belsley NA, Pitman MB, Lauwers GY, Brugge WR, Deshpande V (2008). Serous cystadenoma of the pancreas: limitations and pitfalls of endoscopic ultrasound-guided fine-needle aspiration biopsy. Cancer 114: 102-110.
230. Ben-Haim M, Roayaie S, Ye MQ, Thung SN, Emre S, Fishbein TA et al. (1999). Hepatic epithelioid hemangioendothelioma: resection or transplantation, which and when? Liver Transpl Surg 5: 526-531.
231. Bendelow J, Apps E, Jones LE, Poston GJ (2008). Carcinoid syndrome. Eur J Surg Oncol 34: 289-296.
232. Benediktsdottir K, Lundell L, Thulin A (1981). Premalignant lesions of the periampullary region. Report of two cases. Ann Chir Gynaecol 70: 86-89.
233. Benjamin E, Wright DH (1980). Adenocarcinoma of the pancreas of childhood: a report of two cases. Histopathology 4: 87-104.
234. Berardi RS (1972). Carcinoid tumors of the colon (exclusive of the rectum): review of the literature. Dis Colon Rectum 15: 383-391.
235. Berge T, Lundberg S (1977). Cancer in Malmo. Acta Pathol Microbiol Scand S250: 140-149.
235A. Berger AC, Farma J, Scott WJ, Freedman G, Weiner L, Cheng JD, Wang H, Goldberg M (2005). Complete response to neoadjuvant chemoradiotherapy in esophageal carcinoma is associated with significantly improved survival. J Clin Oncol 23: 4330-4337.
236. Berger KL, Nicholson SA, Dehdashti F, Siegel BA (2000). FDG PET evaluation of mucinous neoplasms: correlation of FDG uptake with histopathologic features. AJR Am J Roentgenol 174: 1005-1008.
237. Bergmann F, Esposito I, Michalski CW, Herpel E, Friess H, Schirmacher P (2007). Early undifferentiated pancreatic carcinoma with osteoclastlike giant cells: direct evidence for ductal evolution. Am J Surg Pathol 31: 1919-1925.
238. Bergquist A, Broome U (2001). Hepatobiliary and extra-hepatic malignancies in primary sclerosing cholangitis. Best Pract Res Clin Gastroenterol 15: 643-656.
239. Bergquist A, Glaumann H, Persson B, Broome U (1998). Risk factors and clinical presentation of hepatobiliary carcinoma in patients with primary sclerosing cholangitis: a case-control study. Hepatology 27: 311-316.
240. Bergquist A, Glaumann H, Stal P, Wang GS, Broome U (2001). Biliary dysplasia, cell proliferation and nuclear DNA-fragmentation in primary sclerosing cholangitis with and without cholangiocarcinoma. J Intern Med 249: 69-75.
241. Berna MJ, Annibale B, Marignani M, Luong TV, Corleto V, Pace A et al. (2008). A prospective study of gastric carcinoids and enterochromaffin-like cell changes in multiple endocrine neoplasia type 1 and Zollinger-Ellison syndrome: identification of risk factors. J Clin Endocrinol Metab 93: 1582-1591.
242. Bernasconi B, Karamitopoulou-Diamantis E, Tornillo L, Lugli A, Di Vizio D, Dirnhofer S et al. (2008). Chromosomal instability in gastric mucosa-associated lymphoid tissue lymphomas: a fluorescent in situ hybridization study using a tissue microarray approach. Hum Pathol 39: 536-542.
243. Bernick PE, Klimstra DS, Shia J, Minsky B, Saltz L, Shi W et al. (2004). Neuroendocrine carcinomas of the colon and rectum. Dis Colon Rectum 47: 163-169.
244. Bertagnolli MM, Niedzwiecki D, Compton CC, Hahn HP, Hall M, Damas B et al. (2009). Microsatellite instability predicts improved response to adjuvant therapy with irinotecan, fluorouracil, and leucovorin in stage III colon cancer: Cancer and Leukemia Group B Protocol 89803. J Clin Oncol 27: 1814-1821.
245. Bertario L, Russo A, Sala P, Eboli M, Giarola M, D'amico F et al. (2001). Genotype and phenotype factors as determinants of desmoid tumors in patients with familial adenomatous polyposis. Int J Cancer 95: 102-107.
246. Bertoni F, Cazzaniga G, Bosshard G, Roggero E, Barbazza R, de Boni M et al. (1997). Immunoglobulin heavy chain diversity genes rearrangement pattern indicates that MALT-type gastric lymphoma B cells have undergone an antigen selection process. Br J Haematol 97: 830-836.
247. Bertoni G, Sassatelli R, Nigrisoli E, Pennazio M, Tansini P, Arrigoni A et al. (1999). Dysplastic changes in gastric fundic gland polyps of patients with familial adenomatous polyposis. Ital J Gastroenterol Hepatol 31: 192-197.
248. Bertram P, Treutner KH, Rubben A, Hauptmann S, Schumpelick V (1995). Invasive squamous-cell carcinoma in giant anorectal condyloma (Buschke-Lowenstein tumor). Langenbecks Arch Chir 380: 115-118.
249. Berx G, Cleton-Jansen AM, Nollet F, de Leeuw WJ, van de Vijver M, Cornelisse C et al. (1995). E-cadherin is a tumour/invasion suppressor gene mutated in human lobular breast cancers. EMBO J 14: 6107-6115.
250. Bettini R, Boninsegna L, Mantovani W, Capelli P, Bassi C, Pederzoli P et al. (2008). Prognostic factors at diagnosis and value of WHO classification in a mono-institutional series of 180 non-functioning pancreatic endocrine tumours. Ann Oncol 19: 903-908.
251. Bettini R, Falconi M, Crippa S, Capelli P, Boninsegna L, Pederzoli P (2007). Ampullary somatostatinomas and jejunal gastrointestinal stromal tumor in a patient with Von Recklinghausen's disease. World J Gastroenterol 13: 2761-2763.
252. Beveridge IG, Swain DJ, Groves CJ, Saunders BP, Windsor AC, Talbot IC et al. (2004). Large villous adenomas arising in ileal pouches in familial adenomatous polyposis: report of two cases. Dis Colon Rectum 47: 123-126.
253. Bhathal PS, Hughes NR, Goodman ZD (1996). The so-called bile duct adenoma is a peribiliary gland hamartoma. Am J Surg Pathol 20: 858-864.
254. Biankin AV, Biankin SA, Kench JG, Morey AL, Lee CS, Head DR et al. (2002). Aberrant p16(INK4A) and DPC4/Smad4 expression in intraductal papillary mucinous tumours of the pancreas is associated with invasive ductal adenocarcinoma. Gut 50: 861-868.
255. Bibeau F, Chateau MC, Guiu M, Assenat

E, Azria D, Lavaill R et al. (2008). Small cell carcinoma with concomitant adenocarcinoma arising in a Barrett's oesophagus: report of a case with a favourable behaviour. Virchows Arch 452: 103-107.

256. Bickel A, Eitan A, Tsilman B, Cohen HI (1999). Low-grade B cell lymphoma of mucosa-associated lymphoid tissue (MALT) arising in the gallbladder. Hepatogastroenterology 46: 1643-1646.

257. Bickenbach K, Galka E, Roggin KK (2009). Molecular mechanisms of cholangiocarcinogenesis: are biliary intraepithelial neoplasia and intraductal papillary neoplasms of the bile duct precursors to cholangiocarcinoma? Surg Oncol Clin N Am 18: 215-24, vii.

258. Bilimoria KY, Bentrem DJ, Rock CE, Stewart AK, Ko CY, Halverson A (2009). Outcomes and prognostic factors for squamous-cell carcinoma of the anal canal: analysis of patients from the National Cancer Data Base. Dis Colon Rectum 52: 624-631.

259. Billings SD, Meisner LF, Cummings OW, Tejada E (2000). Synovial sarcoma of the upper digestive tract: a report of two cases with demonstration of the X;18 translocation by fluorescence in situ hybridization. Mod Pathol 13: 68-76.

260. Bioulac-Sage P, Laumonier H, Couchy G, Le Bail B., Sa Cunha A., Rullier A et al. (2009). Hepatocellular adenoma management and phenotypic classification: the Bordeaux experience. Hepatology 50: 481-489.

261. Bioulac-Sage P, Laumonier H, Cubel G, Rossi JZ, Balabaud C (2010). Hepatic resection for inflammatory hepatocellular adenomas: pathological identification of micronodules expressing inflammatory proteins. Liver Int 30: 149-154.

262. Bioulac-Sage P, Laumonier H, Laurent C, Blanc JF, Balabaud C (2008). Benign and malignant vascular tumors of the liver in adults. Semin Liver Dis 28: 302-314.

263. Bioulac-Sage P, Laumonier H, Rullier A, Cubel G, Laurent C, Zucman-Rossi J et al. (2009). Over-expression of glutamine synthetase in focal nodular hyperplasia: a novel easy diagnostic tool in surgical pathology. Liver Int 29: 459-465.

264. Bioulac-Sage P, Rebouissou S, Sa Cunha A., Jeannot E, Lepreux S, Blanc JF et al. (2005). Clinical, morphologic, and molecular features defining so-called telangiectatic focal nodular hyperplasias of the liver. Gastroenterology 128: 1211-1218.

265. Bioulac-Sage P, Rebouissou S, Thomas C, Blanc JF, Saric J, Sa CA et al. (2007). Hepatocellular adenoma subtype classification using molecular markers and immunohistochemistry. Hepatology 46: 740-748.

266. Bisgaard ML, Fenger K, Bulow S, Niebuhr E, Mohr J (1994). Familial adenomatous polyposis (FAP): frequency, penetrance, and mutation rate. Hum Mutat 3: 121-125.

267. Bishop AE, Hamid QA, Adams C, Bretherton-Watt D, Jones PM, Denny P et al. (1989). Expression of tachykinins by ileal and lung carcinoid tumors assessed by combined in situ hybridization, immunocytochemistry, and radioimmunoassay. Cancer 63: 1129-1137.

268. Bisig B, Copie-Bergman C, Baia M, Gaulard P, Delbecque K, Fassotte MF et al. (2009). Primary mucosa-associated lymphoid tissue lymphoma of the gallbladder: report of a case harboring API2/MALT1 gene fusion. Hum Pathol 40: 1504-1509.

269. Bisogno G, Pilz T, Perilongo G, Ferrari A, Harms D, Ninfo V et al. (2002). Undifferentiated sarcoma of the liver in childhood: a curable disease. Cancer 94: 252-257.

270. Bittinger A, Altekruger I, Barth P (1995). Clear cell carcinoma of the gallbladder. A histological and immunohistochemical study. Pathol

Res Pract 191: 1259-1265.

271. Bjelakovic G, Nikolova D, Simonetti RG, Gluud C (2008). Systematic review: primary and secondary prevention of gastrointestinal cancers with antioxidant supplements. Aliment Pharmacol Ther 28: 689-703.

272. Bjork J, Akerbrant H, Iselius L, Bergman A, Engwall Y, Wahlstrom J et al. (2001). Periampullary adenomas and adenocarcinomas in familial adenomatous polyposis: cumulative risks and APC gene mutations. Gastroenterology 121: 1127-1135.

273. Blackford A, Serrano OK, Wolfgang CL, Parmigiani G, Jones S, Zhang X et al. (2009). SMAD4 gene mutations are associated with poor prognosis in pancreatic cancer. Clin Cancer Res 15: 4674-4679.

274. Blackman E, Nash SV (1985). Diagnosis of duodenal and ampullary epithelial neoplasms by endoscopic biopsy: a clinicopathologic and immunohistochemical study. Hum Pathol 16: 901-910.

275. Blackshaw G, Lewis WG, Hopper AN, Morgan MA, Al-Khyatt W, Edwards P et al. (2008). Prospective comparison of endosonography, computed tomography, and histopathological stage of junctional oesophagogastric cancer. Clin Radiol 63: 1092-1098.

276. Blair V, Martin I, Shaw D, Winship I, Kerr D, Arnold J et al. (2006). Hereditary diffuse gastric cancer: diagnosis and management. Clin Gastroenterol Hepatol 4: 262-275.

277. Blaker H, Helmchen B, Bonisch A, Aulmann S, Penzel R, Otto HF et al. (2004). Mutational activation of the RAS-RAF-MAPK and the Wnt pathway in small intestinal adenocarcinomas. Scand J Gastroenterol 39: 748-753.

278. Blanchard P, Quero L, Hennequin C (2009). [Prognostic and predictive factors of oesophageal carcinoma]. Bull Cancer 96: 379-389.

279. Blandamura S, Parenti A, Famengo B, Canesso A, Moschino P, Pasquali C et al. (2007). Three cases of pancreatic serous cystadenoma and endocrine tumour. J Clin Pathol 60: 278-282.

280. Blaschuk OW, Sullivan R, David S, Pouliot Y (1990). Identification of a cadherin cell adhesion recognition sequence. Dev Biol 139: 227-229.

281. Bloch MJ, Iozzo RV, Edmunds LH, Jr., Brooks JJ (1987). Polypoid synovial sarcoma of the esophagus. Gastroenterology 92: 229-233.

282. Blomjous JG, Hop WC, Langenhorst BL, ten Kate FJ, Eykenboom WM, Tilanus HW (1992). Adenocarcinoma of the gastric cardia. Recurrence and survival after resection. Cancer 70: 569-574.

283. Bloomston M, Chanona-Vilchis J, Ellison EC, Ramirez NC, Frankel WL (2006). Carcinosarcoma of the pancreas arising in a mucinous cystic neoplasm. Am Surg 72: 351-355.

284. Bloomston M, Walker M, Frankel WL (2006). Radical resection in signet ring carcinoma of the ampulla of Vater: report of an 11-year survivor. Am Surg 72: 193-195.

285. Blot WJ, McLaughlin JK, Fraumeni JF (2006). Esophageal cancer. In: Cancer Epidemiology and Prevention. Schottenfeld D, Fraumeni JF, eds. Oxford University Press: New York, pp. 697-706.

286. Bluemke DA, Cameron JL, Hruban RH, Pitt HA, Siegelman SS, Soyer P et al. (1995). Potentially resectable pancreatic adenocarcinoma: spiral CT assessment with surgical and pathologic correlation. Radiology 197: 381-385.

287. Blum MG, Bilimoria KY, Wayne JD, de Hoyos AL, Talamonti MS, Adley B (2007). Surgical considerations for the management and resection of esophageal gastrointestinal stromal tumors. Ann Thorac Surg 84: 1717-1723.

287A. Blumenthal GM, Dennis PA (2008). PTEN hamartoma tumor syndromes. Eur J Hum Genet 16: 1289-1300.

288. Bluteau O, Jeannot E, Bioulac-Sage P, Marques JM, Blanc JF, Bui H et al. (2002). Bi-allelic inactivation of TCF1 in hepatic adenomas. Nat Genet 32: 312-315.

289. Boberg KM, Bergquist A, Mitchell S, Pares A, Rosina F, Broome U et al. (2002). Cholangiocarcinoma in primary sclerosing cholangitis: risk factors and clinical presentation. Scand J Gastroenterol 37: 1205-1211.

290. Boberg KM, Jebsen P, Clausen OP, Foss A, Aabakken L, Schrumpf E (2006). Diagnostic benefit of biliary brush cytology in cholangiocarcinoma in primary sclerosing cholangitis. J Hepatol 45: 568-574.

291. Bodmer WF, Bailey CJ, Bodmer J, Bussey HJ, Ellis A, Gorman P et al. (1987). Localization of the gene for familial adenomatous polyposis on chromosome 5. Nature 328: 614-616.

292. Boey J, Choi TK, Wong J, Ong GB (1981). The surgical management of anorectal malignant melanoma. Aust N Z J Surg 51: 132-136.

293. Boffetta P, Hashibe M (2006). Alcohol and cancer. Lancet Oncol 7: 149-156.

294. Bogomoletz WV, Molas G, Gayet B, Potet F (1989). Superficial squamous cell carcinoma of the esophagus. A report of 76 cases and review of the literature. Am J Surg Pathol 13: 535-546.

295. Boland CR (2005). Evolution of the nomenclature for the hereditary colorectal cancer syndromes. Fam Cancer 4: 211-218.

296. Boland CR, Thibodeau SN, Hamilton SR, Sidransky D, Eshleman JR, Burt RW et al. (1998). A National Cancer Institute Workshop on Microsatellite Instability for cancer detection and familial predisposition: development of international criteria for the determination of microsatellite instability in colorectal cancer. Cancer Res 58: 5248-5257.

297. Boman BM, Huang E (2008). Human colon cancer stem cells: a new paradigm in gastrointestinal oncology. J Clin Oncol 26: 2828-2838.

298. Boman BM, Moertel CG, O'Connell MJ, Scott M, Weiland LH, Beart RW et al. (1984). Carcinoma of the anal canal. A clinical and pathologic study of 188 cases. Cancer 54: 114-125.

299. Boman F, Bossard C, Fabre M, Diab N, Bonnevalle M, Boccon-Gibod L (2004). Mesenchymal hamartomas of the liver may be associated with increased serum alpha foetoprotein concentrations and mimic hepatoblastomas. Eur J Pediatr Surg 14: 63-66.

300. Bonatti H, Hoefer D, Rogatsch H, Margreiter R, Larcher C, Antretter H (2005). Successful management of recurrent Epstein-Barr virus-associated multilocular leiomyosarcoma after cardiac transplantation. Transplant Proc 37: 1839-1844.

301. Boor PJ, Swanson MR (1979). Papillary-cystic neoplasm of the pancreas. Am J Surg Pathol 3: 69-75.

302. Boparai KS, Dekker E, van Eeden S, Polak MM, Bartelsman JF, Mathus-Vliegen EM et al. (2008). Hyperplastic polyps and sessile serrated adenomas as a phenotypic expression of MYH-associated polyposis. Gastroenterology 135: 2014-2018.

303. Borch K, Ahren B, Ahlman H, Falkmer S, Granerus G, Grimelius L (2005). Gastric carcinoids: biologic behavior and prognosis after differentiated treatment in relation to type. Ann Surg 242: 64-73.

304. Bordi C, D'Adda T, Azzoni C, Canavese G, Brandi ML (1998). Gastrointestinal endocrine tumors: recent developments. Endocr Pathol 9:

99-115.

305. Bordi C, D'Adda T, Azzoni C, Pilato FP, Caruana P (1995). Hypergastrinemia and gastric enterochromaffin-like cells. Am J Surg Pathol 19 Suppl 1: S8-19.

306. Bordi C, Falchetti A, Azzoni C, D'Adda T, Canavese G, Guariglia A et al. (1997). Aggressive forms of gastric neuroendocrine tumors in multiple endocrine neoplasia type I. Am J Surg Pathol 21: 1075-1082.

307. Bornstein-Quevedo L, Gamboa-Dominguez A (2001). Carcinoid tumors of the duodenum and ampulla of vater: a clinicomorphologic, immunohistochemical, and cell kinetic comparison. Hum Pathol 32: 1252-1256.

308. Borrmann R (1926). Geshwulste des Magens und Duodenums. In: Handbuch der Speziellen Pathologischen Anatomie und Histologie. Henke F, Lubarsch O, eds. Springer-Verlag: Berlin, pp. 865-

309. Borscheri N, Roessner A, Rocken C (2001). Canalicular immunostaining of neprilysin (CD10) as a diagnostic marker for hepatocellular carcinomas. Am J Surg Pathol 25: 1297-1303.

310. Borzio M, Bruno S, Roncalli M, Mels GC, Ramella G, Borzio F et al. (1995). Liver cell dysplasia is a major risk factor for hepatocellular carcinoma in cirrhosis: a prospective study. Gastroenterology 108: 812-817.

311. Borzio M, Trere D, Borzio F, Ferrari AR, Bruno S, Roncalli M et al. (1998). Hepatocyte proliferation rate is a powerful parameter for predicting hepatocellular carcinoma development in liver cirrhosis. Mol Pathol 51: 96-101.

312. Bosman FT (2001). Dysplasia classification: pathology in disgrace? J Pathol 194: 143-144.

313. Bostanoglu S, Otan E, Akturan S, Hamamci EO, Bostanoglu A, Gokce A et al. (2009). Frantz's tumor (solid pseudopapillary tumor) of the pancreas. A case report. JOP 10: 209-211.

314. Boucher E, Forner A, Reig M, Bruix J (2009). New drugs for the treatment of hepatocellular carcinoma. Liver Int 29 Suppl 1: 148-158.

315. Bourdeaut F, Freneaux P, Thuille B, Lellouch-Tubiana A, Nicolas A, Couturier J et al. (2007). hSNF5/INI1-deficient tumours and rhabdoid tumours are convergent but not fully overlapping entities. J Pathol 211: 323-330.

316. Bouvard V, Baan R, Straif K, Grosse Y, Secretan B, El Ghissassi F et al. (2009). A review of human carcinogens—Part B: biological agents. Lancet Oncol 10: 321-322.

317. Bouzourene H, Haefliger T, Delacretaz F, Saraga E (1999). The role of Helicobacter pylori in primary gastric MALT lymphoma. Histopathology 34: 118-123.

318. Bove KE, Soukup S, Ballard ET, Ryckman F (1996). Hepatoblastoma in a child with trisomy 18: cytogenetics, liver anomalies, and literature review. Pediatr Pathol Lab Med 16: 253-262.

319. Boyle P, Levin B (eds) (2008). World Cancer Report. IARC: Lyon, France.

320. Bradbury PA, Zhai R, Hopkins J, Kulke MH, Heist RS, Singh S et al. (2009). Matrix metalloproteinase 1, 3 and 12 polymorphisms and esophageal adenocarcinoma risk and prognosis. Carcinogenesis 30: 793-798.

321. Bradley RF, Stewart JH, Russell GB, Levine EA, Geisinger KR (2006). Pseudomyxoma peritonei of appendiceal origin: a clinicopathologic analysis of 101 patients uniformly treated at a single institution, with literature review. Am J Surg Pathol 30: 551-559.

322. Brady MS, Kavolius JP, Quan SH (1995). Anorectal melanoma. A 64-year experience at Memorial Sloan-Kettering Cancer Center. Dis Colon Rectum 38: 146-151.

323. Brainard JA, Goldblum JR (1997). Stromal tumors of the jejunum and ileum: a clin-

icopathologic study of 39 cases. Am J Surg Pathol 21: 407-416.

324. Brancatelli G, Federle MP, Vullierme MP, Lagalla R, Midiri M, Vilgrain V (2006). CT and MR imaging evaluation of hepatic adenoma. J Comput Assist Tomogr 30: 745-750.

325. Bras-Goncalves RA, Rosty C, Laurent-Puig P, Soulie P, Dutrillaux B, Poupon MF (2000). Sensitivity to CPT-11 of xenografted human colorectal cancers as a function of microsatellite instability and p53 status. Br J Cancer 82: 913-923.

326. Brat DJ, Hahn SA, Griffin CA, Yeo CJ, Kern SE, Hruban RH (1997). The structural basis of molecular genetic deletions. An integration of classical cytogenetic and molecular analyses in pancreatic adenocarcinoma. Am J Pathol 150: 383-391.

327. Brat DJ, Lillemoe KD, Yeo CJ, Warfield PB, Hruban RH (1998). Progression of pancreatic intraductal neoplasias to infiltrating adenocarcinoma of the pancreas. Am J Surg Pathol 22: 163-169.

328. Braun MS, Richman SD, Quirke P, Daly C, Adlard JW, Elliott F et al. (2008). Predictive biomarkers of chemotherapy efficacy in colorectal cancer: results from the UK MRC FOCUS trial. J Clin Oncol 26: 2690-2698.

329. Brenner B, Shah MA, Gonen M, Klimstra DS, Shia J, Kelsen DP (2004). Small-cell carcinoma of the gastrointestinal tract: a retrospective study of 64 cases. Br J Cancer 90: 1720-1726.

330. Brenner H, Arndt V, Bode G, Stegmaier C, Ziegler H, Stumer T (2002). Risk of gastric cancer among smokers infected with Helicobacter pylori. Int J Cancer 98: 446-449.

331. Brennetot C, Duval A, Hamelin R, Pinto M, Oliveira C, Seruca R et al. (2003). Frequent Ki-ras mutations in gastric tumors of the MSI phenotype. Gastroenterology 125: 1282.

332. Brensinger JD, Laken SJ, Luce MC, Powell SM, Vance GH, Ahnen DJ et al. (1998). Variable phenotype of familial adenomatous polyposis in pedigrees with 3' mutation in the APC gene. Gut 43: 548-552.

333. Bressac B, Kew M, Wands J, Ozturk M (1991). Selective G to T mutations of p53 gene in hepatocellular carcinoma from southern Africa. Nature 350: 429-431.

334. Bridge MF, Perzin KH (1975). Primary adenocarcinoma of the jejunum and ileum. A clinicopathologic study. Cancer 36: 1876-1887.

335. Briggs JC, Ibrahim NB (1983). Oat cell carcinomas of the oesophagus: a clinico-pathological study of 23 cases. Histopathology 7: 261-277.

336. Brockie E, Anand A, Albores Saavedra J (1998). Progression of atypical ductal hyperplasia/carcinoma in situ of the pancreas to invasive adenocarcinoma. Ann Diagn Pathol 2: 286-292.

336A. Broderick P, Carvajal-Carmona L, Pittman AM, Webb E, Howarth K, Rowan A et al. (2007). A genome-wide association study shows that common alleles of SMAD7 influence colorectal cancer risk. Nat Genet 39: 1315-1319

337. Brody JR, Costantino CL, Potoczek M, Cozzitorto J, McCue P, Yeo CJ et al. (2009). Adenosquamous carcinoma of the pancreas harbors KRAS2, DPC4 and TP53 molecular alterations similar to pancreatic ductal adenocarcinoma. Mod Pathol 22: 651-659.

338. Broicher K, Hienz HA (1974). [Carcinoid syndrome in primary esophageal tumor]. Z Gastroenterol 12 Suppl: 377-384.

339. Bronner CE, Baker SM, Morrison PT, Warren G, Smith LG, Lescoe MK et al. (1994). Mutation in the DNA mismatch repair gene homologue hMLH1 is associated with hereditary non-polyposis colon cancer. Nature 368: 258-261.

340. Brooks PJ, Enoch MA, Goldman D, Li TK, Yokoyama A (2009). The alcohol flushing

response: an unrecognized risk factor for esophageal cancer from alcohol consumption. PLoS Med 6: e50-

341. Brooks-Wilson AR, Kaurah P, Suriano G, Leach S, Senz J, Grehan N et al. (2004). Germline E-cadherin mutations in hereditary diffuse gastric cancer: assessment of 42 new families and review of genetic screening criteria. J Med Genet 41: 508-517.

342. Broome U, Lofberg R, Veress B, Eriksson LS (1995). Primary sclerosing cholangitis and ulcerative colitis: evidence for increased neoplastic potential. Hepatology 22: 1404-1408.

343. Brosens LA, van Hattem A, Hylind LM, Iacobuzio-Donahue C, Romans KE, Axilbund J et al. (2007). Risk of colorectal cancer in juvenile polyposis. Gut 56: 965-967.

344. Brosens LA, van Hattem WA, Jansen M, de Leng WW, Giardiello FM, Offerhaus GJ (2007). Gastrointestinal polyposis syndromes. Curr Mol Med 7: 29-46.

345. Brosens LA, van Hattem WA, Kools MC, Ezendam C, Morsink FH, de Leng WW et al. (2009). No TGFBRII germline mutations in juvenile polyposis patients without SMAD4 or BMPR1A mutation. Gut 58: 154-156.

345A. Brotto M, Finegold MJ (2002). Distinct patterns of p27/KIP 1 gene expression in hepatoblastoma and prognostic implications with correlation before and after chemotherapy. Hum.Pathol 33: 198-205.

346. Broughan TA, Leslie JD, Soto JM, Hermann RE (1986). Pancreatic islet cell tumors. Surgery 99: 671-678.

347. Brown LM, Devesa SS, Chow WH (2008). Incidence of adenocarcinoma of the esophagus among white Americans by sex, stage, and age. J Natl Cancer Inst 100: 1184-1187.

348. Brown WM, III, Henderson JM, Kennedy JC (1990). Carcinoid tumor of the bile duct. A case report and literature review. Am Surg 56: 343-346.

349. Brownstein MH, Wolf M, Bikowski JB (1978). Cowden's disease: a cutaneous marker of breast cancer. Cancer 41: 2393-2398.

350. Brucher BL, Geddert H, Langner C, Hofler H, Fink U, Siewert JR et al. (2006). Hypermethylation of hMLH1, HPP1, p14(ARF), p16(INK4A) and APC in primary adenocarcinomas of the small bowel. Int J Cancer 119: 1298-1302.

351. Brueckl WM, Heinze E, Milsmann C, Wein A, Koebnick C, Jung A et al. (2004). Prognostic significance of microsatellite instability in curatively resected adenocarcinoma of the small intestine. Cancer Lett 203: 181-190.

352. Bruix J, Sherman M (2005). Management of hepatocellular carcinoma. Hepatology 42: 1208-1236.

353. Brune K, Abe T, Canto M, O'Malley L, Klein AP, Maitra A et al. (2006). Multifocal neoplastic precursor lesions associated with lobular atrophy of the pancreas in patients having a strong family history of pancreatic cancer. Am J Surg Pathol 30: 1067-1076.

354. Brune KA, Lau B, Palmisano E, Canto M, Goggins MG, Hruban RH et al. (2010). Importance of age of onset in pancreatic cancer kindreds. J Natl Cancer Inst 102: 119-126.

355. Bucher P, Gervaz P, Ris F, Oulhaci W, Egger JF, Morel P (2005). Surgical treatment of appendiceal adenocarcinoid (goblet cell carcinoid). World J Surg 29: 1436-1439.

356. Bucher P, Gervaz P, Ris F, Oulhaci W, Inan I, Morel P (2006). Laparoscopic versus open resection for appendix carcinoid. Surg Endosc 20: 967-970.

357. Buchino JJ, Castello FM, Nagaraj HS (1984). Pancreatoblastoma. A histochemical and ultrastructural analysis. Cancer 53: 963-969.

358. Buchler M, Malfertheiner P, Baczako K,

Krautzberger W, Beger HG (1985). A metastatic endocrine-neurogenic tumor of the ampulla of Vater with multiple endocrine immunoreaction—malignant paraganglioma? Digestion 31: 54-59.

359. Buckley JA, Fishman EK (1998). CT evaluation of small bowel neoplasms: spectrum of disease. Radiographics 18: 379-392.

360. Buecher B, Baert-Desurmont S, Leborgne J, Humeau B, Olschwang S, Frebourg T (2008). Duodenal adenocarcinoma and Mut Y human homologue-associated polyposis. Eur J Gastroenterol Hepatol 20: 1024-1027.

361. Buetow PC, Buck JL, Pantongrag-Brown L, Marshall WH, Ros PR, Levine MS et al. (1997). Undifferentiated (embryonal) sarcoma of the liver: pathologic basis of imaging findings in 28 cases. Radiology 203: 779-783.

362. Buetow PC, Rao P, Thompson LD (1998). From the Archives of the AFIP. Mucinous cystic neoplasms of the pancreas: radiologic-pathologic correlation. Radiographics 18: 433-449.

363. Bugra D, Alper A, Goksen Y, Emre A (1991). Villous tumors of the duodenum. Hepatogastroenterology 38: 84-85.

364. Bulow C, Bulow S (1997). Is screening for thyroid carcinoma indicated in familial adenomatous polyposis? The Leeds Castle Polyposis Group. Int J Colorectal Dis 12: 240-242.

365. Bulow S (1987). Familial polyposis coli. Dan Med Bull 34: 1-15.

366. Bulow S, Skov OP, Poulsen SS, Kirkegaard P (1988). Is epidermal growth factor involved in development of duodenal polyps in familial polyposis coli? Am J Gastroenterol 83: 404-406.

367. Buritica C, Serrano M, Zuluaga A, Arrabal M, Regauer S, Nogales FF (2007). Mixed epithelial and stromal tumour of the kidney with luteinised ovarian stroma. J Clin Pathol 60: 98-100.

368. Burke AB, Shekitka KM, Sobin LH (1991). Small cell carcinomas of the large intestine. Am J Clin Pathol 95: 315-321.

369. Burke AP, Helwig EB (1989). Gangliocytic paraganglioma. Am J Clin Pathol 92: 1-9.

370. Burke AP, Sobin LH, Federspiel BH, Shekitka KM, Helwig EB (1990). Carcinoid tumors of the duodenum. A clinicopathologic study of 99 cases. Arch Pathol Lab Med 114: 700-704.

371. Burke AP, Sobin LH, Federspiel BH, Shekitka KM, Helwig EB (1990). Goblet cell carcinoids and related tumors of the vermiform appendix. Am J Clin Pathol 94: 27-35.

372. Burke AP, Sobin LH, Shekitka KM, Federspiel BH, Helwig EB (1990). Somatostatin-producing duodenal carcinoids in patients with von Recklinghausen's neurofibromatosis. A predilection for black patients. Cancer 65: 1591-1595.

373. Burke AP, Thomas RM, Elsayed AM, Sobin LH (1997). Carcinoids of the jejunum and ileum: an immunohistochemical and clinicopathologic study of 167 cases. Cancer 79: 1086-1093.

374. Burke C (2001). Risk stratification for periampullary carcinoma in patients with familial adenomatous polyposis: does theodore know what to do now? Gastroenterology 121: 1246-1248.

375. Burke CA, Beck GJ, Church JM, van Stolk RU (1999). The natural history of untreated duodenal and ampullary adenomas in patients with familial adenomatous polyposis followed in an endoscopic surveillance program. Gastrointest Endosc 49: 358-364.

376. Burns PN, Wilson SR (2007). Focal liver masses: enhancement patterns on contrast-enhanced images—concordance of US scans with CT scans and MR images. Radiology 242:

162-174.

377. Burns WA, Matthews MJ, Hamosh M, Weide GV, Blum R, Johnson FB (1974). Lipase-secreting acinar cell carcinoma of the pancreas with polyarthropathy. A light and electron microscopic, histochemical, and biochemical study. Cancer 33: 1002-1009.

378. Burt R, Neklason DW (2005). Genetic testing for inherited colon cancer. Gastroenterology 128: 1696-1716.

379. Burt RW, Bishop DT, Lynch HT, Rozen P, Winawer SJ (1990). Risk and surveillance of individuals with heritable factors for colorectal cancer. WHO Collaborating Centre for the Prevention of Colorectal Cancer. Bull World Health Organ 68: 655-665.

380. Burt RW, Leppert MF, Slattery ML, Samowitz WS, Spirio LN, Kerber RA et al. (2004). Genetic testing and phenotype in a large kindred with attenuated familial adenomatous polyposis. Gastroenterology 127: 444-451.

381. Burt RW, Samowitz WS (1996). Serrated adenomatous polyposis: a new syndrome? Gastroenterology 110: 950-952.

382. Buskens CJ, Sivula A, van Rees BP, Haglund C, Offerhaus GJ, van Lanschot JJ et al. (2003). Comparison of cyclooxygenase 2 expression in adenocarcinomas of the gastric cardia and distal oesophagus. Gut 52: 1678-1683.

383. Buskens CJ, van Rees BP, Sivula A, Reitsma JB, Haglund C, Bosma PJ et al. (2002). Prognostic significance of elevated cyclooxygenase 2 expression in patients with adenocarcinoma of the esophagus. Gastroenterology 122: 1800-1807.

384. Bussey HJ (ed) (1975). Familial Polyposis Coli. Family Studies, Histopathology, Differential Diagnosis and Results of Treatment. The John Hopkins University Press: Baltimore.

385. Bussey HJ, Veale AM, Morson BC (1978). Genetics of gastrointestinal polyposis. Gastroenterology 74: 1325-1330.

386. Butler MG, Dasouki MJ, Zhou XP, Talebizadeh Z, Brown M, Takahashi TN et al. (2005). Subset of individuals with autism spectrum disorders and extreme macrocephaly associated with germline PTEN tumour suppressor gene mutations. J Med Genet 42: 318-321.

387. Buttar NS, Wang KK, Sebo TJ, Riehle DM, Krishnadath KK, Lutzke LS et al. (2001). Extent of high-grade dysplasia in Barrett's esophagus correlates with risk of adenocarcinoma. Gastroenterology 120: 1630-1639.

388. Butterworth AS, Higgins JP, Pharoah P (2006). Relative and absolute risk of colorectal cancer for individuals with a family history: a meta-analysis. Eur J Cancer 42: 216-227.

389. Cadden I, Johnston BT, Turner G, McCance D, Ardill J, McGinty A (2007). An evaluation of cyclooxygenase-2 as a prognostic biomarker in mid-gut carcinoid tumours. Neuroendocrinology 86: 104-111.

390. Cadiot G, Laurent-Puig P, Thuille B, Lehy T, Mignon M, Olschwang S (1993). Is the multiple endocrine neoplasia type 1 gene a suppressor for fundic argyrophil tumors in the Zollinger-Ellison syndrome? Gastroenterology 105: 579-582.

391. Cahill DP, Lengauer C, Yu J, Riggins GJ, Willson JK, Markowitz SD et al. (1998). Mutations of mitotic checkpoint genes in human cancers. Nature 392: 300-303.

392. Cai YC, Banner B, Glickman J, Odze RD (2001). Cytokeratin 7 and 20 and thyroid transcription factor 1 can help distinguish pulmonary from gastrointestinal carcinoid and pancreatic endocrine tumors. Hum Pathol 32: 1087-1093.

393. Cakmak A, Karakayali F, Bayar S, Unal E, Akyol C, Kocaoglu H (2009). Pseudomyxoma retroperitonei presenting with a skin fistula. Turk J Gastroenterol 20: 79-80.

394. Calabrese P, Tavare S, Shibata D (2004). Pretumor progression: clonal evolution of human stem cell populations. Am J Pathol 164: 1337-1346.
395. Calcagno DQ, Leal MF, Seabra AD, Khayat AS, Chen ES, Demachki S et al. (2006). Interrelationship between chromosome 8 aneuploidy, C-MYC amplification and increased expression in individuals from northern Brazil with gastric adenocarcinoma. World J Gastroenterol 12: 6207-6211.
396. Caldarola VT, Jackman RJ, Moertel CG, Dockerty MB (1964). Carcinoid tumours of the rectum. Am J Surg 107: 844-849.
397. Caldas C, Carneiro F, Lynch HT, Yokota J, Wiesner GL, Powell SM et al. (1999). Familial gastric cancer: overview and guidelines for management. J Med Genet 36: 873-880.
398. Caldas C, Hahn SA, da Costa LT, Redston MS, Schutte M, Seymour AB et al. (1994). Frequent somatic mutations and homozygous deletions of the *p16* (*MTS1*) gene in pancreatic adenocarcinoma. Nat Genet 8: 27-32.
399. Caldas C, Hahn SA, Hruban RH, Redston MS, Yeo CJ, Kern SE (1994). Detection of *K-ras* mutations in the stool of patients with pancreatic adenocarcinoma and pancreatic ductal hyperplasia. Cancer Res 54: 3568-3573.
400. Calhoun ES, Jones JB, Ashfaq R, Adsay V, Baker SJ, Valentine V et al. (2003). BRAF and FBXW7 (CDC4, FBW7, AGO, SEL10) mutations in distinct subsets of pancreatic cancer: potential therapeutic targets. Am J Pathol 163: 1255-1260.
401. Calva-Cerqueira D, Chinnathambi S, Pechman B, Bair J, Larsen-Haidle J, Howe JR (2009). The rate of germline mutations and large deletions of *SMAD4* and *BMPR1A* in juvenile polyposis. Clin Genet 75: 79-85.
402. Cameron AJ, Souto EO, Smyrk TC (2002). Small adenocarcinomas of the esophagogastric junction: association with intestinal metaplasia and dysplasia. Am J Gastroenterol 97: 1375-1380.
403. Campana D, Nori F, Pezzilli R, Piscitelli L, Santini D, Brocchi E et al. (2008). Gastric endocrine tumors type I: treatment with long-acting somatostatin analogs. Endocr Relat Cancer 15: 337-342.
404. Campoli PM, Ejima FH, Cardoso DM, Silva OQ, Santana Filho JB, Queiroz Barreto PA et al. (2006). Metastatic cancer to the stomach. Gastric Cancer 9: 19-25.
405. Canavese G, Azzoni C, Pizzi S, Corleto VD, Pasquali C, Davoli C et al. (2001). p27: a potential main inhibitor of cell proliferation in digestive endocrine tumors but not a marker of benign behavior. Hum Pathol 32: 1094-1101.
406. Cannon ME, Carpenter SL, Elta GH, Nostrant TT, Kochman ML, Ginsberg GG et al. (1999). EUS compared with CT, magnetic resonance imaging, and angiography and the influence of biliary stenting on staging accuracy of ampullary neoplasms. Gastrointest Endosc 50: 27-33.
407. Canto MI, Goggins M, Hruban RH, Petersen GM, Giardiello FM, Yeo C et al. (2006). Screening for early pancreatic neoplasia in high-risk individuals: a prospective controlled study. Clin Gastroenterol Hepatol 4: 766-781.
408. Cantrell BB, Cubilla AL, Erlandson RA, Fortner J, Fitzgerald PJ (1981). Acinar cell cystadenocarcinoma of human pancreas. Cancer 47: 410-416.
409. Cao D, Antonescu C, Wong G, Winter J, Maitra A, Adsay NV et al. (2006). Positive immunohistochemical staining of KIT in solid-pseudopapillary neoplasms of the pancreas is not associated with KIT/PDGFRA mutations. Mod Pathol 19: 1157-1163.
410. Cao D, Maitra A, Saavedra JA, Klimstra DS, Adsay NV, Hruban RH (2005). Expression of novel markers of pancreatic ductal adenocarcinoma in pancreatic nonductal neoplasms: additional evidence of different genetic pathways. Mod Pathol 18: 752-761.
411. Capella C, Frigerio B, Cornaggia M, Solcia E, Pinzon-Trujillo Y, Chejfec G (1984). Gastric parietal cell carcinoma—a newly recognized entity: light microscopic and ultrastructural features. Histopathology 8: 813-824.
412. Capella C, Polak JM, Timson CM, Frigerio B, Solcia E (1980). Gastric carcinoids of argyrophil ECL cells. Ultrastruct Pathol 1: 411-418.
413. Capella C, Riva C, Rindi G, Sessa F, Usellini L, Chiaravalli A et al. (1991). Histopathology, hormone products and clinicopathologic profile of endocrine tumours of the upper small intestine. A study of 44 cases. Endocr Pathol 2: 92-110.
414. Capella G, Cronauer-Mitra S, Pienado MA, Perucho M (1991). Frequency and spectrum of mutations at codons 12 and 13 of the *c-K-ras* gene in human tumors. Environ Health Perspect 93: 125-131.
415. Capelle LG, Van Grieken NC, Lingsma HF, Steyerberg EW, Klokman WJ, Bruno MJ et al. (2010). Risk and epidemiological time trends of gastric cancer in Lynch syndrome carriers in the Netherlands. Gastroenterology 138: 487-492.
416. Cappell MS (2008). Reducing the incidence and mortality of colon cancer: mass screening and colonoscopic polypectomy. Gastroenterol Clin North Am 37: 129-viii.
417. Cappellari JO, Geisinger KR, Albertson DA, Wolfman NT, Kute TE (1990). Malignant papillary cystic tumor of the pancreas. Cancer 66: 193-198.
418. Capurro M, Wanless IR, Sherman M, Deboer G, Shi W, Miyoshi E et al. (2003). Glypican-3: a novel serum and histochemical marker for hepatocellular carcinoma. Gastroenterology 125: 89-97.
419. Carbone A, Gloghini A (2005). AIDS-related lymphomas: from pathogenesis to pathology. Br J Haematol 130: 662-670.
420. Carbone A, Gloghini A, Gaidano G, Cilia AM, Bassi P, Polito P et al. (1995). AIDS-related Burkitt's lymphoma. Morphologic and immunophenotypic study of biopsy specimens. Am J Clin Pathol 103: 561-567.
421. Carbone PP, Kaplan HS, Musshoff K, Smithers DW, Tubiana M (1971). Report of the Committee on Hodgkin's Disease Staging Classification. Cancer Res 31: 1860-1861.
422. Cardoso J, Molenaar L, de Menezes RX, van Leerdam M, Rosenberg C, Moslein G et al. (2006). Chromosomal instability in MYH- and APC-mutant adenomatous polyps. Cancer Res 66: 2514-2519.
423. Cario E, Runzi M, Metz K, Layer P, Goebell H (1997). Diagnostic dilemma in pancreatic lymphoma. Case report and review. Int J Pancreatol 22: 67-71.
424. Carlson GJ, Nivatvongs S, Snover DC (1984). Colorectal polyps in Cowden's disease (multiple hamartoma syndrome). Am J Surg Pathol 8: 763-770.
425. Carmack SW, Genta RM, Graham DY, Lauwers GY (2009). Management of gastric polyps: a pathology-based guide for gastroenterologists. Nat Rev Gastroenterol Hepatol 6: 331-341.
426. Carneiro F (1997). Classification of gastric carcinomas. Curr Diagn Pathol 4: 51-59.
427. Carneiro F, David L, Seruca R, Castedo S, Nesland JM, Sobrinho-Simoes M (1993). Hyperplastic polyposis and diffuse carcinoma of the stomach. A study of a family. Cancer 72: 323-329.
428. Carneiro F, Huntsman DG, Smyrk TC, Owen DA, Seruca R, Pharoah P et al. (2004). Model of the early development of diffuse gastric cancer in E-cadherin mutation carriers and its implications for patient screening. J Pathol 203: 681-687.
429. Carneiro F, Oliveira C, Leite M, Seruca R (2008). Molecular targets and biological modifiers in gastric cancer. Semin Diagn Pathol 25: 274-287.
430. Carneiro F, Oliveira C, Suriano G, Seruca R (2008). Molecular pathology of familial gastric cancer, with an emphasis on hereditary diffuse gastric cancer. J Clin Pathol 61: 25-30.
431. Carneiro F, Seixas M, Sobrinho-Simoes M (1995). New elements for an updated classification of the carcinomas of the stomach. Pathol Res Pract 191: 571-584.
432. Carneiro F, Sobrinho-Simoes M (1996). Metastatic pattern of gastric carcinoma. Hum Pathol 27: 213-214.
433. Carneiro F, Sobrinho-Simoes M (1996). Signet ring cell carcinoma in hyperplastic polyp. Scand J Gastroenterol 31: 95-96.
434. Carney CP, Jones L, Woolson RF, Noyes R, Jr., Doebbeling BN (2003). Relationship between depression and pancreatic cancer in the general population. Psychosom Med 65: 884-888.
435. Carney JA (1999). Gastric stromal sarcoma, pulmonary chondroma, and extra-adrenal paraganglioma (Carney Triad): natural history, adrenocortical component, and possible familial occurrence. Mayo Clin Proc 74: 543-552.
436. Carney JA, Go VL, Sizemore GW, Hayles AB (1976). Alimentary-tract ganglioneuromatosis. A major component of the syndrome of multiple endocrine neoplasia, type 2b. N Engl J Med 295: 1287-1291.
437. Carney JA, Sizemore GW, Hayles AB (1978). Multiple endocrine neoplasia, type 2b. Pathobiol Annu 8: 105-153.
438. Carr NJ, Emory TS, Sobin LH (2002). Epithelial neoplasms of the appendix and colorectum: an analysis of cell proliferation, apoptosis, and expression of p53, CD44, bcl-2. Arch Pathol Lab Med 126: 837-841.
439. Carr NJ, Mahajan H, Tan KL, Hawkins NJ, Ward RL (2009). Serrated and non-serrated polyps of the colorectum: their prevalence in an unselected case series and correlation of BRAF mutation analysis with the diagnosis of sessile serrated adenoma. J Clin Pathol 62: 516-518.
440. Carr NJ, Sobin LH (1995). Epithelial non-carcinoid tumors and tumor-like lesions of the appendix. Cancer 76: 2383-2384.
441. Carr NJ, Sobin LH (1996). Unusual tumors of the appendix and pseudomyxoma peritonei. Semin Diagn Pathol 13: 314-325.
442. Carstens HB, Ghazi C, Carnighan RH, Brewer MS (1986). Primary malignant melanoma of the common bile duct. Hum Pathol 17: 1282-1285.
443. Carstens PH, Cressman FKJr (1989). Malignant oncocytic carcinoid of the pancreas. Ultrastruct Pathol 13: 69-75.
444. Carta M, Maresi E, Giuffre M, Catalano G, Piro E, Siracusa F et al. (2005). Congenital hepatic mesenchymal hamartoma associated with mesenchymal stem villous hyperplasia of the placenta: case report. J Pediatr Surg 40: e37-e39.
445. Carter KJ, Schaffer HA, Ritchie WP, Jr. (1984). Early gastric cancer. Ann Surg 199: 604-609.
446. Carter PS, Sheffield JP, Shepherd N, Melcher DH, Jenkins D, Ewings P et al. (1994). Interobserver variation in the reporting of the histopathological grading of anal intraepithelial neoplasia. J Clin Pathol 47: 1032-1034.
447. Caruso ML, Pilato FP, D'Adda T, Baggi MT, Fucci L, Valentini AM et al. (1989). Composite carcinoid-adenocarcinoma of the stomach associated with multiple gastric carcinoids and nonantral gastric atrophy. Cancer 64: 1534-1539.
447A. Carvalho B, Buffart TE, Reis RM, Mons T, Moutinho C, Silva P et al. (2006). Mixed gastric carcinomas show similar chromosomal aberrations in both their diffuse and glandular components. Cell Oncol 28: 283-294.
448. Cary NR, Barron DJ, McGoldrick JP, Wells FC (1993). Combined oesophageal adenocarcinoma and carcinoid in Barrett's oesophagitis: potential role of enterochromaffin-like cells in oesophageal malignancy. Thorax 48: 404-405.
449. Casadei R, D'Ambra M, Pezzilli R, Ricci C, Calculli L, Lega S et al. (2008). Solid serous microcystic tumor of the pancreas. JOP 9: 538-540.
450. Caspari R, Olschwang S, Friedl W, Mandl M, Boisson C, Boker T et al. (1995). Familial adenomatous polyposis: desmoid tumours and lack of ophthalmic lesions (CHRPE) associated with APC mutations beyond codon 1444. Hum Mol Genet 4: 337-340.
451. Casson AG, Zheng Z, Evans SC, Geldenhuys L, van Zanten SV, Veugelers PJ et al. (2005). Cyclin D1 polymorphism (G870A) and risk for esophageal adenocarcinoma. Cancer 104: 730-739.
452. Casson AG, Zheng Z, Evans SC, Veugelers PJ, Porter GA, Guernsey DL (2005). Polymorphisms in DNA repair genes in the molecular pathogenesis of esophageal (Barrett) adenocarcinoma. Carcinogenesis 26: 1536-1541.
453. Casson AG, Zheng Z, Porter GA, Guernsey DL (2006). Genetic polymorphisms of microsomal epoxide hydroxylase and glutathione S-transferases M1, T1 and P1, interactions with smoking, and risk for esophageal (Barrett) adenocarcinoma. Cancer Detect Prev 30: 423-431.
454. Castella EM, Ariza A, Ojanguren I, Mate JL, Roca X, Fernandez-Vasalo A et al. (1996). Differential expression of CD44v6 in adenocarcinoma of the pancreas: an immunohistochemical study. Virchows Arch 429: 191-195.
455. Castroagudin JF, Gonzalez-Quintela A, Fraga M, Forteza J, Barrio E (1999). Presentation of T-cell-rich B-cell lymphoma mimicking acute hepatitis. Hepatogastroenterology 46: 1710-1713.
456. Catalano MF, Linder JD, Chak A, Sivak MV, Jr., Raijman I, Geenen JE et al. (2004). Endoscopic management of adenoma of the major duodenal papilla. Gastrointest Endosc 59: 225-232.
457. Cattell RB, Pyrtek LJ (1950). Premalignant lesions of the ampulla of Vater. Surg Gynecol Obstet 90: 21-30.
458. Cavallini A, Falconi M, Bortesi L, Crippa S, Barugola G, Butturini G (2009). Pancreatoblastoma in adults: a review of the literature. Pancreatology 9: 73-80.
459. Cavard C, Audebourg A, Letourneur F, Audard V, Beuvon F, Cagnard N et al. (2009). Gene expression profiling provides insights into the pathways involved in solid pseudopapillary neoplasm of the pancreas. J Pathol 218: 201-209.
460. Cellier C, Delabesse E, Helmer C, Patey N, Matuchansky C, Jabri B et al. (2000). Refractory sprue, coeliac disease, and enteropathy-associated T-cell lymphoma. French Coeliac Disease Study Group. Lancet 356: 203-208.
461. Cellier C, Patey N, Mauvieux L, Jabri B, Delabesse E, Cervoni JP et al. (1998). Abnormal intestinal intraepithelial lymphocytes in refractory sprue. Gastroenterology 114: 471-481.
462. Censini S, Lange C, Xiang Z, Crabtree JE, Ghiara P, Borodovsky M et al. (1996). cag, a pathogenicity island of *Helicobacter pylori*, encodes type I-specific and disease-associated

virulence factors. Proc Natl Acad Sci U S A 93: 14648-14653.

463. Cetta F, Montalto G, Petracci M (1997). Hepatoblastoma and *APC* gene mutation in familial adenomatous polyposis. Gut 41: 417-

464. Cetta F, Toti P, Petracci M, Montalto G, Disanto A, Lore F et al. (1997). Thyroid carcinoma associated with familial adenomatous polyposis. Histopathology 31: 231-236.

465. Chadwick B, Willmore-Payne C, Tripp S, Layfield LJ, Hirschowitz S, Holden J (2009). Histologic, immunohistochemical, and molecular classification of 52 IPMNs of the pancreas. Appl Immunohistochem Mol Morphol 17: 31-39.

466. Chak A, Falk G, Grady WM, Kinnard M, Elston R, Mittal S et al. (2009). Assessment of familiality, obesity, and other risk factors for early age of cancer diagnosis in adenocarcinomas of the esophagus and gastroesophageal junction. Am J Gastroenterol 104: 1913-1921.

467. Chak A, Lee T, Kinnard MF, Brock W, Faulx A, Willis J et al. (2002). Familial aggregation of Barrett's oesophagus, oesophageal adenocarcinoma, and oesophagogastric junctional adenocarcinoma in Caucasian adults. Gut 51: 323-328.

468. Chamberlain RS, Blumgart LH (1999). Carcinoid tumors of the extrahepatic bile duct. A rare cause of malignant biliary obstruction. Cancer 86: 1959-1965.

469. Chambers WM, Warren BF, Jewell DP, Mortensen NJ (2005). Cancer surveillance in ulcerative colitis. Br J Surg 92: 928-936.

470. Chan AO (2006). E-cadherin in gastric cancer. World J Gastroenterol 12: 199-203.

471. Chan AO, Kim SG, Bedeir A, Issa JP, Hamilton SR, Rashid A (2003). CpG island methylation in carcinoid and pancreatic endocrine tumors. Oncogene 22: 924-934.

472. Chan AO, Soliman AS, Zhang Q, Rashid A, Bedeir A, Houlihan PS et al. (2005). Differing DNA methylation patterns and gene mutation frequencies in colorectal carcinomas from Middle Eastern countries. Clin Cancer Res 11: 8281-8287.

473. Chan G, Horton PJ, Thyssen S, Lamarche M, Nahal A, Hill DJ et al. (2007). Malignant transformation of a solitary fibrous tumor of the liver and intractable hypoglycemia. J Hepatobiliary Pancreat Surg 14: 595-599.

474. Chan JY, Phoo MS, Clement MV, Pervaiz S, Lee SC (2008). Resveratrol displays converse dose-related effects on 5-fluorouracil-evoked colon cancer cell apoptosis: the roles of caspase-6 and p53. Cancer Biol Ther 7: 1305-1312.

475. Chan KM, Yu MC, Lee WC, Jan YY, Chen MF (2007). Adenosquamous/squamous cell carcinoma of the gallbladder. J Surg Oncol 95: 129-134.

476. Chan TL, Curtis LC, Leung SY, Farrington SM, Ho JW, Chan AS et al. (2001). Early-onset colorectal cancer with stable microsatellite DNA and near-diploid chromosomes. Oncogene 20: 4871-4876.

477. Chandrasekharappa SC, Guru SC, Manickam P, Olufemi SE, Collins FS, Emmert-Buck MR et al. (1997). Positional cloning of the gene for multiple endocrine neoplasia-type 1. Science 276: 404-407.

478. Chandrasoma P (2005). Controversies of the cardiac mucosa and Barrett's oesophagus. Histopathology 46: 361-373.

479. Chandrasoma PT, Der R, Ma Y, Dalton P, Taira M (2000). Histology of the gastroesophageal junction: an autopsy study. Am J Surg Pathol 24: 402-409.

480. Chandrasoma PT, Der R, Ma Y, Peters J, Demeester T (2003). Histologic classification of patients based on mapping biopsies of the gastroesophageal junction. Am J Surg Pathol 27: 929-936.

480A. Chang F, Deere H, Mahadeva U, George S (2008). Histopathologic examination and reporting of esophageal carcinomas following preoperative neoadjuvant therapy: practical guidelines and current issues. Am J Clin Pathol 129: 252-262.

481. Chang GJ, Gonzalez RJ, Skibber JM, Eng C, Das P, Rodriguez-Bigas MA (2009). A twenty-year experience with adenocarcinoma of the anal canal. Dis Colon Rectum 52: 1375-1380.

482. Chang HJ, Jee CD, Kim WH (2002). Mutation and altered expression of beta-catenin during gallbladder carcinogenesis. Am J Surg Pathol 26: 758-766.

483. Chang HJ, Jin SY, Park C, Park YN, Jang JJ, Park CK et al. (2006). Mesenchymal hamartomas of the liver: comparison of clinicopathologic features between cystic and solid forms. J Korean Med Sci 21: 63-68.

484. Chang MH, Chen CJ, Lai MS, Hsu HM, Wu TC, Kong MS et al. (1997). Universal hepatitis B vaccination in Taiwan and the incidence of hepatocellular carcinoma in children. Taiwan Childhood Hepatoma Study Group. N Engl J Med 336: 1855-1859.

485. Chanvitan A, Nekarda H, Casson AG (1995). Prognostic value of DNA index, S-phase fraction and p53 protein accumulation after surgical resection of esophageal squamous-cell carcinomas in Thailand. Int J Cancer 63: 381-386.

486. Chapman CJ, Dunn-Walters DK, Stevenson FK, Hussell T, Isaacson PG, Spencer J (1996). Sequence analysis of immunoglobulin variable region genes that encode autoantibodies expressed by lymphomas of mucosa associated lymphoid tissue. Clin Mol Pathol 49: M29-M32.

487. Chapman PD, Church W, Burn J, Gunn A (1989). Congenital hypertrophy of retinal pigment epithelium: a sign of familial adenomatous polyposis. BMJ 298: 353-354.

488. Chapman RW (1999). Risk factors for biliary tract carcinogenesis. Ann Oncol 10 Suppl 4: 308-311.

489. Charames GS, Ramyar L, Mitri A, Berk T, Cheng H, Jung J et al. (2008). A large novel deletion in the *APC* promoter region causes gene silencing and leads to classical familial adenomatous polyposis in a Manitoba Mennonite kindred. Hum Genet 124: 535-541.

490. Chari ST, Leibson CL, Rabe KG, Ransom J, de Andrade M, Petersen GM (2005). Probability of pancreatic cancer following diabetes: a population-based study. Gastroenterology 129: 504-511.

491. Chari ST, Takahashi N, Levy MJ, Smyrk TC, Clain JE, Pearson RK et al. (2009). A diagnostic strategy to distinguish autoimmune pancreatitis from pancreatic cancer. Clin Gastroenterol Hepatol 7: 1097-1103.

492. Chari ST, Yadav D, Smyrk TC, Dimagno EP, Miller LJ, Raimondo M et al. (2002). Study of recurrence after surgical resection of intraductal papillary mucinous neoplasm of the pancreas. Gastroenterology 123: 1500-1507.

493. Charlton A, Blair V, Shaw D, Parry S, Guilford P, Martin IG (2004). Hereditary diffuse gastric cancer: predominance of multiple foci of signet ring cell carcinoma in distal stomach and transitional zone. Gut 53: 814-820.

494. Chatelain D, de Lajarte-Thirouard AS, Tiret E, Flejou JF (2002). Adenocarcinoma of the upper esophagus arising in heterotopic gastric mucosa: common pathogenesis with Barrett's adenocarcinoma? Virchows Arch 441: 406-411.

495. Chatelain D, Hammel P, O'Toole D, Terris B, Vilgrain V, Palazzo L et al. (2002). Macrocystic form of serous pancreatic cystadenoma. Am J Gastroenterol 97: 2566-2571.

496. Chatelain D, Paye F, Mourra N, Scoazec JY, Baudrimont M, Parc R et al. (2002). Unilocular acinar cell cystadenoma of the pancreas an unusual acinar cell tumor. Am J Clin Pathol 118: 211-214.

497. Chatila R, Fiedler PN, Vender RJ (1996). Primary lymphoma of the gallbladder; case report and review of the literature. Am J Gastroenterol 91: 2242-2244.

498. Chaturvedi AK, Madeleine MM, Biggar RJ, Engels EA (2009). Risk of human papillomavirus-associated cancers among persons with AIDS. J Natl Cancer Inst 101: 1120-1130.

499. Chaudhary HB, Bhanot P, Logrono R (2005). Phenotypic diversity of intrahepatic and extrahepatic cholangiocarcinoma on aspiration cytology and core needle biopsy: case series and review of the literature. Cancer 105: 220-228.

499A. Cheadle JP, Sampson JR (2003). Exposing the MYtH about base excision repair and human inherited disease. Hum Mol Genet 12: R159-R165

500. Chejfec G, Gould VE (1977). Malignant gastric neuroendogrinomas. Ultrastructural and biochemical characterization of their secretory activity. Hum Pathol 8: 433-440.

501. Chen C, Cook LS, Li XY, Hallagan S, Madeleine MM, Daling JR et al. (1999). CYP2D6 genotype and the incidence of anal and vulvar cancer. Cancer Epidemiol Biomarkers Prev 8: 317-321.

502. Chen C, Madeleine MM, Lubinski C, Weiss NS, Tickman EW, Daling JR (1996). Glutathione S-transferase M1 genotypes and the risk of anal cancer: a population-based case-control study. Cancer Epidemiol Biomarkers Prev 5: 985-991.

503. Chen J, Baithun SI (1985). Morphological study of 391 cases of exocrine pancreatic tumours with special reference to the classification of exocrine pancreatic carcinoma. J Pathol 146: 17-29.

504. Chen J, Baithun SI, Pollock DJ, Berry CL (1988). Argyrophilic and hormone immunoreactive cells in normal and hyperplastic pancreatic ducts and exocrine pancreatic carcinoma. Virchows Arch A Pathol Anat Histopathol 413: 399-405.

505. Chen J, Cheong JH, Yun MJ, Kim J, Lim JS, Hyung WJ et al. (2005). Improvement in preoperative staging of gastric adenocarcinoma with positron emission tomography. Cancer 103: 2383-2390.

506. Chen LT, Lin JT, Tai JJ, Chen GH, Yeh HZ, Yang SS et al. (2005). Long-term results of anti-*Helicobacter pylori* therapy in early-stage gastric high-grade transformed MALT lymphoma. J Natl Cancer Inst 97: 1345-1353.

507. Chen MF, Jan YY, Hwang TL, Jeng LB, Yeh TS (2000). Impact of concomitant hepatolithiasis on patients with peripheral cholangiocarcinoma. Dig Dis Sci 45: 312-316.

508. Chen MF, Jan YY, Jeng LB, Hwang TL, Wang CS, Chen SC et al. (1999). Intrahepatic cholangiocarcinoma in Taiwan. J Hepatobiliary Pancreat Surg 6: 136-141.

509. Chen S, Wang W, Lee S, Nafa K, Lee J, Romans K et al. (2006). Prediction of germline mutations and cancer risk in the Lynch syndrome. JAMA 296: 1479-1487.

510. Chen TC, Nakanuma Y, Zen Y, Chen MF, Jan YY, Yeh TS et al. (2001). Intraductal papillary neoplasia of the liver associated with hepatolithiasis. Hepatology 34: 651-658.

511. Chen TC, Ng KF, Kuo T (2001). Intrahepatic cholangiocarcinoma with lymphoepithelioma-like component. Mod Pathol 14: 527-532.

512. Chen YW, Hu XT, Liang AC, Au WY, So CC, Wong ML et al. (2006). High BCL6 expression predicts better prognosis, independent of BCL6 translocation status, translocation partner, or BCL6-deregulating mutations, in gastric lymphoma. Blood 108: 2373-2383.

513. Chen YW, Yen SH, Chen SY, Huang PI, Shiau CY, Liu YM et al. (2007). Anus-preservation treatment for anal cancer: retrospective analysis at a single institution. J Surg Oncol 96: 374-380.

514. Chen ZM, Ritter JH, Wang HL (2005). Differential expression of alpha-methylacyl coenzyme A racemase in adenocarcinomas of the small and large intestines. Am J Surg Pathol 29: 890-896.

515. Chen ZM, Scudiere JR, Abraham SC, Montgomery E (2009). Pyloric gland adenoma: an entity distinct from gastric foveolar type adenoma. Am J Surg Pathol 33: 186-193.

516. Chen ZM, Wang HL (2004). Alteration of cytokeratin 7 and cytokeratin 20 expression profile is uniquely associated with tumorigenesis of primary adenocarcinoma of the small intestine. Am J Surg Pathol 28: 1352-1359.

517. Cheng JQ, Ruggeri B, Klein WM, Sonoda G, Altomare DA, Watson DK et al. (1996). Amplification of AKT2 in human pancreatic cells and inhibition of AKT2 expression and tumorigenicity by antisense RNA. Proc Natl Acad Sci U S A 93: 3636-3641.

518. Cheng Y, Zhang J, Li Y, Wang Y, Gong J (2007). Proteome analysis of human gastric cardia adenocarcinoma by laser capture microdissection. BMC Cancer 7: 191-

519. Chetritt J, Sagan C, Heymann MF, Le Bodic MF (1996). [Immunohistochemical study of 17 cases of rectal neuroendocrine tumors]. Ann Pathol 16: 98-103.

520. Chetty R, Bhathal PS, Slavin JL (1993). Prolapse-induced inflammatory polyps of the colorectum and anal transitional zone. Histopathology 23: 63-67.

521. Chetty R, Clark SP, Pitson GA (1993). Primary small cell carcinoma of the pancreas. Pathology 25: 240-242.

522. Chetty R, Serra S (2009). Intraductal tubular adenoma (pyloric gland-type) of the pancreas: a reappraisal and possible relationship with gastric-type intraductal papillary mucinous neoplasm. Histopathology 55: 270-276.

523. Cheuk W, Chan JK (2001). Thyroid transcription factor-1 is of limited value in practical distinction between pulmonary and extrapulmonary small cell carcinomas. Am J Surg Pathol 25: 545-546.

524. Cheuk W, Chan JK, Shek TW, Chang JH, Tsou MH, Yuen NW et al. (2001). Inflammatory pseudotumor-like follicular dendritic cell tumor: a distinctive low-grade malignant intra-abdominal neoplasm with consistent Epstein-Barr virus association. Am J Surg Pathol 25: 721-731.

525. Chiaravalli AM, Klersy C, Tava F, Manca R, Fiocca R, Capella C et al. (2009). Lower- and higher-grade subtypes of diffuse gastric cancer. Hum Pathol 40: 1591-1599.

526. Chijiiwa K, Ohtani K, Noshiro H, Yamasaki T, Shimizu S, Yamaguchi K et al. (2002). Cholangiocellular carcinoma depending on the kind of intrahepatic calculi in patients with hepatolithiasis. Hepatogastroenterology 49: 96-99.

527. Chino O, Kijima H, Shimada H, Mizutani K, Nishi T, Tanaka H et al. (2001). Esophageal squamous cell carcinoma with lymphoid stroma: report of 3 cases with immunohistochemical analyses. Gastrointest Endosc 54: 513-517.

528. Chirieac LR, Shen L, Catalano PJ, Issa JP, Hamilton SR (2005). Phenotype of microsatellite-stable colorectal carcinomas with CpG island methylation. Am J Surg Pathol 29: 429-436.

528A. Chirieac LR, Swisher SG, Ajani JA, Komaki RR, Correa AM, Morris JS, Roth JA, Rashid A, Hamilton SR, Wu TT (2005). Posttherapy pathologic stage predicts survival in

patients with esophageal carcinoma receiving preoperative chemoradiation. Cancer 103: 1347-1355.
529. Chittal SM, Ra PM (1989). Carcinoid of the cystic duct. Histopathology 15: 643-646.
530. Chiu BC, Weisenburger DD (2003). An update of the epidemiology of non-Hodgkin's lymphoma. Clin Lymphoma 4: 161-168.
531. Cho NL, Redston M, Zauber AG, Carothers AM, Hornick J, Wilton A et al. (2008). Aberrant crypt foci in the adenoma prevention with celecoxib trial. Cancer Prev Res 1: 21-31.
532. Choi BI, Han JK, Hong ST, Lee KH (2004). Clonorchiasis and cholangiocarcinoma: etiologic relationship and imaging diagnosis. Clin Microbiol Rev 17: 540-552.
533. Choi BI, Kim KW, Han MC, Kim YI, Kim CW (1988). Solid and papillary epithelial neoplasms of the pancreas: CT findings. Radiology 166: 413-416.
534. Choi D, Lim JH, Lee KT, Lee JK, Choi SH, Heo JS et al. (2006). Cholangiocarcinoma and *Clonorchis sinensis* infection: a case-control study in Korea. J Hepatol 44: 1066-1073.
535. Choi DW, Oh SN, Baek SJ, Ahn SH, Chang YJ, Jeong WS et al. (2002). Endoscopically observed lower esophageal capillary patterns. Korean J Intern Med 17: 245-248.
536. Choi SW, Choi JR, Chung YJ, Kim KM, Rhyu MG (2000). Prognostic implications of microsatellite genotypes in gastric carcinoma. Int J Cancer 89: 378-383.
537. Chong FK, Graham JH, Madoff IM (1979). Mucin-producing carcinoid ("composite tumor") of upper third of esophagus: a variant of carcinoid tumor. Cancer 44: 1853-1859.
538. Chong JM, Fukayama M, Shiozawa Y, Hayashi Y, Funata N, Takizawa T et al. (1996). Fibrillary inclusions in neoplastic and fetal acinar cells of the pancreas. Virchows Arch 428: 261-266.
539. Chong Y, Shin JJ, Cho MY, Cui Y, Kim HY, Park KH (2008). Synchronous primary gastric mantle cell lymphoma and early gastric carcinoma: a case report. Pathol Res Pract 204: 407-411.
540. Chott A, Haedicke W, Mosberger I, Fodinger M, Winkler K, Mannhalter C et al. (1998). Most CD56+ intestinal lymphomas are CD8+CD5-T-cell lymphomas of monomorphic small to medium size histology. Am J Pathol 153: 1483-1490.
541. Chott A, Klöppel G, Buxbaum P, Heitz PU (1987). Neuron specific enolase demonstration in the diagnosis of a solid-cystic (papillary cystic) tumour of the pancreas. Virchows Arch A Pathol Anat Histopathol 410: 397-402.
542. Chott A, Vesely M, Simonitsch I, Mosberger I, Hanak H (1999). Classification of intestinal T-cell neoplasms and their differential diagnosis. Am J Clin Pathol 111: S68-S74.
543. Chou P, Mangkornkanok M, Gonzalez-Crussi F (1990). Undifferentiated (embryonal) sarcoma of the liver: ultrastructure, immunohistochemistry, and DNA ploidy analysis of two cases. Pediatr Pathol 10: 549-562.
544. Chow E, Lipton L, Lynch E, D'Souza R, Aragona C, Hodgkin L et al. (2006). Hyperplastic polyposis syndrome: phenotypic presentations and the role of MBD4 and MYH. Gastroenterology 131: 30-39.
545. Chow JS, Chen CC, Ahsan H, Neugut AI (1996). A population-based study of the incidence of malignant small bowel tumours: SEER, 1973-1990. Int J Epidemiol 25: 722-728.
546. Chow WH, Blot WJ, Vaughan TL, Risch HA, Gammon MD, Stanford JL et al. (1998). Body mass index and risk of adenocarcinomas of the esophagus and gastric cardia. J Natl Cancer Inst 90: 150-155.
547. Chow WH, Finkle WD, McLaughlin JK, Frankl H, Ziel HK, Fraumeni JF, Jr. (1995). The relation of gastroesophageal reflux disease and its treatment to adenocarcinomas of the esophagus and gastric cardia. JAMA 274: 474-477.
548. Christison-Lagay ER, Burrows PE, Alomari A, Dubois J, Kozakewich HP, Lane TS et al. (2007). Hepatic hemangiomas: subtype classification and development of a clinical practice algorithm and registry. J Pediatr Surg 42: 62-67.
549. Christodoulopoulos JB, Klotz AP (1961). Carcinoid syndrome with primary carcinoid tumor of the stomach. Gastroenterology 40: 429-440.
550. Christopoulos C, Balatsos V, Rotas E, Karoumpalis I, Papavasileiou D, Kontogeorgos G et al. (2009). The syndrome of gastric carcinoid and hyperparathyroidism: a family study and literature review. Eur J Endocrinol 160: 689-694.
551. Chu P, Wu E, Weiss LM (2000). Cytokeratin 7 and cytokeratin 20 expression in epithelial neoplasms: a survey of 435 cases. Mod Pathol 13: 962-972.
552. Chu PG, Ishizawa S, Wu E, Weiss LM (2002). Hepatocyte antigen as a marker of hepatocellular carcinoma: an immunohistochemical comparison to carcinoembryonic antigen, CD10, and alpha-fetoprotein. Am J Surg Pathol 26: 978-988.
553. Chu PG, Schwarz RE, Lau SK, Yen Y, Weiss LM (2005). Immunohistochemical staining in the diagnosis of pancreatobiliary and ampulla of Vater adenocarcinoma: application of CDX2, CK17, MUC1, and MUC2. Am J Surg Pathol 29: 359-367.
554. Chuah SK, Hu TH, Kuo CM, Chiu KW, Kuo CH, Wu KL et al. (2005). Upper gastrointestinal carcinoid tumors incidentally found by endoscopic examinations. World J Gastroenterol 11: 7028-7032.
555. Chuang SS, Chang ST, Chuang WY, Huang WT, Hsieh PP, Tsou MH et al. (2009). NK-cell lineage predicts poor survival in primary intestinal NK-cell and T-cell lymphomas. Am J Surg Pathol 33: 1230-1240.
556. Chuang SS, Liao YL, Liu H, Lin SH, Hsieh PP, Huang WT et al. (2008). The phenotype of intraepithelial lymphocytes in Taiwanese enteropathy-associated T-cell lymphoma is distinct from that of the West. Histopathology 53: 234-236.
557. Chuma M, Sakamoto M, Yamazaki K, Ohta T, Ohki M, Asaka M et al. (2003). Expression profiling in multistage hepatocarcinogenesis: identification of HSP70 as a molecular marker of early hepatocellular carcinoma. Hepatology 37: 198-207.
558. Chun YS, Lindor NM, Smyrk TC, Petersen BT, Burgart LJ, Guilford PJ et al. (2001). Germline E-cadherin gene mutations: is prophylactic total gastrectomy indicated? Cancer 92: 181-187.
559. Chung CH, Wilentz RE, Polak MM, Ramsoekh TB, Noorduyn LA, Gouma DJ et al. (1996). Clinical significance of *K-ras* oncogene activation in ampullary neoplasms. J Clin Pathol 49: 460-464.
560. Chung DC, Smith AP, Louis DN, Graeme-Cook F, Warshaw AL, Arnold A (1997). A novel pancreatic endocrine tumor suppressor gene locus on chromosome 3p with clinical prognostic implications. J Clin Invest 100: 404-410.
561. Chung JJ, Kim MJ, Kie JH, Kim KW (2005). Mucosa-associated lymphoid tissue lymphoma of the esophagus coexistent with bronchus-associated lymphoid tissue lymphoma of the lung. Yonsei Med J 46: 562-566.
562. Chung SM, Hruban RH, Iacobuzio-Donahue CA, Adsay NV, Zee SY, Klimstra DS (2005). Analysis of molecular alterations and differentiation pathways in intraductal oncocytic papillary neoplasm of the pancreas. Mod Pathol 18: 277A-288A.
563. Cicin I, Ozyilmaz F, Karagol H, Yalcin F, Uzunoglu S, Kaplan M (2009). Massive upper gastrointestinal bleeding from pure metastatic choriocarcinoma in patient with mixed germ cell tumor with subclinical intestinal metastasis. Urology 73: 443-447.
564. Cingolani N, Shaco-Levy R, Farruggio A, Klimstra DS, Rosai J (2000). Alpha-fetoprotein production by pancreatic tumors exhibiting acinar cell differentiation: study of five cases, one arising in a mediastinal teratoma. Hum Pathol 31: 938-944.
565. Clairotte A, Ringenbach F, Laithier V, Aubert D, Kantelip B (2006). [Malignant rhabdoid tumor of the liver with spontaneous rupture: a case report]. Ann Pathol 26: 122-125.
566. Clark S. (ed.) (2008). A Guide to Cancer Genetics In Clinical Practice. TFM Publishing Ltd: Shrewsbury.
567. Clark GW, Smyrk TC, Burdiles P, Hoeft SF, Peters JH, Kiyabu M et al. (1994). Is Barrett's metaplasia the source of adenocarcinomas of the cardia? Arch Surg 129: 609-614.
568. Clark MA, Hartley A, Geh JI (2004). Cancer of the anal canal. Lancet Oncol 5: 149-157.
569. Clark SK, Phillips RK (1996). Desmoids in familial adenomatous polyposis. Br J Surg 83: 1494-1504.
570. Clarke MR, Baker EE, Weyant RJ, Hill L, Carty SE (1997). Proliferative activity in pancreatic endocrine tumors: association with function, metastases, and survival. Endocr Pathol 8: 181-187.
571. Cleary SP, Cotterchio M, Jenkins MA, Kim H, Bristow R, Green R et al. (2009). Germline MutY human homologue mutations and colorectal cancer: a multisite case-control study. Gastroenterology 136: 1251-1260.
572. Coburn MC, Pricolo VE, DeLuca FG, Bland KI (1995). Malignant potential in intestinal juvenile polyposis syndromes. Ann Surg Oncol 2: 386-391.
573. Cochet B, Carrel J, Desbaillets L, Widgren S (1979). Peutz-Jeghers syndrome associated with gastrointestinal carcinoma. Report of two cases in a family. Gut 20: 169-175.
574. Coffin CM, Hornick JL, Fletcher CD (2007). Inflammatory myofibroblastic tumor: comparison of clinicopathologic, histologic, and immunohistochemical features including ALK expression in atypical and aggressive cases. Am J Surg Pathol 31: 509-520.
575. Coggi G, Bosari S, Roncalli M, Graziani D, Bossi P, Viale G et al. (1997). p53 protein accumulation and *p53* gene mutation in esophageal carcinoma. A molecular and immunohistochemical study with clinicopathologic correlations. Cancer 79: 425-432.
576. Cohen JI, Kimura H, Nakamura S, Ko YH, Jaffe ES (2009). Epstein-Barr virus-associated lymphoproliferative disease in non-immunocompromised hosts: a status report and summary of an international meeting, 8-9 September 2008. Ann Oncol 20: 1472-1482.
577. Cohen PR, Kohn SR, Kurzrock R (1991). Association of sebaceous gland tumors and internal malignancy: the Muir-Torre syndrome. Am J Med 90: 606-613.
578. Colarian J, Pietruk T, LaFave L, Calzada R (1990). Adenocarcinoma of the ampulla of vater associated with neurofibromatosis. J Clin Gastroenterol 12: 118-119.
579. Cole BF, Baron JA, Sandler RS, Haile RW, Ahnen DJ, Bresalier RS et al. (2007). Folic acid for the prevention of colorectal adenomas: a randomized clinical trial. JAMA 297: 2351-2359.
580. Colebatch A, Hitchins M, Williams R, Meagher A, Hawkins NJ, Ward RL (2006). The role of MYH and microsatellite instability in the development of sporadic colorectal cancer. Br J Cancer 95: 1239-1243.
581. Collins BT, Cramer HM (1996). Fine-needle aspiration cytology of islet cell tumors. Diagn Cytopathol 15: 37-45.
582. Colliver DW, Crawford NP, Eichenberger MR, Zacharius W, Petras RE, Stromberg AJ et al. (2006). Molecular profiling of ulcerative colitis-associated neoplastic progression. Exp Mol Pathol 80: 1-10.
583. Colombo P, Arizzi C, Roncalli M (2004). Acinar cell cystadenocarcinoma of the pancreas: report of rare case and review of the literature. Hum Pathol 35: 1568-1571.
584. Colonna J, Plaza JA, Frankel WL, Yearsley M, Bloomston M, Marsh WL (2008). Serous cystadenoma of the pancreas: clinical and pathological features in 33 patients. Pancreatology 8: 135-141.
584A. Colvin M, Delis A, Bracamonte E, Villar H, Leon LR Jr (2009). Infiltrating adenocarcinoma arising in a villous adenoma of the anal canal. World J Gastroenterol 15: 3560-3564.
585. Compagno J, Oertel JE (1978). Microcystic adenomas of the pancreas (glycogen-rich cystadenomas): a clinicopathologic study of 34 cases. Am J Clin Pathol 69: 289-298.
586. Comper F, Antonello D, Beghelli S, Gobbo S, Montagna L, Pederzoli P et al. (2009). Expression pattern of claudins 5 and 7 distinguishes solid-pseudopapillary from pancreatoblastoma, acinar cell and endocrine tumors of the pancreas. Am J Surg Pathol 33: 768-774.
587. Conias S, Strutton G, Stephenson G (1998). Adult cutaneous Langerhans cell histiocytosis. Australas J Dermatol 39: 106-108.
588. Conley CR, Scheithauer BW, van Heerden JA, Weiland LH (1987). Diffuse intraductal papillary adenocarcinoma of the pancreas. Ann Surg 205: 246-249.
589. Conlon KC, Klimstra DS, Brennan MF (1996). Long-term survival after curative resection for pancreatic ductal adenocarcinoma. Clinicopathologic analysis of 5-year survivors. Ann Surg 223: 273-279.
590. Connolly MM, Dawson PJ, Michelassi F, Moossa AR, Lowenstein F (1987). Survival in 1001 patients with carcinoma of the pancreas. Ann Surg 206: 366-373.
591. Conran RM, Hitchcock CL, Waclawiw MA, Stocker JT, Ishak KG (1992). Hepatoblastoma: the prognostic significance of histologic type. Pediatr Pathol 12: 167-183.
592. Cook MB, Dawsey SM, Freedman ND, Inskip PD, Wichner SM, Quraishi SM et al. (2009). Sex disparities in cancer incidence by period and age. Cancer Epidemiol Biomarkers Prev 18: 1174-1182.
593. Cooke CB, Krenacs L, Stetler-Stevenson M, Greiner TC, Raffeld M, Kingma DW et al. (1996). Hepatosplenic T-cell lymphoma: a distinct clinicopathologic entity of cytotoxic gamma delta T-cell origin. Blood 88: 4265-4274.
594. Cooney BS, Levine MS, Schnall MD (1995). Metastatic thyroid carcinoma presenting as an expansile intraluminal esophageal mass. Abdom Imaging 20: 20-22.
595. Cooper WN, Luharia A, Evans GA, Raza H, Haire AC, Grundy R et al. (2005). Molecular subtypes and phenotypic expression of Beckwith-Wiedemann syndrome. Eur J Hum Genet 13: 1025-1032.
596. Coppens E, El Nakadi I, Nagy N, Zalcman M (2003). Primary Hodgkin's lymphoma of the esophagus. AJR Am J Roentgenol 180: 1335-1337.
597. Corless CL, Fletcher JA, Heinrich MC (2004). Biology of gastrointestinal stromal tumors. J Clin Oncol 22: 3813-3825.
598. Cormier RT, Hong KH, Halberg RB, Hawkins TL, Richardson P, Mulherkar R et al. (1997). Secretory phospholipase Pla2g2a confers resistance to intestinal tumorigenesis. Nat Genet 17: 88-91.
599. Cornes JS (1961). Multiple lymphoma-

tous polyposis of the gastrointestinal tract. Cancer 14: 249-257.
600. Cornette J, Festen S, van den Hoonaard TL, Steegers EA (2009). Mesenchymal hamartoma of the liver: a benign tumor with deceptive prognosis in the perinatal period. Case report and review of the literature. Fetal Diagn Ther 25: 196-202.
601. Correa P (1988). A human model of gastric carcinogenesis. Cancer Res 48: 3554-3560.
602. Correa P (1992). Human gastric carcinogenesis: a multistep and multifactorial process—First American Cancer Society Award Lecture on Cancer Epidemiology and Prevention. Cancer Res 52: 6735-6740.
603. Correa P, Houghton J (2007). Carcinogenesis of *Helicobacter pylori*. Gastroenterology 133: 659-672.
604. Correa P, Miller MJ (1998). Carcinogenesis, apoptosis and cell proliferation. Br Med Bull 54: 151-162.
605. Corrin B, Gilby ED, Jones NF, Patrick J (1973). Oat cell carcinoma of the pancreas with ectopic ACTH secretion. Cancer 31: 1523-1527.
606. Cortina R, McCormick J, Kolm P, Perry RR (1995). Management and prognosis of adenocarcinoma of the appendix. Dis Colon Rectum 38: 848-852.
607. Costa MJ (1994). Pseudomyxoma peritonei. Histologic predictors of patient survival. Arch Pathol Lab Med 118: 1215-1219.
608. Costi R, Caruana P, Sarli L, Violi V, Roncoroni L, Bordi C (2001). Ampullary adenocarcinoma in neurofibromatosis type 1. Case report and literature review. Mod Pathol 14: 1169-1174.
609. Couch FJ, Johnson MR, Rabe K, Boardman L, McWilliams R, de Andrade M et al. (2005). Germ line Fanconi anemia complementation group C mutations and pancreatic cancer. Cancer Res 65: 383-386.
610. Cox CL, Butts DR, Roberts MP, Wessels RA, Bailey HR (1997). Development of invasive adenocarcinoma in a long-standing Kock continent ileostomy: report of a case. Dis Colon Rectum 40: 500-503.
611. Cox KL, Frates RC, Jr., Wong A, Gandhi G (1980). Hereditary generalized juvenile polyposis associated with pulmonary arteriovenous malformation. Gastroenterology 78: 1566-1570.
612. Craanen ME, Blok P, Dekker W, Ferwerda J, Tytgat GN (1992). Subtypes of intestinal metaplasia and *Helicobacter pylori*. Gut 33: 597-600.
613. Crafa P, Milione M, Azzoni C, Pilato FP, Pizzi S, Bordi C (2003). Pleomorph poorly differentiated endocrine carcinoma of the rectum. Virchows Arch 442: 605-610.
614. Craig JR, Peters RL, and Edmondson HA (eds) (1989). Tumours of the Liver and Intrahepatic Bile Ducts. Armed Forces Institute of Pathology: Washington, DC.
615. Crane SJ, Richard LG, III, Romero Y, Zinsmeister AR, Talley NJ (2008). Adenocarcinoma of the esophagogastric junction may arise from short-segment Barrett's esophagus. Am J Gastroenterol 103: 493-494.
616. Crespi M, Munoz N, Grassi A, Qiong S, Jing WK, Jien LJ (1984). Precursor lesions of oesophageal cancer in a low-risk population in China: comparison with high-risk populations. Int J Cancer 34: 599-602.
617. Crippa S, Angelini C, Mussi C, Bonardi C, Romano F, Sartori P et al. (2006). Surgical treatment of metastatic tumors to the pancreas: a single center experience and review of the literature. World J Surg 30: 1536-1542.
618. Crippa S, Salvia R, Warshaw AL, Dominguez I, Bassi C, Falconi M et al. (2008). Mucinous cystic neoplasm of the pancreas is not an aggressive entity: lessons from 163 resected patients. Ann Surg 247: 571-579.
619. Crist WM, Anderson JR, Meza JL, Fryer C, Raney RB, Ruymann FB et al. (2001). Intergroup rhabdomyosarcoma study-IV: results for patients with nonmetastatic disease. J Clin Oncol 19: 3091-3102.
620. Crocetti E, Paci E (2003). Malignant carcinoids in the USA, SEER 1992-1999. An epidemiological study with 6830 cases. Eur J Cancer Prev 12: 191-194.
621. Croitoru ME, Cleary SP, Di NN, Manno M, Selander T, Aronson M et al. (2004). Association between biallelic and monoallelic germline *MYH* gene mutations and colorectal cancer risk. J Natl Cancer Inst 96: 1631-1634.
622. Cromwell DM, Moore RD, Brensinger JD, Petersen GM, Bass EB, Giardiello FM (1998). Cost analysis of alternative approaches to colorectal screening in familial adenomatous polyposis. Gastroenterology 114: 893-901.
623. Crook T, Wrede D, Tidy J, Scholefield J, Crawford L, Vousden KH (1991). Status of *c-myc, p53* and retinoblastoma genes in human papillomavirus positive and negative squamous cell carcinomas of the anus. Oncogene 6: 1251-1257.
624. Crook T, Wrede D, Tidy JA, Mason WP, Evans DJ, Vousden KH (1992). Clonal p53 mutation in primary cervical cancer: association with human-papillomavirus-negative tumours. Lancet 339: 1070-1073.
625. Crowe DR, Eloubeidi MA, Chhieng DC, Jhala NC, Jhala D, Eltoum IA (2006). Fine-needle aspiration biopsy of hepatic lesions: computerized tomographic-guided versus endoscopic ultrasound-guided FNA. Cancer 108: 180-185.
626. Crump M, Gospodarowicz M, Shepherd FA (1999). Lymphoma of the gastrointestinal tract. Semin Oncol 26: 324-337.
627. Cubilla AL, Fitzgerald PJ (1976). Morphological lesions associated with human primary invasive nonendocrine pancreas cancer. Cancer Res 36: 2690-2698.
628. Cubilla AL, Fitzgerald PJ (eds) (1984). Tumours of the Exocrine Pancreas. Armed Forces Institute of Pathology: Washington, DC.
629. Cui R, Kamatani Y, Takahashi A, Usami M, Hosono N, Kawaguchi T et al. (2009). Functional variants in ADH1B and ALDH2 coupled with alcohol and smoking synergistically enhance esophageal cancer risk. Gastroenterology 137: 1768-1775.
630. Cuilliere P, Lazure T, Bui M, Fabre M, Buffet C, Gayral F et al. (2002). Solid adenoma with exclusive hepatocellular differentiation: a new variant among pancreatic benign neoplasms? Virchows Arch 441: 519-522.
630A. Cunningham D, Allum WH, Stenning SP, Thompson SP, van de Velde CJ, Nicolson M, Scarffe JH, Lofts FJ, Falk SJ, Iveson TJ, Smith DB, Langley RE, Verma M, Weeden S, Chua YJ (2006). Perioperative chemotherapy versus surgery alone for resectable gastroesophageal cancer. NEJM 355: 11-20
631. Cunningham SC, Alexander HR (2007). Porcelain gallbladder and cancer: ethnicity explains a discrepant literature? Am J Med 120: e17-e18.
632. Cunningham SC, Kamangar F, Kim MP, Hammoud S, Haque R, Maitra A et al. (2005). Survival after gastric adenocarcinoma resection: eighteen-year experience at a single institution. J Gastrointest Surg 9: 718-725.
633. Cupisti K, Hoppner W, Dotzenrath C, Simon D, Berndt I, Roher HD et al. (2000). Lack of *MEN1* gene mutations in 27 sporadic insulinomas. Eur J Clin Invest 30: 325-329.
634. Curado MP, Edwards B, Shin HR, Storm H, Ferlay J, Heanue M et al. (eds) (2007). Cancer Incidence in Five Continents. IARC: Lyon, France.
635. Curia MC, Zuckermann M, De LL, Catalano T, Lattanzio R, Aceto G et al. (2008). Sporadic childhood hepatoblastomas show activation of beta-catenin, mismatch repair defects and p53 mutations. Mod Pathol 21: 7-14.
636. Curvers WL, Kiesslich R, Bergman JJ (2008). Novel imaging modalities in the detection of oesophageal neoplasia. Best Pract Res Clin Gastroenterol 22: 687-720.
637. Czene K, Lichtenstein P, Hemminki K (2002). Environmental and heritable causes of cancer among 9.6 million individuals in the Swedish Family-Cancer Database. Int J Cancer 99: 260-266.
638. D'Adda T, Annibale B, Delle FG, Bordi C (1996). Oxyntic endocrine cells of hypergastrinaemic patients. Differential response to antrectomy or octreotide. Gut 38: 668-674.
639. D'Adda T, Candidus S, Denk H, Bordi C, Hofler H (1999). Gastric neuroendocrine neoplasms: tumour clonality and malignancy-associated large X-chromosomal deletions. J Pathol 189: 394-401.
640. D'Adda T, Keller G, Bordi C, Hofler H (1999). Loss of heterozygosity in 11q13-14 regions in gastric neuroendocrine tumors not associated with multiple endocrine neoplasia type 1 syndrome. Lab Invest 79: 671-677.
641. D'Adda T, Pizzi S, Azzoni C, Bottarelli L, Crafa P, Pasquali C et al. (2002). Different patterns of 11q allelic losses in digestive endocrine tumors. Hum Pathol 33: 322-329.
642. D'Elios MM, Appelmelk BJ, Amedei A, Bergman MP, Del Prete G (2004). Gastric autoimmunity: the role of *Helicobacter pylori* and molecular mimicry. Trends Mol Med 10: 316-323.
643. Dahia PL, Aguiar RC, Alberta J, Kum JB, Caron S, Sill H et al. (1999). PTEN is inversely correlated with the cell survival factor Akt/PKB and is inactivated via multiple mechanismsin haematological malignancies. Hum Mol Genet 8: 185-193.
644. Daigo Y, Nakamura Y (2008). From cancer genomics to thoracic oncology: discovery of new biomarkers and therapeutic targets for lung and esophageal carcinoma. Gen Thorac Cardiovasc Surg 56: 43-53.
645. Daigo Y, Nishiwaki T, Kawasoe T, Tamari M, Tsuchiya E, Nakamura Y (1999). Molecular cloning of a candidate tumor suppressor gene, DLC1, from chromosome 3p21.3. Cancer Res 59: 1966-1972.
646. Daimaru Y, Kido H, Hashimoto H, Enjoji M (1988). Benign schwannoma of the gastrointestinal tract: a clinicopathologic and immunohistochemical study. Hum Pathol 19: 257-264.
647. Dalerba P, Dylla SJ, Park IK, Liu R, Wang X, Cho RW et al. (2007). Phenotypic characterization of human colorectal cancer stem cells. Proc Natl Acad Sci U S A 104: 10158-10163.
648. Daley D, Lewis S, Platzer P, MacMillen M, Willis J, Elston RC et al. (2008). Identification of susceptibility genes for cancer in a genomewide scan: results from the colon neoplasia sibling study. Am J Hum Genet 82: 723-736.
649. Daling JR, Madeleine MM, Johnson LG, Schwartz SM, Shera KA, Wurscher MA et al. (2004). Human papillomavirus, smoking, and sexual practices in the etiology of anal cancer. Cancer 101: 270-280.
650. Daling JR, Weiss NS, Hislop TG, Maden C, Coates RJ, Sherman KJ et al. (1987). Sexual practices, sexually transmitted diseases, and the incidence of anal cancer. N Engl J Med 317: 973-977.
651. Dalle I, Sciot R, De Vos R, Aerts R, van Damme B, Desmet V et al. (2000). Malignant angiomyolipoma of the liver: a hitherto unreported variant. Histopathology 36: 443-450.
652. Dammacco F, Gatti P, Sansonno D (1998). Hepatitis C virus infection, mixed cryoglobulinemia, and non-Hodgkin's lymphoma: an emerging picture. Leuk Lymphoma 31: 463-476.
653. Darmstadt GL (1996). Perianal lymphangioma circumscriptum mistaken for genital warts. Pediatrics 98: 461-463.
654. Das A, Neugut AI, Cooper GS, Chak A (2004). Association of ampullary and colorectal malignancies. Cancer 100: 524-530.
655. Datz C, Graziadei IW, Dietze O, Jaschke W, Konigsrainer A, Sandhofer F et al. (2001). Massive progression of diffuse hepatic lymphangiomatosis after liver resection and rapid deterioration after liver transplantation. Am J Gastroenterol 96: 1278-1281.
656. Daum S, Cellier C, Mulder CJ (2005). Refractory coeliac disease. Best Pract Res Clin Gastroenterol 19: 413-424.
657. Daum S, Ipczynski R, Schumann M, Wahnschaffe U, Zeitz M, Ullrich R (2009). High rates of complications and substantial mortality in both types of refractory sprue. Eur J Gastroenterol Hepatol 21: 66-70.
658. DAVIS GH, ZOLLINGER RW (1960). Metastatic melanoma of the stomach. Am J Surg 99: 94-96.
659. Davis GL, Kissane JM, Ishak KG (1969). Embryonal rhabdomyosarcoma (sarcoma botryoides) of the biliary tree. Report of five cases and a review of the literature. Cancer 24: 333-342.
660. Davis RI, Sloan JM, Hood JM, Maxwell P (1988). Carcinoma of the extrahepatic biliary tract: a clinicopathological and immunohistochemical study. Histopathology 12: 623-631.
661. Dawsey SM, Lewin KJ, Wang GQ, Liu FS, Nieberg RK, Yu Y et al. (1994). Squamous esophageal histology and subsequent risk of squamous cell carcinoma of the esophagus. A prospective follow-up study from Linxian, China. Cancer 74: 1686-1692.
662. Dawson PM, Hershman MJ, Wood CB (1985). Metastatic carcinoma of the breast in the anal canal. Postgrad Med J 61: 1081-
663. Day DW, Jass JR, Price AB, Shepherd NA, Sloan JM, Talbot IC et al. (2003). Epithelial tumours of the small intestine. In: Morson & Dawson's Gastrointestinal Pathology. Morson & Dawson's Gastrointestinal Pathology. Blackwell Scientific Publications: Oxford, pp. 359-375.
664. Day DW, Jass JR, Price AB, Shepherd NA, Sloan JM, Talbot IC et al. (2003). Inflammatory disorders of the small intestine. In: Morson & Dawson's Gastrointestinal Pathology. Morson & Dawson's Gastrointestinal Pathology. Blackwell Scientific Publications: Oxford, pp. 288-323.
665. Day JD, Digiuseppe JA, Yeo C, Lai-Goldman M, Anderson SM, Goodman SN et al. (1996). Immunohistochemical evaluation of HER-2/neu expression in pancreatic adenocarcinoma and pancreatic intraepithelial neoplasms. Hum Pathol 27: 119-124.
666. Dayal Y, Tallberg KA, Nunnemacher G, DeLellis RA, Wolfe HJ (1986). Duodenal carcinoids in patients with and without neurofibromatosis. A comparative study. Am J Surg Pathol 10: 348-357.
667. de Chadarevian JP, Pawel BR, Faerber EN, Weintraub WH (1994). Undifferentiated (embryonal) sarcoma arising in conjunction with mesenchymal hamartoma of the liver. Mod Pathol 7: 490-493.
668. De Jong AE, Morreau H, Van Puijenbroek M, Eilers PH, Wijnen J, Nagengast FM et al. (2004). The role of mismatch repair gene defects in the development of adenomas in patients with HNPCC. Gastroenterology 126: 42-48.
669. De Jong AE, Van Puijenbroek M, Hendriks Y, Tops C, Wijnen J, Ausems MG et al. (2004). Microsatellite instability, immunohistochemistry, and additional PMS2 staining in suspected hereditary nonpolyposis colorectal cancer. Clin Cancer Res 10: 972-980.

670. de Jong MM, Nolte IM, te Meerman GJ, van der Graaf WT, De Vries EG, Sijmons RH et al. (2002). Low-penetrance genes and their involvement in colorectal cancer susceptibility. Cancer Epidemiol Biomarkers Prev 11: 1332-1352.
671. de Leng WW, Jansen M, Carvalho R, Polak M, Musler AR, Milne AN et al. (2007). Genetic defects underlying Peutz-Jeghers syndrome (PJS) and exclusion of the polarity-associated *MARK/Par1* gene family as potential PJS candidates. Clin Genet 72: 568-573.
672. de Leng WW, Jansen M, Keller JJ, de GM, Milne AN, Morsink FH et al. (2007). Peutz-Jeghers syndrome polyps are polyclonal with expanded progenitor cell compartment. Gut 56: 1475-1476.
673. de Miranda NF, Nielsen M, Pereira D, Van Puijenbroek M, Vasen HF, Hes FJ et al. (2009). MUTYH-associated polyposis carcinomas frequently lose HLA class I expression - a common event amongst DNA-repair-deficient colorectal cancers. J Pathol 219: 69-76.
674. De Palma GD, Masone S, Rega M, Simeoli I, Donisi M, Addeo P et al. (2006). Metastatic tumors to the stomach: clinical and endoscopic features. World J Gastroenterol 12: 7326-7328.
675. De Quay N, Cerottini JP, Albe X, Saraga E, Givel JC, Caplin S (1999). Prognosis in Duke's B colorectal carcinoma: the Jass classification revisited. Eur J Surg 165: 588-592.
676. De Simone P, Mainente P, Bedin N (2000). Gallbladder melanoma mimicking acute acalculous cholecystitis. Surg Endosc 14: 593-
677. De Vita S., Sacco C, Sansonno D, Gloghini A, Dammacco F, Crovatto M et al. (1997). Characterization of overt B-cell lymphomas in patients with hepatitis C virus infection. Blood 90: 776-782.
678. de vos tot Nederveen Cappel WH, Offerhaus GJ, Van Puijenbroek M, Caspers E, Gruis NA, De Snoo FA et al. (2003). Pancreatic carcinoma in carriers of a specific 19 base pair deletion of CDKN2A/p16 (p16-leiden). Clin Cancer Res 9: 3598-3605.
679. de Vries AC, Haringsma J, de Vries RA, ter Borg F, Nagtzaam NM, Steyerberg EW et al. (2009). The use of clinical, histologic, and serologic parameters to predict the intragastric extent of intestinal metaplasia: a recommendation for routine practice. Gastrointest Endosc 70: 18-25.
680. De IM, Brugieres L, Zimmermann A, Keeling J, Brock P, Maibach R et al. (2008). Hepatoblastoma with a low serum alpha-fetoprotein level at diagnosis: the SIOPEL group experience. Eur J Cancer 44: 545-550.
681. Deans GT, Spence RA (1995). Neoplastic lesions of the appendix. Br J Surg 82: 299-306.
682. Debas HT, Mulvihill SJ (1994). Neuroendocrine gut neoplasms. Important lessons from uncommon tumors. Arch Surg 129: 965-971.
683. Debelenko LV, Emmert-Buck MR, Zhuang Z, Epshteyn E, Moskaluk CA, Jensen RT et al. (1997). The multiple endocrine neoplasia type I gene locus is involved in the pathogenesis of type II gastric carcinoids. Gastroenterology 113: 773-781.
684. Debelenko LV, Zhuang Z, Emmert-Buck MR, Chandrasekharappa SC, Manickam P, Guru SC et al. (1997). Allelic deletions on chromosome 11q13 in multiple endocrine neoplasia type 1-associated and sporadic gastrinomas and pancreatic endocrine tumors. Cancer Res 57: 2238-2243.
685. Defrain C, Chang CY, Srikureja W, Nguyen PT, Gu M (2005). Cytologic features and diagnostic pitfalls of primary ampullary tumors by endoscopic ultrasound-guided fine-needle aspiration biopsy. Cancer 105: 289-297.
686. Dehner LP, Ewing SL, Sumner HW (1975). Infantile mesenchymal hamartoma of the liver. Histologic and ultrastructural observations. Arch Pathol 99: 379-382.
687. Dehner LP, Ishak KG (1971). Vascular tumors of the liver in infants and children. A study of 30 cases and review of the literature. Arch Pathol 92: 101-111.
688. Deinert K, Kiesslich R, Vieth M, Neurath MF, Neuhaus H (2007). In-vivo microvascular imaging of early squamous-cell cancer of the esophagus by confocal laser endomicroscopy. Endoscopy 39: 366-368.
689. Delcore R, Jr., Cheung LY, Friesen SR (1988). Outcome of lymph node involvement in patients with the Zollinger-Ellison syndrome. Ann Surg 208: 291-298.
690. Deleeuw RJ, Zettl A, Klinker E, Haralambieva E, Trottier M, Chari R et al. (2007). Whole-genome analysis and HLA genotyping of enteropathy-type T-cell lymphoma reveals 2 distinct lymphoma subtypes. Gastroenterology 132: 1902-1911.
691. DeLellis RA, Lloyd RV, Heitz PU, and Eng C (eds) (2004). WHO Classification of Tumours of Endocrine Organs. IARC: Lyon, France.
692. Delnatte C, Sanlaville D, Mougenot JF, Vermeesch JR, Houdayer C, Blois MC et al. (2006). Contiguous gene deletion within chromosome arm 10q is associated with juvenile polyposis of infancy, reflecting cooperation between the *BMPR1A* and *PTEN* tumor-suppressor genes. Am J Hum Genet 78: 1066-1074.
693. DeMaioribus CA, Lally KP, Sim K, Isaacs H, Mahour GH (1990). Mesenchymal hamartoma of the liver. A 35-year review. Arch Surg 125: 598-600.
694. Demetris AJ, Minervini M, Raikow RB, Lee RG (1997). Hepatic epithelioid hemangioendothelioma: biological questions based on pattern of recurrence in an allograft and tumor immunophenotype. Am J Surg Pathol 21: 263-270.
695. den Bakker MA, den Bakker AJ, Beenen R, Mulder AH, Eulderink F (1998). Subtotal liver calcification due to epithelioid hemangioendothelioma. Pathol Res Pract 194: 189-194.
696. Deng YF, Lin Q, Zhang SH, Ling YM, He JK, Chen XF (2008). Malignant angiomyolipoma in the liver: a case report with pathological and molecular analysis. Pathol Res Pract 204: 911-918.
697. Dent GA, Feldman JM (1984). Pseudocystic liver metastases in patients with carcinoid tumors: report of three cases. Am J Clin Pathol 82: 275-279.
698. Des GG, Schischmanoff O, Nicolas P, Perret GY, Morere JF, Uzzan B (2009). Does microsatellite instability predict the efficacy of adjuvant chemotherapy in colorectal cancer? A systematic review with meta-analysis. Eur J Cancer 45: 1890-1896.
699. Deschner EE, Lipkin M (1975). Proliferative patterns in colonic mucosa in familial polyposis. Cancer 35: 413-418.
700. Deshpande V, Mino-Kenudson M, Brugge WR, Pitman MB, Fernandez-del CC, Warshaw AL et al. (2005). Endoscopic ultrasound guided fine needle aspiration biopsy of autoimmune pancreatitis: diagnostic criteria and pitfalls. Am J Surg Pathol 29: 1464-1471.
701. Deshpande V, Muzikansky A, Fernandez del Castillo C (2003). Cytokeratin 19 is a powerful predictor of survival in pancreatic endocrine tumors. Mod Pathol 16: 272A-
702. Deshpande V, Sainani NI, Chung RT, Pratt DS, Mentha G, Rubbia-Brandt L et al. (2009). IgG4-associated cholangitis: a comparative histological and immunophenotypic study with primary sclerosing cholangitis on liver biopsy material. Mod Pathol 22: 1287-1295.
703. Detlefsen S, Mohr DA, Vyberg M, Klöppel G (2009). Diagnosis of autoimmune pancreatitis by core needle biopsy: application of six microscopic criteria. Virchows Arch 454: 531-539.
704. Detlefsen S, Sipos B, Feyerabend B, Klöppel G (2005). Pancreatic fibrosis associated with age and ductal papillary hyperplasia. Virchows Arch 447: 800-805.
705. Deugnier YM, Charalambous P, Le QD, Turlin B, Searle J, Brissot P et al. (1993). Preneoplastic significance of hepatic iron-free foci in genetic hemochromatosis: a study of 185 patients. Hepatology 18: 1363-1369.
706. Devaney K, Goodman ZD, Ishak KG (1994). Hepatobiliary cystadenoma and cystadenocarcinoma. A light microscopic and immunohistochemical study of 70 patients. Am J Surg Pathol 18: 1078-1091.
707. Devon KM, Brown CJ, Burnstein M, McLeod RS (2009). Cancer of the anus complicating perianal Crohn's disease. Dis Colon Rectum 52: 211-216.
708. Devor EJ, Buechley RW (1979). Gallbladder cancer in Hispanic New Mexicans II Familial occurrence in two northern New Mexico Kindreds. Can J Genet Cytol 1: 139-145.
709. DeWitt J, Jowell P, Leblanc J, McHenry L, McGreevy K, Cramer H et al. (2005). EUS-guided FNA of pancreatic metastases: a multicenter experience. Gastrointest Endosc 61: 689-696.
710. Deziel DJ, Saclarides TJ, Marshall JS, Yaremko LM (1991). Appendiceal Kaposi's sarcoma: a cause of right lower quadrant pain in the acquired immune deficiency syndrome. Am J Gastroenterol 86: 901-903.
711. Dhebri AR, Connor S, Campbell F, Ghaneh P, Sutton R, Neoptolemos JP (2004). Diagnosis, treatment and outcome of pancreatoblastoma. Pancreatology 4: 441-451.
712. Di Bisceglie AM (2009). Hepatitis B and hepatocellular carcinoma. Hepatology 49: S56-S60.
713. Di Cristofano A, Pesce B, Cordon-Cardo C, Pandolfi PP (1998). Pten is essential for embryonic development and tumour suppression. Nat Genet 19: 348-355.
714. Di Gregorio C, Frattini M, Maffei S, Ponti G, Losi L, Pedroni M et al. (2006). Immunohistochemical expression of MYH protein can be used to identify patients with MYH-associated polyposis. Gastroenterology 131: 439-444.
715. di Martino E, Hardie LJ, Wild CP, Gong YY, Olliver JR, Gough MD et al. (2007). The NAD(P)H:quinone oxidoreductase I C609T polymorphism modifies the risk of Barrett esophagus and esophageal adenocarcinoma. Genet Med 9: 341-347.
716. di Sant'Agnese PA (1991). Acinar cell carcinoma of the pancreas. Ultrastruct Pathol 15: 573-577.
717. Di Tommaso L, Destro A, Seok JY, Balladore E, Terracciano L, Sangiovanni A et al. (2009). The application of markers (HSP70 GPC3 and GS) in liver biopsies is useful for detection of hepatocellular carcinoma. J Hepatol 50: 746-754.
718. Di Tommaso L, Franchi G, Park YN, Fiamengo B, Destro A, Morenghi E et al. (2007). Diagnostic value of HSP70, glypican 3, and glutamine synthetase in hepatocellular nodules in cirrhosis. Hepatology 45: 725-734.
719. Dial PF, Braasch JW, Rossi RL, Lee AK, Jin GL (1985). Management of nonfunctioning islet cell tumors of the pancreas. Surg Clin North Am 65: 291-299.
720. Diamanti A, Colistro F, Calce A, Devito R, Ferretti F, Minozzi A et al. (2006). Clinical value of immunoglobulin A antitransglutaminase assay in the diagnosis of celiac disease. Pediatrics 118: e1696-e1700.
721. Diebold-Berger S, Vaiton JC, Pache JC, d'Amore ES (1995). Undifferentiated carcinoma of the gallbladder. Report of a case with immunohistochemical findings. Arch Pathol Lab Med 119: 279-282.
722. Dighe S, Swift I, Brown G (2008). CT staging of colon cancer. Clin Radiol 63: 1372-1379.
723. Ding SJ, Li Y, Tan YX, Jiang MR, Tian B, Liu YK et al. (2004). From proteomic analysis to clinical significance: overexpression of cytokeratin 19 correlates with hepatocellular carcinoma metastasis. Mol Cell Proteomics 3: 73-81.
724. Diosdado B, Buffart TE, Watkins R, Carvalho B, Ylstra B, Tijssen M et al. (2009). High resolution array comparative genomic hybridization in sporadic and coeliac disease-related small bowel adenocarcinomas. J Clin Oncol. 16:1391-1401.
725. DiSibio G, French SW (2008). Metastatic patterns of cancers: results from a large autopsy study. Arch Pathol Lab Med 132: 931-939.
726. Dixon MF, Genta RM, Yardley JH, Correa P (1996). Classification and grading of gastritis. The updated Sydney System. International Workshop on the Histopathology of Gastritis, Houston 1994. Am J Surg Pathol 20: 1161-1181.
727. Doglioni C, Wotherspoon AC, Moschini A, De BM, Isaacson PG (1992). High incidence of primary gastric lymphoma in northeastern Italy. Lancet 339: 834-835.
728. Doherty MA, McIntyre M, Arnott SJ (1984). Oat cell carcinoma of esophagus: a report of six British patients with a review of the literature. Int J Radiat Oncol Biol Phys 10: 147-152.
729. Doki Y, Shiozaki H, Tahara H, Kobayashi K, Miyata M, Oka H et al. (1993). Prognostic value of DNA ploidy in squamous cell carcinoma of esophagus. Analyzed with improved flow cytometric measurement. Cancer 72: 1813-1818.
730. Dokmak S, Paradis V, Vilgrain V, Sauvanet A, Farges O, Valla D et al. (2009). A single-center surgical experience of 122 patients with single and multiple hepatocellular adenomas. Gastroenterology 137: 1698-1705.
731. Dolcetti R, Viel A, Doglioni C, Russo A, Guidoboni M, Capozzi E et al. (1999). High prevalence of activated intraepithelial cytotoxic T lymphocytes and increased neoplastic cell apoptosis in colorectal carcinomas with microsatellite instability. Am J Pathol 154: 1805-1813.
732. Domingo E, Niessen RC, Oliveira C, Alhopuro P, Moutinho C, Espin E et al. (2005). BRAF-V600E is not involved in the colorectal tumorigenesis of HNPCC in patients with functional *MLH1* and *MSH2* genes. Oncogene 24: 3995-3998.
733. Domizio P, Owen RA, Shepherd NA, Talbot IC, Norton AJ (1993). Primary lymphoma of the small intestine. A clinicopathological study of 119 cases. Am J Surg Pathol 17: 429-442.
734. Domizio P, Talbot IC, Spigelman AD, Williams CB, Phillips RK (1990). Upper gastrointestinal pathology in familial adenomatous polyposis: results from a prospective study of 102 patients. J Clin Pathol 43: 738-743.
735. Donow C, Pipeleers-Marichal M, Schroder S, Stamm B, Heitz PU, Klöppel G (1991). Surgical pathology of gastrinoma. Site, size, multicentricity, association with multiple endocrine neoplasia type 1, and malignancy. Cancer 68: 1329-1334.
736. Dorer R, Odze RD (2006). AMACR immunostaining is useful in detecting dysplastic epithelium in Barrett's esophagus, ulcerative colitis, and Crohn's disease. Am J Surg Pathol 30: 871-877.
736A. Dorland (2007). Dorland's illustrated medical dictionary. 31st ed. Philadelphia, PA: WB Saunders.

737. dos Santos NR, Seruca R, Constancia M, Seixas M, Sobrinho-Simoes M (1996). Microsatellite instability at multiple loci in gastric carcinoma: clinicopathologic implications and prognosis. Gastroenterology 110: 38-44.
738. Dove-Edwin I, De Jong AE, Adams J, Mesher D, Lipton L, Sasieni P et al. (2006). Prospective results of surveillance colonoscopy in dominant familial colorectal cancer with and without Lynch syndrome. Gastroenterology 130: 1995-2000.
739. Dowen SE, Crnogorac-Jurcevic T, Gangeswaran R, Hansen M, Eloranta JJ, Bhakta V et al. (2005). Expression of S100P and its novel binding partner S100PBPR in early pancreatic cancer. Am J Pathol 166: 81-92.
740. Downs-Kelly E, Mendelin JE, Bennett AE, Castilla E, Henricks WH, Schoenfield L et al. (2008). Poor interobserver agreement in the distinction of high-grade dysplasia and adenocarcinoma in pretreatment Barrett's esophagus biopsies. Am J Gastroenterol 103: 2333-2340.
741. Drut R, Jones MC (1988). Congenital pancreatoblastoma in Beckwith-Wiedemann syndrome: an emerging association. Pediatr Pathol 8: 331-339.
742. Du M, Diss TC, Xu C, Peng H, Isaacson PG, Pan L (1996). Ongoing mutation in MALT lymphoma immunoglobulin gene suggests that antigen stimulation plays a role in the clonal expansion. Leukemia 10: 1190-1197.
743. Duarte I, Llanos O, Domke H, Harz C, Valdivieso V (1993). Metaplasia and precursor lesions of gallbladder carcinoma. Frequency, distribution, and probability of detection in routine histologic samples. Cancer 72: 1878-1884.
744. Duff P, Greene VP (1985). Pregnancy complicated by solid-papillary epithelial tumor of the pancreas, pulmonary embolism, and pulmonary embolectomy. Am J Obstet Gynecol 152: 80-81.
745. Duffy A, Capanu M, Abou-Alfa GK, Huitzil D, Jarnagin W, Fong Y et al. (2008). Gallbladder cancer (GBC): 10-year experience at Memorial Sloan-Kettering Cancer Centre (MSKCC). J Surg Oncol 98: 485-489.
746. Dujardin F, Beaussart P, de MA, Rosset P, Waynberger E, Mulleman D et al. (2009). Primary neuroendocrine tumor of the sacrum: case report and review of the literature. Skeletal Radiol 38: 819-823.
747. Dulai GS, Guha S, Kahn KL, Gornbein J, Weinstein WM (2002). Preoperative prevalence of Barrett's esophagus in esophageal adenocarcinoma: a systematic review. Gastroenterology 122: 26-33.
748. Dumas A, Thung SN, Lin CS (1998). Diffuse hyperplasia of the peribiliary glands. Arch Pathol Lab Med 122: 87-89.
749. Dunbar KB, Okolo P, III, Montgomery E, Canto MI (2009). Confocal laser endomicroscopy in Barrett's esophagus and endoscopically inapparent Barrett's neoplasia: a prospective, randomized, double-blind, controlled, crossover trial. Gastrointest Endosc 70: 645-654.
750. Dunlop MG (2002). Guidance on gastrointestinal surveillance for hereditary non-polyposis colorectal cancer, familial adenomatous polypolis, juvenile polyposis, and Peutz-Jeghers syndrome. Gut 51 Suppl 5: V21-V27.
751. Dunn J, Garde J, Dolan K, Gosney JR, Sutton R, Meltzer SJ et al. (1999). Multiple target sites of allelic imbalance on chromosome 17 in Barrett's oesophageal cancer. Oncogene 18: 987-993.
752. Dunn JL, Longnecker DS (1995). Pancreatoblastoma in an older adult. Arch Pathol Lab Med 119: 547-551.
753. Durno C, Monga N, Bapat B, Berk T, Cohen Z, Gallinger S (2007). Does early colectomy increase desmoid risk in familial adenomatous polyposis? Clin Gastroenterol Hepatol 5: 1190-1194.
754. Duval JV, Savas L, Banner BF (2000). Expression of cytokeratins 7 and 20 in carcinomas of the extrahepatic biliary tract, pancreas, and gallbladder. Arch Pathol Lab Med 124: 1196-1200.
755. Dyson N, Howley PM, Munger K, Harlow E (1989). The human papilloma virus-16 E7 oncoprotein is able to bind to the retinoblastoma gene product. Science 243: 934-937.
756. Easson AM, Barron PT, Cripps C, Hill G, Guindi M, Michaud C (1996). Calcification in colorectal hepatic metastases correlates with longer survival. J Surg Oncol 63: 221-225.
757. East JE, Saunders BP, Jass JR (2008). Sporadic and syndromic hyperplastic polyps and serrated adenomas of the colon: classification, molecular genetics, natural history, and clinical management. Gastroenterol Clin North Am 37: 25-46.
758. Ebata T, Kamiya J, Nishio H, Nagasaka T, Nimura Y, Nagino M (2009). The concept of perihilar cholangiocarcinoma is valid. Br J Surg 96: 926-934.
759. Eckhauser FE, Cheung PS, Vinik AI, Strodel WE, Lloyd RV, Thompson NW (1986). Nonfunctioning malignant neuroendocrine tumors of the pancreas. Surgery 100: 978-988.
760. Economopoulos N, Kelekis NL, Argentos S, Tsompanlioti C, Patapis P, Nikolaou I et al. (2008). Bright-dark ring sign in MR imaging of hepatic epithelioid hemangioendothelioma. J Magn Reson Imaging 27: 908-912.
761. Edden Y, Shih SS, Wexner SD (2009). Solitary rectal ulcer syndrome and stercoral ulcers. Gastroenterol Clin North Am 38: 541-545.
762. Edge SB, Byrd DR, Compton CC, Fritz AG, Greene FL, and Trotti A (eds) (2009). AJCC Cancer Staging Manual. Springer: New York.
763. Edmonds P, Merino MJ, Livolsi VA, Duray PH (1984). Adenocarcinoid (mucinous carcinoid) of the appendix. Gastroenterology 86: 302-309.
764. Edwards JM, Hillier VF, Lawson RA, Moussalli H, Hasleton PS (1989). Squamous carcinoma of the oesophagus: histological criteria and their prognostic significance. Br J Cancer 59: 429-433.
765. Efremidis SC, Hytiroglou P, Matsui O (2007). Enhancement patterns and signal-intensity characteristics of small hepatocellular carcinoma in cirrhosis: pathologic basis and diagnostic challenges. Eur Radiol 17: 2969-2982.
766. Egawa N, Maillet B, Schroder S, Mukai K, Klöppel G (1994). Serous oligocystic and ill-demarcated adenoma of the pancreas: a variant of serous cystic adenoma. Virchows Arch 424: 13-17.
767. Eguchi H, Herschenhous N, Kuzushita N, Moss SF (2003). *Helicobacter pylori* increases proteasome-mediated degradation of p27(kip1) in gastric epithelial cells. Cancer Res 63: 4739-4746.
768. Eguchi H, Ishikawa O, Ohigashi H, Tomimaru Y, Sasaki Y, Yamada T et al. (2006). Patients with pancreatic intraductal papillary mucinous neoplasms are at high risk of colorectal cancer development. Surgery 139: 749-754.
769. Eguchi T, Nakanishi Y, Shimoda T, Iwasaki M, Igaki H, Tachimori Y et al. (2006). Histopathological criteria for additional treatment after endoscopic mucosal resection for esophageal cancer: analysis of 464 surgically resected cases. Mod Pathol 19: 475-480.
770. Eidt S, Stolte M, Fischer R (1994). *Helicobacter pylori* gastritis and primary gastric non-Hodgkin's lymphomas. J Clin Pathol 47: 436-439.
771. Ekbom A, Helmick CG, Zack M, Holmberg L, Adami HO (1992). Survival and causes of death in patients with inflammatory bowel disease: a population-based study. Gastroenterology 103: 954-960.
772. Ekeblad S, Skogseid B, Dunder K, Oberg K, Eriksson B (2008). Prognostic factors and survival in 324 patients with pancreatic endocrine tumor treated at a single institution. Clin Cancer Res 14: 7798-7803.
773. Ekstrom AM, Serafini M, Nyren O, Hansson LE, Ye W, Wolk A (2000). Dietary antioxidant intake and the risk of cardia cancer and noncardia cancer of the intestinal and diffuse types: a population-based case-control study in Sweden. Int J Cancer 87: 133-140.
774. El Rassi ZS, Mohsine RM, Berger F, Thierry P, Partensky CC (2004). Endocrine tumors of the extrahepatic bile ducts. Pathological and clinical aspects, surgical management and outcome. Hepatogastroenterology 51: 1295-1300.
775. El-Bahrawy MA, Rowan A, Horncastle D, Tomlinson I, Theis BA, Russell RC et al. (2008). E-cadherin/catenin complex status in solid pseudopapillary tumor of the pancreas. Am J Surg Pathol 32: 1-7.
776. El-Omar EM (2001). The importance of interleukin 1beta in *Helicobacter pylori* associated disease. Gut 48: 743-747.
777. El-Omar EM, Carrington M, Chow WH, McColl KE, Bream JH, Young HA et al. (2000). Interleukin-1 polymorphisms associated with increased risk of gastric cancer. Nature 404: 398-402.
778. El-Omar EM, Carrington M, Chow WH, McColl KE, Bream JH, Young HA et al. (2001). The role of interleukin-1 polymorphisms in the pathogenesis of gastric cancer. Nature 412: 99-
779. El-Rifai W, Sarlomo-Rikala M, Andersson LC, Knuutila S, Miettinen M (2000). DNA sequence copy number changes in gastrointestinal stromal tumors: tumor progression and prognostic significance. Cancer Res 60: 3899-3903.
780. El-Serag H (2008). The association between obesity and GERD: a review of the epidemiological evidence. Dig Dis Sci 53: 2307-2312.
781. El-Serag HB, Hampel H, Javadi F (2006). The association between diabetes and hepatocellular carcinoma: a systematic review of epidemiologic evidence. Clin Gastroenterol Hepatol 4: 369-380.
782. El-Zimaity HM, Ramchatesingh J, Saeed MA, Graham DY (2001). Gastric intestinal metaplasia: subtypes and natural history. J Clin Pathol 54: 679-683.
783. Elliott GB, Fisher BK (1967). Perianal keratoacanthoma. Arch Dermatol 95: 81-82.
784. Ellis A, Field JK, Field EA, Friedmann PS, Fryer A, Howard P et al. (1994). Tylosis associated with carcinoma of the oesophagus and oral leukoplakia in a large Liverpool family—a review of six generations. Eur J Cancer B Oral Oncol 30B: 102-112.
785. Eloubeidi MA, Chen VK, Jhala NC, Eltoum IE, Jhala D, Chhieng DC et al. (2004). Endoscopic ultrasound-guided fine needle aspiration biopsy of suspected cholangiocarcinoma. Clin Gastroenterol Hepatol 2: 209-213.
786. Elsayed AM, Albahra M, Nzeako UC, Sobin LH (1996). Malignant melanomas in the small intestine: a study of 103 patients. Am J Gastroenterol 91: 1001-1006.
787. Elstrom R, Guan L, Baker G, Nakhoda K, Vergilio JA, Zhuang H et al. (2003). Utility of FDG-PET scanning in lymphoma by WHO classification. Blood 101: 3875-3876.
788. Emerson RE, Randolph ML, Cramer HM (2006). Endoscopic ultrasound-guided fine-needle aspiration cytology diagnosis of intraductal papillary mucinous neoplasm of the pancreas is highly predictive of pancreatic neoplasia. Diagn Cytopathol 34: 457-462.
789. Endo EG, Walton DS, Albert DM (1996). Neonatal hepatoblastoma metastatic to the choroid and iris. Arch Ophthalmol 114: 757-761.
790. Endo K, Ashida K, Miyake N, Terada T (2001). E-cadherin gene mutations in human intrahepatic cholangiocarcinoma. J Pathol 193: 310-317.
791. Endo M, Takeshita K, Yoshida M (1986). How can we diagnose the early stage of esophageal cancer? Endoscopic diagnosis. Endoscopy 18 Suppl 3: 11-18.
792. Endoh Y, Tamura G, Motoyama T, Ajioka Y, Watanabe H (1999). Well-differentiated adenocarcinoma mimicking complete-type intestinal metaplasia in the stomach. Hum Pathol 30: 826-832.
793. Eng C (1997). Cowden syndrome. J Genet Counsel 6: 181-191.
794. Eng C, Murday V, Seal S, Mohammed S, Hodgson SV, Chaudary MA et al. (1994). Cowden syndrome and Lhermitte-Duclos disease in a family: a single genetic syndrome with pleiotropy? J Med Genet 31: 458-461.
795. Eng C, Peacocke M (1998). PTEN and inherited hamartoma-cancer syndromes. Nat Genet 19: 223
796. Eng C, Spechler SJ, Ruben R, Li FP (1993). Familial Barrett esophagus and adenocarcinoma of the gastroesophageal junction. Cancer Epidemiol Biomarkers Prev 2: 397-399.
797. Enzan H, Himeno H, Iwamura S, Onishi S, Saibara T, Yamamoto Y et al. (1994). Alpha-smooth muscle actin-positive perisinusoidal stromal cells in human hepatocellular carcinoma. Hepatology 19: 895-903.
798. Enzinger PC, Mayer RJ (2003). Esophageal cancer. N Engl J Med 349: 2241-2252.
799. Epplein M, Nomura AM, Hankin JH, Blaser MJ, Perez-Perez G, Stemmermann GN et al. (2008). Association of *Helicobacter pylori* infection and diet on the risk of gastric cancer: a case-control study in Hawaii. Cancer Causes Control 19: 869-877.
800. Erdogan D, Lamers WH, Offerhaus GJ, Busch OR, Gouma DJ, van Gulik TM (2006). Cystadenomas with ovarian stroma in liver and pancreas: an evolving concept. Dig Surg 23: 186-191.
801. Erickson LA, Papouchado B, Dimashkieh H, Zhang S, Nakamura N, Lloyd RV (2004). Cdx2 as a marker for neuroendocrine tumors of unknown primary sites. Endocr Pathol 15: 247-252.
802. Eriguchi N, Aoyagi S, Jimi A (2003). Signet-ring cell carcinoma of the ampulla of Vater: report of a case. Surg Today 33: 467-469.
803. Eriguchi N, Aoyagi S, Noritomi T, Imamura M, Sato S, Fujiki K et al. (2000). Adenoendocrine cell carcinoma of the gallbladder. J Hepatobiliary Pancreat Surg 7: 97-101.
804. Espinosa A, Berga C, Martin-Paredero V, Sanchez V, Diaz J, Segura J et al. (1998). Hemangiopericytoma ischiorectal. Report of a case. J Cardiovasc Surg (Torino) 39: 577-581.
805. Espinosa I, Lee CH, Kim MK, Rouse BT, Subramanian S, Montgomery K et al. (2008). A novel monoclonal antibody against DOG1 is a sensitive and specific marker for gastrointestinal stromal tumors. Am J Surg Pathol 32: 210-218.
806. Esquivel J, Sugarbaker PH (2000). Clinical presentation of the Pseudomyxoma peritonei syndrome. Br J Surg 87: 1414-1418.
807. Evans JP, Burke W, Chen R, Bennett RL, Schmidt RA, Dellinger EP et al. (1995). Familial pancreatic adenocarcinoma: association with diabetes and early molecular diagnosis. J Med Genet 32: 330-335.
808. Everett SM, Axon AT (1997). Early gastric cancer in Europe. Gut 41: 142-150.
809. Everhart CW, Jr., Holtzapple PG, Humphries TJ (1983). Barrett's esophagus: inherited epithelium or inherited reflux? J Clin Gastroenterol 5: 357-358.

810. Fabre A, Sauvanet A, Flejou JF, Belghiti J, Palazzo L, Ruszniewski P et al. (2001). Intraductal acinar cell carcinoma of the pancreas. Virchows Arch 438: 312-315.
811. Fabre A, Tansey DK, Dave U, Wright M, Teare JP, Rosin DR et al. (2003). Adenocarcinoma in situ arising from the submucosal oesophageal mucous glands. Eur J Gastroenterol Hepatol 15: 1047-1049.
812. Fadare O, DeMartini SD (2006). Eosinophilic dysplasia of the gallbladder: a hitherto undescribed variant identified in association with a "porcelain" gallbladder. Diagn Pathol 1: 15
813. Fagih M, Serra S, Chetty R (2007). Paucicellular infiltrating ductal carcinoma of pancreas: an unusual variant. Ann Diagn Pathol 11: 46-48.
814. Fahmy N, King JF (1993). Barrett's esophagus: an acquired condition with genetic predisposition. Am J Gastroenterol 88: 1262-1265.
815. Fahy BN, Tang LH, Klimstra D, Wong WD, Guillem JG, Paty PB et al. (2007). Carcinoid of the rectum risk stratification (CaRRs): a strategy for preoperative outcome assessment. Ann Surg Oncol 14: 1735-1743.
816. Falconi M, Salvia R, Bassi C, Zamboni G, Talamini G, Pederzoli P (2001). Clinicopathological features and treatment of intraductal papillary mucinous tumour of the pancreas. Br J Surg 88: 376-381.
817. Falk GW, Rice TW, Goldblum JR, Richter JE (1999). Jumbo biopsy forceps protocol still misses unsuspected cancer in Barrett's esophagus with high-grade dysplasia. Gastrointest Endosc 49: 170-176.
818. Fan Z, van de RM, Montgomery K, Rouse RV (2003). Hep par 1 antibody stain for the differential diagnosis of hepatocellular carcinoma: 676 tumors tested using tissue microarrays and conventional tissue sections. Mod Pathol 16: 137-144.
819. Farcet JP, Gaulard P, Marolleau JP, Le Couedic JP, Henni T, Gourdin MF et al. (1990). Hepatosplenic T-cell lymphoma: sinusal/sinusoidal localization of malignant cells expressing the T-cell receptor gamma delta. Blood 75: 2213-2219.
820. Fareed KR, Kaye P, Soomro IN, Ilyas M, Martin S, Parsons SL et al. (2009). Biomarkers of response to therapy in oesophago-gastric cancer. Gut 58: 127-143.
821. Farinha P, Gascoyne RD (2005). Molecular pathogenesis of mucosa-associated lymphoid tissue lymphoma. J Clin Oncol 23: 6370-6378.
822. Farrington SM, Tenesa A, Barnetson R, Wiltshire A, Prendergast J, Porteous M et al. (2005). Germline susceptibility to colorectal cancer due to base-excision repair gene defects. Am J Hum Genet 77: 112-119.
823. Farrow DC, Vaughan TL, Sweeney C, Gammon MD, Chow WH, Risch HA et al. (2000). Gastroesophageal reflux disease, use of H2 receptor antagonists, and risk of esophageal and gastric cancer. Cancer Causes Control 11: 231-238.
824. Fasano M, Theise ND, Nalesnik M, Goswami S, Garcia de Davila MT, Finegold MJ et al. (1998). Immunohistochemical evaluation of hepatoblastomas with use of the hepatocyte-specific marker, hepatocyte paraffin 1, and the polyclonal anti-carcinoembryonic antigen. Mod Pathol 11: 934-938.
825. Fattovich G, Stroffolini T, Zagni I, Donato F (2004). Hepatocellular carcinoma in cirrhosis: incidence and risk factors. Gastroenterology 127: S35-S50.
826. Fava M, Foradori G, Cruz F, Guzman S (1991). Papillomatosis of the common bile duct associated with ampullary carcinoma. AJR Am J Roentgenol 156: 405-406.
827. Favini F, Massimino M, Esposito V, Maestri L, Fava G, Spreafico F (2008). Rectal burkitt lymphoma in childhood. J Pediatr Hematol Oncol 30: 176-178.
828. Feakins RM, Nickols CD, Bidd H, Walton SJ (2003). Abnormal expression of pRb, p16, and cyclin D1 in gastric adenocarcinoma and its lymph node metastases: relationship with pathological features and survival. Hum Pathol 34: 1276-1282.
829. Fearon ER, Vogelstein B (1990). A genetic model for colorectal tumorigenesis. Cell 61: 759-767.
830. Feczko PJ, Collins DD, Mezwa DG (1993). Metastatic disease involving the gastrointestinal tract. Radiol Clin North Am 31: 1359-1373.
831. Federspiel BH, Burke AP, Sobin LH, Shekitka KM (1990). Rectal and colonic carcinoids. A clinicopathologic study of 84 cases. Cancer 65: 135-140.
832. Fendrich V, Ramerth R, Waldmann J, Maschuw K, Langer P, Bartsch DK et al. (2009). Sonic hedgehog and pancreatic-duodenal homeobox 1 expression distinguish between duodenal and pancreatic gastrinomas. Endocr Relat Cancer 16: 613-622.
833. Fendrich V, Waldmann J, Esni F, Ramaswamy A, Mullendore M, Buchholz M et al. (2007). Snail and Sonic Hedgehog activation in neuroendocrine tumors of the ileum. Endocr Relat Cancer 14: 865-874.
834. Fenger C (1989). Surgical pathology of the anal canal: a review of the recent literature on the anatomy and pathology. In: Progress in Surgical Pathology. Fenoglio-Preiser CM, Wolff M, Rilke F, eds. Springer-Verlag: Berlin, pp. 237-260.
835. Fenger C (1997). Anal canal (Chapter 24). In: Histology for Pathologists, Second Edition. Sternberg SS, ed. Lippincott Raven: New York.
836. Fenger C, Filipe MI (1981). Mucin histochemistry of the anal canal epithelium. Studies of normal anal mucosa and mucosa adjacent to carcinoma. Histochem J 13: 921-930.
837. Fenger C, Frisch M, Jass JJ, Williams GT, Hilden J (2000). Anal cancer subtype reproducibility study. Virchows Arch 436: 229-233.
838. Fenger C, Lyon H (1982). Endocrine cells and melanin-containing cells in the anal canal epithelium. Histochem J 14: 631-639.
839. Fenger C, Nielsen VT (1986). Intraepithelial neoplasia in the anal canal. The appearance and relation to genital neoplasia. Acta Pathol Microbiol Immunol Scand A 94: 343-349.
840. Fenger C, Schroder HD (1990). Neuronal hyperplasia in the anal canal. Histopathology 16: 481-485.
841. Ferguson HR, Wild CP, Anderson LA, Murphy SJ, Johnston BT, Murray LJ et al. (2008). Cyclooxygenase-2 and inducible nitric oxide synthase gene polymorphisms and risk of reflux esophagitis, Barrett's esophagus, and esophageal adenocarcinoma. Cancer Epidemiol Biomarkers Prev 17: 727-731.
842. Ferlay J, Bray F, Pisani P, Parkin M (2004). Cancer incidence, Mortality and Prevalence Worldwide. Globocan 2002. IARC CancerBase No. 5. IARC, Lyon.
842A. Ferlay J, Shin H-R, Bray F, Forman D, Mathers C and Parkin DM (2010). Globocan 2008: Cancer Incidence and Mortality Worldwide. IARC CancerBase No. 10, 1027-5614. IARC, Lyon.
843. Ferluga D, Luzar B, Gadzijev EM (2003). Follicular lymphoma of the gallbladder and extrahepatic bile ducts. Virchows Arch 442: 136-140.
844. Fernandez E, La Vecchia C, D'Avanzo B, Negri E, Franceschi S (1994). Family history and the risk of liver, gallbladder, and pancreatic cancer. Cancer Epidemiol Biomarkers Prev 3: 209-212.
845. Ferrandez A, Samowitz W, Disario JA, Burt RW (2004). Phenotypic characteristics and risk of cancer development in hyperplastic polyposis: case series and literature review. Am J Gastroenterol 99: 2012-2018.
846. Ferrell LD, Beckstead JH (1991). Paneth-like cells in an adenoma and adenocarcinoma in the ampulla of Vater. Arch Pathol Lab Med 115: 956-958.
847. Ferreri AJ, Freschi M, Dell'Oro S, Viale E, Villa E, Ponzoni M (2001). Prognostic significance of the histopathologic recognition of low- and high-grade components in stage I-II B-cell gastric lymphomas. Am J Surg Pathol 25: 95-102.
848. Ferrone CR, Kattan MW, Tomlinson JS, Thayer SP, Brennan MF, Warshaw AL (2005). Validation of a postresection pancreatic adenocarcinoma nomogram for disease-specific survival. J Clin Oncol 23: 7529-7535.
849. Ferrone CR, Tang LH, D'Angelica M, Dematteo RP, Blumgart LH, Klimstra DS et al. (2007). Extrahepatic bile duct carcinoid tumors: malignant biliary obstruction with a good prognosis. J Am Coll Surg 205: 357-361.
850. Ferrone CR, Tang LH, Tomlinson J, Gonen M, Hochwald SN, Brennan MF et al. (2007). Determining prognosis in patients with pancreatic endocrine neoplasms: can the WHO classification system be simplified? J Clin Oncol 25: 5609-5615.
851. Ferrucci PF, Zucca E (2007). Primary gastric lymphoma pathogenesis and treatment: what has changed over the past 10 years? Br J Haematol 136: 521-538.
852. Fetsch JF, Laskin WB, Lefkowitz M, Kindblom LG, Meis-Kindblom JM (1996). Aggressive angiomyxoma: a clinicopathologic study of 29 female patients. Cancer 78: 79-90.
853. Fielding JW, Roginski C, Ellis DJ, Jones BG, Powell J, Waterhouse JA et al. (1984). Clinicopathological staging of gastric cancer. Br J Surg 71: 677-680.
854. Fife J, Raniga S, Hider PN, Frizelle FA (2009). Folic Acid Supplementation and Colorectal Cancer Risk; A Meta-analysis. Colorectal Dis -
855. Figueiredo C, Machado JC, Pharoah P, Seruca R, Sousa S, Carvalho R et al. (2002). *Helicobacter pylori* and interleukin 1 genotyping: an opportunity to identify high-risk individuals for gastric carcinoma. J Natl Cancer Inst 94: 1680-1687.
856. Figueiredo C, van Doorn LJ, Nogueira C, Soares JM, Pinho C, Figueira P et al. (2001). *Helicobacter pylori* genotypes are associated with clinical outcome in Portuguese patients and show a high prevalence of infections with multiple strains. Scand J Gastroenterol 36: 128-135.
857. Filipe MI, Jass JR (1986). Intestinal metaplasia subtypes and cancer risk. In: Gastric Carcinoma. Filipe MI, Jass JR, eds. Churchill Livingstone: London, pp. 87-115.
858. Filipe MI, Munoz N, Matko I, Kato I, Pompe-Kirn V, Jutersek A et al. (1994). Intestinal metaplasia types and the risk of gastric cancer: a cohort study in Slovenia. Int J Cancer 57: 324-329.
859. Filipe MI, Potet F, Bogomoletz WV, Dawson PA, Fabiani B, Chauveinc P et al. (1985). Incomplete sulphomucin-secreting intestinal metaplasia for gastric cancer. Preliminary data from a prospective study from three centres. Gut 26: 1319-1326.
860. Finegold MJ, Egler RA, Goss JA, Guillerman RP, Karpen SJ, Krishnamurthy R et al. (2008). Liver tumors: pediatric population. Liver Transpl 14: 1545-1556.
861. Finegold MJ, Lopez-Terrada DH, Bowen J, Washington MK, Qualman SJ (2007). Protocol for the examination of specimens from pediatric patients with hepatoblastoma. Arch Pathol Lab Med 131: 520-529.
862. Fink D, Nebel S, Aebi S, Zheng H, Kim HK, Christen RD et al. (1997). Expression of the DNA mismatch repair proteins hMLH1 and hPMS2 in normal human tissues. Br J Cancer 76: 890-893.
863. Fiocca R, Mastracci L, Riddell R, Takubo K, Vieth M, Yerian L et al. (2010). Development of consensus guidelines for the histologic recognition of microscopic esophagitis in patients with gastroesophageal reflux disease: the Esohisto project. Hum Pathol 41: 223-231.
864. Fiocca R, Rindi G, Capella C, Grimelius L, Polak JM, Schwartz TW et al. (1987). Glucagon, glicentin, proglucagon, PYY, PP and proPP-icosapeptide immunoreactivities of rectal carcinoid tumors and related non-tumor cells. Regul Pept 17: 9-29.
865. Fiocca R, Villani L, Tenti P, Solcia E, Cornaggia M, Frigerio B et al. (1987). Characterization of four main cell types in gastric cancer: foveolar, mucopeptic, intestinal columnar and goblet cells. An histopathologic, histochemical and ultrastructural study of "early" and "advanced" tumours. Pathol Res Pract 182: 308-325.
866. Fischbach W, Kestel W, Kirchner T, Mossner J, Wilms K (1992). Malignant lymphomas of the upper gastrointestinal tract. Results of a prospective study in 103 patients. Cancer 70: 1075-1080.
867. Fischer HP, Zhou H (2003). [Pathogenesis and histomorphology of ampullary carcinomas and their precursor lesions. Review and individual findings]. Pathologe 24: 196-203.
868. Fischer L, Kleeff J, Esposito I, Hinz U, Zimmermann A, Friess H et al. (2008). Clinical outcome and long-term survival in 118 consecutive patients with neuroendocrine tumours of the pancreas. Br J Surg 95: 627-635.
869. Fishel R, Lescoe MK, Rao MR, Copeland NG, Jenkins NA, Garber J et al. (1993). The human mutator gene homolog MSH2 and its association with hereditary nonpolyposis colon cancer. Cell 75: 1027-1038.
870. Fitzgerald RC, Caldas C (2006). Familial gastric cancer - clinical management. Best Pract Res Clin Gastroenterol 20: 735-743.
871. Fitzgerald RC, Hardwick R, Huntsman D, Carneiro F, Guilford P, Blair V et al. (on behalf of the International Gastric Cancer Linkage Consortium) (2010). Hereditary diffuse gastric cancer: updated consensus guidelines for clinical management and directions for future research. J Med Genet 47: 436-444.
872. Flanagan FL, Dehdashti F, Siegel BA, Trask DD, Sundaresan SR, Patterson GA et al. (1997). Staging of esophageal cancer with 18F-fluorodeoxyglucose positron emission tomography. AJR Am J Roentgenol 168: 417-424.
873. Flejou JF, Barge J, Menu Y, Degott C, Bismuth H, Potet F et al. (1985). Liver adenomatosis. An entity distinct from liver adenoma? Gastroenterology 89: 1132-1138.
874. Flejou JF, Gratio V, Muzeau F, Hamelin R (1999). p53 abnormalities in adenocarcinoma of the gastric cardia and antrum. Mol Pathol 52: 263-268.
875. Fleming ID, Cooper JS, Henson DE, Hutter RV, Kennedy BJ, Murphy GP et al. (eds) (1997). AJCC Cancer Staging Manual. Lippincott: Philadelphia.
876. Fleming KA, Boberg KM, Glaumann H, Bergquist A, Smith D, Clausen OP (2001). Biliary dysplasia as a marker of cholangiocarcinoma in primary sclerosing cholangitis. J Hepatol 34: 360-365.
877. Fokkema IF, den Dunnen JT, Taschner PE (2005). LOVD: easy creation of a locus-specific sequence variation database using an

"LSDB-in-a-box" approach. Hum Mutat 26: 63-68.
877A. Folsom AR, Pankow JS, Peacock JM, Bielinski SJ, Heiss G, Boerwinkle E (2008). Variation in TCF7L2 and increased risk of colon cancer: the Atherosclerosis Risk in Communities (ARIC) Study. Diabetes Care 31: 905-909
878. Fong PC, Boss DS, Yap TA, Tutt A, Wu P, Mergui-Roelvink M et al. (2009). Inhibition of poly(ADP-ribose) polymerase in tumors from BRCA mutation carriers. N Engl J Med 361: 123-134.
879. Forcet C, Billaud M (2007). Dialogue between LKB1 and AMPK: a hot topic at the cellular pole. Sci STKE 2007: e51-
880. Forcet C, Etienne-Manneville S, Gaude H, Fournier L, Debilly S, Salmi M et al. (2005). Functional analysis of Peutz-Jeghers mutations reveals that the LKB1 C-terminal region exerts a crucial role in regulating both the AMPK pathway and the cell polarity. Hum Mol Genet 14: 1283-1292.
881. Ford D, Easton DF, Bishop DT, Narod SA, Goldgar DE (1994). Risks of cancer in BRCA1-mutation carriers. Breast Cancer Linkage Consortium. Lancet 343: 692-695.
882. Forman D, Newell DG, Fullerton F, Yarnell JW, Stacey AR, Wald N et al. (1991). Association between infection with *Helicobacter pylori* and risk of gastric cancer: evidence from a prospective investigation. BMJ 302: 1302-1305.
882A. Forte A, De SR, Leonetti G, Manfredelli S, Urbano V, Bezzi M (2008). Dietary chemoprevention of colorectal cancer. Ann Ital Chir 79: 261-267.
883. Fossmark R, Jianu CS, Martinsen TC, Qvigstad G, Syversen U, Waldum HL (2008). Serum gastrin and chromogranin A levels in patients with fundic gland polyps caused by long-term proton-pump inhibition. Scand J Gastroenterol 43: 20-24.
884. Foster DR, Foster DB (1980). Gall-bladder polyps in Peutz-Jeghers syndrome. Postgrad Med J 56: 373-376.
885. Francalanci P, Diomedi-Camassei F, Purificato C, Santorelli FM, Giannotti A, Dominici C et al. (2003). Malignant pancreatic endocrine tumor in a child with tuberous sclerosis. Am J Surg Pathol 27: 1386-1389.
886. Franceschi S, De Vuyst H (2009). Human papillomavirus vaccines and anal carcinoma. Curr Opin HIV AIDS 4: 57-63.
887. Franceschi S, Montella M, Polesel J, La Vecchia C, Crispo A, Dal Maso L et al. (2006). Hepatitis viruses, alcohol, and tobacco in the etiology of hepatocellular carcinoma in Italy. Cancer Epidemiol Biomarkers Prev 15: 683-689.
888. Franco AT, Israel DA, Washington MK, Krishna U, Fox JG, Rogers AB et al. (2005). Activation of beta-catenin by carcinogenic *Helicobacter pylori*. Proc Natl Acad Sci U S A 102: 10646-10651.
889. Fredricks JR, Bejarano PA (2008). Primary malignant melanoma of the esophagus with separate foci of melanoma in situ and atypical melanocytic hyperplasia in a patient positive for human immunodeficiency virus: a case report and review of the literature. Arch Pathol Lab Med 132: 1675-1678.
890. Freeman HJ (2008). Colorectal cancer risk in Crohn's disease. World J Gastroenterol 14: 1810-1811.
891. Fretzayas A, Moustaki M, Kitsiou S, Nychtari G, Alexopoulou E (2009). Long-term follow-up of a multifocal hepatic mesenchymal hamartoma producing a-fetoprotein. Pediatr Surg Int 25: 381-384.
892. Friberg B, Svensson C, Goldman S, Glimelius B (1998). The Swedish National Care Programme for Anal Carcinoma—implementation and overall results. Acta Oncol 37: 25-32.
893. Friedl W, Kruse R, Uhlhaas S, Stolte M, Schartmann B, Keller KM et al. (1999). Frequent 4-bp deletion in exon 9 of the *SMAD4/MADH4* gene in familial juvenile polyposis patients. Genes Chromosomes Cancer 25: 403-406.
894. Friedl W, Uhlhaas S, Schulmann K, Stolte M, Loff S, Back W et al. (2002). Juvenile polyposis: massive gastric polyposis is more common in *MADH4* mutation carriers than in *BMPR1A* mutation carriers. Hum Genet 111: 108-111.
895. Friedlander MA, Stier E, Lin O (2004). Anorectal cytology as a screening tool for anal squamous lesions: cytologic, anoscopic, and histologic correlation. Cancer 102: 19-26.
896. Friedman HD (1990). Nonmucinous, glycogen-poor cystadenocarcinoma of the pancreas. Arch Pathol Lab Med 114: 888-891.
897. Friess H, Wang L, Zhu Z, Gerber R, Schroder M, Fukuda A et al. (1999). Growth factor receptors are differentially expressed in cancers of the papilla of vater and pancreas. Ann Surg 230: 767-774.
898. Frisch M, Fenger C, van den Brule AJ, Sorensen P, Meijer CJ, Walboomers JM et al. (1999). Variants of squamous cell carcinoma of the anal canal and perianal skin and their relation to human papillomaviruses. Cancer Res 59: 753-757.
899. Frisch M, Glimelius B, van den Brule AJ, Wohlfahrt J, Meijer CJ, Walboomers JM et al. (1998). Benign anal lesions, inflammatory bowel disease and risk for high-risk human papillomavirus-positive and -negative anal carcinoma. Br J Cancer 78: 1534-1538.
900. Frisch M, Glimelius B, van den Brule AJ, Wohlfahrt J, Meijer CJ, Walboomers JM et al. (1997). Sexually transmitted infection as a cause of anal cancer. N Engl J Med 337: 1350-1358.
901. Frisch M, Glimelius B, Wohlfahrt J, Adami HO, Melbye M (1999). Tobacco smoking as a risk factor in anal carcinoma: an antiestrogenic mechanism? J Natl Cancer Inst 91: 708-715.
902. Frisch M, Goodman MT (2000). Human papillomavirus-associated carcinomas in Hawaii and the mainland U.S. Cancer 88: 1464-1469.
903. Frisch M, Melbye M, Moller H (1993). Trends in incidence of anal cancer in Denmark. BMJ 306: 419-422.
904. Frisch M, Olsen JH, Bautz A, Melbye M (1994). Benign anal lesions and the risk of anal cancer. N Engl J Med 331: 300-302.
904A. Fritz A, Percy C, Jack A, Shanmugaratnam K, Sobin L, Parkin DM, Whelan S (eds) (2000). International Classification of Diseases for Oncology. Third edition. Geneva: World Health Organization.
905. Froelicher P, Miller G (1986). The European experience with esophageal cancer limited to the mucosa and submucosa. Gastrointest Endosc 32: 88-90.
906. Frossard JL, Amouyal P, Amouyal G, Palazzo L, Amaris J, Soldan M et al. (2003). Performance of endosonography-guided fine needle aspiration and biopsy in the diagnosis of pancreatic cystic lesions. Am J Gastroenterol 98: 1516-1524.
907. Fujii H, Aotake T, Horiuchi T, Chiba Y, Imamura Y, Tanaka K (2001). Small cell carcinoma of the gallbladder: a case report and review of 53 cases in the literature. Hepatogastroenterology 48: 1588-1593.
908. Fujii H, Inagaki M, Kasai S, Miyokawa N, Tokusashi Y, Gabrielson E et al. (1997). Genetic progression and heterogeneity in intraductal papillary-mucinous neoplasms of the pancreas. Am J Pathol 151: 1447-1454.
909. Fujii T, Kawai T, Saito K, Hishima T, Hayashi Y, Imura J et al. (1999). *MEN1* gene mutations in sporadic neuroendocrine tumors of foregut derivation. Pathol Int 49: 968-973.
910. Fujii T, Zen Y, Harada K, Niwa H, Masuda S, Kaizaki Y et al. (2008). Participation of liver cancer stem/progenitor cells in tumorigenesis of scirrhous hepatocellular carcinoma—human and cell culture study. Hum Pathol 39: 1185-1196.
911. Fujii T, Zen Y, Sato Y, Sasaki M, Enomae M, Minato H et al. (2008). Podoplanin is a useful diagnostic marker for epithelioid hemangioendothelioma of the liver. Mod Pathol 21: 125-130.
912. Fujiki K, Duerr EM, Kikuchi H, Ng A, Xavier RJ, Mizukami Y et al. (2008). Hoxc6 is overexpressed in gastrointestinal carcinoids and interacts with JunD to regulate tumor growth. Gastroenterology 135: 907-916.
913. Fujimori M, Ikeda S, Shimizu Y, Okajima M, Asahara T (2001). Accumulation of beta-catenin protein and mutations in exon 3 of beta-catenin gene in gastrointestinal carcinoid tumor. Cancer Res 61: 6656-6659.
914. Fujisawa S, Motomura S, Fujimaki K, Tanabe J, Tomita N, Hara M et al. (1999). Primary esophageal T cell lymphoma. Leuk Lymphoma 33: 199-202.
915. Fujiwara I, Yashiro M, Kubo N, Maeda K, Hirakawa K (2008). Ulcerative colitis-associated colorectal cancer is frequently associated with the microsatellite instability pathway. Dis Colon Rectum 51: 1387-1394.
916. Fujiwara T, Stolker JM, Watanabe T, Rashid A, Longo P, Eshleman JR et al. (1998). Accumulated clonal genetic alterations in familial and sporadic colorectal carcinomas with widespread instability in microsatellite sequences. Am J Pathol 153: 1063-1078.
917. Fukase K, Kato M, Kikuchi S, Inoue K, Uemura N, Okamoto S et al. (2008). Effect of eradication of *Helicobacter pylori* on incidence of metachronous gastric carcinoma after endoscopic resection of early gastric cancer: an open-label, randomised controlled trial. Lancet 372: 392-397.
918. Fukino K, Iido A, Teramoto A, Sakamoto G, Kasumi F, Nakamura Y et al. (1999). Frequent allelic loss at the TOC locus on 17q25.1 in primary breast cancers. Genes Chromosomes Cancer 24: 345-350.
919. Fukushima N, Fukayama M (2007). Mucinous cystic neoplasms of the pancreas: pathology and molecular genetics. J Hepatobiliary Pancreat Surg 14: 238-242.
920. Fukushima N, Mukai K (1999). Pancreatic neoplasms with abundant mucus production: emphasis on intraductal papillary-mucinous tumors and mucinous cystic tumors. Adv Anat Pathol 6: 65-77.
921. Fukushima N, Sato N, Prasad N, Leach SD, Hruban RH, Goggins M (2004). Characterization of gene expression in mucinous cystic neoplasms of the pancreas using oligonucleotide microarrays. Oncogene 23: 9042-9051.
922. Fukushima N, Sato N, Ueki T, Rosty C, Walter KM, Wilentz RE et al. (2002). Aberrant methylation of preproenkephalin and p16 genes in pancreatic intraepithelial neoplasia and pancreatic ductal adenocarcinoma. Am J Pathol 160: 1573-1581.
923. Fung JW, Lam KS (1995). Neurofibromatosis and insulinoma. Postgrad Med J 71: 485-486.
924. Furlan D, Cerutti R, Genasetti A, Pelosi G, Uccella S, La Rosa S et al. (2003). Microallelotyping defines the monoclonal or the polyclonal origin of mixed and collision endocrine-exocrine tumors of the gut. Lab Invest 83: 963-971.
925. Furlan D, Cerutti R, Uccella S, La Rosa S, Rigoli E, Genasetti A et al. (2004). Different molecular profiles characterize well-differentiated endocrine tumors and poorly differentiated endocrine carcinomas of the gastroenteropancreatic tract. Clin Cancer Res 10: 947-957.
926. Furnari FB, Huang HJ, Cavenee WK (1998). The phosphoinositol phosphatase activity of PTEN mediates a serum-sensitive G1 growth arrest in glioma cells. Cancer Res 58: 5002-5008.
927. Furnari FB, Lin H, Huang HS, Cavenee WK (1997). Growth suppression of glioma cells by PTEN requires a functional phosphatase catalytic domain. Proc Natl Acad Sci U S A 94: 12479-12484.
928. Furukawa T, Fujisaki R, Yoshida Y, Kanai N, Sunamura M, Abe T et al. (2005). Distinct progression pathways involving the dysfunction of DUSP6/MKP-3 in pancreatic intraepithelial neoplasia and intraductal papillary-mucinous neoplasms of the pancreas. Mod Pathol 18: 1034-1042.
929. Furukawa T, Klöppel G, Volkan AN, Albores-Saavedra J, Fukushima N, Horii A et al. (2005). Classification of types of intraductal papillary-mucinous neoplasm of the pancreas: a consensus study. Virchows Arch 447: 794-799.
930. Furukawa T, Oohashi K, Yamao K, Naitoh Y, Hirooka Y, Taki T et al. (1997). Intraductal ultrasonography of the pancreas: development and clinical potential. Endoscopy 29: 561-569.
931. Furukawa T, Takahashi T, Kobari M, Matsuno S (1992). The mucus-hypersecreting tumor of the pancreas. Development and extension visualized by three-dimensional computerized mapping. Cancer 70: 1505-1513.
932. Gadacz TR, McFadden DW, Gabrielson EW, Ullah A, Berman JJ (1990). Adenocarcinoma of the ileostomy: the latent risk of cancer after colectomy for ulcerative colitis and familial polyposis. Surgery 107: 698-703.
933. Gaffey MJ, Mills SE, Lack EE (1990). Neuroendocrine carcinoma of the colon and rectum. A clinicopathologic, ultrastructural, and immunohistochemical study of 24 cases. Am J Surg Pathol 14: 1010-1023.
934. Galanis C, Zamani A, Cameron JL, Campbell KA, Lillemoe KD, Caparrelli D et al. (2007). Resected serous cystic neoplasms of the pancreas: a review of 158 patients with recommendations for treatment. J Gastrointest Surg 11: 820-826.
935. Galbut DL, Markowitz AM (1980). Insulinoma: diagnosis, surgical management and long-term follow-up. Review of 41 cases. Am J Surg 139: 682-690.
936. Galiatsatos P, Foulkes WD (2006). Familial adenomatous polyposis. Am J Gastroenterol 101: 385-398.
936A. Galipeau PC, Prevo LJ, Sanchez CA, Longton GM, Reid BJ (1999). Clonal expansion and loss of heterozygosity at chromosomes 9p and 17p in premalignant esophageal (Barrett's) tissue. J Natl Cancer Inst 91: 2087–2095.
937. Gall FP, Kessler H, Hermanek P (1991). Surgical treatment of ductal pancreatic carcinoma. Eur J Surg Oncol 17: 173-181.
938. Gallione CJ, Repetto GM, Legius E, Rustgi AK, Schelley SL, Tejpar S et al. (2004). A combined syndrome of juvenile polyposis and hereditary haemorrhagic telangiectasia associated with mutations in MADH4 (SMAD4). Lancet 363: 852-859.
939. Galon J, Costes A, Sanchez-Cabo F, Kirilovsky A, Mlecnik B, Lagorce-Pages C et al. (2006). Type, density, and location of immune cells within human colorectal tumors predict clinical outcome. Science 313: 1960-1964.
940. Gangi S, Fletcher JG, Nathan MA, Christensen JA, Harmsen WS, Crownhart BS et al. (2004). Time interval between abnormalities seen on CT and the clinical diagnosis of pancreatic cancer: retrospective review of CT scans obtained before diagnosis. AJR Am J Roentgenol 182: 897-903.
941. Ganne-Carrie N, Chastang C, Chapel F, Munz C, Pateron D, Sibony M et al. (1996).

Predictive score for the development of hepatocellular carcinoma and additional value of liver large cell dysplasia in Western patients with cirrhosis. Hepatology 23: 1112-1118.

942. Garas G, Bramston B, Edmunds SE (2000). Malignant melanoma metastatic to the common bile duct. J Gastroenterol Hepatol 15: 1348-1351.

943. Garbrecht N, Anlauf M, Schmitt A, Henopp T, Sipos B, Raffel A et al. (2008). Somatostatin-producing neuroendocrine tumors of the duodenum and pancreas: incidence, types, biological behavior, association with inherited syndromes, and functional activity. Endocr Relat Cancer 15: 229-241.

944. Garcea G, Ong SL, Rajesh A, Neal CP, Pollard CA, Berry DP et al. (2008). Cystic lesions of the pancreas. A diagnostic and management dilemma. Pancreatology 8: 236-251.

945. Garcia Rego JA, Valbuena RL, Alvarez GA, Santiago Freijanes MP, Suarez Penaranda JM, Rois Soto JM (1991). Pancreatic mucinous cystadenocarcinoma with pseudosarcomatous mural nodules. A report of a case with immunohistochemical study. Cancer 67: 494-498.

946. Gardiner GW, Lajoie G, Keith R (1992). Hepatoid adenocarcinoma of the papilla of Vater. Histopathology 20: 541-544.

947. Gardner EJ (1962). Follow-up study of a family group exhibiting dominant inheritance for a syndrome including intestinal polyps, osteomas, fibromas and epidermal cysts. Am J Hum Genet 14: 376-390.

948. Gardner EJ, Richards RC (1953). Multiple cutaneous and subcutaneous lesions occurring simultaneously with hereditary polyposis and osteomatosis. Am J Hum Genet 5: 139-147.

949. Garwood RA, Sawyer MD, Ledesma EJ, Foley E, Claridge JA (2005). A case and review of bowel perforation secondary to metastatic lung cancer. Am Surg 71: 110-116.

950. Gascoyne RD, Adomat SA, Krajewski S, Krajewska M, Horsman DE, Tolcher AW et al. (1997). Prognostic significance of Bcl-2 protein expression and Bcl-2 gene rearrangement in diffuse aggressive non-Hodgkin's lymphoma. Blood 90: 244-251.

951. Gassmann P, Haier J, Schluter K, Domikowsky B, Wendel C, Wiesner U et al. (2009). CXCR4 regulates the early extravasation of metastatic tumor cells in vivo. Neoplasia 11: 651-661.

952. Gatalica Z, Torlakovic E (2008). Pathology of the hereditary colorectal carcinoma. Fam Cancer 7: 15-26.

953. Gatenby PA, Caygill CP, Ramus JR, Charlett A, Fitzgerald RC, Watson A (2007). Short segment columnar-lined oesophagus: an underestimated cancer risk? A large cohort study of the relationship between Barrett's columnar-lined oesophagus segment length and adenocarcinoma risk. Eur J Gastroenterol Hepatol 19: 969-975.

954. Gatof D, Chen YK, Shah RJ (2004). Primary squamous cell carcinoma of the bile duct diagnosed by transpapillary cholangioscopy: case report and review. Gastrointest Endosc 60: 300-304.

955. Gayther SA, Gorringe KL, Ramus SJ, Huntsman D, Roviello F, Grehan N et al. (1998). Identification of germ-line E-cadherin mutations in gastric cancer families of European origin. Cancer Res 58: 4086-4089.

955A. Gebski V, Burmeister B, Smithers BM, Foo K, Zalcberg J, Simes J (2007). Survival benefits from neoadjuvant chemoradiotherapy or chemotherapy in oesophageal carcinoma: a meta-analysis. Lancet Oncol 8: 226-234.

956. Geers C, Moulin P, Gigot JF, Weynand B, Deprez P, Rahier J et al. (2006). Solid and pseudopapillary tumor of the pancreas—review

and new insights into pathogenesis. Am J Surg Pathol 30: 1243-1249.

957. Geisinger KR, Levine EA, Shen P, Bradley RF (2007). Pleuropulmonary involvement in pseudomyxoma peritonei: morphologic assessment and literature review. Am J Clin Pathol 127: 135-143.

958. Gelfand MD (1983). Barrett esophagus in sexagenarian identical twins. J Clin Gastroenterol 5: 251-253.

959. Gembala RB, Hare JL, Meilahn J (1993). Intraabdominal metastatic thymoma. AJR Am J Roentgenol 161: 1331-

960. Gence A, Sahin C, Celayir AC, Yavuz H (2008). Primary Burkitt lymphoma presenting as a solitary rectal polyp in a child. Pediatr Surg Int 24: 1215-1217.

961. Genna M, Leopardi F, Fambri P, Postorino A (1997). [Neurogenic tumors of the ano-rectal region]. Ann Ital Chir 68: 351-353.

962. Genta RM, Rugge M (1999). Gastric precancerous lesions: heading for an international consensus. Gut 45 Suppl 1: I5-I8.

963. Geoffray A, Couanet D, Montagne JP, Leclere J, Flamant F (1987). Ultrasonography and computed tomography for diagnosis and follow-up of biliary duct rhabdomyosarcomas in children. Pediatr Radiol 17: 127-131.

964. George JC, Cohen MD, Tarver RD, Rosales RN (1994). Ruptured cystic mesenchymal hamartoma: an unusual cause of neonatal ascites. Pediatr Radiol 24: 304-305.

965. Ger R, Reuben J (1968). Squamous-cell carcinoma of the anal canal: a metastatic lesion. Dis Colon Rectum 11: 213-219.

966. Gerard JP, Romestaing P, Ardiet JM, Trillet L, V, Rocher FP, Baron MH et al. (1995). [Current treatment of cancers of the anal canal]. Ann Chir 49: 363-368.

967. Gerber MA, Thung SN, Bodenheimer HC, Jr., Kapelman B, Schaffner F (1986). Characteristic histologic triad in liver adjacent to metastatic neoplasm. Liver 6: 85-88.

968. Gerdes B, Wild A, Wittenberg J, Barth P, Ramaswamy A, Kersting M et al. (2003). Tumor-suppressing pathways in cystic pancreatic tumors. Pancreas 26: 42-48.

969. Gervaz P, Efron J, Poza AA, Chun SW, Pham TT, Woodhouse S et al. (2001). Loss of heterozygosity and HIV infection in patients with anal squamous-cell carcinoma. Dis Colon Rectum 44: 1503-1508.

970. Gervaz P, Scholl B, Mainguene C, Poitry S, Gillet M, Wexner S (2000). Angiogenesis of liver metastases: role of sinusoidal endothelial cells. Dis Colon Rectum 43: 980-986.

971. Ghadimi BM, Schrock E, Walker RL, Wangsa D, Jauho A, Meltzer PS et al. (1999). Specific chromosomal aberrations and amplification of the AIB1 nuclear receptor coactivator gene in pancreatic carcinomas. Am J Pathol 154: 525-536.

972. Ghotli ZA, Serra S, Chetty R (2007). Clear cell (glycogen rich) gastric adenocarcinoma: a distinct tubulo-papillary variant with a predilection for the cardia/gastro-oesophageal region. Pathology 39: 466-469.

973. Giannitrapani L, Soresi M, La Spada E., Cervello M, D'Alessandro N, Montalto G (2006). Sex hormones and risk of liver tumor. Ann N Y Acad Sci 1089: 228-236.

974. Giardiello FM, Brensinger JD, Luce MC, Petersen GM, Cayouette MC, Krush AJ et al. (1997). Phenotypic expression of disease in families that have mutations in the 5' region of the adenomatous polyposis coli gene. Ann Intern Med 126: 514-519.

975. Giardiello FM, Brensinger JD, Petersen GM (2001). AGA technical review on hereditary colorectal cancer and genetic testing. Gastroenterology 121: 198-213.

976. Giardiello FM, Brensinger JD, Petersen

GM, Luce MC, Hylind LM, Bacon JA et al. (1997). The use and interpretation of commercial APC gene testing for familial adenomatous polyposis. N Engl J Med 336: 823-827.

977. Giardiello FM, Brensinger JD, Tersmette AC, Goodman SN, Petersen GM, Booker SV et al. (2000). Very high risk of cancer in familial Peutz-Jeghers syndrome. Gastroenterology 119: 1447-1453.

978. Giardiello FM, Hamilton SR, Kern SE, Offerhaus GJ, Green PA, Celano P et al. (1991). Colorectal neoplasia in juvenile polyposis or juvenile polyps. Arch Dis Child 66: 971-975.

979. Giardiello FM, Krush AJ, Petersen GM, Booker SV, Kerr M, Tong LL et al. (1994). Phenotypic variability of familial adenomatous polyposis in 11 unrelated families with identical APC gene mutation. Gastroenterology 106: 1542-1547.

980. Giardiello FM, Petersen GM, Brensinger JD, Luce MC, Cayouette MC, Bacon J et al. (1996). Hepatoblastoma and APC gene mutation in familial adenomatous polyposis. Gut 39: 867-869.

981. Giardiello FM, Petersen GM, Piantadosi S, Gruber SB, Traboulsi EI, Offerhaus GJ et al. (1997). APC gene mutations and extraintestinal phenotype of familial adenomatous polyposis. Gut 40: 521-525.

982. Giardiello FM, Trimbath JD (2006). Peutz-Jeghers syndrome and management recommendations. Clin Gastroenterol Hepatol 4: 408-415.

983. Giardiello FM, Welsh SB, Hamilton SR, Offerhaus GJ, Gittelsohn AM, Booker SV et al. (1987). Increased risk of cancer in the Peutz-Jeghers syndrome. N Engl J Med 316: 1511-1514.

984. Gibson GE, Ahmed I (2001). Perianal and genital basal cell carcinoma: A clinicopathologic review of 51 cases. J Am Acad Dermatol 45: 68-71.

985. Gibson JA, Hornick JL (2009). Mucosal Schwann cell "hamartoma": clinicopathologic study of 26 neural colorectal polyps distinct from neurofibromas and mucosal neuromas. Am J Surg Pathol 33: 781-787.

986. Giercksky KE, Halse J, Mathisen W, Gjone E, Flatmark A (1980). Endocrine tumors of the pancreas. Scand J Gastroenterol 15: 129-135.

987. Gifaldi AS, Petros JG, Wolfe GR (1992). Metastatic breast carcinoma presenting as persistent diarrhea. J Surg Oncol 51: 211-215.

988. Gill SS, Heuman DM, Mihas AA (2001). Small intestinal neoplasms. J Clin Gastroenterol 33: 267-282.

989. Gillen CD, Walmsley RS, Prior P, Andrews HA, Allan RN (1994). Ulcerative colitis and Crohn's disease: a comparison of the colorectal cancer risk in extensive colitis. Gut 35: 1590-1592.

990. Gillen CD, Wilson CA, Walmsley RS, Sanders DS, O'Dwyer ST, Allan RN (1995). Occult small bowel adenocarcinoma complicating Crohn's disease: a report of three cases. Postgrad Med J 71: 172-174.

991. Gilloteaux J, Combetta J (2005). Carcinoma in situ of the cystic duct. Ultrastruct Pathol 29: 79-84.

992. Gimm O, ttie-Bitach T, Lees JA, Vekemans M, Eng C (2000). Expression of the PTEN tumour suppressor protein during human development. Hum Mol Genet 9: 1633-1639.

993. Gisbertz IA, Jonkers DM, Arends JW, Bot FJ, Stockbrugger RW, Vrints LW et al. (1997). Specific detection of Helicobacter pylori and non-Helicobacter pylori flora in small- and large-cell primary gastric B-cell non-Hodgkin's lymphoma. Ann Oncol 8 Suppl 2: 33-36.

994. Gleason BC, Hornick JL (2008). Inflammatory myofibroblastic tumours: where are

we now? J Clin Pathol 61: 428-437.

995. Gledhill A, Hall PA, Cruse JP, Pollock DJ (1986). Enteroendocrine cell hyperplasia, carcinoid tumours and adenocarcinoma in long-standing ulcerative colitis. Histopathology 10: 501-508.

996. Gleeson CM, Sloan JM, McManus DT, Maxwell P, Arthur K, McGuigan JA et al. (1998). Comparison of p53 and DNA content abnormalities in adenocarcinoma of the oesophagus and gastric cardia. Br J Cancer 77: 277-286.

997. Glickman JN, Chen YY, Wang HH, Antonioli DA, Odze RD (2001). Phenotypic characteristics of a distinctive multilayered epithelium suggests that it is a precursor in the development of Barrett's esophagus. Am J Surg Pathol 25: 569-578.

998. Glickman MH, Hart MJ, White TT (1980). Insulinoma in Seattle: 39 cases in 30 years. Am J Surg 140: 119-125.

999. Goatly A, Bacon CM, Nakamura S, Ye H, Kim I, Brown PJ et al. (2008). FOXP1 abnormalities in lymphoma: translocation breakpoint mapping reveals insights into deregulated transcriptional control. Mod Pathol 21: 902-911.

1000. Gobet R (2009). Alternative management of bladder exstrophy. Curr Opin Urol 19: 424-426.

1001. Goddard MJ, Lonsdale RN (1992). The histogenesis of appendiceal carcinoid tumours. Histopathology 20: 345-349.

1002. Godwin JD (1975). Carcinoid tumors. An analysis of 2,837 cases. Cancer 36: 560-569.

1003. Goebel SU, Heppner C, Burns AL, Marx SJ, Spiegel AM, Zhuang Z et al. (2000). Genotype/phenotype correlation of multiple endocrine neoplasia type 1 gene mutations in sporadic gastrinomas. J Clin Endocrinol Metab 85: 116-123.

1004. Goede AC, Caplin ME, Winslet MC (2003). Carcinoid tumour of the appendix. Br J Surg 90: 1317-1322.

1005. Goedert M, Otten U, Suda K, Heitz PU, Stalder GA, Obrecht JP et al. (1980). Dopamine, norepinephrine and serotonin production by an intestinal carcinoid tumor. Cancer 45: 104-107.

1006. Goetz M, Toermer T, Vieth M, Dunbar K, Hoffman A, Galle PR et al. (2009). Simultaneous confocal laser endomicroscopy and chromoendoscopy with topical cresyl violet. Gastrointest Endosc 70: 959-968.

1007. Goggins M, Offerhaus GJ, Hilgers W, Griffin CA, Shekher M, Tang D et al. (1998). Pancreatic adenocarcinomas with DNA replication errors (RER+) are associated with wild-type K-ras and characteristic histopathology. Poor differentiation, a syncytial growth pattern, and pushing borders suggest RER+. Am J Pathol 152: 1501-1507.

1008. Goggins M, Schutte M, Lu J, Moskaluk CA, Weinstein CL, Petersen GM et al. (1996). Germline BRCA2 gene mutations in patients with apparently sporadic pancreatic carcinomas. Cancer Res 56: 5360-5364.

1009. Goggins M, Shekher M, Turnacioglu K, Yeo CJ, Hruban RH, Kern SE (1998). Genetic alterations of the transforming growth factor beta receptor genes in pancreatic and biliary adenocarcinomas. Cancer Res 58: 5329-5332.

1010. Goh BK, Tan YM, Chung YF, Chow PK, Cheow PC, Wong WK et al. (2006). A review of mucinous cystic neoplasms of the pancreas defined by ovarian-type stroma: clinicopathological features of 344 patients. World J Surg 30: 2236-2245.

1011. Goldblum JR, Appelman HD (1995). Stromal tumors of the duodenum. A histologic and immunohistochemical study of 20 cases. Am J Surg Pathol 19: 71-80.

1012. Goldblum JR, Hart WR (1998). Perianal Paget's disease: a histologic and immunohistochemical study of 11 cases with and without

associated rectal adenocarcinoma. Am J Surg Pathol 22: 170-179.
1013. Goldblum JR, Rice TW, Zuccaro G, Richter JE (1996). Granular cell tumors of the esophagus: a clinical and pathologic study of 13 cases. Ann Thorac Surg 62: 860-865.
1014. Goldfarb WB, Bennett D, Monafo W (1963). Carcinoma in heterotopic gastric pancreas. Ann Surg 158: 56-58.
1015. Goldie SJ, Kuntz KM, Weinstein MC, Freedberg KA, Welton ML, Palefsky JM (1999). The clinical effectiveness and cost-effectiveness of screening for anal squamous intraepithelial lesions in homosexual and bisexual HIV-positive men. JAMA 281: 1822-1829.
1016. Goldman S, Auer G, Erhardt K, Seligson U (1987). Prognostic significance of clinical stage, histologic grade, and nuclear DNA content in squamous-cell carcinoma of the anus. Dis Colon Rectum 30: 444-448.
1017. Goldstein AM, Fraser MC, Struewing JP, Hussussian CJ, Ranade K, Zametkin DP et al. (1995). Increased risk of pancreatic cancer in melanoma-prone kindreds with p16INK4 mutations. N Engl J Med 333: 970-974.
1018. Goldstein J, Benharroch D, Sion-Vardy N, Arish A, Levy I, Maor E (1994). Solid cystic and papillary tumor of the pancreas with oncocytic differentiation. J Surg Oncol 56: 63-67.
1019. Goldstein NS (2006). Small colonic microsatellite unstable adenocarcinomas and high-grade epithelial dysplasias in sessile serrated adenoma polypectomy specimens: a study of eight cases. Am J Clin Pathol 125: 132-145.
1020. Goldstein NS, Bassi D (2001). Cytokeratins 7, 17, and 20 reactivity in pancreatic and ampulla of vater adenocarcinomas. Percentage of positivity and distribution is affected by the cut-point threshold. Am J Clin Pathol 115: 695-702.
1021. Goldstein NS, Bhanot P, Odish E, Hunter S (2003). Hyperplastic-like colon polyps that preceded microsatellite-unstable adenocarcinomas. Am J Clin Pathol 119: 778-796.
1022. Goldstein NS, Hart J (1999). Histologic features associated with lymph node metastasis in stage T1 and superficial T2 rectal adenocarcinomas in abdominoperineal resection specimens. Identifying a subset of patients for whom treatment with adjuvant therapy or completion abdominoperineal resection should be considered after local excision. Am J Clin Pathol 111: 51-58.
1023. Golioto M, McGrath K (2001). Primary lymphoma of the esophagus in a chronically immunosuppressed patient with hepatitis C infection: case report and review of the literature. Am J Med Sci 321: 203-205.
1024. Gonzalez CA, Jakszyn P, Pera G, Agudo A, Bingham S, Palli D et al. (2006). Meat intake and risk of stomach and esophageal adenocarcinoma within the European Prospective Investigation Into Cancer and Nutrition (EPIC). J Natl Cancer Inst 98: 345-354.
1025. Gonzalez CA, Pera G, Agudo A, Palli D, Krogh V, Vineis P et al. (2003). Smoking and the risk of gastric cancer in the European Prospective Investigation Into Cancer and Nutrition (EPIC). Int J Cancer 107: 629-634.
1026. Gonzalez-Crussi F (1991). Undifferentiated small cell ("anaplastic") hepatoblastoma. Pediatr Pathol 11: 155-161.
1027. Gonzalez-Crussi F, Goldschmidt RA, Hsueh W, Trujillo YP (1982). Infantile sarcoma with intracytoplasmic filamentous inclusions: distinctive tumor of possible histiocytic origin. Cancer 49: 2365-2375.
1028. Goodman ZD, Albores-Saavedra J, Lundblad DM (1984). Somatostatinoma of the cystic duct. Cancer 53: 498-502.
1029. Goodman ZD, Ishak KG (1984). Angiomyolipomas of the liver. Am J Surg Pathol 8: 745-750.
1030. Goodman ZD, Ishak KG, Langloss JM, Sesterhenn IA, Rabin L (1985). Combined hepatocellular-cholangiocarcinoma. A histologic and immunohistochemical study. Cancer 55: 124-135.
1031. Goodnight J, Venook A, Ames M, Taylor C, Gilden R, Figlin RA (1996). Practice guidelines for esophageal cancer. Cancer J Sci Am 2: S37-S43.
1032. Gopez EV, Mourelatos Z, Rosato EF, Livolsi VA (1997). Acute appendicitis secondary to metastatic bronchogenic adenocarcinoma. Am Surg 63: 778-780.
1033. Gordon DL, Lo MC, Schwartz MA (1971). Carcinoid of the pancreas. Am J Med 51: 412-415.
1034. Gore RM, Mehta UK, Berlin JW, Rao V, Newmark GM (2006). Diagnosis and staging of small bowel tumours. Cancer Imaging 6: 209-212.
1035. Gornicka B, Ziarkiewicz-Wroblewska B, Michalowicz B, Pawlak J, Wroblewski T, Krawczyk M et al. (2001). Immature hepatic tumor of bimodal differentiation in a young adult patient: a novel lesion expressing beta-catenin and mimicking a distinct phase of hepatogenesis. J Hepatol 34: 955-961.
1036. Gortz B, Roth J, Krahenmann A, de Krijger RR, Muletta-Feurer S, Rutimann K et al. (1999). Mutations and allelic deletions of the *MEN1* gene are associated with a subset of sporadic endocrine pancreatic and neuroendocrine tumors and not restricted to foregut neoplasms. Am J Pathol 154: 429-436.
1037. Gorunova L, Johansson B, Dawiskiba S, ndren-Sandberg A, Jin Y, Mandahl N et al. (1995). Massive cytogenetic heterogeneity in a pancreatic carcinoma: fifty-four karyotypically unrelated clones. Genes Chromosomes Cancer 14: 259-266.
1038. Goseki N, Koike M, Yoshida M (1992). Histopathologic characteristics of early stage esophageal carcinoma. A comparative study with gastric carcinoma. Cancer 69: 1088-1093.
1039. Goseki N, Takizawa T, Koike M (1992). Differences in the mode of the extension of gastric cancer classified by histological type: new histological classification of gastric carcinoma. Gut 33: 606-612.
1040. Gotchall J, Traweek ST, Stenzel P (1987). Benign oncocytic endocrine tumor of the pancreas in a patient with polyarteritis nodosa. Hum Pathol 18: 967-969.
1041. Gotoda T, Yanagisawa A, Sasako M, Ono H, Nakanishi Y, Shimoda T et al. (2000). Incidence of lymph node metastasis from early gastric cancer: estimation with a large number of cases at two large centers. Gastric Cancer 3: 219-225.
1042. Gottlieb CA, Meiri E, Maeda KM (1990). Rectal non-Hodgkin's lymphoma: a clinicopathologic study and review. Henry Ford Hosp Med J 38: 255-258.
1043. Govindarajan A, Baxter NN (2008). Lymph node evaluation in early-stage colon cancer. Clin Colorectal Cancer 7: 240-246.
1044. Grabenbauer GG, Lahmer G, Distel L, Niedobitek G (2006). Tumor-infiltrating cytotoxic T cells but not regulatory T cells predict outcome in anal squamous cell carcinoma. Clin Cancer Res 12: 3355-3360.
1045. Grabowski P, Schonfelder J, hnert-Hilger G, Foss HD, Heine B, Schindler I et al. (2002). Expression of neuroendocrine markers: a signature of human undifferentiated carcinoma of the colon and rectum. Virchows Arch 441: 256-263.
1046. Grady WM, Carethers JM (2008). Genomic and epigenetic instability in colorectal cancer pathogenesis. Gastroenterology 135: 1079-1099.
1047. Grady WM, Willis J, Guilford PJ, Dunbier AK, Toro TT, Lynch H et al. (2000). Methylation of the CDH1 promoter as the second genetic hit in hereditary diffuse gastric cancer. Nat Genet 26: 16-17.
1048. Graham DY (2003). The changing epidemiology of GERD: geography and *Helicobacter pylori*. Am J Gastroenterol 98: 1462-1470.
1049. Grama D, Skogseid B, Wilander E, Eriksson B, Martensson H, Cedermark B et al. (1992). Pancreatic tumors in multiple endocrine neoplasia type 1: clinical presentation and surgical treatment. World J Surg 16: 611-618.
1050. Granier G, Marty-Double C (2007). [Gastrointestinal adenocarcinomas with a choriocarcinomatous component: 2 cases and a review of 120 cases in the literature]. Gastroenterol Clin Biol 31: 854-857.
1051. Grapin C, Audry G, Josset P, Patte C, Sorrel DE, Gruner M (1994). Histiocytosis X revealed by complex anal fistula. Eur J Pediatr Surg 4: 184-185.
1052. Grau MV, Baron JA, Sandler RS, Wallace K, Haile RW, Church TR et al. (2007). Prolonged effect of calcium supplementation on risk of colorectal adenomas in a randomized trial. J Natl Cancer Inst 99: 129-136.
1053. Gray SG, Eriksson T, Ekstrom C, Holm S, von SD, Kogner P et al. (2000). Altered expression of members of the IGF-axis in hepatoblastomas. Br J Cancer 82: 1561-1567.
1054. Gray SG, Hartmann W, Eriksson T, Ekstrom C, Holm S, Kytola S et al. (2000). Expression of genes involved with cell cycle control, cell growth and chromatin modification are altered in hepatoblastomas. Int J Mol Med 6: 161-169.
1055. Green BT, Rockey DC (2001). Duodenal somatostatinoma presenting with complete somatostatinoma syndrome. J Clin Gastroenterol 33: 415-417.
1056. Green LK (1990). Hematogenous metastases to the stomach. A review of 67 cases. Cancer 65: 1596-1600.
1057. Green PH, O'Toole KM, Weinberg LM, Goldfarb JP (1981). Early gastric cancer. Gastroenterology 81: 247-256.
1058. Green PHR, Stavropoulos SN, Panagi SG, Goldstein SL, Mcmahon DJ, Absan H et al. (2001). Characteristics of adult celiac disease in the USA: results of a national survey. Am J Gastroenterol 96: 126-131.
1059. Greenberg RE, Bank S, Stark B (1990). Adenocarcinoma of the pancreas producing pancreatitis and pancreatic abscess. Pancreas 5: 108-113.
1060. Greene FL, Page DL, Fleming ID (eds) (2002). AJCC Cancer Staging Manual. Springer: New York.
1061. Greenson JK, Huang SC, Herron C, Moreno V, Bonner JD, Tomsho LP et al. (2009). Pathologic predictors of microsatellite instability in colorectal cancer. Am J Surg Pathol 33: 126-133.
1062. Greenstein AJ, Balasubramanian S, Harpaz N, Rizwan M, Sachar DB (1997). Carcinoid tumor and inflammatory bowel disease: a study of eleven cases and review of the literature. Am J Gastroenterol 92: 682-685.
1063. Greenstein AJ, Sachar DB, Smith H, Janowitz HD, Aufses AH, Jr. (1981). A comparison of cancer risk in Crohn's disease and ulcerative colitis. Cancer 48: 2742-2745.
1064. Griesser GH, Schumacher U, Elfeldt R, Horny HP (1985). Adenosquamous carcinoma of the ileum. Report of a case and review of the literature. Virchows Arch A Pathol Anat Histopathol 406: 483-487.
1065. Griffin CA, Hruban RH, Long PP, Morsberger LA, Douna-Issa F, Yeo CJ (1994). Chromosome abnormalities in pancreatic adenocarcinoma. Genes Chromosomes Cancer 9: 93-100.
1066. Griffin CA, Hruban RH, Morsberger LA, Ellingham T, Long PP, Jaffee EM et al. (1995). Consistent chromosome abnormalities in adenocarcinoma of the pancreas. Cancer Res 55: 2394-2399.
1067. Grigioni WF, D'errico A, Milani M, Villanacci V, Avellini C, Miglioli M et al. (1984). Early gastric cancer. Clinico-pathological analysis of 125 cases of early gastric cancer (EGC). Acta Pathol Jpn 34: 979-989.
1068. Grimelius L, Hultquist GT, Stenkvist B (1975). Cytological differentiation of asymptomatic pancreatic islet cell tumours in autopsy material. Virchows Arch A Pathol Anat Histol 365: 275-288.
1069. Groden J, Thliveris A, Samowitz W, Carlson M, Gelbert L, Albertsen H et al. (1991). Identification and characterization of the familial adenomatous polyposis coli gene. Cell 66: 589-600.
1070. Groisman GM, Polak-Charcon S (1998). Fibroepithelial polyps of the anus: a histologic, immunohistochemical, and ultrastructural study, including comparison with the normal anal subepithelial layer. Am J Surg Pathol 22: 70-76.
1071. Groisman GM, Polak-Charcon S (2008). Fibroblastic polyp of the colon and colonic perineurioma: 2 names for a single entity? Am J Surg Pathol 32: 1088-1094.
1072. Grove A, Vyberg B, Vyberg M (1991). Focal fatty change of the liver. A review and a case associated with continuous ambulatory peritoneal dialysis. Virchows Arch A Pathol Anat Histopathol 419: 69-75.
1073. Groves FD, Linet MS, Travis LB, Devesa SS (2000). Cancer surveillance series: non-Hodgkin's lymphoma incidence by histologic subtype in the United States from 1978 through 1995. J Natl Cancer Inst 92: 1240-1251.
1074. Grozinsky-Glasberg S, Kaltsas G, Gur C, Gal E, Thomas D, Fichman S et al. (2008). Long-acting somatostatin analogues are an effective treatment for type 1 gastric carcinoid tumours. Eur J Endocrinol 159: 475-482.
1075. Grunhage F, Jungck M, Lamberti C, Schulte-Witte H, Plassmann D, Becker U et al. (2008). Contribution of common monoallelic *MUTYH* gene variants in German patients with familial colorectal cancer. Cancer Biomark 4: 55-61.
1076. Grunwald GB (1993). The structural and functional analysis of cadherin calcium-dependent cell adhesion molecules. Curr Opin Cell Biol 5: 797-805.
1077. Grussendorf-Conen EI (1997). Anogenital premalignant and malignant tumors (including Buschke-Lowenstein tumors). Clin Dermatol 15: 377-388.
1078. Gu J, Tamura M, Yamada KM (1998). Tumor suppressor PTEN inhibits integrin- and growth factor-mediated mitogen-activated protein (MAP) kinase signaling pathways. J Cell Biol 143: 1375-1383.
1079. Guanrei Y, Sunglian Q (1987). Incidence rate of adenocarcinoma of the gastric cardia, and endoscopic classification of early cardial carcinoma in Henan Province, the People's Republic of China. Endoscopy 19: 7-10.
1080. Guglielmi A, Ruzzenente A, Campagnaro T, Pachera S, Valdegamberi A, Nicoli P et al. (2009). Intrahepatic cholangiocarcinoma: prognostic factors after surgical resection. World J Surg 33: 1247-1254.
1081. Guilford P, Hopkins J, Harraway J, McLeod M, McLeod N, Harawira P et al. (1998). E-cadherin germline mutations in familial gastric cancer. Nature 392: 402-405.
1082. Guilford PJ, Hopkins JB, Grady WM, Markowitz SD, Willis J, Lynch H et al. (1999). E-cadherin germline mutations define an inherited cancer syndrome dominated by diffuse gastric

cancer. Hum Mutat 14: 249-255.
1083. Guindi M, Riddell RH (2001). The pathology of epithelial pre-malignancy of the gastrointestinal tract. Best Pract Res Clin Gastroenterol 15: 191-210.
1084. Gunes D, Uysal KM, Cecen E, Cakmakci H, Ozer E, Akgur FM et al. (2008). Stromal-predominant mesenchymal hamartoma of the liver with elevated serum alpha-fetoprotein level. Pediatr Hematol Oncol 25: 685-692.
1085. Guo KJ, Yamaguchi K, Enjoji M (1988). Undifferentiated carcinoma of the gallbladder. A clinicopathologic, histochemical, and immunohistochemical study of 21 patients with a poor prognosis. Cancer 61: 1872-1879.
1086. Guo Y, Chen Z, Zhang L, Zhou F, Shi S, Feng X et al. (2008). Distinctive microRNA profiles relating to patient survival in esophageal squamous cell carcinoma. Cancer Res 68: 26-33.
1087. Gupta A, Subhas G, Mittal VK, Jacobs MJ (2009). Pancreatic schwannoma: literature review. J Surg Educ 66: 168-173.
1088. Gupta AK, Schoen RE (2009). Aberrant crypt foci: are they intermediate endpoints of colon carcinogenesis in humans? Curr Opin Gastroenterol 25: 59-65.
1089. Gupta NM, Goenka MK, Jindal A, Behera A, Vaiphei K (1996). Primary lymphoma of the esophagus. J Clin Gastroenterol 23: 203-206.
1090. Gupta RA, DuBois RN (2002). Cyclooxygenase-2 inhibitor therapy for the prevention of esophageal adenocarcinoma in Barrett's esophagus. J Natl Cancer Inst 94: 406-407.
1091. Gurbuz Y, Klöppel G (2004). Differentiation pathways in duodenal and ampullary carcinomas: a comparative study on mucin and trefoil peptide expression, including gastric and colon carcinomas. Virchows Arch 444: 536-541.
1092. Gusani NJ, Marsh JW, Nalesnik MA, Tublin ME, Gamblin TC (2008). Carcinoid of the extra-hepatic bile duct: a case report with long-term follow-up and review of literature. Am Surg 74: 87-90.
1093. Gustafsson BI, Siddique L, Chan A, Dong M, Drozdov I, Kidd M et al. (2008). Uncommon cancers of the small intestine, appendix and colon: an analysis of SEER 1973-2004, and current diagnosis and therapy. Int J Oncol 33: 1121-1131.
1094. Gutierrez-Gonzalez L, Wright NA (2008). Biology of intestinal metaplasia in 2008: more than a simple phenotypic alteration. Dig Liver Dis 40: 510-522.
1095. Gyde SN, Prior P, Allan RN, Stevens A, Jewell DP, Truelove SC et al. (1988). Colorectal cancer in ulcerative colitis: a cohort study of primary referrals from three centres. Gut 29: 206-217.
1096. Haas JE, Feusner JH, Finegold MJ (2001). Small cell undifferentiated histology in hepatoblastoma may be unfavorable. Cancer 92: 3130-3134.
1097. Haas JE, Muczynski KA, Krailo M, Ablin A, Land V, Vietti TJ et al. (1989). Histopathology and prognosis in childhood hepatoblastoma and hepatocarcinoma. Cancer 64: 1082-1095.
1098. Haas M, Dimmler A, Hohenberger W, Grabenbauer GG, Niedobitek G, Distel LV (2009). Stromal regulatory T-cells are associated with a favourable prognosis in gastric cancer of the cardia. BMC Gastroenterol 9: 65-
1099. Hagihara P, Vazquez MD, Parker JC, Jr., Griffen WO (1976). Carcinoma of anal-ductal origin: report of a case. Dis Colon Rectum 19: 694-701.
1100. Hahn SA, Schutte M, Hoque AT, Moskaluk CA, da Costa LT, Rozenblum E et al. (1996). *DPC4*, a candidate tumor suppressor gene at human chromosome 18q21.1. Science 271: 350-353.
1101. Hakanson R, Ekelund M, Sunlder F (1984). Activation and proliferation of gastric endocrine cells. In: Evolution and Tumor Pathology of the Neuroendocrine System. Falkmer S, Hakanson R, Sunlder F, eds. Elsevier: Amsterdam, pp. 371-398.
1102. Half E, Arber N (2009). Colon cancer: preventive agents and the present status of chemoprevention. Expert Opin Pharmacother 10: 211-219.
1103. Hameed O, Xu H, Saddeghi S, Maluf H (2007). Hepatoid carcinoma of the pancreas: a case report and literature review of a heterogeneous group of tumors. Am J Surg Pathol 31: 146-152.
1104. Hamelin R, Chalastanis A, Colas C, El BJ, Mercier D, Schreurs AS et al. (2008). [Clinical and molecular consequences of microsatellite instability in human cancers]. Bull Cancer 95: 121-132.
1105. Hamid QA, Bishop AE, Rode J, Dhillon AP, Rosenberg BF, Reed RJ et al. (1986). Duodenal gangliocytic paragangliomas: a study of 10 cases with immunocytochemical neuroendocrine markers. Hum Pathol 17: 1151-1157.
1106. Hamilton SR, Aaltonen LA (eds) (2000). WHO Classification of Tumours of the Digestive System. IARC: Lyon, France.
1107. Hamilton SR, Aaltonen LA (2010). Anus. In: AJCC cancer staging manual. Hamilton SR, Aaltonen LA, eds. Springer: New York, pp.
1108. Hamilton SR, Liu B, Parsons RE, Papadopoulos N, Jen J, Powell SM et al. (1995). The molecular basis of Turcot's syndrome. N Engl J Med 332: 839-847.
1109. Hammel PR, Vilgrain V, Terris B, Penfornis A, Sauvanet A, Correas JM et al. (2000). Pancreatic involvement in von Hippel-Lindau disease. The Groupe Francophone d'Etude de la Maladie de von Hippel-Lindau. Gastroenterology 119: 1087-1095.
1110. Hammond EH, Yowell RL, Flinner RL (1998). Neuroendocrine carcinomas: role of immunocytochemistry and electron microscopy. Hum Pathol 29: 1367-1371.
1111. Hampel H, Abraham NS, El-Serag HB (2005). Meta-analysis: obesity and the risk for gastroesophageal reflux disease and its complications. Ann Intern Med 143: 199-211.
1112. Han HJ, Maruyama M, Baba S, Park JG, Nakamura Y (1995). Genomic structure of human mismatch repair gene, *hMLH1*, and its mutation analysis in patients with hereditary non-polyposis colorectal cancer (HNPCC). Hum Mol Genet 4: 237-242.
1113. Han HS, Lee SY, Lee KY, Hong SN, Kim JH, Sung IK et al. (2009). Unclassified mucin phenotype of gastric adenocarcinoma exhibits the highest invasiveness. J Gastroenterol Hepatol 24: 658-666.
1114. Hanada K, Itoh M, Fujii K, Tsuchida A, Ooishi H, Kajiyama G (1996). K-ras and p53 mutations in stage I gallbladder carcinoma with an anomalous junction of the pancreaticobiliary duct. Cancer 77: 452-458.
1115. Hanada M, Nakano K, Ii Y, Yamashita H (1984). Carcinosarcoma of the esophagus with osseous and cartilagenous production. A combined study of keratin immunohistochemistry and electron microscopy. Acta Pathol Jpn 34: 669-678.
1116. Handra-Luca A, Condroyer C, de MC, Tepper M, Flejou JF, Thomas G et al. (2005). Vessels' morphology in SMAD4 and BMPR1A-related juvenile polyposis. Am J Med Genet A 138A: 113-117.
1117. Handra-Luca A, Couvelard A, Sauvanet A, Flejou JF, Degott C (2004). Mucinous cystadenoma with mesenchymal over-growth: a new variant among pancreatic mucinous cystadenomas? Virchows Arch 445: 203-205.
1118. Hans CP, Weisenburger DD, Greiner TC, Gascoyne RD, Delabie J, Ott G et al. (2004). Confirmation of the molecular classification of diffuse large B-cell lymphoma by immunohistochemistry using a tissue microarray. Blood 103: 275-282.
1119. Hanssen AM, Fryns JP (1995). Cowden syndrome. J Med Genet 32: 117-119.
1120. Haque S, Gopaldas RR, Plymyer MR, Glantz AI (2005). Pancreatic mass of unusual etiology: case report of metastatic disease after a prolonged lag phase. Am Surg 71: 1082-1085.
1121. Haraguchi M, Kinoshita H, Koori M, Tsuneoka N, Kosaka T, Ito Y et al. (2007). Multiple rectal carcinoids with diffuse ganglioneuromatosis. World J Surg Oncol 5: 19-
1122. Haramis AP, Begthel H, van den Born M, van Es J, Jonkheer S, Offerhaus GJ et al. (2004). De novo crypt formation and juvenile polyposis on BMP inhibition in mouse intestine. Science 303: 1684-1686.
1123. Haratake J, Hashimoto H (1995). An immunohistochemical analysis of 13 cases with combined hepatocellular and cholangiocellular carcinoma. Liver 15: 9-15.
1124. Haratake J, Yamada H, Horie A, Inokuma T (1992). Giant cell tumor-like cholangiocarcinoma associated with systemic cholelithiasis. Cancer 69: 2444-2448.
1125. Harewood GC, Baron TH, Stadheim LM, Kipp BR, Sebo TJ, Salomao DR (2004). Prospective, blinded assessment of factors influencing the accuracy of biliary cytology interpretation. Am J Gastroenterol 99: 1464-1469.
1126. Harris NL, Jaffe ES, Stein H, Banks PM, Chan JK, Cleary ML et al. (1994). A revised European-American classification of lymphoid neoplasms: a proposal from the International Lymphoma Study Group. Blood 84: 1361-1392.
1127. Hartel M, Wente MN, Sido B, Friess H, Buchler MW (2005). Carcinoid of the ampulla of Vater. J Gastroenterol Hepatol 20: 676-681.
1128. Hartmann EM, Ott G, Rosenwald A (2009). Molecular outcome prediction in mantle cell lymphoma. Future Oncol 5: 63-73.
1129. Haruta H, Hosoya Y, Sakuma K, Shibusawa H, Satoh K, Yamamoto H et al. (2008). Clinicopathological study of lymph-node metastasis in 1,389 patients with early gastric cancer: assessment of indications for endoscopic resection. J Dig Dis 9: 213-218.
1130. Hasegawa Y, Ishida Y, Kato K, Ijiri R, Miyake T, Nishimata S et al. (2003). Pancreatoblastoma. A case report with special emphasis on squamoid corpuscles with optically clear nuclei rich in biotin. Acta Cytol 47: 679-684.
1131. Hassan I, You YN, Shyyan R, Dozois EJ, Smyrk TC, Okuno SH et al. (2008). Surgically managed gastrointestinal stromal tumors: a comparative and prognostic analysis. Ann Surg Oncol 15: 52-59.
1132. Hassan MO, Gogate PA (1993). Malignant mixed exocrine-endocrine tumor of the pancreas with unusual intracytoplasmic inclusions. Ultrastruct Pathol 17: 483-493.
1133. Hassan R, Laszik ZG, Lerner M, Raffeld M, Postier R, Brackett D (2005). Mesothelin is overexpressed in pancreaticobiliary adenocarcinomas but not in normal pancreas and chronic pancreatitis. Am J Clin Pathol 124: 838-845.
1134. Hatano B, Ohshima K, Katoh A, Kanda M, Kawasaki C, Tsuchiya T et al. (2002). Non-HTLV-1-associated primary gastric T-cell lymphomas show cytotoxic activity: clinicopathological, immunohistochemical characteristics and TIA-1 expression in 31 cases. Histopathology 41: 421-436.
1135. Hatch GF, III, Wertheimer-Hatch L, Hatch KF, Davis GB, Blanchard DK, Foster RS, Jr. et al. (2000). Tumors of the esophagus. World J Surg 24: 401-411.
1136. Hattori Y, Odagiri H, Nakatani H, Miyagawa K, Naito K, Sakamoto H et al. (1990). *K-sam*, an amplified gene in stomach cancer, is a member of the heparin-binding growth factor receptor genes. Proc Natl Acad Sci U S A 87: 5983-5987.
1137. Hauso O, Gustafsson BI, Kidd M, Waldum HL, Drozdov I, Chan AK et al. (2008). Neuroendocrine tumor epidemiology: contrasting Norway and North America. Cancer 113: 2655-2664.
1138. Hawkins NJ, Gorman P, Tomlinson IP, Bullpitt P, Ward RL (2000). Colorectal carcinomas arising in the hyperplastic polyposis syndrome progress through the chromosomal instability pathway. Am J Pathol 157: 385-392.
1139. Haworth AC, Manley PN, Groll A, Pace R (1989). Bile duct carcinoma and biliary tract dysplasia in chronic ulcerative colitis. Arch Pathol Lab Med 113: 434-436.
1140. Hayashi I, Muto Y, Fujii Y, Morimatsu M (1987). Mucoepidermoid carcinoma of the stomach. J Surg Oncol 34: 94-99.
1141. Hayashi K, Yokozaki H, Goodison S, Oue N, Suzuki T, Lotan R et al. (2001). Inactivation of retinoic acid receptor beta by promoter CpG hypermethylation in gastric cancer. Differentiation 68: 13-21.
1142. Hayashi M, Matsui O, Ueda K, Kawamori Y, Kadoya M, Yoshikawa J et al. (1999). Correlation between the blood supply and grade of malignancy of hepatocellular nodules associated with liver cirrhosis: evaluation by CT during intraarterial injection of contrast medium. AJR Am J Roentgenol 172: 969-976.
1143. Hayashi Y, Inagaki K, Hirota S, Yoshikawa T, Ikawa H (1999). Epithelioid hemangioendothelioma with marked liver deformity and secondary Budd-Chiari syndrome: pathological and radiological correlation. Pathol Int 49: 547-552.
1144. Hayes-Jordan A, Andrassy R (2009). Rhabdomyosarcoma in children. Curr Opin Pediatr 21: 373-378.
1145. He TC, Sparks AB, Rago C, Hermeking H, Zawel L, da Costa LT et al. (1998). Identification of c-MYC as a target of the APC pathway. Science 281: 1509-1512.
1146. Hearle N, Schumacher V, Menko FH, Olschwang S, Boardman LA, Gille JJ et al. (2006). Frequency and spectrum of cancers in the Peutz-Jeghers syndrome. Clin Cancer Res 12: 3209-3215.
1147. Hearle NC, Rudd MF, Lim W, Murday V, Lim AG, Phillips RK et al. (2006). Exonic STK11 deletions are not a rare cause of Peutz-Jeghers syndrome. J Med Genet 43: e15-
1148. Hebbard PC, MacMillan A, Huntsman D, Kaurah P, Carneiro F, Wen X et al. (2009). Prophylactic total gastrectomy (PTG) for hereditary diffuse gastric cancer (HDGC): the Newfoundland experience with 23 patients. Ann Surg Oncol 16: 1890-1895.
1149. Heerema-McKenney A, Leuschner I, Smith N, Sennesh J, Finegold MJ (2005). Nested stromal epithelial tumor of the liver: six cases of a distinctive pediatric neoplasm with frequent calcifications and association with cushing syndrome. Am J Surg Pathol 29: 10-20.
1150. Heidet L, Boye E, Cai Y, Sado Y, Zhang X, Flejou JF et al. (1998). Somatic deletion of the 5' ends of both the COL4A5 and COL4A6 genes in a sporadic leiomyoma of the esophagus. Am J Pathol 152: 673-678.
1151. Heidet L, Dahan K, Zhou J, Xu Z, Cochat P, Gould JD et al. (1995). Deletions of both alpha 5(IV) and alpha 6(IV) collagen genes in Alport syndrome and in Alport syndrome associated with smooth muscle tumours. Hum Mol Genet 4: 99-108.
1152. Heidl G, Langhans P, Krieg V, Mellin W, Schilke R, Bunte H (1993). Comparative studies of cardia carcinoma and infracardial gastric car-

cinoma. J Cancer Res Clin Oncol 120: 91-94.
1153. Heinrich MC, Rubin BP, Longley BJ, Fletcher JA (2002). Biology and genetic aspects of gastrointestinal stromal tumors: KIT activation and cytogenetic alterations. Hum Pathol 33: 484-495.
1154. Heise W, Arasteh K, Mostertz P, Skorde J, Schmidt W, Obst C et al. (1997). Malignant gastrointestinal lymphomas in patients with AIDS. Digestion 58: 218-224.
1155. Heitman SJ, Ronksley PE, Hilsden RJ, Manns BJ, Rostom A, Hemmelgarn BR (2009). Prevalence of Adenomas and Colorectal Cancer in Average Risk Individuals: A Systematic Review and Meta-Analysis. Clin Gastroenterol Hepatol 7: 1272-1278.
1156. Heitz PU (1984). Pancreatic endocrine tumors. In: Pancreatic pathology. Klöppel G, Heitz PU, eds. Churchill Livingstone: Edinburgh/New York, pp. 206-232.
1157. Helicobacter and Cancer Collaborative Group (2001). Gastric cancer and *Helicobacter pylori*: a combined analysis of 12 case control studies nested within prospective cohorts. Gut 49: 347-353.
1158. Helmberger TK, Ros PR, Mergo PJ, Tomczak R, Reiser MF (1999). Pediatric liver neoplasms: a radiologic-pathologic correlation. Eur Radiol 9: 1339-1347.
1159. Hemminki A, Markie D, Tomlinson I, Avizienyte E, Roth S, Loukola A et al. (1998). A serine/threonine kinase gene defective in Peutz-Jeghers syndrome. Nature 391: 184-187.
1160. Hemminki A, Tomlinson I, Markie D, Jarvinen H, Sistonen P, Bjorkqvist AM et al. (1997). Localization of a susceptibility locus for Peutz-Jeghers syndrome to 19p using comparative genomic hybridization and targeted linkage analysis. Nat Genet 15: 87-90.
1161. Hemminki K, Li X (2001). Incidence trends and risk factors of carcinoid tumors: a nationwide epidemiologic study from Sweden. Cancer 92: 2204-2210.
1162. Hemminki K, Li X (2003). Familial and second primary pancreatic cancers: a nationwide epidemiologic study from Sweden. Int J Cancer 103: 525-530.
1163. Hemminki K, Li X (2003). Familial liver and gall bladder cancer: a nationwide epidemiological study from Sweden. Gut 52: 592-596.
1164. Hemminki K, Li X, Sundquist J, Sundquist K (2008). Cancer risks in ulcerative colitis patients. Int J Cancer 123: 1417-1421.
1165. Hempen PM, Zhang L, Bansal RK, Iacobuzio-Donahue CA, Murphy KM, Maitra A et al. (2003). Evidence of selection for clones having genetic inactivation of the activin A type II receptor (ACVR2) gene in gastrointestinal cancers. Cancer Res 63: 994-999.
1166. Hendriks YM, De Jong AE, Morreau H, Tops CM, Vasen HF, Wijnen JT et al. (2006). Diagnostic approach and management of Lynch syndrome (hereditary nonpolyposis colorectal carcinoma): a guide for clinicians. CA Cancer J Clin 56: 213-225.
1167. Henke AC, Kelley CM, Jensen CS, Timmerman TG (2001). Fine-needle aspiration cytology of pancreatoblastoma. Diagn Cytopathol 25: 118-121.
1168. Henne-Bruns D, Vogel I, Luttges J, Klöppel G, Kremer B (1998). Ductal adenocarcinoma of the pancreas head: survival after regional versus extended lymphadenectomy. Hepatogastroenterology 45: 855-866.
1169. Hennies HC, Hagedorn M, Reis A (1995). Palmoplantar keratoderma in association with carcinoma of the esophagus maps to chromosome 17q distal to the keratin gene cluster. Genomics 29: 537-540.
1170. Henson DE, Albores-Saavedra J, Corle D (1992). Carcinoma of the extrahepatic bile ducts. Histologic types, stage of disease, grade, and survival rates. Cancer 70: 1498-1501.
1171. Henson DE, Albores-Saavedra J, Corle D (1992). Carcinoma of the gallbladder. Histologic types, stage of disease, grade, and survival rates. Cancer 70: 1493-1497.
1172. Henson DE, Albores-Saavedra J, Schwartz AM, Batich K (2009). Field cancerization in derivatives of the embryonic foregut : an observation based on epidemiological patterns. In: Clinical utility of molecular signatures in cancer fields. Dakubo GD, ed. Nova Science:
1173. Henson DE, Schwartz AM, Nsouli H, Albores-Saavedra J (2009). Carcinomas of the pancreas, gallbladder, extrahepatic bile ducts, and ampulla of vater share a field for carcinogenesis: a population-based study. Arch Pathol Lab Med 133: 67-71.
1174. Herbertson RA, Scarsbrook AF, Lee ST, Tebbutt N, Scott AM (2009). Established, emerging and future roles of PET/CT in the management of colorectal cancer. Clin Radiol 64: 225-237.
1175. Herman JM, Swartz MJ, Hsu CC, Winter J, Pawlik TM, Sugar E et al. (2008). Analysis of fluorouracil-based adjuvant chemotherapy and radiation after pancreaticoduodenectomy for ductal adenocarcinoma of the pancreas: results of a large, prospectively collected database at the Johns Hopkins Hospital. J Clin Oncol 26: 3503-3510.
1176. Hermanek P (1991). Staging of exocrine pancreatic carcinoma. Eur J Surg Oncol 17: 167-172.
1177. Hernandez L, Fest T, Cazorla M, Teruya-Feldstein J, Bosch F, Peinado MA et al. (1996). *p53* gene mutations and protein overexpression are associated with aggressive variants of mantle cell lymphomas. Blood 87: 3351-3359.
1178. Hernegger GS, Moore HG, Guillem JG (2002). Attenuated familial adenomatous polyposis: an evolving and poorly understood entity. Dis Colon Rectum 45: 127-134.
1179. Hes FJ, Nielsen M, Bik EC, Konvalinka D, Wijnen JT, Bakker E et al. (2008). Somatic APC mosaicism: an underestimated cause of polyposis coli. Gut 57: 71-76.
1180. Heselmeyer K, du MS, Blegen H, Friberg B, Svensson C, Schrock E et al. (1997). A recurrent pattern of chromosomal aberrations and immunophenotypic appearance defines anal squamous cell carcinomas. Br J Cancer 76: 1271-1278.
1181. Hessman O, Lindberg D, Einarsson A, Lillhager P, Carling T, Grimelius L et al. (1999). Genetic alterations on 3p, 11q13, and 18q in nonfamilial and MEN 1-associated pancreatic endocrine tumors. Genes Chromosomes Cancer 26: 258-264.
1182. Hessman O, Lindberg D, Skogseid B, Carling T, Hellman P, Rastad J et al. (1998). Mutation of the multiple endocrine neoplasia type 1 gene in nonfamilial, malignant tumors of the endocrine pancreas. Cancer Res 58: 377-379.
1183. Heymann MF, Fiche M, Dubois-Gordeeff A, Chetritt J, Cloarec D, Guiberteau B et al. (1997). Endocrine cell carcinoma (carcinoid tumour) of the gallbladder producing pancreatic polypeptide and somatostatin. Histopathology 30: 606-607.
1184. Hibi K, Kondo K, Akiyama S, Ito K, Takagi H (1995). Frequent genetic instability in small intestinal carcinomas. Jpn J Cancer Res 86: 357-360.
1185. Hibi T, Ojima H, Sakamoto Y, Kosuge T, Shimada K, Sano T et al. (2006). A solid pseudopapillary tumor arising from the greater omentum followed by multiple metastases with increasing malignant potential. J Gastroenterol 41: 276-281.
1186. Hibi Y, Fukushima N, Tsuchida A, Sofuni A, Itoi T, Moriyasu F et al. (2007). Pancreatic juice cytology and subclassification of intraductal papillary mucinous neoplasms of the pancreas. Pancreas 34: 197-204.
1187. Hidaka E, Yanagisawa A, Seki M, Setoguchi T, Kato Y (2001). Genetic alterations and growth pattern in biliary duct carcinomas: loss of heterozygosity at chromosome 5q bears a close relation with polypoid growth. Gut 48: 656-659.
1188. Higashi D, Futami K, Kawahara K, Kamitani T, Seki K, Naritomi K et al. (2007). Study of colorectal cancer with Crohn's disease. Anticancer Res 27: 3771-3774.
1189. Higashi M, Yonezawa S, Ho JJ, Tanaka S, Irimura T, Kim YS et al. (1999). Expression of MUC1 and MUC2 mucin antigens in intrahepatic bile duct tumors: its relationship with a new morphological classification of cholangiocarcinoma. Hepatology 30: 1347-1355.
1190. Higgins GA, Recant L, Fischman AB (1979). The glucagonoma syndrome: surgically curable diabetes. Am J Surg 137: 142-148.
1191. Higham AD, Bishop LA, Dimaline R, Blackmore CG, Dobbins AC, Varro A et al. (1999). Mutations of RegIalpha are associated with enterochromaffin-like cell tumor development in patients with hypergastrinemia. Gastroenterology 116: 1310-1318.
1192. Higuchi T, Sugihara K, Jass JR (2005). Demographic and pathological characteristics of serrated polyps of colorectum. Histopathology 47: 32-40.
1193. Hilgers W, Groot KB, Geradts J, Tang DJ, Yeo CJ, Hruban RH et al. (2000). Genomic FHIT analysis in RER+ and RER- adenocarcinomas of the pancreas. Genes Chromosomes Cancer 27: 239-243.
1194. Hill DA, Swanson PE, Anderson K, Covinsky MH, Finn LS, Ruchelli ED et al. (2005). Desmoplastic nested spindle cell tumor of liver: report of four cases of a proposed new entity. Am J Surg Pathol 29: 1-9.
1195. Hillman LC, Chiragakis L, Clarke AC, Kaushik SP, Kaye GL (2003). Barrett's esophagus: Macroscopic markers and the prediction of dysplasia and adenocarcinoma. J Gastroenterol Hepatol 18: 526-533.
1196. Hippelainen M, Eskelinen M, Lipponen P, Chang F, Syrjanen K (1993). Mitotic activity index, volume corrected mitotic index and human papilloma-virus suggestive morphology are not prognostic factors in carcinoma of the oesophagus. Anticancer Res 13: 677-681.
1197. Hirabayashi K, Nakamura N, Kajiwara H, Hori S, Kawaguchi Y, Yamashita T et al. (2009). Perivascular epithelioid cell tumor (PEComa) of the pancreas: immunoelectron microscopy and review of the literature. Pathol Int 59: 650-655.
1198. Hirano H, Okimura A, Nakasho K, Nishigami T, Uematsu K, Tamura K (2004). Familial adenomatous polyposis associated with colon carcinoma, desmoid tumour, gallbladder carcinoma, and endometrioid carcinoma: a case report. Histopathology 45: 642-643.
1199. Hirano K, Yamashita K, Yamashita N, Nakatsumi Y, Esumi H, Kawashima A et al. (2002). Non-Hodgkin's lymphoma in a patient with probable hereditary nonpolyposis colon cancer: report of a case and review of the literature. Dis Colon Rectum 45: 273-279.
1200. Hirasawa T, Gotoda T, Miyata S, Kato Y, Shimoda T, Taniguchi H et al. (2009). Incidence of lymph node metastasis and the feasibility of endoscopic resection for undifferentiated-type early gastric cancer. Gastric Cancer 12: 148-152.
1201. Hirata D, Yamabuki T, Miki D, Ito T, Tsuchiya E, Fujita M et al. (2009). Involvement of epithelial cell transforming sequence-2 oncoantigen in lung and esophageal cancer progression. Clin Cancer Res 15: 256-266.
1202. Hirata K, Sato T, Mukaiya M, Yamashiro K, Kimura M, Sasaki K et al. (1997). Results of 1001 pancreatic resections for invasive ductal adenocarcinoma of the pancreas. Arch Surg 132: 771-776.
1203. Hirata Y, Sakamoto N, Yamamoto H, Matsukura S, Imura H, Okada S (1976). Gastric carcinoid with ectopic production of ACTH and beta-MSH. Cancer 37: 377-385.
1204. Hirono S, Tani M, Kawai M, Ina S, Nishioka R, Miyazawa M et al. (2009). Treatment strategy for intraductal papillary mucinous neoplasm of the pancreas based on malignant predictive factors. Arch Surg 144: 345-349.
1205. Hirono S, Tani M, Terasawa H, Kawai M, Ina S, Uchiyama K et al. (2008). A collision tumor composed of cancers of the bile duct and ampulla of Vater—immunohistochemical analysis of a rare entity of double cancer. Hepatogastroenterology 55: 861-864.
1206. Hirota S, Isozaki K, Moriyama Y, Hashimoto K, Nishida T, Ishiguro S et al. (1998). Gain-of-function mutations of c-kit in human gastrointestinal stromal tumors. Science 279: 577-580.
1207. Hirota WK, Loughney TM, Lazas DJ, Maydonovitch CL, Rholl V, Wong RK (1999). Specialized intestinal metaplasia, dysplasia, and cancer of the esophagus and esophagogastric junction: prevalence and clinical data. Gastroenterology 116: 277-285.
1208. Hirschman BA, Pollock BH, Tomlinson GE (2005). The spectrum of APC mutations in children with hepatoblastoma from familial adenomatous polyposis kindreds. J Pediatr 147: 263-266.
1209. Hisa T, Nobukawa B, Suda K, Ohkubo H, Shiozawa S, Ishigame H et al. (2007). Intraductal carcinoma with complex fusion of tubular glands without macroscopic mucus in main pancreatic duct: dilemma in classification. Pathol Int 57: 741-745.
1210. Hisamichi S, Sugawara N (1984). Mass screening for gastric cancer by X-ray examination. Jpn J Clin Oncol 14: 211-223.
1211. Hisamori S, Nagayama S, Kita S, Kawamura J, Yoshizawa A, Sakai Y (2009). Rapid progression of submucosal invasive micropapillary carcinoma of the colon in progressive systemic sclerosis: report of a case. Jpn J Clin Oncol 39: 399-405.
1212. Hitchins MP, Ward RL (2009). Constitutional (germline) MLH1 epimutation as an aetiological mechanism for hereditary non-polyposis colorectal cancer. J Med Genet 46: 793-802.
1213. Hitchins MP, Wong JJ, Suthers G, Suter CM, Martin DI, Hawkins NJ et al. (2007). Inheritance of a cancer-associated MLH1 germline epimutation. N Engl J Med 356: 697-705.
1214. Hoang MP, Hruban RH, Albores-Saavedra J (2001). Clear cell endocrine pancreatic tumor mimicking renal cell carcinoma: a distinctive neoplasm of von Hippel-Lindau disease. Am J Surg Pathol 25: 602-609.
1215. Hoang MP, Murakata LA, Katabi N, Henson DE, Albores-Saavedra J (2002). Invasive papillary carcinomas of the extrahepatic bile ducts: a clinicopathologic and immunohistochemical study of 13 cases. Mod Pathol 15: 1251-1258.
1216. Hoang MP, Murakata LA, Padilla-Rodriguez AL, Albores-Saavedra J (2001). Metaplastic lesions of the extrahepatic bile ducts: a morphologic and immunohistochemical study. Mod Pathol 14: 1119-1125.
1217. Hobbs CM, Lowry MA, Owen D, Sobin LH (2001). Anal gland carcinoma. Cancer 92: 2045-2049.
1218. Hobbs RD, Stewart AF, Ravin ND, Carter D (1984). Hypercalcemia in small cell carcinoma of the pancreas. Cancer 53: 1552-1554.
1219. Hochwald SN, Zee S, Conlon KC, Colleoni R, Louie O, Brennan MF et al. (2002).

Prognostic factors in pancreatic endocrine neoplasms: an analysis of 136 cases with a proposal for low-grade and intermediate-grade groups. J Clin Oncol 20: 2633-2642.
1220. Hock YL, Scott KW, Grace RH (1993). Mixed adenocarcinoma/carcinoid tumour of large bowel in a patient with Crohn's disease. J Clin Pathol 46: 183-185.
1221. Hoda SA, Hajdu SI (1992). Small cell carcinoma of the esophagus. Cytology and immunohistology in four cases. Acta Cytol 36: 113-120.
1222. Hofler H, Klöppel G, Heitz PU (1984). Combined production of mucus, amines and peptides by goblet-cell carcinoids of the appendix and ileum. Pathol Res Pract 178: 555-561.
1223. Hofler H, Langer R, Ott K, Keller G (2007). Prediction of response to neoadjuvant chemotherapy in carcinomas of the upper gastrointestinal tract. Recent Results Cancer Res 176: 33-36.
1224. Hofler H, Ruhri C, Putz B, Wirnsberger G, Hauser H (1988). Oncogene expression in endocrine pancreatic tumors. Virchows Arch B Cell Pathol Incl Mol Pathol 55: 355-361.
1225. Hofmann JW, Fox PS, Wilson SD (1973). Duodenal wall tumors and the Zollinger-Ellison syndrome. Surgical management. Arch Surg 107: 334-339.
1226. Hofting I, Pott G, Stolte M (1993). [The syndrome of juvenile polyposis]. Leber Magen Darm 23: 107-108.
1227. Holen KD, Klimstra DS, Hummer A, Gonen M, Conlon K, Brennan M et al. (2002). Clinical characteristics and outcomes from an institutional series of acinar cell carcinoma of the pancreas and related tumors. J Clin Oncol 20: 4673-4678.
1228. Hollstein M, Marion MJ, Lehman T, Welsh J, Harris CC, Martel-Planche G et al. (1994). p53 mutations at A:T base pairs in angiosarcomas of vinyl chloride-exposed factory workers. Carcinogenesis 15: 1-3.
1229. Holly EA, Chaliha I, Bracci PM, Gautam M (2004). Signs and symptoms of pancreatic cancer: a population-based case-control study in the San Francisco Bay area. Clin Gastroenterol Hepatol 2: 510-517.
1230. Holm R, Tanum G, Karlsen F, Nesland JM (1994). Prevalence and physical state of human papillomavirus DNA in anal carcinomas. Mod Pathol 7: 449-453.
1231. Holmes F, Borek D, Owen-Kummer M, Hassanein R, Fishback J, Behbehani A et al. (1988). Anal cancer in women. Gastroenterology 95: 107-111.
1232. Honda S, Haruta M, Sugawara W, Sasaki F, Ohira M, Matsunaga T et al. (2008). The methylation status of RASSF1A promoter predicts responsiveness to chemotherapy and eventual cure in hepatoblastoma patients. Int J Cancer 123: 1117-1125.
1233. Honda T, Tamura G, Waki T, Kawata S, Terashima M, Nishizuka S et al. (2004). Demethylation of MAGE promoters during gastric cancer progression. Br J Cancer 90: 838-843.
1234. Hoorens A, Gebhard F, Kraft K, Lemoine NR, Klöppel G (1994). Pancreatoblastoma in an adult: its separation from acinar cell carcinoma. Virchows Arch 424: 485-490.
1235. Hoorens A, Lemoine NR, McLellan E, Morohoshi T, Kamisawa T, Heitz PU et al. (1993). Pancreatic acinar cell carcinoma. An analysis of cell lineage markers, p53 expression, and Ki-ras mutation. Am J Pathol 143: 685-698.
1236. Hoorens A, Prenzel K, Lemoine NR, Klöppel G (1998). Undifferentiated carcinoma of the pancreas: analysis of intermediate filament profile and Ki-ras mutations provides evidence of a ductal origin. J Pathol 185: 53-60.
1237. Hoots BE, Palefsky JM, Pimenta JM, Smith JS (2009). Human papillomavirus type distribution in anal cancer and anal intraepithelial lesions. Int J Cancer 124: 2375-2383.
1238. Horie A, Haratake J, Jimi A, Matsumoto M, Ishii N, Tsutsumi Y (1987). Pancreatoblastoma in Japan, with differential diagnosis from papillary cystic tumor (ductuloacinar adenoma) of the pancreas. Acta Pathol Jpn 37: 47-63.
1239. Horiuchi A, Watanabe Y, Yoshida M, Yamamoto Y, Kawachi K (2007). Metastatic osteosarcoma in the jejunum with intussusception: report of a case. Surg Today 37: 440-442.
1240. Horner MJ, Ries LAG, Krapcho M, Neyman N, Aminou R, Howlader N et al. (eds) (2009). SEER Cancer Statistics Review, 1975-2006, National Cancer Institute. Bethesda, MD, http://seer.cancer.gov/csr/1975_2006/, based on November 2008 SEER data submission, posted to the SEER web site.
1241. Hornick JL, Fletcher CD (2005). Intestinal perineuriomas: clinicopathologic definition of a new anatomic subset in a series of 10 cases. Am J Surg Pathol 29: 859-865.
1242. Hornick JL, Lauwers GY, Odze RD (2005). Immunohistochemistry can help distinguish metastatic pancreatic adenocarcinomas from bile duct adenomas and hamartomas of the liver. Am J Surg Pathol 29: 381-389.
1243. Horsch D, Fink T, Goke B, Arnold R, Buchler M, Weihe E (1994). Distribution and chemical phenotypes of neuroendocrine cells in the human anal canal. Regul Pept 54: 527-542.
1244. Horton JD, Lee S, Brown SR, Bader J, Meier DE (2009). Survival trends in children with hepatoblastoma. Pediatr Surg Int 25: 407-412.
1245. Horton KM, Jones B, Bayless TM, Lazenby AJ, Fishman EK (1994). Mucinous adenocarcinoma at the ileocecal valve mimicking Crohn's disease. Dig Dis Sci 39: 2276-2281.
1246. Hosaka S, Nakamura N, Akamatsu T, Fujisawa T, Ogiwara Y, Kiyosawa K et al. (2002). A case of primary low grade mucosa associated lymphoid tissue (MALT) lymphoma of the oesophagus. Gut 51: 281-284.
1247. Hosokawa O, Tsuda S, Kidani E, Watanabe K, Tanigawa Y, Shirasaki S et al. (1998). Diagnosis of gastric cancer up to three years after negative upper gastrointestinal endoscopy. Endoscopy 30: 669-674.
1248. Hosonuma K, Sato K, Honma M, Kashiwabara K, Takahashi H, Takagi H et al. (2008). Small-cell carcinoma of the extrahepatic bile duct: a case report and review of the literature. Hepatol Int 2: 129-132.
1249. Hough DM, Stephens DH, Johnson CD, Binkovitz LA (1994). Pancreatic lesions in von Hippel-Lindau disease: prevalence, clinical significance, and CT findings. AJR Am J Roentgenol 162: 1091-1094.
1250. Houghton J, Stoicov C, Nomura S, Rogers AB, Carlson J, Li H et al. (2004). Gastric cancer originating from bone marrow-derived cells. Science 306: 1568-1571.
1251. Houlston RS, Peto J (2004). The search for low-penetrance cancer susceptibility alleles. Oncogene 23: 6471-6476.
1251A. Houlston RS, Tomlinson IP (2001). Polymorphisms and colorectal tumor risk. Gastroenterology 121(2): 282-301
1251B. Houlston RS, Webb E, Broderick P, Pittman AM, Di Bernardo MC, Lubbe S (2008). Meta-analysis of genome-wide association data identifies four new susceptibility loci for colorectal cancer. Net Genet 40: 1426-1435
1252. House MG, Gonen M, Jarnagin WR, D'Angelica M, Dematteo RP, Fong Y et al. (2007). Prognostic significance of pathologic nodal status in patients with resected pancreatic cancer. J Gastrointest Surg 11: 1549-1555.
1253. Howard JM, Hess W (eds) (2002). History of the Pancreas: Mysteries of a Hidden Organ. Kluwer Academic/Penum Publishers: New York, NY.
1254. Howe JR, Bair JL, Sayed MG, Anderson ME, Mitros FA, Petersen GM et al. (2001). Germline mutations of the gene encoding bone morphogenetic protein receptor 1A in juvenile polyposis. Nat Genet 28: 184-187.
1255. Howe JR, Haidle JL, Lal G, Bair J, Song C, Pechman B et al. (2007). ENG mutations in MADH4/BMPR1A mutation negative patients with juvenile polyposis. Clin Genet 71: 91-92.
1256. Howe JR, Karnell LH, Menck HR, Scott-Conner C (1999). The American College of Surgeons Commission on Cancer and the American Cancer Society. Adenocarcinoma of the small bowel: review of the National Cancer Data Base, 1985-1995. Cancer 86: 2693-2706.
1257. Howe JR, Klimstra DS, Cordon-Cardo C, Paty PB, Park PY, Brennan MF (1997). K-ras mutation in adenomas and carcinomas of the ampulla of vater. Clin Cancer Res 3: 129-133.
1258. Howe JR, Mitros FA, Summers RW (1998). The risk of gastrointestinal carcinoma in familial juvenile polyposis. Ann Surg Oncol 5: 751-756.
1259. Howe JR, Ringold JC, Hughes JH, Summers RW (1999). Direct genetic testing for Smad4 mutations in patients at risk for juvenile polyposis. Surgery 126: 162-170.
1260. Howe JR, Ringold JC, Summers RW, Mitros FA, Nishimura DY, Stone EM (1998). A gene for familial juvenile polyposis maps to chromosome 18q21.1. Am J Hum Genet 62: 1129-1136.
1261. Howe JR, Roth S, Ringold JC, Summers RW, Jarvinen HJ, Sistonen P et al. (1998). Mutations in the *SMAD4/DPC4* gene in juvenile polyposis. Science 280: 1086-1088.
1262. Howel-Evans W, McConnell RB, Clarke CA, Sheppard PM (1958). Carcinoma of the oesophagus with keratosis palmaris et plantaris (tylosis): a study of two families. Q J Med 27: 413-429.
1263. Howell WM, Leung ST, Jones DB, Nakshabendi I, Hall MA, Lanchbury JS et al. (1995). HLA-DRB, -DQA, and -DQB polymorphism in celiac disease and enteropathy-associated T-cell lymphoma. Common features and additional risk factors for malignancy. Hum Immunol 43: 29-37.
1264. Howlett NG, Taniguchi T, Olson S, Cox B, Waisfisz Q, De Die-Smulders C et al. (2002). Biallelic inactivation of BRCA2 in Fanconi anemia. Science 297: 606-609.
1265. Hristov AC, Young RH, Vang R, Yemelyanova AV, Seidman JD, Ronnett BM (2007). Ovarian metastases of appendiceal tumors with goblet cell carcinoidlike and signet ring cell patterns: a report of 30 cases. Am J Surg Pathol 31: 1502-1511.
1266. Hruban RH, Adsay NV (2009). Molecular classification of neoplasms of the pancreas. Hum Pathol 40: 612-623.
1267. Hruban RH, Iacobuzio-Donahue C, Wilentz RE, Goggins M, Kern SE (2001). Molecular pathology of pancreatic cancer. Cancer J 7: 251-258.
1268. Hruban RH, Maitra A, Kern SE, Goggins M (2007). Precursors to pancreatic cancer. Gastroenterol Clin North Am 36: 831-49.
1269. Hruban RH, Petersen GM, Ha PK, Kern SE (1998). Genetics of pancreatic cancer. From genes to families. Surg Oncol Clin N Am 7: 1-23.
1270. Hruban RH, Pitman MB, and Klimstra DS (eds) (2007). Tumors of the Pancreas. Armed Forces Institute of Pathology: Washington, DC.
1271. Hruban RH, Takaori K, Klimstra DS, Adsay NV, Albores-Saavedra J, Biankin AV et al. (2004). An illustrated consensus on the classification of pancreatic intraepithelial neoplasia and intraductal papillary mucinous neoplasms. Am J Surg Pathol 28: 977-987.
1272. Hsu HC, Chen CC, Huang GT, Lee PH (1996). Clonal Epstein-Barr virus associated cholangiocarcinoma with lymphoepithelioma-like component. Hum Pathol 27: 848-850.
1273. Hsu JT, Yeh CN, Chen YR, Chen HM, Hwang TL, Jan YY et al. (2005). Adenosquamous carcinoma of the pancreas. Digestion 72: 104-108.
1274. Hu B, Gong B, Zhou DY (2003). Association of anomalous pancreaticobiliary ductal junction with gallbladder carcinoma in Chinese patients: an ERCP study. Gastrointest Endosc 57: 541-545.
1275. Hua Z, Zhang YC, Hu XM, Jia ZG (2003). Loss of DPC4 expression and its correlation with clinicopathological parameters in pancreatic carcinoma. World J Gastroenterol 9: 2764-2767.
1276. Huang CB, Eng HL, Chuang JH, Cheng YF, Chen WJ (1997). Primary Burkitt's lymphoma of the liver: report of a case with long-term survival after surgical resection and combination chemotherapy. J Pediatr Hematol Oncol 19: 135-138.
1277. Huang CS, O'Brien MJ, Yang S, Farraye FA (2004). Hyperplastic polyps, serrated adenomas, and the serrated polyp neoplasia pathway. Am J Gastroenterol 99: 2242-2255.
1278. Huang KH, Chen JH, Wu CW, Lo SS, Hsieh MC, Li AF et al. (2009). Factors affecting recurrence in node-negative advanced gastric cancer. J Gastroenterol Hepatol 24: 1522-1526.
1279. Huang L, Lang D, Geradts J, Obara T, Klein-Szanto AJ, Lynch HT et al. (1996). Molecular and immunochemical analyses of RB1 and cyclin D1 in human ductal pancreatic carcinomas and cell lines. Mol Carcinog 15: 85-95.
1280. Huang SC, Erdman SH (2009). Pediatric juvenile polyposis syndromes: an update. Curr Gastroenterol Rep 11: 211-219.
1281. Huang WS, Lin PY, Lee IL, Chin CC, Wang JY, Yang WG (2007). Metastatic Merkel cell carcinoma in the rectum: report of a case. Dis Colon Rectum 50: 1992-1995.
1282. Huang WT, Chuang SS, Huang CC, Lu CL, Eng HL (2007). Primary diffuse large B-cell lymphoma of the gallbladder with cholelithiasis masquerading as acute cholecystitis: case report and literature review. N Z Med J 120: U2470
1283. Huber J, Sovinz P, Freidl T, Jahnel J, Lackner H, Hollwarth M et al. (2008). Long term survival in two children with rhabdomyosarcoma of the biliary tract. Klin Padiatr 220: 378-379.
1284. Hubert C, Sempoux C, Berquin A, Deprez P, Jamar F, Gigot JF (2005). Bile duct carcinoid tumors: an uncommon disease but with a good prognosis? Hepatogastroenterology 52: 1042-1047.
1285. Hughes K, Kelty S, Martin R (2004). Hepatoid carcinoma of the pancreas. Am Surg 70: 1030-1033.
1286. Humar B, Fukuzawa R, Blair V, Dunbier A, More H, Charlton A et al. (2007). Destabilized adhesion in the gastric proliferative zone and c-Src kinase activation mark the development of early diffuse gastric cancer. Cancer Res 67: 2480-2489.
1287. Humar B, Guilford P (2009). Hereditary diffuse gastric cancer: a manifestation of lost cell polarity. Cancer Sci 100: 1151-1157.
1288. Huncharek M, Muscat J (1995). Small cell carcinoma of the esophagus. The Massachusetts General Hospital experience, 1978 to 1993. Chest 107: 179-181.
1289. Hunt SJ, Anderson WD (1990). Malignant rhabdoid tumor of the liver. A distinct clinicopathologic entity. Am J Clin Pathol 94: 645-648.
1290. Huntsman DG, Carneiro F, Lewis FR, MacLeod PM, Hayashi A, Monaghan KG et al. (2001). Early gastric cancer in young, asymptomatic carriers of germ-line E-cadherin mutations. N Engl J Med 344: 1904-1909.

1291. Hurtuk MG, Hughes C, Shoup M, Aranha GV (2009). Does lymph node ratio impact survival in resected periampullary malignancies? Am J Surg 197: 348-352.

1292. Husemann B (1989). Cardia carcinoma considered as a distinct clinical entity. Br J Surg 76: 136-139.

1293. Hussein NR, Mohammadi M, Talebkhan Y, Doraghi M, Letley DP, Muhammad MK et al. (2008). Differences in virulence markers between *Helicobacter pylori* strains from Iraq and those from Iran: potential importance of regional differences in *H. pylori*-associated disease. J Clin Microbiol 46: 1774-1779.

1294. Hussell T, Isaacson PG, Crabtree JE, Spencer J (1993). The response of cells from low-grade B-cell gastric lymphomas of mucosa-associated lymphoid tissue to *Helicobacter pylori*. Lancet 342: 571-574.

1295. Hwang S, Lee SG, Lee YJ, Han DJ, Kim SC, Kwon SH et al. (2008). Radical surgical resection for carcinoid tumors of the ampulla. J Gastrointest Surg 12: 713-717.

1296. Hyman NH, Anderson P, Blasyk H (2004). Hyperplastic polyposis and the risk of colorectal cancer. Dis Colon Rectum 47: 2101-2104.

1297. Hytiroglou P, Kotoula V, Thung SN, Tsokos M, Fiel MI, Papadimitriou CS (1998). Telomerase activity in precancerous hepatic nodules. Cancer 82: 1831-1838.

1298. Hytiroglou P, Park YN, Krinsky G, Theise ND (2007). Hepatic precancerous lesions and small hepatocellular carcinoma. Gastroenterol Clin North Am 36: 867-87, vii.

1299. Hytiroglou P, Theise ND, Schwartz M, Mor E, Miller C, Thung SN (1995). Macroregenerative nodules in a series of adult cirrhotic liver explants: issues of classification and nomenclature. Hepatology 21: 703-708.

1300. Iacobuzio-Donahue CA, Fu B, Yachida S, Luo M, Abe H, Henderson CM et al. (2009). *DPC4* gene status of the primary carcinoma correlates with patterns of failure in patients with pancreatic cancer. J Clin Oncol 27: 1806-1813.

1301. Iacobuzio-Donahue CA, Klimstra DS, Adsay NV, Wilentz RE, Argani P, Sohn TA et al. (2000). Dpc-4 protein is expressed in virtually all human intraductal papillary mucinous neoplasms of the pancreas: comparison with conventional ductal adenocarcinomas. Am J Pathol 157: 755-761.

1302. Iacobuzio-Donahue CA, Wilentz RE, Argani P, Yeo CJ, Cameron JL, Kern SE et al. (2000). Dpc4 protein in mucinous cystic neoplasms of the pancreas: frequent loss of expression in invasive carcinomas suggests a role in genetic progression. Am J Surg Pathol 24: 1544-1548.

1303. Ichikawa A, Kinoshita T, Watanabe T, Kato H, Nagai H, Tsushita K et al. (1997). Mutations of the *p53* gene as a prognostic factor in aggressive B-cell lymphoma. N Engl J Med 337: 529-534.

1304. Ida S, Okajima H, Hayashida S, Takeichi T, Asonuma K, Baba H et al. (2009). Undifferentiated sarcoma of the liver. Am J Surg 198: e7-e9.

1305. Ide H, Nakamura T, Hayashi K, Endo T, Kobayashi A, Eguchi R et al. (1994). Esophageal squamous cell carcinoma: pathology and prognosis. World J Surg 18: 321-330.

1306. Idelevich E, Kashtan H, Mavor E, Brenner B (2006). Small bowel obstruction caused by secondary tumors. Surg Oncol 15: 29-32.

1307. Igarashi A, Maruo Y, Ito T, Ohsawa K, Serizawa A, Yabe M et al. (2001). Huge cystic lymphangioma of the pancreas: report of a case. Surg Today 31: 743-746.

1308. Ihamaki T, Kekki M, Sipponen P, Siurala M (1985). The sequelae and course of chronic gastritis during a 30- to 34-year bioptic follow-up study. Scand J Gastroenterol 20: 485-491.

1309. Iida M, Yao T, Itoh H, Ohsato K, Watanabe H (1981). Endoscopic features of adenoma of the duodenal papilla in familial polyposis of the colon. Gastrointest Endosc 27: 6-8.

1310. Iida Y, Tsutsumi Y (1992). Small cell (endocrine cell) carcinoma of the gallbladder with squamous and adenocarcinomatous components. Acta Pathol Jpn 42: 119-125.

1311. Ikeda Y, Kosugi S, Nishikura K, Ohashi M, Kanda T, Kobayashi T et al. (2007). Gastric carcinosarcoma presenting as a huge epigastric mass. Gastric Cancer 10: 63-68.

1312. Ikeda Y, Ozawa S, Ando N, Kitagawa Y, Ueda M, Kitajima M (1996). Meanings of c-erbB and int-2 amplification in superficial esophageal squamous cell carcinomas. Ann Thorac Surg 62: 835-838.

1313. Ikeguchi M, Saito H, Katano K, Tsujitani S, Maeta M, Kaibara N (1997). Clinicopathologic significance of the expression of mutated p53 protein and the proliferative activity of cancer cells in patients with esophageal squamous cell carcinoma. J Am Coll Surg 185: 398-403.

1314. Ikeguchi M, Saito H, Kondo A, Tsujitani S, Maeta M, Kaibara N (1999). Mutated p53 protein expression and proliferative activity in advanced gastric cancer. Hepatogastroenterology 46: 2648-2653.

1315. Iliszko M, Czauderna P, Babinska M, Stoba C, Roszkiewicz A, Limon J (1998). Cytogenetic findings in an embryonal sarcoma of the liver. Cancer Genet Cytogenet 102: 142-144.

1316. Ilyas M, Straub J, Tomlinson IP, Bodmer WF (1999). Genetic pathways in colorectal and other cancers. Eur J Cancer 35: 1986-2002.

1317. Imai K, Yamamoto H (2008). Carcinogenesis and microsatellite instability: the interrelationship between genetics and epigenetics. Carcinogenesis 29: 673-680.

1318. Imai M, Hoshi T, Ogawa K (1994). K-ras codon 12 mutations in biliary tract tumors detected by polymerase chain reaction denaturing gradient gel electrophoresis. Cancer 73: 2727-2733.

1319. Imai T, Kubo T, Watanabe H (1971). Chronic gastritis in Japanese with reference to high incidence of gastric carcinoma. J Natl Cancer Inst 47: 179-195.

1320. Imai T, Sannohe Y, Okano H (1978). Oat cell carcinoma (apudoma) of the esophagus: a case report. Cancer 41: 358-364.

1321. Imai Y, Kawabe T, Takahashi M, Matsumura M, Komatsu Y, Hamada E et al. (1994). A case of primary gastric choriocarcinoma and a review of the Japanese literature. J Gastroenterol 29: 642-646.

1322. Imam H, Eriksson B, Oberg K (2000). Expression of CD44 variant isoforms and association to the benign form of endocrine pancreatic tumours. Ann Oncol 11: 295-300.

1323. Imashuku S (2007). Systemic type Epstein-Barr virus-related lymphoproliferative diseases in children and young adults: challenges for pediatric hemato-oncologists and infectious disease specialists. Pediatr Hematol Oncol 24: 563-568.

1324. In't Hof KH, van der Wal HC, Kazemier G, Lange JF (2008). Carcinoid tumour of the appendix: an analysis of 1,485 consecutive emergency appendectomies. J Gastrointest Surg 12: 1436-1438.

1325. Inagaki H, Nakamura T, Li C, Sugiyama T, Asaka M, Kodaira J et al. (2004). Gastric MALT lymphomas are divided into three groups based on responsiveness to *Helicobacter pylori* eradication and detection of *API2-MALT1* fusion. Am J Surg Pathol 28: 1560-1567.

1326. Inagawa S, Shimazaki J, Hori M, Yoshimi F, Adachi S, Kawamoto T et al. (2001). Hepatoid adenocarcinoma of the stomach. Gastric Cancer 4: 43-52.

1327. Inai K, Kobuke T, Yonehara S, Tokuoka S (1989). Duodenal gangliocytic paraganglioma with lymph node metastasis in a 17-year-old boy. Cancer 63: 2540-2545.

1328. Indinnimeo M, Cicchini C, Memeo L, Stazi A, Provenza C, Ricci F et al. (2002). Correlation between chromogranin-A expression and pathological variables in human colon carcinoma. Anticancer Res 22: 395-398.

1329. Inoki K, Corradetti MN, Guan KL (2005). Dysregulation of the TSC-mTOR pathway in human disease. Nat Genet 37: 19-24.

1330. Inoue H, Furukawa T, Sunamura M, Takeda K, Matsuno S, Horii A (2001). Exclusion of SMAD4 mutation as an early genetic change in human pancreatic ductal tumorigenesis. Genes Chromosomes Cancer 31: 295-299.

1331. International Agency for Research on Cancer (2002). IARC Monographs on the Evaluation of the Carcinogenic Risks to Humans Vol 82. Some Traditional Herbal Medicines, Some Mycotoxins, Naphthalene and Styrene. IARC: Lyon, France.

1332. International Agency for Research on Cancer (2003). IARC Handbooks on Cancer Prevention. Fruit and Vegetables. IARC: Lyon, France.

1333. International Agency for Research on Cancer (2004). IARC Monographs on the Evaluation of the Carcinogenic Risks to Humans Vol 83. Tobacco Smoke and Involuntary Smoking. IARC: Lyon, France.

1334. International Agency for Research on Cancer (2007). IARC Monographs on the Evaluation of the Carcinogenic Risks to Humans Vol 89. Smokeless Tobacco and Some Tobacco-specific N-Nitrosamines. IARC: Lyon, France.

1335. International Working Party (1995). Terminology of nodular hepatocellular lesions. International Working Party. Hepatology 22: 983-993.

1336. Ioachim HL, Antonescu C, Giancotti F, Dorsett B, Weinstein MA (1997). EBV-associated anorectal lymphomas in patients with acquired immune deficiency syndrome. Am J Surg Pathol 21: 997-1006.

1337. Ioachim HL, Dorsett B, Cronin W, Maya M, Wahl S (1991). Acquired immunodeficiency syndrome-associated lymphomas: clinical, pathologic, immunologic, and viral characteristics of 111 cases. Hum Pathol 22: 659-673.

1338. Iodice S, Gandini S, Maisonneuve P, Lowenfels AB (2008). Tobacco and the risk of pancreatic cancer: a review and meta-analysis. Langenbecks Arch Surg 393: 535-545.

1339. Ireland AP, Shibata DK, Chandrasoma P, Lord RV, Peters JH, DeMeester TR (2000). Clinical significance of p53 mutations in adenocarcinoma of the esophagus and cardia. Ann Surg 231: 179-187.

1340. Isaacson P (1981). Crypt cell carcinoma of the appendix (so-called adenocarcinoid tumor). Am J Surg Pathol 5: 213-224.

1341. Isaacson PG (1999). Gastrointestinal lymphomas of T- and B-cell types. Mod Pathol 12: 151-158.

1342. Isaacson PG, Dogan A, Price SK, Spencer J (1989). Immunoproliferative small-intestinal disease. An immunohistochemical study. Am J Surg Pathol 13: 1023-1033.

1343. Isaacson PG, MacLennan KA, Subbuswamy SG (1984). Multiple lymphomatous polyposis of the gastrointestinal tract. Histopathology 8: 641-656.

1344. Isaacson PG, Norton AJ (eds) (1994). Extranodal Lymphomas. Churchill Livingstone: New York, NY.

1345. Isaacson PG, O'Connor NT, Spencer J, Bevan DH, Connolly CE, Kirkham N et al. (1985). Malignant histiocytosis of the intestine: a T-cell lymphoma. Lancet 2: 688-691.

1346. Isaacson PG, Wotherspoon AC, Diss T,

Pan LX (1991). Follicular colonization in B-cell lymphoma of mucosa-associated lymphoid tissue. Am J Surg Pathol 15: 819-828.

1347. Isaji S, Kawarada Y, Uemoto S (2004). Classification of pancreatic cancer: comparison of Japanese and UICC classifications. Pancreas 28: 231-234.

1348. Iseki M, Suzuki T, Koizumi Y, Hirose M, Laskin WB, Nakazawa S et al. (1986). Alpha-fetoprotein-producing pancreatoblastoma. A case report. Cancer 57: 1833-1835.

1349. Ishak KG, Anthony PP, and Sobin LH (eds) (1999). Histological Typing of Tumours of the Liver. Springer: Berlin, Heidelberg, New York, Tokyo.

1350. Ishak KG, Goodman ZD, and Stocker JT (eds) (2001). Tumors of the Liver and Intrahepatic Bile Ducts. Armed Forces Institute of Pathology: Washington, DC.

1351. Ishak KG, Sesterhenn IA, Goodman ZD, Rabin L, Stromeyer FW (1984). Epithelioid hemangioendothelioma of the liver: a clinicopathologic and follow-up study of 32 cases. Hum Pathol 15: 839-852.

1352. Ishida M, Egawa S, Aoki T, Sakata N, Mikami Y, Motoi F et al. (2007). Characteristic clinicopathological features of the types of intraductal papillary-mucinous neoplasms of the pancreas. Pancreas 35: 348-352.

1353. Ishida M, Kushima R, Chano T, Okabe H (2007). Immunohistochemical demonstration of the type III intermediate filament peripherin in human rectal mucosae and well-differentiated endocrine neoplasms. Oncol Rep 18: 633-637.

1354. Ishigami S, Natsugoe S, Miyazono F, Hata Y, Uenosono Y, Sumikura S et al. (2004). Clinical merit of subdividing gastric cancer according to invasion of the muscularis propria. Hepatogastroenterology 51: 869-871.

1355. Ishiguro H, Kato K, Kishimoto T, Nagai Y, Takahashi T, Sasano H et al. (2003). Expression of steroidogenic enzymes by luteinizing cells in the ovarian-type stroma of a mucin-producing cystic tumour of the pancreas. Histopathology 43: 97-98.

1356. Ishihara A, Sanda T, Takanari H, Yatani R, Liu PI (1989). Elastase-1-secreting acinar cell carcinoma of the pancreas. A cytologic, electron microscopic and histochemical study. Acta Cytol 33: 157-163.

1357. Ishihara M, Mehregan DR, Hashimoto K, Yotsumoto S, Toi Y, Pietruk T et al. (1998). Staining of eccrine and apocrine neoplasms and metastatic adenocarcinoma with IKH-4, a monoclonal antibody specific for the eccrine gland. J Cutan Pathol 25: 100-105.

1358. Ishikawa N, Takano A, Yasui W, Inai K, Nishimura H, Ito H et al. (2007). Cancer-testis antigen lymphocyte antigen 6 complex locus K is a serologic biomarker and a therapeutic target for lung and esophageal carcinomas. Cancer Res 67: 11601-11611.

1359. Ishikawa O, Ishiguro S, Ohhigashi H, Sasaki Y, Yasuda T, Imaoka S et al. (1990). Solid and papillary neoplasm arising from an ectopic pancreas in the mesocolon. Am J Gastroenterol 85: 597-601.

1360. Ishikawa O, Ohigashi H, Imaoka S, Furukawa H, Sasaki Y, Fujita M et al. (1992). Preoperative indications for extended pancreatectomy for locally advanced pancreas cancer involving the portal vein. Ann Surg 215: 231-236.

1361. Ishikura H, Kirimoto K, Shamoto M, Miyamoto Y, Yamagiwa H, Itoh Y et al. (1986). Hepatoid adenocarcinomas of the stomach. An analysis of seven cases. Cancer 58: 119-126.

1362. Ishwaran H, Blackstone EH, pperson-Hansen C, Rice TW (2009). A novel approach to cancer staging: application to esophageal cancer. Biostatistics 10: 603-620.

1363. Islam HK, Fujioka Y, Tomidokoro T, Sugiura H, Takahashi T, Kondo S et al. (1999).

Immunohistochemical analysis of expression of molecular biologic factors in intraductal papillary-mucinous tumors of pancreas—diagnostic and biologic significance. Hepatogastroenterology 46: 2599-2605.

1364. Itatsu K, Zen Y, Ohira S, Ishikawa A, Sato Y, Harada K et al. (2007). Immunohistochemical analysis of the progression of flat and papillary preneoplastic lesions in intrahepatic cholangiocarcinogenesis in hepatolithiasis. Liver Int 27: 1174-1184.

1365. Itoh T, Kishi K, Tojo M, Kitajima N, Kinoshita Y, Inatome T et al. (1992). Acinar cell carcinoma of the pancreas with elevated serum alpha-fetoprotein levels: a case report and a review of 28 cases reported in Japan. Gastroenterol Jpn 27: 785-791.

1366. Iwafuchi M, Watanabe H, Ajioka Y, Shimoda T, Iwashita A, Ito S (1990). Immunohistochemical and ultrastructural studies of twelve argentaffin and six argyrophil carcinoids of the appendix vermiformis. Hum Pathol 21: 773-780.

1367. Iwafuchi M, Watanabe H, Ishihara N, Enjoji M, Iwashita A, Yanaihara N et al. (1987). Neoplastic endocrine cells in carcinomas of the small intestine: histochemical and immunohistochemical studies of 24 tumors. Hum Pathol 18: 185-194.

1368. Iwama T, Konishi M, Iijima T, Yoshinaga K, Tominaga T, Koike M et al. (1999). Somatic mutation of the *APC* gene in thyroid carcinoma associated with familial adenomatous polyposis. Jpn J Cancer Res 90: 372-376.

1369. Iwamura Y, Futagawa T, Kaneko M, Nakagawa K, Kawai K, Yamashita K et al. (1992). Co-deletions of the retinoblastoma gene and Wilms' tumor gene and rearrangement of the Krev-1 gene in a human insulinoma. Jpn J Clin Oncol 22: 6-9.

1370. Iwashita A, Watanabe H, Enjoji M (1989). Argyrophil and argentaffin cells in adenomas of the colon and rectum. Fukuoka Igaku Zasshi 80: 114-124.

1371. Iwata T, Kurita N, Nishioka M, Miyamoto H, Wakatsuki S, Sano T et al. (2007). p53 and MIB-1 expression of esophageal carcinoma concominant with achalasia. Hepatogastroenterology 54: 1430-1432.

1372. Iwaya T, Maesawa C, Ogasawara S, Tamura G (1998). Tylosis esophageal cancer locus on chromosome 17q25.1 is commonly deleted in sporadic human esophageal cancer. Gastroenterology 114: 1206-1210.

1373. Iype S, Mirza TA, Propper DJ, Bhattacharya S, Feakins RM, Kocher HM (2009). Neuroendocrine tumours of the gallbladder: three cases and a review of the literature. Postgrad Med J 85: 213-218.

1374. Izumo A, Yamaguchi K, Eguchi T, Nishiyama K, Yamamoto H, Yonemasu H et al. (2003). Mucinous cystic tumor of the pancreas: immunohistochemical assessment of "ovarian-type stroma". Oncol Rep 10: 515-525.

1375. Izzo JG, Malhotra U, Wu TT, Ensor J, Luthra R, Lee JH et al. (2006). Association of activated transcription factor nuclear factor kappab with chemoradiation resistance and poor outcome in esophageal carcinoma. J Clin Oncol 24: 748-754.

1376. JACKSON SH, Varley H (1952). Carcinoma of the pancreas associated with fat-necrosis. Lancet 2: 962-967.

1376A. Jaeger E, Webb E, Howarth K, Carvajal-Carmona L, Rowan A, Broderick P (2008). Common genetic variants at the *CRAC1* (*HMPS*) locus on chromosome 15q13.3 influence colorectal cancer risk. Nat Genet 40: 26-28

1377. Jaffe ES (1987). Malignant lymphomas: pathology of hepatic involvement. Semin Liver Dis 7: 257-268.

1378. Jagelman DG, DeCosse JJ, Bussey HJ (1988). Upper gastrointestinal cancer in familial adenomatous polyposis. Lancet 1: 1149-1151.

1379. Jain S, Lobo DN, Clelland CA, Williams CB (2000). Carcinoid tumour in a caecal duplication cyst. Dig Surg 17: 281-283.

1380. Jakobovitz O, Nass D, DeMarco L, Barbosa AJ, Simoni FB, Rechavi G et al. (1996). Carcinoid tumors frequently display genetic abnormalities involving chromosome 11. J Clin Endocrinol Metab 81: 3164-3167.

1381. Jalving M, Koornstra JJ, Boersma-van EW, de JS, Karrenbeld A, Hollema H et al. (2003). Dysplasia in fundic gland polyps is associated with nuclear beta-catenin expression and relatively high cell turnover rates. Scand J Gastroenterol 38: 916-922.

1382. James JA, Milligan DW, Morgan GJ, Crocker J (1998). Familial pancreatic lymphoma. J Clin Pathol 51: 80-82.

1383. Janka GE (2007). Hemophagocytic syndromes. Blood Rev 21: 245-253.

1384. Jankowski JA, Odze RD (2009). Biomarkers in gastroenterology: between hope and hype comes histopathology. Am J Gastroenterol 104: 1093-1096.

1385. Jansen M, de Leng WW, Baas AF, Myoshi H, Mathus-Vliegen L, Taketo MM et al. (2006). Mucosal prolapse in the pathogenesis of Peutz-Jeghers polyposis. Gut 55: 1-5.

1386. Jansen M, Ten Klooster JP, Offerhaus GJ, Clevers H (2009). LKB1 and AMPK family signaling: the intimate link between cell polarity and energy metabolism. Physiol Rev 89: 777-798.

1387. Japan Esophageal Society (eds) (2009). Guideline for Diagnosis and Treatment of Esophageal Cancer. Kanehara Shuppan: Tokyo.

1388. Japan Esophageal Society (2009). Japanese classification of esophageal cancer, tenth edition: part I. Esophagus 6: 1-25.

1389. Japanese Research Society for Gastric Cancer (1995). Group Classification of Gastric Biopsy Specimens. In: Japanese Classification of Gastric Carcinoma. Nishi M, Omori Y, Miwa K, eds. Kanehara: Tokyo, pp. 74-76.

1390. Japanese Research Society for Gastric Cancer (eds) (1995). Japanese Classification of Gastric Carcinoma. Kanehara: Tokyo.

1391. Japanese Society for Cancer of the Colon and Rectum (2009). Japanese Classification of Colorectal Carcinoma. Kanehara: Tokyo.

1392. Japanese Society for Cancer of the Colon and Rectum (2009). Japanese Classification of Colorectal Carcinoma. Kanehara: Tokyo. English ED ?

1393. Jaques DP, Coit DG, Casper ES, Brennan MF (1995). Hepatic metastases from soft-tissue sarcoma. Ann Surg 221: 392-397.

1394. Jaramillo E, Tamura S, Mitomi H (2005). Endoscopic appearance of serrated adenomas in the colon. Endoscopy 37: 254-260.

1395. Jarvinen HJ (1985). Time and type of prophylactic surgery for familial adenomatosis coli. Ann Surg 202: 93-97.

1396. Jass JR (1983). A classification of gastric dysplasia. Histopathology 7: 181-193.

1397. Jass JR (1994). Juvenile polyposis. In: Familial adenomatous polyposis and other polyposis syndromes. Phillips RK, Spigelman AD, Thomson JP, eds. Edward Arnold: London, pp. 203-

1398. Jass JR (2004). HNPCC and sporadic MSI-H colorectal cancer: a review of the morphological similarities and differences. Fam Cancer 3: 93-100.

1399. Jass JR (2005). Serrated adenoma of the colorectum and the DNA-methylator phenotype. Nat Clin Pract Oncol 2: 398-405.

1400. Jass JR (2007). Classification of colorectal cancer based on correlation of clinical, morphological and molecular features. Histopathology 50: 113-130.

1401. Jass JR (2007). Gastrointestinal polyposes: clinical, pathological and molecular features. Gastroenterol Clin North Am 36: 927-946.

1402. Jass JR, Do KA, Simms LA, Iino H, Wynter C, Pillay SP et al. (1998). Morphology of sporadic colorectal cancer with DNA replication errors. Gut 42: 673-679.

1403. Jass JR, Iino H, Ruszkiewicz A, Painter D, Solomon MJ, Koorey DJ et al. (2000). Neoplastic progression occurs through mutator pathways in hyperplastic polyposis of the colorectum. Gut 47: 43-49.

1404. Jass JR, Smith M (1992). Sialic acid and epithelial differentiation in colorectal polyps and cancer—a morphological, mucin and lectin histochemical study. Pathology 24: 233-242.

1405. Jass JR, Stewart SM, Stewart J, Lane MR (1994). Hereditary non-polyposis colorectal cancer—morphologies, genes and mutations. Mutat Res 310: 125-133.

1406. Jass JR, Whitehall VL, Young J, Leggett BA (2002). Emerging concepts in colorectal neoplasia. Gastroenterology 123: 862-876.

1407. Jass JR, Williams CB, Bussey HJ, Morson BC (1988). Juvenile polyposis—a precancerous condition. Histopathology 13: 619-630.

1408. Jawhari A, Jordan S, Poole S, Browne P, Pignatelli M, Farthing MJ (1997). Abnormal immunoreactivity of the E-cadherin-catenin complex in gastric carcinoma: relationship with patient survival. Gastroenterology 112: 46-54.

1409. Jayaram A, Finegold MJ, Parham DM, Jasty R (2007). Successful management of rhabdoid tumor of the liver. J Pediatr Hematol Oncol 29: 406-408.

1410. Jeannot E, Poussin K, Chiche L, Bacq Y, Sturm N, Scoazec JY et al. (2007). Association of CYP1B1 germ line mutations with hepatocyte nuclear factor 1alpha-mutated hepatocellular adenoma. Cancer Res 67: 2611-2616.

1411. Jeghers H, McKusick VA, Katz KH (1949). Generalized intestinal polyposis and melanin spots of the oral mucosa, lips and digits; a syndrome of diagnostic significance. N Engl J Med 241: 1031-1036.

1412. Jelic TM, Barreta TM, Yu M, Frame JN, Estallila OC, Mellen PF et al. (2004). Primary, extranodal, follicular non-Hodgkin lymphoma of the gallbladder: case report and a review of the literature. Leuk Lymphoma 45: 381-387.

1413. Jemal A, Siegel R, Ward E, Hao Y, Xu J, Thun MJ (2009). Cancer statistics, 2009. CA Cancer J Clin 59: 225-249.

1414. Jen J, Powell SM, Papadopoulos N, Smith KJ, Hamilton SR, Vogelstein B et al. (1994). Molecular determinants of dysplasia in colorectal lesions. Cancer Res 54: 5523-5526.

1415. Jenkins GJ, Doak SH, Parry JM, D'Souza FR, Griffiths AP, Baxter JN (2002). Genetic pathways involved in the progression of Barrett's metaplasia to adenocarcinoma. Br J Surg 89: 824-837.

1416. Jenkins MA, Hayashi S, O'Shea AM, Burgart LJ, Smyrk TC, Shimizu D et al. (2007). Pathology features in Bethesda guidelines predict colorectal cancer microsatellite instability: a population-based study. Gastroenterology 133: 48-56.

1417. Jenne DE, Reimann H, Nezu J, Friedel W, Loff S, Jeschke R et al. (1998). Peutz-Jeghers syndrome is caused by mutations in a novel serine threonine kinase. Nat Genet 18: 38-43.

1418. Jensen RT (1993). Gastrinoma as a model for prolonged hypergastrinemia in man. In: Gastrin. Walsh JH, ed. Raven Press: New York, pp. 373-393.

1419. Jensen RT (1999). Pancreatic endocrine tumors: recent advances. Ann Oncol 10 Suppl 4: 170-176.

1420. Jeon WJ, Chae HB, Park SM, Youn SJ, Choi JW, Kim SH (2006). [A case of primary small cell carcinoma arising from the common bile duct]. Korean J Gastroenterol 48: 438-442.

1421. Jeong YJ, Lee MR, Kim JC, Hwang PH, Moon WS, Chung MJ (2008). Carcinosarcoma of the rectosigmoid colon in a 13-year-old girl. Pathol Int 58: 445-450.

1422. Jess T, Loftus EV, Jr., Velayos FS, Harmsen WS, Zinsmeister AR, Smyrk TC et al. (2006). Risk of intestinal cancer in inflammatory bowel disease: a population-based study from olmsted county, Minnesota. Gastroenterology 130: 1039-1046.

1423. Jetmore AB, Ray JE, Gathright JB, Jr., McMullen KM, Hicks TC, Timmcke AE (1992). Rectal carcinoids: the most frequent carcinoid tumor. Dis Colon Rectum 35: 717-725.

1424. Ji H, Ramsey MR, Hayes DN, Fan C, McNamara K, Kozlowski P et al. (2007). LKB1 modulates lung cancer differentiation and metastasis. Nature 448: 807-810.

1425. Ji J, Hemminki K (2006). Familial risk for esophageal cancer: an updated epidemiologic study from Sweden. Clin Gastroenterol Hepatol 4: 840-845.

1426. Jiang BG, Sun LL, Yu WL, Tang ZH, Zong M, Zhang YJ (2009). Retrospective analysis of histopathologic prognostic factors after hepatectomy for intrahepatic cholangiocarcinoma. Cancer J 15: 257-261.

1427. Jiang SX, Mikami T, Umezawa A, Saegusa M, Kameya T, Okayasu I (2006). Gastric large cell neuroendocrine carcinomas: a distinct clinicopathologic entity. Am J Surg Pathol 30: 945-953.

1428. Jiang W, Zhang YJ, Kahn SM, Hollstein MC, Santella RM, Lu SH et al. (1993). Altered expression of the cyclin D1 and retinoblastoma genes in human esophageal cancer. Proc Natl Acad Sci U S A 90: 9026-9030.

1429. Jiao YF, Nakamura S, Arai T, Sugai T, Uesugi N, Habano W et al. (2003). Adenoma, adenocarcinoma and mixed carcinoid-adenocarcinoma arising in a small lesion of the colon. Pathol Int 53: 457-462.

1430. Jimenez RE, Warshaw AL, Z'graggen K, Hartwig W, Taylor DZ, Compton CC et al. (1999). Sequential accumulation of K-ras mutations and p53 overexpression in the progression of pancreatic mucinous cystic neoplasms to malignancy. Ann Surg 230: 501-509.

1431. Jimenez W, Paszat L, Kupets R, Wilton A, Tinmouth J (2009). Presumed previous human papillomavirus (HPV) related gynecological cancer in women diagnosed with anal cancer in the province of Ontario. Gynecol Oncol 114: 395-398.

1432. Jinfeng M, Kimura W, Sakurai F, Moriya T, Takeshita A, Hirai I (2002). Histopathological study of intraductal papillary mucinous tumor of the pancreas: special reference to the roles of Survivin and p53 in tumorigenesis of IPMT. Int J Gastrointest Cancer 32: 73-81.

1433. Jochem VJ, Fuerst PA, Fromkes JJ (1992). Familial Barrett's esophagus associated with adenocarcinoma. Gastroenterology 102: 1400-1402.

1434. Johannsdottir JT, Jonasson JG, Bergthorsson JT, Amundadottir LT, Magnusson J, Egilsson V et al. (2000). The effect of mismatch repair deficiency on tumourigenesis; microsatellite instability affecting genes containing short repeated sequences. Int J Oncol 16: 133-139.

1435. Johns LE, Houlston RS (2001). A systematic review and meta-analysis of familial colorectal cancer risk. Am J Gastroenterol 96: 2992-3003.

1436. Johnson LG, Madeleine MM, Newcomer LM, Schwartz SM, Daling JR (2004). Anal cancer incidence and survival: the surveillance, epidemiology, and end results experience, 1973-2000. Cancer 101: 281-288.

1437. Johnson V, Volikos E, Halford SE, Eftekhar Sadat ET, Popat S, Talbot I et al. (2005). Exon 3 beta-catenin mutations are specifically associated with colorectal carcinomas in hereditary non-polyposis colorectal cancer syndrome. Gut 54: 264-267.

1438. Johnston J, Helwig EB (1981). Granular cell tumors of the gastrointestinal tract and perianal region: a study of 74 cases. Dig Dis Sci 26: 807-816.

1439. Jones AM, Thirlwell C, Howarth KM, Graham T, Chambers W, Segditsas S et al. (2007). Analysis of copy number changes suggests chromosomal instability in a minority of large colorectal adenomas. J Pathol 213: 249-256.

1440. Jones EA, Morson BC (1984). Mucinous adenocarcinoma in anorectal fistulae. Histopathology 8: 279-292.

1441. Jones K, Pacella J, Wasty F (2007). Hodgkin's disease of the oesophagus: a literature review. Australas Radiol 51: 489-491.

1442. Jones N, Vogt S, Nielsen M, Christian D, Wark PA, Eccles D et al. (2009). Increased colorectal cancer incidence in obligate carriers of heterozygous mutations in MUTYH. Gastroenterology 137: 489-94, 494.

1443. Jones S, Hruban RH, Kamiyama M, Borges M, Zhang X, Parsons DW et al. (2009). Exomic sequencing identifies PALB2 as a pancreatic cancer susceptibility gene. Science 324: 217

1444. Jones S, Zhang X, Parsons DW, Lin JC, Leary RJ, Angenendt P et al. (2008). Core signaling pathways in human pancreatic cancers revealed by global genomic analyses. Science 321: 1801-1806.

1445. Jones WF, Sheikh MY, McClave SA (1997). AIDS-related non-Hodgkin's lymphoma of the pancreas. Am J Gastroenterol 92: 335-338.

1446. Jonkers YM, Claessen SM, Perren A, Schmitt AM, Hofland LJ, de HW et al. (2007). DNA copy number status is a powerful predictor of poor survival in endocrine pancreatic tumor patients. Endocr Relat Cancer 14: 769-779.

1447. Jonsson T, Johannsson JH, Hallgrimsson JG (1989). Carcinoid tumors of the appendix in children younger than 16 years. A retrospective clinical and pathologic study. Acta Chir Scand 155: 113-116.

1448. Jorgensen LJ, Hansen AB, Burcharth F, Philipsen E, Horn T (1992). Solid and papillary neoplasm of the pancreas. Ultrastruct Pathol 16: 659-666.

1449. Joshi SW, Merchant NH, Jambhekar NA (1997). Primary multilocular cystic undifferentiated (embryonal) sarcoma of the liver in childhood resembling hydatid cyst of the liver. Br J Radiol 70: 314-316.

1450. Judkins AR (2007). Immunohistochemistry of INI1 expression: a new tool for old challenges in CNS and soft tissue pathology. Adv Anat Pathol 14: 335-339.

1451. Jun SR, Lee JM, Han JK, Choi BI (2006). High-grade neuroendocrine carcinomas of the gallbladder and bile duct: Report of four cases with pathological correlation. J Comput Assist Tomogr 30: 604-609.

1452. Jung SW, Sugimoto M, Graham DY, Yamaoka Y (2009). homB status of *Helicobacter pylori* as a novel marker to distinguish gastric cancer from duodenal ulcer. J Clin Microbiol 47: 3241-3245.

1453. Kabbani W, Houlihan PS, Luthra R, Hamilton SR, Rashid A (2002). Mucinous and nonmucinous appendiceal adenocarcinomas: different clinicopathological features but similar genetic alterations. Mod Pathol 15: 599-605.

1454. Kader HA, Ruchelli E, Maller ES (1998).

Langerhans' cell histiocytosis with stool retention caused by a perianal mass. J Pediatr Gastroenterol Nutr 26: 226-228.

1455. Kahl P, Buettner R, Friedrichs N, Merkelbach-Bruse S, Wenzel J, Carl HL (2007). Kaposi's sarcoma of the gastrointestinal tract: report of two cases and review of the literature. Pathol Res Pract 203: 227-231.

1456. Kaiho T, Tanaka T, Tsuchiya S, Miura M, Saigusa N, Yanagisawa S et al. (1999). A case of classical carcinoid tumor of the gallbladder: review of the Japanese published works. Hepatogastroenterology 46: 2189-2195.

1457. Kaiser A, Jurowich C, Schonekas H, Gebhardt C, Wunsch PH (2002). The adenoma-carcinoma sequence applies to epithelial tumours of the papilla of Vater. Z Gastroenterol 40: 913-920.

1458. Kakar S, Gown AM, Goodman ZD, Ferrell LD (2007). Best practices in diagnostic immunohistochemistry: hepatocellular carcinoma versus metastatic neoplasms. Arch Pathol Lab Med 131: 1648-1654.

1459. Kakeji Y, Korenaga D, Tsujitani S, Baba H, Anai H, Maehara Y et al. (1993). Gastric cancer with p53 overexpression has high potential for metastasising to lymph nodes. Br J Cancer 67: 589-593.

1460. Kakinoki R, Kushima R, Matsubara A, Saito Y, Okabe H, Fujiyama Y et al. (2009). Re-evaluation of histogenesis of gastric carcinomas: a comparative histopathological study between *Helicobacter pylori*-negative and *H. pylori*-positive cases. Dig Dis Sci 54: 614-620.

1461. Kala Z, Valek V, Hlavsa J, Hana K, Vanova A (2007). The role of CT and endoscopic ultrasound in pre-operative staging of pancreatic cancer. Eur J Radiol 62: 166-169.

1462. Kalish RJ, Clancy PE, Orringer MB, Appelman HD (1984). Clinical, epidemiologic, and morphologic comparison between adenocarcinomas arising in Barrett's esophageal mucosa and in the gastric cardia. Gastroenterology 86: 461-467.

1463. Kallakury BV, Bui HX, delRosario A, Wallace J, Solis OG, Ross JS (1993). Primary gastric adenosarcoma. Arch Pathol Lab Med 117: 299-301.

1464. Kamata S, Nose K, Sawai T, Hasegawa T, Kuroda S, Sasaki T et al. (2003). Fetal mesenchymal hamartoma of the liver: report of a case. J Pediatr Surg 38: 639-641.

1465. Kambara T, Simms LA, Whitehall VL, Spring KJ, Wynter CV, Walsh MD et al. (2004). BRAF mutation is associated with DNA methylation in serrated polyps and cancers of the colorectum. Gut 53: 1137-1144.

1466. Kamisawa T, Fukayama M, Koike M, Tabata I, Okamoto A (1987). So-called "papillary and cystic neoplasm of the pancreas." An immunohistochemical and ultrastructural study. Acta Pathol Jpn 37: 785-794.

1467. Kamisawa T, Tu Y, Egawa N, Ishiwata J, Tsuruta K, Okamoto A et al. (2002). Ductal and acinar differentiation in pancreatic endocrine tumors. Dig Dis Sci 47: 2254-2261.

1468. Kamisawa T, Tu Y, Egawa N, Nakajima H, Tsuruta K, Okamoto A (2005). Malignancies associated with intraductal papillary mucinous neoplasm of the pancreas. World J Gastroenterol 11: 5688-5690.

1469. Kan Z, Ivancev K, Lunderquist A, McCuskey PA, McCuskey RS, Wallace S (1995). In vivo microscopy of hepatic metastases: dynamic observation of tumor cell invasion and interaction with Kupffer cells. Hepatology 21: 487-494.

1470. Kanai N, Nagaki S, Tanaka T (1987). Clear cell carcinoma of the pancreas. Acta Pathol Jpn 37: 1521-1526.

1471. Kaneko S, Yoshimura T (2001). Time trend analysis of gastric cancer incidence in

Japan by histological types, 1975-1989. Br J Cancer 84: 400-405.

1472. Kang H, O'Connell JB, Leonardi MJ, Maggard MA, McGory ML, Ko CY (2007). Rare tumors of the colon and rectum: a national review. Int J Colorectal Dis 22: 183-189.

1473. Kang KP, Lee HS, Kim N, Kang HM, Park YS, Lee DH et al. (2009). Role of intestinal metaplasia subtyping in the risk of gastric cancer in Korea. J Gastroenterol Hepatol 24: 140-148.

1474. Kanhouwa S, Burns W, Matthews M, Chisholm R (1975). Anaplastic carcinoma of the lung with metastasis to the anus: report of a case. Dis Colon Rectum 18: 42-48.

1475. Kaplan KJ, Goodman ZD, Ishak KG (2001). Eosinophilic granuloma of the liver: a characteristic lesion with relationship to visceral larva migrans. Am J Surg Pathol 25: 1316-1321.

1476. Kappas AM, Fatouros M, Roukos DH (2004). Is it time to change surgical strategy for gastric cancer in the United States? Ann Surg Oncol 11: 727-730.

1477. Kapse N, Goh V (2009). Functional imaging of colorectal cancer: positron emission tomography, magnetic resonance imaging, and computed tomography. Clin Colorectal Cancer 8: 77-87.

1478. Karanjawala ZE, Illei PB, Ashfaq R, Infante JR, Murphy K, Pandey A et al. (2008). New markers of pancreatic cancer identified through differential gene expression analyses: claudin 18 and annexin A8. Am J Surg Pathol 32: 188-196.

1479. Karaoglanoglu N, Eroglu A, Turkyilmaz A, Gursan N (2005). Oesophageal adenoid cystic carcinoma and its management options. Int J Clin Pract 59: 1101-1103.

1480. Karasawa Y, Sakaguchi M, Minami S, Kitano K, Kawa S, Aoki Y et al. (2001). Duodenal somatostatinoma and erythrocytosis in a patient with von Hippel-Lindau disease type 2A. Intern Med 40: 38-43.

1481. Karat D, O'Hanlon DM, Hayes N, Scott D, Raimes SA, Griffin SM (1995). Prospective study of *Helicobacter pylori* infection in primary gastric lymphoma. Br J Surg 82: 1369-1370.

1482. Kardon DE, Thompson LD, Przygodzki RM, Heffess CS (2001). Adenosquamous carcinoma of the pancreas: a clinicopathologic series of 25 cases. Mod Pathol 14: 443-451.

1483. Karhunen PJ (1985). Hepatic pseudolipoma. J Clin Pathol 38: 877-879.

1484. Karhunen PJ (1986). Benign hepatic tumours and tumour like conditions in men. J Clin Pathol 39: 183-188.

1485. Karnak I, Senocak ME, Ciftci AO, Caglar M, Bingol-Kologlu M, Tanyel FC et al. (2001). Inflammatory myofibroblastic tumor in children: diagnosis and treatment. J Pediatr Surg 36: 908-912.

1486. Karoui M, Tresallet C, Brouquet A, Radvanyi H, Penna C (2007). [Colorectal carcinogenesis. 2. Underlying epigenetic and genetic alterations and molecular classification of colorectal cancers]. J Chir (Paris) 144: 97-104.

1487. Karpelowsky JS, Pansini A, Lazarus C, Rode H, Millar AJ (2008). Difficulties in the management of mesenchymal hamartomas. Pediatr Surg Int 24: 1171-1175.

1488. Kartheuser A, Stangherlin P, Brandt D, Remue C, Sempoux C (2006). Restorative proctocolectomy and ileal pouch-anal anastomosis for familial adenomatous polyposis revisited. Fam Cancer 5: 241-260.

1489. Kassahun WT, Hauss J (2008). Management of combined hepatocellular and cholangiocarcinoma. Int J Clin Pract 62: 1271-1278.

1490. Kassam A, Mandel K (2008). Metastatic hepatic epithelioid hemangioendothelioma in a teenage girl. J Pediatr Hematol Oncol 30: 550-552.

1491. Kastrinos F, Mukherjee B, Tayob N, Wang F, Sparr J, Raymond VM et al. (2009). Risk of pancreatic cancer in families with Lynch syndrome. JAMA 302: 1790-1795.

1492. Katabi N, Albores-Saavedra J (2003). The extrahepatic bile duct lesions in end-stage primary sclerosing cholangitis. Am J Surg Pathol 27: 349-355.

1493. Katabi N, Klimstra DS (2008). Intraductal papillary mucinous neoplasms of the pancreas: clinical and pathological features and diagnostic approach. J Clin Pathol 61: 1303-1313.

1494. Katajisto P, Vallenius T, Vaahtomeri K, Ekman N, Udd L, Tiainen M et al. (2007). The LKB1 tumor suppressor kinase in human disease. Biochim Biophys Acta 1775: 63-75.

1495. Kato H, Naganuma T, Iizawa Y, Kitagawa M, Tanaka M, Isaji S (2008). Primary non-Hodgkin's lymphoma of the gallbladder diagnosed by laparoscopic cholecystectomy. J Hepatobiliary Pancreat Surg 15: 659-663.

1496. Kato H, Tachimori Y, Watanabe H, Iizuka T (1993). Evaluation of the new (1987) TNM classification for thoracic esophageal tumors. Int J Cancer 53: 220-223.

1497. Kato H, Tachimori Y, Watanabe H, Itabashi M, Hirota T, Yamaguchi H et al. (1992). Intramural metastasis of thoracic esophageal carcinoma. Int J Cancer 50: 49-52.

1498. Kato T, Terashima T, Tomida S, Yamaguchi T, Kawamura H, Kimura N et al. (2005). Cytokeratin 20-positive large cell neuroendocrine carcinoma of the colon. Pathol Int 55: 524-529.

1499. Katzenstein HM, Kletzel M, Reynolds M, Superina R, Gonzalez-Crussi F (2003). Metastatic malignant rhabdoid tumor of the liver treated with tandem high-dose therapy and autologous peripheral blood stem cell rescue. Med Pediatr Oncol 40: 199-201.

1500. Kaurah P, Fitzgerald R, Dwerryhouse S, Huntsman DG (2010). Pregnancy after prophylactic total gastrectomy. Fam Cancer. In press.

1501. Kaurah P, MacMillan A, Boyd N, Senz J, De Luca A, Chun N et al. (2007). Founder and recurrent CDH1 mutations in families with hereditary diffuse gastric cancer. JAMA 297: 2360-2372.

1502. Kavin H, Yaremko L, Valaitis J, Chowdhury L (1996). Chronic esophagitis evolving to verrucous squamous cell carcinoma: possible role of exogenous chemical carcinogens. Gastroenterology 110: 904-914.

1503. Kawahira H, Kobayashi S, Kaneko K, Asano T, Ochiai T (2000). p53 protein expression in intraductal papillary mucinous tumors (IPMT) of the pancreas as an indicator of tumor malignancy. Hepatogastroenterology 47: 973-977.

1504. Kawamoto K, Matsuo T, Jubashi T, Ikeda T, Tomita S (1985). Primary pancreatic carcinoma in childhood. Pancreatoblastoma. Acta Pathol Jpn 35: 137-143.

1505. Kawamoto S, Hiraoka T, Kanemitsu K, Kimura M, Miyauchi Y, Takeya M (1992). Alpha-fetoprotein-producing pancreatic cancer—a case report and review of 28 cases. Hepatogastroenterology 39: 282-286.

1506. Kawamoto S, Lawler LP, Horton KM, Eng J, Hruban RH, Fishman EK (2006). MDCT of intraductal papillary mucinous neoplasm of the pancreas: evaluation of features predictive of invasive carcinoma. AJR Am J Roentgenol 186: 687-695.

1507. Kawamoto S, Siegelman SS, Bluemke DA, Hruban RH, Fishman EK (2009). Focal fatty infiltration in the head of the pancreas: evaluation with multidetector computed tomography with multiplanar reformation imaging. J Comput Assist Tomogr 33: 90-95.

1508. Kawanishi K, Shiozaki H, Doki Y, Sakita I, Inoue M, Yano M et al. (1999). Prognostic significance of heat shock proteins 27 and 70 in patients with squamous cell carcinoma of the esophagus. Cancer 85: 1649-1657.

1509. Kayahara M, Nakagawara H, Kitagawa H, Ohta T (2007). The nature of neural invasion by pancreatic cancer. Pancreas 35: 218-223.

1510. Ke E, Patel BB, Liu T, Li XM, Haluszka O, Hoffman JP et al. (2009). Proteomic analyses of pancreatic cyst fluids. Pancreas 38: e33-e42.

1511. Keating S, Taylor GP (1985). Undifferentiated (embryonal) sarcoma of the liver: ultrastructural and immunohistochemical similarities with malignant fibrous histiocytoma. Hum Pathol 16: 693-699.

1512. Keeney S, Bauer TL (2006). Epidemiology of adenocarcinoma of the esophagogastric junction. Surg Oncol Clin N Am 15: 687-696.

1513. Keller G, Vogelsang H, Becker I, Hutter J, Ott K, Candidus S et al. (1999). Diffuse type gastric and lobular breast carcinoma in a familial gastric cancer patient with an E-cadherin germline mutation. Am J Pathol 155: 337-342.

1514. Keller G, Vogelsang H, Becker I, Plaschke S, Ott K, Suriano G et al. (2004). Germline mutations of the E-cadherin (CDH1) and TP53 genes, rather than of RUNX3 and HPP1, contribute to genetic predisposition in German gastric cancer patients. J Med Genet 41: e89

1515. Keller JJ, Westerman AM, de Rooij FW, Wilson JH, van Dekken H, Giardiello FM et al. (2002). Molecular genetic evidence of an association between nasal polyposis and the Peutz-Jeghers syndrome. Ann Intern Med 136: 855-856.

1516. Kelsell DP, Risk JM, Leigh IM, Stevens HP, Ellis A, Hennies HC et al. (1996). Close mapping of the focal non-epidermolytic palmoplantar keratoderma (PPK) locus associated with oesophageal cancer (TOC). Hum Mol Genet 5: 857-860.

1517. Kemp Z, Carvajal-Carmona L, Spain S, Barclay E, Gorman M, Martin L et al. (2006). Evidence for a colorectal cancer susceptibility locus on chromosome 3q21-q24 from a high-density SNP genome-wide linkage scan. Hum Mol Genet 15: 2903-2910.

1518. Kemp Z, Rowan A, Chambers W, Wortham N, Halford S, Sieber O et al. (2005). CDC4 mutations occur in a subset of colorectal cancers but are not predicted to cause loss of function and are not associated with chromosomal instability. Cancer Res 65: 11361-11366.

1519. Kemp ZE, Carvajal-Carmona LG, Barclay E, Gorman M, Martin L, Wood W et al. (2006). Evidence of linkage to chromosome 9q22.33 in colorectal cancer kindreds from the United Kingdom. Cancer Res 66: 5003-5006.

1520. Kenmochi K, Sugihara S, Kojiro M (1987). Relationship of histologic grade of hepatocellular carcinoma (HCC) to tumor size, and demonstration of tumor cells of multiple different grades in single small HCC. Liver 7: 18-26.

1521. Kenny BD, Sloan JM, Hamilton PW, Watt PC, Johnston CF, Buchanan KD (1989). The role of morphometry in predicting prognosis in pancreatic islet cell tumors. Cancer 64: 460-465.

1522. Kent RBI, van Heerden JA, Weiland LH (1981). Nonfunctioning islet cell tumors. Ann Surg 193: 185-190.

1523. Kerr NJ, Chun YH, Yun K, Heathcott RW, Reeve AE, Sullivan MJ (2002). Pancreatoblastoma is associated with chromosome 11p loss of heterozygosity and IGF2 overexpression. Med Pediatr Oncol 39: 52-54.

1524. Kessler KJ, Kerlakian GM, Welling RE (1996). Perineal and perirectal sarcomas: report of two cases. Dis Colon Rectum 39: 468-472.

1525. Keswani RN, Noffsinger A, Waxman I, Bissonnette M (2006). Clinical use of p53 in Barrett's esophagus. Cancer Epidemiol Biomarkers Prev 15: 1243-1249.

1526. Kets CM, Van Krieken JH, van Erp PE, Feuth T, Jacobs YH, Brunner HG et al. (2008). Is early-onset microsatellite and chromosomally stable colorectal cancer a hallmark of a genetic susceptibility syndrome? Int J Cancer 122: 796-801.

1527. Keung YK, Cobos E, Trowers E (1997). Primary pancreatic lymphoma associated with short bowel syndrome: review of carcinogenesis of gastrointestinal malignancies. Leuk Lymphoma 26: 405-408.

1528. Kew MC, Asare GA (2007). Dietary iron overload in the African and hepatocellular carcinoma. Liver Int 27: 735-741.

1529. Key C, Meisner A (2007). Cancers of the esophagus, stomach, and small intestine. In: Surveillance, Epidemiology, and End Results (SEER) Survival Monograph: Cancer Survival Among Adults-US SEER Program, 1988-2001: Patient and Tumor Characteristics. Ries LAG, ed. National Cancer Institute: Bethesda, MD, pp.

1530. Khan MN, Moran BJ (2007). Four percent of patients undergoing colorectal cancer surgery may have synchronous appendiceal neoplasia. Dis Colon Rectum 50: 1856-1859.

1531. Khan SA, Taylor-Robinson SD, Toledano MB, Beck A, Elliott P, Thomas HC (2002). Changing international trends in mortality rates for liver, biliary and pancreatic tumours. J Hepatol 37: 806-813.

1532. Khayyata S, Basturk O, Adsay NV (2005). Invasive micropapillary carcinomas of the ampullo-pancreatobiliary region and their association with tumor-infiltrating neutrophils. Mod Pathol 18: 1504-1511.

1533. Kheir SM, Halpern NB (1984). Paraganglioma of the duodenum in association with congenital neurofibromatosis. Possible relationship. Cancer 53: 2491-2496.

1534. Khorana AA, Fine RL (2004). Pancreatic cancer and thromboembolic disease. Lancet Oncol 5: 655-663.

1535. Khunamornpong S, Lerwill MF, Siriaunkgul S, Suprasert P, Pojchamarnwiputh S, Chiangmai WN et al. (2008). Carcinoma of extrahepatic bile ducts and gallbladder metastatic to the ovary: a report of 16 cases. Int J Gynecol Pathol 27: 366-379.

1536. Kiani B, Ferrell LD, Qualman S, Frankel WL (2006). Immunohistochemical analysis of embryonal sarcoma of the liver. Appl Immunohistochem Mol Morphol 14: 193-197.

1537. Kidd M, Modlin IM, Shapiro MD, Camp RL, Mane SM, Usinger W et al. (2007). CTGF, intestinal stellate cells and carcinoid fibrogenesis. World J Gastroenterol 13: 5208-5216.

1538. Kiesslich R, Gossner L, Goetz M, Dahlmann A, Vieth M, Stolte M et al. (2006). In vivo histology of Barrett's esophagus and associated neoplasia by confocal laser endomicroscopy. Clin Gastroenterol Hepatol 4: 979-987.

1539. Kijima H, Takeshita T, Suzuki H, Tanahashi T, Suto A, Izumika H et al. (1999). Carcinosarcoma of the ampulla of Vater: a case report with immunohistochemical and ultrastructural studies. Am J Gastroenterol 94: 3055-3059.

1540. Kijima H, Watanabe H, Iwafuchi M, Ishihara N (1989). Histogenesis of gallbladder carcinoma from investigation of early carcinoma and microcarcinoma. Acta Pathol Jpn 39: 235-244.

1541. Kikuchi-Yanoshita R, Konishi M, Ito S, Seki M, Tanaka K, Maeda Y et al. (1992). Genetic changes of both p53 alleles associated with the conversion from colorectal adenoma to early carcinoma in familial adenomatous polyposis and non-familial adenomatous polyposis patients. Cancer Res 52: 3965-3971.

1542. Killinger WA, Jr., Rice TW, Adelstein DJ, Medendorp SV, Zuccaro G, Kirby TJ et al. (1996). Stage II esophageal carcinoma: the significance of T and N. J Thorac Cardiovasc Surg 111: 935-940.

1543. Kim DH, Lee HI, Nam ES, Shin HS, Sohn JH, Park CH et al. (2000). Reduced expression of the cell-cycle inhibitor p27Kip1 is associated with progression and lymph node metastasis of gastric carcinoma. Histopathology 36: 245-251.

1544. Kim DH, Song MH, Kim DH (2006). Malignant carcinoid tumor of the common bile duct: report of a case. Surg Today 36: 485-489.

1545. Kim DY, Kim KH, Jung SE, Lee SC, Park KW, Kim WK (2002). Undifferentiated (embryonal) sarcoma of the liver: combination treatment by surgery and chemotherapy. J Pediatr Surg 37: 1419-1423.

1546. Kim dH, Nagano Y, Choi IS, White JA, Yao JC, Rashid A (2008). Allelic alterations in well-differentiated neuroendocrine tumors (carcinoid tumors) identified by genome-wide single nucleotide polymorphism analysis and comparison with pancreatic endocrine tumors. Genes Chromosomes Cancer 47: 84-92.

1547. Kim GE, Thung SN, Tsui WM, Ferrell LD (2006). Hepatic cavernous hemangioma: under-recognized associated histologic features. Liver Int 26: 334-338.

1548. Kim H, Jen J, Vogelstein B, Hamilton SR (1994). Clinical and pathological characteristics of sporadic colorectal carcinomas with DNA replication errors in microsatellite sequences. Am J Pathol 145: 148-156.

1549. Kim H, Oh BK, Roncalli M, Park C, Yoon SM, Yoo JE et al. (2009). Large liver cell change in hepatitis B virus-related liver cirrhosis. Hepatology 50: 752-762.

1550. Kim H, Park C, Han KH, Choi J, Kim YB, Kim JK et al. (2004). Primary liver carcinoma of intermediate (hepatocyte-cholangiocyte) phenotype. J Hepatol 40: 298-304.

1551. Kim HJ, Lee DH, Ko YT, Lim JW, Kim HC, Kim KW (2008). CT of serous cystadenoma of the pancreas and mimicking masses. AJR Am J Roentgenol 190: 406-412.

1552. Kim IJ, Park JH, Kang HC, Shin Y, Park HW, Park HR et al. (2003). Mutational analysis of BRAF and K-ras in gastric cancers: absence of BRAF mutations in gastric cancers. Hum Genet 114: 118-120.

1553. Kim JH, Moon WS, Kang MJ, Park MJ, Lee DG (2001). Sarcomatoid carcinoma of the colon: a case report. J Korean Med Sci 16: 657-660.

1554. Kim KM, Calabrese P, Tavare S, Shibata D (2004). Enhanced stem cell survival in familial adenomatous polyposis. Am J Pathol 164: 1369-1377.

1555. Kim KM, Kim MJ, Cho BK, Choi SW, Rhyu MG (2002). Genetic evidence for the multistep progression of mixed glandular-neuroendocrine gastric carcinomas. Virchows Arch 440: 85-93.

1556. Kim L, Liao J, Zhang M, Talamonti M, Bentrem D, Rao S et al. (2008). Clear cell carcinoma of the pancreas: histopathologic features and a unique biomarker: hepatocyte nuclear factor-1beta. Mod Pathol 21: 1075-1083.

1557. Kim R, Weissfeld JL, Reynolds JC, Kuller LH (1997). Etiology of Barrett's metaplasia and esophageal adenocarcinoma. Cancer Epidemiol Biomarkers Prev 6: 369-377.

1558. Kim SG, Wu TT, Lee JH, Yun YK, Issa JP, Hamilton SR et al. (2003). Comparison of epigenetic and genetic alterations in mucinous cystic neoplasm and serous microcystic adenoma of pancreas. Mod Pathol 16: 1086-1094.

1559. Kim SH, Kim WS, Cheon JE, Yoon HK, Kang GH, Kim IO et al. (2007). Radiological spectrum of hepatic mesenchymal hamartoma in children. Korean J Radiol 8: 498-505.

1560. Kim SH, Park YN, Yoon DS, Lee SJ, Yu JS, Noh TW (2000). Composite neuroendocrine and adenocarcinoma of the common bile duct associated with Clonorchis sinensis: a case report. Hepatogastroenterology 47: 942-944.

1561. Kim T, Grobmyer SR, Liu C, Hochwald SN (2007). Primary presacral neuroendocrine tumor associated with imperforate anus. World J Surg Oncol 5: 115-

1562. Kim TK, Jang HJ, Burns PN, Murphy-Lavallee J, Wilson SR (2008). Focal nodular hyperplasia and hepatic adenoma: differentiation with low-mechanical-index contrast-enhanced sonography. AJR Am J Roentgenol 190: 58-66.

1563. Kim YH, Lee JH, Yang SK, Kim TI, Kim JS, Kim HJ et al. (2005). Primary colon lymphoma in Korea: a KASID (Korean Association for the Study of Intestinal Diseases) Study. Dig Dis Sci 50: 2243-2247.

1564. Kim YI, Kim ST, Lee GK, Choi BI (1990). Papillary cystic tumor of the liver. A case report with ultrastructural observation. Cancer 65: 2740-2746.

1565. Kimura H, Nakajima T, Kagawa K, Deguchi T, Kakusui M, Katagishi T et al. (1998). Angiogenesis in hepatocellular carcinoma as evaluated by CD34 immunohistochemistry. Liver 18: 14-19.

1566. Kimura W, Futakawa N, Yamagata S, Wada Y, Kuroda A, Muto T et al. (1994). Different clinicopathologic findings in two histologic types of carcinoma of papilla of Vater. Jpn J Cancer Res 85: 161-166.

1567. Kimura W, Kuroda A, Morioka Y (1991). Clinical pathology of endocrine tumors of the pancreas. Analysis of autopsy cases. Dig Dis Sci 36: 933-942.

1568. Kimura W, Ohtsubo K (1988). Incidence, sites of origin, and immunohistochemical and histochemical characteristics of atypical epithelium and minute carcinoma of the papilla of Vater. Cancer 61: 1394-1402.

1569. Kin M, Torimura T, Ueno T, Inuzuka S, Tanikawa K (1994). Sinusoidal capillarization in small hepatocellular carcinoma. Pathol Int 44: 771-778.

1570. Kindblom LG, Remotti HE, Aldenborg F, Meis-Kindblom JM (1998). Gastrointestinal pacemaker cell tumor (GIPACT): gastrointestinal stromal tumors show phenotypic characteristics of the interstitial cells of Cajal. Am J Pathol 152: 1259-1269.

1571. King JC, Ng TT, White SC, Cortina G, Reber HA, Hines OJ (2009). Pancreatic serous cystadenocarcinoma: a case report and review of the literature. J Gastrointest Surg 13: 1864-1868.

1572. Kinzler KW, Nilbert MC, Su LK, Vogelstein B, Bryan TM, Levy DB et al. (1991). Identification of FAP locus genes from chromosome 5q21. Science 253: 661-665.

1572A. Kipp BR, Stadheim LM, Halling SA, Pochron NL, Harmsen S, Nagorney DM et al. (2004). A comparison of routine cytology and fluorescence in situ hybridization for the detection of malignant bile duct strictures. Am J Gastroenterol 99: 1675–1681.

1573. Kirchner T, Reu S (2008). [Development of molecular-pathologic entities of colorectal cancer]. Pathologe 29 Suppl 2: 264-269.

1574. Kirk CM, Lewin D, Lazarchick J (1999). Primary hepatic B-cell lymphoma of mucosa-associated lymphoid tissue. Arch Pathol Lab Med 123: 716-719.

1575. Kiss A, Szepesi A, Lotz G, Nagy P, Schaff Z (1998). Expression of transforming growth factor-alpha in hepatoblastoma. Cancer 83: 690-697.

1576. Kitagami H, Kondo S, Hirano S, Kawakami H, Egawa S, Tanaka M (2007). Acinar cell carcinoma of the pancreas: clinical analysis of 115 patients from Pancreatic Cancer Registry of Japan Pancreas Society. Pancreas 35: 42-46.

1577. Kitagawa H, Ohta T, Makino I, Tani T, Tajima H, Nakagawara H et al. (2008).

Carcinomas of the ventral and dorsal pancreas exhibit different patterns of lymphatic spread. Front Biosci 13: 2728-2735.
1578. Kitagawa Y, Ueda M, Ando N, Ozawa S, Shimizu N, Kitajima M (1996). Further evidence for prognostic significance of epidermal growth factor receptor gene amplification in patients with esophageal squamous cell carcinoma. Clin Cancer Res 2: 909-914.
1579. Kitagawa Y, Unger TA, Taylor S, Kozarek RA, Traverso LW (2003). Mucus is a predictor of better prognosis and survival in patients with intraductal papillary mucinous tumor of the pancreas. J Gastrointest Surg 7: 12-18.
1580. Kitago M, Ueda M, Aiura K, Suzuki K, Hoshimoto S, Takahashi S et al. (2004). Comparison of K-ras point mutation distributions in intraductal papillary-mucinous tumors and ductal adenocarcinoma of the pancreas. Int J Cancer 110: 177-182.
1581. Kitakata H, Nemoto-Sasaki Y, Takahashi Y, Kondo T, Mai M, Mukaida N (2002). Essential roles of tumor necrosis factor receptor p55 in liver metastasis of intrasplenic administration of colon 26 cells. Cancer Res 62: 6682-6687.
1582. Kitamoto Y, Hasegawa M, Ishikawa H, Saito J, Yamakawa M, Kojima M et al. (2003). Mucosa-associated lymphoid tissue lymphoma of the esophagus: a case report. J Clin Gastroenterol 36: 414-416.
1583. Kitamura H, Yazawa T, Sato H, Okudela K, Shimoyamada H (2009). Small cell lung cancer: significance of RB alterations and TTF-1 expression in its carcinogenesis, phenotype, and biology. Endocr Pathol 20: 101-107.
1584. Klapper W, Hoster E, Determann O, Oschlies I, van der Laak J, Berger F et al. (2009). Ki-67 as a prognostic marker in mantle cell lymphoma-consensus guidelines of the pathology panel of the European MCL Network. J Hematop 2:103-111.
1585. Klas JV, Rothenberger DA, Wong WD, Madoff RD (1999). Malignant tumors of the anal canal: the spectrum of disease, treatment, and outcomes. Cancer 85: 1686-1693.
1586. Klein A, Clemens J, Cameron J (1989). Periampullary neoplasms in von Recklinghausen's disease. Surgery 106: 815-819.
1587. Klein AP, Beaty TH, Bailey-Wilson JE, Brune KA, Hruban RH, Petersen GM (2002). Evidence for a major gene influencing risk of pancreatic cancer. Genet Epidemiol 23: 133-149.
1588. Klein AP, Brune KA, Petersen GM, Goggins M, Tersmette AC, Offerhaus GJ et al. (2004). Prospective risk of pancreatic cancer in familial pancreatic cancer kindreds. Cancer Res 64: 2634-2638.
1589. Klein KA, Stephens DH, Welch TJ (1998). CT characteristics of metastatic disease of the pancreas. Radiographics 18: 369-378.
1590. Kletter GB, Sweetser DA, Wallace SF, Sawin RS, Rutledge JC, Geyer JR (2007). Adrenocorticotropin-secreting pancreatoblastoma. J Pediatr Endocrinol Metab 20: 639-642.
1591. Klimstra DS (1994). Pathologic prognostic factors in esophageal carcinoma. Semin Oncol 21: 425-430.
1592. Klimstra DS (1998). Cell lineage in pancreatic neoplasms. In: Pancreatic Cancer: Advances in Molecular Pathology, Diagnosis and Clinical Management. Sarkar FH, Dugan MC, eds. Eaton Publishing Company/BioTechniques Books: Natick, MA.
1593. Klimstra DS (2005). Cystic, mucin-producing neoplasms of the pancreas: the distinguishing features of mucinous cystic neoplasms and intraductal papillary mucinous neoplasms. Semin Diagn Pathol 22: 318-329.
1594. Klimstra DS (2007). Nonductal neoplasms of the pancreas. Mod Pathol 20 Suppl 1: S94-112.
1595. Klimstra DS, Adsay NV (2001). Acinar cell carcinoma of the pancreas. A case associated with the lipase hypersecretion syndrome. Pathol Case Rev 6: 121-126.
1596. Klimstra DS, Adsay NV (2008). Tumors of the pancreas and ampulla of Vater. In: Surgical Pathology of the GI Tract, Liver, Biliary Tract, and Pancreas. Odze RD, Goldblum JR, eds. Saunders Elsevier: Philadelphia, pp. 909-960.
1597. Klimstra DS, Adsay NV, Dhall D, Shimizu M, Cymes K, Basturk O et al. (2007). Intraductal tubular carcinoma of the pancreas: clinicopathologic and immunohistochemical analysis of 18 cases. Mod Pathol 20: 285A-
1598. Klimstra DS, Heffess CS, Oertel JE, Rosai J (1992). Acinar cell carcinoma of the pancreas. A clinicopathologic study of 28 cases. Am J Surg Pathol 16: 815-837.
1599. Klimstra DS, Modlin IR, Adsay NV, Chetty R, Deshpande V, Gonen M et al. (2010). Pathology reporting of neuroendocrine tumors: application of the Delphic Consensus Process to the development of a minimum pathology data set. Am J Surg Pathol 34:300-313.
1600. Klimstra DS, Pitman MB, Hruban RH (2009). An algorithmic approach to the diagnosis of pancreatic neoplasms. Arch Pathol Lab Med 133: 454-464.
1601. Klimstra DS, Rosai J, Heffess CS (1994). Mixed acinar-endocrine carcinomas of the pancreas. Am J Surg Pathol 18: 765-778.
1602. Klimstra DS, Wenig BM, Adair CF, Heffess CS (1995). Pancreatoblastoma. A clinicopathologic study and review of the literature. Am J Surg Pathol 19: 1371-1389.
1603. Klimstra DS, Wenig BM, Heffess CS (2000). Solid-pseudopapillary tumor of the pancreas: a typically cystic carcinoma of low malignant potential. Semin Diagn Pathol 17: 66-80.
1604. Klöppel G (1994). Pancreatic, nonendocrine tumours. In: Pancreatic Pathology. Klöppel G, Heitz PU, eds. Churchill Livingstone: Edinburgh, pp. 79-113.
1605. Klöppel G (1998). Clinicopathologic view of intraductal papillary-mucinous tumor of the pancreas. Hepatogastroenterology 45: 1981-1985.
1606. Klöppel G, Adsay NV (2009). Chronic pancreatitis and the differential diagnosis versus pancreatic cancer. Arch Pathol Lab Med 133: 382-387.
1607. Klöppel G, Clemens A (1996). The biological relevance of gastric neuroendocrine tumors. Yale J Biol Med 69: 69-74.
1608. Klöppel G, Couvelard A, Perren A, Komminoth P, McNicol AM, Nilsson O et al. (2009). ENETS Consensus Guidelines for the Standards of Care in Neuroendocrine Tumors: towards a standardized approach to the diagnosis of gastroenteropancreatic neuroendocrine tumors and their prognostic stratification. Neuroendocrinology 90: 162-166.
1609. Klöppel G, Heitz PU (1988). Pancreatic endocrine tumors. Pathol Res Pract 183: 155-168.
1610. Klöppel G, Kosmahl M (2001). Cystic lesions and neoplasms of the pancreas. The features are becoming clearer. Pancreatology 1: 648-655.
1611. Klöppel G, Kosmahl M (2006). Is the intraductal papillary mucinous neoplasia of the biliary tract a counterpart of pancreatic papillary mucinous neoplasm? J Hepatol 44: 249-250.
1612. Klöppel G, Lingenthal G, von BM, Kern HF (1985). Histological and fine structural features of pancreatic ductal adenocarcinomas in relation to growth and prognosis: studies in xenografted tumours and clinico-histopathological correlation in a series of 75 cases. Histopathology 9: 841-856.
1613. Klöppel G, Lohse T, Bosslet K, Ruckert K (1987). Ductal adenocarcinoma of the head of the pancreas: incidence of tumor involvement beyond the Whipple resection line. Histological and immunocytochemical analysis of 37 total pancreatectomy specimens. Pancreas 2: 170-175.
1614. Klöppel G, Maurer R, Hofmann E, Luthold K, Oscarson J, Forsby N et al. (1991). Solid-cystic (papillary-cystic) tumours within and outside the pancreas in men: report of two patients. Virchows Arch A Pathol Anat Histopathol 418: 179-183.
1615. Klöppel G, Morohoshi T, John HD, Oehmichen W, Opitz K, Angelkort A et al. (1981). Solid and cystic acinar cell tumour of the pancreas. A tumour in young women with favourable prognosis. Virchows Arch A Pathol Anat Histol 392: 171-183.
1616. Klöppel G, Rindi G, Anlauf M, Perren A, Komminoth P (2007). Site-specific biology and pathology of gastroenteropancreatic neuroendocrine tumors. Virchows Arch 451 Suppl 1: S9-27.
1617. Klöppel G, Solcia E, Longnecker DS, Capella C, and Sobin LH (eds) (1996). Histological Typing of Tumours of the Exocrine Pancreas. Springer-Verlag: Berlin.
1618. Knight BK, Hayes MM (1987). Mixed adenocarcinoma and carcinoid tumour of the colon. A report of 4 cases with postulates on histogenesis. S Afr Med J 72: 708-710.
1619. Knudsen AL, Bisgaard ML, Bulow S (2003). Attenuated familial adenomatous polyposis (AFAP). A review of the literature. Fam Cancer 2: 43-55.
1620. Ko YH, Kim CW, Park CS, Jang HK, Lee SS, Kim SH et al. (1998). REAL classification of malignant lymphomas in the Republic of Korea: incidence of recently recognized entities and changes in clinicopathologic features. Hematolymphoreticular Study Group of the Korean Society of Pathologists. Revised European-American lymphoma. Cancer 83: 806-812.
1621. Kobayashi M, Ikeda K, Saitoh S, Suzuki F, Tsubota A, Suzuki Y et al. (2000). Incidence of primary cholangiocellular carcinoma of the liver in Japanese patients with hepatitis C virus-related cirrhosis. Cancer 88: 2471-2477.
1621A. Kobayashi Y, Nakanishi Y, Taniguchi H, Sekine S, Igaki H, Tachimori Y et al. (2009). Histological diversity in basaloid squamous cell carcinoma of the esophagus. Dis Esophagus 22: 231–238.
1622. Koch P, del VF, Berdel WE, Willich NA, Reers B, Hiddemann W et al. (2001). Primary gastrointestinal non-Hodgkin's lymphoma: I. Anatomic and histologic distribution, clinical features, and survival data of 371 patients registered in the German Multicenter Study GIT NHL 01/92. J Clin Oncol 19: 3861-3873.
1623. Kodach LL, Wiercinska E, de Miranda NF, Bleuming SA, Musler AR, Peppelenbosch MP et al. (2008). The bone morphogenetic protein pathway is inactivated in the majority of sporadic colorectal cancers. Gastroenterology 134: 1332-1341.
1624. Kodama I, Kofuji K, Yano S, Shinozaki K, Murakami N, Hori H et al. (1998). Lymph node metastasis and lymphadenectomy for carcinoma in the gastric cardia: clinical experience. Int Surg 83: 205-209.
1625. Kodama M, Kitadai Y, Shishido T, Shimamoto M, Fukumoto A, Masuda H et al. (2008). Primary follicular lymphoma of the gastrointestinal tract: a retrospective case series. Endoscopy 40: 343-346.
1626. Kodama T, Ohshima K, Nomura K, Taniwaki M, Nakamura N, Nakamura S et al. (2005). Lymphomatous polyposis of the gastrointestinal tract, including mantle cell lymphoma, follicular lymphoma and mucosa-associated lymphoid tissue lymphoma. Histopathology 47: 467-478.
1627. Koffron A, Rao S, Ferrario M, Abecassis M (2004). Intrahepatic biliary cystadenoma: role of cyst fluid analysis and surgical management in the laparoscopic era. Surgery 136: 926-936.
1628. Kohashi K, Oda Y, Yamamoto H, Tamiya S, Izumi T, Ohta S et al. (2007). Highly aggressive behavior of malignant rhabdoid tumor: a special reference to *SMARCB1/INI1* gene alterations using molecular genetic analysis including quantitative real-time PCR. J Cancer Res Clin Oncol 133: 817-824.
1629. Kohno S, Ohshima K, Yoneda S, Kodama T, Shirakusa T, Kikuchi M (2003). Clinicopathological analysis of 143 primary malignant lymphomas in the small and large intestines based on the new WHO classification. Histopathology 43: 135-143.
1630. Koito K, Namieno T, Ichimura T, Yama N, Hareyama M, Morita K et al. (1998). Mucin-producing pancreatic tumors: comparison of MR cholangiopancreatography with endoscopic retrograde cholangiopancreatography. Radiology 208: 231-237.
1631. Koito K, Namieno T, Nagakawa T, Hirokawa N, Ichimura T, Syonai T et al. (2001). Pancreas: imaging diagnosis with color/power Doppler ultrasonography, endoscopic ultrasonography, and intraductal ultrasonography. Eur J Radiol 38: 94-104.
1632. Kojima M, Nakamura S, Ohno Y, Sugihara S, Sakata N, Masawa N (2004). Hepatic angiomyolipoma resembling an inflammatory pseudotumor of the liver. A case report. Pathol Res Pract 200: 713-716.
1633. Kojiro M (eds) (2006). Pathology of Hepatocellular Carcinoma. Blackwell: Malden, MA.
1634. Kojiro M, Sugihara S, Kakizoe S, Nakashima O, Kiyomatsu K (1989). Hepatocellular carcinoma with sarcomatous change: a special reference to the relationship with anticancer therapy. Cancer Chemother Pharmacol 23 Suppl: S4-S8.
1635. Kolodner RD, Hall NR, Lipford J, Kane MF, Morrison PT, Finan PJ et al. (1995). Structure of the human MLH1 locus and analysis of a large hereditary nonpolyposis colorectal carcinoma kindred for mlh1 mutations. Cancer Res 55: 242-248.
1636. Kolodner RD, Hall NR, Lipford J, Kane MF, Rao MR, Morrison P et al. (1994). Structure of the human MSH2 locus and analysis of two Muir-Torre kindreds for msh2 mutations. Genomics 24: 516-526.
1637. Komorowski RA, Cohen EB (1981). Villous tumors of the duodenum: a clinicopathologic study. Cancer 47: 1377-1386.
1638. Komuta M, Spee B, Vander Borght S, De Vos R, Verslype C, Aerts R et al. (2008). Clinicopathological study on cholangiolocellular carcinoma suggesting hepatic progenitor cell origin. Hepatology 47: 1544-1556.
1639. Konda A, Duffy MC (2008). Surveillance of patients at increased risk of colon cancer: inflammatory bowel disease and other conditions. Gastroenterol Clin North Am 37: 191-213.
1640. Kondo E, Furukawa T, Yoshinaga K, Kijima H, Semba S, Yatsuoka T et al. (2000). Not hMSH2 but hMLH1 is frequently silenced by hypermethylation in endometrial cancer but rarely silenced in pancreatic cancer with microsatellite instability. Int J Oncol 17: 535-541.
1641. Kondo F (2009). Histological features of early hepatocellular carcinomas and their developmental process: for daily practical clinical application : Hepatocellular carcinoma. Hepatol Int 3: 283-293.
1642. Kondo F, Wada K, Nagato Y, Nakajima T, Kondo Y, Hirooka N et al. (1989). Biopsy diag-

nosis of well-differentiated hepatocellular carcinoma based on new morphologic criteria. Hepatology 9: 751-755.

1643. Kondo H, Sugano K, Fukayama N, Kyogoku A, Nose H, Shimada K et al. (1994). Detection of point mutations in the K-ras oncogene at codon 12 in pure pancreatic juice for diagnosis of pancreatic carcinoma. Cancer 73: 1589-1594.

1644. Kondo K (2002). Duodenogastric reflux and gastric stump carcinoma. Gastric Cancer 5: 16-22.

1645. Kondo Y, Kanai Y, Sakamoto M, Mizokami M, Ueda R, Hirohashi S (2000). Genetic instability and aberrant DNA methylation in chronic hepatitis and cirrhosis—A comprehensive study of loss of heterozygosity and microsatellite instability at 39 loci and DNA hypermethylation on 8 CpG islands in microdissected specimens from patients with hepatocellular carcinoma. Hepatology 32: 970-979.

1646. Konigsrainer I, Glatzle J, Klöppel G, Konigsrainer A, Wehrmann M (2008). Intraductal and cystic tubulopapillary adenocarcinoma of the pancreas—a possible variant of intraductal tubular carcinoma. Pancreas 36: 92-95.

1647. Konishi E, Nakashima Y, Smyrk TC, Masuda S (2003). Clear cell carcinoid tumor of the gallbladder. A case without von Hippel-Lindau disease. Arch Pathol Lab Med 127: 745-747.

1648. Konishi T, Watanabe T, Kishimoto J, Kotake K, Muto T, Nagawa H (2007). Prognosis and risk factors of metastasis in colorectal carcinoids: results of a nationwide registry over 15 years. Gut 56: 863-868.

1649. Konopke R, Distler M, Ludwig S, Kersting S (2008). Location of liver metastases reflects the site of the primary colorectal carcinoma. Scand J Gastroenterol 43: 192-195.

1650. Koo LC, Mang OW, Ho JH (1997). An ecological study of trends in cancer incidence and dietary changes in Hong Kong. Nutr Cancer 28: 289-301.

1651. Koppert LB, Wijnhoven BP, van Dekken H, Tilanus HW, Dinjens WN (2005). The molecular biology of esophageal adenocarcinoma. J Surg Oncol 92: 169-190.

1652. Kosmahl M, Egawa N, Schroder S, Carneiro F, Luttges J, Klöppel G (2002). Mucinous nonneoplastic cyst of the pancreas: a novel nonneoplastic cystic change? Mod Pathol 15: 154-158.

1653. Kosmahl M, Pauser U, Anlauf M, Klöppel G (2005). Pancreatic ductal adenocarcinomas with cystic features: neither rare nor uniform. Mod Pathol 18: 1157-1164.

1654. Kosmahl M, Pauser U, Anlauf M, Sipos B, Peters K, Luttges J et al. (2005). [Cystic pancreas tumors and their classification: features old and new]. Pathologe 26: 22-30.

1655. Kosmahl M, Pauser U, Peters K, Sipos B, Luttges J, Kremer B et al. (2004). Cystic neoplasms of the pancreas and tumor-like lesions with cystic features: a review of 418 cases and a classification proposal. Virchows Arch 445: 168-178.

1656. Kosmahl M, Seada LS, Janig U, Harms D, Klöppel G (2000). Solid-pseudopapillary tumor of the pancreas: its origin revisited. Virchows Arch 436: 473-480.

1657. Kosmahl M, Wagner J, Peters K, Sipos B, Klöppel G (2004). Serous cystic neoplasms of the pancreas: an immunohistochemical analysis revealing alpha-inhibin, neuron-specific enolase, and MUC6 as new markers. Am J Surg Pathol 28: 339-346.

1658. Kotoula V, Hytiroglou P, Pyrpasopoulou A, Saxena R, Thung SN, Papadimitriou CS (2002). Expression of human telomerase reverse transcriptase in regenerative and precancerous lesions of cirrhotic livers. Liver 22: 57-69.

1659. Koura AN, Giacco GG, Curley SA, Skibber JM, Feig BW, Ellis LM (1997). Carcinoid tumors of the rectum: effect of size, histopathology, and surgical treatment on metastasis free survival. Cancer 79: 1294-1298.

1660. Kovacs K, Asa SL (eds) (1998). Functional Endocrine Pathology. Blackwell Science Inc.: Oxford, Boston.

1661. Kozma L, Kiss I, Hajdu J, Szentkereszty Z, Szakall S, Ember I (2001). C-myc amplification and cluster analysis in human gastric carcinoma. Anticancer Res 21: 707-710.

1662. Kozuka S, Sassa R, Taki T, Masamoto K, Nagasawa S, Saga S et al. (1979). Relation of pancreatic duct hyperplasia to carcinoma. Cancer 43: 1418-1428.

1663. Kozuka S, Tsubone M, Yamaguchi A, Hachisuka K (1981). Adenomatous residue in cancerous papilla of Vater. Gut 22: 1031-1034.

1664. Kriege M, Brekelmans CT, Boetes C, Besnard PE, Zonderland HM, Obdeijn IM et al. (2004). Efficacy of MRI and mammography for breast-cancer screening in women with a familial or genetic predisposition. N Engl J Med 351: 427-437.

1665. Krishna NB, Mehra M, Reddy AV, Agarwal B (2009). EUS/EUS-FNA for suspected pancreatic cancer: influence of chronic pancreatitis and clinical presentation with or without obstructive jaundice on performance characteristics. Gastrointest Endosc 70: 70-79.

1666. Kruse R, Rutten A, Lamberti C, Hosseiny-Malayeri HR, Wang Y, Ruelfs C et al. (1998). Muir-Torre phenotype has a frequency of DNA mismatch-repair-gene mutations similar to that in hereditary nonpolyposis colorectal cancer families defined by the Amsterdam criteria. Am J Hum Genet 63: 63-70.

1667. Ku GY, Minsky BD, Rusch VW, Bains M, Kelsen DP, Ilson DH (2008). Small-cell carcinoma of the esophagus and gastroesophageal junction: review of the Memorial Sloan-Kettering experience. Ann Oncol 19: 533-537.

1668. Kubicka S, Kuhnel F, Flemming P, Hain B, Kezmic N, Rudolph KL et al. (2001). K-ras mutations in the bile of patients with primary sclerosing cholangitis. Gut 48: 403-408.

1669. Kubo A, Corley DA (2006). Body mass index and adenocarcinomas of the esophagus or gastric cardia: a systematic review and meta-analysis. Cancer Epidemiol Biomarkers Prev 15: 872-878.

1670. Kubo H, Chijiiwa Y, Akahoshi K, Hamada S, Matsui N, Nawata H (1999). Pre-operative staging of ampullary tumours by endoscopic ultrasound. Br J Radiol 72: 443-447.

1671. Kudo M (2008). Hepatocellular carcinoma 2009 and beyond: from the surveillance to molecular targeted therapy. Oncology 75 Suppl 1: 1-12.

1671A. Kudo M (2010). The 2008 Okuda lecture: Management of hepatocellular carcinoma: from surveillance to molecular targeted therapy. J Gastroenterol Hepatol 25: 439-452.

1672. Kudo M, Okanoue T (2007). Management of hepatocellular carcinoma in Japan: consensus-based clinical practice manual proposed by the Japan Society of Hepatology. Oncology 72 Suppl 1: 2-15.

1673. Kuerer H, Shim H, Pertsemlidis D, Unger P (1997). Functioning pancreatic acinar cell carcinoma: immunohistochemical and ultrastructural analyses. Am J Clin Oncol 20: 101-107.

1674. Kuhlmann KF, de Castro SM, Wesseling JG, ten Kate FJ, Offerhaus GJ, Busch OR et al. (2004). Surgical treatment of pancreatic adenocarcinoma; actual survival and prognostic factors in 343 patients. Eur J Cancer 40: 549-558.

1675. Kuhn Y, Koscielny A, Glowka T, Hirner A, Kalff JC, Standop J (2009). Postresection survival outcomes of pancreatic cancer according to demographic factors and socio-economic status. Eur J Surg Oncol 36: 496-500.

1676. Kumagai Y, Kawada K, Yamazaki S, Iida M, Momma K, Odajima H et al. (2009). Endocytoscopic observation for esophageal squamous cell carcinoma: can biopsy histology be omitted? Dis Esophagus 22: 505-512.

1677. Kumar S, Fend F, Quintanilla-Martinez L, Kingma DW, Sorbara L, Raffeld M et al. (2000). Epstein-Barr virus-positive primary gastrointestinal Hodgkin's disease: association with inflammatory bowel disease and immunosuppression. Am J Surg Pathol 24: 66-73.

1678. Kuniyasu H, Yasui W, Kitadai Y, Yokozaki H, Ito H, Tahara E (1992). Frequent amplification of the c-met gene in scirrhous type stomach cancer. Biochem Biophys Res Commun 189: 227-232.

1679. Kunke D, Bryja V, Mygland L, Arenas E, Krauss S (2009). Inhibition of canonical Wnt signaling promotes gliogenesis in P0-NSCs. Biochem Biophys Res Commun 386: 628-633.

1680. Kuo TT, Su IJ, Chien CH (1984). Solid and papillary neoplasm of the pancreas. Report of three cases from Taiwan. Cancer 54: 1469-1474.

1681. Kuo YH, Wang JH, Lu SN, Hung CH, Wei YC, Hu TH et al. (2009). Natural course of hepatic focal nodular hyperplasia: a long-term follow-up study with sonography. J Clin Ultrasound 37: 132-137.

1682. Kuopio T, Ekfors TO, Nikkanen V, Nevalainen TJ (1995). Acinar cell carcinoma of the pancreas. Report of three cases. APMIS 103: 69-78.

1683. Kurahashi H, Takami K, Oue T, Kusafuka T, Okada A, Tawa A et al. (1995). Biallelic inactivation of the APC gene in hepatoblastoma. Cancer Res 55: 5007-5011.

1684. Kuraoka K, Hoshino E, Tsuchida T, Fujisaki J, Takahashi H, Fujita R (2009). Early esophageal cancer can be detected by screening endoscopy assisted with narrow-band imaging (NBI). Hepatogastroenterology 56: 63-66.

1685. Kuraoka K, Taniyama K, Fujitaka T, Nakatsuka H, Nakayama H, Yasui W (2003). Small cell carcinoma of the extrahepatic bile duct: case report and immunohistochemical analysis. Pathol Int 53: 887-891.

1686. Kurita M, Komatsu H, Hata Y, Shiina S, Ota S, Terano A et al. (1994). Pseudomyxoma peritonei due to adenocarcinoma of the lung: case report. J Gastroenterol 29: 344-348.

1687. Kuroda N, Oonishi K, Ohara M, Hirouchi T, Mizuno K, Hayashi Y et al. (2007). Invasive micropapillary carcinoma of the colon: an immunohistochemical study. Med Mol Morphol 40: 226-230.

1688. Kurogi M, Nakashima O, Miyaaki H, Fujimoto M, Kojiro M (2006). Clinicopathological study of scirrhous hepatocellular carcinoma. J Gastroenterol Hepatol 21: 1470-1477.

1689. Kurose K, Araki T, Matsunaka T, Takada Y, Emi M (1999). Variant manifestation of Cowden disease in Japan: hamartomatous polyposis of the digestive tract with mutation of the PTEN gene. Am J Hum Genet 64: 308-310.

1690. Kurtz RC, Sternberg SS, Miller HH, DeCosse JJ (1987). Upper gastrointestinal neoplasia in familial polyposis. Dig Dis Sci 32: 459-465.

1691. Kurzawski G, Suchy J, Kladny J, Grabowska E, Mierzejewski M, Jakubowska A et al. (2004). The NOD2 3020insC mutation and the risk of colorectal cancer. Cancer Res 64: 1604-1606.

1692. Kushima R, Hattori T (1993). Histogenesis and characteristics of gastric-type adenocarcinomas in the stomach. J Cancer Res Clin Oncol 120: 103-111.

1693. Kushima R, Remmele W, Stolte M, Borchard F (1996). Pyloric gland type adenoma of the gallbladder with squamoid spindle cell metaplasia. Pathol Res Pract 192: 963-969.

1694. Kushima R, Vieth M, Borchard F, Stolte M, Mukaisho K, Hattori T (2006). Gastric-type well-differentiated adenocarcinoma and pyloric gland adenoma of the stomach. Gastric Cancer 9: 177-184.

1695. Kusumoto H, Yoshitake H, Mochida K, Kumashiro R, Sano C, Inutsuka S (1992). Adenocarcinoma in Meckel's diverticulum: report of a case and review of 30 cases in the English and Japanese literature. Am J Gastroenterol 87: 910-913.

1696. Kuwano H (1998). Peculiar histopathologic features of esophageal cancer. Surg Today 28: 573-575.

1697. Kuwano H, Nishimura Y, Ohts H, Kato H, Kitagawa Y, Tamai S et al. (2008). Guidelines for diagnosis and treatment of carcinoma of the esophagus. April 2007 edition: part I. Edited by the Japan Esophageal Society. Esophagus 5: 61-73.

1698. Kvist N, Jacobsen O, Kvist HK, Norgaard P, Ockelmann HH, Schou G et al. (1989). Malignancy in ulcerative colitis. Scand J Gastroenterol 24: 497-506.

1699. Kwaan MR, Goldberg JE, Bleday R (2008). Rectal carcinoid tumors: review of results after endoscopic and surgical therapy. Arch Surg 143: 471-475.

1700. Kwak EL, Jankowski J, Thayer SP, Lauwers GY, Brannigan BW, Harris PL et al. (2006). Epidermal growth factor receptor kinase domain mutations in esophageal and pancreatic adenocarcinomas. Clin Cancer Res 12: 4283-4287.

1701. Kwekkeboom DJ, Krenning EP (1996). Somatostatin receptor scintigraphy in patients with carcinoid tumors. World J Surg 20: 157-161.

1702. Ky A, Sohn N, Weinstein MA, Korelitz BI (1998). Carcinoma arising in anorectal fistulas of Crohn's disease. Dis Colon Rectum 41: 992-996.

1703. La Rosa S, Chiaravalli AM, Capella C, Uccella S, Sessa F (1997). Immunohistochemical localization of acidic fibroblast growth factor in normal human enterochromaffin cells and related gastrointestinal tumours. Virchows Arch 430: 117-124.

1704. La Rosa S, Franzi F, Marchet S, Finzi G, Clerici M, Vigetti D et al. (2009). The monoclonal anti-BCL10 antibody (clone 331.1) is a sensitive and specific marker of pancreatic acinar cell carcinoma and pancreatic metaplasia. Virchows Arch 454: 133-142.

1705. La Rosa S, Klersy C, Uccella S, Dainese L, Albarello L, Sonzogni A et al. (2009). Improved histologic and clinicopathologic criteria for prognostic evaluation of pancreatic endocrine tumors. Hum Pathol 40: 30-40.

1706. La Rosa S, Rigoli E, Uccella S, Chiaravalli AM, Capella C (2004). CDX2 as a marker of intestinal EC-cells and related well-differentiated endocrine tumors. Virchows Arch 445: 248-254.

1707. La Rosa S, Sessa F, Capella C, Riva C, Leone BE, Klersy C et al. (1996). Prognostic criteria in nonfunctioning pancreatic endocrine tumours. Virchows Arch 429: 323-333.

1708. La Rosa S, Uccella S, Billo P, Facco C, Sessa F, Capella C (1999). Immunohistochemical localization of alpha- and betaA-subunits of inhibin/activin in human normal endocrine cells and related tumors of the digestive system. Virchows Arch 434: 29-36.

1709. La Rosa S, Uccella S, Capella C, Chiaravalli A, Sessa F (1998). Localization of acidic fibroblast growth factor, fibroblast growth factor receptor-4, transforming growth factor alpha, and epidermal growth receptor in human endocrine cells of the gut and related tumors: an immunohistochemical study. Appl Immunohistochem 6: 199-208.

1710. Labate AM, Klimstra DL, Zakowski MF (1997). Comparative cytologic features of pancreatic acinar cell carcinoma and islet cell tumor. Diagn Cytopathol 16: 112-116.

1711. Laberge JM, Patenaude Y, Desilets V, Cartier L, Khalife S, Jutras L et al. (2005). Large hepatic mesenchymal hamartoma leading to mid-trimester fetal demise. Fetal Diagn Ther 20: 141-145.

1712. Lack EE (1986). Mesenchymal hamartoma of the liver. A clinical and pathologic study of nine cases. Am J Pediatr Hematol Oncol 8: 91-98.

1713. Lack EE, Cassady JR, Levey R, Vawter GF (1983). Tumors of the exocrine pancreas in children and adolescents. A clinical and pathologic study of eight cases. Am J Surg Pathol 7: 319-327.

1714. Lack EE, Perez-Atayde AR, Schuster SR (1981). Botryoid rhabdomyosarcoma of the biliary tract. Am J Surg Pathol 5: 643-652.

1715. Lack EE, Schloo BL, Azumi N, Travis WD, Grier HE, Kozakewich HP (1991). Undifferentiated (embryonal) sarcoma of the liver. Clinical and pathologic study of 16 cases with emphasis on immunohistochemical features. Am J Surg Pathol 15: 1-16.

1716. Ladeira MS, Rodrigues MA, Salvadori DM, Queiroz DM, Freire-Maia DV (2004). DNA damage in patients infected by *Helicobacter pylori*. Cancer Epidemiol Biomarkers Prev 13: 631-637.

1717. Laffan TA, Horton KM, Klein AP, Berlanstein B, Siegelman SS, Kawamoto S et al. (2008). Prevalence of unsuspected pancreatic cysts on MDCT. AJR Am J Roentgenol 191: 802-807.

1718. Lagarde SM, ten Kate FJ, Richel DJ, Offerhaus GJ, van Lanschot JJ (2007). Molecular prognostic factors in adenocarcinoma of the esophagus and gastroesophageal junction. Ann Surg Oncol 14: 977-991.

1719. Lage P, Cravo M, Sousa R, Chaves P, Salazar M, Fonseca R et al. (2004). Management of Portuguese patients with hyperplastic polyposis and screening of at-risk first-degree relatives: a contribution for future guidelines based on a clinical study. Am J Gastroenterol 99: 1779-1784.

1720. Lagergren J (2005). Adenocarcinoma of oesophagus: what exactly is the size of the problem and who is at risk? Gut 54 Suppl 1: i1-i5.

1721. Lagergren J, Bergstrom R, Lindgren A, Nyren O (1999). Symptomatic gastroesophageal reflux as a risk factor for esophageal adenocarcinoma. N Engl J Med 340: 825-831.

1722. Lagergren J, Ye W, Bergstrom R, Nyren O (2000). Utility of endoscopic screening for upper gastrointestinal adenocarcinoma. JAMA 284: 961-962.

1723. Lai EC, Lau WY (2005). Intraductal papillary mucinous neoplasms of the pancreas. Surgeon 3: 317-324.

1724. Lai MD, Luo MJ, Yao JE, Chen PH (1998). Anal cancer in Chinese: human papillomavirus infection and altered expression of p53. World J Gastroenterol 4: 298-302.

1725. Laitio M (1983). Carcinoma of extrahepatic bile ducts. A histopathologic study. Pathol Res Pract 178: 67-72.

1726. Lakatos PL, Miheller P (2010). Is there an increased risk of lymphoma and malignancies under anti-TNF therapy in IBD? Curr Drug Targets 11: 179-186.

1727. Laken SJ, Papadopoulos N, Petersen GM, Gruber SB, Hamilton SR, Giardiello FM et al. (1999). Analysis of masked mutations in familial adenomatous polyposis. Proc Natl Acad Sci U S A 96: 2322-2326.

1728. Lal A, Bourtsos EP, De Frias DV, Nemcek AA, Nayar R (2004). Microcystic adenoma of the pancreas: clinical, radiologic, and cytologic features. Cancer 102: 288-294.

1729. Lal A, Okonkwo A, Schindler S, De Frias D, Nayar R (2004). Role of biliary brush cytology in primary sclerosing cholangitis. Acta Cytol 48: 9-12.

1730. Lam KY, Law SY, So MK, Fok M, Ma LT, Wong J (1996). Prognostic implication of proliferative markers MIB-1 and PC10 in esophageal squamous cell carcinoma. Cancer 77: 7-13.

1731. Lam KY, Leung CY, Ho JW (1996). Sarcomatoid carcinoma of the small intestine. Aust N Z J Surg 66: 636-639.

1732. Lambert R (1999). Diagnosis of esophagogastric tumors: a trend toward virtual biopsy. Endoscopy 31: 38-46.

1733. Lambert R (1999). The role of endoscopy in the prevention of esophagogastric cancer. Endoscopy 31: 180-199.

1734. Lambert R, Kudo SE, Vieth M, Allen JI, Fujii H, Fujii T et al. (2009). Pragmatic classification of superficial neoplastic colorectal lesions. Gastrointest Endosc 70: 1182-1199.

1735. Lamps LW, Folpe AL (2003). The diagnostic value of hepatocyte paraffin antibody 1 in differentiating hepatocellular neoplasms from nonhepatic tumors: a review. Adv Anat Pathol 10: 39-43.

1736. Lanas A (2009). Nonsteroidal antiinflammatory drugs and cyclooxygenase inhibition in the gastrointestinal tract: a trip from peptic ulcer to colon cancer. Am J Med Sci 338: 96-106.

1737. Lance P, Hamilton SR (2008). Sporadic aberrant crypt foci are not a surrogate endpoint for colorectal adenoma prevention. Cancer Prev Res 1: 4-8.

1738. Landry CS, Brock G, Scoggins CR, McMasters KM, Martin RC (2008). A proposed staging system for rectal carcinoid tumors based on an analysis of 4701 patients. Surgery 144: 460-466.

1739. Langan JE, Cole CG, Huckle EJ, Byrne S, McRonald FE, Rowbottom L et al. (2004). Novel microsatellite markers and single nucleotide polymorphisms refine the tylosis with oesophageal cancer (TOC) minimal region on 17q25 to 42.5 kb: sequencing does not identify the causative gene. Hum Genet 114: 534-540.

1739A.Langer R, Ott K, Specht K, Becker K, Lordick F, Burian M, Herrmann K, Schrattenholz A, Cahill MA, Schwaiger M, Hofler H, Wester HJ (2008). Protein expression profiling in esophageal adenocarcinoma patients indicates association of heat-shock protein 27 expression and chemotherapy response. Clin Cancer Res 14: 8279-8287.

1739B.Langer R, Ott K, Feith M, Lordick F, Siewert JR, Becker K (2009).Prognostic significance of histopathological tumor regression after neoadjuvant chemotherapy in esophageal adenocarcinomas. Mod Pathol 22: 1555-1563.

1740. Langer R, Von Rahden BH, Nahrig J, Von WC, Reiter R, Feith M et al. (2006). Prognostic significance of expression patterns of c-erbB-2, p53, p16INK4A, p27KIP1, cyclin D1 and epidermal growth factor receptor in oesophageal adenocarcinoma: a tissue microarray study. J Clin Pathol 59: 631-634.

1741. Lansiaux A, Bras-Goncalves RA, Rosty C, Laurent-Puig P, Poupon MF, Bailly C (2001). Topoisomerase I-DNA covalent complexes in human colorectal cancer xenografts with different p53 and microsatellite instability status: relation with their sensitivity to CTP-11. Anticancer Res 21: 471-476.

1742. Lanuti M, Liu G, Goodwin JM, Zhai R, Fuchs BC, Asomaning K et al. (2008). A functional epidermal growth factor (EGF) polymorphism, EGF serum levels, and esophageal adenocarcinoma risk and outcome. Clin Cancer Res 14: 3216-3222.

1743. Lanza G, Ferracin M, Gafa R, Veronese A, Spizzo R, Pichiorri F et al. (2007). mRNA/microRNA gene expression profile in microsatellite unstable colorectal cancer. Mol Cancer 6: 54

1744. Lapner PC, Chou S, Jimenez C (1997). Perianal fetal rhabdomyoma: case report. Pediatr Surg Int 12: 544-547.

1745. Larraza-Hernandez O, Henson DE, Albores-Saavedra J (1984). The ultrastructure of gallbladder carcinoma. Acta Morphol Hung 32: 279-293.

1746. Larsson C, Skogseid B, Oberg K, Nakamura Y, Nordenskjold M (1988). Multiple endocrine neoplasia type 1 gene maps to chromosome 11 and is lost in insulinoma. Nature 332: 85-87.

1747. Larsson LI, Grimelius L, Hakanson R, Rehfeld JF, Stadil F, Holst J et al. (1975). Mixed endocrine pancreatic tumors producing several peptide hormones. Am J Pathol 79: 271-284.

1748. Larsson LI, Schwartz T, Lundqvist G, Chance RE, Sundler F, Rehfeld JF et al. (1976). Occurrence of human pancreatic polypeptide in pancreatic endocrine tumors. Possible implication in the watery diarrhea syndrome. Am J Pathol 85: 675-684.

1749. Lashner BA, Riddell RH, Winans CS (1986). Ganglioneuromatosis of the colon and extensive glycogenic acanthosis in Cowden's disease. Dig Dis Sci 31: 213-216.

1750. Lasota J, Miettinen M (2008). Clinical significance of oncogenic KIT and PDGFRA mutations in gastrointestinal stromal tumours. Histopathology 53: 245-266.

1751. Lasota J, Wang ZF, Sobin LH, Miettinen M (2009). Gain-of-function PDGFRA mutations, earlier reported in gastrointestinal stromal tumors, are common in small intestinal inflammatory fibroid polyps. A study of 60 cases. Mod Pathol 22: 1049-1056.

1752. Latchford AR, Sturt NJ, Neale K, Rogers PA, Phillips RK (2006). A 10-year review of surgery for desmoid disease associated with familial adenomatous polyposis. Br J Surg 93: 1258-1264.

1753. Latif F, Tory K, Gnarra J, Yao M, Duh FM, Orcutt ML et al. (1993). Identification of the von Hippel-Lindau disease tumor suppressor gene. Science 260: 1317-1320.

1754. Latulippe E, Klimstra D (2001). Retinoblastoma (Rb) protein expression in colorectal high grade neuroendocrine carcinoma. Mod Pathol 14: 89A-

1755. Lau CP, Leung WK (2008). Caecal metastasis from a primary small-cell lung carcinoma. Hong Kong Med J 14: 152-153.

1756. Laucirica R, Schwartz MR, Ramzy I (1992). Fine needle aspiration of pancreatic cystic epithelial neoplasms. Acta Cytol 36: 881-886.

1757. Laumonier H, Bioulac-Sage P, Laurent C, Zucman-Rossi J, Balabaud C, Trillaud H (2008). Hepatocellular adenomas: magnetic resonance imaging features as a function of molecular pathological classification. Hepatology 48: 808-818.

1758. Laurén P (1965). The two histological main types of gastric carcinoma: diffuse and so-called intestinal-type carcinoma. An attempt at a histo-clinical classification. Acta Pathol Microbiol Scand 64: 31-49.

1759. Laurent-Puig P, Zucman-Rossi J (2006). Genetics of hepatocellular tumors. Oncogene 25: 3778-3786.

1760. Lauwers GY (2009). Epithelial neoplasms of the stomach. In: Surgical pathology of the GI tract, Liver, Biliary tract and Pancreas. Odze RD, Goldblum JR, eds. Saunders: Philadelphia, pp.

1761. Lauwers GY, Forcione DG, Nishioka NS, Deshpande V, Lisovsky MY, Brugge WR et al. (2009). Novel endoscopic therapeutic modalities for superficial neoplasms arising in Barrett's esophagus: a primer for surgical pathologists. Mod Pathol 22: 489-498.

1762. Lauwers GY, Grant LD, Donnelly WH, Meloni AM, Foss RM, Sanberg AA et al. (1997). Hepatic undifferentiated (embryonal) sarcoma arising in a mesenchymal hamartoma. Am J Surg Pathol 21: 1248-1254.

1763. Lauwers GY, Grant LD, Scott GV, Carr NJ, Sobin LH (1998). Spindle cell squamous carcinoma of the esophagus: analysis of ploidy and tumor proliferative activity in a series of 13 cases. Hum Pathol 29: 863-868.

1764. Lauwers GY, Shimizu M, Correa P, Riddell RH, Kato Y, Lewin KJ et al. (1999). Evaluation of gastric biopsies for neoplasia: differences between Japanese and Western pathologists. Am J Surg Pathol 23: 511-518.

1765. Law SY, Fok M, Lam KY, Loke SL, Ma LT, Wong J (1994). Small cell carcinoma of the esophagus. Cancer 73: 2894-2899.

1766. Law SY, Fok M, Wong J (1996). Pattern of recurrence after oesophageal resection for cancer: clinical implications. Br J Surg 83: 107-111.

1767. Lawrence W, Jr., Anderson JR, Gehan EA, Maurer H (1997). Pretreatment TNM staging of childhood rhabdomyosarcoma: a report of the Intergroup Rhabdomyosarcoma Study Group. Children's Cancer Study Group. Pediatric Oncology Group. Cancer 80: 1165-1170.

1768. Layfield LJ, Bentz J (2008). Giant-cell containing neoplasms of the pancreas: an aspiration cytology study. Diagn Cytopathol 36: 238-244.

1769. Layfield LJ, Cramer H (2005). Primary sclerosing cholangitis as a cause of false positive bile duct brushing cytology: report of two cases. Diagn Cytopathol 32: 119-124.

1770. Le Bodic MF, Heymann MF, Lecomte M, Berger N, Berger F, Louvel A et al. (1996). Immunohistochemical study of 100 pancreatic tumors in 28 patients with multiple endocrine neoplasia, type I. Am J Surg Pathol 20: 1378-1384.

1771. Le Borgne J, de Calan L, Partensky C (1999). Cystadenomas and cystadenocarcinomas of the pancreas: a multiinstitutional retrospective study of 398 cases. French Surgical Association. Ann Surg 230: 152-161.

1772. Le Quesne LP, Nabarro JD, Kurtz A, Zweig S (1979). The management of insulin tumours of the pancreas. Br J Surg 66: 373-378.

1773. Leach FS, Nicolaides NC, Papadopoulos N, Liu B, Jen J, Parsons R et al. (1993). Mutations of a mutS homolog in hereditary nonpolyposis colorectal cancer. Cell 75: 1215-1225.

1774. Leach FS, Polyak K, Burrell M, Johnson KA, Hill D, Dunlop MG et al. (1996). Expression of the human mismatch repair gene *hMSH2* in normal and neoplastic tissues. Cancer Res 56: 235-240.

1775. Learmonth GM, Price SK, Visser AE, Emms M (1985). Papillary and cystic neoplasm of the pancreas—an acinar cell tumour? Histopathology 9: 63-79.

1776. Lecuit M, Abachin E, Martin A, Poyart C, Pochart P, Suarez F et al. (2004). Immunoproliferative small intestinal disease associated with Campylobacter jejuni. N Engl J Med 350: 239-248.

1777. Lee B, Cook G, John L, Harrington K, Nutting C (2008). Follicular thyroid carcinoma metastasis to the esophagus detected by 18FDG PET/CT. Thyroid 18: 267-271.

1778. Lee CH, Chang CJ, Lin YJ, Yeh CN, Chen MF, Hsieh SY (2009). Viral hepatitis-associated intrahepatic cholangiocarcinoma shares common disease processes with hepatocellular carcinoma. Br J Cancer 100: 1765-1770.

1779. Lee CJ, Scheiman J, Anderson MA, Hines OJ, Reber HA, Farrell J et al. (2008). Risk of malignancy in resected cystic tumors of the pancreas < or = 3 cm in size: is it safe to observe

asymptomatic patients? A multi-institutional report. J Gastrointest Surg 12: 234-242.
1780. Lee CS, Pirdas A (1995). Epidermal growth factor receptor immunoreactivity in gallbladder and extrahepatic biliary tract tumours. Pathol Res Pract 191: 1087-1091.
1781. Lee HE, Chae SW, Lee YJ, Kim MA, Lee HS, Lee BL et al. (2008). Prognostic implications of type and density of tumour-infiltrating lymphocytes in gastric cancer. Br J Cancer 99: 1704-1711.
1782. Lee HK, Lee HS, Yang HK, Kim WH, Lee KU, Choe KJ et al. (2003). Prognostic significance of Bcl-2 and p53 expression in gastric cancer. Int J Colorectal Dis 18: 518-525.
1783. Lee HS, Choi SI, Lee HK, Kim HS, Yang HK, Kang GH et al. (2002). Distinct clinical features and outcomes of gastric cancers with microsatellite instability. Mod Pathol 15: 632-640.
1784. Lee JH, Abraham SC, Kim HS, Nam JH, Choi C, Lee MC et al. (2002). Inverse relationship between *APC* gene mutation in gastric adenomas and development of adenocarcinoma. Am J Pathol 161: 611-618.
1785. Lee MJ, Lee HS, Kim WH, Choi Y, Yang M (2003). Expression of mucins and cytokeratins in primary carcinomas of the digestive system. Mod Pathol 16: 403-410.
1786. Lee OJ, Kim HJ, Kim JR, Watanabe H (2009). The prognostic significance of the mucin phenotype of gastric adenocarcinoma and its relationship with histologic classifications. Oncol Rep 21: 387-393.
1787. Lee RG, Tsamandas AC, Demetris AJ (1997). Large cell change (liver cell dysplasia) and hepatocellular carcinoma in cirrhosis: matched case-control study, pathological analysis, and pathogenetic hypothesis. Hepatology 26: 1415-1422.
1788. Lee SA, Kang D, Shim KN, Choe JW, Hong WS, Choi H (2003). Effect of diet and *Helicobacter pylori* infection to the risk of early gastric cancer. J Epidemiol 13: 162-168.
1789. Lee SS, Jang JJ, Cho KJ, Khang SK, Kim CW (1997). Epstein-Barr virus-associated primary gastrointestinal lymphoma in non-immunocompromised patients in Korea. Histopathology 30: 234-242.
1790. Lee SS, Kim MH, Lee SK, Jang SJ, Song MH, Kim KP et al. (2004). Clinicopathologic review of 58 patients with biliary papillomatosis. Cancer 100: 783-793.
1791. Lee TY, Lee SS, Jung SW, Jeon SH, Yun SC, Oh HC et al. (2008). Hepatitis B virus infection and intrahepatic cholangiocarcinoma in Korea: a case-control study. Am J Gastroenterol 103: 1716-1720.
1792. Lee WA (2005). Mucinous cystadenoma of the pancreas with predominant stroma creating a solid tumor. World J Surg Oncol 3: 59-
1793. Lee YY, Wilczynski SP, Chumakov A, Chih D, Koeffler HP (1994). Carcinoma of the vulva: HPV and p53 mutations. Oncogene 9: 1655-1659.
1794. Leeuwenburgh I, Haringsma J, van Dekken H, Scholten P, Siersema PD, Kuipers EJ (2006). Long-term risk of oesophagitis, Barrett's oesophagus and oesophageal cancer in achalasia patients. Scand J Gastroenterol Suppl 7-10.
1795. Lefevre JH, Rodrigue CM, Mourra N, Bennis M, Flejou JF, Parc R et al. (2006). Implication of MYH in colorectal polyposis. Ann Surg 244: 874-879.
1796. Leggett BA, Devereaux B, Biden K, Searle J, Young J, Jass J (2001). Hyperplastic polyposis: association with colorectal cancer. Am J Surg Pathol 25: 177-184.
1797. Lehmann FS, Beglinger C, Schnabel K, Terracciano L (1999). Progressive development of diffuse liver hemangiomatosis. J Hepatol 30: 951-954.
1798. Lehy T, Cadiot G, Mignon M, Ruszniewski P, Bonfils S (1992). Influence of multiple endocrine neoplasia type 1 on gastric endocrine cells in patients with the Zollinger-Ellison syndrome. Gut 33: 1275-1279.
1799. Leja J, Essaghir A, Essand M, Wester K, Oberg K, Totterman TH et al. (2009). Novel markers for enterochromaffin cells and gastrointestinal neuroendocrine carcinomas. Mod Pathol 22: 261-272.
1800. Lemrow SM, Perdue DG, Stewart SL, Richardson LC, Jim MA, French HT et al. (2008). Gallbladder cancer incidence among American Indians and Alaska Natives, US, 1999-2004. Cancer 113: 1266-1273.
1801. Lennard-Jones JE, Melville DM, Morson BC, Ritchie JK, Williams CB (1990). Precancer and cancer in extensive ulcerative colitis: findings among 401 patients over 22 years. Gut 31: 800-806.
1802. Lens M, Bataille V, Krivokapic Z (2009). Melanoma of the small intestine. Lancet Oncol 10: 516-521.
1803. Leong AS, Sormunen RT, Tsui WM, Liew CT (1998). Hep Par 1 and selected antibodies in the immunohistological distinction of hepatocellular carcinoma from cholangiocarcinoma, combined tumours and metastatic carcinoma. Histopathology 33: 318-324.
1804. Leopoldo S, Lorena B, Cinzia A, Gabriella DC, Angela LB, Renato C et al. (2008). Two subtypes of mucinous adenocarcinoma of the colorectum: clinicopathological and genetic features. Ann Surg Oncol 15: 1429-1439.
1805. Lepisto A, Kiviluoto T, Halttunen J, Jarvinen HJ (2009). Surveillance and treatment of duodenal adenomatosis in familial adenomatous polyposis. Endoscopy 41: 504-509.
1806. Leppert M, Dobbs M, Scambler P, O'Connell P, Nakamura Y, Stauffer D et al. (1987). The gene for familial polyposis coli maps to the long arm of chromosome 5. Science 238: 1411-1413.
1807. Lepreux S, Laurent C, Blanc JF, Trillaud H, Le BB, Trouette H et al. (2003). The identification of small nodules in liver adenomatosis. J Hepatol 39: 77-85.
1808. Lerut JP, Orlando G, Adam R, Schiavo M, Klempnauer J, Mirza D et al. (2007). The place of liver transplantation in the treatment of hepatic epitheloid hemangioendothelioma: report of the European liver transplant registry. Ann Surg 246: 949-957.
1808A. Leucci E, Cocco M, Onnis A, De Falco G, van Cleef P, Bellan C (2008). MYC translocation-negative classical Burkitt lymphoma cases: an alternative pathogenetic mechanism involving miRNA deregulation. J Pathol 216:440-450.
1809. Leung AC, Wong VC, Yang LC, Chan PL, Daigo Y, Nakamura Y et al. (2008). Frequent decreased expression of candidate tumor suppressor gene, *DEC1*, and its anchorage-independent growth properties and impact on global gene expression in esophageal carcinoma. Int J Cancer 122: 587-594.
1810. Leung WK, Lin SR, Ching JY, To KF, Ng EK, Chan FK et al. (2004). Factors predicting progression of gastric intestinal metaplasia: results of a randomised trial on *Helicobacter pylori* eradication. Gut 53: 1244-1249.
1811. Leuschner I, Schmidt D, Harms D (1990). Undifferentiated sarcoma of the liver in childhood: morphology, flow cytometry, and literature review. Hum Pathol 21: 68-76.
1812. Levey JM, Banner B, Darrah J, Bonkovsky HL (1994). Inflammatory cloacogenic polyp: three cases and literature review. Am J Gastroenterol 89: 438-441.
1813. Levi E, Klimstra DS, Andea A, Basturk O, Adsay NV (2004). MUC1 and MUC2 in pancreatic neoplasia. J Clin Pathol 57: 456-462.
1814. Levi F, Lucchini F, Negri E, La Vecchia C (2003). Pancreatic cancer mortality in Europe: the leveling of an epidemic. Pancreas 27: 139-142.
1815. Levi GS, Harpaz N (2006). Intestinal low-grade tubuloglandular adenocarcinoma in inflammatory bowel disease. Am J Surg Pathol 30: 1022-1029.
1816. Levin B, Lieberman DA, McFarland B, Andrews KS, Brooks D, Bond J et al. (2008). Screening and surveillance for the early detection of colorectal cancer and adenomatous polyps, 2008: a joint guideline from the American Cancer Society, the US Multi-Society Task Force on Colorectal Cancer, and the American College of Radiology. Gastroenterology 134: 1570-1595.
1817. Levine AM (1992). Acquired immunodeficiency syndrome-related lymphoma. Blood 80: 8-20.
1818. Levine DA, Bogomolniy F, Yee CJ, Lash A, Barakat RR, Borgen PI et al. (2005). Frequent mutation of the *PIK3CA* gene in ovarian and breast cancers. Clin Cancer Res 11: 2875-2878.
1819. Levy P, Bougaran J, Gayet B (1997). [Diffuse peritoneal carcinosis of pseudo-papillary and solid tumor of the pancreas. Role of abdominal injury]. Gastroenterol Clin Biol 21: 789-793.
1820. Lewandrowski K, Warshaw A, Compton C (1992). Macrocystic serous cystadenoma of the pancreas: a morphologic variant differing from microcystic adenoma. Hum Pathol 23: 871-875.
1821. Lewandrowski KB, Southern JF, Pins MR, Compton CC, Warshaw AL (1993). Cyst fluid analysis in the differential diagnosis of pancreatic cysts. A comparison of pseudocysts, serous cystadenomas, mucinous cystic neoplasms, and mucinous cystadenocarcinoma. Ann Surg 217: 41-47.
1822. Lewin KJ, Appelman HD (1996). Carcinoma of the stomach. In: Tumors of the esophagus and stomach. Lewin KJ, Appelman HD, eds. Armed Forces Institute of Pathology: Washington, pp. 245-330.
1823. Lewin KJ, Appelman HD (eds) (1996). Tumors of the Esophagus and Stomach. Armed Forces Institute of Pathology: Washington, DC.
1824. Lewin M, Handra-Luca A, Arrive L, Wendum D, Paradis V, Bridel E et al. (2006). Liver adenomatosis: classification of MR imaging features and comparison with pathologic findings. Radiology 241: 433-440.
1825. Lewis JH, Shorb PE, Nochomovitz LE (1985). Benign duodenal villous adenoma obstructing the ampulla of Vater: a surgical dilemma. South Med J 78: 1507-1511.
1826. Lewis JT, Talwalkar JA, Rosen CB, Smyrk TC, Abraham SC (2007). Prevalence and risk factors for gallbladder neoplasia in patients with primary sclerosing cholangitis: evidence for a metaplasia-dysplasia-carcinoma sequence. Am J Surg Pathol 31: 907-913.
1827. Lewis JT, Wang KK, Abraham SC (2008). Muscularis mucosae duplication and the musculo-fibrous anomaly in endoscopic mucosal resections for barrett esophagus: implications for staging of adenocarcinoma. Am J Surg Pathol 32: 566-571.
1828. Ley C, Mohar A, Guarner J, Herrera-Goepfert R, Figueroa LS, Halperin D et al. (2004). *Helicobacter pylori* eradication and gastric preneoplastic conditions: a randomized, double-blind, placebo-controlled trial. Cancer Epidemiol Biomarkers Prev 13: 4-10.
1829. Li B, Lei W, Shao K, Zhang C, Chen Z, Shi S et al. (2007). Characteristics and prognosis of primary malignant melanoma of the esophagus. Melanoma Res 17: 239-242.
1830. Li DM, Sun H (1997). TEP1, encoded by a candidate tumor suppressor locus, is a novel protein tyrosine phosphatase regulated by transforming growth factor beta. Cancer Res 57: 2124-2129.
1831. Li GM (2008). Mechanisms and functions of DNA mismatch repair. Cell Res 18: 85-98.
1832. Li H, Zhang Q, Xu L, Chen Y, Wei Y, Zhou G (2009). Factors predictive of prognosis after esophagectomy for squamous cell cancer. J Thorac Cardiovasc Surg 137: 55-59.
1833. Li J, Simpson L, Takahashi M, Miliaresis C, Myers MP, Tonks N et al. (1998). The *PTEN/MMAC1* tumor suppressor induces cell death that is rescued by the AKT/protein kinase B oncogene. Cancer Res 58: 5667-5672.
1834. Li J, Yen C, Liaw D, Podsypanina K, Bose S, Wang SI et al. (1997). *PTEN*, a putative protein tyrosine phosphatase gene mutated in human brain, breast, and prostate cancer. Science 275: 1943-1947.
1835. Li QL, Ito K, Sakakura C, Fukamachi H, Inoue K, Chi XZ et al. (2002). Causal relationship between the loss of RUNX3 expression and gastric cancer. Cell 109: 113-124.
1836. Li SC, Hamilton SR (1998). Malignant tumors in the rectum simulating solitary rectal ulcer syndrome in endoscopic biopsy specimens. Am J Surg Pathol 22: 106-112.
1837. Li T, Ji Y, Zhi XT, Wang L, Yang XR, Shi GM et al. (2009). A comparison of hepatic mucinous cystic neoplasms with biliary intraductal papillary neoplasms. Clin Gastroenterol Hepatol 7: 586-593.
1838. Li TJ, Zhang YX, Wen J, Cowan DF, Hart J, Xiao SY (2004). Basaloid squamous cell carcinoma of the esophagus with or without adenoid cystic features. Arch Pathol Lab Med 128: 1124-1130.
1838A. Li X, Galipeau PC, Sanchez CA, Blount PL, Maley CC, Arnaudo J et al. (2008). Single nucleotide polymorphism-based genome-wide chromosome copy change, loss of heterozygosity, and aneuploidy in Barrett's esophagus neoplastic progression. Cancer Prev Res (Phila Pa) 1: 413–423.
1839. Li YL, Tian Z, Wu DY, Fu BY, Xin Y (2005). Loss of heterozygosity on 10q23.3 and mutation of tumor suppressor gene *PTEN* in gastric cancer and precancerous lesions. World J Gastroenterol 11: 285-288.
1840. Liang JJ, Alrawi S, Fuller GN, Tan D (2008). Carcinoid tumors arising in tailgut cysts may be associated with estrogen receptor status: case report and review of the literature. Int J Clin Exp Pathol 1: 539-543.
1841. Liang TJ, Heller T (2004). Pathogenesis of hepatitis C-associated hepatocellular carcinoma. Gastroenterology 127: S62-S71.
1842. Liaw D, Marsh DJ, Li J, Dahia PL, Wang SI, Zheng Z et al. (1997). Germline mutations of the *PTEN* gene in Cowden disease, an inherited breast and thyroid cancer syndrome. Nat Genet 16: 64-67.
1843. Libbrecht L, Cassiman D, Verslype C, Maleux G, Van Hees D, Pirenne J et al. (2006). Clinicopathological features of focal nodular hyperplasia-like nodules in 130 cirrhotic explant livers. Am J Gastroenterol 101: 2341-2346.
1844. Libshitz HI, Lindell MM, Dodd GD (1982). Metastases to the hollow viscera. Radiol Clin North Am 20: 487-499.
1845. Lieber MR, Lack EE, Roberts JR, Jr., Merino MJ, Patterson K, Restrepo C et al. (1987). Solid and papillary epithelial neoplasm of the pancreas. An ultrastructural and immunocytochemical study of six cases. Am J Surg Pathol 11: 85-93.
1846. Liede A, Karlan BY, Narod SA (2004). Cancer risks for male carriers of germline mutations in BRCA1 or BRCA2: a review of the literature. J Clin Oncol 22: 735-742.
1847. Lievre A, Laurent-Puig P (2009). Genetics: Predictive value of *KRAS* mutations in chemoresistant CRC. Nat Rev Clin Oncol 6: 306-307.
1848. Ligato S, Furmaga W, Cartun RW, Hull D, Tsongalis GJ (2005). Primary carcinoid tumor

of the common hepatic duct: A rare case with immunohistochemical and molecular findings. Oncol Rep 13: 543-546.
1849. Ligato S, Mandich D, Cartun RW (2008). Utility of glypican-3 in differentiating hepatocellular carcinoma from other primary and metastatic lesions in FNA of the liver: an immunocytochemical study. Mod Pathol 21: 626-631.
1850. Ligneau B, Lombard-Bohas C, Partensky C, Valette PJ, Calender A, Dumortier J et al. (2001). Cystic endocrine tumors of the pancreas: clinical, radiologic, and histopathologic features in 13 cases. Am J Surg Pathol 25: 752-760.
1851. Ligtenberg MJ, Kuiper RP, Chan TL, Goossens M, Hebeda KM, Voorendt M et al. (2009). Heritable somatic methylation and inactivation of MSH2 in families with Lynch syndrome due to deletion of the 3' exons of TACSTD1. Nat Genet 41: 112-117.
1852. Lim CH, Treanor D, Dixon MF, Axon AT (2007). Low-grade dysplasia in Barrett's esophagus has a high risk of progression. Endoscopy 39: 581-587.
1853. Lim JE, Chien MW, Earle CC (2003). Prognostic factors following curative resection for pancreatic adenocarcinoma: a population-based, linked database analysis of 396 patients. Ann Surg 237: 74-85.
1854. Lim JS, Yun MJ, Kim MJ, Hyung WJ, Park MS, Choi JY et al. (2006). CT and PET in stomach cancer: preoperative staging and monitoring of response to therapy. Radiographics 26: 143-156.
1855. Lim MK, Ju YH, Franceschi S, Oh JK, Kong HJ, Hwang SS et al. (2006). *Clonorchis sinensis* infection and increasing risk of cholangiocarcinoma in the Republic of Korea. Am J Trop Med Hyg 75: 93-96.
1856. Lim SH, Yang HW, Kim A, Cha SW, Jung SH, Go H et al. (2007). Adenosquamous carcinoma of extrahepatic bile duct: a case report. Korean J Intern Med 22: 206-210.
1857. Lin AY, Gridley G, Tucker M (1995). Benign anal lesions and anal cancer. N Engl J Med 332: 190-191.
1858. Lin DC, Du XL, Wang MR (2009). Protein alterations in ESCC and clinical implications: a review. Dis Esophagus 22: 9-20.
1859. Lin F, Staerkel G (2003). Cytologic criteria for well differentiated adenocarcinoma of the pancreas in fine-needle aspiration biopsy specimens. Cancer 99: 44-50.
1860. Lin LW, Yang JJ, Lin XY, Xue ES, He YM, Gao SD et al. (2007). Effect of fatty liver background on contrast-enhanced ultrasonographic appearance of focal nodular hyperplasia. Hepatobiliary Pancreat Dis Int 6: 610-615.
1861. Lindblom A, Tannergard P, Werelius B, Nordenskjold M (1993). Genetic mapping of a second locus predisposing to hereditary nonpolyposis colon cancer. Nat Genet 5: 279-282.
1862. Lindor NM (2009). Familial colorectal cancer type X: the other half of hereditary nonpolyposis colon cancer syndrome. Surg Oncol Clin N Am 18: 637-645.
1863. Lindor NM (2009). Hereditary colorectal cancer: MYH-associated polyposis and other newly identified disorders. Best Pract Res Clin Gastroenterol 23: 75-87.
1864. Lindor NM, Rabe K, Petersen GM, Haile R, Casey G, Baron J et al. (2005). Lower cancer incidence in Amsterdam-I criteria families without mismatch repair deficiency: familial colorectal cancer type X. JAMA 293: 1979-1985.
1865. Linos DA, Dozois RR, Dahlin DC, Bartholomew LG (1981). Does Peutz-Jeghers syndrome predispose to gastrointestinal malignancy? A later look. Arch Surg 116: 1182-1184.
1866. Lipkin SM, Wang V, Jacoby R, Banerjee-Basu S, Baxevanis AD, Lynch HT et al. (2000). *MLH3*: a DNA mismatch repair gene associated with mammalian microsatellite instability. Nat Genet 24: 27-35.
1867. Lipton L, Halford SE, Johnson V, Novelli MR, Jones A, Cummings C et al. (2003). Carcinogenesis in MYH-associated polyposis follows a distinct genetic pathway. Cancer Res 63: 7595-7599.
1868. Lisovsky M, Patel K, Cymes K, Chase D, Bhuiya T, Morgenstern N (2007). Immunophenotypic characterization of anal gland carcinoma: loss of p63 and cytokeratin 5/6. Arch Pathol Lab Med 131: 1304-1311.
1869. Liu B, Nicolaides NC, Markowitz S, Willson JK, Parsons RE, Jen J et al. (1995). Mismatch repair gene defects in sporadic colorectal cancers with microsatellite instability. Nat Genet 9: 48-55.
1870. Liu B, Parsons R, Papadopoulos N, Nicolaides NC, Lynch HT, Watson P et al. (1996). Analysis of mismatch repair genes in hereditary non-polyposis colorectal cancer patients. Nat Med 2: 169-174.
1871. Liu B, Parsons RE, Hamilton SR, Petersen GM, Lynch HT, Watson P et al. (1994). hMSH2 mutations in hereditary nonpolyposis colorectal cancer kindreds. Cancer Res 54: 4590-4594.
1872. Liu H, Ye H, Ruskone-Fourmestraux A, De JD, Pileri S, Thiede C et al. (2002). T(11;18) is a marker for all stage gastric MALT lymphomas that will not respond to *H. pylori* eradication. Gastroenterology 122: 1286-1294.
1873. Liu Q, Ohshima K, Masuda Y, Kikuchi M (1995). Detection of the Epstein-Barr virus in primary gastric lymphoma by in situ hybridization. Pathol Int 45: 131-136.
1874. Liu TH, Zhu Y, Cui QC, Cai LX, Ye SF, Zhong SX et al. (1992). Nonfunctioning pancreatic endocrine tumors. An immunohistochemical and electron microscopic analysis of 26 cases. Pathol Res Pract 188: 191-198.
1875. Lloyd KM, DENNIS M (1963). Cowden's disease. A possible new symptom complex with multiple system involvement. Ann Intern Med 58: 136-142.
1876. Lloyd RV, Mervak T, Schmidt K, Warner TF, Wilson BS (1984). Immunohistochemical detection of chromogranin and neuron-specific enolase in pancreatic endocrine neoplasms. Am J Surg Pathol 8: 607-614.
1877. Loane J, Kealy WF, Mulcahy G (1998). Perianal hidradenoma papilliferum occurring in a male: a case report. Ir J Med Sci 167: 26-27.
1878. Lobert PF, Appelman HD (1981). Inflammatory cloacogenic polyp. A unique inflammatory lesion of the anal transitional zone. Am J Surg Pathol 5: 761-766.
1879. Lock MR, Thomson JP (1977). Fissure-in-ano: the initial management and prognosis. Br J Surg 64: 355-358.
1880. Loddenkemper C (2009). Diagnostic standards in the pathology of inflammatory bowel disease. Dig Dis 27: 576-583.
1881. Loddenkemper C, Longerich T, Hummel M, Ernestus K, Anagnostopoulos I, Dienes HP et al. (2007). Frequency and diagnostic patterns of lymphomas in liver biopsies with respect to the WHO classification. Virchows Arch 450: 493-502.
1882. Loffeld RJ (2009). Colorectal adenomas in patients presenting with inflammatory bowel disease. Neth J Med 67: 21-24.
1883. Loftus EV, Jr., Olivares-Pakzad BA, Batts KP, Adkins MC, Stephens DH, Sarr MG et al. (1996). Intraductal papillary-mucinous tumors of the pancreas: clinicopathologic features, outcome, and nomenclature. Members of the Pancreas Clinic, and Pancreatic Surgeons of Mayo Clinic. Gastroenterology 110: 1909-1918.
1884. Logrono R, Rampy BA, Adegboyega PA (2002). Fine needle aspiration cytology of hepatobiliary cystadenoma with mesenchymal stroma. Cancer 96: 37-42.
1885. Lohmann DR, Funk A, Niedermeyer HP, Haupel S, Hofler H (1993). Identification of p53 gene mutations in gastrointestinal and pancreatic carcinoids by nonradioisotopic SSCA. Virchows Arch B Cell Pathol Incl Mol Pathol 64: 293-296.
1886. Lohr M, Klöppel G, Maisonneuve P, Lowenfels AB, Luttges J (2005). Frequency of K-ras mutations in pancreatic intraductal neoplasias associated with pancreatic ductal adenocarcinoma and chronic pancreatitis: a meta-analysis. Neoplasia 7: 17-23.
1887. Loke TK, Lo SS, Chan CS (1997). Case report: Krukenberg tumours arising from a primary duodenojejunal adenocarcinoma. Clin Radiol 52: 154-155.
1888. Lollgen RM, Hessman O, Szabo E, Westin G, Akerstrom G (2001). Chromosome 18 deletions are common events in classical midgut carcinoid tumors. Int J Cancer 92: 812-815.
1889. Lomo LC, Blount PL, Sanchez CA, Li X, Galipeau PC, Cowan DS et al. (2006). Crypt dysplasia with surface maturation: a clinical, pathologic, and molecular study of a Barrett's esophagus cohort. Am J Surg Pathol 30: 423-435.
1890. Lonardo F, Cubilla AL, Klimstra DS (1996). Microadenocarcinoma of the pancreas—morphologic pattern or pathologic entity? A reevaluation of the original series. Am J Surg Pathol 20: 1385-1393.
1891. Longacre TA, Fenoglio-Preiser CM (1990). Mixed hyperplastic adenomatous polyps/serrated adenomas. A distinct form of colorectal neoplasia. Am J Surg Pathol 14: 524-537.
1892. Longacre TA, Kong CS, Welton ML (2008). Diagnostic problems in anal pathology. Adv Anat Pathol 15: 263-278.
1893. Longnecker DS (1998). Observations on the etiology and pathogenesis of intraductal papillary-mucinous neoplasms of the pancreas. Hepatogastroenterology 45: 1973-1980.
1894. Longnecker DS, Tosteson TD, Karagas MF, Mott LA (1998). Incidence of pancreatic intraductal papillary-mucinous carcinomas in Japanese and Caucasians in SEER data. Pancreas 17: 446-
1895. Longy M, Lacombe D (1996). Cowden disease. Report of a family and review. Ann Genet 39: 35-42.
1896. Loos M, Bergmann F, Bauer A, Hoheisel JD, Esposito I, Kleeff J et al. (2007). Solid type clear cell carcinoma of the pancreas: differential diagnosis of an unusual case and review of the literature. Virchows Arch 450: 719-726.
1897. Lopez-Terrada D, Gunaratne PH, Adesina AM, Pulliam J, Hoang DM, Nguyen Y et al. (2009). Histologic subtypes of hepatoblastoma are characterized by differential canonical Wnt and Notch pathway activation in DLK+ precursors. Hum Pathol 40: 783-794.
1898. Lordick F, Ott K, Krause BJ, Weber WA, Becker K, Stein HJ et al. (2007). PET to assess early metabolic response and to guide treatment of adenocarcinoma of the oesophagogastric junction: the MUNICON phase II trial. Lancet Oncol 8: 797-805.
1899. Louie DC, Offit K, Jaslow R, Parsa NZ, Murty VV, Schluger A et al. (1995). p53 overexpression as a marker of poor prognosis in mantle cell lymphomas with t(11;14)(q13;q32). Blood 86: 2892-2899.
1900. Louis DN, Ohgaki H, Wiestler OD, and Cavenee WK (eds) (2007). WHO Classification of Tumours of the Central Nervous System. IARC: Lyon, France.
1901. Lowenfels AB, Maisonneuve P, Dimagno EP, Elitsur Y, Gates LK, Jr., Perrault J et al. (1997). Hereditary pancreatitis and the risk of pancreatic cancer. International Hereditary Pancreatitis Study Group. J Natl Cancer Inst 89: 442-446.
1902. Lowenfels AB, Maisonneuve P, Whitcomb DC, Lerch MM, Dimagno EP (2001). Cigarette smoking as a risk factor for pancreatic cancer in patients with hereditary pancreatitis. JAMA 286: 169-170.
1903. Lowitt MH, Kariniemi AL, Niemi KM, Kao GF (1996). Cutaneous malacoplakia: a report of two cases and review of the literature. J Am Acad Dermatol 34: 325-332.
1904. Lu D, Vohra P, Chu PG, Woda B, Rock KL, Jiang Z (2009). An oncofetal protein IMP3: a new molecular marker for the detection of esophageal adenocarcinoma and high-grade dysplasia. Am J Surg Pathol 33: 521-525.
1905. Lu YK, Li YM, Gu YZ (1987). Cancer of esophagus and esophagogastric junction: analysis of results of 1,025 resections after 5 to 20 years. Ann Thorac Surg 43: 176-181.
1906. Lubbe SJ, Di Bernardo MC, Chandler IP, Houlston RS (2009). Clinical implications of the colorectal cancer risk associated with MUTYH mutation. J Clin Oncol 27: 3975-3980.
1907. Lubensky I (2002). Endocrine pancreas. In: Endocrine Pathology. Livolsi VA, Asa SL, eds. Churchill Livingstone: Philadelphia, pp. 205-235.
1908. Lubensky IA, Debelenko LV, Zhuang Z, Emmert-Buck MR, Dong Q, Chandrasekharappa S et al. (1996). Allelic deletions on chromosome 11q13 in multiple tumors from individual MEN1 patients. Cancer Res 56: 5272-5278.
1909. Lubensky IA, Pack S, Ault D, Vortmeyer AO, Libutti SK, Choyke PL et al. (1998). Multiple neuroendocrine tumors of the pancreas in von Hippel-Lindau disease patients: histopathological and molecular genetic analysis. Am J Pathol 153: 223-231.
1910. Ludwig J, Wahlstrom HE, Batts KP, Wiesner RH (1992). Papillary bile duct dysplasia in primary sclerosing cholangitis. Gastroenterology 102: 2134-2138.
1911. Lugli A, Tornillo L, Mirlacher M, Bundi M, Sauter G, Terracciano LM (2004). Hepatocyte paraffin 1 expression in human normal and neoplastic tissues: tissue microarray analysis on 3,940 tissue samples. Am J Clin Pathol 122: 721-727.
1912. Lukas Z, Dvorak K, Kroupova I, Valaskova I, Habanec B (2006). Immunohistochemical and genetic analysis of osteoclastic giant cell tumor of the pancreas. Pancreas 32: 325-329.
1913. Luna-Perez P, Rodriguez DF, Lujan L, Alvarado I, Kelly J, Rojas ME et al. (1998). Colorectal sarcoma: analysis of failure patterns. J Surg Oncol 69: 36-40.
1914. Lundqvist M, Wilander E (1987). A study of the histopathogenesis of carcinoid tumors of the small intestine and appendix. Cancer 60: 201-206.
1915. Lunniss PJ, Sheffield JP, Talbot IC, Thomson JP, Phillips RK (1995). Persistence of idiopathic anal fistula may be related to epithelialization. Br J Surg 82: 32-33.
1916. Luong TV, Salvagni S, Bordi C (2005). Presacral carcinoid tumour. Review of the literature and report of a clinically malignant case. Dig Liver Dis 37: 278-281.
1917. Lurje G, Manegold PC, Ning Y, Pohl A, Zhang W, Lenz HJ (2009). Thymidylate synthase gene variations: predictive and prognostic markers. Mol Cancer Ther -
1917A.Luthra MG, Ajani JA, Izzo J, Ensor J, Wu TT, Rashid A, Zhang L, Phan A, Fukami N, Luthra R (2007). Decreased expression of gene cluster at chromosome 1q21 defines molecular subgroups of chemoradiotherapy response in esophageal cancers. Clin Cancer Res 13: 912-919.
1917B. Luthra R, Wu TT, Luthra MG, Izzo J, Lopez-Alvarez E, Zhang L, Bailey J, Lee JH, Bresalier R, Rashid A, Swisher SG, Ajani JA (2006). Gene expression profiling of localized

esophageal carcinomas: association with pathologic response to preoperative chemoradiation. J Clin Oncol 24: 259-267
1918. Luttges J, Feyerabend B, Buchelt T, Pacena M, Klöppel G (2002). The mucin profile of noninvasive and invasive mucinous cystic neoplasms of the pancreas. Am J Surg Pathol 26: 466-471.
1919. Luttges J, Mentzel T, Hubner G, Klöppel G (1999). Solitary fibrous tumour of the pancreas: a new member of the small group of mesenchymal pancreatic tumours. Virchows Arch 435: 37-42.
1920. Luttges J, Pierre E, Zamboni G, Weh G, Lietz H, Kussmann J et al. (1997). [Malignant non-epithelial tumors of the pancreas]. Pathologe 18: 233-237.
1921. Luttges J, Schemm S, Vogel I, Hedderich J, Kremer B, Klöppel G (2000). The grade of pancreatic ductal carcinoma is an independent prognostic factor and is superior to the immunohistochemical assessment of proliferation. J Pathol 191: 154-161.
1922. Luttges J, Vogel I, Menke M, Henne-Bruns D, Kremer B, Klöppel G (1998). Clear cell carcinoma of the pancreas: an adenocarcinoma with ductal phenotype. Histopathology 32: 444-448.
1923. Luttges J, Vogel I, Menke M, Henne-Bruns D, Kremer B, Klöppel G (1998). The retroperitoneal resection margin and vessel involvement are important factors determining survival after pancreaticoduodenectomy for ductal adenocarcinoma of the head of the pancreas. Virchows Arch 433: 237-242.
1924. Lyda MH, Fenoglio-Preiser CM (1998). Adenoma-carcinoid tumors of the colon. Arch Pathol Lab Med 122: 262-265.
1925. Lynch ED, Ostermeyer EA, Lee MK, Arena JF, Ji H, Dann J et al. (1997). Inherited mutations in PTEN that are associated with breast cancer, Cowden disease, and juvenile polyposis. Am J Hum Genet 61: 1254-1260.
1926. Lynch HT, Fitzsimmons ML, Smyrk TC, Lanspa SJ, Watson P, McClellan J et al. (1990). Familial pancreatic cancer: clinicopathologic study of 18 nuclear families. Am J Gastroenterol 85: 54-60.
1927. Lynch HT, Fusaro L, Smyrk TC, Watson P, Lanspa S, Lynch JF (1995). Medical genetic study of eight pancreatic cancer-prone families. Cancer Invest 13: 141-149.
1928. Lynch HT, Fusaro RM (1991). Pancreatic cancer and the familial atypical multiple mole melanoma (FAMMM) syndrome. Pancreas 6: 127-131.
1929. Lynch HT, Grady W, Suriano G, Huntsman D (2005). Gastric cancer: new genetic developments. J Surg Oncol 90: 114-133.
1930. Lynch HT, Lynch PM, Lanspa SJ, Snyder CL, Lynch JF, Boland CR (2009). Review of the Lynch syndrome: history, molecular genetics, screening, differential diagnosis, and medicolegal ramifications. Clin Genet 76: 1-18.
1931. Lynch HT, Silva E, Wirtzfeld D, Hebbard P, Lynch J, Huntsman DG (2008). Hereditary diffuse gastric cancer: prophylactic surgical oncology implications. Surg Clin North Am 88: 759-778.
1932. Lynch HT, Smyrk T, Kern SE, Hruban RH, Lightdale CJ, Lemon SJ et al. (1996). Familial pancreatic cancer: a review. Semin Oncol 23: 251-275.
1933. Lynch HT, Smyrk TC, Watson P, Lanspa SJ, Lynch JF, Lynch PM et al. (1993). Genetics, natural history, tumor spectrum, and pathology of hereditary nonpolyposis colorectal cancer: an updated review. Gastroenterology 104: 1535-1549.
1934. Lyss AP (1988). Appendiceal malignancies. Semin Oncol 15: 129-137.
1935. MacDonald RA (1956). A study of 356 carcinoids of the gastrointestinal tract; report of four new cases of the carcinoid syndrome. Am J Med 21: 867-878.
1936. MacGillivray DC, Heaton RB, Rushin JM, Cruess DF (1992). Distant metastasis from a carcinoid tumor of the appendix less than one centimeter in size. Surgery 111: 466-471.
1937. Machado JC, Carneiro F, Beck S, Rossi S, Lopes J, Taveira GA (1998). E-cadherin expression is correlated with the isolated cell/diffuse histotype and with the features of biological aggressiveness of gastric carcinoma. Int J Surg Pathol 6: 135-144.
1938. Machado JC, Carneiro F, Ribeiro P, Blin N, Sobrinho-Simoes M (1996). pS2 protein expression in gastric carcinoma. An immunohistochemical and immunoradiometric study. Eur J Cancer 32A: 1585-1590.
1939. Machado JC, Nogueira AM, Carneiro F, Reis CA, Sobrinho-Simoes M (2000). Gastric carcinoma exhibits distinct types of cell differentiation: an immunohistochemical study of trefoil peptides (TFF1 and TFF2) and mucins (MUC1, MUC2, MUC5AC, and MUC6). J Pathol 190: 437-443.
1940. Machado JC, Oliveira C, Carvalho R, Soares P, Berx G, Caldas C et al. (2001). E-cadherin gene (*CDH1*) promoter methylation as the second hit in sporadic diffuse gastric carcinoma. Oncogene 20: 1525-1528.
1941. Machado JC, Soares P, Carneiro F, Rocha A, Beck S, Blin N et al. (1999). E-cadherin gene mutations provide a genetic basis for the phenotypic divergence of mixed gastric carcinomas. Lab Invest 79: 459-465.
1942. Macpherson N, Lesack D, Klasa R, Horsman D, Connors JM, Barnett M et al. (1999). Small noncleaved, non-Burkitt's (Burkit-Like) lymphoma: cytogenetics predict outcome and reflect clinical presentation. J Clin Oncol 17: 1558-1567.
1943. Madeleine MM, Newcomer LM (2007). Cancer of the Anus. In: SEER Survival Monograph: Cancer Survival Among Adults: U.S. SEER Program, 1988-2001, Patient and Tumor Characteristics. Ries LAG, Young JL, Keel GE, Eisner MP, Lin YD, Horner JM, eds. National Cancer Institute, SEER Program: Bethesda, MD, pp. 43-48.
1944. Madsen JA, Tallini G, Glusac EJ, Salem RR, Braverman I, Robert ME (1999). Biliary tract obstruction secondary to mycosis fungoides: a case report. J Clin Gastroenterol 28: 56-60.
1945. Madura JA, Jarman BT, Doherty MG, Yum MN, Howard TJ (1999). Adenosquamous carcinoma of the pancreas. Arch Surg 134: 599-603.
1946. Madura JA, Wiebke EA, Howard TJ, Cummings OW, Hull MT, Sherman S et al. (1997). Mucin-hypersecreting intraductal neoplasms of the pancreas: a precursor to cystic pancreatic malignancies. Surgery 122: 786-792.
1947. Maeda M, Nagawa H, Maeda T, Koike H, Kasai H (1998). Alcohol consumption enhances liver metastasis in colorectal carcinoma patients. Cancer 83: 1483-1488.
1948. Maeda T, Kajiyama K, Adachi E, Takenaka K, Sugimachi K, Tsuneyoshi M (1996). The expression of cytokeratins 7, 19, and 20 in primary and metastatic carcinomas of the liver. Mod Pathol 9: 901-909.
1949. Maehama T, Dixon JE (1998). The tumor suppressor, PTEN/MMAC1, dephosphorylates the lipid second messenger, phosphatidylinositol 3,4,5-trisphosphate. J Biol Chem 273: 13375-13378.
1950. Maes M, Depardieu C, Dargent JL, Hermans M, Verhaeghe JL, Delabie J et al. (1997). Primary low-grade B-cell lymphoma of MALT-type occurring in the liver: a study of two cases. J Hepatol 27: 922-927.
1951. Maggard MA, O'Connell JB, Ko CY (2004). Updated population-based review of carcinoid tumors. Ann Surg 240: 117-122.
1952. Maglinte DT, Reyes BL (1997). Small bowel cancer. Radiologic diagnosis. Radiol Clin North Am 35: 361-380.
1953. Mahdavi J, Sonden B, Hurtig M, Olfat FO, Forsberg L, Roche N et al. (2002). *Helicobacter pylori* SabA adhesin in persistent infection and chronic inflammation. Science 297: 573-578.
1954. Mahmoud NN, Boolbol SK, Bilinski RT, Martucci C, Chadburn A, Bertagnolli MM (1997). *APC* gene mutation is associated with a dominant-negative effect upon intestinal cell migration. Cancer Res 57: 5045-5050.
1955. Maire F, Hammel P, Terris B, Olschwang S, O'Toole D, Sauvanet A et al. (2002). Intraductal papillary and mucinous pancreatic tumour: a new extracolonic tumour in familial adenomatous polyposis. Gut 51: 446-449.
1956. Maitra A, Adsay NV, Argani P, Iacobuzio-Donahue C, De MA, Cameron JL et al. (2003). Multicomponent analysis of the pancreatic adenocarcinoma progression model using a pancreatic intraepithelial neoplasia tissue microarray. Mod Pathol 16: 902-912.
1957. Maitra A, Krueger JE, Tascilar M, Offerhaus GJ, Angeles-Angeles A, Klimstra DS et al. (2000). Carcinoid tumors of the extrahepatic bile ducts: a study of seven cases. Am J Surg Pathol 24: 1501-1510.
1958. Maitra A, Tascilar M, Hruban RH, Offerhaus GJ, Albores-Saavedra J (2001). Small cell carcinoma of the gallbladder: a clinicopathologic, immunohistochemical, and molecular pathology study of 12 cases. Am J Surg Pathol 25: 595-601.
1959. Makhlouf HR, Ahrens W, Agarwal B, Dow N, Marshalleck JJ, Lee EL et al. (2008). Synovial sarcoma of the stomach: a clinicopathologic, immunohistochemical, and molecular genetic study of 10 cases. Am J Surg Pathol 32: 275-281.
1960. Makhlouf HR, Burke AP, Sobin LH (1999). Carcinoid tumors of the ampulla of Vater: a comparison with duodenal carcinoid tumors. Cancer 85: 1241-1249.
1961. Makhlouf HR, Ishak KG, Goodman ZD (1999). Epithelioid hemangioendothelioma of the liver: a clinicopathologic study of 137 cases. Cancer 85: 562-582.
1962. Makhlouf HR, Ishak KG, Shekar R, Sesterhenn IA, Young DY, Fanburg-Smith JC (2002). Melanoma markers in angiomyolipoma of the liver and kidney: a comparative study. Arch Pathol Lab Med 126: 49-55.
1963. Makinen MJ (2007). Colorectal serrated adenocarcinoma. Histopathology 50: 131-150.
1964. Makino A, Serra S, Chetty R (2006). Composite adenocarcinoma and large cell neuroendocrine carcinoma of the rectum. Virchows Arch 448: 644-647.
1965. Malamut G, Afchain P, Verkarre V, Lecomte T, Amiot A, Damotte D et al. (2009). Presentation and long-term follow-up of refractory celiac disease: comparison of type I with type II. Gastroenterology 136: 81-90.
1966. Malats N, Porta M, Pinol JL, Corominas JM, Rifa J, Real FX (1995). Ki-ras mutations as a prognostic factor in extrahepatic bile system cancer. PANK-ras I Project Investigators. J Clin Oncol 13: 1679-1686.
1967. Malhi H, Gores GJ (2006). Cholangiocarcinoma: modern advances in understanding a deadly old disease. J Hepatol 45: 856-867.
1968. Mallory SB (1995). Cowden syndrome (multiple hamartoma syndrome). Dermatol Clin 13: 27-31.
1969. Mandal RV, Forcione DG, Brugge WR, Nishioka NS, Mino-Kenudson M, Lauwers GY (2009). Effect of tumor characteristics and duplication of the muscularis mucosae on the endoscopic staging of superficial Barrett esophagus-related neoplasia. Am J Surg Pathol 33: 620-625.
1970. Mandal S, Kawatra V, Khurana N (2008). Mucinous cystadenocarcinoma arising in mature cystic teratoma ovary and associated pseudomyxoma peritonei: report of a case. Arch Gynecol Obstet 278: 265-267.
1971. Mandard AM, Chasle J, Marnay J, Villedieu B, Bianco C, Roussel A et al. (1981). Autopsy findings in 111 cases of esophageal cancer. Cancer 48: 329-335.
1971A.Mandard AM, Dalibard F, Mandard JC, Marnay J, Henry-Amar M, Petiot JF, Roussel A, Jacob JH, Segol P, Samama G (1994). Pathologic assessment of tumor regression after preoperative chemoradiotherapy of esophageal carcinoma. Clinicopathologic correlations. Cancer 73: 2680-2686
1972. Mandujano-Vera G, ngeles-Angeles A, de lC-H, Sansores-Perez M, Larriva-Sahd J (1995). Gastrinoma of the common bile duct: immunohistochemical and ultrastructural study of a case. J Clin Gastroenterol 20: 321-324.
1972A. Mani, H, Climent, F, Colomo, L, Pittaluga, S, Raffeld, M, and Jaffe, E S (2010). Primary gall bladder lymphomas: clinicopathological observations and biological implications. Am J Surg Pathol. In press.
1973. Mannick EE, Bravo LE, Zarama G, Realpe JL, Zhang XJ, Ruiz B et al. (1996). Inducible nitric oxide synthase, nitrotyrosine, and apoptosis in *Helicobacter pylori* gastritis: effect of antibiotics and antioxidants. Cancer Res 56: 3238-3243.
1974. Mao C, Domenico DR, Kim K, Hanson DJ, Howard JM (1995). Observations on the developmental patterns and the consequences of pancreatic exocrine adenocarcinoma. Findings of 154 autopsies. Arch Surg 130: 125-134.
1975. Marchesa P, Fazio VW, Church JM, McGannon E (1997). Adrenal masses in patients with familial adenomatous polyposis. Dis Colon Rectum 40: 1023-1028.
1976. Marchesa P, Fazio VW, Oliart S, Goldblum JR, Lavery IC, Milsom JW (1997). Long-term outcome of patients with perianal Paget's disease. Ann Surg Oncol 4: 475-480.
1977. Marchio A, Terris B, Meddeb M, Pineau P, Duverger A, Tiollais P et al. (2001). Chromosomal abnormalities in liver cell dysplasia detected by comparative genomic hybridisation. Mol Pathol 54: 270-274.
1978. Markowitz S, Wang J, Myeroff L, Parsons R, Sun L, Lutterbaugh J et al. (1995). Inactivation of the type II TGF-beta receptor in colon cancer cells with microsatellite instability. Science 268: 1336-1338.
1979. Marsh DJ, Coulon V, Lunetta KL, Rocca-Serra P, Dahia PL, Zheng Z et al. (1998). Mutation spectrum and genotype-phenotype analyses in Cowden disease and Bannayan-Zonana syndrome, two hamartoma syndromes with germline *PTEN* mutation. Hum Mol Genet 7: 507-515.
1980. Marsh DJ, Dahia PL, Caron S, Kum JB, Frayling IM, Tomlinson IP et al. (1998). Germline *PTEN* mutations in Cowden syndrome-like families. J Med Genet 35: 881-885.
1980A. Marsh DJ, Dahia PL, Coulon V, Zheng Z, Dorion-Bonnet F, Call KM et al. (1998). Allelic imbalance, including deletion of PTEN/MMACI, at the Cowden disease locus on 10q22-23, in hamartomas from patients with Cowden syndrome and germline PTEN mutation. Genes Chromosomes Cancer 21: 61-69.
1981. Marsh DJ, Dahia PL, Zheng Z, Liaw D, Parsons R, Gorlin RJ et al. (1997). Germline mutations in PTEN are present in Bannayan-Zonana syndrome. Nat Genet 16: 333-334.
1982. Marsh DJ, Kum JB, Lunetta KL, Bennett MJ, Gorlin RJ, Ahmed SF et al. (1999). PTEN

mutation spectrum and genotype-phenotype correlations in Bannayan-Riley-Ruvalcaba syndrome suggest a single entity with Cowden syndrome. Hum Mol Genet 8: 1461-1472.
1983. Marsh DJ, Roth S, Lunetta KL, Hemminki A, Dahia PL, Sistonen P et al. (1997). Exclusion of PTEN and 10q22-24 as the susceptibility locus for juvenile polyposis syndrome. Cancer Res 57: 5017-5021.
1984. Marsh DJ, Trahair TN, Martin JL, Chee WY, Walker J, Kirk EP et al. (2008). Rapamycin treatment for a child with germline PTEN mutation. Nat Clin Pract Oncol 5: 357-361.
1984A.Marshall JR (2008). Prevention of colorectal cancer: diet, chemoprevention, and lifestyle. Gastroenterol Clin North Am 37: 73-82.
1985. Martellucci J, Naldini G, Colosimo C, Cionini L, Rossi M (2009). Accuracy of endoanal ultrasound in the follow-up assessment for squamous cell carcinoma of the anal canal treated with radiochemotherapy. Surg Endosc 23: 1054-1057.
1986. Martensson H, Nobin A, Sundler F, Falkmer S (1985). Endocrine tumors of the ileum. Cytochemical and clinical aspects. Pathol Res Pract 180: 356-363.
1987. Martignoni G, Pea M, Reghellin D, Zamboni G, Bonetti F (2008). PEComas: the past, the present and the future. Virchows Arch 452: 119-132.
1988. Martignoni ME, Friess H, Lubke D, Uhl W, Maurer C, Muller M et al. (1999). Study of a primary gastrinoma in the common hepatic duct - a case report. Digestion 60: 187-190.
1989. Martin IG, Dixon MF, Sue-Ling H, Axon AT, Johnston D (1994). Goseki histological grading of gastric cancer is an important predictor of outcome. Gut 35: 758-763.
1990. Martinez F, Haase GM, Koep LJ, Akers DR (1982). Rhabdomyosarcoma of the biliary tree: the case for aggressive surgery. J Pediatr Surg 17: 508-511.
1991. Martinez ME, Baron JA, Lieberman DA, Schatzkin A, Lanza E, Winawer SJ et al. (2009). A pooled analysis of advanced colorectal neoplasia diagnoses after colonoscopic polypectomy. Gastroenterology 136: 832-841.
1992. Maru D, Wu TT, Canada A, Houlihan PS, Hamilton SR, Rashid A (2004). Loss of chromosome 18q and DPC4 (Smad4) mutations in appendiceal adenocarcinomas. Oncogene 23: 859-864.
1993. Maru DM, Khurana H, Rashid A, Correa AM, Anandasabapathy S, Krishnan S et al. (2008). Retrospective study of clinicopathologic features and prognosis of high-grade neuroendocrine carcinoma of the esophagus. Am J Surg Pathol 32: 1404-1411.
1994. Marubashi S, Yano H, Monden T, Tateishi H, Kanoh T, Iwazawa T et al. (1999). Primary squamous cell carcinoma of the stomach. Gastric Cancer 2: 136-141.
1995. Marudanayagam R, Williams GT, Rees BI (2006). Review of the pathological results of 2660 appendicectomy specimens. J Gastroenterol 41: 745-749.
1996. Maruyama H, Nakatsuji N, Sugihara S, Atsumi M, Shimamoto K, Hayashi K et al. (1997). Anaplastic Ki-1-positive large cell lymphoma of the pancreas: a case report and review of the literature. Jpn J Clin Oncol 27: 51-57.
1997. Masaki T, Sheffield JP, Talbot IC, Williams CB (1994). Non-polypoid adenoma of the large intestine. Int J Colorectal Dis 9: 180-183.
1998. Mascarello JT, Krous HF (1992). Second report of a translocation involving 19q13.4 in a mesenchymal hamartoma of the liver. Cancer Genet Cytogenet 58: 141-142.
1999. Matano S, Nakamura S, Annen Y, Hattori N, Kiyohara K, Kakuta K et al. (1998). Primary hepatic lymphoma in a patient with chronic hepatitis B. Am J Gastroenterol 93: 2301-2302.
2000. Mathieu D, Kobeiter H, Maison P, Rahmouni A, Cherqui D, Zafrani ES et al. (2000). Oral contraceptive use and focal nodular hyperplasia of the liver. Gastroenterology 118: 560-564.
2001. Matos JM, Schmidt CM, Turrini O, Agaram NP, Niedergethmann M, Saeger HD et al. (2009). Pancreatic acinar cell carcinoma: a multi-institutional study. J Gastrointest Surg 13: 1495-1502.
2002. Matsubara M, Shiozawa T, Tachibana R, Hondo T, Osasda K, Kawaguchi K et al. (2005). Primary retroperitoneal mucinous cystadenoma of borderline malignancy: a case report and review of the literature. Int J Gynecol Pathol 24: 218-223.
2003. Matsubayashi H, Matsunaga K, Sasaki K, Yamaguchi Y, Hasuike N, Ono H (2008). Small carcinoid tumor of papilla of the Vater with lymph node metastases. J Gastrointest Cancer 39: 61-65.
2004. Matsui K, Jin XM, Kitagawa M, Miwa A (1998). Clinicopathologic features of neuroendocrine carcinomas of the stomach: appraisal of small cell and large cell variants. Arch Pathol Lab Med 122: 1010-1017.
2005. Matsumoto T, Iida M, Nakamura S, Hizawa K, Yao T, Tsuneyoshi M et al. (2000). Natural history of ampullary adenoma in familial adenomatous polyposis: reconfirmation of benign nature during extended surveillance. Am J Gastroenterol 95: 1557-1562.
2006. Matsumoto T, Mizuno M, Shimizu M, Manabe T, Iida M, Fujishima M (1999). Serrated adenoma of the colorectum: colonoscopic and histologic features. Gastrointest Endosc 49: 736-742.
2007. Matsunou H, Konishi F (1990). Papillary-cystic neoplasm of the pancreas. A clinicopathologic study concerning the tumor aging and malignancy of nine cases. Cancer 65: 283-291.
2008. Matsunou H, Konishi F, Hori H, Ikeda T, Sasaki K, Hirose Y et al. (1996). Characteristics of Epstein-Barr virus-associated gastric carcinoma with lymphoid stroma in Japan. Cancer 77: 1998-2004.
2009. Matsunou H, Konishi F, Yamamichi N, Takayanagi N, Mukai M (1990). Solid, infiltrating variety of papillary cystic neoplasm of the pancreas. Cancer 65: 2747-2757.
2010. Matsuura H, Sugimachi K, Ueo H, Kuwano H, Koga Y, Okamura T (1986). Malignant potentiality of squamous cell carcinoma of the esophagus predictable by DNA analysis. Cancer 57: 1810-1814.
2011. Maxwell P, Davis RI, Sloan JM (1993). Carcinoembryonic antigen (CEA) in benign and malignant epithelium of the gall bladder, extrahepatic bile ducts, and ampulla of Vater. J Pathol 170: 73-76.
2012. May A, Nachbar L, Pohl J, Ell C (2007). Endoscopic interventions in the small bowel using double balloon enteroscopy: feasibility and limitations. Am J Gastroenterol 102: 527-535.
2013. May R, Riehl TE, Hunt C, Sureban SM, Anant S, Houchen CW (2008). Identification of a novel putative gastrointestinal stem cell and adenoma stem cell marker, doublecortin and CaM kinase-like-1, following radiation injury and in adenomatous polyposis coli/multiple intestinal neoplasia mice. Stem Cells 26: 630-637.
2014. Mayer B, Johnson JP, Leitl F, Jauch KW, Heiss MM, Schildberg FW et al. (1993). E-cadherin expression in primary and metastatic gastric cancer: down-regulation correlates with cellular dedifferentiation and glandular disintegration. Cancer Res 53: 1690-1695.
2015. Mayo SC, Pawlik TM (2009). Current management of colorectal hepatic metastasis. Expert Rev Gastroenterol Hepatol 3: 131-144.
2016. McCarthy DM, Hruban RH, Argani P, Howe JR, Conlon KC, Brennan MF et al. (2003). Role of the *DPC4* tumor suppressor gene in adenocarcinoma of the ampulla of Vater: analysis of 140 cases. Mod Pathol 16: 272-278.
2017. McCarthy JH, Aga R (1988). A fallopian tube lesion of borderline malignancy associated with pseudo-myxoma peritonei. Histopathology 13: 223-225.
2018. McClave SA, Boyce HW, Jr., Gottfried MR (1987). Early diagnosis of columnar-lined esophagus: a new endoscopic diagnostic criterion. Gastrointest Endosc 33: 413-416.
2019. McCluggage WG, Mackel E, McCusker G (1996). Primary low grade malignant lymphoma of mucosa-associated lymphoid tissue of gallbladder. Histopathology 29: 285-287.
2020. McColl I, Busxhey HJ, Veale AM, Morson BC (1964). Juvenile polyposis coli. Proc R Soc Med 57: 896-897.
2021. McGarrity TJ, Amos C (2006). Peutz-Jeghers syndrome: clinicopathology and molecular alterations. Cell Mol Life Sci 63: 2135-2144.
2022. McGlynn KA, Tarone RE, El-Serag HB (2006). A comparison of trends in the incidence of hepatocellular carcinoma and intrahepatic cholangiocarcinoma in the United States. Cancer Epidemiol Biomarkers Prev 15: 1198-1203.
2023. McGory ML, Maggard MA, Kang H, O'Connell JB, Ko CY (2005). Malignancies of the appendix: beyond case series reports. Dis Colon Rectum 48: 2264-2271.
2024. McGregor DK, Wu TT, Rashid A, Luthra R, Hamilton SR (2004). Reduced expression of cytokeratin 20 in colorectal carcinomas with high levels of microsatellite instability. Am J Surg Pathol 28: 712-718.
2025. McKenna BJ, Appelman HD (2002). Dysplasia can be a pain in the gut. Pathology 34: 518-528.
2026. McLaughlin CC, Baptiste MS, Schymura MJ, Nasca PC, Zdeb MS (2006). Maternal and infant birth characteristics and hepatoblastoma. Am J Epidemiol 163: 818-828.
2027. McLean CA, Pedersen JS (1991). Endocrine cell carcinoma of the gallbladder. Histopathology 19: 173-176.
2028. McLemore EC, Pockaj BA, Reynolds C, Gray RJ, Hernandez JL, Grant CS et al. (2005). Breast cancer: presentation and intervention in women with gastrointestinal metastasis and carcinomatosis. Ann Surg Oncol 12: 886-894.
2029. McNeely B, Owen DA, Pezim M (1992). Multiple microcarcinoids arising in chronic ulcerative colitis. Am J Clin Pathol 98: 112-116.
2030. McRonald FE, Liloglou T, Xinarianos G, Hill L, Rowbottom L, Langan JE et al. (2006). Down-regulation of the cytoglobin gene, located on 17q25, in tylosis with oesophageal cancer (TOC): evidence for trans-allele repression. Hum Mol Genet 15: 1271-1277.
2031. McShane LM, Altman DG, Sauerbrei W, Taube SE, Gion M, Clark GM (2005). REporting recommendations for tumour MARKer prognostic studies (REMARK). Br J Cancer 93: 387-391.
2032. Medeiros F, Corless CL, Duensing A, Hornick JL, Oliveira AM, Heinrich MC et al. (2004). KIT-negative gastrointestinal stromal tumors: proof of concept and therapeutic implications. Am J Surg Pathol 28: 889-894.
2033. Medeiros F, Nascimento AF, Crum CP (2005). Early vulvar squamous neoplasia: advances in classification, diagnosis, and differential diagnosis. Adv Anat Pathol 12: 20-26.
2034. Mehenni H, Gehrig C, Nezu J, Oku A, Shimane M, Rossier C et al. (1998). Loss of LKB1 kinase activity in Peutz-Jeghers syndrome, and evidence for allelic and locus heterogeneity. Am J Hum Genet 63: 1641-1650.
2035. Mehra S, Chung-Park M (2005). Gallbladder paraganglioma: a case report with review of the literature. Arch Pathol Lab Med 129: 523-526.
2036. Melbye M, Cote TR, Kessler L, Gail M, Biggar RJ (1994). High incidence of anal cancer among AIDS patients. The AIDS/Cancer Working Group. Lancet 343: 636-639.
2037. Melbye M, Rabkin C, Frisch M, Biggar RJ (1994). Changing patterns of anal cancer incidence in the United States, 1940-1989. Am J Epidemiol 139: 772-780.
2038. Mellemkjaer L, Johansen C, Gridley G, Linet MS, Kjaer SK, Olsen JH (2000). Crohn's disease and cancer risk (Denmark). Cancer Causes Control 11: 145-150.
2039. Mellemkjaer L, Olsen JH, Frisch M, Johansen C, Gridley G, McLaughlin JK (1995). Cancer in patients with ulcerative colitis. Int J Cancer 60: 330-333.
2040. Melo CR, Melo IS, Schmitt FC, Fagundes R, Amendola D (1993). Multicentric granular cell tumor of the colon: report of a patient with 52 tumors. Am J Gastroenterol 88: 1785-1787.
2041. Memeo L, Pecorello I, Ciardi A, Aiello E, De QA, Di TU (1999). Primary non-Hodgkin's lymphoma of the liver. Acta Oncol 38: 655-658.
2042. Mendelsohn G, Diamond MP (1984). Familial ganglioneuromatous polyposis of the large bowel. Report of a family with associated juvenile polyposis. Am J Surg Pathol 8: 515-520.
2043. Mendez-Sanchez N, King-Martinez AC, Ramos MH, Pichardo-Bahena R, Uribe M (2004). The Amerindian's genes in the Mexican population are associated with development of gallstone disease. Am J Gastroenterol 99: 2166-2170.
2044. Mendoza-Marin M, Hoang MP, Albores-Saavedra J (2002). Malignant stromal tumor of the gallbladder with interstitial cells of Cajal phenotype. Arch Pathol Lab Med 126: 481-483.
2045. Meng F, Yamagiwa Y, Ueno Y, Patel T (2006). Over-expression of interleukin-6 enhances cell survival and transformed cell growth in human malignant cholangiocytes. J Hepatol 44: 1055-1065.
2046. Mennigen R, Tuebergen D, Koehler G, Sauerland C, Senninger N, Bruewer M (2008). Endoscopic ultrasound with conventional probe and miniprobe in preoperative staging of esophageal cancer. J Gastrointest Surg 12: 256-262.
2047. Mention JJ, Ben AM, Begue B, Barbe U, Verkarre V, Asnafi V et al. (2003). Interleukin 15: a key to disrupted intraepithelial lymphocyte homeostasis and lymphomagenesis in celiac disease. Gastroenterology 125: 730-745.
2048. Menuck LS, Amberg JR (1975). Metastatic disease involving the stomach. Am J Dig Dis 20: 903-913.
2049. Menzel J, Hoepffner N, Sulkowski U, Reimer P, Heinecke A, Poremba C et al. (1999). Polypoid tumors of the major duodenal papilla: preoperative staging with intraductal US, EUS, and CT—a prospective, histopathologically controlled study. Gastrointest Endosc 49: 349-357.
2050. Menzel J, Poremba C, Dietl KH, Bocker W, Domschke W (1999). Tumors of the papilla of Vater—inadequate diagnostic impact of endoscopic forceps biopsies taken prior to and following sphincterotomy. Ann Oncol 10: 1227-1231.
2051. Mera R, Fontham ET, Bravo LE, Bravo JC, Piazuelo MB, Camargo MC et al. (2005). Long term follow up of patients treated for *Helicobacter pylori* infection. Gut 54: 1536-1540.
2052. Merchant SH, VanderJagt T, Lathrop S, Amin MB (2006). Sporadic duodenal bulb gastrin-cell tumors: association with *Helicobacter pylori* gastritis and long-term use of proton pump inhibitors. Am J Surg Pathol 30: 1581-1587.
2052A. Merriam-Webster (2002). Merriam-Webster's Medical Desk Dictionary, Revised Edition. Springfield, Mass.: Merriam-Webster.
2053. Metaxas G, Tangalos A, Pappa P, Papageorgiou I (2009). Mucinous cystic neoplasms of the mesentery: a case report and

review of the literature. World J Surg Oncol 7: 47
2054. Meurs-Szojda MM, Terhaar sive Droste JS, Kuik DJ, Mulder CJ, Felt-Bersma RJ (2008). Diverticulosis and diverticulitis form no risk for polyps and colorectal neoplasia in 4,241 colonoscopies. Int J Colorectal Dis 23: 979-984.
2055. Meyerhardt JA, Giovannucci EL, Holmes MD, Chan AT, Chan JA, Colditz GA et al. (2006). Physical activity and survival after colorectal cancer diagnosis. J Clin Oncol 24: 3527-3534.
2056. Meyerhardt JA, Niedzwiecki D, Hollis D, Saltz LB, Hu FB, Mayer RJ et al. (2007). Association of dietary patterns with cancer recurrence and survival in patients with stage III colon cancer. JAMA 298: 754-764.
2057. Meyers RL (2007). Tumors of the liver in children. Surg Oncol 16: 195-203.
2058. Meyskens FL, Jr., McLaren CE, Pelot D, Fujikawa-Brooks S, Carpenter PM, Hawk E et al. (2008). Difluoromethylornithine plus sulindac for the prevention of sporadic colorectal adenomas: a randomized placebo-controlled, double-blind trial. Cancer Prev Res 1: 32-38.
2059. Micchelli ST, Vivekanandan P, Boitnott JK, Pawlik TM, Choti MA, Torbenson M (2008). Malignant transformation of hepatic adenomas. Mod Pathol 21: 491-497.
2060. Michaels PJ, Brachtel EF, Bounds BC, Brugge WR, Pitman MB (2006). Intraductal papillary mucinous neoplasm of the pancreas: cytologic features predict histologic grade. Cancer 108: 163-173.
2061. Michelassi F, Testa G, Pomidor WJ, Lashner BA, Block GE (1993). Adenocarcinoma complicating Crohn's disease. Dis Colon Rectum 36: 654-661.
2062. Middeldorp A, Van Puijenbroek M, Nielsen M, Corver WE, Jordanova ES, ter Haar N et al. (2008). High frequency of copy-neutral LOH in MUTYH-associated polyposis carcinomas. J Pathol 216: 25-31.
2063. Miettinen M, Fetsch JF (2000). Distribution of keratins in normal endothelial cells and a spectrum of vascular tumors: implications in tumor diagnosis. Hum Pathol 31: 1062-1067.
2064. Miettinen M, Furlong M, Sarlomo-Rikala M, Burke A, Sobin LH, Lasota J (2001). Gastrointestinal stromal tumors, intramural leiomyomas, and leiomyosarcomas in the rectum and anus: a clinicopathologic, immunohistochemical, and molecular genetic study of 144 cases. Am J Surg Pathol 25: 1121-1133.
2065. Miettinen M, Kahlos T (1989). Undifferentiated (embryonal) sarcoma of the liver. Epithelial features as shown by immunohistochemical analysis and electron microscopic examination. Cancer 64: 2096-2103.
2066. Miettinen M, Lasota J (2006). Gastrointestinal stromal tumors: review on morphology, molecular pathology, prognosis, and differential diagnosis. Arch Pathol Lab Med 130: 1466-1478.
2067. Miettinen M, Lasota J, Sobin LH (2005). Gastrointestinal stromal tumors of the stomach in children and young adults: a clinicopathologic, immunohistochemical, and molecular genetic study of 44 cases with long-term follow-up and review of the literature. Am J Surg Pathol 29: 1373-1381.
2068. Miettinen M, Makhlouf H, Sobin LH, Lasota J (2006). Gastrointestinal stromal tumors of the jejunum and ileum: a clinicopathologic, immunohistochemical, and molecular genetic study of 906 cases before imatinib with long-term follow-up. Am J Surg Pathol 30: 477-489.
2069. Miettinen M, Makhlouf HR, Sobin LH, Lasota J (2009). Plexiform fibromyxoma: a distinctive benign gastric antral neoplasm not to be confused with a myxoid GIST. Am J Surg Pathol 33: 1624-1632.
2070. Miettinen M, Paal E, Lasota J, Sobin LH (2002). Gastrointestinal glomus tumors: a clinicopathologic, immunohistochemical, and molecular genetic study of 32 cases. Am J Surg Pathol 26: 301-311.
2071. Miettinen M, Partanen S, Fraki O, Kivilaakso E (1987). Papillary cystic tumor of the pancreas. An analysis of cellular differentiation by electron microscopy and immunohistochemistry. Am J Surg Pathol 11: 855-865.
2072. Miettinen M, Sarlomo-Rikala M, Sobin LH (2001). Mesenchymal tumors of muscularis mucosae of colon and rectum are benign leiomyomas that should be separated from gastrointestinal stromal tumors—a clinicopathologic and immunohistochemical study of eighty-eight cases. Mod Pathol 14: 950-956.
2073. Miettinen M, Sarlomo-Rikala M, Sobin LH, Lasota J (2000). Esophageal stromal tumors: a clinicopathologic, immunohistochemical, and molecular genetic study of 17 cases and comparison with esophageal leiomyomas and leiomyosarcomas. Am J Surg Pathol 24: 211-222.
2074. Miettinen M, Sarlomo-Rikala M, Sobin LH, Lasota J (2000). Gastrointestinal stromal tumors and leiomyosarcomas in the colon: a clinicopathologic, immunohistochemical, and molecular genetic study of 44 cases. Am J Surg Pathol 24: 1339-1352.
2075. Miettinen M, Shekitka KM, Sobin LH (2001). Schwannomas in the colon and rectum: a clinicopathologic and immunohistochemical study of 20 cases. Am J Surg Pathol 25: 846-855.
2076. Miettinen M, Sobin LH (2001). Gastrointestinal stromal tumors in the appendix: a clinicopathologic and immunohistochemical study of four cases. Am J Surg Pathol 25: 1433-1437.
2077. Miettinen M, Sobin LH, Lasota J (2005). Gastrointestinal stromal tumors of the stomach: a clinicopathologic, immunohistochemical, and molecular genetic study of 1765 cases with long-term follow-up. Am J Surg Pathol 29: 52-68.
2078. Miettinen M, Sobin LH, Lasota J (2009). True smooth muscle tumors of the small intestine: a clinicopathologic, immunhistochemical, and molecular genetic study of 25 cases. Am J Surg Pathol 33: 430-436.
2079. Miettinen M, Wang ZF, Lasota J (2009). DOG1 antibody in the differential diagnosis of gastrointestinal stromal tumors: a study of 1840 cases. Am J Surg Pathol 33: 1401-1408.
2080. Miki K, Fujishiro M, Kodashima S, Yahagi N (2009). Long-term results of gastric cancer screening using the serum pepsinogen test method among an asymptomatic middle-aged Japanese population. Dig Endosc 21: 78-81.
2081. Mills SE, Allen MS, Jr., Cohen AR (1983). Small-cell undifferentiated carcinoma of the colon. A clinicopathological study of five cases and their association with colonic adenomas. Am J Surg Pathol 7: 643-651.
2082. Minaguchi T, Waite KA, Eng C (2006). Nuclear localization of PTEN is regulated by Ca(2+) through a tyrosil phosphorylation-independent conformational modification in major vault protein. Cancer Res 66: 11677-11682.
2083. Minamoto T, Mai M, Watanabe K, Ooi A, Kitamura T, Takahashi Y et al. (1990). Medullary carcinoma with lymphocytic infiltration of the stomach. Clinicopathologic study of 27 cases and immunohistochemical analysis of the subpopulations of infiltrating lymphocytes in the tumor. Cancer 66: 945-952.
2084. Ming SC (eds) (1973). Tumors of the Esophagus and Stomach. Armed Forces Institute of Pathology: Washington, DC.
2085. Ming SC (1977). Gastric carcinoma. A pathobiological classification. Cancer 39: 2475-2485.
2086. Ming SC, Hirota T (1998). Malignant Epithelial Tumors of the Stomach. In: Pathology of the Gastrointestinal Tract. Ming SC, Goldman H (eds). Williams & Wilkins: Baltimore, pp.
2087. Mingazzini PL, Malchiodi AF, Blandamura V (1982). Villous adenoma of the duodenum: cellular composition and histochemical findings. Histopathology 6: 235-244.
2088. Mingoli A, Brachini G, Petroni R, Antoniozzi A, Cavaliere F, Simonelli L et al. (2005). Squamous and adenosquamous cell carcinomas of the gallbladder. J Exp Clin Cancer Res 24: 143-150.
2089. Minguez B, Tovar V, Chiang D, Villanueva A, Llovet JM (2009). Pathogenesis of hepatocellular carcinoma and molecular therapies. Curr Opin Gastroenterol 25: 186-194.
2090. Misdraji J, Burgart LJ, Lauwers GY (2004). Defective mismatch repair in the pathogenesis of low-grade appendiceal mucinous neoplasms and adenocarcinomas. Mod Pathol 17: 1447-1454.
2091. Misdraji J, Fernandez del Castillo C, Ferry JA (1997). Follicle center lymphoma of the ampulla of Vater presenting with jaundice: report of a case. Am J Surg Pathol 21: 484-488.
2092. Misdraji J, Yantiss RK, Graeme-Cook FM, Balis UJ, Young RH (2003). Appendiceal mucinous neoplasms: a clinicopathologic analysis of 107 cases. Am J Surg Pathol 27: 1089-1103.
2093. Misumi A, Murakami A, Harada K, Baba K, Akagi M (1989). Definition of carcinoma of the gastric cardia. Langenbecks Arch Chir 374: 221-226.
2094. Mitani Y, Oue N, Hamai Y, Aung PP, Matsumura S, Nakayama H et al. (2005). Histone H3 acetylation is associated with reduced p21(WAF1/CIP1) expression by gastric carcinoma. J Pathol 205: 65-73.
2095. Mitchell DI, Char G, McDonald A, Scott P (1995). Plexiform neurofibroma: a rare cause of obstructive jaundice. West Indian Med J 44: 146-147.
2096. Mitchell H, English DR, Elliott F, Gengos M, Barrett JH, Giles GG et al. (2008). Immunoblotting using multiple antigens is essential to demonstrate the true risk of *Helicobacter pylori* infection for gastric cancer. Aliment Pharmacol Ther 28: 903-910.
2097. Mitropoulos FA, Angelopoulou MK, Siakantaris MP, Rassidakis G, Vayiopoulos GA, Papalampros E et al. (2000). Primary non-Hodgkin's lymphoma of the gall bladder. Leuk Lymphoma 40: 123-131.
2098. Mitsunaga S, Hasebe T, Kinoshita T, Konishi M, Takahashi S, Gotohda N et al. (2007). Detail histologic analysis of nerve plexus invasion in invasive ductal carcinoma of the pancreas and its prognostic impact. Am J Surg Pathol 31: 1636-1644.
2099. Miura S, Yoshidome H, Shida T, Kimura F, Shimizu H, Otsuka M et al. (2008). Clinical implications of unusual NeuroD and mASH1 expression in a patient with primary large-cell neuroendocrine carcinoma of the duodenum: report of a case. Surg Today 38: 857-861.
2100. Miwa W, Yasuda J, Murakami Y, Yashima K, Sugano K, Sekine T et al. (1996). Isolation of DNA sequences amplified at chromosome 19q13.1-q13.2 including the AKT2 locus in human pancreatic cancer. Biochem Biophys Res Commun 225: 968-974.
2101. Miyahara R, Niwa Y, Matsuura T, Maeda O, Ando T, Ohmiya N et al. (2007). Prevalence and prognosis of gastric cancer detected by screening in a large Japanese population: data from a single institute over 30 years. J Gastroenterol Hepatol 22: 1435-1442.
2102. Miyaki M, Konishi M, Kikuchi-Yanoshita R, Enomoto M, Tanaka K, Takahashi H et al. (1993). Coexistence of somatic and germ-line mutations of *APC* gene in desmoid tumors from patients with familial adenomatous polyposis. Cancer Res 53: 5079-5082.
2103. Miyamoto H, Kurita N, Nishioka M, Ando T, Tashiro T, Hirokawa M et al. (2006). Poorly differentiated neuroendocrine cell carcinoma of the rectum: report of a case and literal review. J Med Invest 53: 317-320.
2104. Miyata H, Doki Y, Yasuda T, Yamasaki M, Higuchi I, Makari Y et al. (2008). Evaluation of clinical significance of 18F-fluorodeoxyglucose positron emission tomography in superficial squamous cell carcinomas of the thoracic esophagus. Dis Esophagus 21: 144-150.
2105. Miyazaki K, Date K, Imamura S, Ogawa Y, Nakayama F (1989). Familial occurrence of anomalous pancreaticobiliary duct union associated with gallbladder neoplasms. Am J Gastroenterol 84: 176-181.
2106. Miyazaki T, Kato H, Masuda N, Nakajima M, Manda R, Fukuchi M et al. (2004). Mucosa-associated lymphoid tissue lymphoma of the esophagus: case report and review of the literature. Hepatogastroenterology 51: 750-753.
2107. Miyazawa M, Torii T, Toshimitsu Y, Kamizasa N, Suzuki T, Shinozuka N et al. (2006). Alpha-fetoprotein-producing clear cell carcinoma of the extrahepatic bile ducts. J Clin Gastroenterol 40: 555-557.
2108. Mizobuchi S, Tachimori Y, Kato H, Watanabe H, Nakanishi Y, Ochiai A (1997). Metastatic esophageal tumors from distant primary lesions: report of three esophagectomies and study of 1835 autopsy cases. Jpn J Clin Oncol 27: 410-414.
2109. Mizukami Y, Kono K, Kawaguchi Y, Akaike H, Kamimura K, Sugai H et al. (2008). Localisation pattern of Foxp3+ regulatory T cells is associated with clinical behaviour in gastric cancer. Br J Cancer 98: 148-153.
2110. Mo JQ, Dimashkieh HH, Bove KE (2004). GLUT1 endothelial reactivity distinguishes hepatic infantile hemangioma from congenital hepatic vascular malformation with associated capillary proliferation. Hum Pathol 35: 200-209.
2111. Modlin IM, Champaneria MC, Chan AK, Kidd M (2007). A three-decade analysis of 3,911 small intestinal neuroendocrine tumors: the rapid pace of no progress. Am J Gastroenterol 102: 1464-1473.
2112. Modlin IM, Kidd M, Latich I, Zikusoka MN, Eick GN, Mane SM et al. (2006). Genetic differentiation of appendiceal tumor malignancy: a guide for the perplexed. Ann Surg 244: 52-60.
2113. Modlin IM, Lye KD, Kidd M (2003). A 5-decade analysis of 13,715 carcinoid tumors. Cancer 97: 934-959.
2114. Modlin IM, Moss SF, Chung DC, Jensen RT, Snyderwine E (2008). Priorities for improving the management of gastroenteropancreatic neuroendocrine tumors. J Natl Cancer Inst 100: 1282-1289.
2115. Modlin IM, Sandor A (1997). An analysis of 8305 cases of carcinoid tumors. Cancer 79: 813-829.
2116. Modlin IM, Shapiro MD, Kidd M (2005). An analysis of rare carcinoid tumors: clarifying these clinical conundrums. World J Surg 29: 92-101.
2117. Moertel CG, Dockerty MB (1973). Familial occurrence of metastasizing carcinoid tumors. Ann Intern Med 78: 389-390.
2118. Moertel CG, Dockerty MB, Judd ES (1968). Carcinoid tumors of the vermiform appendix. Cancer 21: 270-278.
2119. Moertel CG, SAUER WG, Dockerty MB, BAGGENSTOSS AH (1961). Life history of the carcinoid tumor of the small intestine. Cancer 14: 901-912.
2120. Moertel CG, Weiland LH, Nagorney DM, Dockerty MB (1987). Carcinoid tumor of the appendix: treatment and prognosis. N Engl J Med 317: 1699-1701.
2121. Moertel CL, Weiland LH, Telander RL

(1990). Carcinoid tumor of the appendix in the first two decades of life. J Pediatr Surg 25: 1073-1075.
2122. Mohler M, Gutzler F, Kallinowski B, Goeser T, Stremmel W (1997). Primary hepatic high-grade non-Hodgkin's lymphoma and chronic hepatitis C infection. Dig Dis Sci 42: 2241-2245.
2123. Mohr VH, Vortmeyer AO, Zhuang Z, Libutti SK, Walther MM, Choyke PL et al. (2000). Histopathology and molecular genetics of multiple cysts and microcystic (serous) adenomas of the pancreas in von Hippel-Lindau patients. Am J Pathol 157: 1615-1621.
2124. Molberg KH, Heffess C, Delgado R, Albores-Saavedra J (1998). Undifferentiated carcinoma with osteoclast-like giant cells of the pancreas and periampullary region. Cancer 82: 1279-1287.
2125. Moll R, Lowe A, Laufer J, Franke WW (1992). Cytokeratin 20 in human carcinomas. A new histodiagnostic marker detected by monoclonal antibodies. Am J Pathol 140: 427-447.
2126. Monges GM, Mathoulin-Portier MP, Acres RB, Houvenaeghel GF, Giovannini MF, Seitz JF et al. (1999). Differential MUC 1 expression in normal and neoplastic human pancreatic tissue. An immunohistochemical study of 60 samples. Am J Clin Pathol 112: 635-640.
2127. Monno S, Nagata A, Homma T, Oguchi H, Kawa S, Kaji R et al. (1984). Exocrine pancreatic cancer with humoral hypercalcemia. Am J Gastroenterol 79: 128-132.
2128. Montalban C, Santon A, Boixeda D, Redondo C, Alvarez I, Calleja JL et al. (2001). Treatment of low grade gastric mucosa-associated lymphoid tissue lymphoma in stage I with *Helicobacter pylori* eradication. Long-term results after sequential histologic and molecular follow-up. Haematologica 86: 609-617.
2129. Montecino M, Stein JL, Stein GS, Lian JB, van Wijnen AJ, Cruzat F et al. (2007). Nucleosome organization and targeting of SWI/SNF chromatin-remodeling complexes: contributions of the DNA sequence. Biochem Cell Biol 85: 419-425.
2130. Montemarano H, Lonergan GJ, Bulas DI, Selby DM (2000). Pancreatoblastoma: imaging findings in 10 patients and review of the literature. Radiology 214: 476-482.
2131. Montero M, Vazquez JL, Rihuete MA, Corton D, Anton L, Soriano D et al. (2003). Serous cystadenoma of the pancreas in a child. J Pediatr Surg 38: E6-E7.
2132. Montesano R, Hainaut P (1998). Molecular precursor lesions in oesophageal cancer. Cancer Surv 32: 53-68.
2133. Montesano R, Hainaut P, Wild CP (1997). Hepatocellular carcinoma: from gene to public health. J Natl Cancer Inst 89: 1844-1851.
2134. Montesano R, Hollstein M, Hainaut P (1996). Genetic alterations in esophageal cancer and their relevance to etiology and pathogenesis: a review. Int J Cancer 69: 225-235.
2135. Montgomery E, Bronner MP, Goldblum JR, Greenson JK, Haber MM, Hart J et al. (2001). Reproducibility of the diagnosis of dysplasia in Barrett esophagus: a reaffirmation. Hum Pathol 32: 368-378.
2136. Montgomery E, Bronner MP, Greenson JK, Haber MM, Hart J, Lamps LW et al. (2002). Are ulcers a marker for invasive carcinoma in Barrett's esophagus? Data from a diagnostic variability study with clinical follow-up. Am J Gastroenterol 97: 27-31.
2137. Moody F, THORBJARNARSON B (1964). Carcinoma of the ampulla of Vater. Am J Surg 107: 572-579.
2138. Moon WK, Kim WS, Kim IO, Yeon KM, Yu IK, Choi BI et al. (1994). Undifferentiated embryonal sarcoma of the liver: US and CT findings. Pediatr Radiol 24: 500-503.
2139. Moons LM, Kuipers EJ, Rygiel AM, Groothuismink AZ, Geldof H, Bode WA et al. (2007). COX-2 CA-haplotype is a risk factor for the development of esophageal adenocarcinoma. Am J Gastroenterol 102: 2373-2379.
2139A.Moore HG, Guillem JG (2002). Anal neoplasms. Surg Clin North Am 82:1233-1251.
2140. Moore PS, Missiaglia E, Antonello D, Zamo A, Zamboni G, Corleto V et al. (2001). Role of disease-causing genes in sporadic pancreatic endocrine tumors: *MEN1* and *VHL*. Genes Chromosomes Cancer 32: 177-181.
2141. Moore PS, Orlandini S, Zamboni G, Capelli P, Rigaud G, Falconi M et al. (2001). Pancreatic tumours: molecular pathways implicated in ductal cancer are involved in ampullary but not in exocrine nonductal or endocrine tumorigenesis. Br J Cancer 84: 253-262.
2142. Moore PS, Zamboni G, Brighenti A, Lissandrini D, Antonello D, Capelli P et al. (2001). Molecular characterization of pancreatic serous microcystic adenomas: evidence for a tumor suppressor gene on chromosome 10q. Am J Pathol 158: 317-321.
2143. Morak M, Schackert HK, Rahner N, Betz B, Ebert M, Walldorf C et al. (2008). Further evidence for heritability of an epimutation in one of 12 cases with MLH1 promoter methylation in blood cells clinically displaying HNPCC. Eur J Hum Genet 16: 804-811.
2144. Morales CP, Souza RF, Spechler SJ (2002). Hallmarks of cancer progression in Barrett's oesophagus. Lancet 360: 1587-1589.
2145. Moran CA, Ishak KG, Goodman ZD (1998). Solitary fibrous tumor of the liver: a clinicopathologic and immunohistochemical study of nine cases. Ann Diagn Pathol 2: 19-24.
2146. Morant R, Bruckner HW (1989). Complete remission of refractory small cell carcinoma of the pancreas with cisplatin and etoposide. Cancer 64: 2007-2009.
2147. Morgner A, Miehlke S, Fischbach W, Schmitt W, Muller-Hermelink H, Greiner A et al. (2001). Complete remission of primary high-grade B-cell gastric lymphoma after cure of *Helicobacter pylori* infection. J Clin Oncol 19: 2041-2048.
2148. Mori M, Iwashita A, Enjoji M (1986). Adenosquamous carcinoma of the stomach. A clinicopathologic analysis of 28 cases. Cancer 57: 333-339.
2149. Mori M, Kitagawa S, Iida M, Sakurai T, Enjoji M, Sugimachi K et al. (1987). Early carcinoma of the gastric cardia. A clinicopathologic study of 21 cases. Cancer 59: 1758-1766.
2150. Mori M, Matsukuma A, Adachi Y, Miyagahara T, Matsuda H, Kuwano H et al. (1989). Small cell carcinoma of the esophagus. Cancer 63: 564-573.
2151. Mori M, Sakaguchi H, Akazawa K, Tsuneyoshi M, Sueishi K, Sugimachi K (1995). Correlation between metastatic site, histological type, and serum tumor markers of gastric carcinoma. Hum Pathol 26: 504-508.
2152. Mori T, Yanagisawa A, Kato Y, Miura K, Nishihira T, Mori S et al. (1994). Accumulation of genetic alterations during esophageal carcinogenesis. Hum Mol Genet 3: 1969-1971.
2153. Morimitsu Y, Hsia CC, Kojiro M, Tabor E (1995). Nodules of less-differentiated tumor within or adjacent to hepatocellular carcinoma: relative expression of transforming growth factor-alpha and its receptor in the different areas of tumor. Hum Pathol 26: 1126-1132.
2154. Morinaga S, Tsumuraya M, Nakajima T, Shimosato Y, Okazaki N (1986). Ciliated-cell adenocarcinoma of the pancreas. Acta Pathol Jpn 36: 1905-1910.
2155. Morishita Y, Tanaka T, Kato K, Kawamori T, Amano K, Funato T et al. (1991). Gastric collision tumor (carcinoid and adenocarcinoma) with gastritis cystica profunda. Arch Pathol Lab Med 115: 1006-1010.
2156. Morita M, Kuwano H, Nakashima T, Taketomi A, Baba H, Saito T et al. (1998). Family aggregation of carcinoma of the hypopharynx and cervical esophagus: special reference to multiplicity of cancer in upper aerodigestive tract. Int J Cancer 76: 468-471.
2157. Morita M, Kuwano H, Ohno S, Sugimachi K, Seo Y, Tomoda H et al. (1994). Multiple occurrence of carcinoma in the upper aerodigestive tract associated with esophageal cancer: reference to smoking, drinking and family history. Int J Cancer 58: 207-210.
2158. Morita T, Tomita N, Ohue M, Sekimoto M, Yamamoto H, Ohnishi T et al. (2002). Molecular analysis of diminutive, flat, depressed colorectal lesions: are they precursors of polypoid adenoma or early stage carcinoma? Gastrointest Endosc 56: 663-671.
2159. Morohoshi T, Held G, Klöppel G (1983). Exocrine pancreatic tumours and their histological classification. A study based on 167 autopsy and 97 surgical cases. Histopathology 7: 645-661.
2160. Morohoshi T, Kanda M, Asanuma K, Klöppel G (1989). Intraductal papillary neoplasms of the pancreas. A clinicopathologic study of six patients. Cancer 64: 1329-1335.
2161. Morohoshi T, Kanda M, Horie A, Chott A, Dreyer T, Klöppel G et al. (1987). Immunocytochemical markers of uncommon pancreatic tumors. Acinar cell carcinoma, pancreatoblastoma, and solid cystic (papillary-cystic) tumor. Cancer 59: 739-747.
2162. Morohoshi T, Sagawa F, Mitsuya T (1990). Pancreatoblastoma with marked elevation of serum alpha-fetoprotein. An autopsy case report with immunocytochemical study. Virchows Arch A Pathol Anat Histopathol 416: 265-270.
2163. Morselli-Labate AM, Pezzilli R (2009). Usefulness of serum IgG4 in the diagnosis and follow up of autoimmune pancreatitis: A systematic literature review and meta-analysis. J Gastroenterol Hepatol 24: 15-36.
2163A. Mosby Inc. (2009). Mosby's dictionary of medicine, nursing & health professions. 8th ed. St. Louis, Mo.: Mosby Elsevier.
2164. Moser AR, Shoemaker AR, Connelly CS, Clipson L, Gould KA, Luongo C et al. (1995). Homozygosity for the Min allele of Apc results in disruption of mouse development prior to gastrulation. Dev Dyn 203: 422-433.
2165. Moskaluk CA, Hruban H, Lietman A, Smyrk T, Fusaro L, Fusaro R et al. (1998). Novel germline p16(INK4) allele (Asp145Cys) in a family with multiple pancreatic carcinomas. Mutations in brief no. 148. Online. Hum Mutat 12: 70-
2166. Mosoia L, Mabrut JY, Adham M, Boillot O, Ducerf C, Partensky C et al. (2008). Hepatic epithelioid hemangioendothelioma: long-term results of surgical management. J Surg Oncol 98: 432-437.
2167. Moss SF, Blaser MJ (2005). Mechanisms of disease: Inflammation and the origins of cancer. Nat Clin Pract Oncol 2: 90-97.
2168. Motola-Kuba D, Zamora-Valdes D, Uribe M, Mendez-Sanchez N (2006). Hepatocellular carcinoma. An overview. Ann Hepatol 5: 16-24.
2169. Motoyama T, Aizawa K, Watanabe H, Fukase M, Saito K (1993). alpha-Fetoprotein producing gastric carcinomas: a comparative study of three different subtypes. Acta Pathol Jpn 43: 654-661.
2170. Movahedi-Lankarani S, Hruban RH, Westra WH, Klimstra DS (2002). Primitive neuroectodermal tumors of the pancreas: a report of seven cases of a rare neoplasm. Am J Surg Pathol 26: 1040-1047.
2171. Moyana TN (1989). Carcinoid tumors arising from Meckel's diverticulum. A clinical, morphologic, and immunohistochemical study. Am J Clin Pathol 91: 52-56.
2172. Moyana TN, Satkunam N (1992). A comparative immunohistochemical study of jejunoileal and appendiceal carcinoids. Implications for histogenesis and pathogenesis. Cancer 70: 1081-1088.
2173. Moyana TN, Xiang J, Senthilselvan A, Kulaga A (2000). The spectrum of neuroendocrine differentiation among gastrointestinal carcinoids: importance of histologic grading, MIB-1, p53, and bcl-2 immunoreactivity. Arch Pathol Lab Med 124: 570-576.
2174. Moynihan MJ, Bast MA, Chan WC, Delabie J, Wickert RS, Wu G et al. (1996). Lymphomatous polyposis. A neoplasm of either follicular mantle or germinal center cell origin. Am J Surg Pathol 20: 442-452.
2175. Mozos A, Royo C, Hartmann E, De JD, Baro C, Valera A et al. (2009). SOX11 expression is highly specific for mantle cell lymphoma and identifies the cyclin D1-negative subtype. Haematologica 94: 1555-1562.
2176. Mueller J, Gansauge S, Mattfeldt T (2003). P53 mutation but not p16/MTS1 mutation occurs in intraductal papillary mucinous tumors of the pancreas. Hepatogastroenterology 50: 541-544.
2177. Muguerza R, Rodriguez A, Formigo E, Montero M, Vazquez JL, Paramo C et al. (2005). Pancreatoblastoma associated with incomplete Beckwith-Wiedemann syndrome: case report and review of the literature. J Pediatr Surg 40: 1341-1344.
2178. Mukai K, Grotting JC, Greider MH, Rosai J (1982). Retrospective study of 77 pancreatic endocrine tumors using the immunoperoxidase method. Am J Surg Pathol 6: 387-399.
2179. Muleris M, Salmon RJ, Girodet J, Zafrani B, Dutrillaux B (1987). Recurrent deletions of chromosomes 11q and 3p in anal canal carcinoma. Int J Cancer 39: 595-598.
2180. Muller G, Dargent JL, Duwel V, D'Olne D, Vanvuchelen J, Haot J et al. (1997). Leukaemia and lymphoma of the appendix presenting as acute appendicitis or acute abdomen. Four case reports with a review of the literature. J Cancer Res Clin Oncol 123: 560-564.
2181. Muller-Hocker J, Zietz CH, Sendelhofert A (2001). Deregulated expression of cell cycle-associated proteins in solid pseudopapillary tumor of the pancreas. Mod Pathol 14: 47-53.
2182. Mulligan RM (1972). Histogenesis and biologic behavior of gastric carcinoma. Pathol Annu 7: 349-415.
2183. Mulrooney DA, Carpenter B, Georgieff M, Angel C, Hunter D, Foker J et al. (2001). Hepatic mesenchymal hamartoma in a neonate: a case report and review of the literature. J Pediatr Hematol Oncol 23: 316-317.
2184. Mundinger GS, Gust S, Micchelli ST, Fishman EK, Hruban RH, Wolfgang CL (2009). Adult pancreatic hemangioma: case report and literature review. Gastroenterol Res Pract 2009: 839730-
2185. Murakami H, Furihata M, Ohtsuki Y, Ogoshi S (1999). Determination of the prognostic significance of cyclin B1 overexpression in patients with esophageal squamous cell carcinoma. Virchows Arch 434: 153-158.
2186. Murakami T (1971). Pathomorphological diagnosis. Definition and gross classification of early gastric cancer. Gann Monogr 11: 53-
2187. Murakami Y, Uemura K, Hayashidani Y, Sudo T, Sueda T (2006). Relapsing acute pancreatitis due to ampullary adenoma in a patient with familial adenomatous polyposis. J Gastroenterol 41: 798-801.
2188. Murakata LA, Ishak KG (2001). Expression of inhibin-alpha by granular cell tumors of the gallbladder and extrahepatic bile ducts. Am J Surg Pathol 25: 1200-1203.
2189. Murakata LA, Ishak KG, Nzeako UC

(2000). Clear cell carcinoma of the liver: a comparative immunohistochemical study with renal clear cell carcinoma. Mod Pathol 13: 874-881.
2190. Murata M, Iwao K, Miyoshi Y, Nagasawa Y, Ohta T, Shibata K et al. (2000). Molecular and biological analysis of carcinoma of the small intestine: beta-catenin gene mutation by interstitial deletion involving exon 3 and replication error phenotype. Am J Gastroenterol 95: 1576-1580.
2191. Murphy EM, Farquharson SM, Moran BJ (2006). Management of an unexpected appendiceal neoplasm. Br J Surg 93: 783-792.
2192. Murphy G, Pfeiffer R, Camargo MC, Rabkin CS (2009). Meta-analysis shows that prevalence of Epstein-Barr virus-positive gastric cancer differs based on sex and anatomic location. Gastroenterology 137: 824-833.
2193. Murray A, Cuevas EC, Jones DB, Wright DH (1995). Study of the immunohistochemistry and T cell clonality of enteropathy-associated T cell lymphoma. Am J Pathol 146: 509-519.
2194. Murray GI, Duncan ME, O'Neil P, McKay JA, Melvin WT, Fothergill JE (1998). Matrix metalloproteinase-1 is associated with poor prognosis in oesophageal cancer. J Pathol 185: 256-261.
2195. Murray L, Sedo A, Scott M, McManus D, Sloan JM, Hardie LJ et al. (2006). TP53 and progression from Barrett's metaplasia to oesophageal adenocarcinoma in a UK population cohort. Gut 55: 1390-1397.
2196. Murthi GV, Paterson L, Azmy A (2003). Chromosomal translocation in mesenchymal hamartoma of liver: what is its significance? J Pediatr Surg 38: 1543-1545.
2197. Musto P (2002). Hepatitis C virus infection and B-cell non-Hodgkin's lymphomas: more than a simple association. Clin Lymphoma 3: 150-160.
2198. Muto M, Takahashi M, Ohtsu A, Ebihara S, Yoshida S, Esumi H (2005). Risk of multiple squamous cell carcinomas both in the esophagus and the head and neck region. Carcinogenesis 26: 1008-1012.
2199. Muto T, Bussey HJ, Morson BC (1975). The evolution of cancer of the colon and rectum. Cancer 36: 2251-2270.
2200. Myers MP, Stolarov JP, Eng C, Li J, Wang SI, Wigler MH et al. (1997). P-TEN, the tumor suppressor from human chromosome 10q23, is a dual-specificity phosphatase. Proc Natl Acad Sci U S A 94: 9052-9057.
2201. Myerson RJ, Karnell LH, Menck HR (1997). The National Cancer Data Base report on carcinoma of the anus. Cancer 80: 805-815.
2202. Nafidi O, Nguyen BN, Roy A (2008). Carcinoid tumor of the common bile duct: a rare complication of von Hippel-Lindau syndrome. World J Gastroenterol 14: 1299-1301.
2203. Nagai E, Ueyama T, Yao T, Tsuneyoshi M (1993). Hepatoid adenocarcinoma of the stomach. A clinicopathologic and immunohistochemical analysis. Cancer 72: 1827-1835.
2204. Nagakawa T, Kayahara M, Ueno K, Ohta T, Konishi I, Miyazaki I (1992). Clinicopathological study on neural invasion to the extrapancreatic nerve plexus in pancreatic cancer. Hepatogastroenterology 39: 51-55.
2205. Nagakawa T, Mori K, Nakano T, Kadoya M, Kobayashi H, Akiyama T et al. (1993). Perineural invasion of carcinoma of the pancreas and biliary tract. Br J Surg 80: 619-621.
2206. Nagar B, Overduin M, Ikura M, Rini JM (1996). Structural basis of calcium-induced E-cadherin rigidification and dimerization. Nature 380: 360-364.
2207. Nagase H, Miyoshi Y, Horii A, Aoki T, Ogawa M, Utsunomiya J et al. (1992). Correlation between the location of germ-line mutations in the *APC* gene and the number of colorectal polyps in familial adenomatous polyposis patients. Cancer Res 52: 4055-4057.
2208. Nagata K, Horinouchi M, Saitou M, Higashi M, Nomoto M, Goto M et al. (2007). Mucin expression profile in pancreatic cancer and the precursor lesions. J Hepatobiliary Pancreat Surg 14: 243-254.
2209. Nagata S, Yamaguchi K, Inoue T, Yamaguchi H, Ito T, Gibo J et al. (2007). Solid pancreatic hamartoma. Pathol Int 57: 276-280.
2210. Nahas CS, Shia J, Joseph R, Schrag D, Minsky BD, Weiser MR et al. (2007). Squamous-cell carcinoma of the rectum: a rare but curable tumor. Dis Colon Rectum 50: 1393-1400.
2211. Nakajima T (2002). Gastric cancer treatment guidelines in Japan. Gastric Cancer 5: 1-5.
2212. Nakamura A, Horinouchi M, Goto M, Nagata K, Sakoda K, Takao S et al. (2002). New classification of pancreatic intraductal papillary-mucinous tumour by mucin expression: its relationship with potential for malignancy. J Pathol 197: 201-210.
2213. Nakamura E, Shimizu M, Itoh T, Manabe T (2001). Secondary tumors of the pancreas: clinicopathological study of 103 autopsy cases of Japanese patients. Pathol Int 51: 686-690.
2214. Nakamura K, Sugano H, Takagi K (1968). Carcinoma of the stomach in incipient phase: its histogenesis and histological appearances. Gann 59: 251-258.
2215. Nakamura M, Miyamoto S, Maeda H, Zhang SC, Sangai T, Ishii G et al. (2004). Low levels of insulin-like growth factor type 1 receptor expression at cancer cell membrane predict liver metastasis in Dukes' C human colorectal cancers. Clin Cancer Res 10: 8434-8441.
2216. Nakamura S, Akazawa K, Yao T, Tsuneyoshi M (1995). A clinicopathologic study of 233 cases with special reference to evaluation with the MIB-1 index. Cancer 76: 1313-1324.
2217. Nakamura S, Aoyagi K, Furuse M, Suekane H, Matsumoto T, Yao T et al. (1998). B-cell monoclonality precedes the development of gastric MALT lymphoma in *Helicobacter pylori*-associated chronic gastritis. Am J Pathol 152: 1271-1279.
2218. Nakamura S, Kino I, Baba S (1988). Cell kinetics analysis of background colonic mucosa of patients with intestinal neoplasms by ex vivo autoradiography. Gut 29: 997-1002.
2219. Nakamura S, Matsumoto T, Iida M, Yao T, Tsuneyoshi M (2003). Primary gastrointestinal lymphoma in Japan: a clinicopathologic analysis of 455 patients with special reference to its time trends. Cancer 97: 2462-2473.
2220. Nakamura S, Matsumoto T, Takeshita M, Kurahara K, Yao T, Tsuneyoshi M et al. (2000). A clinicopathologic study of primary small intestine lymphoma: prognostic significance of mucosa-associated lymphoid tissue-derived lymphoma. Cancer 88: 286-294.
2221. Nakamura S, Matsumoto T, Umeno J, Yanai S, Shono Y, Suekane H et al. (2007). Endoscopic features of intestinal follicular lymphoma: the value of double-balloon enteroscopy. Endoscopy 39 Suppl 1: E26-E27.
2222. Nakamura S, Ueki T, Yao T, Ueyama T, Tsuneyoshi M (1994). Epstein-Barr virus in gastric carcinoma with lymphoid stroma. Special reference to its detection by the polymerase chain reaction and in situ hybridization in 99 tumors, including a morphologic analysis. Cancer 73: 2239-2249.
2223. Nakamura S, Yao T, Aoyagi K, Iida M, Fujishima M, Tsuneyoshi M (1997). *Helicobacter pylori* and primary gastric lymphoma. A histopathologic and immunohistochemical analysis of 237 patients. Cancer 79: 3-11.
2224. Nakamura S, Ye H, Bacon CM, Goatly A, Liu H, Banham AH et al. (2007). Clinical impact of genetic aberrations in gastric MALT lymphoma: a comprehensive analysis using interphase fluorescence in situ hybridisation. Gut 56: 1358-1363.
2225. Nakamura S, Ye H, Bacon CM, Goatly A, Liu H, Kerr L et al. (2008). Translocations involving the immunoglobulin heavy chain gene locus predict better survival in gastric diffuse large B-cell lymphoma. Clin Cancer Res 14: 3002-3010.
2226. Nakamura T, Inagaki H, Seto M, Nakamura S (2003). Gastric low-grade B-cell MALT lymphoma: treatment, response, and genetic alteration. J Gastroenterol 38: 921-929.
2227. Nakamura T, Mohri H, Shimazaki M, Ito Y, Ohnishi T, Nishino Y et al. (1997). Esophageal metastasis from prostate cancer: diagnostic use of reverse transcriptase-polymerase chain reaction for prostate-specific antigen. J Gastroenterol 32: 236-240.
2228. Nakamura T, Nakamura S, Yonezumi M, Seto M, Yokoi T (2000). The t(11; 18)(q21; q21) translocation in *H. pylori*-negative low-grade gastric MALT lymphoma. Am J Gastroenterol 95: 3314-3315.
2229. Nakamura T, Nakamura S, Yonezumi M, Suzuki T, Matsuura A, Yatabe Y et al. (2000). *Helicobacter pylori* and the t(11;18)(q21;q21) translocation in gastric low-grade B-cell lymphoma of mucosa-associated lymphoid tissue type. Jpn J Cancer Res 91: 301-309.
2230. Nakamura T, Seto M, Tajika M, Kawai H, Yokoi T, Yatabe Y et al. (2008). Clinical features and prognosis of gastric MALT lymphoma with special reference to responsiveness to *H. pylori* eradication and *API2-MALT1* status. Am J Gastroenterol 103: 62-70.
2231. Nakanishi Y, Ito T, Kubota K, Takeda H, Yonemori A, Kawakami H et al. (2007). Spindle cell-type undifferentiated carcinoma of the common bile duct of the hepatic hilus: report of a case. Surg Today 37: 708-712.
2232. Nakanishi Y, Ochiai A, Yoshimura K, Kato H, Shimoda T, Yamaguchi H et al. (1998). The clinicopathologic significance of small areas unstained by Lugol's iodine in the mucosa surrounding resected esophageal carcinoma: an analysis of 147 cases. Cancer 82: 1454-1459.
2233. Nakanishi Y, Saka M, Eguchi T, Sekine S, Taniguchi H, Shimoda T (2007). Distribution and significance of the oesophageal and gastric cardiac mucosae: a study of 131 operation specimens. Histopathology 51: 515-519.
2234. Nakanishi Y, Zen Y, Kawakami H, Kubota K, Itoh T, Hirano S et al. (2008). Extrahepatic bile duct carcinoma with extensive intraepithelial spread: a clinicopathological study of 21 cases. Mod Pathol 21: 807-816.
2235. Nakanishi Y, Zen Y, Kondo S, Itoh T, Itatsu K, Nakanuma Y (2008). Expression of cell cycle-related molecules in biliary premalignant lesions: biliary intraepithelial neoplasia and biliary intraductal papillary neoplasm. Hum Pathol 39: 1153-1161.
2236. Nakanuma Y, Hoso M, Sanzen T, Sasaki M (1997). Microstructure and development of the normal and pathologic biliary tract in humans, including blood supply. Microsc Res Tech 38: 552-570.
2237. Nakanuma Y, Sasaki M, Ikeda H, Sato Y, Zen Y, Kosaka K et al. (2008). Pathology of peripheral intrahepatic cholangiocarcinoma with reference to tumorigenesis. Hepatol Res 38: 325-334.
2238. Nakanuma Y, Sasaki M, Ishikawa A, Tsui W, Chen TC, Huang SF (2002). Biliary papillary neoplasm of the liver. Histol Histopathol 17: 851-861.
2239. Nakao A, Harada A, Nonami T, Kaneko T, Inoue S, Takagi H (1995). Clinical significance of portal invasion by pancreatic head carcinoma. Surgery 117: 50-55.
2240. Nakao A, Harada A, Nonami T, Kaneko T, Takagi H (1996). Clinical significance of carcinoma invasion of the extrapancreatic nerve plexus in pancreatic cancer. Pancreas 12: 357-361.
2241. Nakase Y, Sakakura C, Miyagawa K, Kin S, Fukuda K, Yanagisawa A et al. (2005). Frequent loss of *RUNX3* gene expression in remnant stomach cancer and adjacent mucosa with special reference to topography. Br J Cancer 92: 562-569.
2242. Nakashima O, Sugihara S, Kage M, Kojiro M (1995). Pathomorphologic characteristics of small hepatocellular carcinoma: a special reference to small hepatocellular carcinoma with indistinct margins. Hepatology 22: 101-105.
2243. Nakata B, Wang YQ, Yashiro M, Ohira M, Ishikawa T, Nishino H et al. (2003). Negative hMSH2 protein expression in pancreatic carcinoma may predict a better prognosis of patients. Oncol Rep 10: 997-1000.
2244. Nakata B, Yashiro M, Nishioka N, Aya M, Yamada S, Takenaka C et al. (2002). Very low incidence of microsatellite instability in intraductal papillary-mucinous neoplasm of the pancreas. Int J Cancer 102: 655-659.
2245. Nakatsuru S, Yanagisawa A, Furukawa Y, Ichii S, Kato Y, Nakamura Y et al. (1993). Somatic mutations of the *APC* gene in precancerous lesion of the stomach. Hum Mol Genet 2: 1463-1465.
2245A. Nakatsuru S, Yanagisawa A, Ichii S, Tahara E, Kato Y, Nakamura Y et al. (1992). Somatic mutation of the *APC* gene in gastric cancer: frequent mutations in very well differentiated adenocarcinoma and signet-ring cell carcinoma. Hum Mol Genet 1: 559–563.
2246. Nakayama Y, Inoue H, Hamada Y, Takeshita M, Iwasaki H, Maeshiro K et al. (2005). Intraductal tubular adenoma of the pancreas, pyloric gland type: a clinicopathologic and immunohistochemical study of 6 cases. Am J Surg Pathol 29: 607-616.
2247. Nakayama Y, Murayama H, Iwasaki H, Iwanaga S, Kikuchi M, Ikeda S et al. (1997). Gastric carcinosarcoma (sarcomatoid carcinoma) with rhabdomyoblastic and osteoblastic differentiation. Pathol Int 47: 557-563.
2248. Nakeeb A, Pitt HA, Sohn TA, Coleman J, Abrams RA, Piantadosi S et al. (1996). Cholangiocarcinoma. A spectrum of intrahepatic, perihilar, and distal tumors. Ann Surg 224: 463-473.
2249. Namatame K, Ookubo M, Suzuki K, Sagawa H, Nagashima T, Kataba Y et al. (1986). [A clinicopathological study of five cases of adenosquamous carcinoma of the stomach]. Gan No Rinsho 32: 170-175.
2250. Nanashima A, Kinoshita N, Nakanuma Y, Zen Y, Sumida Y, Abo T et al. (2008). Clinicopathological features of "intraductal papillary neoplasm of the bile duct" and patient outcome after surgical resection. Hepatogastroenterology 55: 1167-1173.
2251. Nandurkar S, Talley NJ (1999). Barrett's esophagus: the long and the short of it. Am J Gastroenterol 94: 30-40.
2252. Nara S, Shimada K, Kosuge T, Kanai Y, Hiraoka N (2008). Minimally invasive intraductal papillary-mucinous carcinoma of the pancreas: clinicopathologic study of 104 intraductal papillary-mucinous neoplasms. Am J Surg Pathol 32: 243-255.
2253. Narayanan Menon KV (2006). Primary sclerosing cholangitis, chronic ulcerative colitis, and bile duct dysplasia—Case presentation. Liver Transpl 12: S14-
2254. Nassar H, Albores-Saavedra J, Klimstra DS (2005). High-grade neuroendocrine carcinoma of the ampulla of Vater: a clinicopathologic and immunohistochemical analysis of 14 cases. Am J Surg Pathol 29: 588-594.
2255. Natarajan S, Theise ND, Thung SN, Antonio L, Paronetto F, Hytiroglou P (1997). Large-cell change of hepatocytes in cirrhosis may represent a reaction to prolonged cholestasis. Am J Surg Pathol 21: 312-318.

2256. Naunheim KS, Zeitels J, Kaplan EL, Sugimoto J, Shen KL, Lee CH et al. (1983). Rectal carcinoid tumors—treatment and prognosis. Surgery 94: 670-676.
2257. Navarro JT, Ribera JM, Mate JL, Granada I, Junca J, Batlle M et al. (2003). Hepatosplenic T-gammadelta lymphoma in a patient with Crohn's disease treated with azathioprine. Leuk Lymphoma 44: 531-533.
2258. Nawgiri RS, Nagle JA, Wilbur DC, Pitman MB (2007). Cytomorphology and B72.3 labeling of benign and malignant ductal epithelium in pancreatic lesions compared to gastrointestinal epithelium. Diagn Cytopathol 35: 300-305.
2259. Nawroz IM (1987). Malignant carcinoid tumour of oesophagus. Histopathology 11: 879-880.
2260. Neef B, Kunzig B, Sinn I, Kieninger G, von GU (1997). [Primary pancreatic lymphoma. A rare cause of pain-free icterus]. Dtsch Med Wochenschr 122: 12-17.
2261. Nehal KS, Levine VJ, Ashinoff R (1998). Basal cell carcinoma of the genitalia. Dermatol Surg 24: 1361-1363.
2262. Nelen MR, Kremer H, Konings IB, Schoute F, van Essen AJ, Koch R et al. (1999). Novel PTEN mutations in patients with Cowden disease: absence of clear genotype-phenotype correlations. Eur J Hum Genet 7: 267-273.
2263. Nelen MR, Padberg GW, Peeters EA, Lin AY, van den Helm B, Frants RR et al. (1996). Localization of the gene for Cowden disease to chromosome 10q22-23. Nat Genet 13: 114-116.
2264. Nelen MR, van Staveren WC, Peeters EA, Hassel MB, Gorlin RJ, Hamm H et al. (1997). Germline mutations in the *PTEN/MMAC1* gene in patients with Cowden disease. Hum Mol Genet 6: 1383-1387.
2265. Nemolato S, Fanni D, Naccarato AG, Ravarino A, Bevilacqua G, Faa G (2008). Lymphoepitelioma-like hepatocellular carcinoma: a case report and a review of the literature. World J Gastroenterol 14: 4694-4696.
2266. Neoptolemos JP, Dunn JA, Stocken DD, Almond J, Link K, Beger H et al. (2001). Adjuvant chemoradiotherapy and chemotherapy in resectable pancreatic cancer: a randomised controlled trial. Lancet 358: 1576-1585.
2267. Neoptolemos JP, Stocken DD, Dunn JA, Almond J, Beger HG, Pederzoli P et al. (2001). Influence of resection margins on survival for patients with pancreatic cancer treated by adjuvant chemoradiation and/or chemotherapy in the ESPAC-1 randomized controlled trial. Ann Surg 234: 758-768.
2268. Neoptolemos JP, Stocken DD, Friess H, Bassi C, Dunn JA, Hickey H et al. (2004). A randomized trial of chemoradiotherapy and chemotherapy after resection of pancreatic cancer. N Engl J Med 350: 1200-1210.
2269. Neugut AI, Jacobson JS, Suh S, Mukherjee R, Arber N (1998). The epidemiology of cancer of the small bowel. Cancer Epidemiol Biomarkers Prev 7: 243-251.
2270. Neuman HB, Park J, Weiser MR (2010). Randomized clinical trials in colon cancer. Surg Oncol Clin N Am 19: 183-204.
2271. Newman DH, Doerhoff CR, Bunt TJ (1984). Villous adenoma of the duodenum. Am Surg 50: 26-28.
2272. Ng FC, Ang HK, Chng HC (1993). Adenosquamous carcinoma of the ileum—a case report. Singapore Med J 34: 361-362.
2273. Ng SB, Turner EH, Robertson PD, Flygare SD, Bigham AW, Lee C et al. (2009). Targeted capture and massively parallel sequencing of 12 human exomes. Nature 461: 272-276.
2274. Nguyen BN, Flejou JF, Terris B, Belghiti J, Degott C (1999). Focal nodular hyperplasia of the liver: a comprehensive pathologic study of 305 lesions and recognition of new histologic forms. Am J Surg Pathol 23: 1441-1454.
2275. Nguyen NQ, Leong RW (2008). Current application of confocal endomicroscopy in gastrointestinal disorders. J Gastroenterol Hepatol 23: 1483-1491.
2276. Nguyen TT, Gorman B, Shields D, Goodman Z (2008). Malignant hepatic angiomyolipoma: report of a case and review of literature. Am J Surg Pathol 32: 793-798.
2277. Ni Y, Zbuk KM, Sadler T, Patocs A, Lobo G, Edelman E et al. (2008). Germline mutations and variants in the succinate dehydrogenase genes in Cowden and Cowden-like syndromes. Am J Hum Genet 83: 261-268.
2278. Nicol K, Savell V, Moore J, Teot L, Spunt SL, Qualman S (2007). Distinguishing undifferentiated embryonal sarcoma of the liver from biliary tract rhabdomyosarcoma: a Children's Oncology Group study. Pediatr Dev Pathol 10: 89-97.
2279. Nicolaides NC, Carter KC, Shell BK, Papadopoulos N, Vogelstein B, Kinzler KW (1995). Genomic organization of the human *PMS2* gene family. Genomics 30: 195-206.
2280. Nicolaides NC, Palombo F, Kinzler KW, Vogelstein B, Jiricny J (1996). Molecular cloning of the N-terminus of GTBP. Genomics 31: 395-397.
2281. Nicolaides NC, Papadopoulos N, Liu B, Wei YF, Carter KC, Ruben SM et al. (1994). Mutations of two PMS homologues in hereditary nonpolyposis colon cancer. Nature 371: 75-80.
2282. Nielsen GP, Isaksson HJ, Finnbogason H, Gunnlaugsson GH (1991). Adenocarcinoma of the vermiform appendix. A population study. APMIS 99: 653-656.
2283. Nielsen M, de Miranda NF, Van Puijenbroek M, Jordanova ES, Middeldorp A, van Wezel T et al. (2009). Colorectal carcinomas in MUTYH-associated polyposis display histopathological similarities to microsatellite unstable carcinomas. BMC Cancer 9: 184-
2284. Nielsen M, Franken PF, Reinards TH, Weiss MM, Wagner A, van der Klift H et al. (2005). Multiplicity in polyp count and extracolonic manifestations in 40 Dutch patients with MYH associated polyposis coli (MAP). J Med Genet 42: e54
2285. Nielsen M, Joerink-van de Beld MC, Jones N, Vogt S, Tops CM, Vasen HF et al. (2009). Analysis of MUTYH genotypes and colorectal phenotypes in patients With MUTYH-associated polyposis. Gastroenterology 136: 471-476.
2286. Nielsen M, Poley JW, Verhoef S, Van Puijenbroek M, Weiss MM, Burger GT et al. (2006). Duodenal carcinoma in MUTYH-associated polyposis. J Clin Pathol 59: 1212-1215.
2287. Nielsen OV, Jensen SL (1981). Basal cell carcinoma of the anus-a clinical study of 34 cases. Br J Surg 68: 856-857.
2288. Nielsen SN, Wold LE (1986). Adenocarcinoma of jejunum in association with nontropical sprue. Arch Pathol Lab Med 110: 822-824.
2289. Nies C, Zielke A, Hasse C, Ruschoff J, Rothmund M (1992). Carcinoid tumors of Meckel's diverticula. Report of two cases and review of the literature. Dis Colon Rectum 35: 589-596.
2290. Nieuwenhuis MH, Vasen HF (2007). Correlations between mutation site in APC and phenotype of familial adenomatous polyposis (FAP): a review of the literature. Crit Rev Oncol Hematol 61: 153-161.
2291. Nilsson B, Bumming P, Meis-Kindblom JM, Oden A, Dortok A, Gustavsson B et al. (2005). Gastrointestinal stromal tumors: the incidence, prevalence, clinical course, and prognostication in the preimatinib mesylate era—a population-based study in western Sweden. Cancer 103: 821-829.
2292. Nilsson PJ, Lenander C, Rubio C, Auer G, Ljungqvist O, Glimelius B (2006). Prognostic significance of Cyclin A in epidermoid anal cancer. Oncol Rep 16: 443-449.
2293. Nilsson PJ, Rubio C, Lenander C, Auer G, Glimelius B (2005). Tumour budding detected by laminin-5 {gamma}2-chain immunohistochemistry is of prognostic value in epidermoid anal cancer. Ann Oncol 16: 893-898.
2294. Nishigami T, Yamada M, Nakasho K, Yamamura M, Satomi M, Uematsu K et al. (1996). Carcinoid tumor of the gall bladder. Intern Med 35: 953-956.
2295. Nishihara K, Nagai E, Izumi Y, Yamaguchi K, Tsuneyoshi M (1994). Adenosquamous carcinoma of the gallbladder: a clinicopathological, immunohistochemical and flow-cytometric study of twenty cases. Jpn J Cancer Res 85: 389-399.
2296. Nishihara K, Nagai E, Tsuneyoshi M, Nagashima M (1994). Small-cell carcinoma combined with adenocarcinoma of the gallbladder. A case report with immunohistochemical and flow cytometric studies. Arch Pathol Lab Med 118: 177-181.
2297. Nishihara K, Nagoshi M, Tsuneyoshi M, Yamaguchi K, Hayashi I (1993). Papillary cystic tumors of the pancreas. Assessment of their malignant potential. Cancer 71: 82-92.
2298. Nishihara K, Tsuneyoshi M (1993). Undifferentiated spindle cell carcinoma of the gallbladder: a clinicopathologic, immunohistochemical, and flow cytometric study of 11 cases. Hum Pathol 24: 1298-1305.
2299. Nishihara K, Tsuneyoshi M, Shimura H, Yasunami Y (1994). Three synchronous carcinomas of the papilla of Vater, common bile duct and pancreas. Pathol Int 44: 325-332.
2300. Nishihara K, Yamaguchi K, Hashimoto H, Enjoji M (1991). Tubular adenoma of the gallbladder with squamoid spindle cell metaplasia. Report of three cases with immunohistochemical study. Acta Pathol Jpn 41: 41-45.
2301. Nishikura K, Watanabe H (1997). Gastric microcarcinoma. Its histopathological characteristics. In: Progress in Gastric Cancer Research. Siewert JR, Roder JD, eds. Monduzzi Editore: Bologna, Italy, pp. 251-256.
2302. Nishimata H, Setoyama S, Nishimata Y (1992). Natural history of gastric cancer in cardia. Stom Intest 27: 25-38.
2303. Nishimata S, Kato K, Tanaka M, Ijiri R, Toyoda Y, Kigasawa H et al. (2005). Expression pattern of keratin subclasses in pancreatoblastoma with special emphasis on squamoid corpuscles. Pathol Int 55: 297-302.
2304. Nishio J, Iwasaki H, Sakashita N, Haraoka S, Isayama T, Naito M et al. (2003). Undifferentiated (embryonal) sarcoma of the liver in middle-aged adults: smooth muscle differentiation determined by immunohistochemistry and electron microscopy. Hum Pathol 34: 246-252.
2305. Nishisho I, Nakamura Y, Miyoshi Y, Miki Y, Ando H, Horii A et al. (1991). Mutations of chromosome 5q21 genes in FAP and colorectal cancer patients. Science 253: 665-669.
2306. Nishiwaki T, Daigo Y, Kawasoe T, Nakamura Y (2000). Isolation and mutational analysis of a novel human cDNA, DEC1 (deleted in esophageal cancer 1), derived from the tumor suppressor locus in 9q32. Genes Chromosomes Cancer 27: 169-176.
2307. Nishizuka S, Tamura G, Terashima M, Satodate R (1998). Loss of heterozygosity during the development and progression of differentiated adenocarcinoma of the stomach. J Pathol 185: 38-43.
2308. Nitecki SS, Wolff BG, Schlinkert R, Sarr MG (1994). The natural history of surgically treated primary adenocarcinoma of the appendix. Ann Surg 219: 51-57.
2309. Noda Y, Watanabe H, Iida M, Narisawa R, Kurosaki I, Iwafuchi M et al. (1992). Histologic follow-up of ampullary adenomas in patients with familial adenomatosis coli. Cancer 70: 1847-1856.
2310. Noel JC, Hermans P, Andre J, Fayt I, Simonart T, Verhest A et al. (1996). Herpesvirus-like DNA sequences and Kaposi's sarcoma: relationship with epidemiology, clinical spectrum, and histologic features. Cancer 77: 2132-2136.
2311. Nogueira AM, Machado JC, Carneiro F, Reis CA, Gott P, Sobrinho-Simoes M (1999). Patterns of expression of trefoil peptides and mucins in gastric polyps with and without malignant transformation. J Pathol 187: 541-548.
2312. Nogueira C, Figueiredo C, Carneiro F, Gomes AT, Barreira R, Figueira P et al. (2001). *Helicobacter pylori* genotypes may determine gastric histopathology. Am J Pathol 158: 647-654.
2313. Nojima T, Kojima T, Kato H, Sato T, Koito K, Nagashima K (1992). Alpha-fetoprotein-producing acinar cell carcinoma of the pancreas. Hum Pathol 23: 828-830.
2314. Nojima T, Nakamura F, Ishikura M, Inoue K, Nagashima K, Kato H (1993). Pleomorphic carcinoma of the pancreas with osteoclast-like giant cells. Int J Pancreatol 14: 275-281.
2315. Nokubi M, Kawanowa K, Kawata H, Hanatsuka K, Hosoya Y (2004). Extremely well-differentiated adenocarcinoma of the gastric cardia: a unique case with columnar cells and laminated stones. Pathol Int 54: 854-860.
2316. Nomura A, Stemmermann GN, Chyou PH, Kato I, Perez-Perez GI, Blaser MJ (1991). *Helicobacter pylori* infection and gastric carcinoma among Japanese Americans in Hawaii. N Engl J Med 325: 1132-1136.
2317. Nonaka D, Kusamura S, Baratti D, Casali P, Younan R, Deraco M (2006). CDX-2 expression in pseudomyxoma peritonei: a clinicopathological study of 42 cases. Histopathology 49: 381-387.
2318. Nonomura A, Kono N, Mizukami Y, Nakanuma Y, Matsubara F (1992). Duct-acinar-islet cell tumor of the pancreas. Ultrastruct Pathol 16: 317-329.
2319. Nordback IH, Hruban RH, Cameron JL (1992). Second primary lesions in the biliary tree after successful resection of ampullary carcinoma. Surgery 112: 111-115.
2320. Norder H, Courouce AM, Coursaget P, Echevarria JM, Lee SD, Mushahwar IK et al. (2004). Genetic diversity of hepatitis B virus strains derived worldwide: genotypes, subgenotypes, and HBsAg subtypes. Intervirology 47: 289-309.
2321. Normanno N, Tejpar S, Morgillo F, De Luca A, Van Cutsem E, Ciardiello F (2009). Implications for KRAS status and EGFR-targeted therapies in metastatic CRC. Nat Rev Clin Oncol 6: 519-527.
2322. Norton JA, Ham CM, Van Dam J, Jeffrey RB, Longacre TA, Huntsman DG et al. (2007). CDH1 truncating mutations in the E-cadherin gene: an indication for total gastrectomy to treat hereditary diffuse gastric cancer. Ann Surg 245: 873-879.
2323. Norton JA, Melcher ML, Gibril F, Jensen RT (2004). Gastric carcinoid tumors in multiple endocrine neoplasia-1 patients with Zollinger-Ellison syndrome can be symptomatic, demonstrate aggressive growth, and require surgical treatment. Surgery 136: 1267-1274.
2324. Notohara K, Hamazaki S, Tsukayama C, Nakamoto S, Kawabata K, Mizobuchi K et al. (2000). Solid-pseudopapillary tumor of the pancreas: immunohistochemical localization of neuroendocrine markers and CD10. Am J Surg Pathol 24: 1361-1371.
2325. Nowak MA, Guerriere-Kovach P, Pathan A, Campbell TE, Deppisch LM (1998). Perianal Paget's disease: distinguishing primary and sec-

ondary lesions using immunohistochemical studies including gross cystic disease fluid protein-15 and cytokeratin 20 expression. Arch Pathol Lab Med 122: 1077-1081.
2326. Nucci MR, Robinson CR, Longo P, Campbell P, Hamilton SR (1997). Phenotypic and genotypic characteristics of aberrant crypt foci in human colorectal mucosa. Hum Pathol 28: 1396-1407.
2327. Nudo CG, Yoshida EM, Bain VG, Marleau D, Wong P, Marotta PJ et al. (2008). Liver transplantation for hepatic epithelioid hemangioendothelioma: the Canadian multicentre experience. Can J Gastroenterol 22: 821-824.
2328. Nugent KP, Spigelman AD, Talbot IC, Phillips RK (1994). Gallbladder dysplasia in patients with familial adenomatous polyposis. Br J Surg 81: 291-292.
2329. Nystrom-Lahti M, Wu Y, Moisio AL, Hofstra RM, Osinga J, Mecklin JP et al. (1996). DNA mismatch repair gene mutations in 55 kindreds with verified or putative hereditary nonpolyposis colorectal cancer. Hum Mol Genet 5: 763-769.
2330. O'Briain DS, Kennedy MJ, Daly PA, O'Brien AA, Tanner WA, Rogers P et al. (1989). Multiple lymphomatous polyposis of the gastrointestinal tract. A clinicopathologically distinctive form of non-Hodgkin's lymphoma of B-cell centrocytic type. Am J Surg Pathol 13: 691-699.
2331. O'Brien CA, Pollett A, Gallinger S, Dick JE (2007). A human colon cancer cell capable of initiating tumour growth in immunodeficient mice. Nature 445: 106-110.
2332. O'Brien MJ (2007). Hyperplastic and serrated polyps of the colorectum. Gastroenterol Clin North Am 36: 947-968.
2333. O'Brien MJ, Yang S, Clebanoff JL, Mulcahy E, Farraye FA, Amorosino M et al. (2004). Hyperplastic (serrated) polyps of the colorectum: relationship of CpG island methylator phenotype and K-ras mutation to location and histologic subtype. Am J Surg Pathol 28: 423-434.
2334. O'Byrne KJ, Goggins MG, McDonald GS, Daly PA, Kelleher DP, Weir DG (1994). A metastatic neuroendocrine anaplastic small cell tumor in a patient with multiple endocrine neoplasia type 1 syndrome. Assessment of disease status and response to doxorubicin, cyclophosphamide, etoposide chemotherapy through scintigraphic imaging with 111In-pentetreotide. Cancer 74: 2374-2378.
2335. O'Connell FP, Wang HH, Odze RD (2005). Utility of immunohistochemistry in distinguishing primary adenocarcinomas from metastatic breast carcinomas in the gastrointestinal tract. Arch Pathol Lab Med 129: 338-347.
2336. O'Connell JB, Maggard MA, Manunga J, Jr., Tomlinson JS, Reber HA, Ko CY et al. (2008). Survival after resection of ampullary carcinoma: a national population-based study. Ann Surg Oncol 15: 1820-1827.
2337. O'Connell JT, Tomlinson JS, Roberts AA, McGonigle KF, Barsky SH (2002). Pseudomyxoma peritonei is a disease of MUC2-expressing goblet cells. Am J Pathol 161: 551-564.
2338. O'Connor TP, Wade TP, Sunwoo YC, Reimers HJ, Palmer DC, Silverberg AB et al. (1992). Small cell undifferentiated carcinoma of the pancreas. Report of a patient with tumor marker studies. Cancer 70: 1514-1519.
2339. O'Kane AM, O'Donnell ME, Shah R, Carey DP, Lee J (2008). Small cell carcinoma of the appendix. World J Surg Oncol 6: 4-
2340. O'Shea AM, Cleary SP, Croitoru MA, Kim H, Berk T, Monga N et al. (2008). Pathological features of colorectal carcinomas in MYH-associated polyposis. Histopathology 53: 184-194.
2341. Oates JA, Sjoerdsma A (1962). A unique syndrome associated with secretion of 5-hydroxytryptophan by metastatic gastric carcinoids. Am J Med 32: 333-342.
2342. Oberg A, Stenling R, Tavelin B, Lindmark G (1998). Are lymph node micrometastases of any clinical significance in Dukes Stages A and B colorectal cancer? Dis Colon Rectum 41: 1244-1249.
2343. Oberg K, Astrup L, Eriksson B, Falkmer SE, Falkmer UG, Gustafsen J et al. (2004). Guidelines for the management of gastroenteropancreatic neuroendocrine tumours (including bronchopulmonary and thymic neoplasms). Part I-general overview. Acta Oncol 43: 617-625.
2344. Oberg K, Astrup L, Eriksson B, Falkmer SE, Falkmer UG, Gustafsen J et al. (2004). Guidelines for the management of gastroenteropancreatic neuroendocrine tumours (including bronchopulmonary and thymic neoplasms). Part II-specific NE tumour types. Acta Oncol 43: 626-636.
2345. Oberg K, Jelic S (2009). Neuroendocrine gastroenteropancreatic tumors: ESMO clinical recommendation for diagnosis, treatment and follow-up. Ann Oncol 20 Suppl 4: 150-153.
2346. Oda, Kondo H, Yamao T, Saito D, Ono H, Gotoda T et al. (2001). Metastatic tumors to the stomach: analysis of 54 patients diagnosed at endoscopy and 347 autopsy cases. Endoscopy 33: 507-510.
2347. Oda H, Imai Y, Nakatsuru Y, Hata J, Ishikawa T (1996). Somatic mutations of the *APC* gene in sporadic hepatoblastomas. Cancer Res 56: 3320-3323.
2348. Oda N, Tsujino T, Tsuda T, Yoshida K, Nakayama H, Yasui W et al. (1990). DNA ploidy pattern and amplification of *ERBB* and *ERBB2* genes in human gastric carcinomas. Virchows Arch B Cell Pathol Incl Mol Pathol 58: 273-277.
2349. Oda T, Tsuda H, Scarpa A, Sakamoto M, Hirohashi S (1992). Mutation pattern of the *p53* gene as a diagnostic marker for multiple hepatocellular carcinoma. Cancer Res 52: 3674-3678.
2350. Odenbreit S, Swoboda K, Barwig I, Ruhl S, Boren T, Koletzko S et al. (2009). Outer membrane protein expression profile in *Helicobacter pylori* clinical isolates. Infect Immun 77: 3782-3790
2351. Odze R, Gallinger S, So K, Antonioli D (1994). Duodenal adenomas in familial adenomatous polyposis: relation of cell differentiation and mucin histochemical features to growth pattern. Mod Pathol 7: 376-384.
2351A. Odze RD, Maley C (2009). Neoplasia without dysplasia: Lessons from Barrett oesophagus and other tubal gut neoplasms. Arch Pathol Lab Med 134:896-906.
2352. Odze RD (2005). Pathology of the gastroesophageal junction. Semin Diagn Pathol 22: 256-265.
2353. Odze RD (2006). Diagnosis and grading of dysplasia in Barrett's oesophagus. J Clin Pathol 59: 1029-1038.
2354. Odze RD (2009). Barrett esophagus: histology and pathology for the clinician. Nat Rev Gastroenterol Hepatol 6: 478-490.
2355. Odze RD, Medline P, Cohen Z (1994). Adenocarcinoma arising in an appendix involved with chronic ulcerative colitis. Am J Gastroenterol 89: 1905-1907.
2356. Oertel JE, Mendelsohn G, Compagno J (1982). Solid and papillary epithelial neoplasms of the pancreas. In: Pancreatic Tumours in Children. Humphrey GB, Grindey GB, Dehner LP, Acton RT, Pysher TJ, eds. Martinus Nijhoff: Den Haag, pp. 161-171.
2357. Oettle H, Post S, Neuhaus P, Gellert K, Langrehr J, Ridwelski K et al. (2007). Adjuvant chemotherapy with gemcitabine vs observation in patients undergoing curative-intent resection of pancreatic cancer: a randomized controlled trial. JAMA 297: 267-277.
2358. Oettling G, Franz HB (1998). Mapping of androgen, estrogen and progesterone receptors in the anal continence organ. Eur J Obstet Gynecol Reprod Biol 77: 211-216.
2359. Offerhaus GJ, Giardiello FM, Krush AJ, Booker SV, Tersmette AC, Kelley NC et al. (1992). The risk of upper gastrointestinal cancer in familial adenomatous polyposis. Gastroenterology 102: 1980-1982.
2360. Ogawa T, Yoshida T, Tsuruta T, Tokuyama W, Adachi S, Kikuchi M et al. (2009). Tumor budding is predictive of lymphatic involvement and lymph node metastases in submucosal invasive colorectal adenocarcinomas and in non-polypoid compared with polypoid growths. Scand J Gastroenterol 44: 605-614.
2361. Ogino S, Nosho K, Kirkner GJ, Kawasaki T, Meyerhardt JA, Loda M et al. (2009). CpG island methylator phenotype, microsatellite instability, BRAF mutation and clinical outcome in colon cancer. Gut 58: 90-96.
2362. Ogino S, Nosho K, Kirkner GJ, Shima K, Irahara N, Kure S et al. (2009). PIK3CA mutation is associated with poor prognosis among patients with curatively resected colon cancer. J Clin Oncol 27: 1477-1484.
2363. Ogiwara H, Sugimoto M, Ohno T, Vilaichone RK, Mahachai V, Graham DY et al. (2009). Role of deletion located between the intermediate and middle regions of the *Helicobacter pylori vacA* gene in cases of gastroduodenal diseases. J Clin Microbiol 47: 3493-3500.
2364. Oguzkurt L, Karabulut N, Cakmakci E, Besim A (1997). Primary non-Hodgkin's lymphoma of the esophagus. Abdom Imaging 22: 8-10.
2365. Oh C, Jemerin EE (1965). Benign adenomatous polyps of the papilla of Vater. Surgery 57: 495-503.
2366. Oh HC, Kim MH, Hwang CY, Lee TY, Lee SS, Seo DW et al. (2008). Cystic lesions of the pancreas: challenging issues in clinical practice. Am J Gastroenterol 103: 229-239.
2367. Ohgaki H, Hernandez-Boussard T, Kleihues P, Hainaut P (1999). p53 germline mutations and the molecular basis of the Li-Fraumeni syndrome. In: Molecular biology in cancer medicine. Kurzrock R, Talpaz M, eds. Martin Dunitz Ltd: London, pp. 477-492.
2368. Ohike N, Jurgensen A, Pipeleers-Marichal M, Klöppel G (2003). Mixed ductal-endocrine carcinomas of the pancreas and ductal adenocarcinomas with scattered endocrine cells: characterization of the endocrine cells. Virchows Arch 442: 258-265.
2369. Ohike N, Kosmahl M, Klöppel G (2004). Mixed acinar-endocrine carcinoma of the pancreas. A clinicopathological study and comparison with acinar-cell carcinoma. Virchows Arch 445: 231-235.
2370. Ohike N, Yamochi T, Shiokawa A, Yoshida T, Yamazaki T, Date Y et al. (2008). A peculiar variant of pancreatoblastoma in an adult. Pancreas 36: 320-322.
2371. Ohmori K, Kinoshita H, Shiraha Y, Satake K (1976). Pancreatic duct obstruction by a benign polypoid adenoma of the ampulla of Vater. Am J Surg 132: 662-663.
2372. Ohmori T, Furuya K, Okada K, Tabei R, Tao S (1993). Adenoendocrine cell carcinoma of the gallbladder: a histochemical and immunohistochemical study. Acta Pathol Jpn 43: 268-274.
2373. Ohmoto K, Honda T, Hirokawa M, Mitsui Y, Iguchi Y, Kuboki M et al. (2002). Spontaneous regression of focal nodular hyperplasia of the liver. J Gastroenterol 37: 849-853.
2374. Ohnishi Y, Akashi T, Kuniyoshi M, Fukutomi M, Yokota M, Iguchi H et al. (1999). [A case of adult T cell leukemia (lymphoma type) involving the pancreas]. Nippon Shokakibyo Gakkai Zasshi 96: 64-69.
2375. Ohshima K, Kimura H, Yoshino T, Kim CW, Ko YH, Lee SS et al. (2008). Proposed categorization of pathological states of EBV-associated T/natural killer-cell lymphoproliferative disorder (LPD) in children and young adults: overlap with chronic active EBV infection and infantile fulminant EBV T-LPD. Pathol Int 58: 209-217.
2376. Ohshio G, Imamura T, Okada N, Wang ZH, Yamaki K, Kyogoku T et al. (1996). Immunohistochemical study of metallothionein in pancreatic carcinomas. J Cancer Res Clin Oncol 122: 351-355.
2377. Ohta H, Noguchi Y, Takagi K, Nishi M, Kajitani T, Kato Y (1987). Early gastric carcinoma with special reference to macroscopic classification. Cancer 60: 1099-1106.
2378. Ohtani T, Shirai Y, Tsukada K, Hatakeyama K, Muto T (1994). The association between extrahepatic biliary carcinoma and the junction of the cystic duct and the biliary tree. Eur J Surg 160: 37-40.
2379. Ohuchida K, Mizumoto K, Miyasaka Y, Yu J, Cui L, Yamaguchi H et al. (2007). Overexpression of S100A2 in pancreatic cancer correlates with progression and poor prognosis. J Pathol 213: 275-282.
2380. Oien KA (2009). Pathologic evaluation of unknown primary cancer. Semin Oncol 36: 8-37.
2381. Oikawa T, Ojima H, Yamasaki S, Takayama T, Hirohashi S, Sakamoto M (2005). Multistep and multicentric development of hepatocellular carcinoma: histological analysis of 980 resected nodules. J Hepatol 42: 225-229.
2382. Oka T, Ayabe H, Kawahara K, Tagawa Y, Hara S, Tsuji H et al. (1993). Esophagectomy for metastatic carcinoma of the esophagus from lung cancer. Cancer 71: 2958-2961.
2383. Okabayashi T, Hanazaki K (2008). Surgical outcome of adenosquamous carcinoma of the pancreas. World J Gastroenterol 14: 6765-6770.
2384. Okabayashi T, Kobayashi M, Nishimori I, Sugimoto T, Namikawa T, Onishi S et al. (2008). Clinicopathological features and medical management of early gastric cancer. Am J Surg 195: 229-232.
2385. Okamoto H, Miura K, Ogawara T, Fujii H, Matsumoto Y (2003). Small-cell carcinoma manifesting systemic lymphadenopathy combined with adenocarcinoma in the gallbladder: aggressiveness and sensitivity to chemotherapy. J Gastroenterol 38: 801-805.
2386. Okamura D, Ohtsuka M, Kimura F, Shimizu H, Yoshidome H, Kato A et al. (2008). Ezrin expression is associated with hepatocellular carcinoma possibly derived from progenitor cells and early recurrence after surgical resection. Mod Pathol 21: 847-855.
2387. Okon K, Zazula M, Rudzki Z, Papla B, Osuch C, Stachura J (2004). CDX-2 expression is reduced in colorectal carcinomas with solid growth pattern and proximal location, but is largely independent of MSI status. Pol J Pathol 55: 9-14.
2388. Oku T, Ono K, Nagamachi Y, Misu K, Senmaru N, Fujita M et al. (2008). [Pedunculated carcinoid tumor of the gallbladder—analysis of the relationship between location and morphology in carcinoid tumor of the gallbladder]. Nippon Shokakibyo Gakkai Zasshi 105: 397-403.
2389. Okuda K (1997). Hepatitis C virus and hepatocellular carcinoma. In: Liver Cancer. Okuda K, Tabor E, eds. Churchill Livingstone: New York, pp. 39-50.
2390. Okuda K, Nakanuma Y, Miyazaki M (2002). Cholangiocarcinoma: recent progress. Part 1: epidemiology and etiology. J Gastroenterol Hepatol 17: 1049-1055.
2391. Oliveira C, de Bruin J, Nabais S, Ligtenberg M, Moutinho C, Nagengast FM et al. (2004). Intragenic deletion of *CDH1* as the inactivating mechanism of the wild-type allele in an HDGC tumour. Oncogene 23: 2236-2240.

2392. Oliveira C, Ferreira P, Nabais S, Campos L, Ferreira A, Cirnes L et al. (2004). E-Cadherin (*CDH1*) and *p53* rather than *SMAD4* and *Caspase-10* germline mutations contribute to genetic predisposition in Portuguese gastric cancer patients. Eur J Cancer 40: 1897-1903.
2393. Oliveira C, Pinto M, Duval A, Brennetot C, Domingo E, Espin E et al. (2003). *BRAF* mutations characterize colon but not gastric cancer with mismatch repair deficiency. Oncogene 22: 9192-9196.
2394. Oliveira C, Senz J, Kaurah P, Pinheiro H, Sanges R, Haegert A et al. (2009). Germline *CDH1* deletions in hereditary diffuse gastric cancer families. Hum Mol Genet 18: 1545-1555.
2395. Oliveira C, Seruca R, Carneiro F (2006). Genetics, pathology, and clinics of familial gastric cancer. Int J Surg Pathol 14: 21-33.
2396. Oliveira C, Seruca R, Carneiro F (2009). Hereditary gastric cancer. Best Pract Res Clin Gastroenterol 23: 147-157.
2397. Oliveira C, Sousa S, Pinheiro H, Karam R, Bordeira-Carrico R, Senz J et al. (2009). Quantification of epigenetic and genetic second hits in *CDH1* during hereditary diffuse gastric cancer syndrome progression. Gastroenterology 136: 2137-2148.
2398. Ollila S, Dermadi BD, Jiricny J, Nystrom M (2008). Mechanisms of pathogenicity in human *MSH2* missense mutants. Hum Mutat 29: 1355-1363.
2399. Olschwang S, Serova-Sinilnikova OM, Lenoir GM, Thomas G (1998). *PTEN* germ-line mutations in juvenile polyposis coli. Nat Genet 18: 12-14.
2400. Olsen BS (1987). Giant appendicular neurofibroma. A light and immunohistochemical study. Histopathology 11: 851-855.
2401. Olsen BS, Holck S (1987). Neurogenous hyperplasia leading to appendiceal obliteration: an immunohistochemical study of 237 cases. Histopathology 11: 843-849.
2402. Ono A, Tanoue S, Yamada Y, Takaji Y, Okada F, Matsumoto S et al. (2009). Primary malignant lymphoma of the gallbladder: a case report and literature review. Br J Radiol 82: e15-e19.
2403. Ono J, Sakamoto H, Sakoda K, Yagi Y, Hagio S, Sato E et al. (1984). Acinar cell carcinoma of the pancreas with elevated serum alpha-fetoprotein. Int Surg 69: 361-364.
2404. Ono S, Fujishiro M, Niimi K, Goto O, Kodashima S, Yamamichi N et al. (2009). Long-term outcomes of endoscopic submucosal dissection for superficial esophageal squamous cell neoplasms. Gastrointest Endosc 70: 860-866.
2405. Ooi A, Nakanishi I, Itoh T, Ueda H, Mai M (1991). Predominant Paneth cell differentiation in an intestinal type gastric cancer. Pathol Res Pract 187: 220-225.
2406. Ordonez NG (2001). Pancreatic acinar cell carcinoma. Adv Anat Pathol 8: 144-159.
2407. Orlando CA, Bowman RL, Loose JH (1991). Multicentric papillary-cystic neoplasm of the pancreas. Arch Pathol Lab Med 115: 958-960.
2408. Orloff MS, Eng C (2008). Genetic and phenotypic heterogeneity in the *PTEN* hamartoma tumour syndrome. Oncogene 27: 5387-5397.
2409. Ormsby AH, Petras RE, Henricks WH, Rice TW, Rybicki LA, Richter JE et al. (2002). Observer variation in the diagnosis of superficial oesophageal adenocarcinoma. Gut 51: 671-676.
2410. Ortega AE, Klipfel N, Kelso R, Petrone P, Roman I, Diaz A et al. (2008). Changing concepts in the pathogenesis, evaluation, and management of solitary rectal ulcer syndrome. Am Surg 74: 967-972.
2411. Ortiz-Hidalgo C, de Leon Bojorge B, Albores-Saavedra J (2000). Stromal tumor of the gallbladder with phenotype of interstitial cells of Cajal: a previously unrecognized neoplasm. Am J Surg Pathol 24: 1420-1423.
2412. Osada T, Sakamoto M, Nagawa H, Yamamoto J, Matsuno Y, Iwamatsu A et al. (1999). Acquisition of glutamine synthetase expression in human hepatocarcinogenesis: relation to disease recurrence and possible regulation by ubiquitin-dependent proteolysis. Cancer 85: 819-831.
2413. Osborn NK, Keate RF, Trastek VF, Nguyen CC (2003). Verrucous carcinoma of the esophagus: clinicopathophysiologic features and treatment of a rare entity. Dig Dis Sci 48: 465-474.
2414. Othman M, Basturk O, Groisman G, Krasinskas A, Adsay NV (2007). Squamoid cyst of pancreatic ducts: A distinct type of cystic lesion in the pancreas. Am J Surg Pathol 31: 291-297.
2415. Ott G, Katzenberger T, Greiner A, Kalla J, Rosenwald A, Heinrich U et al. (1997). The t(11;18)(q21;q21) chromosome translocation is a frequent and specific aberration in low-grade but not high-grade malignant non-Hodgkin's lymphomas of the mucosa-associated lymphoid tissue (MALT-) type. Cancer Res 57: 3944-3948.
2416. Ott G, Kirchner T, Seidl S, Muller-Hermelink HK (1993). Primary gastric lymphoma is rarely associated with Epstein-Barr virus. Virchows Arch B Cell Pathol Incl Mol Pathol 64: 287-291.
2417. Ott K, Bader FG, Lordick F, Feith M, Bartels H, Siewert JR (2009). Surgical factors influence the outcome after Ivor-Lewis esophagectomy with intrathoracic anastomosis for adenocarcinoma of the esophagogastric junction: a consecutive series of 240 patients at an experienced center. Ann Surg Oncol 16: 1017-1025.
2418. Otter R, Bieger R, Kluin PM, Hermans J, Willemze R (1989). Primary gastrointestinal non-Hodgkin's lymphoma in a population-based registry. Br J Cancer 60: 745-750.
2419. Ou J, Niessen RC, Vonk J, Westers H, Hofstra RM, Sijmons RH (2008). A database to support the interpretation of human mismatch repair gene variants. Hum Mutat 29: 1337-1341.
2420. Overbeek LI, Ligtenberg MJ, Willems RW, Hermens RP, Blokx WA, Dubois SV et al. (2008). Interpretation of immunohistochemistry for mismatch repair proteins is only reliable in a specialized setting. Am J Surg Pathol 32: 1246-1251.
2421. Oyama T, Yamamoto K, Asano N, Oshiro A, Suzuki R, Kagami Y et al. (2007). Age-related EBV-associated B-cell lymphoproliferative disorders constitute a distinct clinicopathologic group: a study of 96 patients. Clin Cancer Res 13: 5124-5132.
2422. Ozaki H, Hiraoka T, Mizumoto R, Matsuno S, Matsumoto Y, Nakayama T et al. (1999). The prognostic significance of lymph node metastasis and intrapancreatic perineural invasion in pancreatic cancer after curative resection. Surg Today 29: 16-22.
2423. Ozaki S, Harada K, Sanzen T, Watanabe K, Tsui W, Nakanuma Y (1999). In situ nucleic acid detection of human telomerase in intrahepatic cholangiocarcinoma and its preneoplastic lesion. Hepatology 30: 914-919.
2424. Ozaki S, Ogasahara K, Kosaka M, Inoshita T, Wakatsuki S, Uehara H et al. (1998). Hepatosplenic gamma delta T-cell lymphoma associated with hepatitis B virus infection. J Med Invest 44: 215-217.
2425. Ozawa K, Kinoshita M, Kagata Y, Matsubara O (2003). A case of double carcinoid tumors of the gallbladder. Dig Dis Sci 48: 1760-1761.
2426. Ozcelik H, Schmocker B, Di NN, Shi XH, Langer B, Moore M et al. (1997). Germline *BRCA2* 6174delT mutations in Ashkenazi Jewish pancreatic cancer patients. Nat Genet 16: 17-18.
2427. Ozturk M (1999). Genetic aspects of hepatocellular carcinogenesis. Semin Liver Dis 19: 235-242.
2428. Paal E, Thompson LD, Frommelt RA, Przygodzki RM, Heffess CS (2001). A clinicopathologic and immunohistochemical study of 35 anaplastic carcinomas of the pancreas with a review of the literature. Ann Diagn Pathol 5: 129-140.
2429. Paal E, Thompson LD, Przygodzki RM, Bratthauer GL, Heffess CS (1999). A clinicopathologic and immunohistochemical study of 22 intraductal papillary mucinous neoplasms of the pancreas, with a review of the literature. Mod Pathol 12: 518-528.
2430. Pachera S, Nishio H, Takahashi Y, Yokoyama Y, Oda K, Ebata T et al. (2008). Undifferentiated embryonal sarcoma of the liver: case report and literature survey. J Hepatobiliary Pancreat Surg 15: 536-544.
2431. Padberg B, Schroder S, Capella C, Frilling A, Klöppel G, Heitz PU (1995). Multiple endocrine neoplasia type 1 (MEN 1) revisited. Virchows Arch 426: 541-548.
2432. Padberg GW, Schot JD, Vielvoye GJ, Bots GT, de Beer FC (1991). Lhermitte-Duclos disease and Cowden disease: a single phakomatosis. Ann Neurol 29: 517-523.
2433. Paggi S, Radaelli F, Amato A, Meucci G, Mandelli G, Imperiali G et al. (2009). The impact of narrow band imaging in screening colonoscopy: a randomized controlled trial. Clin Gastroenterol Hepatol 7: 1049-1054.
2434. Pai RK, Beck AH, Norton JA, Longacre TA (2009). Appendiceal Mucinous Neoplasms: Clinicopathologic Study of 116 Cases With Analysis of Factors Predicting Recurrence. Am J Surg Pathol 33: 1425-1439.
2435. Pai RK, Longacre TA (2005). Appendiceal mucinous tumors and pseudomyxoma peritonei: histologic features, diagnostic problems, and proposed classification. Adv Anat Pathol 12: 291-311.
2436. Pairojkul C, Shirai T, Hirohashi S, Thamavit W, Bhudhisawat W, Uttaravicien T et al. (1991). Multistage carcinogenesis of liver-fluke-associated cholangiocarcinoma in Thailand. Princess Takamatsu Symp 22: 77-86.
2437. Palefsky JM (1994). Anal human papillomavirus infection and anal cancer in HIV-positive individuals: an emerging problem. AIDS 8: 283-295.
2438. Palefsky JM, Holly EA, Ralston ML, Jay N, Berry JM, Darragh TM (1998). High incidence of anal high-grade squamous intra-epithelial lesions among HIV-positive and HIV-negative homosexual and bisexual men. AIDS 12: 495-503.
2439. Palli D, Galli M, Caporaso NE, Cipriani F, Decarli A, Saieva C et al. (1994). Family history and risk of stomach cancer in Italy. Cancer Epidemiol Biomarkers Prev 3: 15-18.
2440. Palli D, Masala G, del GG, Plebani M, Basso D, Berti D et al. (2007). CagA+ *Helicobacter pylori* infection and gastric cancer risk in the EPIC-EURGAST study. Int J Cancer 120: 859-867.
2441. Palombo F, Gallinari P, Iaccarino I, Lettieri T, Hughes M, D'Arrigo A et al. (1995). GTBP, a 160-kilodalton protein essential for mismatch-binding activity in human cells. Science 268: 1912-1914.
2442. Pande R, Sunga A, Levea C, Wilding GE, Bshara W, Reid M et al. (2008). Significance of signet-ring cells in patients with colorectal cancer. Dis Colon Rectum 51: 50-55.
2443. Paner GP, Thompson KS, Reyes CV (2000). Hepatoid carcinoma of the pancreas. Cancer 88: 1582-1589.
2444. Panizo-Santos A, Sola I, Lozano M, de AE, Pardo J (2000). Metastatic osteosarcoma presenting as a small-bowel polyp. A case report and review of the literature. Arch Pathol Lab Med 124: 1682-1684.
2445. Panzuto F, Nasoni S, Falconi M, Corleto VD, Capurso G, Cassetta S et al. (2005). Prognostic factors and survival in endocrine tumor patients: comparison between gastrointestinal and pancreatic localization. Endocr Relat Cancer 12: 1083-1092.
2446. Papadopoulos N, Nicolaides NC, Wei YF, Ruben SM, Carter KC, Rosen CA et al. (1994). Mutation of a mutL homolog in hereditary colon cancer. Science 263: 1625-1629.
2447. Papaemmanuil E, Carvajal-Carmona L, Sellick GS, Kemp Z, Webb E, Spain S et al. (2008). Deciphering the genetics of hereditary non-syndromic colorectal cancer. Eur J Hum Genet 16: 1477-1486.
2448. Papaxoinis G, Papageorgiou S, Rontogianni D, Kaloutsi V, Fountzilas G, Pavlidis N et al. (2006). Primary gastrointestinal non-Hodgkin's lymphoma: a clinicopathologic study of 128 cases in Greece. A Hellenic Cooperative Oncology Group study (HeCOG). Leuk Lymphoma 47: 2140-2146.
2449. Pape UF, Jann H, Muller-Nordhorn J, Bockelbrink A, Berndt U, Willich SN et al. (2008). Prognostic relevance of a novel TNM classification system for upper gastroenteropancreatic neuroendocrine tumors. Cancer 113: 256-265.
2450. Papotti M, Bongiovanni M, Volante M, Allia E, Landolfi S, Helboe L et al. (2002). Expression of somatostatin receptor types 1-5 in 81 cases of gastrointestinal and pancreatic endocrine tumors. A correlative immunohistochemical and reverse-transcriptase polymerase chain reaction analysis. Virchows Arch 440: 461-475.
2451. Papotti M, Cassoni P, Sapino A, Passarino G, Krueger JE, Albores-Saavedra J (2000). Large cell neuroendocrine carcinoma of the gallbladder: report of two cases. Am J Surg Pathol 24: 1424-1428.
2452. Papotti M, Cassoni P, Taraglio S, Bussolati G (1999). Oncocytic and oncocytoid tumors of the exocrine pancreas, liver, and gastrointestinal tract. Semin Diagn Pathol 16: 126-134.
2453. Papotti M, Cassoni P, Volante M, Deghenghi R, Muccioli G, Ghigo E (2001). Ghrelin-producing endocrine tumors of the stomach and intestine. J Clin Endocrinol Metab 86: 5052-5059.
2454. Papotti M, Galliano D, Monga G (1990). Signet-ring cell carcinoid of the gallbladder. Histopathology 17: 255-259.
2455. Papotti M, Sambataro D, Marchesa P, Negro F (1997). A combined hepatocellular/cholangiocellular carcinoma with sarcomatoid features. Liver 17: 47-52.
2456. Paradis V, Benzekri A, Dargere D, Bieche I, Laurendeau I, Vilgrain V et al. (2004). Telangiectatic focal nodular hyperplasia: a variant of hepatocellular adenoma. Gastroenterology 126: 1323-1329.
2457. Paradis V, Bieche I, Dargere D, Laurendeau I, Nectoux J, Degott C et al. (2003). A quantitative gene expression study suggests a role for angiopoietins in focal nodular hyperplasia. Gastroenterology 124: 651-659.
2458. Paradis V, Champault A, Ronot M, Deschamps L, Valla DC, Vidaud D et al. (2007). Telangiectatic adenoma: an entity associated with increased body mass index and inflammation. Hepatology 46: 140-146.
2459. Paradis V, Laurent A, Flejou JF, Vidaud M, Bedossa P (1997). Evidence for the polyclonal nature of focal nodular hyperplasia of the liver by the study of X-chromosome inactivation. Hepatology 26: 891-895.
2460. Paraf F, Flejou JF, Pignon JP, Fekete F,

Potet F (1995). Surgical pathology of adenocarcinoma arising in Barrett's esophagus. Analysis of 67 cases. Am J Surg Pathol 19: 183-191.

2461. Parc Y, Piquard A, Dozois RR, Parc R, Tiret E (2004). Long-term outcome of familial adenomatous polyposis patients after restorative coloproctectomy. Ann Surg 239: 378-382.

2462. Parente F, Cernuschi M, Orlando G, Rizzardini G, Lazzarin A, Bianchi PG (1991). Kaposi's sarcoma and AIDS: frequency of gastrointestinal involvement and its effect on survival. A prospective study in a heterogeneous population. Scand J Gastroenterol 26: 1007-1012.

2463. Parfitt JR, Bella AJ, Izawa JI, Wehrli BM (2006). Malignant neoplasm of perivascular epithelioid cells of the liver. Arch Pathol Lab Med 130: 1219-1222.

2464. Parfitt JR, Shepherd NA (2008). Polypoid mucosal prolapse complicating low rectal adenomas: beware the inflammatory cloacogenic polyp! Histopathology 53: 91-96.

2465. Parham DM, Kelly DR, Donnelly WH, Douglass EC (1991). Immunohistochemical and ultrastructural spectrum of hepatic sarcomas of childhood: evidence for a common histogenesis. Mod Pathol 4: 648-653.

2466. Parham DM, Weeks DA, Beckwith JB (1994). The clinicopathologic spectrum of putative extrarenal rhabdoid tumors. An analysis of 42 cases studied with immunohistochemistry or electron microscopy. Am J Surg Pathol 18: 1010-1029.

2467. Park do Y, Lauwers GY (2008). Gastric polyps: classification and management. Arch Pathol Lab Med 132: 633-640.

2468. Park do Y, Srivastava A, Kim GH, Mino-Kenudson M, Deshpande V, Zukerberg LR et al. (2008). Adenomatous and foveolar gastric dysplasia: distinct patterns of mucin expression and background intestinal metaplasia. Am J Surg Pathol 32: 524-533.

2469. Park DH, Kim HS, Kim WH, Kim TI, Kim YH, Park DI et al. (2008). Clinicopathologic characteristics and malignant potential of colorectal flat neoplasia compared with that of polypoid neoplasia. Dis Colon Rectum 51: 43-49.

2470. Park DI, Rhee PL, Kim JE, Hyun JG, Kim YH, Son HJ et al. (2001). Risk factors suggesting malignant transformation of gastric adenoma: univariate and multivariate analysis. Endoscopy 33: 501-506.

2471. Park DY, Srivastava A, Kim GH, Mino-Kenudson M, Deshpande V, Zukerberg LR et al. (2010). CDX2 expression in the intestinal-type gastric epithelial neoplasia: frequency and significance. Mod Pathol 23: 54-61.

2472. Park IJ, Choi GS, Lim KH, Kang BM, Jun SH (2008). Different patterns of lymphatic spread of sigmoid, rectosigmoid, and rectal cancers. Ann Surg Oncol 15: 3478-3483.

2473. Park S, Lee J, Ko YH, Han A, Jun HJ, Lee SC et al. (2007). The impact of Epstein-Barr virus status on clinical outcome in diffuse large B-cell lymphoma. Blood 110: 972-978.

2474. Park SJ, Lee KY, Kim SY (2008). Clinical Significance of Lymph Node Micrometastasis in Stage I and II Colon Cancer. Cancer Res Treat 40: 75-80.

2475. Park SY, Kim BH, Kim JH, Lee S, Kang GH (2007). Panels of immunohistochemical markers help determine primary sites of metastatic adenocarcinoma. Arch Pathol Lab Med 131: 1561-1567.

2476. Park WS, Pham T, Wang C, Pack S, Mueller E, Mueller J et al. (1998). Loss of heterozygosity and microsatellite instability in nonneoplastic mucosa from patients with chronic ulcerative colitis. Int J Mol Med 2: 221-224.

2477. Park YH, Kim WS, Kang HJ, Na II, Ryoo BY, Yang SH et al. (2006). Gastric Burkitt lymphoma is a distinct subtype that has superior outcomes to other types of Burkitt lymphoma/leukemia. Ann Hematol 85: 285-290.

2478. Park YN, Kojiro M, Di TL, Dhillon AP, Kondo F, Nakano M et al. (2007). Ductular reaction is helpful in defining early stromal invasion, small hepatocellular carcinomas, and dysplastic nodules. Cancer 109: 915-923.

2479. Park YN, Roncalli M (2006). Large liver cell dysplasia: a controversial entity. J Hepatol 45: 734-743.

2480. Park YN, Yang CP, Fernandez GJ, Cubukcu O, Thung SN, Theise ND (1998). Neoangiogenesis and sinusoidal "capillarization" in dysplastic nodules of the liver. Am J Surg Pathol 22: 656-662.

2481. Parker GM, Stollman NH, Rogers A (1996). Adenomatous polyposis coli presenting as adenocarcinoma of the appendix. Am J Gastroenterol 91: 801-802.

2482. Parker JA, Kalnins VI, Deck JH, Cohen Z, Berk T, Cullen JB et al. (1990). Histopathological features of congenital fundus lesions in familial adenomatous polyposis. Can J Ophthalmol 25: 159-163.

2483. Parkin DM (2006). The global health burden of infection-associated cancers in the year 2002. Int J Cancer 118: 3030-3044.

2484. Parkin DM, Bray F (2006). Chapter 2: The burden of HPV-related cancers. Vaccine 24 Suppl 3: 11-25.

2485. Parkin DM, Ferlay J, Hamdi-Chérif M, Sitas F, Thomas JO, Wabinga H et al. (eds) (2009). Cancer in Africa. IARC: Lyon, France.

2486. Parkin DM, Ohshima H, Srivatanakul P, Vatanasapt V (1993). Cholangiocarcinoma: epidemiology, mechanisms of carcinogenesis and prevention. Cancer Epidemiol Biomarkers Prev 2: 537-544.

2487. Parkin DM, Srivatanakul P, Khlat M, Chenvidhya D, Chotiwan P, Insiripong S et al. (1991). Liver cancer in Thailand. I. A case-control study of cholangiocarcinoma. Int J Cancer 48: 323-328.

2488. Parkin DM, Whelan SL, Ferlay J, Raymond L, and Young J (eds) (1997). Cancer Incidence in Five Continents. IARC: Lyon, France.

2489. Parkin DM, Whelan SL, Ferlay J, and Storm H (eds) (2005). Cancer Incidence in Five Continents. IARCPress: Lyon.

2490. Parks TG (1970). Mucus-secreting adenocarcinoma of anal gland origin. Br J Surg 57: 434-436.

2491. Parsonnet J, Friedman GD, Vandersteen DP, Chang Y, Vogelman JH, Orentreich N et al. (1991). Helicobacter pylori infection and the risk of gastric carcinoma. N Engl J Med 325: 1127-1131.

2492. Parsonnet J, Hansen S, Rodriguez L, Gelb AB, Warnke RA, Jellum E et al. (1994). Helicobacter pylori infection and gastric lymphoma. N Engl J Med 330: 1267-1271.

2493. Parsons DW, Wang TL, Samuels Y, Bardelli A, Cummins JM, DeLong L et al. (2005). Colorectal cancer: mutations in a signalling pathway. Nature 436: 792-

2494. Parwani AV, Geradts J, Caspers E, Offerhaus GJ, Yeo CJ, Cameron JL et al. (2003). Immunohistochemical and genetic analysis of non-small cell and small cell gallbladder carcinoma and their precursor lesions. Mod Pathol 16: 299-308.

2495. Pascal RR, Clearfield HR (1987). Mucoepidermoid (adenosquamous) carcinoma arising in Barrett's esophagus. Dig Dis Sci 32: 428-432.

2496. Pasquinelli G, Preda P, Martinelli GN, Galassi A, Santini D, Venza E (1995). Filamentous inclusions in nonneoplastic and neoplastic pancreas: an ultrastructural and immunogold labeling study. Ultrastruct Pathol 19: 495-500.

2497. Passik SD, Breitbart WS (1996). Depression in patients with pancreatic carcinoma. Diagnostic and treatment issues. Cancer 78: 615-626.

2498. Patel P, Hanson DL, Sullivan PS, Novak RM, Moorman AC, Tong TC et al. (2008). Incidence of types of cancer among HIV-infected persons compared with the general population in the United States, 1992-2003. Ann Intern Med 148: 728-736.

2499. Patel T (2001). Increasing incidence and mortality of primary intrahepatic cholangiocarcinoma in the United States. Hepatology 33: 1353-1357.

2500. Patil KK, Omojola MF, Khurana P, Iyengar JK (1992). Embryonal rhabdomyosarcoma within a choledochal cyst. Can Assoc Radiol J 43: 145-148.

2501. Pauli RM, Pauli ME, Hall JG (1980). Gardner syndrome and periampullary malignancy. Am J Med Genet 6: 205-219.

2502. Paulson TG, Galipeau PC, Xu L, Kissel HD, Li X, Blount PL et al. (2008). p16 mutation spectrum in the premalignant condition Barrett's esophagus. PLoS One 3: e3809-

2503. Pauser U, Kosmahl M, Kruslin B, Klimstra DS, Klöppel G (2005). Pancreatic solid and cystic hamartoma in adults: characterization of a new tumorous lesion. Am J Surg Pathol 29: 797-800.

2504. Pavlick AC, Gerdes H, Portlock CS (1997). Endoscopic ultrasound in the evaluation of gastric small lymphocytic mucosa-associated lymphoid tumors. J Clin Oncol 15: 1761-1766.

2505. Pawlik TM, Gleisner AL, Cameron JL, Winter JM, Assumpcao L, Lillemoe KD et al. (2007). Prognostic relevance of lymph node ratio following pancreaticoduodenectomy for pancreatic cancer. Surgery 141: 610-618.

2506. Payan MJ, Xerri L, Moncada K, Bastid C, Agostini S, Sastre B et al. (1990). Villous adenoma of the main pancreatic duct: a potentially malignant tumor? Am J Gastroenterol 85: 459-463.

2507. Pech O, May A, Gunter E, Gossner L, Ell C (2006). The impact of endoscopic ultrasound and computed tomography on the TNM staging of early cancer in Barrett's esophagus. Am J Gastroenterol 101: 2223-2229.

2508. Pech O, Rabenstein T, Manner H, Petrone MC, Pohl J, Vieth M et al. (2008). Confocal laser endomicroscopy for in vivo diagnosis of early squamous cell carcinoma in the esophagus. Clin Gastroenterol Hepatol 6: 89-94.

2509. Peers F, Bosch X, Kaldor J, Linsell A, Pluijmen M (1987). Aflatoxin exposure, hepatitis B virus infection and liver cancer in Swaziland. Int J Cancer 39: 545-553.

2510. Peiffert D, Bey P, Pernot M, Guillemin F, Luporsi E, Hoffstetter S et al. (1997). Conservative treatment by irradiation of epidermoid cancers of the anal canal: prognostic factors of tumoral control and complications. Int J Radiat Oncol Biol Phys 37: 313-324.

2511. Peiffert D, Bey P, Pernot M, Hoffstetter S, Marchal C, Beckendorf V et al. (1997). Conservative treatment by irradiation of epidermoid carcinomas of the anal margin. Int J Radiat Oncol Biol Phys 39: 57-66.

2512. Pelaez-Luna M, Chari ST, Smyrk TC, Takahashi N, Clain JE, Levy MJ et al. (2007). Do consensus indications for resection in branch duct intraductal papillary mucinous neoplasm predict malignancy? A study of 147 patients. Am J Gastroenterol 102: 1759-1764.

2513. Pellegata NS, Sessa F, Renault B, Bonato M, Leone BE, Solcia E et al. (1994). K-ras and p53 gene mutations in pancreatic cancer: ductal and nonductal tumors progress through different genetic lesions. Cancer Res 54: 1556-1560.

2514. Pelosi G, Bresaola E, Bogina G, Pasini F,

Rodella S, Castelli P et al. (1996). Endocrine tumors of the pancreas: Ki-67 immunoreactivity on paraffin sections is an independent predictor for malignancy: a comparative study with proliferating-cell nuclear antigen and progesterone receptor protein immunostaining, mitotic index, and other clinicopathologic variables. Hum Pathol 27: 1124-1134.

2515. Peltomaki P, Aaltonen LA, Sistonen P, Pylkkanen L, Mecklin JP, Jarvinen H et al. (1993). Genetic mapping of a locus predisposing to human colorectal cancer. Science 260: 810-812.

2516. Peltomaki P, Lothe RA, Aaltonen LA, Pylkkanen L, Nystrom-Lahti M, Seruca R et al. (1993). Microsatellite instability is associated with tumors that characterize the hereditary nonpolyposis colorectal carcinoma syndrome. Cancer Res 53: 5853-5855.

2517. Peltomaki P, Vasen H (2004). Mutations associated with HNPCC predisposition — Update of ICG-HNPCC/INSiGHT mutation database. Dis Markers 20: 269-276.

2518. Peng HQ, Darwin P, Papadimitriou JC, Drachenberg CB (2006). Liver metastases of pancreatic acinar cell carcinoma with marked nuclear atypia and pleomorphism diagnosed by EUS FNA cytology: a case report with emphasis on FNA cytological findings. Cytojournal 3: 29

2519. Penn I (1986). Cancers of the anogenital region in renal transplant recipients. Analysis of 65 cases. Cancer 58: 611-616.

2520. Pennazio M, Rondonotti E, de FR (2008). Capsule endoscopy in neoplastic diseases. World J Gastroenterol 14: 5245-5253.

2521. Pera M, Manterola C, Vidal O, Grande L (2005). Epidemiology of esophageal adenocarcinoma. J Surg Oncol 92: 151-159.

2522. Pereira-Lima JE, Lichtenfels E, Barbosa FS, Zettler CG, Kulczynski JM (2003). Prevalence study of metastases in cirrhotic livers. Hepatogastroenterology 50: 1490-1495.

2523. Perez-Montiel MD, Frankel WL, Suster S (2003). Neuroendocrine carcinomas of the pancreas with 'Rhabdoid' features. Am J Surg Pathol 27: 642-649.

2524. Perigny M, Hammel P, Corcos O, Larochelle O, Giraud S, Richard S et al. (2009). Pancreatic endocrine microadenomatosis in patients with von Hippel-Lindau disease: characterization by VHL/HIF pathway proteins expression. Am J Surg Pathol 33: 739-748.

2525. Perilongo G, Shafford E, Maibach R, Aronson D, Brugieres L, Brock P et al. (2004). Risk-adapted treatment for childhood hepatoblastoma. final report of the second study of the International Society of Paediatric Oncology— SIOPEL 2. Eur J Cancer 40: 411-421.

2526. Perini MV, Herman P, D'Albuquerque LA, Saad WA (2008). Solitary fibrous tumor of the liver: report of a rare case and review of the literature. Int J Surg 6: 396-399.

2527. Perkins JT, Blackstone MO, Riddell RH (1985). Adenomatous polyposis coli and multiple endocrine neoplasia type 2b. A pathogenetic relationship. Cancer 55: 375-381.

2528. Perren A, Anlauf M, Komminoth P (2007). Molecular profiles of gastroenteropancreatic endocrine tumors. Virchows Arch 451 Suppl 1: S39-S46.

2529. Perren A, Barghorn A, Schmid S, Saremaslani P, Roth J, Heitz PU et al. (2002). Absence of somatic SDHD mutations in sporadic neuroendocrine tumors and detection of two germline variants in paraganglioma patients. Oncogene 21: 7605-7608.

2530. Perren A, Komminoth P, Saremaslani P, Matter C, Feurer S, Lees JA et al. (2000). Mutation and expression analyses reveal differential subcellular compartmentalization of PTEN in endocrine pancreatic tumors compared to normal islet cells. Am J Pathol 157: 1097-1103.

2531. Perrone T, Sibley RK, Rosai J (1985). Duodenal gangliocytic paraganglioma. An immunohistochemical and ultrastructural study and a hypothesis concerning its origin. Am J Surg Pathol 9: 31-41.

2532. Persson PG, Bernell O, Leijonmarck CE, Farahmand BY, Hellers G, Ahlbom A (1996). Survival and cause-specific mortality in inflammatory bowel disease: a population-based cohort study. Gastroenterology 110: 1339-1345.

2533. Perzin KH, Bridge MF (1981). Adenomas of the small intestine: a clinicopathologic review of 51 cases and a study of their relationship to carcinoma. Cancer 48: 799-819.

2534. Perzin KH, Bridge MF (1982). Adenomatous and carcinomatous changes in hamartomatous polyps of the small intestine (Peutz-Jeghers syndrome): report of a case and review of the literature. Cancer 49: 971-983.

2535. Peters JH, Hoeft SF, Heimbucher J, Bremner RM, DeMeester TR, Bremner CG et al. (1994). Selection of patients for curative or palliative resection of esophageal cancer based on preoperative endoscopic ultrasonography. Arch Surg 129: 534-539.

2536. Peters U, Askling J, Gridley G, Ekbom A, Linet M (2003). Causes of death in patients with celiac disease in a population-based Swedish cohort. Arch Intern Med 163: 1566-1572.

2536A.Peters U, Chatterjee N, Yeager M, Chanock SJ, Schoen RE, McGlynn KA et al. (2004). Association of genetic variants in the calcium-sensing receptor with risk of colorectal adenoma. Cancer Epidemiol Biomarkers Prev 13: 2181-2186

2537. Petersen GM, Slack J, Nakamura Y (1991). Screening guidelines and premorbid diagnosis of familial adenomatous polyposis using linkage. Gastroenterology 100: 1658-1664.

2538. Peutz JL (1921). [A very remarkable case of familial polyposis of mucous membrane of intestinal tract and accompanied by peculiar pigmentations of skin and mucous membrane]. Netherlands Tijdschrift voor Geneeskunde 10: 134-146.

2539. Pham BN, Villanueva RP (1989). Ganglioneuromatous proliferation associated with juvenile polyposis coli. Arch Pathol Lab Med 113: 91-94.

2540. Phan TG, Hersch M, Zagami AS (1999). Guillain-Barre syndrome and adenocarcinoma of the gall bladder: a paraneoplastic phenomenon? Muscle Nerve 22: 141-142.

2541. Pharoah PD, Guilford P, Caldas C (2001). Incidence of gastric cancer and breast cancer in CDH1 (E-cadherin) mutation carriers from hereditary diffuse gastric cancer families. Gastroenterology 121: 1348-1353.

2542. Phelan CM, Lancaster JM, Tonin P, Gumbs C, Cochran C, Carter R et al. (1996). Mutation analysis of the BRCA2 gene in 49 site-specific breast cancer families. Nat Genet 13: 120-122.

2543. Phukan RK, Narain K, Zomawia E, Hazarika NC, Mahanta J (2006). Dietary habits and stomach cancer in Mizoram, India. J Gastroenterol 41: 418-424.

2544. Picciocchi A, Coppola R, Pallavicini F, Riccioni ME, Ciletti S, Marino-Cosentino LM et al. (1998). Major liver resection for non-Hodgkin's lymphoma in an HIV-positive patient: report of a case. Surg Today 28: 1257-1260.

2545. Picelli S, Vandrovcova J, Jones S, Djureinovic T, Skoglund J, Zhou XL et al. (2008). Genome-wide linkage scan for colorectal cancer susceptibility genes supports linkage to chromosome 3q. BMC Cancer 8: 87-

2546. Pickhardt PJ, Kim DH (2009). Colorectal cancer screening with CT colonography: key concepts regarding polyp prevalence, size, histology, morphology, and natural history. AJR Am J Roentgenol 193: 40-46.

2547. Pickhardt PJ, Levy AD, Rohrmann CA, Jr., Kende AI (2002). Primary neoplasms of the appendix manifesting as acute appendicitis: CT findings with pathologic comparison. Radiology 224: 775-781.

2548. Pickren JW, Tsukada Y, Lane WW (1982). Liver metastases: analysis of autopsy data. In: Liver Metastases. Weiss L, Gilbert HA, eds. Hall Medical Publishers: Boston, pp. 2-18.

2549. Picus D, Balfe DM, Koehler RE, Roper CL, Owen JW (1983). Computed tomography in the staging of esophageal carcinoma. Radiology 146: 433-438.

2550. Pignatelli M, Ansari TW, Gunter P, Liu D, Hirano S, Takeichi M et al. (1994). Loss of membranous E-cadherin expression in pancreatic cancer: correlation with lymph node metastasis, high grade, and advanced stage. J Pathol 174: 243-248.

2551. Pineda M, Castellsague E, Musulen E, Llort G, Frebourg T, Baert-Desurmont S et al. (2008). Non-Hodgkin lymphoma related to hereditary nonpolyposis colorectal cancer in a patient with a novel heterozygous complex deletion in the MSH2 gene. Genes Chromosomes Cancer 47: 326-332.

2552. Pinotti G, Zucca E, Roggero E, Pascarella A, Bertoni F, Savio A et al. (1997). Clinical features, treatment and outcome in a series of 93 patients with low-grade gastric MALT lymphoma. Leuk Lymphoma 26: 527-537.

2553. Pinto M, Wu Y, Mensink RG, Cirnes L, Seruca R, Hofstra RM (2008). Somatic mutations in mismatch repair genes in sporadic gastric carcinomas are not a cause but a consequence of the mutator phenotype. Cancer Genet Cytogenet 180: 110-114.

2554. Pipeleers-Marichal M, Donow C, Heitz PU, Klöppel G (1993). Pathologic aspects of gastrinomas in patients with Zollinger-Ellison syndrome with and without multiple endocrine neoplasia type I. World J Surg 17: 481-488.

2555. Pipeleers-Marichal M, Somers G, Willems G, Foulis A, Imrie C, Bishop AE et al. (1990). Gastrinomas in the duodenums of patients with multiple endocrine neoplasia type 1 and the Zollinger-Ellison syndrome. N Engl J Med 322: 723-727.

2555A.PitBman AM, Naranjo S, Webb E, Broderick P, Lips EH, van Wezel T et al. (2009). The colorectal cancer risk at 18q21 is caused by a novel variant altering SMAD7 expression. Genome Res 19: 987-993

2555A.Pittman AM, Webb E, Carvajal-Carmona L, Howarth K, Di Bernardo MC, Broderick P (2008). Refinement of the basis and impact of common 11q23.1 variation to the risk of developing colorectal cancer. Hum Mol Genet 17: 3720-3727

2556. Pitman MB, Deshpande V (2007). Endoscopic ultrasound-guided fine needle aspiration cytology of the pancreas: a morphological and multimodal approach to the diagnosis of solid and cystic mass lesions. Cytopathology 18: 331-347.

2557. Pitman MB, Faquin WC (2004). The fine-needle aspiration biopsy cytology of pancreatoblastoma. Diagn Cytopathol 31: 402-406.

2558. Pitman MB, Michaels PJ, Deshpande V, Brugge WR, Bounds BC (2008). Cytological and cyst fluid analysis of small (< or =3 cm) branch duct intraductal papillary mucinous neoplasms adds value to patient management decisions. Pancreatology 8: 277-284.

2559. Pitt HA, Dooley WC, Yeo CJ, Cameron JL (1995). Malignancies of the biliary tree. Curr Probl Surg 32: 1-90.

2560. Pizzi S, Azzoni C, Bassi D, Bottarelli L, Milione M, Bordi C (2003). Genetic alterations in poorly differentiated endocrine carcinomas of the gastrointestinal tract. Cancer 98: 1273-1282.

2561. Pizzi S, Azzoni C, Tamburini E, Bottarelli L, Campanini N, D'Adda T et al. (2008). Adenomatous polyposis coli alteration in digestive endocrine tumours: correlation with nuclear translocation of beta-catenin and chromosomal instability. Endocr Relat Cancer 15: 1013-1024.

2562. Pizzi S, D'Adda T, Azzoni C, Rindi G, Grigolato P, Pasquali C et al. (2002). Malignancy-associated allelic losses on the X-chromosome in foregut but not in midgut endocrine tumours. J Pathol 196: 401-407.

2563. Planck M, Ericson K, Piotrowska Z, Halvarsson B, Rambech E, Nilbert M (2003). Microsatellite instability and expression of MLH1 and MSH2 in carcinomas of the small intestine. Cancer 97: 1551-1557.

2564. Platt CC, Haboubi NY, Schofield PF (1991). Primary squamous cell carcinoma of the terminal ileum. J Clin Pathol 44: 253-254.

2565. Plentz RR, Park YN, Lechel A, Kim H, Nellessen F, Langkopf BH et al. (2007). Telomere shortening and inactivation of cell cycle checkpoints characterize human hepatocarcinogenesis. Hepatology 45: 968-976.

2566. Plockinger U, Couvelard A, Falconi M, Sundin A, Salazar R, Christ E et al. (2008). Consensus guidelines for the management of patients with digestive neuroendocrine tumours: well-differentiated tumour/carcinoma of the appendix and goblet cell carcinoma. Neuroendocrinology 87: 20-30.

2567. Plockinger U, Rindi G, Arnold R, Eriksson B, Krenning EP, de Herder WW et al. (2004). Guidelines for the diagnosis and treatment of neuroendocrine gastrointestinal tumours. A consensus statement on behalf of the European Neuroendocrine Tumour Society (ENETS). Neuroendocrinology 80: 394-424.

2568. Plummer M, van Doorn LJ, Franceschi S, Kleter B, Canzian F, Vivas J et al. (2007). Helicobacter pylori cytotoxin-associated genotype and gastric precancerous lesions. J Natl Cancer Inst 99: 1328-1334.

2569. Podsypanina K, Ellenson LH, Nemes A, Gu J, Tamura M, Yamada KM et al. (1999). Mutation of Pten/Mmac1 in mice causes neoplasia in multiple organ systems. Proc Natl Acad Sci U S A 96: 1563-1568.

2570. Polesel J, Zucchetto A, Montella M, Dal ML, Crispo A, La VC et al. (2009). The impact of obesity and diabetes mellitus on the risk of hepatocellular carcinoma. Ann Oncol 20: 353-357.

2571. Poley JW, Kluijt I, Gouma DJ, Harinck F, Wagner A, Aalfs C et al. (2009). The yield of first-time endoscopic ultrasonography in screening individuals at a high risk of developing pancreatic cancer. Am J Gastroenterol 104: 2175-2181.

2572. Polkowski M (2008). Endoscopic diagnosis and treatment of upper gastrointestinal tumors. Endoscopy 40: 862-867.

2573. Pollono DG, Tomarchio S, Berghoff R, Drut R, Urrutia A, Cedola J (1998). Rhabdomyosarcoma of extrahepatic biliary tree: initial treatment with chemotherapy and conservative surgery. Med Pediatr Oncol 30: 290-293.

2574. Polydorides AD, Shia J, Tang (2008). An immunohistochemical panel distinguishes colonization by pancreatic ductal adenocarcinoma from adenomas of ampullary and duodenal mucosa (Abstract). Mod Pathol 21: 132A-

2575. Ponchon T, Berger F, Chavaillon A, Bory R, Lambert R (1989). Contribution of endoscopy to diagnosis and treatment of tumors of the ampulla of Vater. Cancer 64: 161-167.

2575A.Ponti G, Ponz de Leon M, Maffei S, Pedroni M, Losi L, Di Gregorio C (2005). Attenuated familial adenomatous polyposis and Muir–Torre syndrome linked to compound biallelic constitutional MYH gene mutations. Clin Genet 68:442-447.

2575B. Poultsides GA, Reddy S, Cameron JL, Hruban RH, Pawlik TM, Ahuja N et al. (2010). Histopathologic basis for the favorable survival after resection of intraductal papillary mucinous neoplasm-associated invasive adenocarcinoma of the pancreas. Ann Surg 251: 470–476.

2576. Ponzoni M, Ferreri AJ, Pruneri G, Pozzi B, Dell'Oro S, Pigni A et al. (2003). Prognostic value of bcl-6, CD10 and CD38 immunoreactivity in stage I-II gastric lymphomas: identification of a subset of CD10+ large B-cell lymphomas with a favorable outcome. Int J Cancer 106: 288-291.

2577. Popat S, Houlston RS (2005). A systematic review and meta-analysis of the relationship between chromosome 18q genotype, DCC status and colorectal cancer prognosis. Eur J Cancer 41: 2060-2070.

2578. Popat S, Hubner R, Houlston RS (2005). Systematic review of microsatellite instability and colorectal cancer prognosis. J Clin Oncol 23: 609-618.

2579. Popescu RA, Wotherspoon AC, Cunningham D (1998). Local recurrence of a primary pancreatic lymphoma 18 years after complete remission. Hematol Oncol 16: 29-32.

2580. Porter JM, Kalloo AN, Abernathy EC, Yeo CJ (1992). Carcinoid tumor of the gallbladder: laparoscopic resection and review of the literature. Surgery 112: 100-105.

2581. Posen JA (1981). Giant cell tumor of the pancreas of the osteoclastic type associated with a mucous secreting cystadenocarcinoma. Hum Pathol 12: 944-947.

2582. Potter DD, Murray JA, Donohue JH, Burgart LJ, Nagorney DM, van Heerden JA et al. (2004). The role of defective mismatch repair in small bowel adenocarcinoma in celiac disease. Cancer Res 64: 7073-7077.

2583. Poulsen ML, Bisgaard ML (2008). MUTYH Associated Polyposis (MAP). Curr Genomics 9: 420-435.

2583A.Poynter JN, Figueiredo JC, Conti DV, Kennedy K, Gallinger S, Siegmund KD et al. (2007). Variants on 9p24 and 8q24 are associated with risk of colorectal cancer: results from the Colon Cancer Family Registry. Cancer Res 67: 11127-11132

2584. Prabhu RM, Medeiros LJ, Kumar D, Drachenberg CI, Papadimitriou JC, Appelman HD et al. (1998). Primary hepatic low-grade B-cell lymphoma of mucosa-associated lymphoid tissue (MALT) associated with primary biliary cirrhosis. Mod Pathol 11: 404-410.

2585. Prakash S, Sarran L, Socci N, Dematteo RP, Eisenstat J, Greco AM et al. (2005). Gastrointestinal stromal tumors in children and young adults: a clinicopathologic, molecular, and genomic study of 15 cases and review of the literature. J Pediatr Hematol Oncol 27: 179-187.

2586. Prati D (2006). Transmission of hepatitis C virus by blood transfusions and other medical procedures: a global review. J Hepatol 45: 607-616.

2587. Prayson RA, Hart WR, Petras RE (1994). Pseudomyxoma peritonei. A clinicopathologic study of 19 cases with emphasis on site of origin and nature of associated ovarian tumors. Am J Surg Pathol 18: 591-603.

2588. Preston SL, Leedham SJ, Oukrif D, Deheregoda M, Goodlad RA, Poulsom R et al. (2008). The development of duodenal microadenomas in FAP patients: the human correlate of the Min mouse. J Pathol 214: 294-301.

2589. Price AB (1991). The Sydney System: histological division. J Gastroenterol Hepatol 6: 209-222.

2590. Price TN, Thompson GB, Lewis JT, Lloyd RV, Young WF (2009). Zollinger-Ellison Syndrome Due to Primary Gastrinoma of the Extrahepatic Biliary Tree: Three Case Reports and Review of the Literature. Endocr Pract 1-38.

2591. Prinz RA, Dorsch TR, Lawrence AM (1981). Clinical aspects of glucagon-producing islet cell tumors. Am J Gastroenterol 76: 125-131.

2592. Prior A, Whorwell PJ (1986). Familial Barrett's oesophagus? Hepatogastroenterology 33: 86-87.

2593. Pritchard BN, Youngberg GA (1993). Atypical mitotic figures in basal cell carcinoma. A review of 208 cases. Am J Dermatopathol 15: 549-552.

2594. Proctor DD, Fraser JL, Mangano MM, Calkins DR, Rosenberg SJ (1992). Small cell carcinoma of the esophagus in a patient with longstanding primary achalasia. Am J Gastroenterol 87: 664-667.

2595. Prokurat A, Kluge P, Kosciesza A, Perek D, Kappeler A, Zimmermann A (2002). Transitional liver cell tumors (TLCT) in older children and adolescents: a novel group of aggressive hepatic tumors expressing beta-catenin. Med Pediatr Oncol 39: 510-518.

2596. Przygodzki RM, Finkelstein SD, Keohavong P, Zhu D, Bakker A, Swalsky PA et al. (1997). Sporadic and Thorotrast-induced angiosarcomas of the liver manifest frequent and multiple point mutations in K-ras-2. Lab Invest 76: 153-159.

2597. Psyrri A, Papageorgiou S, Economopoulos T (2008). Primary extranodal lymphomas of stomach: clinical presentation, diagnostic pitfalls and management. Ann Oncol 19: 1992-1999.

2598. Pulitzer M, Xu R, Suriawinata AA, Waye JD, Harpaz N (2006). Microcarcinoids in large intestinal adenomas. Am J Surg Pathol 30: 1531-1536.

2599. Puppa G, Caneva A, Colombari R (2009). Venous invasion detection in colorectal cancer: which approach, which technique? J Clin Pathol 62: 102-103.

2600. Puppa G, Colombari R, Pelosi G, Ueno H (2008). Pericolonic tumour deposits in colorectal cancer patients: the challenge is on-going. Histopathology 52: 767-768.

2601. Puppa G, Maisonneuve P, Sonzogni A, Masullo M, Capelli P, Chilosi M et al. (2007). Pathological assessment of pericolonic tumor deposits in advanced colonic carcinoma: relevance to prognosis and tumor staging. Mod Pathol 20: 843-855.

2602. Qi Y, Chiu JF, Wang L, Kwong DL, He QY (2005). Comparative proteomic analysis of esophageal squamous cell carcinoma. Proteomics 5: 2960-2971.

2603. Qiao QL, Zhao YG, Ye ML, Yang YM, Zhao JX, Huang YT et al. (2007). Carcinoma of the ampulla of Vater: factors influencing long-term survival of 127 patients with resection. World J Surg 31: 137-143.

2604. Qiao YL, Dawsey SM, Kamangar F, Fan JH, Abnet CC, Sun XD et al. (2009). Total and cancer mortality after supplementation with vitamins and minerals: follow-up of the Linxian General Population Nutrition Intervention Trial. J Natl Cancer Inst 101: 507-518.

2605. Qiao ZK, Halliday ML, Rankin JG, Coates RA (1988). Relationship between hepatitis B surface antigen prevalence, per capita alcohol consumption and primary liver cancer death rate in 30 countries. J Clin Epidemiol 41: 787-792.

2606. Qin LX, Tang ZY (2004). Recent progress in predictive biomarkers for metastatic recurrence of human hepatocellular carcinoma: a review of the literature. J Cancer Res Clin Oncol 130: 497-513.

2607. Qin Y, Greiner A, Trunk MJ, Schmausser B, Ott MM, Muller-Hermelink HK (1995). Somatic hypermutation in low-grade mucosa-associated lymphoid tissue-type B-cell lymphoma. Blood 86: 3528-3534.

2608. Qiu SL, Yang GR (1988). Precursor lesions of esophageal cancer in high-risk populations in Henan Province, China. Cancer 62: 551-557.

2609. Queiroz DM, Mendes EN, Rocha GA, Oliveira AM, Oliveira CA, Magalhaes PP et al. (1998). cagA-positive Helicobacter pylori and risk for developing gastric carcinoma in Brazil. Int J Cancer 78: 135-139.

2610. Quintanilla-Martinez L, Kumar S, Fend F, Reyes E, Teruya-Feldstein J, Kingma DW et al. (2000). Fulminant EBV(+) T-cell lymphoproliferative disorder following acute/chronic EBV infection: a distinct clinicopathologic syndrome. Blood 96: 443-451.

2611. Raderer M, Puspok A, Birkner T, Streubel B, Chott A (2004). Primary gastric mantle cell lymphoma in a patient with long standing history of Crohn's disease. Leuk Lymphoma 45: 1459-1462.

2612. Radford DM, Ashley SW, Wells SA, Jr., Gerhard DS (1990). Loss of heterozygosity of markers on chromosome 11 in tumors from patients with multiple endocrine neoplasia syndrome type 1. Cancer Res 50: 6529-6533.

2613. Radi MJ, Fenoglio-Preiser CM, Bartow SA, Key CR, Pathak DR (1986). Gastric carcinoma in the young: a clinicopathological and immunohistochemical study. Am J Gastroenterol 81: 747-756.

2614. Radi MJ, Fenoglio-Preiser CM, Chiffelle T (1985). Functioning oncocytic islet-cell carcinoma. Report of a case with electron-microscopic and immunohistochemical confirmation. Am J Surg Pathol 9: 517-524.

2615. Raevaara TE, Korhonen MK, Lohi H, Hampel H, Lynch E, Lonnqvist KE et al. (2005). Functional significance and clinical phenotype of nontruncating mismatch repair variants of MLH1. Gastroenterology 129: 537-549.

2616. Rahemtullah A, Misdraji J, Pitman MB (2003). Adenosquamous carcinoma of the pancreas: cytologic features in 14 cases. Cancer 99: 372-378.

2617. Raina A, Yadav D, Krasinskas AM, McGrath KM, Khalid A, Sanders M et al. (2009). Evaluation and management of autoimmune pancreatitis: experience at a large US center. Am J Gastroenterol 104: 2295-2306.

2618. Rajagopalan H, Jallepalli PV, Rago C, Velculescu VE, Kinzler KW, Vogelstein B et al. (2004). Inactivation of hCDC4 can cause chromosomal instability. Nature 428: 77-81.

2619. Rajaram V, Knezevich S, Bove KE, Perry A, Pfeifer JD (2007). DNA sequence of the translocation breakpoints in undifferentiated embryonal sarcoma arising in mesenchymal hamartoma of the liver harboring the t(11;19)(q11;q13.4) translocation. Genes Chromosomes Cancer 46: 508-513.

2620. Rajvanshi P, Kowdley KV, Hirota WK, Meyers JB, Keeffe EB (2005). Fulminant hepatic failure secondary to neoplastic infiltration of the liver. J Clin Gastroenterol 39: 339-343.

2621. Ramage JK, Davies AH, Ardill J, Bax N, Caplin M, Grossman A et al. (2005). Guidelines for the management of gastroenteropancreatic neuroendocrine (including carcinoid) tumours. Gut 54 Suppl 4: 1-16.

2622. Ramanujam TM, Ramesh JC, Goh DW, Wong KT, Ariffin WA, Kumar G et al. (1999). Malignant transformation of mesenchymal hamartoma of the liver: case report and review of the literature. J Pediatr Surg 34: 1684-1686.

2623. Ramirez-Amador V, Esquivel-Pedraza L, Caballero-Mendoza E, Berumen-Campos J, Orozco-Topete R, ngeles-Angeles A (1999). Oral manifestations as a hallmark of malignant acanthosis nigricans. J Oral Pathol Med 28: 278-281.

2624. Ramnani DM, Wistuba II, Behrens C, Gazdar AF, Sobin LH, Albores-Saavedra J (1999). K-ras and p53 mutations in the pathogenesis of classical and goblet cell carcinoids of the appendix. Cancer 86: 14-21.

2625. Rampado S, Ruol A, Guido M, Zaninotto G, Battaglia G, Costantini M et al. (2007).

Mediastinal carcinosis involving the esophagus in breast cancer: the "breast-esophagus" syndrome: report on 25 cases and guidelines for diagnosis and treatment. Ann Surg 246: 316-322.

2626. Rampertab SD, Forde KA, Green PH (2003). Small bowel neoplasia in coeliac disease. Gut 52: 1211-1214.

2627. Rampino N, Yamamoto H, Ionov Y, Li Y, Sawai H, Reed JC et al. (1997). Somatic frameshift mutations in the BAX gene in colon cancers of the microsatellite mutator phenotype. Science 275: 967-969.

2628. Ramsay AD, Bates AW, Williams S, Sebire NJ (2008). Variable antigen expression in hepatoblastomas. Appl Immunohistochem Mol Morphol 16: 140-147.

2629. Ramuz O, Lelong B, Giovannini M, Delpero JR, Rochaix P, Xerri L et al. (2005). "Sugar" tumor of the pancreas: a rare entity that is diagnosable on preoperative fine-needle biopsies. Virchows Arch 446: 555-559.

2630. Randi G, Franceschi S, La Vecchia C (6 A.D.). Gallbladder cancer worldwide: geographical distribution and risk factors. Int J Cancer 118: 1591-1602.

2631. Raney RB, Jr., Crist W, Hays D, Newton W, Ruymann F, Tefft M et al. (1990). Soft tissue sarcoma of the perineal region in childhood. A report from the Intergroup Rhabdomyosarcoma Studies I and II, 1972 through 1984. Cancer 65: 2787-2792.

2632. Rapiti E, Fioretta G, Verkooijen HM, Zanetti R, Schmidlin F, Shubert H et al. (2008). Increased risk of colon cancer after external radiation therapy for prostate cancer. Int J Cancer 123: 1141-1145.

2633. Rashid A (2002). Cellular and molecular biology of biliary tract cancers. Surg Oncol Clin N Am 11: 995-1009.

2634. Rashid A, Gao YT, Bhakta S, Shen MC, Wang BS, Deng J et al. (2001). Beta-catenin mutations in biliary tract cancers: a population-based study in China. Cancer Res 61: 3406-3409.

2635. Rashid A, Hamilton SR (1997). Genetic alterations in sporadic and Crohn's-associated adenocarcinomas of the small intestine. Gastroenterology 113: 127-135.

2636. Rashid A, Houlihan PS, Booker S, Petersen GM, Giardiello FM, Hamilton SR (2000). Phenotypic and molecular characteristics of hyperplastic polyposis. Gastroenterology 119: 323-332.

2637. Rashid A, Ueki T, Gao YT, Houlihan PS, Wallace C, Wang BS et al. (2002). K-ras mutation, p53 overexpression, and microsatellite instability in biliary tract cancers: a population-based study in China. Clin Cancer Res 8: 3156-3163.

2638. Rauser S, Weis R, Braselmann H, Feith M, Stein HJ, Langer R et al. (2007). Significance of HER2 low-level copy gain in Barrett's cancer: implications for fluorescence in situ hybridization testing in tissues. Clin Cancer Res 13: 5115-5123.

2639. Ravera M, Reggiori A, Cocozza E, Andreata M, Ciantia F (1994). Kaposi's sarcoma and AIDS in Uganda: its frequency and gastrointestinal distribution. Ital J Gastroenterol 26: 329-333.

2640. Rayhan N, Sano T, Qian ZR, Obari AK, Hirokawa M (2005). Histological and immunohistochemical study of composite neuroendocrine-exocrine carcinomas of the stomach. J Med Invest 52: 191-202.

2641. Raza SA, Clifford GM, Franceschi S (2007). Worldwide variation in the relative importance of hepatitis B and hepatitis C viruses in hepatocellular carcinoma: a systematic review. Br J Cancer 96: 1127-1134.

2642. Ready AR, Soul JO, Newman J,

Matthews HR (1989). Malignant carcinoid tumour of the oesophagus. Thorax 44: 594-596.

2643. Reardon W, Zhou XP, Eng C (2001). A novel germline mutation of the PTEN gene in a patient with macrocephaly, ventricular dilatation, and features of VATER association. J Med Genet 38: 820-823.

2644. Rebouissou S, Amessou M, Couchy G, Poussin K, Imbeaud S, Pilati C et al. (2009). Frequent in-frame somatic deletions activate gp130 in inflammatory hepatocellular tumours. Nature 457: 200-204.

2645. Rebouissou S, Bioulac-Sage P, Zucman-Rossi J (2008). Molecular pathogenesis of focal nodular hyperplasia and hepatocellular adenoma. J Hepatol 48: 163-170.

2646. Rebouissou S, Couchy G, Libbrecht L, Balabaud C, Imbeaud S, Auffray C et al. (2008). The beta-catenin pathway is activated in focal nodular hyperplasia but not in cirrhotic FNH-like nodules. J Hepatol 49: 61-71.

2647. Rebouissou S, Imbeaud S, Balabaud C, Boulanger V, Bertrand-Michel J, Terce F et al. (2007). HNF1alpha inactivation promotes lipogenesis in human hepatocellular adenoma independently of SREBP-1 and carbohydrate-response element-binding protein (ChREBP) activation. J Biol Chem 282: 14437-14446.

2648. Recine M, Kaw M, Evans DB, Krishnamurthy S (2004). Fine-needle aspiration cytology of mucinous tumors of the pancreas. Cancer 102: 92-99.

2649. Reddy S, Cameron JL, Scudiere J, Hruban RH, Fishman EK, Ahuja N et al. (2009). Surgical management of solid-pseudopapillary neoplasms of the pancreas (Franz or Hamoudi tumors): a large single-institutional series. J Am Coll Surg 208: 950-957.

2650. Reddy S, Edil BH, Cameron JL, Pawlik TM, Herman JM, Gilson MM et al. (2008). Pancreatic resection of isolated metastases from nonpancreatic primary cancers. Ann Surg Oncol 15: 3199-3206.

2651. Redston MS, Caldas C, Seymour AB, Hruban RH, da CL, Yeo CJ et al. (1994). p53 mutations in pancreatic carcinoma and evidence of common involvement of homocopolymer tracts in DNA microdeletions. Cancer Res 54: 3025-3033.

2652. Regauer S (2006). Extramammary Paget's disease—a proliferation of adnexal origin? Histopathology 48: 723-729.

2653. Reid BJ, Blount PL, Feng Z, Levine DS (2000). Optimizing endoscopic biopsy detection of early cancers in Barrett's high-grade dysplasia. Am J Gastroenterol 95: 3089-3096.

2654. Reid BJ, Haggitt RC, Rubin CE, Roth G, Surawicz CM, Van Belle G et al. (1988). Observer variation in the diagnosis of dysplasia in Barrett's esophagus. Hum Pathol 19: 166-178.

2655. Reid-Lombardo KM, Mathis KL, Wood CM, Harmsen WS, Sarr MG (2009). Frequency of Extrapancreatic Neoplasms in Intraductal Papillary Mucinous Neoplasm of the Pancreas: Implications for Management. Ann Surg 251: 64-69.

2656. Reis CA, David L, Correa P, Carneiro F, de BC, Garcia E et al. (1999). Intestinal metaplasia of human stomach displays distinct patterns of mucin (MUC1, MUC2, MUC5AC, and MUC6) expression. Cancer Res 59: 1003-1007.

2657. Remstein ED, Dogan A, Einerson RR, Paternoster SF, Fink SR, Law M et al. (2006). The incidence and anatomic site specificity of chromosomal translocations in primary extranodal marginal zone B-cell lymphoma of mucosa-associated lymphoid tissue (MALT lymphoma) in North America. Am J Surg Pathol 30: 1546-1553.

2658. Renaut AJ, Douglas PR, Newstead GL (2002). Hyperplastic polyposis of the colon and rectum. Colorectal Dis 4: 213-215.

2659. Renshaw AA, Granter SR (1998). A comparison of A103 and inhibin reactivity in adrenal cortical tumors: distinction from hepatocellular carcinoma and renal tumors. Mod Pathol 11: 1160-1164.

2660. Resnick MB, Gallinger S, Wang HH, Odze RD (1995). Growth factor expression and proliferation kinetics in periampullary neoplasms in familial adenomatous polyposis. Cancer 76: 187-194.

2661. Resnick MB, Jacobs DO, Brodsky GL (1994). Multifocal adenocarcinoma in situ with underlying carcinoid tumor of the gallbladder. Arch Pathol Lab Med 118: 933-934.

2662. Restrepo C, Moreno J, Duque E, Cuello C, Amsel J, Correa P (1978). Juvenile colonic polyposis in Colombia. Dis Colon Rectum 21: 600-612.

2663. Reti A, Pap E, Zalatnai A, Jeney A, Kralovanszky J, Budai B (2009). Co-inhibition of cyclooxygenase-2 and dihydropyrimidine dehydrogenase by non-steroidal anti-inflammatory drugs in tumor cells and xenografts. Anticancer Res 29: 3095-3101.

2664. Rex DK, Bond JH, Winawer S, Levin TR, Burt RW, Johnson DA et al. (2002). Quality in the technical performance of colonoscopy and the continuous quality improvement process for colonoscopy: recommendations of the U.S. Multi-Society Task Force on Colorectal Cancer. Am J Gastroenterol 97: 1296-1308.

2665. Reyes CV, Wang T (1981). Undifferentiated small cell carcinoma of the pancreas: a report of five cases. Cancer 47: 2500-2502.

2666. Reynolds M (1999). Pediatric liver tumors. Semin Surg Oncol 16: 159-172.

2667. Reynolds P, Urayama KY, Von BJ, Feusner J (2004). Birth characteristics and hepatoblastoma risk in young children. Cancer 100: 1070-1076.

2668. Rhead JL, Letley DP, Mohammadi M, Hussein N, Mohagheghi MA, Eshagh HM et al. (2007). A new *Helicobacter pylori* vacuolating cytotoxin determinant, the intermediate region, is associated with gastric cancer. Gastroenterology 133: 926-936.

2669. Ribeiro MB, Greenstein AJ, Heimann TM, Yamazaki Y, Aufses AH, Jr. (1991). Adenocarcinoma of the small intestine in Crohn's disease. Surg Gynecol Obstet 173: 343-349.

2670. Ricci R, Maggiano N, Martini M, Mule AM, Pierconti F, Capelli A et al. (2001). Primary malignant melanoma of the gallbladder in dysplastic naevus syndrome. Virchows Arch 438: 159-165.

2671. Ricci-Vitiani L, Lombardi DG, Pilozzi E, Biffoni M, Todaro M, Peschle C et al. (2007). Identification and expansion of human colon-cancer-initiating cells. Nature 445: 111-115.

2672. Rice TW, Rusch VW, pperson-Hansen C, Allen MS, Chen LQ, Hunter JG et al. (2009). Worldwide esophageal cancer collaboration. Dis Esophagus 22: 1-8.

2673. Richards FM, McKee SA, Rajpar MH, Cole TR, Evans DG, Jankowski JA et al. (1999). Germline E-cadherin gene (*CDH1*) mutations predispose to familial gastric cancer and colorectal cancer. Hum Mol Genet 8: 607-610.

2674. Riddell RH, Goldman H, Ransohoff DF, Appelman HD, Fenoglio CM, Haggitt RC et al. (1983). Dysplasia in inflammatory bowel disease: standardized classification with provisional clinical applications. Hum Pathol 14: 931-968.

2675. Riddell RH, Odze RD (2009). Definition of Barrett's esophagus: time for a rethink—is intestinal metaplasia dead? Am J Gastroenterol 104: 2588-2594.

2676. Rigaud G, Missiaglia E, Moore PS, Zamboni G, Falconi M, Talamini G et al. (2001). High resolution allelotype of nonfunctional pancreatic endocrine tumors: identification of two molecular subgroups with clinical implications. Cancer Res 61: 285-292.

2677. Riikonen P, Tuominen L, Seppa A, Perkkio M (1990). Simultaneous hepatoblastoma in identical male twins. Cancer 66: 2429-2431.

2678. Rijcken FE, Hollema H, Kleibeuker JH (2002). Proximal adenomas in hereditary non-polyposis colorectal cancer are prone to rapid malignant transformation. Gut 50: 382-386.

2679. Rijken AM, van Gulik TM, Polak MM, Sturm PD, Gouma DJ, Offerhaus GJ (1998). Diagnostic and prognostic value of incidence of K-ras codon 12 mutations in resected distal bile duct carcinoma. J Surg Oncol 68: 187-192.

2680. Riley E, Swift M (1980). A family with Peutz-Jeghers syndrome and bilateral breast cancer. Cancer 46: 815-817.

2681. Rimola J, Forner A, Reig M, Vilana R, de Lope CR, Ayuso C et al. (2009). Cholangiocarcinoma in cirrhosis: absence of contrast washout in delayed phases by magnetic resonance imaging avoids misdiagnosis of hepatocellular carcinoma. Hepatology 50: 791-798.

2682. Rindi G, Azzoni C, La Rosa S, Klersy C, Paolotti D, Rappel S et al. (1999). ECL cell tumor and poorly differentiated endocrine carcinoma of the stomach: prognostic evaluation by pathological analysis. Gastroenterology 116: 532-542.

2683. Rindi G, Bordi C, Rappel S, La Rosa S, Stolte M, Solcia E (1996). Gastric carcinoids and neuroendocrine carcinomas: pathogenesis, pathology, and behavior. World J Surg 20: 168-172.

2684. Rindi G, Klöppel G, Alhman H, Caplin M, Couvelard A, de Herder WW et al. (2006). TNM staging of foregut (neuro)endocrine tumors: a consensus proposal including a grading system. Virchows Arch 449: 395-401.

2685. Rindi G, Klöppel G, Couvelard A, Komminoth P, Korner M, Lopes JM et al. (2007). TNM staging of midgut and hindgut (neuro) endocrine tumors: a consensus proposal including a grading system. Virchows Arch 451: 757-762.

2686. Rindi G, Luinetti O, Cornaggia M, Capella C, Solcia E (1993). Three subtypes of gastric argyrophil carcinoid and the gastric neuroendocrine carcinoma: a clinicopathologic study. Gastroenterology 104: 994-1006.

2687. Rindi G, Paolotti D, Fiocca R, Wiedenmann B, Henry JP, Solcia E (2000). Vesicular monoamine transporter 2 as a marker of gastric enterochromaffin-like cell tumors. Virchows Arch 436: 217-223.

2688. Rindi G, Savio A, Torsello A, Zoli M, Locatelli V, Cocchi D et al. (2002). Ghrelin expression in gut endocrine growths. Histochem Cell Biol 117: 521-525.

2689. Riopel MA, Klimstra DS, Godellas CV, Blumgart LH, Westra WH (1997). Intrabiliary growth of metastatic colonic adenocarcinoma: a pattern of intrahepatic spread easily confused with primary neoplasia of the biliary tract. Am J Surg Pathol 21: 1030-1036.

2690. Risk JM, Field EA, Field JK, Whittaker J, Fryer A, Ellis A et al. (1994). Tylosis oesophageal cancer mapped. Nat Genet 8: 319-321.

2691. Risk JM, Mills HS, Garde J, Dunn JR, Evans KE, Hollstein M et al. (1999). The tylosis esophageal cancer (TOC) locus: more than just a familial cancer gene. Dis Esophagus 12: 173-176.

2692. Risk JM, Ruhrberg C, Hennies H, Mills HS, Di CT, Evans KE et al. (1999). Envoplakin, a possible candidate gene for focal NEPPK/esophageal cancer (TOC): the integration of genetic and physical maps of the TOC region on 17q25. Genomics 59: 234-242.

2693. Risques RA, Rabinovitch PS, Brentnall TA (2006). Cancer surveillance in inflammatory bowel disease: new molecular approaches. Curr Opin Gastroenterol 22: 382-390.

2694. Rivera-Hueto F, Rios-Martin JJ, Dominguez-Triano R, Herrerias-Gutierrez JM (1999). Early gastric stump carcinoma with rhabdoid features. Case report. Pathol Res Pract 195: 841-846.

2695. Rizzetto M (2009). Hepatitis D: thirty years after. J Hepatol 50: 1043-1050.

2696. Roberts LJ, Bloomgarden ZT, Marney SR, Jr., Rabin D, Oates JA (1983). Histamine release from a gastric carcinoid: provocation by pentagastrin and inhibition by somatostatin. Gastroenterology 84: 272-275.

2697. Roberts PL, Veidenheimer MC, Cassidy S, Silverman ML (1989). Adenocarcinoma arising in an ileostomy. Report of two cases and review of the literature. Arch Surg 124: 497-499.

2698. Robertson PL, Muraszko KM, Axtell RA (1997). Hepatoblastoma metastatic to brain: prolonged survival after multiple surgical resections of a solitary brain lesion. J Pediatr Hematol Oncol 19: 168-171.

2699. Robey-Cafferty SS, el-Naggar AK, Sahin AA, Bruner JM, Ro JY, Cleary KR (1991). Prognostic factors in esophageal squamous carcinoma. A study of histologic features, blood group expression, and DNA ploidy. Am J Clin Pathol 95: 844-849.

2700. Robins DB, Katz RL, Evans DB, Atkinson EN, Green L (1995). Fine needle aspiration of the pancreas. In quest of accuracy. Acta Cytol 39: 1-10.

2701. Rock CL (2007). Primary dietary prevention: is the fiber story over? Recent Results Cancer Res 174: 171-177.

2702. Roder JD, Bottcher K, Busch R, Wittekind C, Hermanek P, Siewert JR (1998). Classification of regional lymph node metastasis from gastric carcinoma. German Gastric Cancer Study Group. Cancer 82: 621-631.

2703. Rodrigues LR, Teixeira JA, Schmitt FL, Paulsson M, Lindmark-Mansson H (2007). The role of osteopontin in tumor progression and metastasis in breast cancer. Cancer Epidemiol Biomarkers Prev 16: 1087-1097.

2704. Rodriguez JR, Salvia R, Crippa S, Warshaw AL, Bassi C, Falconi M et al. (2007). Branch-duct intraductal papillary mucinous neoplasms: observations in 145 patients who underwent resection. Gastroenterology 133: 72-79.

2705. Roebuck DJ (1998). Interventional radiology in children with hepatobiliary rhabdomyosarcoma. Med Pediatr Oncol 31: 187-188.

2706. Roebuck DJ, Aronson D, Clapuyt P, Czauderna P, de Ville de GJ, Gauthier F et al. (2007). 2005 PRETEXT: a revised staging system for primary malignant liver tumours of childhood developed by the SIOPEL group. Pediatr Radiol 37: 123-132.

2707. Roebuck DJ, Perilongo G (2006). Hepatoblastoma: an oncological review. Pediatr Radiol 36: 183-186.

2708. Roebuck DJ, Yang WT, Lam WW, Stanley P (1998). Hepatobiliary rhabdomyosarcoma in children: diagnostic radiology. Pediatr Radiol 28: 101-108.

2709. Roebuck DJ, Yuen MK, Wong YC, Shing MK, Lee CW, Li CK (2001). Imaging features of pancreatoblastoma. Pediatr Radiol 31: 501-506.

2710. Roedl JB, Halpern EF, Colen RR, Sahani DV, Fischman AJ, Blake MA (2009). Metabolic tumor width parameters as determined on PET/CT predict disease-free survival and treatment response in squamous cell carcinoma of the esophagus. Mol Imaging Biol 11: 54-60.

2711. Rogers LF, Lastra MP, Lin KT, Bennett D (1973). Calcifying mucinous adenocarcinoma of the gallbladder. Am J Gastroenterol 59: 441-445.

2712. Rogers WM, Dobo E, Norton JA, Van DJ, Jeffrey RB, Huntsman DG et al. (2008). Risk-reducing total gastrectomy for germline mutations in E-cadherin (CDH1): pathologic findings with clinical implications. Am J Surg Pathol 32: 799-809.

2713. Roggo A, Wood WC, Ottinger LW (1993). Carcinoid tumors of the appendix. Ann Surg 217: 385-390.

2714. Roh YH, Kim YH, Lee HW, Kim SJ, Roh MS, Jeong JS et al. (2007). The clinicopathologic and immunohistochemical characteristics of ampulla of Vater carcinoma: the intestinal type is associated with a better prognosis. Hepatogastroenterology 54: 1641-1644.

2714A. Rohatgi PR, Swisher SG, Correa AM, Wu TT, Liao Z, Komaki R, Walsh G, Vapociyan A, Lynch PM, Rice DC, Roth JA, Ajani JA (2005). Failure patterns correlate with the proportion of residual carcinoma after preoperative chemoradiotherapy for carcinoma of the esophagus. Cancer 104: 1349-1355.

2715. Rohatiner A, d'Amore F, Coiffier B, Crowther D, Gospodarowicz M, Isaacson P et al. (1994). Report on a workshop convened to discuss the pathological and staging classifications of gastrointestinal tract lymphoma. Ann Oncol 5: 397-400.

2716. Rokkas T, Filipe MI, Sladen GE (1991). Detection of an increased incidence of early gastric cancer in patients with intestinal metaplasia type III who are closely followed up. Gut 32: 1110-1113.

2717. Roldo C, Missiaglia E, Hagan JP, Falconi M, Capelli P, Bersani S et al. (2006). MicroRNA expression abnormalities in pancreatic endocrine and acinar tumors are associated with distinctive pathologic features and clinical behavior. J Clin Oncol 24: 4677-4684.

2718. Romaguera J, Hagemeister FB (2005). Lymphoma of the colon. Curr Opin Gastroenterol 21: 80-84.

2719. Romano A, Quaratino D, Papa G, Di FM, Venuti A (1997). Aminopenicillin allergy. Arch Dis Child 76: 513-517.

2720. Romero Y, Cameron AJ, Locke GR, III, Schaid DJ, Slezak JM, Branch CD et al. (1997). Familial aggregation of gastroesophageal reflux in patients with Barrett's esophagus and esophageal adenocarcinoma. Gastroenterology 113: 1449-1456.

2721. Roncalli M, Roz E, Coggi G, Di Rocco MG, Bossi P, Minola E et al. (1999). The vascular profile of regenerative and dysplastic nodules of the cirrhotic liver: implications for diagnosis and classification. Hepatology 30: 1174-1178.

2722. Ronnett BM, Zahn CM, Kurman RJ, Kass ME, Sugarbaker PH, Shmookler BM (1995). Disseminated peritoneal adenomucinosis and peritoneal mucinous carcinomatosis. A clinicopathologic analysis of 109 cases with emphasis on distinguishing pathologic features, site of origin, prognosis, and relationship to "pseudomyxoma peritonei". Am J Surg Pathol 19: 1390-1408.

2723. Rooks JB, Ory HW, Ishak KG, Strauss LT, Greenspan JR, Hill AP et al. (1979). Epidemiology of hepatocellular adenoma. The role of oral contraceptive use. JAMA 242: 644-648.

2724. Ros PR, Olmsted WW, Dachman AH, Goodman ZD, Ishak KG, Hartman DS (1986). Undifferentiated (embryonal) sarcoma of the liver: radiologic-pathologic correlation. Radiology 161: 141-145.

2725. Rosato FE, Jr., Rosato EL (2008). Current surgical management of intestinal metastases. Semin Oncol 35: 177-182.

2726. Rosch T (1995). Endosonographic staging of gastric cancer: a review of literature results. Gastrointest Endosc Clin N Am 5: 549-557.

2727. Rose PG, Abdul-Karim FW (1997). Isolated appendiceal metastasis in early ovarian carcinoma. J Surg Oncol 64: 246-247.

2728. Rosenbaum SJ, Stergar H, Antoch G, Veit P, Bockisch A, Kuhl H (2006). Staging and follow-up of gastrointestinal tumors with PET/CT. Abdom Imaging 31: 25-35.
2729. Rosenberg J, Welch JP, Pyrtek LJ, Walker M, Trowbridge P (1986). Benign villous adenomas of the ampulla of Vater. Cancer 58: 1563-1568.
2730. Rosenberg JM, Welch JP (1985). Carcinoid tumors of the colon. A study of 72 patients. Am J Surg 149: 775-779.
2731. Rossi DJ, Ylikorkala A, Korsisaari N, Salovaara R, Luukko K, Launonen V et al. (2002). Induction of cyclooxygenase-2 in a mouse model of Peutz-Jeghers polyposis. Proc Natl Acad Sci U S A 99: 12327-12332.
2732. Rossi G, Bertolini F, Sartori G, Bigiani N, Cavazza A, Foroni M et al. (2004). Primary mixed adenocarcinoma and small cell carcinoma of the appendix: a clinicopathologic, immunohistochemical, and molecular study of a hitherto unreported tumor. Am J Surg Pathol 28: 1233-1239.
2733. Rossi G, Valli R, Bertolini F, Sighinolfi P, Losi L, Cavazza A et al. (2003). Does mesoappendix infiltration predict a worse prognosis in incidental neuroendocrine tumors of the appendix? A clinicopathologic and immunohistochemical study of 15 cases. Am J Clin Pathol 120: 706-711.
2734. Rossi S, Kopetz S, Davuluri R, Hamilton SR, Calin GA (2009). MicroRNAs, ultraconserved genes and colorectal cancers. Int J Biochem Cell Biol -
2735. Roth J, Komminoth P, Klöppel G, Heitz PU (1996). Diabetes and the endocrine pancreas. In: Anderson's Pathology. Damjanov I, Linder J, eds. Mosby-Year Book Inc: St. Louis, pp. 2042-2070.
2736. Roth S, Sistonen P, Salovaara R, Hemminki A, Loukola A, Johansson M et al. (1999). *SMAD* genes in juvenile polyposis. Genes Chromosomes Cancer 26: 54-61.
2737. Rousseau DL, Jr., Thomas CR, Jr., Petrelli NJ, Kahlenberg MS (2005). Squamous cell carcinoma of the anal canal. Surg Oncol 14: 121-132.
2738. Rouzbahman M, Serra S, Adsay NV, Bejarano PA, Nakanuma Y, Chetty R (2007). Oncocytic papillary neoplasms of the biliary tract: a clinicopathological, mucin core and Wnt pathway protein analysis of four cases. Pathology 39: 413-418.
2739. Rowland JM (2002). Hepatoblastoma: assessment of criteria for histologic classification. Med Pediatr Oncol 39: 478-483.
2740. Rozenblum E, Schutte M, Goggins M, Hahn SA, Panzer S, Zahurak M et al. (1997). Tumor-suppressive pathways in pancreatic carcinoma. Cancer Res 57: 1731-1734.
2741. Rubbia-Brandt L, Brundler MA, Kerl K, Negro F, Nador RG, Scherrer A et al. (1999). Primary hepatic diffuse large B-cell lymphoma in a patient with chronic hepatitis C. Am J Surg Pathol 23: 1124-1130.
2742. Rubinfeld B, Albert I, Porfiri E, Fiol C, Munemitsu S, Polakis P (1996). Binding of GSK3beta to the APC-beta-catenin complex and regulation of complex assembly. Science 272: 1023-1026.
2742A. Rubio CA, Liu FS, Zhao HZ (1989). Histological classification of intraepithelial neoplasias and microinvasive squamous carcinoma of the esophagus. Am J Surg Pathol 13: 685–690.
2743. Rubio CA, Jonasson J, Nesi G, Mandai K, Pisano R, King A et al. (2005). Extensive intestinal metaplasia in gastric carcinoma and in other lesions requiring surgery: a study of 3,421 gastrectomy specimens from dwellers of the Atlantic and Pacific basins. J Clin Pathol 58: 1271-1277.
2744. Rubio CA, Stemme S, Jaramillo E, Lindblom A (2006). Hyperplastic polyposis coli syndrome and colorectal carcinoma. Endoscopy 38: 266-270.
2745. Ruck P, Kaiserling E (1992). Extracellular matrix in hepatoblastoma: an immunohistochemical investigation. Histopathology 21: 115-126.
2746. Ruck P, Xiao JC, Kaiserling E (1995). Immunoreactivity of sinusoids in hepatoblastoma: an immunohistochemical study using lectin UEA-1 and antibodies against endothelium-associated antigens, including CD34. Histopathology 26: 451-455.
2747. Rucker-Schmidt RL, Sanchez CA, Blount PL, Ayub K, Li X, Rabinovitch PS et al. (2009). Nonadenomatous dysplasia in barrett esophagus: a clinical, pathologic, and DNA content flow cytometric study. Am J Surg Pathol 33: 886-893.
2748. Ruemmele P, Dietmaier W, Terracciano L, Tornillo L, Bataille F, Kaiser A et al. (2009). Histopathologic features and microsatellite instability of cancers of the papilla of vater and their precursor lesions. Am J Surg Pathol 33: 691-704.
2749. Rugge M, Cassaro M, Leandro G, Baffa R, Avellini C, Bufo P et al. (1996). *Helicobacter pylori* in promotion of gastric carcinogenesis. Dig Dis Sci 41: 950-955.
2750. Rugge M, Correa P, Di MF, El-Omar E, Fiocca R, Geboes K et al. (2008). OLGA staging for gastritis: a tutorial. Dig Liver Dis 40: 650-658.
2751. Rugge M, Correa P, Dixon MF, Fiocca R, Hattori T, Lechago J et al. (2002). Gastric mucosal atrophy: interobserver consistency using new criteria for classification and grading. Aliment Pharmacol Ther 16: 1249-1259.
2752. Rugge M, Correa P, Dixon MF, Hattori T, Leandro G, Lewin K et al. (2000). Gastric dysplasia: the Padova international classification. Am J Surg Pathol 24: 167-176.
2753. Rugge M, Correa P, Dixon MF, Hattori T, Leandro G, Lewin K et al. (2000). Gastric dysplasia: the Padova international classification. Am J Surg Pathol 24: 167-176.
2754. Rugge M, Sonego F, Militello C, Guido M, Ninfo V (1992). Primary carcinoid tumor of the cystic and common bile ducts. Am J Surg Pathol 16: 802-807.
2755. Rugge M, Sonego F, Pollice L, Perilongo G, Guido M, Basso G et al. (1998). Hepatoblastoma: DNA nuclear content, proliferative indices, and pathology. Liver 18: 128-133.
2756. Rullier A, Le BB, Fawaz R, Blanc JF, Saric J, Bioulac-Sage P (2000). Cytokeratin 7 and 20 expression in cholangiocarcinomas varies along the biliary tract but still differs from that in colorectal carcinoma metastasis. Am J Surg Pathol 24: 870-876.
2757. Rumilla KM, Erickson LA, Erickson AK, Lloyd RV (2006). Galectin-4 expression in carcinoid tumors. Endocr Pathol 17: 243-249.
2758. Ruo L, Coit DG, Brennan MF, Guillem JG (2002). Long-term follow-up of patients with familial adenomatous polyposis undergoing pancreaticoduodenal surgery. J Gastrointest Surg 6: 671-675.
2759. Ruskone-Fourmestraux A, Dragosics B, Morgner A, Wotherspoon A, De JD (2003). Paris staging system for primary gastrointestinal lymphomas. Gut 52: 912-913.
2760. Rustin RB, Broughan TA, Hermann RE, Grundfest-Broniatowski SF, Petras RE, Hart WR (1988). Papillary cystic epithelial neoplasms of the pancreas. A clinical study of six cases. Arch Surg 121: 1073-1076.
2761. Ruszniewski P, Delle FG, Cadiot G, Komminoth P, Chung D, Kos-Kudla B et al. (2006). Well-differentiated gastric tumors/carcinomas. Neuroendocrinology 84: 158-164.
2762. Ruttman E, Klöppel G, Bommer G, Kiehn M, Heitz PU (1980). Pancreatic glucagonoma with and without syndrome. Immunocytochemical study of 5 tumour cases and review of the literature. Virchows Arch A Pathol Anat Histol 388: 51-67.
2763. Ruymann FB, Raney RB, Jr., Crist WM, Lawrence W, Jr., Lindberg RD, Soule EH (1985). Rhabdomyosarcoma of the biliary tree in childhood. A report from the Intergroup Rhabdomyosarcoma Study. Cancer 56: 575-581.
2764. Ryan A, Razak A, Graham J, Benson A, Rowe D, Haugk B et al. (2007). Desmoplastic small round-cell tumor of the pancreas. J Clin Oncol 25: 1440-1442.
2765. Ryan DP, Schapiro RH, Warshaw AL (1986). Villous tumors of the duodenum. Ann Surg 203: 301-306.
2766. Ryu KW, Choi IJ, Doh YW, Kook MC, Kim CG, Park HJ et al. (2007). Surgical indication for non-curative endoscopic resection in early gastric cancer. Ann Surg Oncol 14: 3428-3434.
2767. Saadat M (2006). Genetic polymorphisms of glutathione S-transferase T1 (*GSTT1*) and susceptibility to gastric cancer: a meta-analysis. Cancer Sci 97: 505-509.
2768. Sabeti PC, Varilly P, Fry B, Lohmueller J, Hostetter E, Cotsapas C et al. (2007). Genome-wide detection and characterization of positive selection in human populations. Nature 449: 913-918.
2769. Sabljak P, Stojakov D, Bjelovic M, Mihaljevic B, Velickovic D, Ebrahimi K et al. (2008). Primary esophageal diffuse large B-cell lymphoma: report of a case. Surg Today 38: 647-650.
2770. Sachatello CR, Hahn IS, Carrington CB (1974). Juvenile gastrointestinal polyposis in a female infant: report of a case and review of the literature of a recently recognized syndrome. Surgery 75: 107-114.
2771. Sadakari Y, Ienaga J, Kobayashi K, Miyasaka Y, Takahata S, Nakamura M et al. (2009). Cyst Size Indicates Malignant Transformation in Branch Duct Intraductal Papillary Mucinous Neoplasm of the Pancreas Without Mural Nodules. Pancreas -
2772. Safioleas M, Agapitos E, Kontzoglou K, Stamatakos M, Safioleas P, Mouzopoulos G et al. (2006). Primary melanoma of the gallbladder: does it exist? Report of a case and review of the literature. World J Gastroenterol 12: 4259-4261.
2773. Safioleas MC, Moulakakis KG, Kontzoglou K, Stamoulis J, Nikou GC, Toubanakis C et al. (2005). Carcinoid tumors of the appendix. Prognostic factors and evaluation of indications for right hemicolectomy. Hepatogastroenterology 52: 123-127.
2774. Sagaert X, de PP, Libbrecht L, Vanhentenrijk V, Verhoef G, Thomas J et al. (2006). Forkhead box protein P1 expression in mucosa-associated lymphoid tissue lymphomas predicts poor prognosis and transformation to diffuse large B-cell lymphoma. J Clin Oncol 24: 2490-2497.
2775. Sahani DV, Shah ZK, Catalano OA, Boland GW, Brugge WR (2008). Radiology of pancreatic adenocarcinoma: current status of imaging. J Gastroenterol Hepatol 23: 23-33.
2776. Sahu KK, Rau AR, Bhat N, Kini JR, Mathai AM (2009). Imprint cytology of pancreatoblastoma: a case report and review of the literature. Diagn Cytopathol 37: 290-292.
2777. Saint Martin MC, Chejfec G (1999). Barrett esophagus-associated small cell carcinoma. Arch Pathol Lab Med 123: 1123-
2778. Sakai Y, Kupelioglu AA, Yanagisawa A, Yamaguchi K, Hidaka E, Matsuya S et al. (2000). Origin of giant cells in osteoclast-like giant cell tumors of the pancreas. Hum Pathol 31: 1223-1229.
2779. Sakamoto K, Kimura N, Tokumura H, Ogasawara T, Moriya T, Sasano H (2005). Hepatoid adenocarcinoma of the gallbladder. Histopathology 47: 649-651.
2780. Sakamoto K, Watanabe M, De La CC, Honda H, Ise H, Mitsui K et al. (2005). Primary invasive micropapillary carcinoma of the colon. Histopathology 47: 479-484.
2781. Sakamoto M, Hirohashi S (1998). Natural history and prognosis of adenomatous hyperplasia and early hepatocellular carcinoma: multi-institutional analysis of 53 nodules followed up for more than 6 months and 141 patients with single early hepatocellular carcinoma treated by surgical resection or percutaneous ethanol injection. Jpn J Clin Oncol 28: 604-608.
2782. Sakamoto M, Hirohashi S, Shimosato Y (1991). Early stages of multistep hepatocarcinogenesis: adenomatous hyperplasia and early hepatocellular carcinoma. Hum Pathol 22: 172-178.
2783. Sakamoto M, Hirohashi S, Tsuda H, Shimosato Y, Makuuchi M, Hosoda Y (1989). Multicentric independent development of hepatocellular carcinoma revealed by analysis of hepatitis B virus integration pattern. Am J Surg Pathol 13: 1064-1067.
2784. Salit IE, Tinmouth J, Chong S, Raboud J, Diong C, Su D et al. (2009). Screening for HIV-associated anal cancer: correlation of HPV genotypes, p16, and E6 transcripts with anal pathology. Cancer Epidemiol Biomarkers Prev 18: 1986-1992.
2785. Salmi TT, Collin P, Korponay-Szabo IR, Laurila K, Partanen J, Huhtala H et al. (2006). Endomysial antibody-negative coeliac disease: clinical characteristics and intestinal autoantibody deposits. Gut 55: 1746-1753.
2786. Salvia R, Crippa S, Falconi M, Bassi C, Guarise A, Scarpa A et al. (2007). Branch-duct intraductal papillary mucinous neoplasms of the pancreas: to operate or not to operate? Gut 56: 1086-1090.
2787. Salvia R, Fernandez-del Castillo C, Bassi C, Thayer SP, Falconi M, Mantovani W et al. (2004). Main-duct intraductal papillary mucinous neoplasms of the pancreas: clinical predictors of malignancy and long-term survival following resection. Ann Surg 239: 678-685.
2788. Samowitz WS, Sweeney C, Herrick J, Albertsen H, Levin TR, Murtaugh MA et al. (2005). Poor survival associated with the BRAF V600E mutation in microsatellite-stable colon cancers. Cancer Res 65: 6063-6069.
2789. Samplaski MK, Rosato EL, Witkiewicz AK, Mastrangelo MJ, Berger AC (2008). Malignant melanoma of the gallbladder: a report of two cases and review of the literature. J Gastrointest Surg 12: 1123-1126.
2790. Sampson JR, Jones N (2009). MUTYH-associated polyposis. Best Pract Res Clin Gastroenterol 23: 209-218.
2791. Samuel LH, Frierson HF, Jr. (1996). Fine needle aspiration cytology of acinar cell carcinoma of the pancreas: a report of two cases. Acta Cytol 40: 585-591.
2792. Sanchez AA, Wu TT, Prieto VG, Rashid A, Hamilton SR, Wang H (2008). Comparison of primary and metastatic malignant melanoma of the esophagus: clinicopathologic review of 10 cases. Arch Pathol Lab Med 132: 1623-1629.
2793. Sanchez-Cespedes M, Parrella P, Esteller M, Nomoto S, Trink B, Engles JM et al. (2002). Inactivation of LKB1/STK11 is a common event in adenocarcinomas of the lung. Cancer Res 62: 3659-3662.
2794. Sanchez-de-Abajo A, de la Hoya M, Van Puijenbroek M, Tosar A, Lopez-Asenjo JA, Diaz-Rubio E et al. (2007). Molecular analysis of colorectal cancer tumors from patients with mismatch repair proficient hereditary nonpolyposis colorectal cancer suggests novel carcinogenic pathways. Clin Cancer Res 13: 5729-5735.
2795. Sanduleanu S, Jonkers D, de Bruine A,

Hameeteman W, Stockbrugger RW (2001). Changes in gastric mucosa and luminal environment during acid-suppressive therapy: a review in depth. Dig Liver Dis 33: 707-719.
2796. Sanoff HK, McLeod HL (2008). Predictive Factors for Response and Toxicity in Chemotherapy: Pharmacogenomics. Semin Colon Rectal Surg 19: 226-230.
2797. Santoro E, Sacchi M, Scutari F, Carboni F, Graziano F (1997). Primary adenocarcinoma of the duodenum: treatment and survival in 89 patients. Hepatogastroenterology 44: 1157-1163.
2798. Santoro IM, Groden J (1997). Alternative splicing of the *APC* gene and its association with terminal differentiation. Cancer Res 57: 488-494.
2799. Santos LD, Chow C, Henderson CJ, Blomberg DN, Merrett ND, Kennerson AR et al. (2002). Serous oligocystic adenoma of the pancreas: a clinicopathological and immunohistochemical study of three cases with ultrastructural findings. Pathology 34: 148-156.
2800. Sanz N, de ML, Florez F, Rollan V (1997). Rhabdomyosarcoma of the biliary tree. Pediatr Surg Int 12: 200-201.
2801. Saqi A, Alexis D, Remotti F, Bhagat G (2005). Usefulness of CDX2 and TTF-1 in differentiating gastrointestinal from pulmonary carcinoids. Am J Clin Pathol 123: 394-404.
2802. Sarbia M (2006). The histological appearance of oesophageal adenocarcinoma—an analysis based on 215 resection specimens. Virchows Arch 448: 532-538.
2803. Sarbia M, Bittinger F, Porschen R, Dutkowski P, Torzewski M, Willers R et al. (1996). The prognostic significance of tumour cell proliferation in squamous cell carcinomas of the oesophagus. Br J Cancer 74: 1012-1016.
2804. Sarbia M, Bittinger F, Porschen R, Dutkowski P, Willers R, Gabbert HE (1995). Prognostic value of histopathologic parameters of esophageal squamous cell carcinoma. Cancer 76: 922-927.
2805. Sarbia M, Geddert H, Klump B, Kiel S, Iskender E, Gabbert HE (2004). Hypermethylation of tumor suppressor genes (*p16INK4A*, *p14ARF* and *APC*) in adenocarcinomas of the upper gastrointestinal tract. Int J Cancer 111: 224-228.
2806. Sarbia M, Porschen R, Borchard F, Horstmann O, Willers R, Gabbert HE (1995). Incidence and prognostic significance of vascular and neural invasion in squamous cell carcinomas of the esophagus. Int J Cancer 61: 333-336.
2807. Sardi A, Singer JA (1987). Insulinoma and gastrinoma in Wermer's disease (MEN I). Arch Surg 122: 835-836.
2808. Sarmiento JM, Wolff BG, Burgart LJ, Frizelle FA, Ilstrup DM (1997). Paget's disease of the perianal region—an aggressive disease? Dis Colon Rectum 40: 1187-1194.
2809. Sarr MG, Carpenter HA, Prabhakar LP, Orchard TF, Hughes S, van Heerden JA et al. (2000). Clinical and pathologic correlation of 84 mucinous cystic neoplasms of the pancreas: can one reliably differentiate benign from malignant (or premalignant) neoplasms? Ann Surg 231: 205-212.
2810. Sartore-Bianchi A, Martini M, Molinari F, Veronese S, Nichelatti M, Artale S et al. (2009). PIK3CA mutations in colorectal cancer are associated with clinical resistance to EGFR-targeted monoclonal antibodies. Cancer Res 69: 1851-1857.
2811. Sasaki M, Ikeda H, Nakanuma Y (2007). Expression profiles of MUC mucins and trefoil factor family (TFF) peptides in the intrahepatic biliary system: physiological distribution and pathological significance. Prog Histochem Cytochem 42: 61-110.
2812. Sasaki M, Nakanuma Y, Kim YS (1996). Characterization of apomucin expression in intrahepatic cholangiocarcinomas and their precursor lesions: an immunohistochemical study. Hepatology 24: 1074-1078.
2813. Sasaki M, Yamaguchi J, Itatsu K, Ikeda H, Nakanuma Y (2008). Over-expression of polycomb group protein EZH2 relates to decreased expression of *p16 INK4a* in cholangiocarcinogenesis in hepatolithiasis. J Pathol 215: 175-183.
2814. Sashiyama H, Abe Y, Sasagawa S, Hanada H (2009). Unusual presentation of appendiceal myxoglobulosis as a right inguinal hernia. J Am Coll Surg 208: 314-315.
2815. Sass DA, Clark K, Grzybicki D, Rabinovitz M, Shaw-Stiffel TA (2007). Diffuse desmoplastic metastatic breast cancer simulating cirrhosis with severe portal hypertension: a case of "pseudocirrhosis". Dig Dis Sci 52: 749-752.
2816. Sata N, Kurogochi A, Endo K, Shimura K, Koizumi M, Nagai H (2007). Follicular lymphoma of the pancreas: a case report and proposed new strategies for diagnosis and surgery of benign or low-grade malignant lesions of the head of the pancreas. JOP 8: 44-49.
2817. Sata N, Tsukahara M, Koizumi M, Yoshizawa K, Kurihara K, Nagai H et al. (2004). Primary small-cell neuroendocrine carcinoma of the duodenum - a case report and review of literature. World J Surg Oncol 2: 28-
2818. Satarug S, Haswell-Elkins MR, Sithithaworn P, Bartsch H, Ohshima H, Tsuda M et al. (1998). Relationships between the synthesis of *N*-nitrosodimethylamine and immune responses to chronic infection with the carcinogenic parasite, *Opisthorchis viverrini*, in men. Carcinogenesis 19: 485-491.
2819. Sato F, Meltzer SJ (2006). CpG island hypermethylation in progression of esophageal and gastric cancer. Cancer 106: 483-493.
2820. Sato M, Ishida H, Konno K, Naganuma H, Hamashima Y, Komatsuda T et al. (2000). Liver tumors in children and young patients: sonographic and color Doppler findings. Abdom Imaging 25: 596-601.
2821. Sato N, Fukushima N, Hruban RH, Goggins M (2008). CpG island methylation profile of pancreatic intraepithelial neoplasia. Mod Pathol 21: 238-244.
2822. Sato N, Rosty C, Jansen M, Fukushima N, Ueki T, Yeo CJ et al. (2001). *STK11/LKB1* Peutz-Jeghers gene inactivation in intraductal papillary-mucinous neoplasms of the pancreas. Am J Pathol 159: 2017-2022.
2823. Sato N, Ueki T, Fukushima N, Iacobuzio-Donahue CA, Yeo CJ, Cameron JL et al. (2002). Aberrant methylation of CpG islands in intraductal papillary mucinous neoplasms of the pancreas. Gastroenterology 123: 365-372.
2824. Sato Y, Ichimura K, Tanaka T, Takata K, Morito T, Sato H et al. (2008). Duodenal follicular lymphomas share common characteristics with mucosa-associated lymphoid tissue lymphomas. J Clin Pathol 61: 377-381.
2825. Sato Y, Shimozono T, Kawano S, Toyoda K, Onoe K, Asada Y et al. (2001). Gastric carcinosarcoma, coexistence of adenosquamous carcinoma and rhabdomyosarcoma: a case report. Histopathology 39: 543-544.
2826. Sato Y, Tominaga H, Tangoku A, Hamanaka Y, Yamashita Y, Suzuki T (1992). Alpha-fetoprotein-producing cancer of the ampulla of Vater. Hepatogastroenterology 39: 566-569.
2827. Satoh K, Ohtani H, Shimosegawa T, Koizumi M, Sawai T, Toyota T (1994). Infrequent stromal expression of gelatinase A and intact basement membrane in intraductal neoplasms of the pancreas. Gastroenterology 107: 1488-1495.
2828. Satoh K, Sasano H, Shimosegawa T, Koizumi M, Yamazaki T, Mochizuki F et al. (1993). An immunohistochemical study of the *c-erbB-2* oncogene product in intraductal mucin-hypersecreting neoplasms and in ductal cell carcinomas of the pancreas. Cancer 72: 51-56.
2829. Saw EC, Yu GS, Wagner G, Heng Y (1997). Synchronous primary neuroendocrine carcinoma and adenocarcinoma in Barrett's esophagus. J Clin Gastroenterol 24: 116-119.
2830. Saxena R, Leake JL, Shafford EA, Davenport M, Mowat AP, Pritchard J et al. (1993). Chemotherapy effects on hepatoblastoma. A histological study. Am J Surg Pathol 17: 1266-1271.
2831. Sayed MG, Ahmed AF, Ringold JR, Anderson ME, Bair JL, Mitros FA et al. (2002). Germline SMAD4 or BMPR1A mutations and phenotype of juvenile polyposis. Ann Surg Oncol 9: 901-906.
2832. Scarpa A, Capelli P, Zamboni G, Oda T, Mukai K, Bonetti F et al. (1993). Neoplasia of the ampulla of Vater. Ki-ras and p53 mutations. Am J Pathol 142: 1163-1172.
2832A. Scarpa A, Mantovani W, Capelli P, Beghelli S, Boninsegna L, Bettini R et al. (2010). Pancreatic endocrine tumors: improved TNM staging and histopathological grading permit a clinically efficient prognostic stratification of patients. Mod Pathol 23: 824-833.
2833. Scarpis M, De MM, Pezzotta MG, Sonnino D, Mosca D, Milani M (1998). Endoscopic resection of esophageal lymphangioma incidentally discovered. Diagn Ther Endosc 4: 141-147.
2834. Scelo G, Boffetta P, Hemminki K, Pukkala E, Olsen JH, Andersen A et al. (2006). Associations between small intestine cancer and other primary cancers: an international population-based study. Int J Cancer 118: 189-196.
2835. Scerpella EG, Villareal AA, Casanova PF, Moreno JN (1996). Primary lymphoma of the liver in AIDS. Report of one new case and review of the literature. J Clin Gastroenterol 22: 51-53.
2836. Scheil-Bertram S, Lorenz D, Ell C, Sheremet E, Fisseler-Eckhoff A (2008). Expression of alpha-methylacyl coenzyme A racemase in the dysplasia carcinoma sequence associated with Barrett's esophagus. Mod Pathol 21: 961-967.
2837. Scheimberg I, Cullinane C, Kelsey A, Malone M (1996). Primary hepatic malignant tumor with rhabdoid features. A histological, immunocytochemical, and electron microscopic study of four cases and a review of the literature. Am J Surg Pathol 20: 1394-1400.
2838. Schildhaus HU, Cavlar T, Binot E, Buttner R, Wardelmann E, Merkelbach-Bruse S (2008). Inflammatory fibroid polyps harbour mutations in the platelet-derived growth factor receptor alpha (*PDGFRA*) gene. J Pathol 216: 176-182.
2839. Schlemper RJ, Dawsey SM, Itabashi M, Iwashita A, Kato Y, Koike M et al. (2000). Differences in diagnostic criteria for esophageal squamous cell carcinoma between Japanese and Western pathologists. Cancer 88: 996-1006.
2840. Schlemper RJ, Itabashi M, Kato Y, Lewin KJ, Riddell RH, Shimoda T et al. (1997). Differences in diagnostic criteria for gastric carcinoma between Japanese and western pathologists. Lancet 349: 1725-1729.
2841. Schlemper RJ, Kato Y, Stolte M (2001). Review of histological classifications of gastrointestinal epithelial neoplasia: differences in diagnosis of early carcinomas between Japanese and Western pathologists. J Gastroenterol 36: 445-456.
2842. Schlemper RJ, Riddell RH, Kato Y, Borchard F, Cooper HS, Dawsey SM et al. (2000). The Vienna classification of gastrointestinal epithelial neoplasia. Gut 47: 251-255.
2843. Schlosnagle DC, Campbell WG, Jr. (1981). The papillary and solid neoplasm of the pancreas: a report of two cases with electron microscopy, one containing neurosecretory granules. Cancer 47: 2603-2610.
2844. Schmidt CM, Matos JM, Bentrem DJ, Talamonti MS, Lillemoe KD, Bilimoria KY (2008). Acinar cell carcinoma of the pancreas in the United States: prognostic factors and comparison to ductal adenocarcinoma. J Gastrointest Surg 12: 2078-2086.
2845. Schmitt AM, Anlauf M, Rousson V, Schmid S, Kofler A, Riniker F et al. (2007). WHO 2004 criteria and CK19 are reliable prognostic markers in pancreatic endocrine tumors. Am J Surg Pathol 31: 1677-1682.
2846. Schmitt AM, Riniker F, Anlauf M, Schmid S, Soltermann A, Moch H et al. (2008). Islet 1 (Isl1) expression is a reliable marker for pancreatic endocrine tumors and their metastases. Am J Surg Pathol 32: 420-425.
2847. Schmutte C, Marinescu RC, Copeland NG, Jenkins NA, Overhauser J, Fishel R (1998). Refined chromosomal localization of the mismatch repair and hereditary nonpolyposis colorectal cancer genes *hMSH2* and *hMSH6*. Cancer Res 58: 5023-5026.
2848. Schnelldorfer T, Sarr MG, Nagorney DM, Zhang L, Smyrk TC, Qin R et al. (2008). Experience with 208 resections for intraductal papillary mucinous neoplasm of the pancreas. Arch Surg 143: 639-646.
2849. Schnelldorfer T, Ware AL, Sarr MG, Smyrk TC, Zhang L, Qin R et al. (2008). Long-term survival after pancreatoduodenectomy for pancreatic adenocarcinoma: is cure possible? Ann Surg 247: 456-462.
2850. Scholefield JH, Castle MT, Watson NF (2005). Malignant transformation of high-grade anal intraepithelial neoplasia. Br J Surg 92: 1133-1136.
2851. Scholefield JH, Johnson J, Hitchcock A, Kocjan G, Smith JH, Smith PA et al. (1998). Guidelines for anal cytology—to make cytological diagnosis and follow up much more reliable. Cytopathology 9: 15-22.
2851A. Scholefield JH, Sonnex C, Talbot IC, Palmer JG, Whatrup C, Miindel A et al. (1989). Anal and cervical intraepithelial neoplasia: possible parallel. Lancet 2: 765–769.
2852. Schonleben F, Qiu W, Bruckman KC, Ciau NT, Li X, Lauerman MH et al. (2007). *BRAF* and *KRAS* gene mutations in intraductal papillary mucinous neoplasm/carcinoma (IPMN/IPMC) of the pancreas. Cancer Lett 249: 242-248.
2853. Schonleben F, Qiu W, Ciau NT, Ho DJ, Li X, Allendorf JD et al. (2006). PIK3CA mutations in intraductal papillary mucinous neoplasm/carcinoma of the pancreas. Clin Cancer Res 12: 3851-3855.
2854. Schottenfeld D, Beebe-Dimmer JL, Vigneau FD (2009). The epidemiology and pathogenesis of neoplasia in the small intestine. Ann Epidemiol 19: 58-69.
2855. Schrader KA, Masciari S, Boyd N, Wiyrick S, Kaurah P, Senz J et al. (2008). Hereditary diffuse gastric cancer: association with lobular breast cancer. Fam Cancer 7: 73-82.
2856. Schrager CA, Schneider D, Gruener AC, Tsou HC, Peacocke M (1998). Clinical and pathological features of breast disease in Cowden's syndrome: an underrecognized syndrome with an increased risk of breast cancer. Hum Pathol 29: 47-53.
2857. Schron DS, Mendelsohn G (1984). Pancreatic carcinoma with duct, endocrine, and acinar differentiation. A histologic, immunocytochemical, and ultrastructural study. Cancer 54: 1766-1770.
2858. Schussler MH, Skoudy A, Ramaekers F, Real FX (1992). Intermediate filaments as differentiation markers of normal pancreas and pancreas cancer. Am J Pathol 140: 559-568.
2859. Schutte M, da Costa LT, Hahn SA, Moskaluk C, Hoque AT, Rozenblum E et al.

(1995). Identification by representational difference analysis of a homozygous deletion in pancreatic carcinoma that lies within the BRCA2 region. Proc Natl Acad Sci U S A 92: 5950-5954.

2860. Schutte M, Hruban RH, Geradts J, Maynard R, Hilgers W, Rabindran SK et al. (1997). Abrogation of the Rb/p16 tumor-suppressive pathway in virtually all pancreatic carcinomas. Cancer Res 57: 3126-3130.

2861. Schwab AL, Tuohy TM, Condie M, Neklason DW, Burt RW (2008). Gonadal mosaicism and familial adenomatous polyposis. Fam Cancer 7: 173-177.

2862. Schwartz S Jr, Yamamoto H, Navarro M, Maestro M, Reventos J, Perucho M (1999). Frameshift mutations at mononucleotide repeats in caspase-5 and other target genes in endometrial and gastrointestinal cancer of the microsatellite mutator phenotype. Cancer Res 59: 2995-3002.

2863. Schweizer J, Bowden PE, Coulombe PA, Langbein L, Lane EB, Magin TM et al. (2006). New consensus nomenclature for mammalian keratins. J Cell Biol 174: 169-174.

2864. Sclafani LM, Reuter VE, Coit DG, Brennan MF (1991). The malignant nature of papillary and cystic neoplasm of the pancreas. Cancer 68: 153-158.

2865. Scoazec JY, Degott C, Reynes M, Benhamou JP, Feldmann G (1989). Epithelioid hemangioendothelioma of the liver: an ultrastructural study. Hum Pathol 20: 673-681.

2866. Scott N, Jamali A, Verbeke C, Ambrose NS, Botterill ID, Jayne DG (2008). Retroperitoneal margin involvement by adenocarcinoma of the caecum and ascending colon: what does it mean? Colorectal Dis 10: 289-293.

2867. Scott NA, Beart RW, Jr., Weiland LH, Cha SS, Lieber MM (1989). Carcinoma of the anal canal and flow cytometric DNA analysis. Br J Cancer 60: 56-58.

2867A. Segen JC (2006). Concise dictionary of modern medicine. New York: McGraw-HillMmedical.

2868. Seidel G, Zahurak M, Iacobuzio-Donahue C, Sohn TA, Adsay NV, Yeo CJ et al. (2002). Almost all infiltrating colloid carcinomas of the pancreas and periampullary region arise from in situ papillary neoplasms: a study of 39 cases. Am J Surg Pathol 26: 56-63.

2869. Seifert E, Schulte F, Stolte M (1992). Adenoma and carcinoma of the duodenum and papilla of Vater: a clinicopathologic study. Am J Gastroenterol 87: 37-42.

2870. Selby DM, Stocker JT, Waclawiw MA, Hitchcock CL, Ishak KG (1994). Infantile hemangioendothelioma of the liver. Hepatology 20: 39-45.

2871. Sellner F (1990). Investigations on the significance of the adenoma-carcinoma sequence in the small bowel. Cancer 66: 702-715.

2872. Selves J (2009). [Histological types and prognostic factors in colorectal cancer]. Med Sci (Paris) 25 Spec No 1: 9-12.

2873. Selves J, Meggetto F, Brousset P, Voigt JJ, Pradere B, Grasset D et al. (1996). Inflammatory pseudotumor of the liver. Evidence for follicular dendritic reticulum cell proliferation associated with clonal Epstein-Barr virus. Am J Surg Pathol 20: 747-753.

2874. Senda E, Fujimoto K, Ohnishi K, Higashida A, Ashida C, Okutani T et al. (2009). Minute ampullary carcinoid tumor with lymph node metastases: a case report and review of literature. World J Surg Oncol 7: 9-

2875. Sendler A, Avril N, Helmberger H, Stollfuss J, Weber W, Bengel F et al. (2000). Preoperative evaluation of pancreatic masses with positron emission tomography using 18F-fluorodeoxyglucose: diagnostic limitations. World J Surg 24: 1121-1129.

2876. Sener SF, Fremgen A, Menck HR, Winchester DP (1999). Pancreatic cancer: a report of treatment and survival trends for 100,313 patients diagnosed from 1985-1995, using the National Cancer Database. J Am Coll Surg 189: 1-7.

2877. Senter L, Clendenning M, Sotamaa K, Hampel H, Green J, Potter JD et al. (2008). The clinical phenotype of Lynch syndrome due to germ-line PMS2 mutations. Gastroenterology 135: 419-428.

2878. Sequens R (1997). Cancer in the anal canal (transitional zone) after restorative proctocolectomy with stapled ileal pouch-anal anastomosis. Int J Colorectal Dis 12: 254-255.

2879. Seremetis MG, Lyons WS, deGuzman VC, Peabody JW, Jr. (1976). Leiomyomata of the esophagus. An analysis of 838 cases. Cancer 38: 2166-2177.

2880. Serra S, Chetty R (2008). Revision 2: an immunohistochemical approach and evaluation of solid pseudopapillary tumour of the pancreas. J Clin Pathol 61: 1153-1159.

2881. Serrano J, Goebel SU, Peghini PL, Lubensky IA, Gibril F, Jensen RT (2000). Alterations in the p16INK4a/CDKN2A tumor suppressor gene in gastrinomas. J Clin Endocrinol Metab 85: 4146-4156.

2882. Service FJ, Dale AJ, Elveback LR, Jiang NS (1976). Insulinoma: clinical and diagnostic features of 60 consecutive cases. Mayo Clin Proc 51: 417-429.

2883. Service FJ, McMahon MM, O'Brien PC, Ballard DJ (1991). Functioning insulinoma—incidence, recurrence, and long-term survival of patients: a 60-year study. Mayo Clin Proc 66: 711-719.

2884. Sessa F, Bonato M, Frigerio B, Capella C, Solcia E, Prat M et al. (1990). Ductal cancers of the pancreas frequently express markers of gastrointestinal epithelial cells. Gastroenterology 98: 1655-1665.

2885. Sessa F, Furlan D, Zampatti C, Carnevali I, Franzi F, Capella C (2007). Prognostic factors for ampullary adenocarcinomas: tumor stage, tumor histology, tumor location, immunohistochemistry and microsatellite instability. Virchows Arch 451: 649-657.

2886. Sessa F, Solcia E, Capella C, Bonato M, Scarpa A, Zamboni G et al. (1994). Intraductal papillary-mucinous tumours represent a distinct group of pancreatic neoplasms: an investigation of tumour cell differentiation and K-ras, p53 and c-erbB-2 abnormalities in 26 patients. Virchows Arch 425: 357-367.

2887. Seth R, Crook S, Ibrahem S, Fadhil W, Jackson D, Ilyas M (2009). Concomitant mutations and splice variants in KRAS and BRAF demonstrate complex perturbation of the Ras/Raf signalling pathway in advanced colorectal cancer. Gut 58: 1234-1241.

2888. Seymour AB, Hruban RH, Redston M, Caldas C, Powell SM, Kinzler KW et al. (1994). Allelotype of pancreatic adenocarcinoma. Cancer Res 54: 2761-2764.

2889. Shackelford DB, Vasquez DS, Corbeil J, Wu S, Leblanc M, Wu CL et al. (2009). mTOR and HIF-1alpha-mediated tumor metabolism in an LKB1 mouse model of Peutz-Jeghers syndrome. Proc Natl Acad Sci U S A 106: 11137-11142.

2890. Shaffer EA (2006). Gallstone disease: Epidemiology of gallbladder stone disease. Best Pract Res Clin Gastroenterol 20: 981-996.

2891. Shafford EA, Pritchard J (1993). Extreme thrombocytosis as a diagnostic clue to hepatoblastoma. Arch Dis Child 69: 171-

2892. Shafizadeh N, Ferrell LD, Kakar S (2008). Utility and limitations of glypican-3 expression for the diagnosis of hepatocellular carcinoma at both ends of the differentiation spectrum. Mod Pathol 21: 1011-1018.

2893. Shafqat A, Merchant M, Malik IA (1996). Clinico-pathological features and survival of patients presenting with hepatic metastases: a retrospective analysis. J Pak Med Assoc 46: 99-102.

2894. Shah SM, Smart DF, Texter EC, Jr., Morris WD (1977). Metastatic melanoma of the stomach: the endoscopic and roentgenographic findings and review of the literature. South Med J 70: 379-381.

2895. Shahabi M, Noori Daloii MR, Langan JE, Rowbottom L, Jahanzad E, Khoshbin E et al. (2004). An investigation of the tylosis with oesophageal cancer (TOC) locus in Iranian patients with oesophageal squamous cell carcinoma. Int J Oncol 25: 389-395.

2896. Shaheen NJ, Richter JE (2009). Barrett's oesophagus. Lancet 373: 850-861.

2897. Shahi KS, Geeta B, Rajput P (2009). Solitary hepatic lymphangioma in a 22-day-old infant. J Pediatr Surg 44: E9-11.

2898. Shaib YH, Davila JA, McGlynn K, El-Serag HB (2004). Rising incidence of intrahepatic cholangiocarcinoma in the United States: a true increase? J Hepatol 40: 472-477.

2899. Shaib YH, El-Serag HB, Davila JA, Morgan R, McGlynn KA (2005). Risk factors of intrahepatic cholangiocarcinoma in the United States: a case-control study. Gastroenterology 128: 620-626.

2900. Shan L, Nakamura Y, Nakamura M, Yokoi T, Tsujimoto M, Arima R et al. (1998). Somatic mutations of multiple endocrine neoplasia type 1 gene in the sporadic endocrine tumors. Lab Invest 78: 471-475.

2901. Shapiro PF, Lifvendahl RA (1931). Tumors of the Extrahepatic Bile-ducts. Ann Surg 94: 61-79.

2902. Sharif K, Ramani P, Lochbuhler H, Grundy R, de Ville de GJ (2006). Recurrent mesenchymal hamartoma associated with 19q translocation. A call for more radical surgical resection. Eur J Pediatr Surg 16: 64-67.

2903. Shariff MI, Cox IJ, Gomaa AI, Khan SA, Gedroyc W, Taylor-Robinson SD (2009). Hepatocellular carcinoma: current trends in worldwide epidemiology, risk factors, diagnosis and therapeutics. Expert Rev Gastroenterol Hepatol 3: 353-367.

2904. Sharma P, Dent J, Armstrong D, Bergman JJ, Gossner L, Hoshihara Y et al. (2006). The development and validation of an endoscopic grading system for Barrett's esophagus: the Prague C & M criteria. Gastroenterology 131: 1392-1399.

2905. Sharma P, Morales TG, Bhattacharyya A, Garewal HS, Sampliner RE (1997). Dysplasia in short-segment Barrett's esophagus: a prospective 3-year follow-up. Am J Gastroenterol 92: 2012-2016.

2906. Sharma P, Morales TG, Sampliner RE (1998). Short segment Barrett's esophagus—the need for standardization of the definition and of endoscopic criteria. Am J Gastroenterol 93: 1033-1036.

2907. Sharma P, Weston AP, Morales T, Topalovski M, Mayo MS, Sampliner RE (2000). Relative risk of dysplasia for patients with intestinal metaplasia in the distal oesophagus and in the gastric cardia. Gut 46: 9-13.

2908. Sharma S, Green KB (2004). The pancreatic duct and its arteriovenous relationship: an underutilized aid in the diagnosis and distinction of pancreatic adenocarcinoma from pancreatic intraepithelial neoplasia. A study of 126 pancreatectomy specimens. Am J Surg Pathol 28: 613-620.

2909. Shashidharan M, Smyrk T, Lin KM, Ternent CA, Thorson AG, Blatchford GJ et al. (1999). Histologic comparison of hereditary nonpolyposis colorectal cancer associated with MSH2 and MLH1 and colorectal cancer from the

general population. Dis Colon Rectum 42: 722-726.

2910. Shaw D, Blair V, Framp A, Harawira P, McLeod M, Guilford P et al. (2005). Chromoendoscopic surveillance in hereditary diffuse gastric cancer: an alternative to prophylactic gastrectomy? Gut 54: 461-468.

2911. Shaw PA, Pringle JH (1992). The demonstration of a subset of carcinoid tumours of the appendix by in situ hybridization using synthetic probes to proglucagon mRNA. J Pathol 167: 375-380.

2912. Shaw RJ, Omar MM, Rokadiya S, Kogera FA, Lowe D, Hall GL et al. (2009). Cytoglobin is upregulated by tumour hypoxia and silenced by promoter hypermethylation in head and neck cancer. Br J Cancer 101: 139-144.

2913. Shek TW, Ng IO, Chan KW (1993). Inflammatory pseudotumor of the liver. Report of four cases and review of the literature. Am J Surg Pathol 17: 231-238.

2914. Shekitka KM, Sobin LH (1994). Ganglioneuromas of the gastrointestinal tract. Relation to Von Recklinghausen disease and other multiple tumor syndromes. Am J Surg Pathol 18: 250-257.

2915. Shelton AA, Lehman RE, Schrock TR, Welton ML (1996). Retrospective review of colorectal cancer in ulcerative colitis at a tertiary center. Arch Surg 131: 806-810.

2916. Shemesh E, Bat L (1985). A prospective evaluation of the upper gastrointestinal tract and periampullary region in patients with Gardner syndrome. Am J Gastroenterol 80: 825-827.

2917. Shen J, Brugge WR, Dimaio CJ, Pitman MB (2009). Molecular analysis of pancreatic cyst fluid: a comparative analysis with current practice of diagnosis. Cancer Cytopathol 117: 217-227.

2918. Shen L, Toyota M, Kondo Y, Lin E, Zhang L, Guo Y et al. (2007). Integrated genetic and epigenetic analysis identifies three different subclasses of colon cancer. Proc Natl Acad Sci U S A 104: 18654-18659.

2919. Shen WH, Balajee AS, Wang J, Wu H, Eng C, Pandolfi PP et al. (2007). Essential role for nuclear PTEN in maintaining chromosomal integrity. Cell 128: 157-170.

2920. Sheng L, Weixia Z, Longhai Y, Jinming Y (2005). Clinical and biologic analysis of pancreatoblastoma. Pancreas 30: 87-90.

2921. Shepherd NA (1995). Pouchitis and neoplasia in the pelvic ileal reservoir. Gastroenterology 109: 1381-1383.

2922. Shepherd NA, Blackshaw AJ, Hall PA, Bostad L, Coates PJ, Lowe DG et al. (1987). Malignant lymphoma with eosinophilia of the gastrointestinal tract. Histopathology 11: 115-130.

2923. Shepherd NA, Bussey HJ, Jass JR (1987). Epithelial misplacement in Peutz-Jeghers polyps. A diagnostic pitfall. Am J Surg Pathol 11: 743-749.

2924. Shepherd NA, Hall PA (1990). Epithelial-mesenchymal interactions can influence the phenotype of carcinoma metastases in the mucosa of the intestine. J Pathol 160: 103-109.

2925. Shepherd NA, Hall PA, Coates PJ, Levison DA (1988). Primary malignant lymphoma of the colon and rectum. A histopathological and immunohistochemical analysis of 45 cases with clinicopathological correlations. Histopathology 12: 235-252.

2926. Shepherd NA, Scholefield JH, Love SB, England J, Northover JM (1990). Prognostic factors in anal squamous carcinoma: a multivariate analysis of clinical, pathological and flow cytometric parameters in 235 cases. Histopathology 16: 545-555.

2927. Sheridan TB, Fenton H, Lewin MR, Burkart AL, Iacobuzio-Donahue CA, Frankel WL et al. (2006). Sessile serrated adenomas with low- and high-grade dysplasia and early carcinomas: an immunohistochemical study of serrated lesions "caught in the act". Am J Clin Pathol 126: 564-571.

2928. Sherman SP, Li CY, Carney JA (1979). Microproliferation of enterochromaffin cells and the origin of carcinoid tumors of the ileum: a light microscopic and immunocytochemical study. Arch Pathol Lab Med 103: 639-641.

2929. Shi C, Hong SM, Lim P, Kamiyama H, Khan M, Anders RA et al. (2009). KRAS2 mutations in human pancreatic acinar-ductal metaplastic lesions are limited to those with PanIN: implications for the human pancreatic cancer cell of origin. Mol Cancer Res 7: 230-236.

2930. Shi C, Klein AP, Goggins M, Maitra A, Canto M, Ali S et al. (2009). Increased Prevalence of Precursor Lesions in Familial Pancreatic Cancer Patients. Clin Cancer Res 15: 7737-7743.

2931. Shi XY, Bhagwandeen B, Leong AS (2008). p16, cyclin D1, Ki-67, and AMACR as markers for dysplasia in Barrett esophagus. Appl Immunohistochem Mol Morphol 16: 447-452.

2932. Shia J, Tang LH, Weiser MR, Brenner B, Adsay NV, Stelow EB et al. (2008). Is nonsmall cell type high-grade neuroendocrine carcinoma of the tubular gastrointestinal tract a distinct disease entity? Am J Surg Pathol 32: 719-731.

2933. Shibahara H, Tamada S, Goto M, Oda K, Nagino M, Nagasaka T et al. (2004). Pathologic features of mucin-producing bile duct tumors: two histopathologic categories as counterparts of pancreatic intraductal papillary-mucinous neoplasms. Am J Surg Pathol 28: 327-338.

2934. Shih CH, Ozawa S, Ando N, Ueda M, Kitajima M (2000). Vascular endothelial growth factor expression predicts outcome and lymph node metastasis in squamous cell carcinoma of the esophagus. Clin Cancer Res 6: 1161-1168.

2935. Shikata K, Kiyohara Y, Kubo M, Yonemoto K, Ninomiya T, Shirota T et al. (2006). A prospective study of dietary salt intake and gastric cancer incidence in a defined Japanese population: the Hisayama study. Int J Cancer 119: 196-201.

2936. Shim KN, Yang SK, Myung SJ, Chang HS, Jung SA, Choe JW et al. (2004). Atypical endoscopic features of rectal carcinoids. Endoscopy 36: 313-316.

2936A. Shim YH, Park HJ, Choi MS, Kim JS, Kim H, Kim JJ, Jang JJ, Yu E (2003). Hypermethylation of the p16 gene and lack of p16 expression in hepatoblastoma. Mod Pathol 16 430-436.

2937. Shimada H, Kitabayashi H, Nabeya Y, Okazumi S, Matsubara H, Funami Y et al. (2003). Treatment response and prognosis of patients after recurrence of esophageal cancer. Surgery 133: 24-31.

2938. Shimada H, Matsubara H, Okazumi S, Isono K, Ochiai T (2008). Improved surgical results in thoracic esophageal squamous cell carcinoma: a 40-year analysis of 792 patients. J Gastrointest Surg 12: 518-526.

2939. Shimada K, Sakamoto Y, Sano T, Kosuge T (2006). Prognostic factors after distal pancreatectomy with extended lymphadenectomy for invasive pancreatic adenocarcinoma of the body and tail. Surgery 139: 288-295.

2940. Shimada K, Sakamoto Y, Sano T, Kosuge T, Hiraoka N (2006). Invasive carcinoma originating in an intraductal papillary mucinous neoplasm of the pancreas: a clinicopathologic comparison with a common type of invasive ductal carcinoma. Pancreas 32: 281-287.

2941. Shimada K, Sakamoto Y, Sano T, Kosuge T, Hiraoka N (2006). Reappraisal of the clinical significance of tumor size in patients with pancreatic ductal carcinoma. Pancreas 33: 233-239.

2942. Shimada-Hiratsuka M, Fukayama M,

Hayashi Y, Ushijima T, Suzuki M, Hishima T et al. (1997). Primary gastric T-cell lymphoma with and without human T-lymphotropic virus type 1. Cancer 80: 292-303.

2943. Shimamura T, Sakamoto M, Ino Y, Sato Y, Shimada K, Kosuge T et al. (2003). Dysadherin overexpression in pancreatic ductal adenocarcinoma reflects tumor aggressiveness: relationship to e-cadherin expression. J Clin Oncol 21: 659-667.

2944. Shimer GR, Helwig EB (1984). Inflammatory fibroid polyps of the intestine. Am J Clin Pathol 81: 708-714.

2945. Shimizu M, Ban S, Odze RD (2007). Squamous dysplasia and other precursor lesions related to esophageal squamous cell carcinoma. Gastroenterol Clin North Am 36: 797-811.

2946. Shimizu M, Nagata K, Yamaguchi H, Kita H (2009). Squamous intraepithelial neoplasia of the esophagus: past, present, and future. J Gastroenterol 44: 103-112.

2947. Shimizu T, Tajiri T, Akimaru K, Arima Y, Yoshida H, Yokomuro S et al. (2006). Combined neuroendocrine cell carcinoma and adenocarcinoma of the gallbladder: report of a case. J Nippon Med Sch 73: 101-105.

2948. Shin HJ, Lahoti S, Sneige N (2002). Endoscopic ultrasound-guided fine-needle aspiration in 179 cases: the M. D. Anderson Cancer Center experience. Cancer 96: 174-180.

2949. Shinagawa T, Tadokoro M, Maeyama S, Maeda C, Yamaguchi S, Morohoshi T et al. (1995). Alpha fetoprotein-producing acinar cell carcinoma of the pancreas showing multiple lines of differentiation. Virchows Arch 426: 419-423.

2950. Shinmura K, Goto M, Tao H, Shimizu S, Otsuki Y, Kobayashi H et al. (2005). A novel STK11 germline mutation in two siblings with Peutz-Jeghers syndrome complicated by primary gastric cancer. Clin Genet 67: 81-86.

2951. Shinozaki H, Ozawa S, Ando N, Tsuruta H, Terada M, Ueda M et al. (1996). Cyclin D1 amplification as a new predictive classification for squamous cell carcinoma of the esophagus, adding gene information. Clin Cancer Res 2: 1155-1161.

2952. Shiono S, Suda K, Nobukawa B, Arakawa A, Yamasaki S, Sasahara N et al. (2006). Pancreatic, hepatic, splenic, and mesenteric mucinous cystic neoplasms (MCN) are lumped together as extra ovarian MCN. Pathol Int 56: 71-77.

2953. Shiota K, Taguchi J, Nakashima O, Nakashima M, Kojiro M (2001). Clinicopathologic study on cholangiolocellular carcinoma. Oncol Rep 8: 263-268.

2954. Shipp MA (1994). Prognostic factors in aggressive non-Hodgkin's lymphoma: who has "high-risk" disease? Blood 83: 1165-1173.

2955. Shiratsuchi H, Saito T, Sakamoto A, Itakura E, Tamiya S, Oshiro Y et al. (2002). Mutation analysis of human cytokeratin 8 gene in malignant rhabdoid tumor: a possible association with intracytoplasmic inclusion body formation. Mod Pathol 15: 146-153.

2956. Shiroshita H, Watanabe H, Ajioka Y, Watanabe G, Nishikura K, Kitano S (2004). Re-evaluation of mucin phenotypes of gastric minute well-differentiated-type adenocarcinomas using a series of HGM, MUC5AC, MUC6, M-GGMC, MUC2 and CD10 stains. Pathol Int 54: 311-321.

2957. Sho M, Nakajima Y, Kanehiro H, Hisanaga M, Nishio K, Nagao M et al. (1998). Pattern of recurrence after resection for intraductal papillary mucinous tumors of the pancreas. World J Surg 22: 874-878.

2958. Shorter NA, Glick RD, Klimstra DS, Brennan MF, Laquaglia MP (2002). Malignant pancreatic tumors in childhood and adolescence: The Memorial Sloan-Kettering experience, 1967 to present. J Pediatr Surg 37: 887-892.

2959. Shousha S (1979). Paneth cell-rich papillary adenocarcinoma and a mucoid adenocarcinoma occurring synchronously in colon: a light and electron microscopic study. Histopathology 3: 489-501.

2960. Shuangshoti S, Thaicharoen A (1994). Hepatocellular adenoma in a beta-thalassemic woman having secondary iron overload. J Med Assoc Thai 77: 108-112.

2961. Sieber OM, Lipton L, Crabtree M, Heinimann K, Fidalgo P, Phillips RK et al. (2003). Multiple colorectal adenomas, classic adenomatous polyposis, and germ-line mutations in MYH. N Engl J Med 348: 791-799.

2962. Siegal A, Swartz A (1986). Malignant carcinoid of oesophagus. Histopathology 10: 761-765.

2963. Siewert JR, Stein HJ (1998). Classification of adenocarcinoma of the oesophagogastric junction. Br J Surg 85: 1457-1459.

2964. Siewert JR, Stein HJ, Feith M (2006). Adenocarcinoma of the esophago-gastric junction. Scand J Surg 95: 260-269.

2965. Sigel JE, Goldblum JR (1998). Neuroendocrine neoplasms arising in inflammatory bowel disease: a report of 14 cases. Mod Pathol 11: 537-542.

2966. Sigel JE, Petras RE, Lashner BA, Fazio VW, Goldblum JR (1999). Intestinal adenocarcinoma in Crohn's disease: a report of 30 cases with a focus on coexisting dysplasia. Am J Surg Pathol 23: 651-655.

2967. Silverman DT, Hoover RN, Brown LM, Swanson GM, Schiffman M, Greenberg RS et al. (2003). Why do Black Americans have a higher risk of pancreatic cancer than White Americans? Epidemiology 14: 45-54.

2968. Silverman JF, Holbrook CT, Pories WJ, Kodroff MB, Joshi VV (1990). Fine needle aspiration cytology of pancreatoblastoma with immunocytochemical and ultrastructural studies. Acta Cytol 34: 632-640.

2969. Siman JH, Engstrand L, Berglund G, Forsgren A, Floren CH (2007). Helicobacter pylori and CagA seropositivity and its association with gastric and oesophageal carcinoma. Scand J Gastroenterol 42: 933-940.

2970. Siman JH, Forsgren A, Berglund G, Floren CH (2001). Tobacco smoking increases the risk for gastric adenocarcinoma among Helicobacter pylori-infected individuals. Scand J Gastroenterol 36: 208-213.

2971. Simchuk EJ, Low DE (2001). Direct esophageal metastasis from a distant primary tumor is a submucosal process: a review of six cases. Dis Esophagus 14: 247-250.

2972. Simpson EL, Dalinka MK (1985). Association of hypertrophic osteoarthropathy with gastrointestinal polyposis. AJR Am J Roentgenol 144: 983-984.

2973. Singh AD, Bergman L, Seregard S (2005). Uveal melanoma: epidemiologic aspects. Ophthalmol Clin North Am 18: 75-84.

2974. Singh B, Mortensen NJ, Warren BF (2007). Histopathological mimicry in mucosal prolapse. Histopathology 50: 97-102.

2975. Sinicrope FA, Sargent DJ (2009). Clinical implications of microsatellite instability in sporadic colon cancers. Curr Opin Oncol 21: 369-373.

2976. Sinkre PA, Murakata L, Rabin L, Hoang MP, Albores-Saavedra J (2001). Clear cell carcinoid tumor of the gallbladder: another distinctive manifestation of von Hippel-Lindau disease. Am J Surg Pathol 25: 1334-1339.

2977. Sinn DH, Chang DK, Kim YH, Rhee PL, Kim JJ, Kim DS et al. (2009). Effectiveness of each Bethesda marker in defining microsatellite instability when screening for Lynch syndrome. Hepatogastroenterology 56: 672-676.

2978. Sinning C, Schaefer N, Standop J, Hirner A, Wolff M (2007). Gastric stump carcinoma -

epidemiology and current concepts in pathogenesis and treatment. Eur J Surg Oncol 33: 133-139.

2979. Sipos B, Frank S, Gress T, Hahn S, Klöppel G (2009). Pancreatic intraepithelial neoplasia revisited and updated. Pancreatology 9: 45-54.

2980. Sipos B, Klöppel G (2005). [Acinar cell carcinomas and pancreatoblastomas: related but not the same]. Pathologe 26: 37-40.

2981. Sitzmann JV, Coleman J, Pitt HA, Zerhouni E, Fishman E, Kaufman SL et al. (1990). Preoperative assessment of malignant hepatic tumors. Am J Surg 159: 137-142.

2982. Sjoblom SM (1988). Clinical presentation and prognosis of gastrointestinal carcinoid tumours. Scand J Gastroenterol 23: 779-787.

2983. Skoglund J, Djureinovic T, Zhou XL, Vandrovcova J, Renkonen E, Iselius L et al. (2006). Linkage analysis in a large Swedish family supports the presence of a susceptibility locus for adenoma and colorectal cancer on chromosome 9q22.32-31.1. J Med Genet 43: e7

2984. Slovis TL, Roebuck DJ (2006). Hepatoblastoma: why so many low-birth-weight infants? Pediatr Radiol 36: 173-174.

2985. Smeenk RM, van Velthuysen ML, Verwaal VJ, Zoetmulder FA (2008). Appendiceal neoplasms and pseudomyxoma peritonei: a population based study. Eur J Surg Oncol 34: 196-201.

2986. Smiley D, Goldberg RI, Phillips RS, Barkin JS (1988). Anal metastasis from colorectal carcinoma. Am J Gastroenterol 83: 460-462.

2987. Smith DP, Spicer J, Smith A, Swift S, Ashworth A (1999). The mouse Peutz-Jeghers syndrome gene LKB1 encodes a nuclear protein kinase. Hum Mol Genet 8: 1479-1485.

2988. Smith JL, Dixon MF (2003). Is subtyping of intestinal metaplasia in the upper gastrointestinal tract a worthwhile exercise? An evaluation of current mucin histochemical stains. Br J Biomed Sci 60: 180-186.

2989. Smith JW, Kemeny N, Caldwell C, Banner P, Sigurdson E, Huvos A (1992). Pseudomyxoma peritonei of appendiceal origin. The Memorial Sloan-Kettering Cancer Center experience. Cancer 70: 396-401.

2990. Smith MG, Hold GL, Tahara E, El-Omar EM (2006). Cellular and molecular aspects of gastric cancer. World J Gastroenterol 12: 2979-2990.

2991. Smith RR, Hamilton SR, Boitnott JK, Rogers EL (1984). The spectrum of carcinoma arising in Barrett's esophagus. A clinicopathologic study of 26 patients. Am J Surg Pathol 8: 563-573.

2992. Sneige N, Ordonez NG, Veanattukalathil S, Samaan NA (1987). Fine-needle aspiration cytology in pancreatic endocrine tumors. Diagn Cytopathol 3: 35-40.

2993. Snover DC (2005). Serrated polyps of the large intestine. Semin Diagn Pathol 22: 301-308.

2994. Snover DC, Jass JR, Fenoglio-Preiser C, Batts KP (2005). Serrated polyps of the large intestine: a morphologic and molecular review of an evolving concept. Am J Clin Pathol 124: 380-391.

2995. Sobel JM, Lai R, Mallery S, Levy MJ, Wiersema MJ, Greenwald BD et al. (2005). The utility of EUS-guided FNA in the diagnosis of metastatic breast cancer to the esophagus and the mediastinum. Gastrointest Endosc 61: 416-420.

2996. Sobin LH, Gospodarowicz MK, and Wittekind C (eds) (2009). TNM Classification of Malignant Tumours. Wiley-Blackwell: Oxford, UK.

2997. Sobol S, Cooperman AM (1978). Villous adenoma of the ampulla of Vater. An unusual cause of biliary colic and obstructive jaundice. Gastroenterology 75: 107-109.

2998. Soga J (2003). Endocrinocarcinomas (carcinoids and their variants) of the duodenum. An evaluation of 927 cases. J Exp Clin Cancer Res 22: 349-363.

2999. Soga J (2003). Primary endocrinomas (carcinoids and variant neoplasms) of the gallbladder. A statistical evaluation of 138 reported cases. J Exp Clin Cancer Res 22: 5-15.

3000. Soga J (2005). Early-stage carcinoids of the gastrointestinal tract: an analysis of 1914 reported cases. Cancer 103: 1587-1595.

3001. Soga J, Tazawa K (1971). Pathologic analysis of carcinoids. Histologic reevaluation of 62 cases. Cancer 28: 990-998.

3002. Soga J, Yakuwa Y, Osaka M (1998). Insulinoma/hypoglycemic syndrome: a statistical evaluation of 1085 reported cases of a Japanese series. J Exp Clin Cancer Res 17: 379-388.

3003. Sogabe M, Taniki T, Fukui Y, Yoshida T, Okamoto K, Okita Y et al. (2006). A patient with esophageal hemangioma treated by endoscopic mucosal resection: a case report and review of the literature. J Med Invest 53: 177-182.

3004. Sohn DK, Choi HS, Chang YS, Huh JM, Kim DH, Kim DY et al. (2004). Granular cell tumor of colon: report of a case and review of literature. World J Gastroenterol 10: 2452-2454.

3005. Sohn TA, Yeo CJ, Cameron JL, Hruban RH, Fukushima N, Campbell KA et al. (2004). Intraductal papillary mucinous neoplasms of the pancreas: an updated experience. Ann Surg 239: 788-797.

3006. Sohn TA, Yeo CJ, Cameron JL, Iacobuzio-Donahue CA, Hruban RH, Lillemoe KD (2001). Intraductal papillary mucinous neoplasms of the pancreas: an increasingly recognized clinicopathologic entity. Ann Surg 234: 313-321.

3007. Sohn TA, Yeo CJ, Cameron JL, Koniaris L, Kaushal S, Abrams RA et al. (2000). Resected adenocarcinoma of the pancreas-616 patients: results, outcomes, and prognostic indicators. J Gastrointest Surg 4: 567-579.

3008. Soini Y, Welsh JA, Ishak KG, Bennett WP (1995). *p53* mutations in primary hepatic angiosarcomas not associated with vinyl chloride exposure. Carcinogenesis 16: 2879-2881.

3009. Solcia E, Bordi C, Creutzfeldt W, Dayal Y, Dayan AD, Falkmer S et al. (1988). Histopathological classification of nonantral gastric endocrine growths in man. Digestion 41: 185-200.

3010. Solcia E, Capella C, Fiocca R, Rindi G, Rosai J (1990). Gastric argyrophil carcinoidosis in patients with Zollinger-Ellison syndrome due to type 1 multiple endocrine neoplasia. A newly recognized association. Am J Surg Pathol 14: 503-513.

3011. Solcia E, Capella C, Fiocca R, Sessa F, La Rosa S, Rindi G (1998). Disorders of the endocrine system. In: Pathology of the gastrointestinal tract. Ming SC, Goldman H, eds. Williams & Wilkins: Baltimore, pp. 295-322.

3012. Solcia E, Capella C, and Klöppel G (eds) (1997). Tumours of the Pancreas. Armed Forces Institute of Pathology: Washington, DC.

3013. Solcia E, Klöppel G, and Sobin LH (eds.) (2000). Histological Typing of Endocrine Tumours. Springer-Verlag: Berlin-New York.

3014. Solcia E, Rindi G, Fiocca R, Villani L, Buffa R, Ambrosiani L et al. (1992). Distinct patterns of chronic gastritis associated with carcinoid and cancer and their role in tumorigenesis. Yale J Biol Med 65: 793-804.

3015. Sole M, Iglesias C, Fernandez-Esparrach G, Colomo L, Pellise M, Gines A (2005). Fine-needle aspiration cytology of intraductal papillary mucinous tumors of the pancreas. Cancer 105: 298-303.

3016. Soliman AS, Bondy ML, Raouf AA, Makram MA, Johnston DA, Levin B (1999). Cancer mortality in Menofeia, Egypt: comparison with US mortality rates. Cancer Causes Control 10: 349-354.

3016A.Sommerer F, Vieth M, Markwarth A, Rohrich K, Vomschloss S, May A (2004). Mutations of *BRAF* and *KRAS2* in the development of Barrett's adenocarcinoma. Oncogene 23:554-558.

3017. Song DE, Park JK, Hur B, Ro JY (2004). Carcinoid tumor arising in a tailgut cyst of the anorectal junction with distant metastasis: a case report and review of the literature. Arch Pathol Lab Med 128: 578-580.

3017A.Song HG, Yoo KS, Ju NR, Park JC, Jung JO, Shin WG, Moon JH, Kim JP, Kim KO, Park CH, Hahn T, Park SH, Kim JH, Lee IJ, Min SK, and Park CK (2006). A case of adenosquamous carcinoma of the papilla of Vater. Korean J Gastroenterol. 48: 132-136.

3018. Songsivilai S, Dharakul T, Kanistanon D (1996). Hepatitis C virus genotypes in patients with hepatocellular carcinoma and cholangiocarcinoma in Thailand. Trans R Soc Trop Med Hyg 90: 505-507.

3019. Songun I, van de Velde CJ, Arends JW, Blok P, Grond AJ, Offerhaus GJ et al. (1999). Classification of gastric carcinoma using the Goseki system provides prognostic information additional to TNM staging. Cancer 85: 2114-2118.

3020. Sonoda I, Imoto I, Inoue J, Shibata T, Shimada Y, Chin K et al. (2004). Frequent silencing of low density lipoprotein receptor-related protein 1B (LRP1B) expression by genetic and epigenetic mechanisms in esophageal squamous cell carcinoma. Cancer Res 64: 3741-3747.

3021. Sonoda Y, Yamaguchi K, Nagai E, Nakamuta M, Ito T, Eguchi T et al. (2003). Small cell carcinoma of the cystic duct: a case report. J Gastrointest Surg 7: 631-634.

3022. Sons HU, Borchard F (1984). Esophageal cancer. Autopsy findings in 171 cases. Arch Pathol Lab Med 108: 983-988.

3023. Sons HU, Borchard F (1986). Cancer of the distal esophagus and cardia. Incidence, tumorous infiltration, and metastatic spread. Ann Surg 203: 188-195.

3024. Soreide K, Nedrebo BS, Reite A, Thorsen K, Korner H (2009). Endoscopy, morphology, morphometry and molecular markers: predicting cancer risk in colorectal adenoma. Expert Rev Mol Diagn 9: 125-137.

3025. Souglakos J, Philips J, Wang R, Marwah S, Silver M, Tzardi M et al. (2009). Prognostic and predictive value of common mutations for treatment response and survival in patients with metastatic colorectal cancer. Br J Cancer 101: 465-472.

3026. Soule JC, Potet F, Mignon FC, Julien M, Bader JP (1976). [Zollinger-Ellison syndrome due to a gastric gastrinoma (author's transl)]. Arch Fr Mal App Dig 65: 215-225.

3027. Souza RF, Appel R, Yin J, Wang S, Smolinski KN, Abraham JM et al. (1996). Microsatellite instability in the insulin-like growth factor II receptor gene in gastrointestinal tumours. Nat Genet 14: 255-257.

3028. Souza RF, Spechler SJ (2005). Concepts in the prevention of adenocarcinoma of the distal esophagus and proximal stomach. CA Cancer J Clin 55: 334-351.

3029. Sowery RD, Jensen C, Morrison KB, Horsman DE, Sorensen PH, Webber EM (2001). Comparative genomic hybridization detects multiple chromosomal amplifications and deletions in undifferentiated embryonal sarcoma of the liver. Cancer Genet Cytogenet 126: 128-133.

3030. Soyer P, Bluemke DA, Hruban RH, Sitzmann JV, Fishman EK (1994). Hepatic metastases from colorectal cancer: detection and false-positive findings with helical CT during arterial portography. Radiology 193: 71-74.

3031. Soyer P, Levesque M, Elias D, Zeitoun G, Roche A (1992). Detection of liver metastases from colorectal cancer: comparison of intraoperative US and CT during arterial portography. Radiology 183: 541-544.

3032. Spano JP, Costagliola D, Katlama C, Mounier N, Oksenhendler E, Khayat D (2008). AIDS-related malignancies: state of the art and therapeutic challenges. J Clin Oncol 26: 4834-4842.

3033. Spechler SJ (1999). The role of gastric carditis in metaplasia and neoplasia at the gastroesophageal junction. Gastroenterology 117: 218-228.

3034. Spechler SJ (2002). Clinical practice. Barrett's Esophagus. N Engl J Med 346: 836-842.

3035. Spechler SJ (2004). Intestinal metaplasia at the gastroesophageal junction. Gastroenterology 126: 567-575.

3036. Spechler SJ, Goyal RK (1996). The columnar-lined esophagus, intestinal metaplasia, and Norman Barrett. Gastroenterology 110: 614-621.

3036A. Spechler SJ, Zeroogian JM, Antonioli DA, Wang HH, Goyal RK (1994). Prevalence of metaplasia at the gastro-oesophageal junction. Lancet 344: 1533–1536.

3037. Spector LG, Johnson KJ, Soler JT, Puumala SE (2008). Perinatal risk factors for hepatoblastoma. Br J Cancer 98: 1570-1573.

3038. Speleman F, De Telder V, De Potter KR, Dal CP, Van Daele S, Benoit Y et al. (1989). Cytogenetic analysis of a mesenchymal hamartoma of the liver. Cancer Genet Cytogenet 40: 29-32.

3039. Spence RW, Burns-Cox CJ (1975). ACTH-secreting 'apudoma' of gallbladder. Gut 16: 473-476.

3040. Spencer J, Cerf-Bensussan N, Jarry A, Brousse N, Guy-Grand D, Krajewski AS et al. (1988). Enteropathy-associated T cell lymphoma (malignant histiocytosis of the intestine) is recognized by a monoclonal antibody (HML-1) that defines a membrane molecule on human mucosal lymphocytes. Am J Pathol 132: 1-5.

3041. Sperti C, Pasquali C, Pedrazzoli S (1997). Ductal adenocarcinoma of the body and tail of the pancreas. J Am Coll Surg 185: 255-259.

3042. Sperti C, Pasquali C, Pedrazzoli S, Guolo P, Liessi G (1997). Expression of mucin-like carcinoma-associated antigen in the cyst fluid differentiates mucinous from nonmucinous pancreatic cysts. Am J Gastroenterol 92: 672-675.

3043. Spigelman AD, Crofton-Sleigh C, Venitt S, Phillips RK (1990). Mutagenicity of bile and duodenal adenomas in familial adenomatous polyposis. Br J Surg 77: 878-881.

3044. Spigelman AD, Farmer KC, James M, Richman PI, Phillips RK (1991). Tumours of the liver, bile ducts, pancreas and duodenum in a single patient with familial adenomatous polyposis. Br J Surg 78: 979-980.

3045. Spigelman AD, Murday V, Phillips RK (1989). Cancer and the Peutz-Jeghers syndrome. Gut 30: 1588-1590.

3046. Spigelman AD, Talbot IC, Penna C, Nugent KP, Phillips RK, Costello C et al. (1994). Evidence for adenoma-carcinoma sequence in the duodenum of patients with familial adenomatous polyposis. The Leeds Castle Polyposis Group (Upper Gastrointestinal Committee). J Clin Pathol 47: 709-710.

3047. Spigelman AD, Williams CB, Talbot IC, Domizio P, Phillips RK (1989). Upper gastrointestinal cancer in patients with familial adenomatous polyposis. Lancet 2: 783-785.

3048. Spirio LN, Samowitz W, Robertson J, Robertson M, Burt RW, Leppert M et al. (1998). Alleles of APC modulate the frequency and classes of mutations that lead to colon polyps. Nat Genet 20: 385-388.

3049. Spring KJ, Zhao ZZ, Karamatic R, Walsh MD, Whitehall VL, Pike T et al. (2006). High prevalence of sessile serrated adenomas with BRAF mutations: a prospective study of patients undergoing colonoscopy. Gastroenterology 131: 1400-1407.

3050. Spunt SL, Lobe TE, Pappo AS, Parham DM, Wharam MD, Jr., Arndt C et al. (2000). Aggressive surgery is unwarranted for biliary tract rhabdomyosarcoma. J Pediatr Surg 35: 309-316.

3051. Squarize CH, Castilho RM, Gutkind JS (2008). Chemoprevention and treatment of experimental Cowden's disease by mTOR inhibition with rapamycin. Cancer Res 68: 7066-7072.

3052. Srivastava A, Hornick JL (2009). Immunohistochemical staining for CDX-2, PDX-1, NESP-55, and TTF-1 can help distinguish gastrointestinal carcinoid tumors from pancreatic endocrine and pulmonary carcinoid tumors. Am J Surg Pathol 33: 626-632.

3053. Stambolic V, Suzuki A, de la Pompa JL, Brothers GM, Mirtsos C, Sasaki T et al. (1998). Negative regulation of PKB/Akt-dependent cell survival by the tumor suppressor PTEN. Cell 95: 29-39.

3054. Stamm B, Burger H, Hollinger A (1987). Acinar cell cystadenocarcinoma of the pancreas. Cancer 60: 2542-2547.

3055. Stamm B, Hedinger CE, Saremaslani P (1986). Duodenal and ampullary carcinoid tumors. A report of 12 cases with pathological characteristics, polypeptide content and relation to the MEN I syndrome and von Recklinghausen's disease (neurofibromatosis). Virchows Arch A Pathol Anat Histopathol 408: 475-489.

3056. Stancu M, Wu TT, Wallace C, Houlihan PS, Hamilton SR, Rashid A (2003). Genetic alterations in goblet cell carcinoids of the vermiform appendix and comparison with gastrointestinal carcinoid tumors. Mod Pathol 16: 1189-1198.

3057. Stang A, Kluttig A (2008). Etiologic insights from surface adjustment of colorectal carcinoma incidences: an analysis of the U.S. SEER data 2000-2004. Am J Gastroenterol 103: 2853-2861.

3058. Starink TM, van der Veen JP, Arwert F, de Waal LP, de Lange GG, Gille JJ et al. (1986). The Cowden syndrome: a clinical and genetic study in 21 patients. Clin Genet 29: 222-233.

3059. Starling JR, Turner JH (1982). Villous adenoma involving the ampulla of Vater: treatment by submucosal resection and double sphincteroplasty. Am Surg 48: 188-190.

3060. Starostik P, Greiner A, Schultz A, Zettl A, Peters K, Rosenwald A et al. (2000). Genetic aberrations common in gastric high-grade large B-cell lymphoma. Blood 95: 1180-1187.

3061. Starostik P, Patzner J, Greiner A, Schwarz S, Kalla J, Ott G et al. (2002). Gastric marginal zone B-cell lymphomas of MALT type develop along 2 distinct pathogenetic pathways. Blood 99: 3-9.

3062. Stavrou GA, Flemming P, Oldhafer KJ (2006). Liver resection for metastasis due to malignant mesenchymal tumours. HPB (Oxford) 8: 110-113.

3063. Steck PA, Pershouse MA, Jasser SA, Yung WK, Lin H, Ligon AH et al. (1997). Identification of a candidate tumour suppressor gene, *MMAC1*, at chromosome 10q23.3 that is mutated in multiple advanced cancers. Nat Genet 15: 356-362.

3064. Steenbergen RD, de WJ, Wilting SM, Brink AA, Snijders PJ, Meijer CJ (2005). HPV-mediated transformation of the anogenital tract. J Clin Virol 32 Suppl 1: S25-S33.

3065. Stefanini P, Carboni M, Patrassi N, Basoli A (1974). Beta-islet cell tumors of the pan-

creas: results of a study on 1,067 cases. Surgery 75: 597-609.
3066. Stein A, Sova Y, Almalah I, Lurie A (1996). The appendix as a metastatic target for male urogenital tumours. Br J Urol 78: 647-648.
3067. Stein HJ, Barlow AP, DeMeester TR, Hinder RA (1992). Complications of gastroesophageal reflux disease. Role of the lower esophageal sphincter, esophageal acid and acid/alkaline exposure, and duodenogastric reflux. Ann Surg 216: 35-43.
3068. Stein HJ, Kauer WK, Feussner H, Siewert JR (1998). Bile reflux in benign and malignant Barrett's esophagus: effect of medical acid suppression and nissen fundoplication. J Gastrointest Surg 2: 333-341.
3069. Steiner MA, Giles HW (2008). Mesenchymal hamartoma of the liver demonstrating peripheral calcification in a 12-year-old boy. Pediatr Radiol 38: 1232-1234.
3070. Stelow EB, Bardales RH, Shami VM, Woon C, Presley A, Mallery S et al. (2006). Cytology of pancreatic acinar cell carcinoma. Diagn Cytopathol 34: 367-372.
3071. Stelow EB, Moskaluk CA, Mills SE (2006). The mismatch repair protein status of colorectal small cell neuroendocrine carcinomas. Am J Surg Pathol 30: 1401-1404.
3072. Stelow EB, Pambuccian SE, Bauer TW, Moskaluk CA, Klimstra DS (2009). Mucus rupture (extrusion) and duct expansion/expansive growth are not diagnostic of minimal invasion when seen with intraductal papillary mucinous neoplasms. Am J Surg Pathol 33: 320-321.
3073. Stelow EB, Shaco-Levy R, Bao F, Garcia J, Klimstra DS (2010). Pancreatic acinar cell carcinomas with prominent ductal differentiation: Mixed acinar ductal carcinoma and mixed acinar endocrine ductal carcinoma. Am J Surg Pathol 34:510-518.
3074. Stelow EB, Shami VM, Abbott TE, Kahaleh M, Adams RB, Bauer TW et al. (2008). The use of fine needle aspiration cytology for the distinction of pancreatic mucinous neoplasia. Am J Clin Pathol 129: 67-74.
3075. Stephen AE, Berger DL (2001). Carcinoma in the porcelain gallbladder: a relationship revisited. Surgery 129: 699-703.
3076. Stephens M, Williams GT, Jasani B, Williams ED (1987). Synchronous duodenal neuroendocrine tumours in von Recklinghausen's disease—a case report of co-existing gangliocytic paraganglioma and somatostatin-rich glandular carcinoid. Histopathology 11: 1331-1340.
3077. Stevens HP, Kelsell DP, Bryant SP, Bishop DT, Spurr NK, Weissenbach J et al. (1996). Linkage of an American pedigree with palmoplantar keratoderma and malignancy (palmoplantar ectodermal dysplasia type III) to 17q24. Literature survey and proposed updated classification of the keratodermas. Arch Dermatol 132: 640-651.
3078. Stewenius J, Adnerhill I, Anderson H, Ekelund GR, Floren CH, Fork FT et al. (1995). Incidence of colorectal cancer and all cause mortality in non-selected patients with ulcerative colitis and indeterminate colitis in Malmo, Sweden. Int J Colorectal Dis 10: 117-122.
3079. Stier EA, Krown SE, Chi DS, Brown CL, Chiao EY, Lin O (2004). Anal dysplasia in HIV-infected women with cervical and vulvar dysplasia. J Low Genit Tract Dis 8: 272-275.
3080. Stinner B, Kisker O, Zielke A, Rothmund M (1996). Surgical management for carcinoid tumors of small bowel, appendix, colon, and rectum. World J Surg 20: 183-188.
3081. Stinner B, Rothmund M (2005). Neuroendocrine tumours (carcinoids) of the appendix. Best Pract Res Clin Gastroenterol 19: 729-738.
3082. Stocker JT (1998). An approach to handling pediatric liver tumors. Am J Clin Pathol 109: S67-S72.
3083. Stocker JT (2001). Hepatic tumors in children. Clin Liver Dis 5: 259-281.
3084. Stocker JT, Conran R, Selby D (1998). Tumor and Pseudotumors of the Liver. In: Pathology of Solid Tumors in Children. Stocker J, Askin F, eds. Chapman & Hall: London, pp. 83-110.
3085. Stocker JT, Ishak KG (1978). Undifferentiated (embryonal) sarcoma of the liver: report of 31 cases. Cancer 42: 336-348.
3086. Stocker JT, Ishak KG (1983). Mesenchymal hamartoma of the liver: report of 30 cases and review of the literature. Pediatr Pathol 1: 245-267.
3087. Stoidis CN, Spyropoulos BG, Misiakos EP, Fountzilas CK, Paraskeva PP, Fotiadis CI (2009). Diffuse anorectal melanoma; review of the current diagnostic and treatment aspects based on a case report. World J Surg Oncol 7: 64
3088. Stojanova A, Penn LZ (2009). The role of INI1/hSNF5 in gene regulation and cancer. Biochem Cell Biol 87: 163-177.
3089. Stolte M (2001). Hyperplastic polyps of the stomach: associations with histologic patterns of gastritis and gastric atrophy. Am J Surg Pathol 25: 1342-1344.
3090. Stolte M (2003). The new Vienna classification of epithelial neoplasia of the gastrointestinal tract: advantages and disadvantages. Virchows Arch 442: 99-106.
3091. Stolte M, Pscherer C (1996). Adenoma-carcinoma sequence in the papilla of Vater. Scand J Gastroenterol 31: 376-382.
3092. Stolte M, Vieth M, Ebert MP (2003). High-grade dysplasia in sporadic fundic gland polyps: clinically relevant or not? Eur J Gastroenterol Hepatol 15: 1153-1156.
3093. Stratakis CA, Carney JA (2009). The triad of paragangliomas, gastric stromal tumours and pulmonary chondromas (Carney triad), and the dyad of paragangliomas and gastric stromal sarcomas (Carney-Stratakis syndrome): molecular genetics and clinical implications. J Intern Med 266: 43-52.
3094. Streubel B, Lamprecht A, Dierlamm J, Cerroni L, Stolte M, Ott G et al. (2003). T(14;18)(q32;q21) involving IGH and MALT1 is a frequent chromosomal aberration in MALT lymphoma. Blood 101: 2335-2339.
3095. Streubel B, Seitz G, Stolte M, Birner P, Chott A, Raderer M (2006). MALT lymphoma associated genetic aberrations occur at different frequencies in primary and secondary intestinal MALT lymphomas. Gut 55: 1581-1585.
3096. Streubel B, Simonitsch-Klupp I, Mullauer L, Lamprecht A, Huber D, Siebert R et al. (2004). Variable frequencies of MALT lymphoma-associated genetic aberrations in MALT lymphomas of different sites. Leukemia 18: 1722-1726.
3097. Streubel B, Vinatzer U, Lamprecht A, Raderer M, Chott A (2005). T(3;14)(p14.1;q32) involving IGH and FOXP1 is a novel recurrent chromosomal aberration in MALT lymphoma. Leukemia 19: 652-658.
3098. Stringer MD, Alizai NK (2005). Mesenchymal hamartoma of the liver: a systematic review. J Pediatr Surg 40: 1681-1690.
3099. Strodel WE, Talpos G, Eckhauser F, Thompson N (1983). Surgical therapy for small-bowel carcinoid tumors. Arch Surg 118: 391-397.
3100. Stromeyer FW, Ishak KG, Gerber MA, Mathew T (1980). Ground-glass cells in hepatocellular carcinoma. Am J Clin Pathol 74: 254-258.
3101. Stubbe TP, Vetner M (1977). Gastric carcinoma I. The reproducibility of a histogenetic classification proposed by Masson, Rember and Mulligan. Acta Pathol Microbiol Scand A 85: 519-527.
3102. Sturm PD, Rauws EA, Hruban RH, Caspers E, Ramsoekh TB, Huibregtse K et al. (1999). Clinical value of K-ras codon 12 analysis and endobiliary brush cytology for the diagnosis of malignant extrahepatic bile duct stenosis. Clin Cancer Res 5: 629-635.
3103. Su GH, Bansal R, Murphy KM, Montgomery E, Yeo CJ, Hruban RH et al. (2001). ACVR1B (ALK4, activin receptor type 1B) gene mutations in pancreatic carcinoma. Proc Natl Acad Sci U S A 98: 3254-3257.
3104. Su GH, Hilgers W, Shekher MC, Tang DJ, Yeo CJ, Hruban RH et al. (1998). Alterations in pancreatic, biliary, and breast carcinomas support *MKK4* as a genetically targeted tumor suppressor gene. Cancer Res 58: 2339-2342.
3105. Su GH, Hruban RH, Bansal RK, Bova GS, Tang DJ, Shekher MC et al. (1999). Germline and somatic mutations of the *STK11/LKB1* Peutz-Jeghers gene in pancreatic and biliary cancers. Am J Pathol 154: 1835-1840.
3106. Su JY, Erikson E, Maller JL (1996). Cloning and characterization of a novel serine/threonine protein kinase expressed in early Xenopus embryos. J Biol Chem 271: 14430-14437.
3107. Su LD, Atayde-Perez A, Sheldon S, Fletcher JA, Weiss SW (1998). Inflammatory myofibroblastic tumor: cytogenetic evidence supporting clonal origin. Mod Pathol 11: 364-368.
3108. Su MC, Wang CC, Chen CC, Hu RH, Wang TH, Kao HL et al. (2006). Nuclear translocation of beta-catenin protein but absence of beta-catenin and APC mutation in gastrointestinal carcinoid tumor. Ann Surg Oncol 13: 1604-1609.
3109. Su MY, Hsu CM, Ho YP, Chen PC, Lin CJ, Chiu CT (2006). Comparative study of conventional colonoscopy, chromoendoscopy, and narrow-band imaging systems in differential diagnosis of neoplastic and nonneoplastic colonic polyps. Am J Gastroenterol 101: 2711-2716.
3110. Suarez S, Sueiro RA, Araujo M, Pardo F, Menendez MD, Pardinas MC et al. (2007). Increased frequency of micronuclei in peripheral blood lymphocytes of subjects infected with *Helicobacter pylori*. Mutat Res 626: 162-170.
3111. Suchy J, Klujszo-Grabowska E, Kladny J, Cybulski C, Wokolorczyk D, Szymanska-Pasternak J et al. (2008). Inflammatory response gene polymorphisms and their relationship with colorectal cancer risk. BMC Cancer 8: 112
3112. Suda K, Hirai S, Matsumoto Y, Mogaki M, Oyama T, Mitsui T et al. (1996). Variant of intraductal carcinoma (with scant mucin production) is of main pancreatic duct origin: a clinicopathological study of four patients. Am J Gastroenterol 91: 798-800.
3113. Sudo T, Murakami Y, Uemura K, Hayashidani Y, Hashimoto Y, Ohge H et al. (2008). Prognostic impact of perineural invasion following pancreatoduodenectomy with lymphadenectomy for ampullary carcinoma. Dig Dis Sci 53: 2281-2286.
3114. Sudo Y, Harada K, Tsuneyama K, Katayanagi K, Zen Y, Nakanuma Y (2001). Oncocytic biliary cystadenocarcinoma is a form of intraductal oncocytic papillary neoplasm of the liver. Mod Pathol 14: 1304-1309.
3115. Suehiro Y, Wong CW, Chirieac LR, Kondo Y, Shen L, Webb CR et al. (2008). Epigenetic-genetic interactions in the APC/WNT, RAS/RAF, and P53 pathways in colorectal carcinoma. Clin Cancer Res 14: 2560-2569.
3116. Suekane H, Iida M, Yao T, Matsumoto T, Masuda Y, Fujishima M (1993). Endoscopic ultrasonography in primary gastric lymphoma: correlation with endoscopic and histologic findings. Gastrointest Endosc 39: 139-145.
3117. Sugarbaker PH (1994). Pseudomyxoma peritonei. A cancer whose biology is characterized by a redistribution phenomenon. Ann Surg 219: 109-111.
3118. Sugawara G, Nagino M, Oda K, Nishio H, Ebata T, Nimura Y (2008). Follicular lymphoma of the extrahepatic bile duct mimicking cholangiocarcinoma. J Hepatobiliary Pancreat Surg 15: 196-199.
3119. Sugawara G, Yamaguchi A, Isogai M, Watanabe Y, Kaneoka Y, Suzuki M (2004). Small cell neuroendocrine carcinoma of the ampulla of Vater with foci of squamous differentiation: a case report. J Hepatobiliary Pancreat Surg 11: 56-60.
3120. Sugawara H, Yasoshima M, Katayanagi K, Kono N, Watanabe Y, Harada K et al. (1998). Relationship between interleukin-6 and proliferation and differentiation in cholangiocarcinoma. Histopathology 33: 145-153.
3121. Sugimachi K, Matsuura H, Kai H, Kanematsu T, Inokuchi K, Jingu K (1986). Prognostic factors of esophageal carcinoma: univariate and multivariate analyses. J Surg Oncol 31: 108-112.
3122. Sugiyama M, Atomi Y (1999). Extrapancreatic neoplasms occur with unusual frequency in patients with intraductal papillary mucinous tumors of the pancreas. Am J Gastroenterol 94: 470-473.
3123. Sugiyama M, Izumisato Y, Abe N, Masaki T, Mori T, Atomi Y (2003). Predictive factors for malignancy in intraductal papillary-mucinous tumours of the pancreas. Br J Surg 90: 1244-1249.
3124. Sugiyama M, Suzuki Y, Abe N, Mori T, Atomi Y (2008). Management of intraductal papillary mucinous neoplasm of the pancreas. J Gastroenterol 43: 181-185.
3125. Sugiyama T, Asaka M, Nakamura T, Nakamura S, Yonezumi S, Seto M (2001). API2-MALT1 chimeric transcript is a predictive marker for the responsiveness of *H. pylori* eradication treatment in low-grade gastric MALT lymphoma. Gastroenterology 120: 1884-1885.
3126. Sugo H, Takamori S, Kojima K, Beppu T, Futagawa S (1999). The significance of p53 mutations as an indicator of the biological behavior of recurrent hepatocellular carcinomas. Surg Today 29: 849-855.
3127. Sulkin TV, O'Neill H, Amin AI, Moran B (2002). CT in pseudomyxoma peritonei: a review of 17 cases. Clin Radiol 57: 608-613.
3128. Sun K, Zhang R, Zhang D, Huang G, Wang L (1996). Prognostic significance of lymph node metastasis in surgical resection of esophageal cancer. Chin Med J (Engl) 109: 89-92.
3129. Sun LF, Ye HL, Zhou QY, Ding KF, Qiu PL, Deng YC et al. (2009). A giant hemolymphangioma of the pancreas in a 20-year-old girl: a report of one case and review of the literature. World J Surg Oncol 7: 31-
3130. Sun MH (2004). Neuroendocrine differentiation in sporadic CRC and hereditary nonpolyosis colorectal cancer. Dis Markers 20: 283-288.
3131. Sun Z, Lu P, Gail MH, Pee D, Zhang Q, Ming L et al. (1999). Increased risk of hepatocellular carcinoma in male hepatitis B surface antigen carriers with chronic hepatitis who have detectable urinary aflatoxin metabolite M1. Hepatology 30: 379-383.
3132. Sunlder F, Eriksson B, Grimelius L, Hakanson R, Lonroth H, Lundell L (1992). Histamine in gastric carcinoid tumors: immunocytochemical evidence. Endocr Pathol 3: 23-27.
3133. Sureban SM, May R, George RJ, Dieckgraefe BK, McLeod HL, Ramalingam S et al. (2008). Knockdown of RNA binding protein musashi-1 leads to tumor regression in vivo. Gastroenterology 134: 1448-1458.
3134. Suriano G, Mulholland D, de Wever O, Ferreira P, Mateus AR, Bruyneel E et al. (2003).

The intracellular E-cadherin germline mutation V832 M lacks the ability to mediate cell-cell adhesion and to suppress invasion. Oncogene 22: 5716-5719.
3135. Suriano G, Oliveira MJ, Huntsman D, Mateus AR, Ferreira P, Casares F et al. (2003). E-cadherin germline missense mutations and cell phenotype: evidence for the independence of cell invasion on the motile capabilities of the cells. Hum Mol Genet 12: 3007-3016.
3136. Suriano G, Yew S, Ferreira P, Senz J, Kaurah P, Ford JM et al. (2005). Characterization of a recurrent germ line mutation of the E-cadherin gene: implications for genetic testing and clinical management. Clin Cancer Res 11: 5401-5409.
3137. Suster S, Huszar M, Herczeg E, Bubis JJ (1987). Adenosquamous carcinoma of the gallbladder with spindle cell features. A light microscopic and immunocytochemical study of a case. Histopathology 11: 209-214.
3138. Suzuki A, de la Pompa JL, Stambolic V, Elia AJ, Sasaki T, del BB, I et al. (1998). High cancer susceptibility and embryonic lethality associated with mutation of the *PTEN* tumor suppressor gene in mice. Curr Biol 8: 1169-1178.
3139. Suzuki M, Takahashi T, Ouchi K, Matsuno S (1989). The development and extension of hepatohilar bile duct carcinoma. A three-dimensional tumor mapping in the intrahepatic biliary tree visualized with the aid of a graphics computer system. Cancer 64: 658-666.
3140. Suzuki N, Price AB, Talbot IC, Wakasa K, Arakawa T, Ishiguro S et al. (2006). Flat colorectal neoplasms and the impact of the revised Vienna Classification on their reporting: a case-control study in UK and Japanese patients. Scand J Gastroenterol 41: 812-819.
3141. Suzuki S, Sakaguchi T, Yokoi Y, Okamoto K, Kurachi K, Tsuchiya Y et al. (2002). Clinicopathological prognostic factors and impact of surgical treatment of mass-forming intrahepatic cholangiocarcinoma. World J Surg 26: 687-693.
3142. Svrcek M, Jourdan F, Sebbagh N, Couvelard A, Chatelain D, Mourra N et al. (2003). Immunohistochemical analysis of adenocarcinoma of the small intestine: a tissue microarray study. J Clin Pathol 56: 898-903.
3143. Swanson PE, Dykoski D, Wick MR, Snover DC (1986). Primary duodenal small-cell neuroendocrine carcinoma with production of vasoactive intestinal polypeptide. Arch Pathol Lab Med 110: 317-320.
3144. Sweet K, Willis J, Zhou XP, Gallione C, Sawada T, Alhopuro P et al. (2005). Molecular classification of patients with unexplained hamartomatous and hyperplastic polyposis. JAMA 294: 2465-2473.
3145. Swerdlow SH, Campo E, Harris NL, Jaffe ES, Pileri SA, Stein H et al. (eds.) (2008). WHO Classification of Tumours of Haematopoietic System and Lymphoid Tissues. IARC: Lyon, France.
3145A. Swisher SG, Hofstetter W, Wu TT, Correa AM, Ajani A, Komaki RR, Chirieac L, Hunt KK, Liao Z, Phan A, Rice DC, Vaporciyan AA, Walsh GL, Roth JA (2005). Proposed revision of the esophageal cancer staging system to accommodate pathologic response (pP) following preoperative chemoradiation (CRT). Ann Surg 241:810-817.
3146. Sy SM, Huen MS, Chen J (2009). PALB2 is an integral component of the BRCA complex required for homologous recombination repair. Proc Natl Acad Sci U S A 106: 7155-7160.
3147. Syracuse DC, Perzin KH, Price JB, Wiedel PD, Mesa-Tejada R (1979). Carcinoid tumors of the appendix. Mesoappendiceal extension and nodal metastases. Ann Surg 190: 58-63.
3148. Syros G, Mehran R, Weisz G, Kittas C, Moses JW, Leon M et al. (2009). Role of PLA2 polymorphism on clinical events after percutaneous coronary intervention. Acute Card Care 11: 88-91.
3149. Szych C, Staebler A, Connolly DC, Wu R, Cho KR, Ronnett BM (1999). Molecular genetic evidence supporting the clonality and appendiceal origin of Pseudomyxoma peritonei in women. Am J Pathol 154: 1849-1855.
3150. Taal BG, Peterse H, Boot H (2000). Clinical presentation, endoscopic features, and treatment of gastric metastases from breast carcinoma. Cancer 89: 2214-2221.
3151. Tachezy R, Jirasek T, Salakova M, Ludvikova V, Kubecova M, Horak L et al. (2007). Human papillomavirus infection and tumours of the anal canal: correlation of histology, PCR detection in paraffin sections and serology. APMIS 115: 195-203.
3152. Tachibana M, Kinugasa S, Dhar DK, Tabara H, Masunaga R, Kotoh T et al. (1999). Prognostic factors in T1 and T2 squamous cell carcinoma of the thoracic esophagus. Arch Surg 134: 50-54.
3153. Tada M, Omata M, Kawai S, Saisho H, Ohto M, Saiki RK et al. (1993). Detection of *ras* gene mutations in pancreatic juice and peripheral blood of patients with pancreatic adenocarcinoma. Cancer Res 53: 2472-2474.
3154. Taege C, Holzhausen H, Gunter G, Flemming P, Rodeck B, Rath FW (1999). [Malignant epithelioid hemangioendothelioma of the liver - a very rare tumor in children]. Pathologe 20: 345-350.
3155. Tajima Y, Nakanishi Y, Ochiai A, Tachimori Y, Kato H, Watanabe H et al. (2000). Histopathologic findings predicting lymph node metastasis and prognosis of patients with superficial esophageal carcinoma: analysis of 240 surgically resected tumors. Cancer 88: 1285-1293.
3156. Tajiri T, Tate G, Inagaki T, Kunimura T, Inoue K, Mitsuya T et al. (2005). Intraductal tubular neoplasms of the pancreas: histogenesis and differentiation. Pancreas 30: 115-121.
3157. Tajiri T, Tate G, Kunimura T, Inoue K, Mitsuya T, Yoshiba M et al. (2004). Histologic and immunohistochemical comparison of intraductal tubular carcinoma, intraductal papillary-mucinous carcinoma, and ductal adenocarcinoma of the pancreas. Pancreas 29: 116-122.
3158. Takada M, Yamamoto M, Saitoh Y (1994). The significance of CD44 in human pancreatic cancer: II. The role of CD44 in human pancreatic adenocarcinoma invasion. Pancreas 9: 753-757.
3159. Takahashi M, Sakayori M, Takahashi S, Kato T, Kaji M, Kawahara M et al. (2004). A novel germline mutation of the *LKB1* gene in a patient with Peutz-Jeghers syndrome with early-onset gastric cancer. J Gastroenterol 39: 1210-1214.
3160. Takahashi Y, Shimizu S, Ishida T, Aita K, Toida S, Fukusato T et al. (2007). Plexiform angiomyxoid myofibroblastic tumor of the stomach. Am J Surg Pathol 31: 724-728.
3161. Takashima M, Ueki T, Nagai E, Yao T, Yamaguchi K, Tanaka M et al. (2000). Carcinoma of the ampulla of Vater associated with or without adenoma: a clinicopathologic analysis of 198 cases with reference to p53 and Ki-67 immunohistochemical expressions. Mod Pathol 13: 1300-1307.
3162. Takata K, Sato Y, Nakamura N, Kikuti YY, Ichimura K, Tanaka T et al. (2009). Duodenal and nodal follicular lymphomas are distinct: the former lacks activation-induced cytidine deaminase and follicular dendritic cells despite ongoing somatic hypermutations. Mod Pathol 22: 940-949.
3163. Takeda S, Nakao A, Ichihara T, Suzuki Y, Nonami T, Harada A et al. (1991). Serum concentration and immunohistochemical localization of SPan-1 antigen in pancreatic cancer. A comparison with CA19-9 antigen. Hepatogastroenterology 38: 143-148.
3164. Takeshita M, Iwashita A, Kurihara K, Ikejiri K, Higashi H, Udoh T et al. (2000). Histologic and immunohistologic findings and prognosis of 40 cases of gastric large B-cell lymphoma. Am J Surg Pathol 24: 1641-1649.
3165. Taketo MM, Edelmann W (2009). Mouse models of colon cancer. Gastroenterology 136: 780-798.
3166. Takeuchi H, Ozawa S, Ando N, Shih CH, Koyanagi K, Ueda M et al. (1997). Altered *p16/MTS1/CDKN2* and cyclin D1/*PRAD-1* gene expression is associated with the prognosis of squamous cell carcinoma of the esophagus. Clin Cancer Res 3: 2229-2236.
3167. Takubo K (ed) (2000). Pathology of the Esophagus. Tokyo, Japan.
3168. Takubo K (2007). Squamous epithelial dysplasia and squamous cell carcinoma. In: Pathology of the esophagus. An atlas and textbook. Pathology of the esophagus. An atlas and textbook. Springer: Tokyo, pp. 145-190.
3169. Takubo K, Aida J, Naomoto Y, Sawabe M, Arai T, Shiraishi H et al. (2009). Cardiac rather than intestinal-type background in endoscopic resection specimens of minute Barrett adenocarcinoma. Hum Pathol 40: 65-74.
3170. Takubo K, Aida J, Sawabe M, Kurosumi M, Arima M, Fujishiro M et al. (2007). Early squamous cell carcinoma of the oesophagus: the Japanese viewpoint. Histopathology 51: 733-742.
3171. Takubo K, Nakamura K, Sawabe M, Arai T, Esaki Y, Miyashita M et al. (1999). Primary undifferentiated small cell carcinoma of the esophagus. Hum Pathol 30: 216-221.
3172. Takubo K, Takai A, Takayama S, Sasajima K, Yamashita K, Fujita K (1987). Intraductal spread of esophageal squamous cell carcinoma. Cancer 59: 1751-1757.
3173. Talamonti MS, Goetz LH, Rao S, Joehl RJ (2002). Primary cancers of the small bowel: analysis of prognostic factors and results of surgical management. Arch Surg 137: 564-570.
3174. Talbot IC, Neoptolemos JP, Shaw DE, Carr-Locke D (1988). The histopathology and staging of carcinoma of the ampulla of Vater. Histopathology 12: 155-165.
3175. Talmon GA, Cohen SM (2006). Mesenchymal hamartoma of the liver with an interstitial deletion involving chromosome band 19q13.4: a theory as to pathogenesis? Arch Pathol Lab Med 130: 1216-1218.
3176. Tam PC, Siu KF, Cheung HC, Ma L, Wong J (1987). Local recurrences after subtotal esophagectomy for squamous cell carcinoma. Ann Surg 205: 189-194.
3177. Tamada S, Shibahara H, Higashi M, Goto M, Batra SK, Imai K et al. (2006). MUC4 is a novel prognostic factor of extrahepatic bile duct carcinoma. Clin Cancer Res 12: 4257-4264.
3178. Tamura G, Maesawa C, Suzuki Y, Tamada H, Satoh M, Ogasawara S et al. (1994). Mutations of the A*PC* gene occur during early stages of gastric adenoma development. Cancer Res 54: 1149-1151.
3179. Tamura M, Gu J, Matsumoto K, Aota S, Parsons R, Yamada KM (1998). Inhibition of cell migration, spreading, and focal adhesions by tumor suppressor PTEN. Science 280: 1614-1617.
3180. Tamura S, Kobayashi K, Seki Y, Matsuyama J, Kagara N, Ukei T et al. (2003). Mucoepidermoid carcinoma of the esophagus treated by endoscopic mucosal resection. Dis Esophagus 16: 265-267.
3181. Tan E, Gouvas N, Nicholls RJ, Ziprin P, Xynos E, Tekkis PP (2009). Diagnostic precision of carcinoembryonic antigen in the detection of recurrence of colorectal cancer. Surg Oncol 18: 15-24.
3182. Tanaka E, Hashimoto Y, Ito T, Okumura T, Kan T, Watanabe G et al. (2005). The clinical significance of Aurora-A/STK15/BTAK expression in human esophageal squamous cell carcinoma. Clin Cancer Res 11: 1827-1834.
3183. Tanaka H, Hiyama T, Okubo Y, Kitada A, Fujimoto I (1994). Primary liver cancer incidence-rates related to hepatitis-C virus infection: a correlational study in Osaka, Japan. Cancer Causes Control 5: 61-65.
3184. Tanaka K, Imoto I, Inoue J, Kozaki K, Tsuda H, Shimada Y et al. (2007). Frequent methylation-associated silencing of a candidate tumor-suppressor, *CRABP1*, in esophageal squamous-cell carcinoma. Oncogene 26: 6456-6468.
3185. Tanaka M, Chari S, Adsay V, Fernandez-del CC, Falconi M, Shimizu M et al. (2006). International consensus guidelines for management of intraductal papillary mucinous neoplasms and mucinous cystic neoplasms of the pancreas. Pancreatology 6: 17-32.
3186. Tanaka M, Wanless IR (1998). Pathology of the liver in Budd-Chiari syndrome: portal vein thrombosis and the histogenesis of veno-centric cirrhosis, veno-portal cirrhosis, and large regenerative nodules. Hepatology 27: 488-496.
3187. Tanaka S, Oka S, Chayama K (2008). Colorectal endoscopic submucosal dissection: present status and future perspective, including its differentiation from endoscopic mucosal resection. J Gastroenterol 43: 641-651.
3188. Tanaka Y, Ijiri R, Yamanaka S, Kato K, Nishihira H, Nishi T et al. (1998). Pancreatoblastoma: optically clear nuclei in squamoid corpuscles are rich in biotin. Mod Pathol 11: 945-949.
3189. Tanaka Y, Kato K, Notohara K, Hojo H, Ijiri R, Miyake T et al. (2001). Frequent beta-catenin mutation and cytoplasmic/nuclear accumulation in pancreatic solid-pseudopapillary neoplasm. Cancer Res 61: 8401-8404.
3190. Tanaka Y, Kato K, Notohara K, Nakatani Y, Miyake T, Ijiri R et al. (2003). Significance of aberrant (cytoplasmic/nuclear) expression of beta-catenin in pancreatoblastoma. J Pathol 199: 185-190.
3191. Tang LH, Aydin H, Brennan MF, Klimstra DS (2005). Clinically aggressive solid pseudopapillary tumors of the pancreas: a report of two cases with components of undifferentiated carcinoma and a comparative clinicopathologic analysis of 34 conventional cases. Am J Surg Pathol 29: 512-519.
3192. Tang LH, Modlin IM, Lawton GP, Kidd M, Chinery R (1996). The role of transforming growth factor alpha in the enterochromaffin-like cell tumor autonomy in an African rodent mastomys. Gastroenterology 111: 1212-1223.
3193. Tang LH, Shia J, Soslow RA, Dhall D, Wong WD, O'Reilly E et al. (2008). Pathologic classification and clinical behavior of the spectrum of goblet cell carcinoid tumors of the appendix. Am J Surg Pathol 32: 1429-1443.
3194. Taniai M, Higuchi H, Burgart LJ, Gores GJ (2002). p16INK4a promoter mutations are frequent in primary sclerosing cholangitis (PSC) and PSC-associated cholangiocarcinoma. Gastroenterology 123: 1090-1098.
3195. Taniere P, Martel-Planche G, Maurici D, Lombard-Bohas C, Scoazec JY, Montesano R et al. (2001). Molecular and clinical differences between adenocarcinomas of the esophagus and of the gastric cardia. Am J Pathol 158: 33-40.
3196. Tanimura A, Yamamoto H, Shibata H, Sano E (1979). Carcinoma in heterotopic gastric pancreas. Acta Pathol Jpn 29: 251-257.
3197. Tanimura M, Matsui I, Abe J, Ikeda H, Kobayashi N, Ohira M et al. (1998). Increased risk of hepatoblastoma among immature children

with a lower birth weight. Cancer Res 58: 3032-3035.
3198. Tanizawa T, Seki T, Nakano M, Kamiyama R (2003). Pseudoinvasion of the colorectal polypoid tumors: serial section study of problematic cases. Pathol Int 53: 584-590.
3199. Tanno S, Nakano Y, Nishikawa T, Nakamura K, Sasajima J, Minoguchi M et al. (2008). Natural history of branch duct intraductal papillary-mucinous neoplasms of the pancreas without mural nodules: long-term follow-up results. Gut 57: 339-343.
3200. Tanno S, Obara T, Fujii T, Izawa T, Mizukami Y, Saitoh Y et al. (1999). alpha-Fetoprotein-producing adenocarcinoma of the pancreas presenting focal hepatoid differentiation. Int J Pancreatol 26: 43-47.
3201. Tantachamrun T, Borvonsombat S, Theetranont C (1979). Gardner's syndrome associated with adenomatous polyp of gall bladder: report of a case. J Med Assoc Thai 62: 441-447.
3202. Tascilar M, Offerhaus GJ, Altink R, Argani P, Sohn TA, Yeo CJ et al. (2001). Immunohistochemical labeling for the Dpc4 gene product is a specific marker for adenocarcinoma in biopsy specimens of the pancreas and bile duct. Am J Clin Pathol 116: 831-837.
3203. Tascilar M, Skinner HG, Rosty C, Sohn T, Wilentz RE, Offerhaus GJ et al. (2001). The SMAD4 protein and prognosis of pancreatic ductal adenocarcinoma. Clin Cancer Res 7: 4115-4121.
3204. Tateishi K, Ohta M, Kanai F, Guleng B, Tanaka Y, Asaoka Y et al. (2006). Dysregulated expression of stem cell factor Bmi1 in precancerous lesions of the gastrointestinal tract. Clin Cancer Res 12: 6960-6966.
3205. Tatli S, Mortele KJ, Levy AD, Glickman JN, Ros PR, Banks PA et al. (2005). CT and MRI features of pure acinar cell carcinoma of the pancreas in adults. AJR Am J Roentgenol 184: 511-519.
3206. Tatsuta M, Iishi H, Okuda S, Taniguchi H (1985). Early adenocarcinoma of the gastric cardia. Oncology 42: 232-235.
3207. Taxy JB, Battifora H (1988). Angiosarcoma of the gastrointestinal tract. A report of three cases. Cancer 62: 210-216.
3208. Taylor BA, Williams GT, Hughes LE, Rhodes J (1989). The histology of anal skin tags in Crohn's disease: an aid to confirmation of the diagnosis. Int J Colorectal Dis 4: 197-199.
3209. Tchana-Sato V, Detry O, Polus M, Thiry A, Detroz B, Maweja S et al. (2006). Carcinoid tumor of the appendix: a consecutive series from 1237 appendectomies. World J Gastroenterol 12: 6699-6701.
3210. te Boekhorst DS, Gerhards MF, van Gulik TM, Gouma DJ (2000). Granular cell tumor at the hepatic duct confluence mimicking Klatskin tumor. A report of two cases and a review of the literature. Dig Surg 17: 299-303.
3211. Telerman A, Gerard B, Van den Heule B, Bleiberg H (1985). Gastrointestinal metastases from extra-abdominal tumors. Endoscopy 17: 99-101.
3212. Temellini F, Bavosi M, Lamarra M, Quagliarini P, Giuliani F (1989). Pancreatic metastasis 25 years after nephrectomy for renal cancer. Tumori 75: 503-504.
3212A.Tenesa A, Farrington SM, Prendergast JG, Porteous ME, Walker M, Haq N et al. (2008). Genome-wide association scan identifies a colorectal cancer susceptibility locus on 11q23 and replicates risk loci at 8q24 and 18q21. Nat Genet 40: 631-637
3213. Terada T, Kitamura Y, Ohta T, Nakanuma Y (1997). Endocrine cells in hepatobiliary cystadenomas and cystadenocarcinomas. Virchows Arch 430: 37-40.
3214. Terada T, Ohta T, Kitamura Y, Ashida K, Matsunaga Y (1998). Cell proliferative activity in intraductal papillary-mucinous neoplasms and invasive ductal adenocarcinomas of the pancreas: an immunohistochemical study. Arch Pathol Lab Med 122: 42-46.
3215. Terada T, Ohta T, Nakanuma Y (1996). Expression of oncogene products, anti-oncogene products and oncofetal antigens in intraductal papillary-mucinous neoplasm of the pancreas. Histopathology 29: 355-361.
3216. Terada T, Ohta T, Sasaki M, Nakanuma Y, Kim YS (1996). Expression of MUC apomucins in normal pancreas and pancreatic tumours. J Pathol 180: 160-165.
3217. Terasawa H, Uchiyama K, Tani M, Kawai M, Tsuji T, Tabuse K et al. (2006). Impact of lymph node metastasis on survival in patients with pathological T1 carcinoma of the ampulla of Vater. J Gastrointest Surg 10: 823-828.
3218. Terhune PG, Heffess CS, Longnecker DS (1994). Only wild-type c-Ki-ras codons 12, 13, and 61 in human pancreatic acinar cell carcinomas. Mol Carcinog 10: 110-114.
3219. Terhune PG, Memoli VA, Longnecker DS (1998). Evaluation of p53 mutation in pancreatic acinar cell carcinomas of humans and transgenic mice. Pancreas 16: 6-12.
3220. Terris B, Ingster O, Rubbia L, Dubois S, Belghiti J, Feldmann G et al. (1997). Interphase cytogenetic analysis reveals numerical chromosome aberrations in large liver cell dysplasia. J Hepatol 27: 313-319.
3221. Terris B, Meddeb M, Marchio A, Danglot G, Flejou JF, Belghiti J et al. (1998). Comparative genomic hybridization analysis of sporadic neuroendocrine tumors of the digestive system. Genes Chromosomes Cancer 22: 50-56.
3222. Terris B, Ponsot P, Paye F, Hammel P, Sauvanet A, Molas G et al. (2000). Intraductal papillary mucinous tumors of the pancreas confined to secondary ducts show less aggressive pathologic features as compared with those involving the main pancreatic duct. Am J Surg Pathol 24: 1372-1377.
3223. Terry P, Lagergren J, Wolk A, Nyren O (2000). Reflux-inducing dietary factors and risk of adenocarcinoma of the esophagus and gastric cardia. Nutr Cancer 38: 186-191.
3224. Tetsu O, McCormick F (1999). Beta-catenin regulates expression of cyclin D1 in colon carcinoma cells. Nature 398: 422-426.
3225. Tezuka K, Yamakawa M, Jingu A, Ikeda Y, Kimura W (2006). An unusual case of undifferentiated carcinoma in situ with osteoclast-like giant cells of the pancreas. Pancreas 33: 304-310.
3226. Thakker RV, Bouloux P, Wooding C, Chotai K, Broad PM, Spurr NK et al. (1989). Association of parathyroid tumors in multiple endocrine neoplasia type 1 with loss of alleles on chromosome 11. N Engl J Med 321: 218-224.
3227. Thamboo TP, Sim R, Tan SY, Yap WM (2006). Primary retroperitoneal mucinous cystadenocarcinoma in a male patient. J Clin Pathol 59: 655-657.
3228. Thayu M, Markowitz JE, Mamula P, Russo PA, Muinos WI, Baldassano RN (2005). Hepatosplenic T-cell lymphoma in an adolescent patient after immunomodulator and biologic therapy for Crohn disease. J Pediatr Gastroenterol Nutr 40: 220-222.
3229. Theise ND (1996). Cirrhosis and hepatocellular neoplasia: more like cousins than like parent and child. Gastroenterology 111: 526-528.
3230. Theise ND, Miller F, Worman HJ, Morris P, Schwartz M, Miller C et al. (1993). Biliary cystadenocarcinoma arising in a liver with fibropolycystic disease. Arch Pathol Lab Med 117: 163-165.
3231. Theise ND, Yao JL, Harada K, Hytiroglou P, Portmann B, Thung SN et al. (2003). Hepatic 'stem cell' malignancies in adults: four cases. Histopathology 43: 263-271.
3232. Theisen J, Stein HJ, Feith M, Kauer WK, Dittler HJ, Pirchi D et al. (2006). Preferred location for the development of esophageal adenocarcinoma within a segment of intestinal metaplasia. Surg Endosc 20: 235-238.
3233. Thibodeau SN, French AJ, Roche PC, Cunningham JM, Tester DJ, Lindor NM et al. (1996). Altered expression of hMSH2 and hMLH1 in tumors with microsatellite instability and genetic alterations in mismatch repair genes. Cancer Res 56: 4836-4840.
3234. Thieblemont C, Bastion Y, Berger F, Rieux C, Salles G, Dumontet C et al. (1997). Mucosa-associated lymphoid tissue gastrointestinal and nongastrointestinal lymphoma behavior: analysis of 108 patients. J Clin Oncol 15: 1624-1630.
3235. Thiede C, Morgner A, Alpen B, Wundisch T, Herrmann J, Ritter M et al. (1997). What role does *Helicobacter pylori* eradication play in gastric MALT and gastric MALT lymphoma? Gastroenterology 113: S61-S64.
3236. Thirlby RC, Kasper CS, Jones RC (1984). Metastatic carcinoid tumor of the appendix. Report of a case and review of the literature. Dis Colon Rectum 27: 42-46.
3237. Thomas RM, Sobin LH (1995). Gastrointestinal cancer. Cancer 75: 154-170.
3238. Thompson IW, Day DW, Wright NA (1987). Subnuclear vacuolated mucous cells: a novel abnormality of simple mucin-secreting cells of non-specialized gastric mucosa and Brunner's glands. Histopathology 11: 1067-1081.
3239. Thompson LD, Becker RC, Przygodzki RM, Adair CF, Heffess CS (1999). Mucinous cystic neoplasm (mucinous cystadenocarcinoma of low-grade malignant potential) of the pancreas: a clinicopathologic study of 130 cases. Am J Surg Pathol 23: 1-16.
3240. Thompson-Fawcett MW, Warren BF, Mortensen NJ (1998). A new look at the anal transitional zone with reference to restorative proctocolectomy and the columnar cuff. Br J Surg 85: 1517-1521.
3241. Thomson BJ (2009). Hepatitis C virus: the growing challenge. Br Med Bull 89: 153-167.
3242. Thorgeirsson SS, Grisham JW (2002). Molecular pathogenesis of human hepatocellular carcinoma. Nat Genet 31: 339-346.
3243. Thorlacius S, Olafsdottir G, Tryggvadottir L, Neuhausen S, Jonasson JG, Tavtigian SV et al. (1996). A single BRCA2 mutation in male and female breast cancer families from Iceland with varied cancer phenotypes. Nat Genet 13: 117-119.
3244. Thung SN, Gerber MA, Sarno E, Popper H (1979). Distribution of five antigens in hepatocellular carcinoma. Lab Invest 41: 101-105.
3245. Thurberg BL, Duray PH, Odze RD (1999). Polypoid dysplasia in Barrett's esophagus: a clinicopathologic, immunohistochemical, and molecular study of five cases. Hum Pathol 30: 745-752.
3246. Tichansky DS, Cagir B, Borrazzo E, Topham A, Palazzo J, Weaver EJ et al. (2002). Risk of second cancers in patients with colorectal carcinoids. Dis Colon Rectum 45: 91-97.
3247. Tiemann K, Heitling U, Kosmahl M, Klöppel G (2007). Solid pseudopapillary neoplasms of the pancreas show an interruption of the Wnt-signaling pathway and express gene products of 11q. Mod Pathol 20: 955-960.
3248. Tiemann K, Kosmahl M, Ohlendorf J, Krams M, Klöppel G (2006). Solid pseudopapillary neoplasms of the pancreas are associated with FLI-1 expression, but not with EWS/FLI-1 translocation. Mod Pathol 19: 1409-1413.
3249. Timmons CF, Dawson DB, Richards CS, Andrews WS, Katz JA (1995). Epstein-Barr virus-associated leiomyosarcomas in liver transplantation recipients. Origin from either donor or recipient tissue. Cancer 76: 1481-1489.
3250. Tischkowitz MD, Sabbaghian N, Hamel N, Borgida A, Rosner C, Taherian N et al. (2009). Analysis of the gene coding for the BRCA2-interacting protein PALB2 in familial and sporadic pancreatic cancer. Gastroenterology 137: 1183-1186.
3251. Todoroki T, Okamura T, Fukao K, Nishimura A, Otsu H, Sato H et al. (1980). Gross appearance of carcinoma of the main hepatic duct and its prognosis. Surg Gynecol Obstet 150: 33-40.
3252. Todoroki T, Sano T, Yamada S, Hirahara N, Toda N, Tsukada K et al. (2007). Clear cell carcinoid tumor of the distal common bile duct. World J Surg Oncol 5: 6-
3253. Toliat MR, Berger W, Ropers HH, Neuhaus P, Wiedenmann B (1997). Mutations in the *MEN I* gene in sporadic neuroendocrine tumours of gastroenteropancreatic system. Lancet 350: 1223-
3254. Toll AD, Mitchell D, Yeo CJ, Hruban RH, Witkiewicz AK (2009). Acinar cell carcinoma with a prominent intraductal growth pattern: case report with review of the literature. Int J Surg Pathol -
3255. Tollefson MK, Libsch KD, Sarr MG, Chari ST, Dimagno EP, Urrutia R et al. (2003). Intraductal papillary mucinous neoplasm: did it exist prior to 1980? Pancreas 26: e55-e58.
3256. Tomassetti P, Campana D, Piscitelli L, Casadei R, Nori F, Brocchi E et al. (2006). Endocrine tumors of the ileum: factors correlated with survival. Neuroendocrinology 83: 380-386.
3257. Tomassetti P, Migliori M, Caletti GC, Fusaroli P, Corinaldesi R, Gullo L (2000). Treatment of type II gastric carcinoid tumors with somatostatin analogues. N Engl J Med 343: 551-554.
3258. Tomaszewska R, Okon K, Nowak K, Stachura J (1998). HER-2/Neu expression as a progression marker in pancreatic intraepithelial neoplasia. Pol J Pathol 49: 83-92.
3259. Tominaga K, Nakanishi Y, Nimura S, Yoshimura K, Sakai Y, Shimoda T (2005). Predictive histopathologic factors for lymph node metastasis in patients with nonpedunculated submucosal invasive colorectal carcinoma. Dis Colon Rectum 48: 92-100.
3260. Tomita N, Tokunaka M, Nakamura N, Takeuchi K, Koike J, Motomura S et al. (2009). Clinicopathological features of lymphoma/leukemia patients carrying both BCL2 and MYC translocations. Haematologica 94: 935-943.
3261. Tomita T, Bhatia P, Gourley W (1981). Mucin producing islet cell adenoma. Hum Pathol 12: 850-853.
3262. Tomita T, Friesen SR, Kimmel JR (1986). Pancreatic polypeptide-secreting islet cell tumor. A follow-up report. Cancer 57: 129-133.
3263. Tomita T, Kimmel JR, Friesen SR, Doull V, Pollock HG (1985). Pancreatic polypeptide in islet cell tumors. Morphologic and functional correlations. Cancer 56: 1649-1657.
3264. Tomizawa M, Saisho H (2007). Insulin-like growth factor (IGF)-II regulates CCAAT/enhancer binding protein alpha expression via phosphatidyl-inositol 3 kinase in human hepatoblastoma cell lines. J Cell Biochem 102: 161-170.
3265. Tomlinson IP, Dunlop M, Campbell H, Zanke B, Gallinger S, Hudson T et al. (2009). COGENT (COlorectal cancer GENeTics): an international consortium to study the role of polymorphic variation on the risk of colorectal cancer. Br J Cancer 102: 447-454.
3265A.Tomlinson IP, Webb E, Carvajal-Carmona L, Broderick P, Howarth K, Pittman AM

et al. (2008). A genome-wide association study identifies colorectal cancer susceptibility loci on chromosomes 10p14 and 8q23.3. Nat Genet 40: 623-630

3265B.Tomlinson I, Webb E, Carvajal-Carmona L, Broderick P, Kemp Z, Spain S (2007). A genome-wide association scan of tag SNPs identifies a susceptibility variant for colorectal cancer at 8q24.21. Net Genet 39: 984-988.

3266. Tomori H, Nagahama M, Miyazato H, Shiraishi M, Muto Y, Toda T (1999). Mucosa-associated lymphoid tissue (MALT) of the gallbladder: a clinicopathological correlation. Int Surg 84: 144-150.

3267. Tong GX, Yu WM, Beaubier NT, Weeden EM, Hamele-Bena D, Mansukhani MM et al. (2009). Expression of PAX8 in normal and neoplastic renal tissues: an immunohistochemical study. Mod Pathol 22: 1218-1227.

3268. Tonnies H, Toliat MR, Ramel C, Pape UF, Neitzel H, Berger W et al. (2001). Analysis of sporadic neuroendocrine tumours of the enteropancreatic system by comparative genomic hybridisation. Gut 48: 536-541.

3269. Toracchio S, Ota H, De JD, Wotherspoon A, Rugge M, Graham DY et al. (2009). Translocation t(11;18)(q21;q21) in gastric B-cell lymphomas. Cancer Sci 100: 881-887.

3270. Torbenson M (2007). Review of the clinicopathologic features of fibrolamellar carcinoma. Adv Anat Pathol 14: 217-223.

3271. Torbenson M, Kannangai R, Abraham S, Sahin F, Choti M, Wang J (2004). Concurrent evaluation of p53, beta-catenin, and alpha-fetoprotein expression in human hepatocellular carcinoma. Am J Clin Pathol 122: 377-382.

3272. Torbenson M, Lee JH, Cruz-Correa M, Ravich W, Rastgar K, Abraham SC et al. (2002). Sporadic fundic gland polyposis: a clinical, histological, and molecular analysis. Mod Pathol 15: 718-723.

3273. Torbenson M, Yeh MM, Abraham SC (2007). Bile duct dysplasia in the setting of chronic hepatitis C and alcohol cirrhosis. Am J Surg Pathol 31: 1410-1413.

3274. Torlakovic E, Skovlund E, Snover DC, Torlakovic G, Nesland JM (2003). Morphologic reappraisal of serrated colorectal polyps. Am J Surg Pathol 27: 65-81.

3275. Torlakovic E, Snover DC (1996). Serrated adenomatous polyposis in humans. Gastroenterology 110: 748-755.

3276. Torlakovic EE, Gomez JD, Driman DK, Parfitt JR, Wang C, Benerjee T et al. (2008). Sessile serrated adenoma (SSA) vs. traditional serrated adenoma (TSA). Am J Surg Pathol 32: 21-29.

3277. Torres C, Turner JR, Wang HH, Richards W, Sugarbaker D, Shahsafaei A et al. (1999). Pathologic prognostic factors in Barrett's associated adenocarcinoma: a follow-up study of 96 patients. Cancer 85: 520-528.

3278. Torzewski M, Sarbia M, Verreet P, Dutkowski P, Heep H, Willers R et al. (1997). Prognostic significance of urokinase-type plasminogen activator expression in squamous cell carcinomas of the esophagus. Clin Cancer Res 3: 2263-2268.

3279. Towfigh S, McFadden DW, Cortina GR, Thompson JE, Jr., Tompkins RK, Chandler C et al. (2001). Porcelain gallbladder is not associated with gallbladder carcinoma. Am Surg 67: 7-10.

3280. Towler MC, Fogarty S, Hawley SA, Pan DA, Martin DM, Morrice NA et al. (2008). A novel short splice variant of the tumour suppressor LKB1 is required for spermiogenesis. Biochem J 416: 1-14.

3281. Toyooka M, Konishi M, Kikuchi-Yanoshita R, Iwama T, Miyaki M (1995). Somatic mutations of the adenomatous polyposis coli gene in gastroduodenal tumors from patients with familial adenomatous polyposis. Cancer Res 55: 3165-3170.

3282. Toyota M, Issa JP (1999). CpG island methylator phenotypes in aging and cancer. Semin Cancer Biol 9: 349-357.

3283. Trabelsi A, Ali AB, Yacoub-Abid LB, Stita W, Mokni M, Korbi S (2008). Primary invasive micropapillary carcinoma of the colon: case report and review of the literature. Pathologica 100: 428-430.

3284. Tracey KJ, O'Brien MJ, Williams LF, Klibaner M, George PK, Saravis CA et al. (1984). Signet ring carcinoma of the pancreas, a rare variant with very high CEA values. Immunohistologic comparison with adenocarcinoma. Dig Dis Sci 29: 573-576.

3285. Trajber HJ, Szego T, de Camargo H, Jr., Mester M, Marujo WC, Roll S (1982). Adenocarcinoma of the gallbladder in two siblings. Cancer 50: 1200-1203.

3286. Tramacere I, Scotti L, Jenab M, Bagnardi V, Bellocco R, Rota M et al. (2009). Alcohol drinking and pancreatic cancer risk: a meta-analysis of the dose-risk relation. Int J Cancer 126: 1474-1486.

3287. Traverso LW, Peralta EA, Ryan JA, Jr., Kozarek RA (1998). Intraductal neoplasms of the pancreas. Am J Surg 175: 426-432.

3288. Travis WD, Brambilla E, Muller-Hermelink HK, and Harris CC (eds.) (2004). WHO Classification of Tumours of the Lung, Pleura, Thymus and Heart. IARC: Lyon, France.

3289. Travis WD, Linnoila RI, Tsokos MG, Hitchcock CL, Cutler GB, Jr., Nieman L et al. (1991). Neuroendocrine tumors of the lung with proposed criteria for large-cell neuroendocrine carcinoma. An ultrastructural, immunohistochemical, and flow cytometric study of 35 cases. Am J Surg Pathol 15: 529-553.

3290. Trede M, Schwall G, Saeger HD (1990). Survival after pancreatoduodenectomy. 118 consecutive resections without an operative mortality. Ann Surg 211: 447-458.

3291. Trentino P, Rapacchietta S, Silvestri F, Marzullo A, Fantini A (1997). Esophageal metastasis from clear cell carcinoma of the kidney. Am J Gastroenterol 92: 1381-1382.

3292. Triantafillidis JK, Nasioulas G, Kosmidis PA (2009). Colorectal cancer and inflammatory bowel disease: epidemiology, risk factors, mechanisms of carcinogenesis and prevention strategies. Anticancer Res 29: 2727-2737.

3293. Trimbath JD, Griffin C, Romans K, Giardiello FM (2003). Attenuated familial adenomatous polyposis presenting as ampullary adenocarcinoma. Gut 52: 903-904.

3294. Trobaugh-Lotrario AD, Tomlinson GE, Finegold MJ, Gore L, Feusner JH (2009). Small cell undifferentiated variant of hepatoblastoma: adverse clinical and molecular features similar to rhabdoid tumors. Pediatr Blood Cancer 52: 328-334.

3295. Trudgill NJ, Kapur KC, Riley SA (1999). Familial clustering of reflux symptoms. Am J Gastroenterol 94: 1172-1178.

3296. Truninger K, Menigatti M, Luz J, Russell A, Haider R, Gebbers JO et al. (2005). Immunohistochemical analysis reveals high frequency of PMS2 defects in colorectal cancer. Gastroenterology 128: 1160-1171.

3297. Truta B, Chen YY, Blanco AM, Deng G, Conrad PG, Kim YH et al. (2008). Tumor histology helps to identify Lynch syndrome among colorectal cancer patients. Fam Cancer 7: 267-274.

3298. Tsang WY, Chan JK, Lee KC, Leung AK, Fu YT (1991). Basaloid-squamous carcinoma of the upper aerodigestive tract and so-called adenoid cystic carcinoma of the oesophagus: the same tumour type? Histopathology 19: 35-46.

3299. Tschang TP, Garza-Garza R, Kissane JM (1977). Pleomorphic carcinoma of the pancreas: an analysis of 15 cases. Cancer 39: 2114-2126.

3300. Tseng JF, Warshaw AL, Sahani DV, Lauwers GY, Rattner DW, Fernandez-del CC (2005). Serous cystadenoma of the pancreas: tumor growth rates and recommendations for treatment. Ann Surg 242: 413-419.

3301. Tsioulias G, Muto T, Kubota Y, Masaki T, Suzuki K, Akasu T et al. (1991). DNA ploidy pattern in rectal carcinoid tumors. Dis Colon Rectum 34: 31-36.

3302. Tsolakis AV, Portela-Gomes GM, Stridsberg M, Grimelius L, Sundin A, Eriksson BK et al. (2004). Malignant gastric ghrelinoma with hyperghrelinemia. J Clin Endocrinol Metab 89: 3739-3744.

3303. Tsou HC, Teng DH, Ping XL, Brancolini V, Davis T, Hu R et al. (1997). The role of *MMAC1* mutations in early-onset breast cancer: causative in association with Cowden syndrome and excluded in *BRCA1*-negative cases. Am J Hum Genet 61: 1036-1043.

3304. Tsuboi K, Shimura T, Suzuki H, Mochiki E, Haga N, Masuda N et al. (2004). Liver metastases of a minute rectal carcinoid less than 5mm in diameter: a case report. Hepatogastroenterology 51: 1330-1332.

3305. Tsuboniwa N, Miki T, Kuroda M, Maeda O, Saiki S, Kinouchi T et al. (1996). Primary adenocarcinoma in an ileal conduit. Int J Urol 3: 64-66.

3306. Tsuchikame N, Ishimaru Y, Ohshima S, Takahashi M (1993). Three familial cases of fundic gland polyposis without polyposis coli. Virchows Arch A Pathol Anat Histopathol 422: 337-340.

3307. Tsuchiya A, Endo Y, Yazawa T, Saito A, Inoue N (2006). Adenoendocrine cell carcinoma of the gallbladder: report of a case. Surg Today 36: 849-852.

3308. Tsuchiya R, Noda T, Harada N, Miyamoto T, Tomioka T, Yamamoto K et al. (1986). Collective review of small carcinomas of the pancreas. Ann Surg 203: 77-81.

3309. Tsui WM, Colombari R, Portmann BC, Bonetti F, Thung SN, Ferrell LD et al. (1999). Hepatic angiomyolipoma: a clinicopathologic study of 30 cases and delineation of unusual morphologic variants. Am J Surg Pathol 23: 34-48.

3310. Tsui WM, Lam PW, Mak CK, Pay KH (2000). Fine-needle aspiration cytologic diagnosis of intrahepatic biliary papillomatosis (intraductal papillary tumor): report of three cases and comparative study with cholangiocarcinoma. Diagn Cytopathol 22: 293-298.

3311. Tsui WM, Loo KT, Chow LT, Tse CC (1993). Biliary adenofibroma. A heretofore unrecognized benign biliary tumor of the liver. Am J Surg Pathol 17: 186-192.

3312. Tsukashita S, Kushima R, Bamba M, Sugihara H, Hattori T (2001). *MUC* gene expression and histogenesis of adenocarcinoma of the stomach. Int J Cancer 94: 166-170.

3313. Tsukuma H, Mishima T, Oshima A (1983). Prospective study of "early" gastric cancer. Int J Cancer 31: 421-426.

3314. Tsukuma H, Tanaka H (1996). Descriptive epidemiology of hepatitis C virus related liver cancer in Japan. In: Hepatitis Type C. Hayashi N, Kiyosawa K, eds. Igaku-Shoin: Tokyo, pp. 112-119.

3315. Tsunoda T, Eto T, Tsurifune T, Tokunaga S, Ishii T, Motojima K et al. (1991). Solid and cystic tumor of the pancreas in an adult male. Acta Pathol Jpn 41: 763-770.

3316. Tsunoda T, Ura K, Eto T, Matsumoto T, Tsuchiya R (1991). UICC and Japanese stage classifications for carcinoma of the pancreas. Int J Pancreatol 8: 205-214.

3317. Tuchmann-Duplessis H (eds.) (1968). Embryologie. Travaux pratiques et enseignement dirige. Masson: Paris.

3318. Tucker JA, Shelburne JD, Benning TL, Yacoub L, Federman M (1994). Filamentous inclusions in acinar cell carcinoma of the pancreas. Ultrastruct Pathol 18: 279-286.

3319. Tung CL, Hsieh PP, Chang JH, Chen RS, Chen YJ, Wang JS (2008). Intestinal T-cell and natural killer-cell lymphomas in Taiwan with special emphasis on 2 distinct cellular types: natural killer-like cytotoxic T cell and true natural killer cell. Hum Pathol 39: 1018-1025.

3320. Turbiner J, Amin MB, Humphrey PA, Srigley JR, de Leval L, Radhakrishnan A et al. (2007). Cystic nephroma and mixed epithelial and stromal tumor of kidney: a detailed clinicopathologic analysis of 34 cases and proposal for renal epithelial and stromal tumor (REST) as a unifying term. Am J Surg Pathol 31: 489-500.

3321. Turcot J, Despres JP, St Pierre F (1959). Malignant tumors of the central nervous system associated with familial polyposis of the colon: report of two cases. Dis Colon Rectum 2: 465-468.

3322. Turner BG, Cizginer S, Agarwal D, Yang J, Pitman MB, Brugge WR (2009). Diagnosis of pancreatic neoplasia with EUS and FNA: a report of accuracy. Gastrointest Endosc 71: 91-98.

3323. Turner PC, Sylla A, Gong YY, Diallo MS, Sutcliffe AE, Hall AJ et al. (2005). Reduction in exposure to carcinogenic aflatoxins by postharvest intervention measures in west Africa: a community-based intervention study. Lancet 365: 1950-1956.

3324. Tworek JA, Appelman HD, Singleton TP, Greenson JK (1997). Stromal tumors of the jejunum and ileum. Mod Pathol 10: 200-209.

3325. Ubiali A, Benetti A, Papotti M, Villanacci V, Rindi G (2001). Genetic alterations in poorly differentiated endocrine colon carcinomas developing in tubulo-villous adenomas: a report of two cases. Virchows Arch 439: 776-781.

3326. Uchida N, Kamada H, Tsutsui K, Ono M, Aritomo Y, Masaki T et al. (2007). Utility of pancreatic duct brushing for diagnosis of pancreatic carcinoma. J Gastroenterol 42: 657-662.

3327. Uchida Y, Tomonari K, Shibata O, Hadama T, Shirabe J, Matsumoto K et al. (1986). Carcinoma in adenoma of the papilla of Vater. Jpn J Surg 16: 371-376.

3328. Uchimura K, Nakamuta M, Osoegawa M, Takeaki S, Nishi H, Iwamoto H et al. (2001). Hepatic epithelioid hemangioendothelioma. J Clin Gastroenterol 32: 431-434.

3329. Uchino S, Tsuda H, Noguchi M, Yokota J, Terada M, Saito T et al. (1992). Frequent loss of heterozygosity at the DCC locus in gastric cancer. Cancer Res 52: 3099-3102.

3330. Uchiyama S, Chijiiwa K, Imamura N, Hiyoshi M, Ohuchida J, Nagano M et al. (2008). Adenoma of the major duodenal papilla with intraductal extension into the lower common bile duct. J Gastrointest Surg 12: 1146-1148.

3331. Udd L, Katajisto P, Rossi DJ, Lepisto A, Lahesmaa AM, Ylikorkala A et al. (2004). Suppression of Peutz-Jeghers polyposis by inhibition of cyclooxygenase-2. Gastroenterology 127: 1030-1037.

3332. Ueda K, Terada T, Nakanuma Y, Matsui O (1992). Vascular supply in adenomatous hyperplasia of the liver and hepatocellular carcinoma: a morphometric study. Hum Pathol 23: 619-626.

3333. Uemura K, Hiyama E, Murakami Y, Kanehiro T, Ohge H, Sueda T et al. (2003). Comparative analysis of K-ras point mutation, telomerase activity, and p53 overexpression in pancreatic tumours. Oncol Rep 10: 277-283.

3334. Uemura N, Nakanishi Y, Kato H, Saito S, Nagino M, Hirohashi S et al. (2009). Transglutaminase 3 as a prognostic biomarker in esophageal cancer revealed by proteomics. Int J Cancer 124: 2106-2115.

3335. Uenishi T, Kubo S, Yamamoto T, Shuto T, Ogawa M, Tanaka H et al. (2003). Cytokeratin 19 expression in hepatocellular carcinoma predicts early postoperative recurrence. Cancer Sci 94: 851-857.

3336. Ueno H, Mochizuki H, Hashiguchi Y, Ishiguro M, Miyoshi M, Kajiwara Y et al. (2007). Extramural cancer deposits without nodal structure in colorectal cancer: optimal categorization for prognostic staging. Am J Clin Pathol 127: 287-294.

3337. Ueyama T, Nagai E, Yao T, Tsuneyoshi M (1993). Vimentin-positive gastric carcinomas with rhabdoid features. A clinicopathologic and immunohistochemical study. Am J Surg Pathol 17: 813-819.

3338. Uka K, Aikata H, Takaki S, Shirakawa H, Jeong SC, Yamashina K et al. (2007). Clinical features and prognosis of patients with extrahepatic metastases from hepatocellular carcinoma. World J Gastroenterol 13: 414-420.

3339. Ukita Y, Kato M, Terada T (2002). Gene amplification and mRNA and protein overexpression of c-erbB-2 (HER-2/neu) in human intrahepatic cholangiocarcinoma as detected by fluorescence in situ hybridization, in situ hybridization, and immunohistochemistry. J Hepatol 36: 780-785.

3340. Ulich T, Cheng L, Lewin KJ (1982). Acinar-endocrine cell tumor of the pancreas. Report of a pancreatic tumor containing both zymogen and neuroendocrine granules. Cancer 50: 2099-2105.

3341. Ullman T, Odze R, Farraye FA (2009). Diagnosis and management of dysplasia in patients with ulcerative colitis and Crohn's disease of the colon. Inflamm Bowel Dis 15: 630-638.

3342. Umar A, Boland CR, Terdiman JP, Syngal S, de la Chapelle A, Ruschoff J et al. (2004). Revised Bethesda Guidelines for hereditary nonpolyposis colorectal cancer (Lynch syndrome) and microsatellite instability. J Natl Cancer Inst 96: 261-268.

3343. Umeyama K, Sowa M, Kamino K, Kato Y, Satake K (1982). Gastric carcinoma in young adults in Japan. Anticancer Res 2: 283-286.

3344. Unal E, Koksal Y, Akcoren Z, Tavl L, Gunel E, Kerimoglu U (2008). Mesenchymal hamartoma of the liver mimicking hepatoblastoma. J Pediatr Hematol Oncol 30: 458-460.

3345. Uribe-Uribe NO, Jimenez-Garduno AM, Henson DE, Albores-Saavedra J (2009). Paraneoplastic sensory neuropathy associated with small cell carcinoma of the gallbladder. Ann Diagn Pathol 13: 124-126.

3346. Uronis HE, Bendell JC (2007). Anal cancer: an overview. Oncologist 12: 524-534.

3347. Usui M, Matsuda S, Suzuki H, Hirata K, Ogura Y, Shiraishi T (2002). Somatostatinoma of the papilla of Vater with multiple gastrointestinal stromal tumors in a patient with von Recklinghausen's disease. J Gastroenterol 37: 947-953.

3348. Vakiani E, Young RH, Carcangiu ML, Klimstra DS (2008). Acinar cell carcinoma of the pancreas metastatic to the ovary: a report of 4 cases. Am J Surg Pathol 32: 1540-1545.

3349. Valbuena JR, Gualco G, Espejo-Plascencia I, Medeiros LJ (2005). Classical Hodgkin lymphoma arising in the rectum. Ann Diagn Pathol 9: 38-42.

3350. Van Biervliet S, Velde SV, De Bruyne R, De Looze D, De Vos M, Van WM (2008). Epstein-Barr virus related lymphoma in inflammatory bowel disease. Acta Gastroenterol Belg 71: 33-35.

3351. van Bokhoven MM, Aarntzen EH, Tan AC (2006). Metastatic melanoma of the common bile duct and ampulla of Vater. Gastrointest Endosc 63: 873-874.

3352. van Dekken H, Alers JC, Riegman PH, Rosenberg C, Tilanus HW, Vissers K (2001). Molecular cytogenetic evaluation of gastric cardia adenocarcinoma and precursor lesions. Am J Pathol 158: 1961-1967.

3353. van Dekken H, Tilanus HW, Hop WC, Dinjens WN, Wink JC, Vissers KJ et al. (2009). Array comparative genomic hybridization, expression array, and protein analysis of critical regions on chromosome arms 1q, 7q, and 8p in adenocarcinomas of the gastroesophageal junction. Cancer Genet Cytogenet 189: 37-42.

3354. van Dekken H, van Marion R, Vissers KJ, Hop WC, Dinjens WN, Tilanus HW et al. (2008). Molecular dissection of the chromosome band 7q21 amplicon in gastroesophageal junction adenocarcinomas identifies cyclin-dependent kinase 6 at both genomic and protein expression levels. Genes Chromosomes Cancer 47: 649-656.

3355. van den Berg W, Tascilar M, Offerhaus GJ, Albores-Saavedra J, Wenig BM, Hruban RH et al. (2000). Pancreatic mucinous cystic neoplasms with sarcomatous stroma: molecular evidence for monoclonal origin with subsequent divergence of the epithelial and sarcomatous components. Mod Pathol 13: 86-91.

3356. van den Bos I, Hussain SM, Dwarkasing RS, Stoop H, Zondervan PE, Krestin GP et al. (2007). Hepatoid adenocarcinoma of the gallbladder: a mimicker of hepatocellular carcinoma. Br J Radiol 80: e317-e320.

3357. Van den Broeck A, Sergeant G, Ectors N, van Steenbergen W, Aerts R, Topal B (2009). Patterns of recurrence after curative resection of pancreatic ductal adenocarcinoma. Eur J Surg Oncol 35: 600-604.

3358. van der Heijden MS, Brody JR, Dezentje DA, Gallmeier E, Cunningham SC, Swartz MJ et al. (2005). In vivo therapeutic responses contingent on Fanconi anemia/BRCA2 status of the tumor. Clin Cancer Res 11: 7508-7515.

3359. van der Heijden MS, Yeo CJ, Hruban RH, Kern SE (2003). Fanconi anemia gene mutations in young-onset pancreatic cancer. Cancer Res 63: 2585-2588.

3360. van der Post RS, Kets CM, Ligtenberg MJ, Van Krieken JH, Hoogerbrugge N (2009). Immunohistochemistry is not an accurate first step towards the molecular diagnosis of MUTYH-associated polyposis. Virchows Arch 454: 25-29.

3360A. van Duijnhoven FJ, Bueno-de-Mesquita HB, Ferrari P, Jenab M, Boshuizen HC, Ros MM et al. (2009). Fruit, vegetables, and colorectal cancer risk: the European Prospective Investigation into Cancer and Nutrition. Am J Clin Nutr 89: 1441-1452.

3361. van Eeden S, de Leng WW, Offerhaus GJ, Morsink FH, Weterman MA, de Krijger RR et al. (2004). Ductuloinsular tumors of the pancreas: endocrine tumors with entrapped nonneoplastic ductules. Am J Surg Pathol 28: 813-820.

3362. van Eeden S, Offerhaus GJ, Hart AA, Boerrigter L, Nederlof PM, Porter E et al. (2007). Goblet cell carcinoid of the appendix: a specific type of carcinoma. Histopathology 51: 763-773.

3363. van Eeden S, Offerhaus GJ, Peterse HL, Dingemans KP, Blaauwgeers HL (2000). Gangliocytic paraganglioma of the appendix. Histopathology 36: 47-49.

3364. van Eeden S, Quaedvlieg PF, Taal BG, Offerhaus GJ, Lamers CB, van Velthuysen ML (2002). Classification of low-grade neuroendocrine tumors of midgut and unknown origin. Hum Pathol 33: 1126-1132.

3365. van Hattem WA, Brosens LA, de Leng WW, Morsink FH, Lens S, Carvalho R et al. (2008). Large genomic deletions of SMAD4, BMPR1A and PTEN in juvenile polyposis. Gut 57: 623-627.

3366. van Heerden JA, Edis AJ, Service FJ (1979). The surgical aspects of insulinomas. Ann Surg 189: 677-682.

3367. van Lieshout EM, Roelofs HM, Dekker S, Mulder CJ, Wobbes T, Jansen JB et al. (1999). Polymorphic expression of the glutathione S-transferase P1 gene and its susceptibility to Barrett's esophagus and esophageal carcinoma. Cancer Res 59: 586-589.

3368. Van Overbeke L, Ectors N, Tack J (2005). What is the role of celiac disease in enteropathy-type intestinal lymphoma? A retrospective study of nine cases. Acta Gastroenterol Belg 68: 419-423.

3369. Van Puijenbroek M, Nielsen M, Tops CM, Halfwerk H, Vasen HF, Weiss MM et al. (2008). Identification of patients with (atypical) MUTYH-associated polyposis by KRAS2 c.34G > T pre-screening followed by MUTYH hotspot analysis in formalin-fixed paraffin-embedded tissue. Clin Cancer Res 14: 139-142.

3370. van Schaik FD, Offerhaus GJ, Schipper ME, Siersema PD, Vleggaar FP, Oldenburg B (2009). Endoscopic and pathological aspects of colitis-associated dysplasia. Nat Rev Gastroenterol Hepatol 6: 671-678.

3371. Van Tornout JM, Buckley JD, Quinn JJ, Feusner JH, Krailo MD, King DR et al. (1997). Timing and magnitude of decline in alpha-fetoprotein levels in treated children with unresectable or metastatic hepatoblastoma are predictors of outcome: a report from the Children's Cancer Group. J Clin Oncol 15: 1190-1197.

3372. Vandendriessche L, Bonhomme A, Breysem L, Smet MH, Uyttebroeck A, Brock P et al. (1996). Mesenchymal hamartoma: radiological differentiation from other possible liver tumors in childhood. J Belge Radiol 79: 74-75.

3373. Vandewoude M, Cornelis A, Wyndaele D, Brussaard C, Kums R (2006). (18)FDG-PET-scan in staging of primary malignant melanoma of the oesophagus: a case report. Acta Gastroenterol Belg 69: 12-14.

3374. Vang R, Gown AM, Farinola M, Barry TS, Wheeler DT, Yemelyanova A et al. (2007). p16 expression in primary ovarian mucinous and endometrioid tumors and metastatic adenocarcinomas in the ovary: utility for identification of metastatic HPV-related endocervical adenocarcinomas. Am J Surg Pathol 31: 653-663.

3375. Vang R, Gown AM, Wu LS, Barry TS, Wheeler DT, Yemelyanova A et al. (2006). Immunohistochemical expression of CDX2 in primary ovarian mucinous tumors and metastatic mucinous carcinomas involving the ovary: comparison with CK20 and correlation with coordinate expression of CK7. Mod Pathol 19: 1421-1428.

3376. VanSaun MN, Lee IK, Washington MK, Matrisian L, Gorden DL (2009). High fat diet induced hepatic steatosis establishes a permissive microenvironment for colorectal metastases and promotes primary dysplasia in a murine model. Am J Pathol 175: 355-364.

3377. Vardaman C, Albores-Saavedra J (1995). Clear cell carcinomas of the gallbladder and extrahepatic bile ducts. Am J Surg Pathol 19: 91-99.

3378. Varis A, Zaika A, Puolakkainen P, Nagy B, Madrigal I, Kokkola A et al. (2004). Coamplified and overexpressed genes at ERBB2 locus in gastric cancer. Int J Cancer 109: 548-553.

3379. Varley JM, McGown G, Thorncroft M, Tricker KJ, Teare MD, Santibanez-Koref MF et al. (1995). An extended Li-Fraumeni kindred with gastric carcinoma and a codon 175 mutation in TP53. J Med Genet 32: 942-945.

3380. Varnholt H, Vauthey JN, Dal CP, Marsh RW, Bhathal PS, Hughes NR et al. (2003). Biliary adenofibroma: a rare neoplasm of bile duct origin with an indolent behavior. Am J Surg Pathol 27: 693-698.

3381. Vartio T, Nickels J, Hockerstedt K, Scheinin TM (1980). Rhabdomyosarcoma of the oesophagus. Light and electron microscopic study of a rare tumor. Virchows Arch A Pathol Anat Histol 386: 357-361.

3382. Vasen HF (2005). Clinical description of the Lynch syndrome [hereditary nonpolyposis colorectal cancer (HNPCC)]. Fam Cancer 4: 219-225.

3383. Vasen HF, Boland CR (2005). Progress in genetic testing, classification, and identification of Lynch syndrome. JAMA 293: 2028-2030.

3384. Vasen HF, Mecklin JP, Khan PM, Lynch HT (1991). The International Collaborative Group on Hereditary Non-Polyposis Colorectal Cancer (ICG-HNPCC). Dis Colon Rectum 34: 424-425.

3385. Vasen HF, Moslein G, Alonso A, Aretz S, Bernstein I, Bertario L et al. (2008). Guidelines for the clinical management of familial adenomatous polyposis (FAP). Gut 57: 704-713.

3386. Vasen HF, Moslein G, Alonso A, Bernstein I, Bertario L, Blanco I et al. (2007). Guidelines for the clinical management of Lynch syndrome (hereditary non-polyposis cancer). J Med Genet 44: 353-362.

3387. Vasen HF, Stormorken A, Menko FH, Nagengast FM, Kleibeuker JH, Griffioen G et al. (2001). MSH2 mutation carriers are at higher risk of cancer than MLH1 mutation carriers: a study of hereditary nonpolyposis colorectal cancer families. J Clin Oncol 19: 4074-4080.

3388. Vasen HF, Watson P, Mecklin JP, Lynch HT (1999). New clinical criteria for hereditary nonpolyposis colorectal cancer (HNPCC, Lynch syndrome) proposed by the International Collaborative group on HNPCC. Gastroenterology 116: 1453-1456.

3389. Velazquez I, Alter BP (2004). Androgens and liver tumors: Fanconi's anemia and non-Fanconi's conditions. Am J Hematol 77: 257-267.

3390. Venkatesh S, Ordonez NG, Ajani J, Schultz PN, Hickey RC, Johnston DA et al. (1990). Islet cell carcinoma of the pancreas. A study of 98 patients. Cancer 65: 354-357.

3391. Venu RP, Rolny P, Geenen JE, Hogan WJ, Komorowski RA, Ferstenberg R (1991). Ampullary tumor caused by metastatic renal cell carcinoma. Dig Dis Sci 36: 376-378.

3392. Verbeek WH, Van De Water JM, Al-Toma A, Oudejans JJ, Mulder CJ, Coupe VM (2008). Incidence of enteropathy—associated T-cell lymphoma: a nation-wide study of a population-based registry in The Netherlands. Scand J Gastroenterol 43: 1322-1328.

3393. Verbeek WH, von Blomberg BM, Coupe VM, Daum S, Mulder CJ, Schreurs MW (2009). Aberrant T-lymphocytes in refractory coeliac disease are not strictly confined to a small intestinal intraepithelial localization. Cytometry B Clin Cytom 76: 367-374.

3394. Veres G, Baldassano RN, Mamula P (2007). Infliximab therapy for pediatric Crohn's disease. Expert Opin Biol Ther 7: 1869-1880.

3395. Verhoef S, van Diemen-Steenvoorde R, Akkersdijk WL, Bax NM, Ariyurek Y, Hermans CJ et al. (1999). Malignant pancreatic tumour within the spectrum of tuberous sclerosis complex in childhood. Eur J Pediatr 158: 284-287.

3396. Verkarre V, Romana SP, Cellier C, Asnafi V, Mention JJ, Barbe U et al. (2003). Recurrent partial trisomy 1q22-q44 in clonal intraepithelial lymphocytes in refractory celiac sprue. Gastroenterology 125: 40-46.

3397. Vermeulen L, Todaro M, de Sousa MF, Sprick MR, Kemper K, Perez AM et al. (2008). Single-cell cloning of colon cancer stem cells reveals a multi-lineage differentiation capacity. Proc Natl Acad Sci U S A 105: 13427-13432.

3398. Vernadakis S, Rallis G, Danias N, Serafimidis C, Christodoulou E, Troullinakis M et al. (2009). Metastatic melanoma of the gallblad-

der: an unusual clinical presentation of acute cholecystitis. World J Gastroenterol 15: 3434-3436.
3399. Veronezi-Gurwell A, Wittchow RJ, Bottles K, Cohen MB (1996). Cytologic features of villous adenoma of the ampullary region. Diagn Cytopathol 14: 145-149.
3400. Vetelainen R, Erdogan D, de Graaf W, ten Kate F, Jansen PL, Gouma DJ et al. (2008). Liver adenomatosis: re-evaluation of aetiology and management. Liver Int 28: 499-508.
3401. Viale G, Doglioni C, Gambacorta M, Zamboni G, Coggi G, Bordi C (1992). Progesterone receptor immunoreactivity in pancreatic endocrine tumors. An immunocytochemical study of 156 neuroendocrine tumors of the pancreas, gastrointestinal and respiratory tracts, and skin. Cancer 70: 2268-2277.
3402. Vianna A, Hayes PC, Moscoso G, Driver M, Portmann B, Westaby D et al. (1987). Normal venous circulation of the gastroesophageal junction. A route to understanding varices. Gastroenterology 93: 876-889.
3403. Vieth M, Grunewald M, Niemeyer C, Stolte M (1998). Adenocarcinoma in an ileal pouch after prior proctocolectomy for carcinoma in a patient with ulcerative pancolitis. Virchows Arch 433: 281-284.
3404. Villanueva A, Chiang DY, Newell P, Peix J, Thung S, Alsinet C et al. (2008). Pivotal role of mTOR signaling in hepatocellular carcinoma. Gastroenterology 135: 1972-83, 1983.
3405. Villanueva RR, Nguyen-Ho P, Nguyen GK (1994). Needle aspiration cytology of acinar-cell carcinoma of the pancreas: report of a case with diagnostic pitfalls and unusual ultrastructural findings. Diagn Cytopathol 10: 362-364.
3406. Vilppula A, Collin P, Maki M, Valve R, Luostarinen M, Krekela I et al. (2008). Undetected coeliac disease in the elderly: a biopsy-proven population-based study. Dig Liver Dis 40: 809-813.
3407. Vinik AI, McLeod MK, Fig LM, Shapiro B, Lloyd RV, Cho K (1989). Clinical features, diagnosis, and localization of carcinoid tumors and their management. Gastroenterol Clin North Am 18: 865-896.
3408. Vogt S, Jones N, Christian D, Engel C, Nielsen M, Kaufmann A et al. (2009). Expanded Extracolonic Tumor Spectrum in MUTYH-Associated Polyposis. Gastroenterology 137: 1976-1985.
3409. Volmar KE, Jones CK, Xie HB (2004). Metastases in the pancreas from nonhematologic neoplasms: report of 20 cases evaluated by fine-needle aspiration. Diagn Cytopathol 31: 216-220.
3410. Volpin E, Sauvanet A, Couvelard A, Belghiti J (2002). Primary malignant melanoma of the esophagus: a case report and review of the literature. Dis Esophagus 15: 244-249.
3411. von Brevern M, Hollstein MC, Risk JM, Garde J, Bennett WP, Harris CC et al. (1998). Loss of heterozygosity in sporadic oesophageal tumors in the tylosis oesophageal cancer (TOC) gene region of chromosome 17q. Oncogene 17: 2101-2105.
3412. von Herbay A, Sieg B, Schurmann G, Hofmann WJ, Betzler M, Otto HF (1991). Proliferative activity of neuroendocrine tumours of the gastroenteropancreatic endocrine system: DNA flow cytometric and immunohistological investigations. Gut 32: 949-953.
3413. von Holzen U, Viehl CT, Hamel CT, Oertli D (2009). Ileal intussusception due to visceral malignant melanoma metastasis. Surgery 145: 339-340.
3414. von Horn H, Tally M, Hall K, Eriksson T, Ekstrom TJ, Gray SG (2001). Expression levels of insulin-like growth factor binding proteins and insulin receptor isoforms in hepatoblastomas. Cancer Lett 162: 253-260.
3415. Von Rahden BH, Stein HJ, Puhringer F, Koch I, Langer R, Piontek G et al. (2005). Coexpression of cyclooxygenases (COX-1, COX-2) and vascular endothelial growth factors (VEGF-A, VEGF-C) in esophageal adenocarcinoma. Cancer Res 65: 5038-5044.
3416. von Schweinitz D, Hecker H, Schmidt-von-Arndt G, Harms D (1997). Prognostic factors and staging systems in childhood hepatoblastoma. Int J Cancer 74: 593-599.
3417. von Schweinitz D, Schmidt D, Fuchs J, Welte K, Pietsch T (1995). Extramedullary hematopoiesis and intratumoral production of cytokines in childhood hepatoblastoma. Pediatr Res 38: 555-563.
3418. von Schweinitz D, Wischmeyer P, Leuschner I, Schmidt D, Wittekind C, Harms D et al. (1994). Clinico-pathological criteria with prognostic relevance in hepatoblastoma. Eur J Cancer 30A: 1052-1058.
3419. Voong KR, Davison J, Pawlik TM, Uy MO, Hsu CC, Winter J et al. (2009). Resected pancreatic adenosquamous carcinoma: clinicopathologic review and evaluation of adjuvant chemotherapy and radiation in 38 patients. Hum Pathol 41: 113-122.
3420. Vortmeyer AO, Kingma DW, Fenton RG, Curti BD, Jaffe ES, Duray PH (1998). Hepatobiliary lymphoepithelioma-like carcinoma associated with Epstein-Barr virus. Am J Clin Pathol 109: 90-95.
3421. Vortmeyer AO, Lubensky IA, Fogt F, Linehan WM, Khettry U, Zhuang Z (1997). Allelic deletion and mutation of the von Hippel-Lindau (VHL) tumor suppressor gene in pancreatic microcystic adenomas. Am J Pathol 151: 951-956.
3422. Vortmeyer AO, Lubensky IA, Merino MJ, Wang CY, Pham T, Furth EE et al. (1997). Concordance of genetic alterations in poorly differentiated colorectal neuroendocrine carcinomas and associated adenocarcinomas. J Natl Cancer Inst 89: 1448-1453.
3423. Wachtel MS, Miller EJ (2005). Focal changes of chronic pancreatitis and duct-arteriovenous relationships: avoiding a diagnostic pitfall. Am J Surg Pathol 29: 1521-1523.
3424. Wada K (2002). *p16* and *p53* gene alterations and accumulations in the malignant evolution of intraductal papillary-mucinous tumors of the pancreas. J Hepatobiliary Pancreat Surg 9: 76-85.
3425. Wada K, Asoh T, Imamura T, Wada K, Tanaka N, Yamaguchi K et al. (1998). Rectal carcinoid tumor associated with the Peutz-Jeghers syndrome. J Gastroenterol 33: 743-746.
3426. Wada R (2009). Proposal of a new hypothesis on the development of colorectal epithelial neoplasia: nonspecific inflammation—colorectal Paneth cell metaplasia—colorectal epithelial neoplasia. Digestion 79 Suppl 1: 9-12.
3427. Wagner LM, Garrett JK, Ballard ET, Hill DA, Perry A, Biegel JA et al. (2007). Malignant rhabdoid tumor mimicking hepatoblastoma: a case report and literature review. Pediatr Dev Pathol 10: 409-415.
3428. Wagner PL, Chen YT, Yantiss RK (2008). Immunohistochemical and molecular features of sporadic and FAP-associated duodenal adenomas of the ampullary and nonampullary mucosa. Am J Surg Pathol 32: 1388-1395.
3429. Wain SL, Kier R, Vollmer RT, Bossen EH (1986). Basaloid-squamous carcinoma of the tongue, hypopharynx, and larynx: report of 10 cases. Hum Pathol 17: 1158-1166.
3430. Wakatsuki K, Yamada Y, Narikiyo M, Ueno M, Takayama T, Tamaki H et al. (2008). Clinicopathological and prognostic significance of mucin phenotype in gastric cancer. J Surg Oncol 98: 124-129.
3431. Walch A, Specht K, Braselmann H, Stein H, Siewert JR, Hopt U et al. (2004). Coamplification and coexpression of GRB7 and ERBB2 is found in high grade intraepithelial neoplasia and in invasive Barrett's carcinoma. Int J Cancer 112: 747-753.
3432. Waldner M, Schimanski CC, Neurath MF (2006). Colon cancer and the immune system: the role of tumor invading T cells. World J Gastroenterol 12: 7233-7238.
3433. Walker NI, Horn MJ, Strong RW, Lynch SV, Cohen J, Ong TH et al. (1992). Undifferentiated (embryonal) sarcoma of the liver. Pathologic findings and long-term survival after complete surgical resection. Cancer 69: 52-59.
3434. Walsh MM, Hytiroglou P, Thung SN, Fiel MI, Siegel D, Emre S et al. (1998). Epithelioid hemangioendothelioma of the liver mimicking Budd-Chiari syndrome. Arch Pathol Lab Med 122: 846-848.
3435. Walsh N, Qizilbash A, Banerjee R, Waugh GA (1987). Biliary neoplasia in Gardner's syndrome. Arch Pathol Lab Med 111: 76-77.
3436. Walterhouse D, Watson A (2007). Optimal management strategies for rhabdomyosarcoma in children. Paediatr Drugs 9: 391-400.
3437. Walther A, Houlston R, Tomlinson I (2008). Association between chromosomal instability and prognosis in colorectal cancer: a meta-analysis. Gut 57: 941-950.
3438. Walther A, Johnstone E, Swanton C, Midgley R, Tomlinson I, Kerr D (2009). Genetic prognostic and predictive markers in colorectal cancer. Nat Rev Cancer 9: 489-499.
3439. Walts AE, Lechago J, Bose S (2006). P16 and Ki67 immunostaining is a useful adjunct in the assessment of biopsies for HPV-associated anal intraepithelial neoplasia. Am J Surg Pathol 30: 795-801.
3440. Wang AY, Ahmad NA (2006). Rectal carcinoids. Curr Opin Gastroenterol 22: 529-535.
3441. Wang DG, Johnston CF, Anderson N, Sloan JM, Buchanan KD (1995). Overexpression of the tumour suppressor gene *p53* is not implicated in neuroendocrine tumour carcinogenesis. J Pathol 175: 397-401.
3442. Wang EH, Ebrahimi SA, Wu AY, Kashefi C, Passaro EJ, Sawicki MP (1998). Mutation of the *MENIN* gene in sporadic pancreatic endocrine tumors. Cancer Res 58: 4417-4420.
3443. Wang FY, Arisawa T, Tahara T, Takahama K, Watanabe M, Hirata I et al. (2008). Aberrant DNA methylation in ulcerative colitis without neoplasia. Hepatogastroenterology 55: 62-65.
3444. Wang HH, Antonioli DA, Goldman H (1986). Comparative features of esophageal and gastric adenocarcinomas: recent changes in type and frequency. Hum Pathol 17: 482-487.
3445. Wang HH, Wu MS, Shun CT, Wang HP, Lin CC, Lin JT (1999). Lymphoepithelioma-like carcinoma of the stomach: a subset of gastric carcinoma with distinct clinicopathological features and high prevalence of Epstein-Barr virus infection. Hepatogastroenterology 46: 1214-1219.
3446. Wang HL, Dhall D (2009). Goblet or signet ring cells: that is the question. Adv Anat Pathol 16: 247-254.
3447. Wang KK, Sampliner RE (2008). Updated guidelines 2008 for the diagnosis, surveillance and therapy of Barrett's esophagus. Am J Gastroenterol 103: 788-797.
3448. Wang L, Baudhuin LM, Boardman LA, Steenblock KJ, Petersen GM, Halling KC et al. (2004). MYH mutations in patients with attenuated and classic polyposis and with young-onset colorectal cancer without polyps. Gastroenterology 127: 9-16.
3449. Wang L, Brune KA, Visvanathan K, Laheru D, Herman J, Wolfgang C et al. (2009). Elevated cancer mortality in the relatives of patients with pancreatic cancer. Cancer Epidemiol Biomarkers Prev 18: 2829-2834.
3450. Wang L, Zhang F, Wu PP, Jiang XC, Zheng L, Yu YY (2006). Disordered beta-catenin expression and E-cadherin/CDH1 promoter methylation in gastric carcinoma. World J Gastroenterol 12: 4228-4231.
3451. Wang LC, Lee HC, Yeung CY, Chan WT, Jiang CB (2009). Gastrointestinal polyps in children. Pediatr Neonatol 50: 196-201.
3452. Wang LM, Kevans D, Mulcahy H, O'Sullivan J, Fennelly D, Hyland J et al. (2009). Tumor budding is a strong and reproducible prognostic marker in T3N0 colorectal cancer. Am J Surg Pathol 33: 134-141.
3453. Wang N, Thuraisingam T, Fallavollita L, Ding A, Radzioch D, Brodt P (2006). The secretory leukocyte protease inhibitor is a type 1 insulin-like growth factor receptor-regulated protein that protects against liver metastasis by attenuating the host proinflammatory response. Cancer Res 66: 3062-3070.
3454. Wanless IR (2002). Benign liver tumors. Clin Liver Dis 6: 513-526.
3455. Wanless IR, Albrecht S, Bilbao J, Frei JV, Heathcote EJ, Roberts EA et al. (1989). Multiple focal nodular hyperplasia of the liver associated with vascular malformations of various organs and neoplasia of the brain: a new syndrome. Mod Pathol 2: 456-462.
3456. Wanless IR, Mawdsley C, Adams R (1985). On the pathogenesis of focal nodular hyperplasia of the liver. Hepatology 5: 1194-1200.
3457. Warfel KA, Hull MT (1992). Hepatoblastomas: an ultrastructural and immunohistochemical study. Ultrastruct Pathol 16: 451-461.
3458. Warshaw AL, Compton CC, Lewandrowski K, Cardenosa G, Mueller PR (1990). Cystic tumors of the pancreas. New clinical, radiologic, and pathologic observations in 67 patients. Ann Surg 212: 432-443.
3459. Wasan HS, Park HS, Liu KC, Mandir NK, Winnett A, Sasieni P et al. (1998). APC in the regulation of intestinal crypt fission. J Pathol 185: 246-255.
3460. Washburn WK, Noda S, Lewis WD, Jenkins RL (1995). Primary malignant melanoma of the biliary tract. Liver Transpl Surg 1: 103-106.
3461. Washington K, McDonagh D (1995). Secondary tumors of the gastrointestinal tract: surgical pathologic findings and comparison with autopsy survey. Mod Pathol 8: 427-433.
3462. Washington MK, Berlin J, Branton P, Burgart LJ, Carter DK, Fitzgibbons PL et al. (2009). Protocol for the examination of specimens from patients with primary carcinoma of the colon and rectum. Arch Pathol Lab Med 133: 1539-1551.
3463. Watanabe H, Enjoji M, Imai T (1976). Gastric carcinoma with lymphoid stroma. Its morphologic characteristics and prognostic correlations. Cancer 38: 232-243.
3464. Watanabe H, Jass JR, and Sobin LH (eds.) (1990). Histological Typing of Oesophageal and Gastric Tumours. Springer-Verlag: Berlin.
3465. Watanabe M, Asaka M, Tanaka J, Kurosawa M, Kasai M, Miyazaki T (1994). Point mutation of *K-ras* gene codon 12 in biliary tract tumors. Gastroenterology 107: 1147-1153.
3466. Watanabe S, Okita K, Harada T, Kodama T, Numa Y, Takemoto T et al. (1983). Morphologic studies of the liver cell dysplasia. Cancer 51: 2197-2205.
3467. Watanabe T, Tada M, Nagai H, Sasaki S, Nakao M (1998). *Helicobacter pylori* infection induces gastric cancer in mongolian gerbils. Gastroenterology 115: 642-648.

3468. Watanapa P, Watanapa WB (2002). Liver fluke-associated cholangiocarcinoma. Br J Surg 89: 962-970.
3469. Watson KJ, Shulkes A, Smallwood RA, Douglas MC, Hurley R, Kalnins R et al. (1985). Watery diarrhea-hypokalemia-achlorhydria syndrome and carcinoma of the esophagus. Gastroenterology 88: 798-803.
3470. Watson P, Lynch HT (1993). Extracolonic cancer in hereditary nonpolyposis colorectal cancer. Cancer 71: 677-685.
3471. Watson P, Vasen HF, Mecklin JP, Bernstein I, Aarnio M, Jarvinen HJ et al. (2008). The risk of extra-colonic, extra-endometrial cancer in the Lynch syndrome. Int J Cancer 123: 444-449.
3472. Watts JL, Morton DG, Bestman J, Kemphues KJ (2000). The *C. elegans* par-4 gene encodes a putative serine-threonine kinase required for establishing embryonic asymmetry. Development 127: 1467-1475.
3473. Waxman I, Konda VJ (2009). Mucosal ablation of Barrett esophagus. Nat Rev Gastroenterol Hepatol 6: 393-401.
3473A. Webb EL, Rudd MF, Sellick GS, El Galta R, Bethke L, Wood W, Fletcher O, Penegar S, Withey L, Qureshi M, Johnson N, Tomlinson I, Gray R, Peto J, Houlston RS (2006). Search for low penetrance alleles for colorectal cancer through a scan of 1467 non-synonymous SNPs in 2575 cases and 2707 controls with validation by kin-cohort analysis of 14,704 first-degree relatives. Hum Mol Genet 15: 3263-3271
3474. Webb JN (1977). Acinar cell neoplasms of the exocrine pancreas. J Clin Pathol 30: 103-112.
3475. Webber EM, Fraser RB, Resch L, Giacomantonio M (1997). Perianal ependymoma presenting in the neonatal period. Pediatr Pathol Lab Med 17: 283-291.
3476. Weber HC, Marsh DJ, Lubensky IA, Lin AY, Eng C (1998). Germline PTEN/MMAC1/-TEP1 mutations and association with gastrointestinal manifestations in Cowden disease. Gastroenterology 114S: G2902.
3477. Weber HC, Venzon DJ, Lin JT, Fishbein VA, Orbuch M, Strader DB et al. (1995). Determinants of metastatic rate and survival in patients with Zollinger-Ellison syndrome: a prospective long-term study. Gastroenterology 108: 1637-1649.
3478. Weckstrom P, Hedrum A, Makridis C, Akerstrom G, Rastad J, Scheibenpflug L et al. (1996). Midgut Carcinoids and Solid Carcinomas of the Intestine: Differences in Endocrine Markers and p53 Mutations. Endocr Pathol 7: 273-279.
3479. Wee A, Nilsson B, Kang JY, Tan LKA, Rauff A (1993). Biliary cystadenocarcinoma arising in a cystadenoma. Report of a case diagnosed by fine needle aspiration cytology. Acta Cytol 37: 966-970.
3480. Weeratunge CN, Bolivar HH, Anstead GM, Lu DH (2004). Primary esophageal lymphoma: a diagnostic challenge in acquired immunodeficiency syndrome—two case reports and review. South Med J 97: 383-387.
3481. Wei J, O'Brien D, Vilgelm A, Piazuelo MB, Correa P, Washington MK et al. (2008). Interaction of *Helicobacter pylori* with gastric epithelial cells is mediated by the p53 protein family. Gastroenterology 134: 1412-1423.
3482. Wei ZG, Tang LF, Chen ZM, Tang HF, Li MJ (2008). Childhood undifferentiated embryonal liver sarcoma: clinical features and immunohistochemistry analysis. J Pediatr Surg 43: 1912-1919.
3483. Weidner N, Flanders DJ, Mitros FA (1984). Mucosal ganglioneuromatosis associated with multiple colonic polyps. Am J Surg Pathol 8: 779-786.
3484. Weihrauch M, Benicke M, Lehnert G, Wittekind C, Wrbitzky R, Tannapfel A (2001). Frequent k- ras -2 mutations and p16(INK4A)methylation in hepatocellular carcinomas in workers exposed to vinyl chloride. Br J Cancer 84: 982-989.
3485. Weisenburger DD, Armitage JO (1996). Mantle cell lymphoma— an entity comes of age. Blood 87: 4483-4494.
3486. WELLMAN KF (1962). Adenocarcinoma of anal duct origin. Can J Surg 5: 311-318.
3487. Welton ML, Sharkey FE, Kahlenberg MS (2004). The etiology and epidemiology of anal cancer. Surg Oncol Clin N Am 13: 263-275.
3488. Welzel TM, Graubard BI, El-Serag HB, Shaib YH, Hsing AW, Davila JA et al. (2007). Risk factors for intrahepatic and extrahepatic cholangiocarcinoma in the United States: a population-based case-control study. Clin Gastroenterol Hepatol 5: 1221-1228.
3489. Welzel TM, McGlynn KA, Hsing AW, O'Brien TR, Pfeiffer RM (2006). Impact of classification of hilar cholangiocarcinomas (Klatskin tumors) on the incidence of intra- and extrahepatic cholangiocarcinoma in the United States. J Natl Cancer Inst 98: 873-875.
3490. Werling RW, Yaziji H, Bacchi CE, Gown AM (2003). CDX2, a highly sensitive and specific marker of adenocarcinomas of intestinal origin: an immunohistochemical survey of 476 primary and metastatic carcinomas. Am J Surg Pathol 27: 303-310.
3491. Werness BA, Levine AJ, Howley PM (1990). Association of human papillomavirus types 16 and 18 E6 proteins with p53. Science 248: 76-79.
3492. Westerman AM, Entius MM, de Baar E, Boor PP, Koole R, van Velthuysen ML et al. (1999). Peutz-Jeghers syndrome: 78-year follow-up of the original family. Lancet 353: 1211-1215.
3493. Westra WH, Sturm P, Drillenburg P, Choti MA, Klimstra DS, Albores-Saavedra J et al. (1998). *K-ras* oncogene mutations in osteoclast-like giant cell tumors of the pancreas and liver: genetic evidence to support origin from the duct epithelium. Am J Surg Pathol 22: 1247-1254.
3494. Wheeler JM, Warren BF, Mortensen NJ, Kim HC, Biddolph SC, Elia G et al. (2002). An insight into the genetic pathway of adenocarcinoma of the small intestine. Gut 50: 218-223.
3495. Whelan AJ, Bartsch D, Goodfellow PJ (1995). Brief report: a familial syndrome of pancreatic cancer and melanoma with a mutation in the *CDKN2* tumor-suppressor gene. N Engl J Med 333: 975-977.
3496. Whitcomb DC, Gorry MC, Preston RA, Furey W, Sossenheimer MJ, Ulrich CD et al. (1996). Hereditary pancreatitis is caused by a mutation in the cationic trypsinogen gene. Nat Genet 14: 141-145.
3497. White R, D'Angelica M, Katabi N, Tang L, Klimstra D, Fong Y et al. (2007). Fate of the remnant pancreas after resection of noninvasive intraductal papillary mucinous neoplasm. J Am Coll Surg 204: 987-993.
3498. White SH, Nazarian NA, Smith AM, Balfour TW (1981). Periampullary adenoma causing pancreatitis. Br Med J (Clin Res Ed) 283: 527-
3499. Whittaker MA, Carr NJ, Midwinter MJ, Badham DP, Higgins B (2000). Acinar morphology in colorectal cancer is associated with survival but is not an independent prognostic variable. Histopathology 36: 439-442.
3500. Wideroff L, Vaughan TL, Farin FM, Gammon MD, Risch H, Stanford JL et al. (2007). GST, NAT1, CYP1A1 polymorphisms and risk of esophageal and gastric adenocarcinomas. Cancer Detect Prev 31: 233-236.
3501. Wienert V, Albrecht O, Gahlen W (1978). [Results of incidence analyses in external hemorrhoids]. Hautarzt 29: 536-540.
3502. Wiesner GL, Daley D, Lewis S, Ticknor C, Platzer P, Lutterbaugh J et al. (2003). A subset of familial colorectal neoplasia kindreds linked to chromosome 9q22.2-31.2. Proc Natl Acad Sci U S A 100: 12961-12965.
3503. Wijn MA, Keller JJ, Giardiello FM, Brand HS (2007). Oral and maxillofacial manifestations of familial adenomatous polyposis. Oral Dis 13: 360-365.
3504. Wijnen J, Khan PM, Vasen H, van der Klift H, Mulder A, van Leeuwen-Cornelisse I et al. (1997). Hereditary nonpolyposis colorectal cancer families not complying with the Amsterdam criteria show extremely low frequency of mismatch-repair-gene mutations. Am J Hum Genet 61: 329-335.
3505. Wijnen JT, Brohet RM, van Eijk R, Jagmohan-Changur S, Middeldorp A, Tops CM et al. (2009). Chromosome 8q23.3 and 11q23.1 variants modify colorectal cancer risk in Lynch syndrome. Gastroenterology 136: 131-137.
3506. Wijnen JT, Vasen HF, Khan PM, Zwinderman AH, van der Klift H, Mulder A et al. (1998). Clinical findings with implications for genetic testing in families with clustering of colorectal cancer. N Engl J Med 339: 511-518.
3507. Wild CP, Hardie LJ (2003). Reflux, Barrett's oesophagus and adenocarcinoma: burning questions. Nat Rev Cancer 3: 676-684.
3508. Wilentz RE, Albores-Saavedra J, Zahurak M, Talamini MA, Yeo CJ, Cameron JL et al. (1999). Pathologic examination accurately predicts prognosis in mucinous cystic neoplasms of the pancreas. Am J Surg Pathol 23: 1320-1327.
3509. Wilentz RE, Geradts J, Maynard R, Offerhaus GJ, Kang M, Goggins M et al. (1998). Inactivation of the *p16 (INK4A)* tumor-suppressor gene in pancreatic duct lesions: loss of intranuclear expression. Cancer Res 58: 4740-4744.
3510. Wilentz RE, Goggins M, Redston M, Marcus VA, Adsay NV, Sohn TA et al. (2000). Genetic, immunohistochemical, and clinical features of medullary carcinoma of the pancreas: A newly described and characterized entity. Am J Pathol 156: 1641-1651.
3511. Wilentz RE, Su GH, Dai JL, Sparks AB, Argani P, Sohn TA et al. (2000). Immunohistochemical labeling for dpc4 mirrors genetic status in pancreatic adenocarcinomas : a new marker of DPC4 inactivation. Am J Pathol 156: 37-43.
3512. Willems S, Carneiro F, Geboes K (2005). Gastric carcinoma with osteoclast-like giant cells and lymphoepithelioma-like carcinoma of the stomach: two of a kind? Histopathology 47: 331-333.
3513. Willert K, Shibamoto S, Nusse R (1999). Wnt-induced dephosphorylation of axin releases beta-catenin from the axin complex. Genes Dev 13: 1768-1773.
3514. Willett CG, Lewandrowski K, Warshaw AL, Efird J, Compton CC (1993). Resection margins in carcinoma of the head of the pancreas. Implications for radiation therapy. Ann Surg 217: 144-148.
3515. Williams AO, Prince DL (1975). Intestinal polyps in the Nigerian African. J Clin Pathol 28: 367-371.
3516. Williams ED, Siebenmann RE, and Sobin LH (eds.) (1980). Histological Typing of Endocrine Tumours. World Health Organization: Geneva.
3517. Williams GR, Talbot IC (1994). Anal carcinoma—a histological review. Histopathology 25: 507-516.
3518. Williams GR, Talbot IC, Leigh IM (1997). Keratin expression in anal carcinoma: an immunohistochemical study. Histopathology 30: 443-450.
3519. Williams LH, Choong D, Johnson SA, Campbell IG (2006). Genetic and epigenetic analysis of *CHEK2* in sporadic breast, colon, and ovarian cancers. Clin Cancer Res 12: 6967-6972.
3520. Willis TG, Jadayel DM, Du MQ, Peng H, Perry AR, Abdul-Rauf M et al. (1999). Bcl10 is involved in t(1;14)(p22;q32) of MALT B cell lymphoma and mutated in multiple tumor types. Cell 96: 35-45.
3521. Wilson DM, Pitts WC, Hintz RL, Rosenfeld RG (1986). Testicular tumors with Peutz-Jeghers syndrome. Cancer 57: 2238-2240.
3522. Wilson MB, Adams DB, Garen PD, Gansler TS (1992). Aspiration cytologic, ultrastructural, and DNA cytometric findings of solid and papillary tumor of the pancreas. Cancer 69: 2235-2243.
3523. Wilson TM, Ewel A, Duguid JR, Eble JN, Lescoe MK, Fishel R et al. (1995). Differential cellular expression of the human MSH2 repair enzyme in small and large intestine. Cancer Res 55: 5146-5150.
3524. Wimmer K, Etzler J (2008). Constitutional mismatch repair-deficiency syndrome: have we so far seen only the tip of an iceberg? Hum Genet 124: 105-122.
3525. Winter JM, Cameron JL, Campbell KA, Arnold MA, Chang DC, Coleman J et al. (2006). 1423 pancreaticoduodenectomies for pancreatic cancer: A single-institution experience. J Gastrointest Surg 10: 1199-1210.
3526. Winter JM, Cameron JL, Lillemoe KD, Campbell KA, Chang D, Riall TS et al. (2006). Periampullary and pancreatic incidentaloma: a single institution's experience with an increasingly common diagnosis. Ann Surg 243: 673-680.
3527. Winter JM, Ting AH, Vilardell F, Gallmeier E, Baylin SB, Hruban RH et al. (2008). Absence of E-cadherin expression distinguishes noncohesive from cohesive pancreatic cancer. Clin Cancer Res 14: 412-418.
3528. Wisnoski NC, Townsend CM, Jr., Nealon WH, Freeman JL, Riall TS (2008). 672 patients with acinar cell carcinoma of the pancreas: a population-based comparison to pancreatic adenocarcinoma. Surgery 144: 141-148.
3529. Wistuba II, Albores-Saavedra J (1999). Genetic abnormalities involved in the pathogenesis of gallbladder carcinoma. J Hepatobiliary Pancreat Surg 6: 237-244.
3530. Wistuba II, Gazdar AF, Roa I, Albores-Saavedra J (1996). p53 protein overexpression in gallbladder carcinoma and its precursor lesions: an immunohistochemical study. Hum Pathol 27: 360-365.
3531. Wistuba II, Miquel JF, Gazdar AF, Albores-Saavedra J (1999). Gallbladder adenomas have molecular abnormalities different from those present in gallbladder carcinomas. Hum Pathol 30: 21-25.
3532. Wistuba II, Sugio K, Hung J, Kishimoto Y, Virmani AK, Roa I et al. (1995). Allele-specific mutations involved in the pathogenesis of endemic gallbladder carcinoma in Chile. Cancer Res 55: 2511-2515.
3533. Witte S (1979). Brush cytology of the papilla of Vater. Scand J Gastroenterol Suppl 54: 55-58.
3534. Wittekind C, Sobin LH (eds.) (1997). TNM Classification of Malignant Tumors. Wiley Press: New York, NY.
3535. Wittekind C, Tannapfel A (2001). Adenoma of the papilla and ampulla—premalignant lesions? Langenbecks Arch Surg 386: 172-175.
3536. Witteman BJ, Janssens AR, Terpstra JL, Eulderink F, Welvaart K, Lamers CB (1991). Villous tumors of the duodenum. Presentation of five cases. Hepatogastroenterology 38: 550-553.
3537. Wolf C, Friedl P, Obrist P, Ensinger C, Gritsch W (1999). Metastasis to the appendix:

sonographic appearance and review of the literature. J Ultrasound Med 18: 23-25.
3538. Wolfsen HC, Wallace MB (2008). Reconsidering Barrett's esophagus: practical applications of biophotonics. Gastroenterology 134: 382-385.
3539. Won OH, Farman J, Krishnan MN, Iyer SK, Vuletin JC (1978). Squamous cell carcinoma of the stomach. Am J Gastroenterol 69: 594-598.
3539A. Wong DJ, Paulson TG, Prevo LJ, Galipeau PC, Longton G, Blount PL et al. (2001). p16(INK4a) lesions are common, early abnormalities that undergo clonal expansion in Barrett's metaplastic epithelium. Cancer Res 61: 8284–8289.
3540. Wong AY, Rahilly MA, Adams W, Lee CS (1998). Mucinous anal gland carcinoma with perianal Pagetoid spread. Pathology 30: 1-3.
3541. Wong BC, Lam SK, Wong WM, Chen JS, Zheng TT, Feng RE et al. (2004). *Helicobacter pylori* eradication to prevent gastric cancer in a high-risk region of China: a randomized controlled trial. JAMA 291: 187-194.
3542. Wong NA, Herbst H, Herrmann K, Kirchner T, Krajewski AS, Moorghen M et al. (2003). Epstein-Barr virus infection in colorectal neoplasms associated with inflammatory bowel disease: detection of the virus in lymphomas but not in adenocarcinomas. J Pathol 201: 312-318.
3543. Wong NA, Young R, Malcomson RD, Nayar AG, Jamieson LA, Save VE et al. (2003). Prognostic indicators for gastrointestinal stromal tumours: a clinicopathological and immunohistochemical study of 108 resected cases of the stomach. Histopathology 43: 118-126.
3544. Wong P, Verselis SJ, Garber JE, Schneider K, DiGianni L, Stockwell DH et al. (2006). Prevalence of early onset colorectal cancer in 397 patients with classic Li-Fraumeni syndrome. Gastroenterology 130: 73-79.
3545. Woo A, Sadana A, Mauger DT, Baker MJ, Berk T, McGarrity TJ (2009). Psychosocial impact of Peutz-Jeghers Syndrome. Fam Cancer 8: 59-65.
3546. Woodford-Richens K, Bevan S, Churchman M, Dowling B, Jones D, Norbury CG et al. (2000). Analysis of genetic and phenotypic heterogeneity in juvenile polyposis. Gut 46: 656-660.
3547. Woods MO, Williams P, Careen A, Edwards L, Bartlett S, McLaughlin JR et al. (2007). A new variant database for mismatch repair genes associated with Lynch syndrome. Hum Mutat 28: 669-673.
3548. World Cancer Research Fund, American Institute for Cancer Research (eds.) (2007). Food, Nutrition, Physical Activity and the Prevention of Cancer: A Global Perspective. Second Expert Report. AICR: Washington, DC.
3549. Wotherspoon AC, Diss TC, Pan L, Singh N, Whelan J, Isaacson PG (1996). Low grade gastric B-cell lymphoma of mucosa associated lymphoid tissue in immunocompromised patients. Histopathology 28: 129-134.
3550. Wotherspoon AC, Doglioni C, Diss TC, Pan L, Moschini A, De BM et al. (1993). Regression of primary low-grade B-cell gastric lymphoma of mucosa-associated lymphoid tissue type after eradication of *Helicobacter pylori*. Lancet 342: 575-577.
3551. Wotherspoon AC, Ortiz-Hidalgo C, Falzon MR, Isaacson PG (1991). *Helicobacter pylori*-associated gastritis and primary B-cell gastric lymphoma. Lancet 338: 1175-1176.
3552. Wrba F, Chott A, Schratter M, Ludvik B, Krisch K, Holzner JH (1988). [Fine-needle puncture cytology of a solid cystic tumor of the pancreas]. Pathologe 9: 340-344.
3553. Wright DH (1995). The major complications of coeliac disease. Baillieres Clin Gastroenterol 9: 351-369.
3554. Wright DH (1997). Enteropathy associated T cell lymphoma. Cancer Surv 30: 249-261.
3555. Wu AH, Tseng CC, Bernstein L (2003). Hiatal hernia, reflux symptoms, body size, and risk of esophageal and gastric adenocarcinoma. Cancer 98: 940-948.
3556. Wu AH, Wan P, Bernstein L (2001). A multiethnic population-based study of smoking, alcohol and body size and risk of adenocarcinomas of the stomach and esophagus (United States). Cancer Causes Control 12: 721-732.
3557. Wu CM, Fishman EK, Hruban RK, Schlott WD, Cameron JL (1999). Serous cystic neoplasm involving the pancreas and liver: an unusual clinical entity. Abdom Imaging 24: 75-77.
3558. Wu CW, Chen GD, Jiang KC, Li AF, Chi CW, Lo SS et al. (2001). A genome-wide study of microsatellite instability in advanced gastric carcinoma. Cancer 92: 92-101.
3559. Wu M, Semba S, Oue N, Ikehara N, Yasui W, Yokozaki H (2004). BRAF/K-ras mutation, microsatellite instability, and promoter hypermethylation of hMLH1/MGMT in human gastric carcinomas. Gastric Cancer 7: 246-253.
3560. Wu MH, Lin MT, Lee PH (2007). Clinicopathological study of gastric metastases. World J Surg 31: 132-136.
3561. Wu TT, Kornacki S, Rashid A, Yardley JH, Hamilton SR (1998). Dysplasia and dysregulation of proliferation in foveolar and surface epithelia of fundic gland polyps from patients with familial adenomatous polyposis. Am J Surg Pathol 22: 293-298.
3561A. Wu TT, Chirieac LR, Abraham SC, Krasinskas AM, Wang H, Rashid A, Correa AM, Hofstetter WL, Ajani JA, Swisher SG (2007). Excellent interobserver agreement on grading the extent of residual carcinoma after preoperative chemoradiation in esophageal and esophagogastric junction carcinoma: a reliable predictor for patient outcome. Am J Surg Pathol 31: 58-64.
3562. Wu X, Dagar V, Algar E, Muscat A, Bandopadhayay P, Ashley D et al. (2008). Rhabdoid tumour: a malignancy of early childhood with variable primary site, histology and clinical behaviour. Pathology 40: 664-670.
3563. Wundisch T, Mosch C, Neubauer A, Stolte M (2006). *Helicobacter pylori* eradication in gastric mucosa-associated lymphoid tissue lymphoma: Results of a 196-patient series. Leuk Lymphoma 47: 2110-2114.
3564. Wundisch T, Neubauer A, Stolte M, Ritter M, Thiede C (2003). B-cell monoclonality is associated with lymphoid follicles in gastritis. Am J Surg Pathol 27: 882-887.
3565. Wundisch T, Thiede C, Morgner A, Dempfle A, Gunther A, Liu H et al. (2005). Long-term follow-up of gastric MALT lymphoma after *Helicobacter pylori* eradication. J Clin Oncol 23: 8018-8024.
3566. Xiangming C, Natsugoe S, Takao S, Hokita S, Tanabe G, Baba M et al. (2000). The cooperative role of p27 with cyclin E in the prognosis of advanced gastric carcinoma. Cancer 89: 1214-1219.
3567. Xiao SY, Wang HL, Hart J, Fleming D, Beard MR (2001). cDNA arrays and immunohistochemistry identification of CD10/CALLA expression in hepatocellular carcinoma. Am J Pathol 159: 1415-1421.
3568. Xie J, Itzkowitz SH (2008). Cancer in inflammatory bowel disease. World J Gastroenterol 14: 378-389.
3569. Xinarianos G, McRonald FE, Risk JM, Bowers NL, Nikolaidis G, Field JK et al. (2006). Frequent genetic and epigenetic abnormalities contribute to the deregulation of cytoglobin in non-small cell lung cancer. Hum Mol Genet 15: 2038-2044.
3570. Xu WS, Chan AC, Lee JM, Liang RH, Ho FC, Srivastava G (1998). Epstein-Barr virus infection and its gene expression in gastric lymphoma of mucosa-associated lymphoid tissue. J Med Virol 56: 342-350.
3571. Xu WS, Ho FC, Ho J, Chan AC, Srivastava G (1997). Pathogenesis of gastric lymphoma: the enigma in Hong Kong. Ann Oncol 8 Suppl 2: 41-44.
3572. Xuan ZX, Ueyama T, Yao T, Tsuneyoshi M (1993). Time trends of early gastric carcinoma. A clinicopathologic analysis of 2846 cases. Cancer 72: 2889-2894.
3573. Yachida S, Iacobuzio-Donahue CA (2009). The pathology and genetics of metastatic pancreatic cancer. Arch Pathol Lab Med 133: 413-422.
3574. Yada S, Matsumoto T, Kudo T, Hirahashi M, Yao T, Mibu R et al. (2005). Colonic obstruction due to giant inflammatory polyposis in a patient with ulcerative colitis. J Gastroenterol 40: 536-539.
3575. Yagihashi S, Sato I, Kaimori M, Matsumoto J, Nagai K (1988). Papillary and cystic tumor of the pancreas. Two cases indistinguishable from islet cell tumor. Cancer 61: 1241-1247.
3576. Yamabuki T, Daigo Y, Kato T, Hayama S, Tsunoda T, Miyamoto M et al. (2006). Genome-wide gene expression profile analysis of esophageal squamous cell carcinomas. Int J Oncol 28: 1375-1384.
3577. Yamabuki T, Takano A, Hayama S, Ishikawa N, Kato T, Miyamoto M et al. (2007). Dikkopf-1 as a novel serologic and prognostic biomarker for lung and esophageal carcinomas. Cancer Res 67: 2517-2525.
3578. Yamada M, Kozuka S, Yamao K, Nakazawa S, Naitoh Y, Tsukamoto Y (1991). Mucin-producing tumor of the pancreas. Cancer 68: 159-168.
3579. Yamada S, Ohira M, Horie H, Ando K, Takayasu H, Suzuki Y et al. (2004). Expression profiling and differential screening between hepatoblastomas and the corresponding normal livers: identification of high expression of the *PLK1* oncogene as a poor-prognostic indicator of hepatoblastomas. Oncogene 23: 5901-5911.
3580. Yamaguchi H, Shimizu M, Ban S, Koyama I, Hatori T, Fujita I et al. (2009). Intraductal tubulopapillary neoplasms of the pancreas distinct from pancreatic intraepithelial neoplasia and intraductal papillary mucinous neoplasms. Am J Surg Pathol 33: 1164-1172.
3581. Yamaguchi K, Chijiiwa K, Saiki S, Shimizu S, Takashima M, Tanaka M (1997). Carcinoma of the extrahepatic bile duct: mode of spread and its prognostic implications. Hepatogastroenterology 44: 1256-1261.
3582. Yamaguchi K, Enjoji M (1988). Carcinoma of the gallbladder. A clinicopathology of 103 patients and a newly proposed staging. Cancer 62: 1425-1432.
3583. Yamaguchi K, Enjoji M (1991). Adenoma of the ampulla of Vater: putative precancerous lesion. Gut 32: 1558-1561.
3584. Yamaguchi K, Enjoji M, Kitamura K (1990). Endoscopic biopsy has limited accuracy in diagnosis of ampullary tumors. Gastrointest Endosc 36: 588-592.
3585. Yamaguchi K, Hirakata R, Kitamura K (1990). Papillary cystic neoplasm of the pancreas: radiological and pathological characteristics in 11 cases. Br J Surg 77: 1000-1003.
3586. Yamaguchi K, Miyagahara T, Tsuneyoshi M, Enjoji M, Horie A, Nakayama I et al. (1989). Papillary cystic tumor of the pancreas: an immunohistochemical and ultrastructural study of 14 patients. Jpn J Clin Oncol 19: 102-111.
3587. Yamaguchi K, Ohuchida J, Ohtsuka T, Nakano K, Tanaka M (2002). Intraductal papillary-mucinous tumor of the pancreas concomitant with ductal carcinoma of the pancreas. Pancreatology 2: 484-490.
3588. Yamaguchi K, Tanaka M (1991). Mucin-hypersecreting tumor of the pancreas with mucin extrusion through an enlarged papilla. Am J Gastroenterol 86: 835-839.
3589. Yamaguchi M, Nakamura N, Suzuki R, Kagami Y, Okamoto M, Ichinohasama R et al. (2008). De novo CD5+ diffuse large B-cell lymphoma: results of a detailed clinicopathological review in 120 patients. Haematologica 93: 1195-1202.
3590. Yamamoto H, Adachi Y, Itoh F, Iku S, Matsuno K, Kusano M et al. (1999). Association of matrilysin expression with recurrence and poor prognosis in human esophageal squamous cell carcinoma. Cancer Res 59: 3313-3316.
3591. Yamamoto H, Itoh F, Nakamura H, Fukushima H, Sasaki S, Perucho M et al. (2001). Genetic and clinical features of human pancreatic ductal adenocarcinomas with widespread microsatellite instability. Cancer Res 61: 3139-3144.
3592. Yamamoto H, Sawai H, Perucho M (1997). Frameshift somatic mutations in gastrointestinal cancer of the microsatellite mutator phenotype. Cancer Res 57: 4420-4426.
3593. Yamamoto J, Abe Y, Nishihara K, Katsumoto F, Takeda S, Abe R et al. (1998). Composite glandular-neuroendocrine carcinoma of the hilar bile duct: report of a case. Surg Today 28: 758-762.
3594. Yamamoto J, Ohshima K, Ikeda S, Iwashita A, Kikuchi M (2003). Primary esophageal small cell carcinoma with concomitant invasive squamous cell carcinoma or carcinoma in situ. Hum Pathol 34: 1108-1115.
3595. Yamamoto M, Nakajo S, Miyoshi N, Nakai S, Tahara E (1989). Endocrine cell carcinoma (carcinoid) of the gallbladder. Am J Surg Pathol 13: 292-302.
3596. Yamamoto M, Takahashi I, Iwamoto T, Mandai K, Tahara E (1984). Endocrine cells in extrahepatic bile duct carcinoma. J Cancer Res Clin Oncol 108: 331-335.
3597. Yamamoto M, Takasaki K, Nakano M, Saito A (1998). Minute nodular intrahepatic cholangiocarcinoma. Cancer 82: 2145-2149.
3598. Yamamoto M, Takasaki K, Yoshikawa T (1999). Lymph node metastasis in intrahepatic cholangiocarcinoma. Jpn J Clin Oncol 29: 147-150.
3599. Yamamoto M, Takasaki K, Yoshikawa T, Ueno K, Nakano M (1998). Does gross appearance indicate prognosis in intrahepatic cholangiocarcinoma? J Surg Oncol 69: 162-167.
3600. Yamamoto N, Tokunaga M, Uemura Y, Tanaka S, Shirahama H, Nakamura T et al. (1994). Epstein-Barr virus and gastric remnant cancer. Cancer 74: 805-809.
3601. Yamamoto T, Uki K, Takeuchi K, Nagashima N, Honjo H, Sakurai N et al. (2003). Early gallbladder carcinoma associated with primary sclerosing cholangitis and ulcerative colitis. J Gastroenterol 38: 704-706.
3602. Yamanaka N, Okamoto E, Ando T, Oriyama T, Fujimoto J, Furukawa K et al. (1995). Clinicopathologic spectrum of resected extraductal mass-forming intrahepatic cholangiocarcinoma. Cancer 76: 2449-2456.
3603. Yamaoka H, Ohtsu K, Sueda T, Yokoyama T, Hiyama E (2006). Diagnostic and prognostic impact of beta-catenin alterations in pediatric liver tumors. Oncol Rep 15: 551-556.
3604. Yamasaki S (2003). Intrahepatic cholangiocarcinoma: macroscopic type and stage classification. J Hepatobiliary Pancreat Surg 10: 288-291.
3605. Yamashita T, Forgues M, Wang W, Kim JW, Ye Q, Jia H et al. (2008). EpCAM and alpha-fetoprotein expression defines novel prognostic subtypes of hepatocellular carcinoma. Cancer Res 68: 1451-1461.
3606. Yamato T, Sasaki M, Hoso M, Sakai J, Ohta H, Watanabe Y et al. (1998). Intrahepatic

cholangiocarcinoma arising in congenital hepatic fibrosis: report of an autopsy case. J Hepatol 28: 717-722.
3607. Yamazaki K, Eyden B (2006). An immunohistochemical and ultrastructural study of pancreatic microcystic serous cyst adenoma with special reference to tumor-associated microvasculature and vascular endothelial growth factor in tumor cells. Ultrastruct Pathol 30: 119-128.
3608. Yan BC, Hart JA (2009). Recent developments in liver pathology. Arch Pathol Lab Med 133: 1078-1086.
3609. Yanagawa N, Tamura G, Honda T, Endoh M, Nishizuka S, Motoyama T (2004). Demethylation of the synuclein gamma gene CpG island in primary gastric cancers and gastric cancer cell lines. Clin Cancer Res 10: 2447-2451.
3610. Yanagi M, Keller G, Mueller J, Walch A, Werner M, Stein HJ et al. (2000). Comparison of loss of heterozygosity and microsatellite instability in adenocarcinomas of the distal esophagus and proximal stomach. Virchows Arch 437: 605-610.
3611. Yanagisawa A, Ohashi K, Hori M, Takagi K, Kitagawa T, Sugano H et al. (1993). Ductectatic-type mucinous cystadenoma and cystadenocarcinoma of the human pancreas: a novel clinicopathological entity. Jpn J Cancer Res 84: 474-479.
3612. Yanagisawa N, Mikami T, Saegusa M, Okayasu I (2001). More frequent beta-catenin exon 3 mutations in gallbladder adenomas than in carcinomas indicate different lineages. Cancer Res 61: 19-22.
3613. Yang GY, Liao J, Cassai ND, Smolka AJ, Sidhu GS (2003). Parietal cell carcinoma of gastric cardia: immunophenotype and ultrastructure. Ultrastruct Pathol 27: 87-94.
3614. Yang GY, Xu KS, Pan ZQ, Zhang ZY, Mi YT, Wang JS et al. (2008). Integrin alpha v beta 6 mediates the potential for colon cancer cells to colonize in and metastasize to the liver. Cancer Sci 99: 879-887.
3615. Yang K, Ulich T, Cheng L, Lewin KJ (1983). The neuroendocrine products of intestinal carcinoids. An immunoperoxidase study of 35 carcinoid tumors stained for serotonin and eight polypeptide hormones. Cancer 51: 1918-1926.
3616. Yang L, Leung AC, Ko JM, Lo PH, Tang JC, Srivastava G et al. (2005). Tumor suppressive role of a 2.4 Mb 9q33-q34 critical region and DEC1 in esophageal squamous cell carcinoma. Oncogene 24: 697-705.
3617. Yang R, Cheung MC, Zhuge Y, Armstrong C, Koniaris LG, Sola JE (2008). Primary Solid Tumors of the Colon and Rectum in the Pediatric Patient: A Review of 270 Cases. J Surg Res -
3618. Yano T, Ishikura H, Wada T, Kishimoto T, Kondo S, Katoh H et al. (1999). Hepatoid adenocarcinoma of the pancreas. Histopathology 35: 90-92.
3619. Yantiss RK, Oh KY, Chen YT, Redston M, Odze RD (2007). Filiform serrated adenomas: a clinicopathologic and immunophenotypic study of 18 cases. Am J Surg Pathol 31: 1238-1245.
3620. Yantiss RK, Panczykowski A, Misdraji J, Hahn HP, Odze RD, Rennert H et al. (2007). A comprehensive study of nondysplastic and dysplastic serrated polyps of the vermiform appendix. Am J Surg Pathol 31: 1742-1753.
3621. Yantiss RK, Shia J, Klimstra DS, Hahn HP, Odze RD, Misdraji J (2009). Prognostic significance of localized extra-appendiceal mucin deposition in appendiceal mucinous neoplasms. Am J Surg Pathol 33: 248-255.
3622. Yantiss RK, Woda BA, Fanger GR, Kalos M, Whalen GF, Tada H et al. (2005). KOC (K homology domain containing protein overexpressed in cancer): a novel molecular marker that distinguishes between benign and malignant lesions of the pancreas. Am J Surg Pathol 29: 188-195.
3623. Yao GY, Zhou JL, Lai MD, Chen XQ, Chen PH (2003). Neuroendocrine markers in adenocarcinomas: an investigation of 356 cases. World J Gastroenterol 9: 858-861.
3624. Yao JC, Hassan M, Phan A, Dagohoy C, Leary C, Mares JE et al. (2008). One hundred years after "carcinoid": epidemiology of and prognostic factors for neuroendocrine tumors in 35,825 cases in the United States. J Clin Oncol 26: 3063-3072.
3625. Yap LB, Neary P (2004). A comparison of wide local excision with abdominoperineal resection in anorectal melanoma. Melanoma Res 14: 147-150.
3626. Yasuda H, Takada T, Amano H, Yoshida M (1998). Surgery for mucin-producing pancreatic tumor. Hepatogastroenterology 45: 2009-2015.
3627. Yasui W, Kudo Y, Semba S, Yokozaki H, Tahara E (1997). Reduced expression of cyclin-dependent kinase inhibitor p27Kip1 is associated with advanced stage and invasiveness of gastric carcinomas. Jpn J Cancer Res 88: 625-629.
3628. Ye H, Gong L, Liu H, Hamoudi RA, Shirali S, Ho L et al. (2005). MALT lymphoma with t(14;18)(q32;q21)/IGH-MALT1 is characterized by strong cytoplasmic MALT1 and BCL10 expression. J Pathol 205: 293-301.
3629. Ye W, Chow WH, Lagergren J, Yin L, Nyren O (2001). Risk of adenocarcinomas of the esophagus and gastric cardia in patients with gastroesophageal reflux diseases and after antireflux surgery. Gastroenterology 121: 1286-1293.
3630. Yeh JJ, Shia J, Hwu WJ, Busam KJ, Paty PB, Guillem JG et al. (2006). The role of abdominoperineal resection as surgical therapy for anorectal melanoma. Ann Surg 244: 1012-1017.
3631. Yeh TS, Jan YY, Chiu CT, Ho YB, Chen TC, Lee KF et al. (2002). Characterisation of oestrogen receptor, progesterone receptor, trefoil factor 1, and epidermal growth factor and its receptor in pancreatic cystic neoplasms and pancreatic ductal adenocarcinoma. Gut 51: 712-716.
3632. Yemelyanova AV, Vang R, Judson K, Wu LS, Ronnett BM (2008). Distinction of primary and metastatic mucinous tumors involving the ovary: analysis of size and laterality data by primary site with reevaluation of an algorithm for tumor classification. Am J Surg Pathol 32: 128-138.
3633. Yen JB, Kong MS, Lin JN (2003). Hepatic mesenchymal hamartoma. J Paediatr Child Health 39: 632-634.
3634. Yeo CJ, Cameron JL, Lillemoe KD, Sitzmann JV, Hruban RH, Goodman SN et al. (1995). Pancreaticoduodenectomy for cancer of the head of the pancreas. 201 patients. Ann Surg 221: 721-731.
3635. Yeoman A, Young J, Arnold J, Jass J, Parry S (2007). Hyperplastic polyposis in the New Zealand population: a condition associated with increased colorectal cancer risk and European ancestry. N Z Med J 120: U2827-
3636. Yeong ML, Wood KP, Scott B, Yun K (1992). Synchronous squamous and glandular neoplasia of the anal canal. J Clin Pathol 45: 261-263.
3637. Yesim G, Gupse T, Zafer U, Ahmet A (2005). Mesenchymal hamartoma of the liver in adulthood: immunohistochemical profiles, clinical and histopathological features in two patients. J Hepatobiliary Pancreat Surg 12: 502-507.
3638. Yettimis E, Trompetas V, Varsamidakis N, Courcoutsakis N, Polymeropoulos V, Kalokairinos E (2003). Pathologic splenic rupture: an unusual presentation of pancreatic cancer. Pancreas 27: 273-274.
3639. Yeung YP, AhChong K, Chung CK, Chun AY (2003). Biliary papillomatosis: report of seven cases and review of English literature. J Hepatobiliary Pancreat Surg 10: 390-395.
3640. Yiannopoulos G, Ravazoula P, Meimaris N, Stavropoulos M, Andonopoulos AP (2002). Dermatomyositis in a patient with adenocarcinoma of the gall bladder. Ann Rheum Dis 61: 663-664.
3641. Ylagan LR, Edmundowicz S, Kasal K, Walsh D, Lu DW (2002). Endoscopic ultrasound guided fine-needle aspiration cytology of pancreatic carcinoma: a 3-year experience and review of the literature. Cancer 96: 362-369.
3642. Ylikorkala A, Avizienyte E, Tomlinson IP, Tiainen M, Roth S, Loukola A et al. (1999). Mutations and impaired function of LKB1 in familial and non-familial Peutz-Jeghers syndrome and a sporadic testicular cancer. Hum Mol Genet 8: 45-51.
3643. Yokoyama A, Watanabe H, Fukuda H, Haneda T, Kato H, Yokoyama T et al. (2002). Multiple cancers associated with esophageal and oropharyngolaryngeal squamous cell carcinoma and the aldehyde dehydrogenase-2 genotype in male Japanese drinkers. Cancer Epidemiol Biomarkers Prev 11: 895-900.
3644. Yonemura Y, Fushida S, Tsugawa K, Ninomiya I, Fonseca L, Yamaguchi A et al. (1993). Correlation of p53 expression and proliferative activity in gastric cancer. Anal Cell Pathol 5: 277-288.
3645. Yonezawa S, Sueyoshi K, Nomoto M, Kitamura H, Nagata K, Arimura Y et al. (1997). *MUC2* gene expression is found in noninvasive tumors but not in invasive tumors of the pancreas and liver: its close relationship with prognosis of the patients. Hum Pathol 28: 344-352.
3646. Yonezawa S, Taira M, Osako M, Kubo M, Tanaka S, Sakoda K et al. (1998). MUC-1 mucin expression in invasive areas of intraductal papillary mucinous tumors of the pancreas. Pathol Int 48: 319-322.
3647. Yoon WJ, Lee JK, Lee KH, Ryu JK, Kim YT, Yoon YB (2008). Cystic neoplasms of the exocrine pancreas: an update of a nationwide survey in Korea. Pancreas 37: 254-258.
3648. Yoshida K, Manabe T, Tsunoda T, Kimoto M, Tadaoka Y, Shimizu M (1996). Early gastric cancer of adenosquamous carcinoma type: report of a case and review of literature. Jpn J Clin Oncol 26: 252-257.
3649. Yoshida N, Nomura K, Wakabayashi N, Konishi H, Nishida K, Taki T et al. (2006). Cytogenetic and clinicopathological characterization by fluorescence in situ hybridization on paraffin-embedded tissue sections of twenty-six cases with malignant lymphoma of small intestine. Scand J Gastroenterol 41: 212-222.
3650. Yoshikawa D, Ojima H, Iwasaki M, Hiraoka N, Kosuge T, Kasai S et al. (2008). Clinicopathological and prognostic significance of EGFR, VEGF, and HER2 expression in cholangiocarcinoma. Br J Cancer 98: 418-425.
3651. Yoshikawa K, Maruyama K (1985). Characteristics of gastric cancer invading to the proper muscle layer—with special reference to mortality and cause of death. Jpn J Clin Oncol 15: 499-503.
3652. Yoshino T, Nakamura S, Matsuno Y, Ochiai A, Yokoi T, Kitadai Y et al. (2006). Epstein-Barr virus involvement is a predictive factor for the resistance to chemoradiotherapy of gastric diffuse large B-cell lymphoma. Cancer Sci 97: 163-166.
3653. Yosry A (2006). Schistosomiasis and neoplasia. Contrib Microbiol 13: 81-100.
3654. You WC, Brown LM, Zhang L, Li JY, Jin ML, Chang YS et al. (2006). Randomized double-blind factorial trial of three treatments to reduce the prevalence of precancerous gastric lesions. J Natl Cancer Inst 98: 974-983.
3655. Younes M, Lebovitz RM, Lechago LV, Lechago J (1993). p53 protein accumulation in Barrett's metaplasia, dysplasia, and carcinoma: a follow-up study. Gastroenterology 105: 1637-1642.
3656. Young J, Jenkins M, Parry S, Young B, Nancarrow D, English D et al. (2007). Serrated pathway colorectal cancer in the population: genetic consideration. Gut 56: 1453-1459.
3657. Young RH, Gilks CB, Scully RE (1991). Mucinous tumors of the appendix associated with mucinous tumors of the ovary and pseudomyxoma peritonei. A clinicopathological analysis of 22 cases supporting an origin in the appendix. Am J Surg Pathol 15: 415-429.
3658. Young RH, Rosenberg AE, Clement PB (1997). Mucin deposits within inguinal hernia sacs: a presenting finding of low-grade mucinous cystic tumors of the appendix. A report of two cases and a review of the literature. Mod Pathol 10: 1228-1232.
3659. Young RH, Welch WR, Dickersin GR, Scully RE (1982). Ovarian sex cord tumor with annular tubules: review of 74 cases including 27 with Peutz-Jeghers syndrome and four with adenoma malignum of the cervix. Cancer 50: 1384-1402.
3660. Yousef F, Cardwell C, Cantwell MM, Galway K, Johnston BT, Murray L (2008). The incidence of esophageal cancer and high-grade dysplasia in Barrett's esophagus: a systematic review and meta-analysis. Am J Epidemiol 168: 237-249.
3661. Youssef EM, Matsuda T, Takada N, Osugi H, Higashino M, Kinoshita H et al. (1995). Prognostic significance of the MIB-1 proliferation index for patients with squamous cell carcinoma of the esophagus. Cancer 76: 358-366.
3662. Yu F, Jensen RT, Lubensky IA, Mahlamaki EH, Zheng YL, Herr AM et al. (2000). Survey of genetic alterations in gastrinomas. Cancer Res 60: 5536-5542.
3663. Yu RS, Chen Y, Jiang B, Wang LH, Xu XF (2008). Primary hepatic sarcomas: CT findings. Eur Radiol 18: 2196-2205.
3664. Yun JP, Zhang MF, Hou JH, Tian QH, Fu J, Liang XM et al. (2007). Primary small cell carcinoma of the esophagus: clinicopathological and immunohistochemical features of 21 cases. BMC Cancer 7: 38-
3665. Yun WK, Ko YH, Kim DS, Kim WS, Rhee PL, Kwak SY et al. (2008). Composite marginal zone B cell lymphoma and enteropathy-type T cell lymphoma of the stomach: a case report. Eur J Gastroenterol Hepatol 20: 791-795.
3666. Yuri T, Danbara N, Shikata N, Fujimoto S, Nakano T, Sakaida N et al. (2004). Malignant rhabdoid tumor of the liver: case report and literature review. Pathol Int 54: 623-629.
3667. Zaanan A, Cuilliere-Dartigues P, Guilloux A, Parc Y, Louvet C, de GA et al. (2009). Impact of p53 expression and microsatellite instability on stage III colon cancer disease-free survival in patients treated by 5-fluorouracil and leucovorin with or without oxaliplatin. Ann Oncol -
3668. Zamboni G, Bonetti F, Castelli P, Balercia G, Pea M, Martignoni G et al. (1994). Mucinous cystic tumor of the pancreas recurring after 11 years as cystadenocarcinoma with foci of choriocarcinoma and osteoclast-like giant cell tumor. Surg Pathol 5: 253-262.
3669. Zamboni G, Bonetti F, Scarpa A, Pelosi G, Doglioni C, Iannucci A et al. (1993). Expression of progesterone receptors in solid-cystic tumour of the pancreas: a clinicopathological and immunohistochemical study of ten cases. Virchows Arch A Pathol Anat Histopathol 423: 425-431.
3670. Zamboni G, Franzin G, Bonetti F, Scarpa A, Chilosi M, Colombari R et al. (1990). Small-cell neuroendocrine carcinoma of the ampullary region. A clinicopathologic, immunohistochemi-

cal, and ultrastructural study of three cases. Am J Surg Pathol 14: 703-713.
3671. Zamboni G, Franzin G, Scarpa A, Bonetti F, Pea M, Mariuzzi GM et al. (1996). Carcinoma-like signet-ring cells in gastric mucosa-associated lymphoid tissue (MALT) lymphoma. Am J Surg Pathol 20: 588-598.
3672. Zamboni G, Pea M, Martignoni G, Zancanaro C, Faccioli G, Gilioli E et al. (1996). Clear cell "sugar" tumor of the pancreas. A novel member of the family of lesions characterized by the presence of perivascular epithelioid cells. Am J Surg Pathol 20: 722-730.
3673. Zamboni G, Scarpa A, Bogina G, Iacono C, Bassi C, Talamini G et al. (1999). Mucinous cystic tumors of the pancreas: clinicopathological features, prognosis, and relationship to other mucinous cystic tumors. Am J Surg Pathol 23: 410-422.
3674. Zamboni G, Terris B, Scarpa A, Kosmahl M, Capelli P, Klimstra DS et al. (2002). Acinar cell cystadenoma of the pancreas: a new entity? Am J Surg Pathol 26: 698-704.
3675. Zambrano E, Reyes-Mugica M, Franchi A, Rosai J (2003). An osteoclast-rich tumor of the gastrointestinal tract with features resembling clear cell sarcoma of soft parts: reports of 6 cases of a GIST simulator. Int J Surg Pathol 11: 75-81.
3676. Zanelli M, Casadei R, Santini D, Gallo C, Verdirame F, La Donna M et al. (1998). Pseudomyxoma peritonei associated with intraductal papillary-mucinous neoplasm of the pancreas. Pancreas 17: 100-102.
3677. Zaninotto G, Rizzetto C, Zambon P, Guzzinati S, Finotti E, Costantini M (2008). Long-term outcome and risk of oesophageal cancer after surgery for achalasia. Br J Surg 95: 1488-1494.
3677A. Zanke BW, Greenwood CM, Rangrej J, Kustra R, Tenesa A, Farrington SM et al. (2007). Genome-wide association scan identifies a colorectal cancer susceptibility locus on chromosome 8q24. Nat Genet 39: 989-994.
3678. Zar N, Holmberg L, Wilander E, Rastad J (1996). Survival in small intestinal adenocarcinoma. Eur J Cancer 32A: 2114-2119.
3679. Zarabi M, LaBach JP (1982). Ganglioneuroma causing acute appendicitis. Hum Pathol 13: 1143-1146.
3680. Zaridze D, Borisova E, Maximovitch D, Chkhikvadze V (2000). Alcohol consumption, smoking and risk of gastric cancer: case-control study from Moscow, Russia. Cancer Causes Control 11: 363-371.
3681. Zaridze D, Brennan P, Boreham J, Boroda A, Karpov R, Lazarev A et al. (2009). Alcohol and cause-specific mortality in Russia: a retrospective case-control study of 48,557 adult deaths. Lancet 373: 2201-2214.
3681A. Zatkova A, Rouillard JM, Hartmann W, Lamb BJ, Kuick R, Eckart M, Von Schweinitz D, Koch A, Fonatsch C, Pietsch T, Hanash SM, Wimmer K (2004). Genes chromosomes Cancer 39:126:137.
3682. Zbar AP, Fenger C, Efron J, Beer-Gabel M, Wexner SD (2002). The pathology and molecular biology of anal intraepithelial neoplasia: comparisons with cervical and vulvar intraepithelial carcinoma. Int J Colorectal Dis 17: 203-215.
3683. Zbuk KM, Eng C (2007). Cancer phenomics: RET and PTEN as illustrative models. Nat Rev Cancer 7: 35-45.
3684. Zbuk KM, Eng C (2007). Hamartomatous polyposis syndromes. Nat Clin Pract Gastroenterol Hepatol 4: 492-502.
3685. Zea-Iriarte WL, Sekine I, Itsuno M, Makiyama K, Naito S, Nakayama T et al. (1996). Carcinoma in gastric hyperplastic polyps. A phenotypic study. Dig Dis Sci 41: 377-386.
3686. Zee S, Hochwald S, Conlon K, Brennan M, Klimstra D (2001). Pleomorphic pancreatic endocrine neoplasms (PENs): a variant comonly confused with adenocarcinoma. Mod Pathol 14: 1212A
3687. Zee SY, Hochwald SN, Conlon KC, Brennan MF, Klimstra DS (2005). Pleomorphic pancreatic endocrine neoplasms: a variant commonly confused with adenocarcinoma. Am J Surg Pathol 29: 1194-1200.
3688. Zen Y, Adsay NV, Bardadin K, Colombari R, Ferrell L, Haga H et al. (2007). Biliary intraepithelial neoplasia: an international interobserver agreement study and proposal for diagnostic criteria. Mod Pathol 20: 701-709.
3689. Zen Y, Aishima S, Ajioka Y, Haratake J, Kage M, Kondo F et al. (2005). Proposal of histological criteria for intraepithelial atypical/proliferative biliary epithelial lesions of the bile duct in hepatolithiasis with respect to cholangiocarcinoma: preliminary report based on interobserver agreement. Pathol Int 55: 180-188.
3690. Zen Y, Fujii T, Itatsu K, Nakamura K, Konishi F, Masuda S et al. (2006). Biliary cystic tumors with bile duct communication: a cystic variant of intraductal papillary neoplasm of the bile duct. Mod Pathol 19: 1243-1254.
3691. Zen Y, Fujii T, Itatsu K, Nakamura K, Minato H, Kasashima S et al. (2006). Biliary papillary tumors share pathological features with intraductal papillary mucinous neoplasm of the pancreas. Hepatology 44: 1333-1343.
3692. Zen Y, Fujii T, Sato Y, Masuda S, Nakanuma Y (2007). Pathological classification of hepatic inflammatory pseudotumor with respect to IgG4-related disease. Mod Pathol 20: 884-894.
3693. Zen Y, Harada K, Sasaki M, Sato Y, Tsuneyama K, Haratake J et al. (2004). IgG4-related sclerosing cholangitis with and without hepatic inflammatory pseudotumor, and sclerosing pancreatitis-associated sclerosing cholangitis: do they belong to a spectrum of sclerosing pancreatitis? Am J Surg Pathol 28: 1193-1203.
3694. Zen Y, Sasaki M, Fujii T, Chen TC, Chen MF, Yeh TS et al. (2006). Different expression patterns of mucin core proteins and cytokeratins during intrahepatic cholangiocarcinogenesis from biliary intraepithelial neoplasia and intraductal papillary neoplasm of the bile duct—an immunohistochemical study of 110 cases of hepatolithiasis. J Hepatol 44: 350-358.
3695. Zen Y, Terahata S, Miyayama S, Mitsui T, Takehara A, Miura S et al. (2006). Multicystic biliary hamartoma: a hitherto undescribed lesion. Hum Pathol 37: 339-344.
3696. Zettl A, deLeeuw R, Haralambieva E, Mueller-Hermelink HK (2007). Enteropathy-type T-cell lymphoma. Am J Clin Pathol 127: 701-706.
3697. Zettl A, Ott G, Makulik A, Katzenberger T, Starostik P, Eichler T et al. (2002). Chromosomal gains at 9q characterize enteropathy-type T-cell lymphoma. Am J Pathol 161: 1635-1645.
3698. Zettl A, Rudiger T, Muller-Hermelink HK (2007). [Enteropathy type T-cell lymphomas: pathology and pathogenesis]. Pathologe 28: 59-64.
3699. Zhang B, Su YP, Ai GP, Liu XH, Wang FC, Cheng TM (2003). Differentially expressed proteins of gamma-ray irradiated mouse intestinal epithelial cells by two-dimensional electrophoresis and MALDI-TOF mass spectrometry. World J Gastroenterol 9: 2726-2731.
3700. Zhang L, Notohara K, Levy MJ, Chari ST, Smyrk TC (2007). IgG4-positive plasma cell infiltration in the diagnosis of autoimmune pancreatitis. Mod Pathol 20: 23-28.
3701. Zhang M, Higashi T (2009). Time trends of liver cancer incidence (1973-2002) in Asia, from cancer incidence in five continents, Vols IV-IX. Jpn J Clin Oncol 39: 275-276.
3702. Zhang X, Huang Q, Goyal RK, Odze RD (2008). DNA ploidy abnormalities in basal and superficial regions of the crypts in Barrett's esophagus and associated neoplastic lesions. Am J Surg Pathol 32: 1327-1335.
3703. Zhao H, Davydova L, Mandich D, Cartun RW, Ligato S (2007). S100A4 protein and mesothelin expression in dysplasia and carcinoma of the extrahepatic bile duct. Am J Clin Pathol 127: 374-379.
3704. Zhao J, de Krijger RR, Meier D, Speel EJ, Saremaslani P, Muletta-Feurer S et al. (2000). Genomic alterations in well-differentiated gastrointestinal and bronchial neuroendocrine tumors (carcinoids): marked differences indicating diversity in molecular pathogenesis. Am J Pathol 157: 1431-1438.
3705. Zheng HC, Li XH, Hara T, Masuda S, Yang XH, Guan YF et al. (2008). Mixed-type gastric carcinomas exhibit more aggressive features and indicate the histogenesis of carcinomas. Virchows Arch 452: 525-534.
3706. Zheng T, Mayne ST, Holford TR, Boyle P, Liu W, Chen Y et al. (1993). The time trend and age-period-cohort effects on incidence of adenocarcinoma of the stomach in Connecticut from 1955-1989. Cancer 72: 330-340.
3707. Zheng W, Sung CJ, Hanna I, DePetris G, Lambert-Messerlian G, Steinhoff M et al. (1997). Alpha and beta subunits of inhibin/activin as sex cord-stromal differentiation markers. Int J Gynecol Pathol 16: 263-271.
3708. Zhong L (2007). Magnetic resonance imaging in the detection of pancreatic neoplasms. J Dig Dis 8: 128-132.
3709. Zhou H, Schaefer N, Wolff M, Fischer HP (2004). Carcinoma of the ampulla of Vater: comparative histologic/immunohistochemical classification and follow-up. Am J Surg Pathol 28: 875-882.
3710. Zhou L, Liu J, Luo F (2006). Serum tumor markers for detection of hepatocellular carcinoma. World J Gastroenterol 12: 1175-1181.
3711. Zhou M, Kort E, Hoekstra P, Westphal M, Magi-Galluzzi C, Sercia L et al. (2009). Adult cystic nephroma and mixed epithelial and stromal tumor of the kidney are the same disease entity: molecular and histologic evidence. Am J Surg Pathol 33: 72-80.
3712. Zhou X, Hampel H, Thiele H, Gorlin RJ, Hennekam RC, Parisi M et al. (2001). Association of germline mutation in the PTEN tumour suppressor gene and Proteus and Proteus-like syndromes. Lancet 358: 210-211.
3713. Zhou XP, Marsh DJ, Morrison CD, Chaudhury AR, Maxwell M, Reifenberger G et al. (2003). Germline inactivation of PTEN and dysregulation of the phosphoinositol-3-kinase/Akt pathway cause human Lhermitte-Duclos disease in adults. Am J Hum Genet 73: 1191-1198.
3714. Zhou XP, Waite KA, Pilarski R, Hampel H, Fernandez MJ, Bos C et al. (2003). Germline PTEN promoter mutations and deletions in Cowden/Bannayan-Riley-Ruvalcaba syndrome result in aberrant PTEN protein and dysregulation of the phosphoinositol-3-kinase/Akt pathway. Am J Hum Genet 73: 404-411.
3715. Zhou YM, Li B, Xu F, Wang B, Li DQ, Liu P et al. (2008). Clinical features of solitary necrotic nodule of the liver. Hepatobiliary Pancreat Dis Int 7: 485-489.
3716. Zhu LC, Sidhu GS, Cassai ND, Yang GC (2005). Fine-needle aspiration cytology of pancreatoblastoma in a young woman: report of a case and review of the literature. Diagn Cytopathol 33: 258-262.
3717. Zhu W, Appelman HD, Greenson JK, Ramsburgh SR, Orringer MB, Chang AC et al. (2009). A histologically defined subset of high-grade dysplasia in Barrett mucosa is predictive of associated carcinoma. Am J Clin Pathol 132: 94-100.
3718. Zhuang Z, Vortmeyer AO, Pack S, Huang S, Pham TA, Wang C et al. (1997). Somatic mutations of the MEN1 tumor suppressor gene in sporadic gastrinomas and insulinomas. Cancer Res 57: 4682-4686.
3719. Zimmermann A (2002). Hepatoblastoma with cholangioblastic features ('cholangioblastic hepatoblastoma') and other liver tumors with bimodal differentiation in young patients. Med Pediatr Oncol 39: 487-491.
3720. Zimmermann A (2005). The emerging family of hepatoblastoma tumours: from ontogenesis to oncogenesis. Eur J Cancer 41: 1503-1514.
3721. Zinner MJ, Shurbaji MS, Cameron JL (1990). Solid and papillary epithelial neoplasms of the pancreas. Surgery 108: 475-480.
3722. Zippel K, Hoksch B, Zieren HU (1997). [A rare stomach tumor—Hodgkin's lymphoma of the stomach]. Chirurg 68: 540-542.
3723. Zisman TL, Rubin DT (2008). Colorectal cancer and dysplasia in inflammatory bowel disease. World J Gastroenterol 14: 2662-2669.
3724. Zitt M, Zitt M, Muller HM (2007). DNA methylation in colorectal cancer—impact on screening and therapy monitoring modalities? Dis Markers 23: 51-71.
3725. Zlobec I, Lugli A (2008). Prognostic and predictive factors in colorectal cancer. J Clin Pathol 61: 561-569.
3726. Zucca E, Bertoni F, Roggero E, Bosshard G, Cazzaniga G, Pedrinis E et al. (1998). Molecular analysis of the progression from *Helicobacter pylori*-associated chronic gastritis to mucosa-associated lymphoid-tissue lymphoma of the stomach. N Engl J Med 338: 804-810.
3727. Zucman-Rossi J, Jeannot E, Nhieu JT, Scoazec JY, Guettier C, Rebouissou S et al. (2006). Genotype-phenotype correlation in hepatocellular adenoma: new classification and relationship with HCC. Hepatology 43: 515-524.
3728. Zwick A, Munir M, Ryan CK, Gian J, Burt RW, Leppert M et al. (1997). Gastric adenocarcinoma and dysplasia in fundic gland polyps of a patient with attenuated adenomatous polyposis coli. Gastroenterology 113: 659-663.

Subject index

GLUL, *see* Glutamine synthetase

Glutamic oxaloacetic transaminase, 83, 87

Glutamic pyruvic transaminase, 83, 87

Glutamine synthetase, 199–203, 216, 235, 256, 257

Glutathione S-transferase (GST), 30, 57, 144

Glycogen synthase kinase 3β (GSK3β), 150, 151

Glycogenic acanthosis, 171

Glycogenosis type 1, 201

Glypican-3 (GPC3), 216, 253, 255–257

Goblet cell carcinoid, 120, 122, 124–126, 128, 264, 274

Goblet-cell rich hyperplastic polyps (GCHP), 160, 161

Goldenhar syndrome, 234

GORD, *see* Gastro-oesophageal reflux disease

Goseki classification, 58

gp130, 203

GPC3, *see* Glypican-3

Granular cell tumour, 16, 35, 46, 74, 182, 193, 264, 277

Granuloma, 193

Granzyme B, 73, 113

Gross cystic disease fluid protein (GCDFP), 80, 189, 192

GSK3β, *see* Glycogen synthase kinase 3β

GST, *see* Glutathione S-transferase

Guillain-Barré syndrome, 267

GWAS, *see* Genome-wide association studies

H

H. pylori, *see* Helicobacter pylori

H2-receptor antagonist, 26

H3, 57

H4, 57

HAART, *see* Highly-active antiretroviral therapy

Haemangioma, 16, 35, 36, 79, 182, 193, 198, 242–244, 253–255, 261, 277, 298

Haemangiopericytoma, 193, 246, 247, 331

Haematemesis, 32, 37

Haematochezia, 135

HAM56, 269

Hamartoma, 10, 96, 132, 167, 171, 331

Hamartomatous polyps, 57, 166, 171

HBsAg, 206, 210, 255

HBV, 205–208, 215, 216, 218, 239, 255

HCA, *see* Hepatocellular adenoma

HCC, *see* Hepatocellular carcinoma

HCV, 205–207, 216–218, 239

HDGC, *see* Hereditary diffuse gastric carcinoma

HDLG, 150, 151

HDV, *see* Hepatitis D virus

Heat shock protein, see HSP

Helicobacter pylori, 26, 41, 43, 49, 50, 54, 57, 61, 64, 69, 71, 73, 102

Hemihypertrophy, 234, 243, 321

Hepatitis B, 205, 206, 213, 215, 239, 255, 257

Hepatitis B surface antigen, *see* HBsAg

Hepatitis B virus, *see* HBV

Hepatitis C, 205, 213, 217, 239

Hepatitis C virus, *see* HCV

Hepatitis D virus (HDV), 207

Hepatobiliary rhabdomyosarcoma, 249

Hepatoblastoma, 149, 150, 195, 228–235, 242, 246, 247, 250, 254–256, 258, 260, 261, 321

Hepatoblastoma, epithelial variants, 196

Hepatoblastoma, mixed epithelial-mesenchymal, 196

Hepatocellular adenoma (HCA), 195, 196, 198, 200–204, 215, 254, 256, 260

Hepatocellular carcinoma (HCC), 195–197, 200, 201–204, *205–216*, 217–219, 225–228, 230, 233, 245, 247, 251–258, 260, 261, 269, 294

Hepatocellular carcinoma, fibrolamellar variant, 196, 205

Hepatocyte nuclear factor 1 α (HNF1α), 201, 202, 204, 245, 256

Hepatocyte-paraffin-1 antibody (Hep-Par1), 80, 89, 118, 209, 225, 226, 253–255, 258, 269, 294

Hepatocyte-specific antigen, *see* HSA

Hepatoid adenocarcinoma, 46, 48, 53, 82, 87, 89, 269

Hepatoid carcinoma, 280, 286, 292, 294

Hepatolithiasis, 217, 218

Hepatomegaly, 208, 239, 241, 251

HepPar1, *see* Hepatocyte-paraffin-1 antibody

HER2, *see* ERBB2

HER3, *see* ERBB3

Hereditary diffuse gastric carcinoma (HDGC), 11, 45, 46, 59, 60–63

Hereditary haemorrhagic telangiectasia (HHT), 143, 166, 167, 198, 244

Hereditary mixed polyposis syndrome (HMPS), 143, 144

Hereditary nonpolyposis colorectal cancer (HNPCC), 142, 152, 153, 156

Hereditary pancreatitis, 281

HGDN, 213, 214, 257

HGIEN, *see* High-grade intraepithelial neoplasia

HHV-8 (human herpesvirus 8), 79, 248

HHT, *see* Hereditary haemorrhagic telangiectasia syndrome

Hibernoma, 245

HIC1, 104

HIF-1 α, *see* Hypoxia-inducible factor α

High-grade anal intraepithelial neoplasia, 186

High-grade dysplasia, 11, 12, 17, 21, 27–29, 31, 46, 55, 56, 82–86, 88, 123, 124, 137, 139, 304, 306–311

High-grade dysplastic nodule, 257

High-grade intraepithelial neoplasia (dysplasia), 21, 22, 55, 83, 139, 154, 217, 253, 269, 270, 271

High-grade MALT lymphoma, 70, 72

High-grade neuroendocrine carcinoma (NEC), 32, 64, 92, 102, 126, 174, 176, 177, 274, 322–326

High-grade squamous intraepithelial lesion (HSIL), 184, 186, 190

Highly-active antiretroviral therapy (HAART), 178, 179

Hilar cholangiocarcinoma, *see* Intrahepatic cholangiocarcinoma

Histamine, 65, 66

HIV, 34, 36, 70, 78, 108, 111, 178, 179, 186, 187, 193, 217, 239, 250, 332

HLA (human leukocyte antigen), 112, 114, 159, 190, 271

HLA-DQ2, 112, 114

HLA-DQ8, 112, 114

HLA-DQB1, 114

HMB45, 37, 91, 116, 182, 189, 190, 245, 253, 255, 331

HMPS, *see* Hereditary mixed polyposis syndrome

HNF1A (HNF1α), *see* 201, 202, 204, 245, 256

HNF1α-inactivated HCA, 201–204, 256

MYB, 290

MYC, 24, 31, 43, 57, 72, 73, 111, 114, 144, 150, 179, 180, 190, 215, 329

Mycotoxins, 19

Myelolipoma, 245

Myeloma, 193

MYH11, 170

Myoblastoma, 193

MYOD1, *see* Myogenin

Myogenin (MYOD), 36, 247, 249, 277

Myxofibrosarcoma, 277

N

N-acetyltransferase 1, 57

NAP1L1, 128

NAT2, 144

NCAM (CD56), 33, 66, 73, 92, 107, 112, 114, 124, 126, 127, 175, 176, 225, 226, 276, 318, 324, 325, 328, 337

NCOA3 (AIB1), 290

NEC (neuroendocrine carcinoma), 13, 14, 16, 23, 32–34, 46, 53, 64–68, 82, 88, 89, 92–94, 96, 102–105, 120, 126, 128, 132, 138, 174–177, 184, 251, 255, 264, 274–276, 280, 293, 322–326

NF, *see* Neurofibromatosis

NEN, *see* Neuroendocrine neoplasms

Neuroendocrine carcinoma, *see* NEC

NEPPK, 23

NET (neuroendocrine tumour), 13, 14, 16, 32–34, 46, 47, 64–68, 82, 92–94, 96, 97, 102–107, 120, 121, 126–128, 132, 133, 174–177, 184, 189, 255, 264, 274–276, 280, 317, 318, 321–326

NET G1, 13, 16, 32, 33, 46, 64, 82, 92, 96, 102, 120, 126, 132, 174, 184, 264, 274, 280, 322

NET G2, 16, 32, 33, 46, 64, 82, 92, 96, 102, 120, 126, 132, 174, 184, 264, 274, 280, 322

Neurilemmoma, 193

Neuroblastoma, 115, 230, 321

Neuroendocrine microadenoma, 280, 322, 323, 325, 326

Neuroendocrine microadenomatosis, 298

Neuroendocrine neoplasms (NEN), 9, 13, 14, 16, 32, 34, 46, 64–68, 82, 92, 94, 96, 102, 104–106, 120, 128, 132, 149, 174, 177, 184, 251, 252, 264, 274, 276, 280, 285, 286, 293, 297, 298, 302, 310, 322, 326, 330, 335

Neuroendocrine tumour, *see* NET

Neurofibroma, 129, 193, 325

Neurofibromatosis (NF), 325

Neurofibromatosis type 1 (NF1), 75, 76, 92, 94, 104, 115, 154, 182, 277, 325

Neuron-specific enolase (NSE), 33, 66, 182, 253, 275, 276, 297, 299, 325, 331

Neurotensin, 103, 175, 323

NFkB, 31

NK-cell lymphoma, 178

NLRP1, 125

N-nitroso compounds, 19

NOD2, 142, 144

Nonfunctioning NETs, 102, 280, 322–326

Non-Hodgkin lymphoma, 70, 109, 110, 178, 251, 253

Noninvasive carcinoma, 12, 22, 27

Noninvasive pancreaticobiliary papillary neoplasm, 11

Noninvasive pancreatobiliary papillary neoplasm with high-grade dysplasia (high-grade intraepithelial neoplasia), 82, 83

Noninvasive pancreatobiliary papillary neoplasm with low-grade dysplasia (low-grade intraepithelial neoplasia), 82, 83

Noninvasive papillary carcinoma, 271

Non-mucinous, glycogen-poor cystadenocarcinoma, 295

Non-steroidal anti-inflammatory drugs (NSAIDs), 27, 134, 135

Nonsyndromic NETs, 322

Notch signalling pathways, 330

NSE, *see* Neuron-specific enolase

Nuclear cell adhesion molecule, *see* NCAM

O

Oesophagitis, 19, 22

Oligocystic serous cystic neoplasms, 309

Oncocytic adenocarcinoma, 53

Oncocytic carcinoma, 295

Oncocytic solid-pseudopapillary neoplasms, 310

Oncocytic-type IPMN, 306–308, 310

Opisthorchis viverrini, 205, 217, 272

Oral contraceptives, 198, 200

Osler-Weber-Rendu syndrome, 79, 166,

Osteoma, 147, 148

Osteopontin, 145

Ovarian cancer, 80, 117, 125, 142

Ovarian-type stroma, 223, 224, 236, 237, 300–303, 309, 315, 337

Oxaliplatin, 145, 146

Oxyntomodulin, 127

P

p16INK4a, *see* CDKN2A

p16-Leiden deletion, 289

p21/WAF1, *see* CDKN1A

p27/KIP1, *see* CDKN1B

p53, see TP53

p63, 33, 191, 269, 292

p73, 50

Paget cells, 189, 190, 192

Paget disease, 183, 184, 191, 192

Paired box gene 8, *see* PAX8

Pale bodies, 210, 211

Pancreatic intraepithelial neoplasia, *see* PanIN

Pancreatic neuroendocrine microadenoma, 280, 322–326

Pancreatic polypeptide, 66, 93, 102, 103, 105, 124, 275, 302, 323, 324

Pancreatic secretory trypsin inhibitor, 316

Pancreatic stone protein, 316

Pancreatobiliary-type IPMN, 307–309, 313

Pancreatoblastoma, 279, 280, 294, 317–321, 325, 334–337

Paneth cell carcinoma, 53

Paneth cell-rich papillary adenocarcinoma, 138

Paneth cells, 27, 29, 56, 84, 85, 88, 101, 124, 139, 267, 270, 276

PanIN (pancreatic intraepithelial neoplasia), 11, 280, 281, 284, 287–291, 293, 304, 307, 309, 310, 314, 315

PanIN-1, 287, 288, 290

PanIN-2, 287, 288, 290

PanIN-3, 280, 281, 284, 287, 288, 290, 293

Papillary adenocarcinoma, 46, 48, 52

Papillary adenoma, 271, 304

Papillary carcinoma, 304

Papillary hidradenoma, 192

Papillary intraductal papillary neoplasm, *see* IPN

Papillary-cystic tumour, 327

Paraganglioma, 75, 76, 97, 277

VHL-associated serous cystic neoplasm, 297, 298

Vienna grading system, 10, 11, 27

Villous adenoma, 82–84, 86, 99, 132, 140, 304

Vimentin, 189, 230, 231, 233, 237, 245, 247, 248, 250, 255, 285, 295, 318, 325, 328, 329, 335

VIP, 32, 93, 280, 323

VIPoma, 280, 322, 323

Vitamin A, 49

Vitamin C, 49

Vitamin D, 134

Vitamin E, 19, 49

VMAT2 (vesicular monoamine transporter 2), 33, 65

Von Gierke disease, 201

Von Hippel-Lindau disease, *see* VHL

Von Meyenburg complex, 222, 260

Von Recklinghausen disease, 91, 92, 94, 104

W

Weibel-Palade bodies, 248

Well-differentiated endocrine carcinoma (WDEC), 13; *see* NET G2

Well-differentiated endocrine tumour (WDET), 13, 14, 32, 92, 102, 133, 274, *see* NET G1

Well-differentiated endocrine tumour/ carcinoma, 64, 126

Well-differentiated hepatocellular carcinoma, 211

WHO classification, 10–13, 16, 46, 52, 82, 96, 120, 180, 184, 189, 190, 264, 267, 273, 280, 322

Wilms tumour, 321

Wnt, 101, 104, 150, 158, 215, 234, 235, 320, 329, 330

WT1, 331

X

Xeroderma pigmentosum group C (XPC) gene, 30

Xeroderma pigmentosum group D, 30

XRCC1 (X-ray repair cross-complementing 1), 30

Y

Yolk sac tumour, 196

Z

Zinc, 19

Zollinger-Ellison syndrome, 64, 102, 275, 335